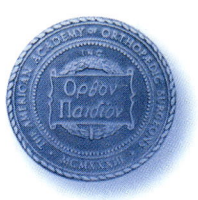

American Academy of Orthopaedic Surgeons

OKU

WITHDRAWN

Orthopaedic Knowledge Update:

7

Home Study Syllabus

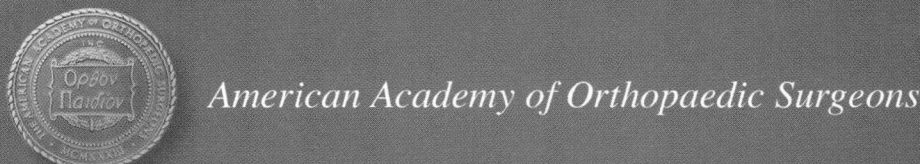

American Academy of Orthopaedic Surgeons

OKU

Orthopaedic Knowledge Update:

Home Study Syllabus

7

Edited by
Kenneth J. Koval, MD

Published 2002
by the American Academy of Orthopaedic Surgeons
6300 North River Road
Rosemont, IL 60018
1-800-626-6726

ISBN 0-89203-256-1

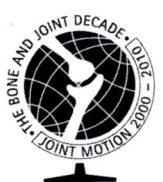

Acknowledgments

Editorial Board, OKU 7

Kenneth J. Koval, MD
Chairman
Associate Professor
Department of Orthopaedics
New York University School of Medicine
New York, New York

Frederick M. Azar, MD
Sports Medicine
Assistant Professor
University of Tennessee - Campbell Clinic
Department of Orthopaedic Surgery
Memphis, Tennessee

Paul E. DiCesare, MD
Basic Science
Associate Professor
Department of Orthopaedics
Hospital for Joint Diseases
New York, New York

Lawrence G. Lenke, MD
Spine
Professor
Department of Orthopedic Surgery
Washington University
St. Louis, Missouri

Jay R. Lieberman, MD
Adult Reconstruction
Associate Professor of Orthopaedic Surgery
Department of Orthopaedic Surgery
University of California, Los Angeles, School of Medicine
Los Angeles, California

Regis J. O'Keefe, MD, PhD
Basic Science
Professor of Orthopaedics
Department of Orthopaedics
University of Rochester School of Medicine
Rochester, New York

Paul Tornetta III, MD
Trauma
Professor and Vice Chairman
Director of Orthopaedic Trauma
Department of Orthopaedic Surgery
Boston University Medical Center
Boston, Massachusetts

Elly Trepman, MD
Foot and Ankle
Associate Professor
Section of Orthopaedic Surgery
Department of Surgery
University of Manitoba
Winnipeg, Manitoba, Canada

Arnold-Peter Weiss, MD
Wrist and Hand
Professor of Hand Surgery
Department of Orthopaedics
Brown Medical School
Providence, Rhode Island

Michael A. Wirth, MD
Shoulder and Elbow
Associate Professor, Orthopaedics
University of Texas Health Science Center
Chief, Shoulder Service
Department of Orthopaedics
Audie Murphy Veterans Hospital
San Antonio, Texas

James G. Wright, MD, MPH, FRCSC
Pediatrics
Robert B. Salter Chair of Paediatric Surgical Research
Program Head, Population Health Sciences
Research Institute
The Hospital for Sick Children
Division of Orthopaedic Surgery
University of Toronto
Toronto, Ontario, Canada

American Academy of Orthopaedic Surgeons

Staff

Mark Wieting
  Vice President, Educational Programs
Marilyn L. Fox, PhD
  Director, Department of Publications
Lisa Claxton Moore
  Senior Editor
Mary Steermann
  Manager, Production and Archives

Sophie Tosta
  Assistant Production Manager
Kathleen Anderson
  Editorial Assistant
Courtney Astle
  Production Assistant
Karen Danca
  Production Assistant

Contributors

Mark F. Abel, MD
Associate Professor of Orthopaedic
    Surgery and Pediatrics
University of Virginia
Charlottesville, Virginia

Brian D. Adams, MD
Professor
Department of Orthopedic Surgery
University of Iowa
Iowa City, Iowa

Benjamin A. Alman, MD, FRCSC
Canadian Research Chair
Associate Professor and Scientist
Division of Orthopaedic Surgery
Program in Developmental Biology
Hospital for Sick Children
University of Toronto
Toronto, Ontario, Canada

Peter C. Amadio, MD
Professor of Orthopedics
Department of Orthopedic Surgery
Mayo Clinic
Rochester, Minnesota

Michael J. Archibeck, MD
New Mexico Orthopaedics
New Mexico Center for Joint
    Replacement Surgery
Albuquerque, New Mexico

Peter F. Armstrong, MD
Professor
Shriners Hospital
Tampa, Florida

David C. Ayers, MD
Chief
Adult Reconstruction Service
Associate Professor of Orthopaedic
    Surgery
State University of New York Upstate
    Medical University
Syracuse, New York

Frederick M. Azar, MD
Assistant Professor
University of Tennessee - Campbell
    Clinic
Department of Orthopaedic Surgery
Memphis, Tennessee

R. Tracy Ballock, MD
Associate Professor of Orthopaedics
    and Pediatrics
Department of Orthopaedics
Case Western Reserve University
Cleveland, Ohio

Mark E. Baratz, MD
Director, Division of Upper Extremity
    Surgery
Associate Professor of Orthopaedic
    Surgery
MCP Hahnemann University School of
    Medicine
Allegheny General Hospital
Pittsburgh, Pennsylvania

Ann E. Barr, PhD, PT
Assistant Professor
Physical Therapy Department
College of Allied Health Professions
Temple University
Philadelphia, Pennsylvania

Robert L. Barrack, MD
Professor of Orthopaedic Surgery
Director, Adult Reconstructive Surgery
Department of Orthopaedic Surgery
Tulane University Health Sciences
    Center
New Orleans, Louisiana

Judith Ford Baumhauer, MD
Associate Professor
Chief of Division of Foot and Ankle
    Surgery
Department of Orthopaedics
University of Rochester School of
    Medicine and Dentistry
Rochester, New York

John A. Bendo, MD
Associate Director, Hospital for Joint
    Diseases Spine Center
Clinical Assistant Professor Orthopedic
    Surgery
New York University School of
    Medicine
Hospital for Joint Diseases
New York, New York

Richard A. Berger, MD
Assistant Professor of Orthopaedics
Rush-Presbyterian Hospital
Department of Orthopaedic Surgery
Rush Medical College
Chicago, Illinois

Steven Bernstein, MD
Orthopaedic Surgeon
Metropolitan Orthopaedics and Sports
    Therapy
Silver Spring, Maryland

Daniel J. Berry, MD
Associate Professor of Orthopedics
Consultant in Orthopedic Surgery
Department of Orthopedic Surgery
Mayo Clinic
Rochester, Minnesota

Mohit Bhandari, MD, MSc
Research Fellow
Department of Orthopaedic Surgery
St. Michael's Hospital
Toronto, Ontario, Canada

Oren G. Blam, MD
Clinical Instructor and Chief Resident
Department of Orthopaedic Surgery
Thomas Jefferson University Hospital
Philadelphia, Pennsylvania

John S. Blanco, MD
Associate Professor or Orthopaedic
    Surgery and Pediatrics
Head, Division of Pediatric
    Orthopaedics
Department of Orthopaedic Surgery
University of Virginia
Charlottesville, Virginia

Mathias P. G. Bostrom, MD
Assistant Attending Surgeon
Hospital for Special Surgery
New York, New York

Joseph A. Buckwalter, MD
Professor and Chair
Department of Orthopaedic Surgery
University of Iowa
Iowa City, Iowa

Susan V. Bukata, MD
Research Fellow, Department of
    Orthopaedics
Department of Orthopaedic Surgery
University of Rochester
Rochester, New York

Robert L. Buly, MD
Assistant Professor of Orthopaedic
    Surgery
Weill Medical College of Cornell
    University
The Hospital for Special Surgery
New York, New York

Corey Burak, MD
Arthroplasty Fellow
Department of Orthopaedic Surgery
Tulane University Medical School
New Orleans, Louisiana

Charles A. Bush-Joseph, MD
Associate Professor
Department of Orthopaedic Surgery
Rush-Presbyterian St. Luke's Medical
    Center
Chicago, Illinois

John J. Callaghan, MD
The Lawrence and Marilyn Dorr Chair
    and Professor
Department of Orthopaedics
University of Iowa
Iowa City, Iowa

Cathy S. Carlson, DVM, PhD
Associate Professor
Department of Veterinary Diagnostic
    Medicine
University of Minnesota
St. Paul, Minnesota

Kristen Lee Carroll, MD
Assistant Professor
Department of Orthopedics, Pediatric
    Orthopedics
University of Utah
Salt Lake City, Utah

Thomas R. Carter, MD
Head of Orthopaedic Surgery
Arizona State University
Tempe, Arizona

Patrick J. Casey, MD
Chief Resident, Emory Orthopaedic
    Residency
Department of Orthopaedic Surgery
Emory University School of Medicine
Atlanta, Georgia

R. Sean Churchill, MD
Acting Instructor
Department of Orthopaedics and Sports
    Medicine
University of Washington School of
    Medicine
Seattle, Washington

Denis R. Clohisy, MD
Associate Professor
Department of Orthopaedic Surgery
University of Minnesota Medical School
    and Cancer Center
Minneapolis, Minnesota

David B. Cohen, MD
Assistant Professor of Orthopaedic
    Surgery
Johns Hopkins University
Baltimore, Maryland

Frances Cuomo, MD
Chief, Shoulder and Elbow Service
Department of Orthopaedics
New York University Hospital for Joint
    Diseases
New York, New York

Diane L. Damiano, PhD
Associate Professor of Neurological
    Surgery
Washington University
St. Louis, Missouri

John R. Dimar II, MD
Associate Clinical Professor
Director of Basic Sciences
Department of Orthopedics
University of Louisville
Louisville, Kentucky

Douglas R. Dirschl, MD
Associate Professor
Department of Orthopaedics
University of North Carolina School of
    Medicine
Chapel Hill, North Carolina

Kenneth A. Egol, MD
Assistant Professor of Orthopaedic
    Surgery
New York University School of
    Medicine
New York University Hospital for Joint
    Diseases
Department of Orthopaedic Surgery
New York, New York

Charles H. Epps, Jr, MD
Professor Emeritus, Orthopaedic
    Surgery
Department of Orthopaedic Surgery
Howard University College of Medicine
Washington, District of Columbia

Gracia Etienne, MD
Attending Physician
Department of Orthopaedics
The John Hopkins Medical Institutions
Baltimore, Maryland

David S. Feldman, MD
Chief, Pediatric Orthopedic Surgery
Department of Orthopedic Surgery
Hospital for Joint Diseases
New York University
New York, New York

Linda R. Ferris, MBBS, BSc (med),
    FRACS
Head of Orthopaedic Unit
Modbury Hospital
Wakefield Orthopaedic Clinic
Adelaide, South Australia

Christopher G. Finkemeier, MD
Assistant Professor
Department of Orthopaedic Surgery
University of California Davis Health
    System
Sacramento, California

Kevin L. Garvin, MD
Professor
Department of Orthopaedic Surgery
University of Nebraska Medical Center
Omaha, Nebraska

Mark J. Geppert, MD
Orthopaedic Surgeon
Orthopaedic and Trauma Specialists
Somersworth, New Hampshire

Bruce L. Gillingham, MD, CDR, MC,
    VSN
Assistant Professor of Surgery
Uniformed Services University of the
    Health Sciences
Department of Orthopaedic Surgery
Naval Medical Center
San Diego, California

Steven D. Glassman, MD
Assistant Professor of Orthopaedic
    Surgery
Department of Orthopaedics
University of Louisville
Louisville, Kentucky

Keith A. Glowacki, MD
Assistant Clinical Professor
Department of Orthopaedic Surgery
Virginia Commonwealth University
Medical College of Virginia
Richmond, Virginia

Guy Grimard, MD, FRCSC
Clinical Associate Professor of Surgery
Department of Surgery
University of Montreal
Montreal, Canada

David J. Hak, MD
Assistant Professor
Department of Orthopaedic Surgery
University of California Davis
Sacramento, California

Christopher Hamill, MD
Assistant Professor of Orthopaedic
    Surgery
Department of Orthopaedic Surgery
State University of New York
Buffalo, New York

Michael R. Hausman, MD
Clinical Associate Professor of
    Orthopaedic Surgery and Plastic
    Surgery
Mount Sinai Medical Center
New York, New York

Alan S. Hilibrand, MD
Assistant Professor of Orthopaedic
    Surgery
The Rothman Institute
Jefferson Medical College
Philadelphia, Pennsylvania

Robert N. Hotchkiss, MD
Chief of Hand Service
Hospital for Special Surgery
New York, New York

Michelle A. James, MD
Assistant Chief of Orthopaedic Surgery
Shriners Hospital for Children,
    Northern California
Sacramento, California

James Kang, MD
Assistant Professor, Division of Spinal
    Surgery
Department of Orthopedic Surgery
University of Pittsburgh Medical
    Center
Pittsburgh, Pennsylvania

Julie A. Katarincic, MD
Instructor, Mayo Medical School
Consultant, Department of Orthopedic
    Surgery
Department of Orthopedics
Mayo Clinic
Rochester, Minnesota

E. Michael Keating, MD
Orthopaedic Surgeon
The Center for Hip and Knee Surgery
Mooresville, Indiana

Paul Khanuja, MD
Attending Surgeon
Department of Orthopaedics
The John Hopkins Medical Institutions
Baltimore, Maryland

Mininder S. Kocher, MD, MPH
Instructor of Orthopaedic Surgery,
    Harvard Medical School
Program in Clinical Effectiveness,
    Harvard School of Public Health
Department of Orthopaedic Surgery
Children's Hospital
Boston, Massachusetts

Kenneth J. Koval, MD
Associate Professor
Department of Orthopaedics
New York University School of
    Medicine
New York, New York

Joseph M. Kowalski, MD, DC
Assistant Professor of Orthopaedic
    Surgery
Department of Orthopaedic Surgery
State University of New York
Buffalo, New York

Scott H. Kozin, MD
Associate Professor
Department of Orthopaedic Surgery
Temple University
Philadelphia, Pennsylvania

Hans J. Kreder, MD, MPH, FRCSC
Associate Professor
Department of Orthopaedic Surgery
University of Toronto
Toronto, Ontario, Canada

Ronald Scott Kvitne, MD
Associate
Department of Orthopaedics
Kerlan-Jobe Orthopaedic Clinic
Los Angeles, California

Hubert Labelle, MD
Clinical Professor of Surgery
Department of Surgery
University of Montreal
Montreal, Canada

Raymond Lambert, MD, FRCPC,
    ABNM
Associate Professor
Faculty of Medicine, University of
    Montreal
Department of Nuclear Medicine
Hôpital Sainte-Justine
Montreal, Quebec, Canada

Gerald J. Lang, MD
Assistant Professor
Department of Orthopedic Surgery
University of Wisconsin
Madison, Wisconsin

Lawrence G. Lenke, MD
Professor
Department of Orthopedic Surgery
Washington University
St. Louis, Missouri

Jay R. Lieberman, MD
Associate Professor of Orthopaedic
    Surgery
Department of Orthopaedic Surgery
University of California, Los Angeles,
    School of Medicine
Los Angeles, California

Jess H. Lonner, MD
Assistant Professor of Orthopaedic
    Surgery
Pennsylvania Orthopaedic Institute
University of Pennsylvania School of
    Medicine
Philadelphia, Pennsylvania

Scott J. Luhmann, MD
Instructor, St. Louis Children's Hospital
Department of Orthopaedic Surgery
Washington University School of
    Medicine
St. Louis, Missouri

William J. Maloney, MD
The Charles F. and Joanne Knight
    Distinguished Professor of
    Orthopaedic Surgery
Chief-of-Service and Head of Joint
    Reconstruction, Barnes-Jewish
    Hospital
Department of Orthopaedic Surgery
Washington University School of
    Medicine
St. Louis, Missouri

Frederick A. Matsen III, MD
Professor and Chairman
Department of Orthopaedics and Sports
    Medicine
University of Washington School of
    Medicine
Seattle, Washington

John A. McAuliffe, MD
Staff Physician
Section of Hand Surgery
Department of Orthopaedic Surgery
Cleveland Clinic, Florida
Fort Lauderdale, Florida

Eric C. McCarty, MD
Assistant Professor
Department of Orthopaedics and
    Rehabilitation
Vanderbilt University Medical Center
Nashville, Tennessee

Amir Mehbod, MD
Department of Orthopaedic Surgery
University of Minnesota
Minneapolis, Minnesota

Charles T. Mehlman, DO, MPH
Director, Musculoskeletal Outcomes
    Research
Assistant Professor Pediatric
    Orthopaedic Surgery
Division of Pediatric Orthopaedic
    Surgery
Children's Hospital Medical Center
Cincinnati, Ohio

James D. Michelson, MD
Professor
Department of Orthopaedics and
    Rehabilitation
University of Vermont
Burlington, Vermont

Mark D. Miller, MD
Associate Professor
Department of Orthopaedic Surgery
University of Virginia
Charlottesville, Virginia

Nancy Hadley Miller, MS, MD
Associate Professor
Department of Orthopedic Surgery
Johns Hopkins School of Medicine
Baltimore, Maryland

Michael B. Millis, MD
Associate Professor of Orthopaedic
    Surgery
Director, Adolescent/Young Adult Hip
    Unit
Children's Hospital
Harvard Medical School
Boston, Massachusetts

Marie-Claude Miron, MD, FRCPC
Clinical Assistant Professor
Department of Radiology
Hôpital Sainte-Justine
Montreal, Quebec, Canada

H. David Moehring, MD
Associate Professor of Orthopaedic
    Surgery
Department of Orthopaedic Trauma
    and Reconstruction
University of California, Davis
Sacramento, California

Michael A. Mont, MD
Associate Professor
Department of Orthopaedics
The John Hopkins Medical Institutions
Baltimore, Maryland

Mark J. R. Moulton, MD
Department of Orthopaedic Spine
    Surgery
Orthopaedic Associates of Muskegon
Muskegon, Michigan

Steven A. Olson, MD
Associate Professor
Chief, Orthopaedic Trauma
Department of Surgery
Duke University
Durham, North Carolina

Norman Y. Otsuka, MD, FRCSC, FACS
Assistant Clinical Professor
UCLA School of Medicine
Attending Pediatric Orthopaedic
    Surgeon
Shriners Hospitals for Children, Los
    Angeles
Los Angeles, California

Erik Thor Otterberg, MD
Adjunct Clinical Instructor
Department of Orthopaedic Surgery
University of Nebraska Medical Center
Omaha, Nebraska

William M. Oxner, MD, FRCSC
Department of Orthopaedic Surgery
University of Pittsburgh
Pittsburgh, Pennsylvannia

Nader Paksima, DO, MPH
Clinical Assistant Professor of
    Orthopaedic Surgery
New York University
Hospital for Joint Diseases
New York, New York

George A. Paletta, Jr, MD
Assistant Professor of Orthopaedic
    Surgery
Chief, Sports Medicine Service
Department of Orthopaedic Surgery
Washington University School of
    Medicine
St. Louis, Missouri

Michael S. Pinzur, MD
Professor of Orthopaedic Surgery and
    Rehabilitation
Department of Orthopaedic Surgery
    and Rehabilitation
Loyola University Medical School
Maywood, Illinois

Kevin D. Plancher, MD
Associate Clinical Professor
Albert Einstein College of Medicine
Director, Plancher Orthopaedic
    Associates
New York, New York

Louis G. Quartararo, MD
Clinical Instructor
Department of Orthopedic Surgery
Thomas Jefferson University, Rothman
    Institute
Philadelphia, Pennsylvania

John J. Regan, MD
Medical Director
Institute for Spinal Disorders
Cedars-Sinai Hospital
Los Angeles, California

Richard A.K. Reynolds, MD, FRCSC,
    FACS
Associate Professor of Orthopedics
Department of Orthopedics
Children's Hospital of Los Angeles
Los Angeles, California

John M. Rhee, MD
Assistant Professor, Orthopaedic
    Surgery
Emory Spine Center
Emory University
Decatur, Georgia

Michael D. Ries, MD
Associate Professor
Chief of Arthroplasty
Department of Orthopaedic Surgery
University of California, San Francisco
San Francisco, California

K. Daniel Riew, MD
Assistant Professor
Department of Orthopaedic Surgery
Barnes-Jewish Hospital at Washington
    University
St. Louis, Missouri

Andrew S. Rokito, MD
Associate Director of Sports Medicine
Department of Orthopaedic Surgery
New York University - Hospital for
    Joint Diseases
New York, New York

Randy N. Rosier, MD, PhD
Chairman and Professor of
    Orthopaedics and Oncology
Department of Orthopaedics
The University of Rochester
Rochester, New York

Kavi Sachar, MD
Hand Surgeon
Hand Surgery Associates
Denver, Colorado

Emil H. Schemitsch, MD, FRCSC
Head, Division of Orthopaedic Surgery
Professor of Surgery
Division of Orthopaedic Surgery
Department of Surgery
St. Michael's Hospital, University of
    Toronto
Toronto, Ontario, Canada

David M. Scher, MD
Clinical Instructor of Orthopaedic
    Surgery
Department of Orthopaedic Surgery
New York University Hospital for Joint
    Diseases
New York, New York

Gregory J. Schmeling, MD
Associate Professor
Director, Division of Orthopaedic
    Trauma
Department of Orthopaedics
Medical College of Wisconsin
Milwaukee, Wisconsin

Christopher C. Schmidt, MD
Hand Surgeon
Department of Orthopedics
Allegheny General Hospital
Philadelphia, Pennsylvania

Perry L. Schoenecker, MD
Professor of Orthopedic Surgery,
    Washington University
Chief of Staff, Shriner's Hospital for
    Children
Shriner's Hospital for Children
St. Louis, Missouri

John Gray Seiler III, MD
Associate Clinical Professor
Orthopaedic Surgery
Georgia Hand and Microsurgery
Atlanta, Georgia

Joel A. Shapiro, MD
Shoulder Fellow
Department of Orthopaedic Surgery
Hospital for Joint Diseases
New York, New York

Stephen H. Sims, MD
Chief of the Fracture Service
Miller Orthopaedic Clinic
Carolinas Medical Center
Charlotte, North Carolina

David L. Skaggs, MD
Assistant Professor of Orthopedic
    Surgery
Department of Orthopedics
Children's Hospital of Los Angeles
Los Angeles, California

Stephen R. Skinner, MD
Chief of Orthopaedics
Shriners Hospital for Children,
    Northern California
Sacramento, California

Kurt P. Spindler, MD
Associate Professor
Department of Orthopaedics and
    Rehabilitation
Vanderbilt University Medical Center
Nashville, Tennessee

Jeffrey M. Spivak, MD
Assistant Professor of Orthopaedic
    Surgery
Department of Orthopaedic Surgery
New York University Hospital for Joint
    Diseases
New York, New York

Michael J. Stuart, MD
Associate Professor
Department of Orthopedic Surgery
Mayo Clinic
Rochester, Minnesota

Nirmal Tejwani, MD
Assistant Professor of Clinical
    Orthopedics
Department of Orthopedic Surgery
New York University Hospital for Joint
    Diseases
New York, New York

H. Thomas Temple, MD
Professor of Orthopaedics and
    Pathology
Chief, Orthopaedic Oncology Division
Department of Orthopaedics and
    Rehabilitation
University of Miami School of Medicine
Miami, Florida

David C. Templeman, MD
Assistant Professor of Orthopaedic
    Surgery, University of Minnesota
Hennepin County Medical Center
Wayzata Orthopedics
Plymouth, Minnesota

Paul Tornetta III, MD
Professor and Vice Chairman
Director of Orthopaedic Trauma
Department of Orthopaedic Surgery
Boston University Medical Center
Boston, Massachusetts

Robert Trousdale, MD
Associate Professor, Mayo Graduate
    School
Department of Orthopedic Surgery
Mayo Clinic
Rochester, Minnesota

Sophie Turpin, MD, FRCPC
Associate Professor
University of Montreal
Department of Nuclear Medicine
Hôpital Sainte-Justine
Montreal, Quebec, Canada

Alexander R. Vaccaro, MD
Professor and Chief of Spinal Surgery
Co-director of the Delaware Valley
    Spinal Cord Injury Center
Department of Orthopaedic Surgery
Thomas Jefferson University Hospital
Philadelphia, Pennsylvania

Michael G. Vitale, MD, MPH
Assistant Professor Orthopaedic
    Surgery
Children's Hospital of New York
New York Presbyterian Hospital
New York, New York

Arthur K. Walling, MD
Clinical Associate Professor
  Orthopaedics, University of South
  Florida
Director, Foot and Ankle Fellowship
Florida Orthopaedic Institute
Tampa, Florida

Daniel C. Wascher, MD
Associate Professor
Department of Orthopaedics
Health Sciences Center
University of New Mexico
Albuquerque, New Mexico

Steven B. Weinfeld, MD
Chief, Foot and Ankle Service
Assistant Professor of Orthopaedic
  Surgery
Mount Sinai Medical Center
New York, New York

Russell E. Windsor, MD
Professor of Orthopaedic Surgery
Sanford Weill Medical School of Cornell
  University
Attending Orthopaedic Surgeon
Hospital for Special Surgery
New York, New York

Brent Wise, MD
Chief, Division of Infectious Diseases
Hospital for Joint Diseases
New York University Medical Center
New York, New York

Philip R. Wolinsky, MD
Clinical Associate Professor
Chief, Orthopedic Trauma Service,
  Bellevue Medical Center
Department of Orthopedic Surgery
New York University Hospital for Joint
  Diseases
New York, New York

Kirkham B. Wood, MD
Associate Professor
Department of Orthopaedic Surgery
University of Minnesota
Minneapolis, Minnesota

Rick W. Wright, MD
Assistant Professor
Department of Orthopaedic Surgery
Washington University School of
  Medicine
St. Louis, Missouri

Ken Yamaguchi, MD
Assistant Professor
Chief, Shoulder and Elbow Service
Department of Orthopaedic Surgery
Washington University School of
  Medicine
St. Louis, Missouri

Table of Contents

American Academy of Orthopaedic Surgeons

Section 3 Upper Extremity

Section Editors
Frederick M. Azar
Paul Tornetta III
Arnold-Peter Weiss
Michael A. Wirth

Preface

I am pleased to present the latest edition of Orthopaedic Knowledge Update, OKU 7, which is the culmination of many months of hard work by a dedicated team of editors. Understanding the process by which OKU 7 was written highlights the commitment of the section editors, selected authors, and AAOS staff. First, a team of section editors was chosen who, over several conference calls, determined the most important topics for inclusion in OKU and selected the key individuals to present the topics in a clear, concise, and unbiased manner. The chapters submitted for each section were then reviewed for content and presentation by a team of reviewers, which included the appropriate section editor and the authors of each chapter. The section editors believed that a team approach to editorial review by experts familiar with each particular section would allow us to identify controversial topics and to ensure that bias would be eliminated. Each chapter was then revised and reviewed a second time by the appropriate section editor. Finally, over a 2-day meeting in Chicago, the entire OKU manuscript was reviewed and edited by the team of Section Editors and myself. It is our hope that OKU 7 provides a comprehensive and useful review of orthopaedic knowledge, incorporating the latest information available.

I am indebted to a number of individuals who worked so hard to make OKU 7 a reality, in particular Marilyn Fox, PhD, AAOS Director of Publications, and Lisa Claxton Moore, Senior Editor, and Kathleen Anderson, Editorial Assistant, who spent many hours on the phone and computer to get the chapters finished and submitted in a timely fashion. I am also grateful for the opportunity to have worked with so many dedicated and knowledgeable Section Editors, who made this endeavor so much more enjoyable. Finally, I am grateful for the honor bestowed upon me by the AAOS leadership, and in particular James Beaty, MD, for recommending me to be the Editor of OKU 7.

Kenneth J. Koval, MD
Editor

Section 1

General Knowledge

Section Editors:
Frederick M. Azar, MD
Paul E. DiCesare, MD
Jay R. Lieberman, MD
Regis J. O'Keefe, MD
James G. Wright, MD

Chapter 1

Soft-Tissue Physiology and Repair

Kurt P. Spindler, MD

Rick W. Wright, MD

Meniscus

Structure and Function

The meniscus is a fibrocartilaginous semicircular "cushion" in a joint. Its function and structure are interdependent at both the macroscopic and microscopic levels. The primary functions of the meniscus are load transmission, shock absorption, and lubrication of the articular surfaces. The normal meniscus is stabilized by its peripheral attachments, especially the anterior and posterior horn along with the meniscal-femoral and meniscal-tibial attachments. There is relatively more motion in the lateral meniscus, which is more circular, than the medial meniscus, which is more C-shaped, partly because of the popliteal hiatus in the posterolateral corner, which does not provide peripheral attachment to the femur and the tibia in this location. The meniscus' vascular supply is from the medial and lateral geniculate arteries. It is this vascular supply with reference to the peripheral versus central location of the meniscus that determines the meniscus' potential for healing and is the predominant reason for excision versus repair. Approximately 10% to 25% of the meniscus (on the periphery or closer to the capsule) has a vascular supply and is considered the "red" zone. The inner central two thirds is avascular and is considered the "white" zone. There is a relatively increased blood supply present at the attachments of the anterior and posterior horns. Previous studies have demonstrated that tears in the red zone or vascular zone will heal whereas tears in the central avascular zone do not heal.

The meniscus is composed of an extracellular matrix, which is a complex, three-dimensional (3-D), interlocking array of ordered collagen fibers with proteoglycan and water, which is responsible for its load-bearing properties. The cells are composed of meniscal fibrochondrocytes with at least two separate populations spatially separated. By dry weight 75% is collagen, 8%

to 13% is noncollagenous protein, and 1% is hexosamine. The principal collagen type is more than 90% type I, with the remainder being small amounts of type II, III, V, and VI. The load-bearing role of the meniscus is determined by the collagen fiber ultrastructure— large collagen fiber bundles predominant in a circumferential orientation and radial collagen bundles run from the periphery toward the center (Fig. 1). There is no organization to the collagen bundles on the superior femoral surface or inferior tibial surface. The meniscus is a viscoelastic structure where the rate of creep depends on the rate of fluid exudation from the tissue and the equilibrium deformation is dependent on the collagen proteoglycan solid matrix and the applied load to this structure.

During normal knee motion, the menisci more closely follow the tibia than the femur. In flexion-extension the lateral meniscus shows greater total anterior-posterior excursion than the medial meniscus. For posterior displacement only the lateral meniscus and medial meniscus are equal. As the knee flexes, the menisci move posteriorly; as the knee extends, the menisci move more anteriorly. The role of the meniscus in maintaining stability in the knee is as follows: it is not a primary stabilizer for anterior-posterior displacement but in an anterior cruciate ligament (ACL)-deficient knee the posterior horns resist anterior displacement. The lateral and medial menisci also may have a proprioceptive role in positional control in alignment. By their relative motion, the menisci position themselves for their primary role in load transmission where they are found to transmit 50% of the compressive load in the ranges of 0° to 90°. The more flexion that is achieved in the knee, the greater the contribution of the meniscus to the transmission of load across the femoral-tibial surface. Total medial meniscectomy has been shown to decrease the contact area 50% to 75%, resulting in supraphysiologic loads for a given surface area on the articular cartilage;

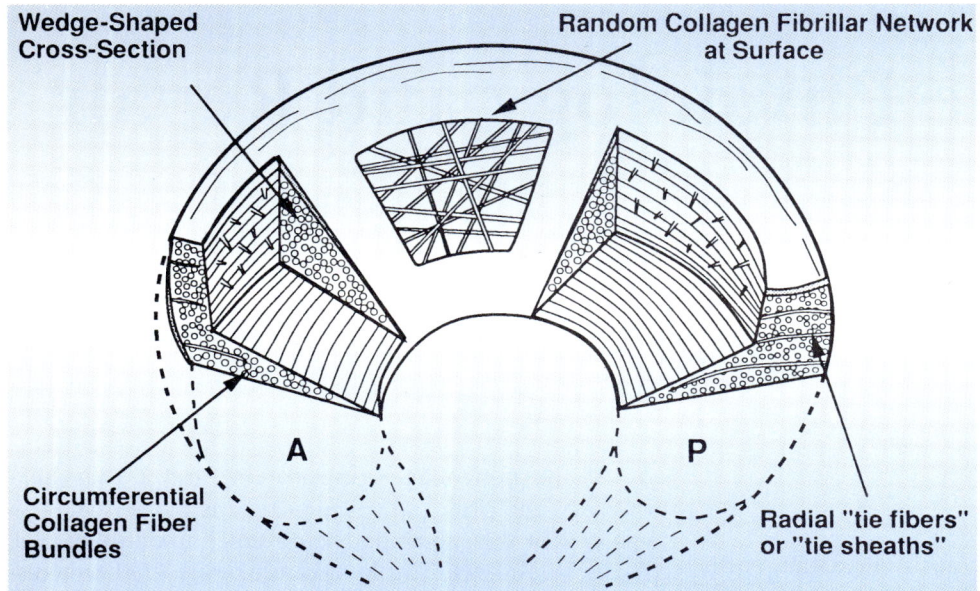

Wedge-Shaped Cross-Section

Random Collagen Fibrillar Network at Surface

Circumferential Collagen Fiber Bundles

A   **P**

Radial "tie fibers" or "tie sheaths"

Figure 1 Collagen fiber ultrastructure of the meniscus. Note the predominant circumferential orientation of the large collagen fiber bundles in the interior of the tissue. The fibers of the surface layer have no preferred orientation. Also within the interior of the meniscus are radially oriented collagen "tie" fibers. (Reproduced with permission from Mow VC, Ratcliffe A, Chern KY, Keily MA: Structure and function relationships of the menisci of the knee, in Mow VC, Arnoczky SP, Jackson DW (eds): Knee Meniscus: Basic and Clinical Foundations. New York, NY, Raven Press, 1992, p 40.)

hence, the subsequent acceleration of degenerative changes. In partial meniscectomy, the remaining rim of the meniscus transmits load; however, if the circumferential collagen fibers of the meniscus have been disrupted (these maintain hoop stresses), it functions similar to total meniscectomy.

Physiologic Responses

The meniscus responds to normal physiologic stresses including immobilization and exercise, the effects of age, and ligamentous injury and reconstruction. During a 12-week period of immobilization, the collagen content of the lateral meniscus has been shown to decrease. However, knee motion, even without weight bearing, can prevent collagen loss in the lateral meniscus. As a result of advancing age, a normal degenerative process occurs within the meniscal tissue and its response to physiologic stress becomes limited due to declining cellularity, decreased noncollagenous proteins and proteoglycans, and an increase in degradative proteases. An increase in calcium pyrophosphate crystal levels, as well as a rise in horizontal cleavage planes and tears within the meniscus, occur with age. Finally, in patients up to 30 years old, the percentage of collagen within the meniscus has been shown to increase.

Remodeling and Regeneration

Remodeling of the meniscus is the accretion of new tissue from an extrinsic source. In a study on partial meniscectomy in canines, some remodeling was found to have occurred in two thirds of the subjects. Regeneration of the meniscus has been demonstrated in animals. In a rabbit model studied after total meniscectomy, the meniscus

will regenerate (if the vascular synovial tissue is exposed); however, if a synovectomy is performed, regeneration does not occur. In the canine model, 83% of the meniscus will show evidence of regrowth or regeneration. In humans, predictable degenerative changes after extensive partial and complete meniscectomy will occur and point to the fact that any regeneration is most likely clinically insignificant.

Tears and Repairs

The natural history of meniscal tears varies with respect to its vascular supply. Traumatic tears in the peripheral vascular zone have the capability for healing, while tears within the central avascular region do not. Stabilization of tears in the peripheral vascular region lead to a high percentage of healing. Investigators have tried to promote healing in the avascular region with the use of a fibrin clot, fibrin glue, endothelial cell growth factor, vascular access channels, and synovial pedicle flaps. The exact role of soluble extrinsic mediators from the blood that may modulate healing as well as cytokines such as platelet-derived growth factor (PDGF), transforming growth factor-beta, endothelial cell growth factor, and fibroblast growth factor are currently being actively investigated. PDGF has been shown in vitro to increase the proliferation of meniscal cells. In the intra-articular environment, a naturally-occurring fibrin clot from surgical bleeding might be rendered ineffective by synovial fluid dissolution. Recombinant growth factors combined with collagen-based biologic scaffolds are under investigation to promote healing within the avascular region of the meniscus. Stable tears that are either partial thickness (not extending through both the femoral and tibial surface of the meniscus) and complete longitudinal tears smaller than 7 mm are considered stable, especially in the setting of an ACL tear and reconstruction, and can be left alone. Complete, unstable tears that are larger than 10 mm warrant treatment whether the decision is repair or excision. Repair rates have clearly been shown to be adversely affected by the presence of an ACL deficiency, with a decreased healing rate and increased incidence of re-tears. Therefore, in order to preserve the meniscal repair, an ACL reconstruction is indicated. Other important factors to consider are the type of tear, whether there is a degenerative component to the tear with multiple cleavage planes within the central body of the meniscus, and whether multiple tears are present. Both outside-in and inside-out techniques have had excellent success rates in short- and long-term reports with prevention of radiographic changes of osteoarthritis.

Meniscal Replacement: Prosthetics and Allografts

Meniscal replacements have used biocompatible prostheses or allografts and bioabsorbable collagen scaffolds. A synthetic prosthetic meniscal replacement has been investigated extensively in animal models. Teflon, Dacron, and carbon fiber have been used in animal models and have failed to duplicate or prevent degenerative changes in the short term. Furthermore, there is a potential for wear debris particles to cause inflammation of the synovial cavity. For these reasons a permanent meniscal prosthesis is not currently available.

Factors to be considered when using allograft menisci are antigenicity, preservation with or without secondary sterilization, and the ability of the graft to remodel into a living meniscus. While animal models have had little immunologic reaction, the antigenicity of human tissue also appears minimal. Cryopreservation is the only technique in which living donor meniscal fibrochondrocytes can survive, with viability at 10% to 40%. However, in animal models, fresh allografts, cryopreserved allografts, and deep frozen allografts all have similar results. Host-cell repopulation proceeds from superficial to the central core of the meniscus. Sterilization methods including ethylene oxide, glutaraldehyde, or gamma radiation can adversely affect graft function. In summary, animal models show reliable peripheral capsule healing and normal gross macroscopic appearance. However, an increased proteoglycan content as well as an increased water content are seen at 6 months, consistent with early degenerative changes. This raises the question about long-term allograft function.

Human allograft meniscal transplantation trials are difficult to interpret due to multiple confounding variables including additional intra-articular procedures. It

appears, however, that the allografts can heal at the periphery and, if properly sized and matched, appear to remain viable in the synovial cavity. The long-term function will clearly depend on the incorporation of living fibrochondrocytes, proper size matching of these meniscal transplants, and secure bony fixation so hoop stresses can be generated and transmitted across the femoral-tibial articular surfaces.

Articular Cartilage
Structure and Function

The principal function of articular cartilage is to provide load transmission via a relatively frictionless articulation surface. This function is dependent on the specific composition and organization of the extracellular matrix that is maintained by the chondrocytes. Articular cartilage is a highly organized viscoelastic material. Articular cartilage is both aneural and devoid of blood and lymphatic vessels. The dense extracellular matrix protects the chondrocytes from immunologic recognition, and that factor along with the lack of blood and lymphatic vessels make articular cartilage an immuno-privileged site. The chondrocytes that populate the extracellular matrix depend on the flux of fluid into and out of the extracellular matrix for their metabolic requirements. The chondrocytes are believed to respond to the mechanical environment by sensing alterations in the pericellular environment. They are metabolically active and maintain the surrounding extracellular matrix. Furthermore, they clearly respond to cytokines present within the synovial fluid.

The extracellular matrix consists of water, proteoglycans, and collagen. Water makes up the majority (approximately 65% to 80%) of wet weight. Ninety-five percent of the collagen is type II with much smaller amounts of other collagens including types IV, VI, IX, X, and XI. The exact functions of these other collagens are unknown, but they are believed to be important in matrix attachment and stabilization and diameter of collagen fibrils. The collagen forms a 3-D network that encases proteoglycan molecules, predominantly keratan sulfate and chondroitin sulfate. Proteoglycan molecules are negatively charged and along with cations attract water. The high water content with the collagen-proteoglycan solid matrix is responsible for its mechanical properties. The rate of deformation or compression of articular cartilage is highly dependent on the rate of exudation of water from the matrix. The limit to deformation is dependent on the structural integrity of the collagen framework.

The ebb and flow of synovial fluid, water, and nutrients into and out of the articular surface is vital for maintenance of normal chondrocyte metabolism and the integrity of the extracellular matrix. Therefore,

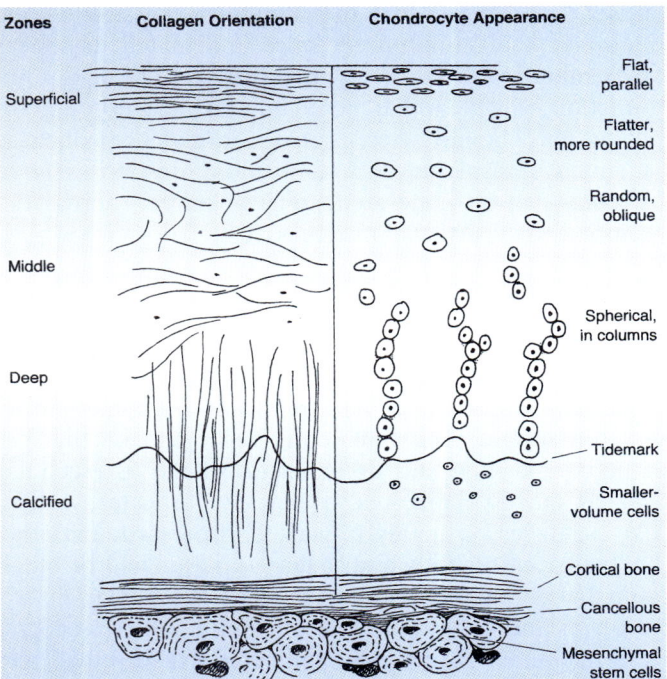

Figure 2 Basic structural anatomy of articular cartilage. *(Reproduced from Browne JE, Branch TP: Surgical alternatives for treatment of articular cartilage lesions. J Am Acad Orthop Surg 2000;8:180-189.)*

active joint motion and application of a physiologic load is required for maintenance of a healthy articular surface. The exact correlation between the minimum and maximum rate of loading and amount of compression necessary to maintain the articular surface is unknown. However, supraphysiologic stresses that occur after the total loss of the meniscus (which decreases contact area by over 50%) result in early degenerative changes. Furthermore, ligamentous insufficiency such as ACL tears with resultant altered joint mechanics after ACL reconstruction also may place supraphysiologic forces on articular cartilage that predispose to early degenerative changes. Finally, genetic differences and/or anatomic alignment may predispose to degenerative changes.

The normal thickness of the articular cartilage correlates with the surface pressure. The higher the peak pressures, the thicker the articular surface, with the area underneath the patella being the thickest in the human body. The basic structural anatomy of the articular cartilage can be divided into four distinct zones, superficial, middle, deep, and calcified, as shown in Figure 2. These layers differ in collagen orientation, cellular morphology, and biomechanically. The collagen orientation changes from parallel to the surface in the superficial layer to a more random, less densely packed array in the middle zone. In the deep and calcified zones the collagen bundles are perpendicular to the joint surface and subchon-

dral bone. The largest collagen fibrils are in the deep zone, which has the highest concentration of proteoglycans and lowest concentration of water. The chondrocytes are arranged in a manner similar to that of the collagen fibrils. In the deepest calcified zone, small, low-volume chondrocytes are randomly arranged. This transitions to a columnar arrangement of spherical cells in the deep zone to a more random array of cells in the middle zone, and finally, to a flat, parallel array of chondrocytes in the superficial zone. The tidemark is a thin basophilic line seen at light microscopy sections of decalcified articular cartilage that corresponds to the boundary between the calcified and uncalcified cartilage.

Injury and Repair

Injuries to the articular surface can be divided into acute and subacute (gradual). Acute injury types include blunt trauma, shear, and thermal (including electrocautery as well as laser). Subacute or gradual types occur as a result of mechanical overload secondary to meniscal loss and/or ligamentous instability, aging, and potentially exercise. Mechanical trauma (blunt, twisting, or impact loading) to the articular cartilage leads to three basic types of tissue damage. Type 1 is the destruction or alteration of the macromolecule framework (that is, loss of matrix or macromolecules, or cell injury without evidence of disruption). Type 2 is the disruption of the articular cartilage alone (chondral fractures or fissuring). Type 3 is disruption of the articular cartilage with penetration into the subchondral bone (for example, an osteochondral fracture). The healing potentials of these lesions are significantly different because the articular cartilage is avascular. Because types 1 and 2 do not penetrate the subchondral bone, there exists an extremely poor to nonexistent potential for healing because an inflammatory component is not elicited and the chondrocytes have limited ability to initiate a repair process. In contrast, type 3 injuries produce an inflammatory response with a fibrin clot and exposure of mesenchymal undifferentiated cells that populate this fibrin clot and produce a reparative tissue. However, this tissue consists primarily of type I collagen and does not have the biomechanical properties of normal articular cartilage. This fibrocartilage is prone to early degenerative changes.

Classification

No uniform classification system exists to define the natural history of articular cartilage lesions as well as results of treatment. Table 1 lists current classification systems. All classification systems prior to that of

TABLE 1 | Classification Systems for Articular Cartilage Lesions

Author	Reference	Surface	Diameter/Size	Location
Outerbridge	*JBJS Br*, 1961	I-IV	$\geq 1/2$ in	Patella, trochlea
Goodfellow	*JBJS Br*, 1976	2 grades	1 cm	Patella
Cassells	*CORR*, 1978	I-VI	1, 2, 4 cm	Patella, trochlea
Hungerford	*JBJS Br*, 1979	5 grades	> 1 cm^2	Patella
Bentley	*CORR*, 1984	I-IV	0.5, 1, 2 cm	Patella
Insall	*Knee*, 1984	I-IV	None	Patella, trochlea
Noyes	*Am J Sports Med*, 1989	3 surface, 2 depths	10, 15, 20, 25, > 25 mm^2	Entire knee
Dougados	*Arthroscopy*, 1994	I-IV	0 to 100% diagram	Entire knee
Curl	*Arthroscopy*, 1997	I-IV, osteochondritis dissecans, articular cartilage fracture fixation	None	Entire knee

Noyes in 1989 were developed for patellofemoral pathology. The Noyes system uses diameter estimates based on probe widths and includes osteochondritis dissecans and articular cartilage fractures. The Dougados system acknowledges the importance of the scale diagram drawn by surgeons but grade III exposed bone was considered unique to this system versus all others. The Curl system modified the Outerbridge classification system but its shortcoming was that it did not define size of lesion. Because there is no single agreed-upon classification system that reproducibly defines depth and size of articular cartilage lesions, natural history and treatment investigations are hindered.

Treatment

Treatment of full-thickness cartilage defects has included (1) débridement, (2) abrasion arthroplasty or microfracture, (3) autologous chondrocyte cell transplantation, (4) periosteum or perichondrium transplantation, (5) mosaicplasty (single or multiple autograft osteochondral transfer) and (6) fresh allograft osteochondral transfer. Evaluation of these treatments requires validated outcome measures and adequate follow-up. Furthermore, treatment needs to control for confounding variables, such as ACL reconstruction, meniscus surgery (excision, repair, replacement), and osteotomy, which clearly have been shown to improve outcomes. These shortcomings have led the International Cartilage Repair Society to develop comprehensive documentation and classification to include the following factors: (1) etiology, (2) defect thickness, (3) size of lesion (cm^2), (4) degree of containment, (5) location(s), (6) ligament integrity, (7) menis-

cus integrity, (8) alignment (normal, varus, valgus), (9) previous management, (10) radiologic assessment, (11) assessment by MRI (fat suppression techniques), and (12) general medical, systemic, or family history issues. With the understanding of significant confounding variables such as ACL reconstruction, as well as the clear scientific value of general and disease-specific validated outcome forms, future studies should at a minimum be prospective, use validated outcome for pretreatment and posttreatment, and stratify for major confounding variables.

Muscle

Structure and Function

The primary role of skeletal muscle is locomotion. The myotendinous junction is the most common site of injury (such as delayed muscle soreness, strains, and traumatic tears or avulsion). The length of muscle fibers may make them susceptible to injuries, especially those fibers that cross two joints. For example, the hamstring, gastrocnemius, and long head of the biceps most frequently undergo strains and/or partial tears.

Understanding muscle physiology requires knowledge of the microscopic and macroscopic anatomy including the motor unit, muscle fiber bundles, individual muscle fibers, myofibrils within fibers, and the contractile unit of the myofibril, the sarcomere (Fig. 3). Muscle contracts in response to input via nerve fibers through the neuromuscular junction (motor end plate) to all the muscle fibers innervated by that nerve fiber. These contractions are "all or none" and these fibers are scattered throughout the muscle. Therefore, the force of contraction is dependent on percentage of motor units firing. In general, smaller muscles (ocular, hand) required for fine motor control have smaller motor units (less muscle fibers per nerve fiber) as compared with larger muscles (hamstrings and gastric), which have much larger motor units. An early component of increase in strength from resistance training is neuromuscular adaptation, which includes firing a higher percentage of motor units.

The characteristics of muscle contraction depend on the type of contraction and muscle fiber types. The types of contraction include isometric (fixed load, no joint motion), concentric (moving a load as joint moves with muscle shortening), eccentric (controlling a load as the joint moves with muscle lengthening), and isokinetic (load varies at constant joint velocity). There are three basic muscle fiber types—type I, type IIA, and type IIB (Table 2). Types I and II are determined by speed of contraction. Type I is slow-twitch and type II is fast-twitch. Type II is further divided by major mode of energy utilization with type IIB being primarily anaerobic. Conversely, type IIA is intermediate between type I and type IIB in both aerobic and anaerobic capacity. Postural muscles and primary movers are type I, and muscles associated with power generation are type II. Most muscles have both types I and II fibers.

Response to Immobilization, Exercise, and Resistance Training

Mammalian skeletal muscle is capable of responding to functional loads such as those caused by disuse, immobilization, and exercise. Muscle quickly adapts to a spectrum of disuse by rapidly losing contractile strength and mass. The profound reduction in strength and mass with bed rest or microgravity is reversible relatively quickly. During immobilization the position of muscle is significant as the muscle positioned in a lengthened position undergoes less reduction in mass versus that in a neutral or shortened state.

The type of exercise, such as aerobic or endurance training (running, biking, swimming, or cross-country skiing) versus resistance training (weight lifting) determines the specific adaptive response. Low loads characterize endurance training with high repetitions requiring oxidative metabolism by muscle. This stimulates mitochondria biogenesis and increased capillary density and results in increased Vo_{2max} and improved fatigue resistance. At a cellular or muscle fiber level, alterations result in mRNA stability, increased protein synthesis, and greater density of mitochondria per muscle cell. It is now known that mitochondrial biogenesis may be initiated by a single episode of exercise.

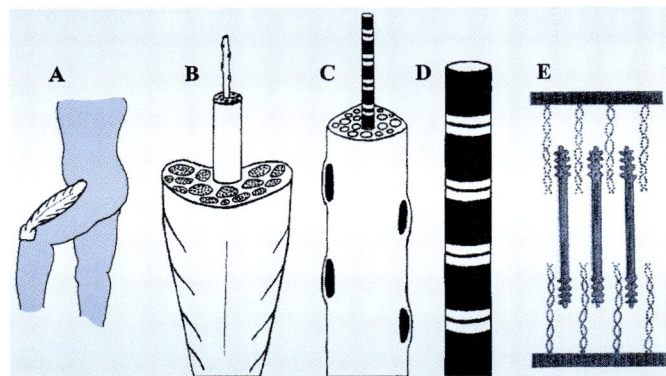

Figure 3 Macroscopic to microscopic view of muscle contracture. **A,** Quadriceps. **B,** Fascicle arrangements within quadriceps. **C,** Muscle cell within fascicle. Muscle cell contains nucleus, mitochondria, and plasma membrane called sarcolemma. **D,** Myofibril within muscle cell. **E,** Sarcomere, smallest contractile unit of myofibril, longitudinally arranged within myofibril.

Injury and Repair

The role of stretching before exercise to prevent muscle injuries has been debated. In a randomized trial of preexercise stretching during warm-up in 1,538 Army recruits during 12 weeks of training, there were no clinically meaningful reductions in risk of exercise-related injuries. Significant factors predictive of injury were fitness and age.

Microscopic muscle injury is characterized by delayed muscle soreness that occurs throughout the muscle fiber as a result of overzealous eccentric activity for which the muscle has not had prior conditioning. Pain typically occurs 12 to 48 hours after activity.

TABLE 2	**Characteristics of Human Skeletal Muscle Fiber Types**		
	Type I	**Type IIA**	**Type IIB**
Other names	Red, slow-twitch	White, fast-twitch	
	Slow oxidative	Fast oxidative glycolytic	Fast glycolytic
Speed of contraction	Slow	Fast	Fast
Strength of contraction	Low	High	High
Fatigability	Fatigue-resistant	Fatigable	Most fatigable
Aerobic capacity	High	Medium	Low
Anaerobic capacity	Low	Medium	High
Motor unit size	Small	Larger	Largest
Capillary density	High	High	Low

(Reproduced from Garrett WE Jr, Best TM: Anatomy, physiology, and mechanics of skeletal muscle, in Simon SR (ed): *Orthopaedic Basic Science*. Rosemont, iL, American Academy of Orthopaedic Surgeons, 1994, pp 89–125.)

These ultrastructural changes to muscle cells are reversible during repair. Clinically apparent muscle strains are partial disruptions usually localized to the myotendinous junction in response to powerful eccentric contractions. The repair process includes inflammatory reaction followed by fibrosis. Clinically the most common sites for injury are hamstrings and gastrocnemius (especially medial head)—both of these muscles cross two joints. Recent studies have focused on pharmacologic ways to promote repair and clinical recovery using anabolic steroids, corticosteroids, nonsteroidal anti-inflammatory drugs (NSAIDs), ultrasound, and hyperbaric oxygen. In a rat model with muscle contusion injury, an anabolic steroid (nandrolone decanoate, 20 mg/kg), a corticosteroid (methylprednisolone acetate, 25 mg/kg) and a control group were compared. Healing (measured by active contractile tension and histology) in the corticosteroid group showed earlier improvement at day 2, but was weaker than the control group by day 7, and the muscle was degenerated at day 14. At day 14 the anabolic steroid group was significantly stronger in twitch. Naproxen (500 mg twice daily for 48 hours) was administered in the presence of delayed onset muscle soreness in a prospective randomized, double-blind trial in moderately trained men. The NSAID did not alter serum creatine kinase, muscle force deficit at 24 hours, visual analog scale pain, and immunohistochemical inflammatory cells. However, at 48 hours, naproxen significantly increased voluntary knee extension torque.

The effect of pulsed ultrasound on regeneration was investigated after a contusion injury. Though satellite cell proliferation was increased in myoregeneration there were no overall morphologic manifestations of muscle regeneration. Two studies investigated the effect of hyperbaric oxygen on muscle injury models. In a prospective randomized, double-blind study of delayed muscle soreness in 66 untrained men (18 to 35 years of age) there was a significant increase in recovery of eccentric quadriceps torque at 96 hours, but no change in visual analog scale pain at any time. In a rabbit model of acute muscle stretch, a group treated with hyperbaric oxygen demonstrated a significant reduction in functional deficit (ankle isometric torque) versus a control group. Morphologic investigation confirmed more complete healing in the treatment group than in the control group.

Muscle lacerations remain a difficult problem clinically because of the paucity of investigations on recovery of function. A mouse model of gastrocnemius laceration studied surgical repair versus short period of immobilization (5 days) on healing, with the repair group showing significant increased recovery of tetanus strength 1 month after injury (81% control repair versus 18% control immobilized). Histologic and immunohistochemical evaluation revealed improved healing with suture repair as evidenced by higher regenerating myofibers, less development of a deep scar, and a more fibrotic scar. The role of cytokines (basic fibroblastic growth factor, insulin-like growth factor, and nerve growth factors) or gene therapy in improving muscle regeneration and repair is currently under investigation.

Ligament

Structure and Function

Ligaments are dense regular connective tissues that consist of short wide bands of tough fibrous tissue, which provide bone-to-bone connections. These tissues have been studied extensively because of their importance in work and sports injuries. Much of the research involving ligaments has focused on the knee. Water is the primary component of ligaments, comprising 60% to 80% of their weight. Collagen is the predominant dry weight component at 70%—type I collagen is the most common type in normal ligament at 90%. Type III collagen, among others, makes up the remaining 10%. Type III collagen is found more commonly in injured ligaments. Elastin makes up 1% of the dry weight except in spine ligaments, where it is found at a higher rate. Elastin allows the ligament to return to its normal length by storing energy during loading. Fibroblasts are found between the rows of collagen fibers; these cellular components of ligaments produce the extracellular matrix. Ligaments exhibit a more interwoven structure than tendons because of their more variable direction of loading. The fibrous structure of ligament collagen is similar to that found in other tissues containing collagen with a polypeptide chain and triple helix formation. Cross-links are crucial to ligament function because they add significant strength to the structure. The extracellular matrix also contains proteoglycans, which store water and affect viscoelastic properties of the structure. Groups of fibers organized as bands or bundles make up the ultrastructure of ligaments. Studies of the ACL demonstrate that separate bands tighten and loosen based on their location and the flexion angle of the knee.

The transition from ligament to bone at its insertion site is complex. Two types of insertion sites are found: direct and indirect, with direct being more common. An example of a direct insertion is the femoral attachment of the medial collateral ligament (MCL). In direct insertions, the collagen deep fibers attach at right angles to the bone through four distinct zones over a distance of 1 mm. Collagen with extracellular matrix and fibroblasts makes up zone 1. Zone 2 is fibrocartilage with cellular changes. Mineralized fibrocartilage is found in zone 3. Zones 2 and 3 are separated by the tidemark or mineralization front. The abrupt transition to bone distinguishes zone 4. In indirect insertions, the superficial layer connects directly to the periosteum while the deep layer anchors to bone by Sharpey fibers (direct-connection collagen of tendon into bone). An example of an indirect insertion is the tibial insertion of the MCL.

Histologic studies have revealed a uniform microvascularity throughout the ligament. This vascular supply originates from the ligament insertions and epiligamentous tissue. The vascular supply is critical in supplying nutritional support for the processes of matrix synthesis and repair. Histologic studies of human and animal ligaments have demonstrated specialized nerve endings in ligaments. The ACL and MCL had been demonstrated to have a nerve supply, which provides proprioceptive pain responses.

The biomechanical properties of ligaments are related to structural and mechanical properties. The structural properties characterize the behavior of the overall bone-ligament-bone complex (load-elongation relationship) and are influenced by the mechanical properties and ligament geometry as well as the insertion site characteristics (Figs. 4 and 5). The mechanical properties of the ligament under tensile loading (stress-strain relationship) are affected by collagen composition and fiber orientation. The structural properties of the ligament complex can be measured by tensile testing and the subsequent load elongation curve. Like the load elongation curve obtained in tendon testing, two regions are noted in the ligament load elongation curve. A low-stiffness region called the toe region is followed by a more linear region with higher stiffness. The nonlinear response is caused by collagen fiber crimp and a lack of uniformity of the individual fiber recruitment. During initial testing, large elongation is noted with small force because of the straightening of the crimp. After the initial crimp is released, larger forces are required to elongate the fibers. Following elongation of the fibers, the ultimate load of the bone-ligament-bone complex is reached and failure occurs. The curve slope can end abruptly or gradually. A gradual failure represents failure of small individual fibers prior to complete ligament disruption. The mechanical properties can also be obtained from the same load elongation curve. The stress-strain curve will demonstrate the modulus of elasticity, tensile strength, ultimate strain, and strain energy density. The ACL and MCL have been extensively studied because of their frequency of injury. The mechanical properties of the ACL and MCL differ significantly. The elastic modulus for the MCL is twice that of the ACL. The MCL has more dense fiber bundles with less crimp than the

ACL. The MCL also has more collagen fibers per unit area than the ACL. Fibril diameter in the MCL is on average higher than that seen in the ACL. It is believed that this factor contributes to a higher resistance to elongation.

Factors Affecting Ligament Properties

An increased prevalence of ACL injury is noted in females. Anatomic features such as intercondylar notch size and shape, femoral or tibial geometry, or pelvic width have been suggested as contributing factors. Gender differences in muscle response to sport-specific activities, such as cutting, jumping, and landing, have also been proposed. Gender differences in ligament properties at the molecular level also may influence these rates. Estrogen's effect on fibroblast proliferation and collagen synthesis has been studied in vitro. Physiologic levels of 17-β estradiol reduce collagen synthesis by more than 40% in isolated ligament cells as compared with controls, and resulted in a significant

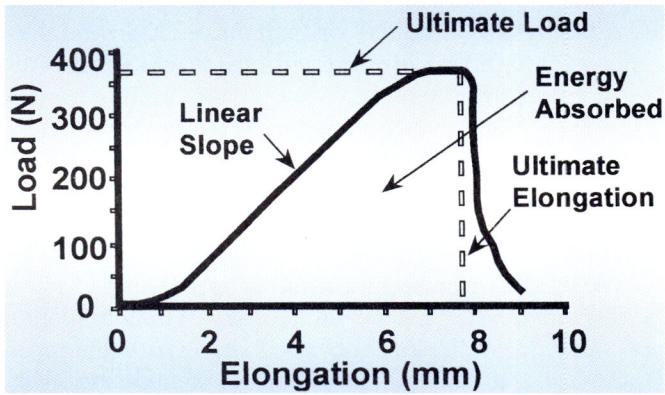

Figure 4 A schematic load-elongation curve for ligament. *(Reproduced with permission from Woo SL-Y, Debski RE, Withrow JD, Janaushek MA: Biomechanics of knee ligaments. Am J Sports Med 1999;27:533-543.)*

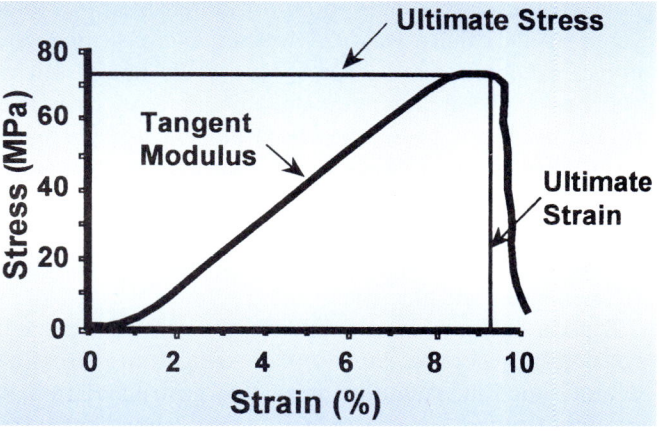

Figure 5 A schematic stress-strain curve resulting from tensile testing of a ligament. *(Reproduced with permission from Woo SL-Y, Debski RE, Withrow JD, Janaushek MA: Biomechanics of knee ligaments. Am J Sports Med 1999;27: 533-543.)*

decrease in proliferation. Reverse transcriptase polymerase estrogen and progesterone receptor expression has been identified in the ACL of humans and rabbits. Ovariectomized rabbits were used to study estrogen's effect on ACL load to failure. Half of the rabbits were given supplemental estrogen and were noted to have a significantly reduced load to failure as compared with controls, who received no estrogen.

Skeletal maturity and age have been demonstrated to affect ligament mechanical and structural properties. Young donors (age 22 to 35 years) demonstrate a significant increase in ligament stiffness and ultimate load. In vitro studies using fibroblast cultures from MCL specimens of physically immature, mature, and senescent rabbits demonstrated declining collagen synthesis with age.

Structural and mechanical properties of ligaments are changed by immobilization. In a study involving rats, the cruciate ligaments demonstrated a 25% decrease in load-to-failure after 4 weeks of immobilization. In a study of the MCL in rabbits, the bone-ligament-bone complex was noted to demonstrate an ultimate load-to-failure decrease of 66% as compared with the opposite nonimmobilized control. The energy absorbed at failure decreased to 16% of the opposite limb. The structural property decrease is caused by a combination of changes. The MCL-tibial insertion demonstrates marked disruption of the deep fiber bone insertions with osteoclastic subperiosteal bone resorption. A slow reversal of these effects is noted with remobilization with the ultimate load and energy absorbed to failure reaching 80% to 90% of control at 1 year. Evaluation of the new bone formation at the ligament insertion site reveals that return to normal is slow. The mechanical properties of the MCL returned to normal after 9 weeks of remobilization. The properties of the bone-ligament-bone complex are also affected by exercise but to a much lesser extent than by immobilization.

Injury and Repair

The healing process of extra-articular ligaments is similar to wound repair in other structures. The ligaments heal by a scar repair process. This process, while a continuum, can be divided into four phases based on biologic events. Phase 1, the inflammatory phase, is marked by hematoma formation and occurs during the first 3 days. Platelets, inflammatory cells, and erythrocytes aggregate at the site of the injury. Cytokines are released and induce angiogenesis and the formation of granulation tissue. Fibroblasts (from the neighboring tissue and the systemic circulation) proliferate near the end of this phase. Early scar formation occurs, composed primarily of type III collagen. During phase 2,

cell proliferation matrix deposition occur. During this time, the fibrin clot organizes and the ligament injury gap is filled with a vascular granulation tissue. Type I collagen synthesis dominates in both the scar area and the adjacent normal ligament. Phases 3 and 4 occur over weeks to months and represent remodeling and maturation of the scar. The cellularity and vascularity at the scar site gradually decrease. The type I and type III collagen ratios begin to approach normal levels. An increase in collagen density occurs and then plateaus. Despite this plateau, the tensile strength gradually increases as a result of matrix changes involving collagen reorganization and cross-linking. Even with this reorganization, the strength of the injured ligament never reaches that of the uninjured ligament. The tensile strength of the healed ligament correlates with the concentration of large-diameter type I collagen fibrils and pyridinoline cross-links. Small-diameter collagen fibrils and decreased cross-link density dominate ligament scarring.

The MCL and other extra-articular ligaments have an intrinsic healing response, which has not been observed in intra-articular ligaments such as the ACL. This difference in healing has been extensively studied and may be a result of a variety of biologic factors. Intra-articular ligaments have a limited blood supply compared with extra-articular ligaments, and the environment inside the joint may not permit the inflammatory phase of healing. Based on this lack of healing response, graft reconstruction of the ACL remains the recommended choice of treatment.

The effect of injury size on healing of the MCL was demonstrated in a rabbit study. An 8-mm gap injury or a 4-mm Z-plasty injury was created. Both injuries healed with histologically similar tissue when evaluated at 40, 78, or 100 weeks. Mechanically, there were significantly decreased structural properties at all intervals. This study suggests there are long-term structural weaknesses in large gap injuries. Collagen fibril diameter has been demonstrated to be similar in healing and grafted ligaments with a predominance of small-diameter fibrils (probably newly synthesized collagen). An in vitro study using rabbit MCL tissue incubated in collagenase for 3 and 6 days demonstrated mean fibril diameter values resembling 40-week scar values. This study demonstrates that collagenase may alter the fibril diameter, and therefore the small fibrils found in healing ligaments and reconstruction grafts may represent the enzymatically reduced endogenous fibrils. Collagen fibril diameter has been studied in a long-term model of the MCL. A consistent pattern of small-diameter fibrils is noted at 40 weeks in the rabbit MCL injury model. An increased number of large-diameter fibrils are noted at 78 and 104 weeks, but 90% of the fibrils are still of small diameter. No rabbits demonstrated the fibril pattern seen in uninjured ligaments. The proteoglycan network is significantly altered in healing ligaments. In the normal ligament, decorin is the most common proteoglycan, representing 80% of the total. In the healing ligament, biglycan is predominant and decorin is barely detected. The proteoglycan-rich matrix accumulates in the injury gap by 3 weeks postinjury and is present for up to 2 years. The increased level of biglycan may interfere with normal collagen remodeling, preventing a return to normal ligamentous tissue.

The effect of ibuprofen on healing of MCL injuries in rabbits has been studied. A 14-day course of ibuprofen did not affect load-to-failure of healing MCL injuries tested at 14 and 28 days as compared with untreated controls. Some evidence exists that hyperbaric oxygen treatment may improve MCL healing. A study using a rat model demonstrated a significant increase in load-to-failure at 6 weeks in rats treated with hyperbaric oxygen as compared with untreated controls.

Tendon

Structure and Function

Tendons are made up of dense regular connective tissue highly specialized to transmit high tensile loads from muscle to bone. Collagen (86% type I and 5% type III of the dry weight) is the major constituent of tendon. Three collagen chains are combined in a collagen molecule and organize into microfibrils and then fibrils. Proteoglycans and glycoproteins with water combine with fibrils in a matrix to form fascicles. The fascicles coalesce to bundles, which are surrounded by the endotenon. The endotenon supports the vascular supply, lymphatics, and nerves. The epitenon and subsequently the paratenon surround a set of bundles and complete the structural anatomy of the tendon.

Fibroblasts align along the fibril subunits, but the tendon is relatively hypocellular. Proteoglycans, although small in concentration, provide an important function. Proteoglycans are extremely hydrophilic and influence the viscoelastic properties of tendons. Decorin is widely distributed and is thought to play a fundamental role in regulating collagen fiber formation in vivo. Decorin is speculated to prevent slippage during tendon deformation, thus increasing the tensile strength of the tendon. Compared with ligaments, deformation is less under an applied load. Thus, tendons are better able to transmit load from muscle to bone, allowing motion during contraction or to resist motion during eccentric contraction. Tendons typically transmit tensile forces but in tendons that wrap around an articular surface, compressive forces are produced.

Tendons in these regions develop a more cartilaginous structure.

Tendons can be divided into two major categories: (1) those that pull in a straight line, are not enclosed in a sheath but are surrounded by the paratenon (Achilles tendon), a loose connective tissue continuous with the tendon, or (2) those that are required to bend, such as the flexor tendons of the hand, that are enclosed by a tendon sheath that directs the tendon path and acts as a pulley. Motion of this type of tendon is assisted by synovial fluid produced by the synovial membrane or epitenon. The vascular supply of these two types of tendons is quite different. Tendons within a sheath receive their vascular supply from the perimysium, the periosteal insertion, and long and short vinculae by way of the proximal mesotendon. In tendons surrounded by the paratenon the vascular supply enters from the periphery into a longitudinal system of capillaries. These tendons also receive blood supply from the perimysium and their osseous insertions.

The mechanical and structural properties of tendons are critical to their ability to generate tensile force. The mechanical properties of the tendon are dependent on the structure of the collagen fibrils. The structural properties of the bone-tendon-muscle unit depend not only on the mechanical properties of the tendon but on its myotendinous junction and bony insertion. The structural properties of the bone-tendon-muscle unit are represented by a load-elongation curve similar to that of ligaments. The load-elongation curve demonstrates an initial toe region where the tendon shows initial stretch without significant force applied secondary to the straightening of the cramped fibrils and orientation of the longitudinal collagen fibers. The toe region is smaller in tendon compared to ligament because the collagen fibers are oriented in a more parallel fashion and therefore less realignment occurs during initial loading. Following the toe region is a more linear region, which represents the elastic modulus of the tendon. Tendon failure occurs abruptly or in a downward curve. The downward curve represents permanent structural changes or irreversible elongation in the tendon. Young animals, which are skeletally immature, demonstrate a more abrupt failure on the load-elongation curve than skeletally mature animals. Viscoelastic properties of tendons affect their function. In isometric contractions, the muscle-tendon unit length remains constant but elongation of the tendon occurs secondary to creep, which allows the muscle to shorten. This improves muscle function during isometric contractions. Preconditioning occurs when the initial cycles of elongation following a period of rest reveal increased energy loss. Following preconditioning, the load elongation cycle is more repeatable. This is why warm-up prior to exercise is critical for appropriate muscle-tendon-bone unit function.

Factors Affecting Tendon Properties

The anatomic location of tendons affects their mechanical and structural properties. Biomechanical and biochemical studies have revealed significant differences between flexor and extensor tendons. In adult miniature swine, the ultimate load to failure of digital flexor tendons is twice that of digital extensor tendons. In addition, on load-elongation curves, hysteresis (energy loss) is twice as large in extensor tendons as compared with flexor tendons. Biochemically the collagen content of digital flexor tendons is higher than that of extensor tendons. Age and maturation increase the difference between the types of tendons.

Exercise has been shown to impart positive effects on the mechanical and structural properties of tendons. The elastic modulus and ultimate load to failure of swine digital extensor tendons has been shown to increase following exercise. Collagen synthesis and fibril diameter both increase following exercise as demonstrated by biochemical studies. Larger fibrils demonstrate improved tensile stress properties due to increased cross-links. In a study of stress-shielded and partially stress-shielded patellar tendons, the stress-shielded tendons demonstrated significantly less tensile strength when tested at 1, 2, 3, and 6 weeks as compared with even the partially stress-shielded tendons. In an in vitro study of the stress-shielded canine digital flexor tendon, a significant decrease was noted in the elastic modulus over an 8-week period. The canine digital flexor tendon demonstrated a significant increase in tensile properties when subjected to cyclic loading, compared with in vitro tendons, which underwent no stress. Exercise has been shown to have a differential effect on different tendons suggesting that some tendons may have the ability to improve their structural properties while others work near their peak capacity. Immobilization of tendon decreases its tensile strength, stiffness, and total weight due to a decrease in cellularity, collagen organization, collagen fibril diameter, and collagen cross-links and an altered proteoglycan and water content. Remobilization results in a slow return to normal of the biochemical and biomechanical properties of the tendon. This process takes much longer than the period of immobilization and points to the need for early mobilization of tendons when possible.

A reduction in tendon vascularity and cellularity is noted with aging. The aging process also results in an increased amount of insoluble collagen, increased maturation of collagen cross-links, increased collagen fibril diameter, reduced collagen turnover, and decreased proteoglycan and water content. These changes, which may become evident by the third decade, result in a weaker, stiffer, and less compliant tendon. Additional degenerative changes in the tendon will increase the possibility of injury. Exercise may help slow these age-related changes.

Fluoroquinolones, a class of widely used antibiotics, have been associated with tendinitis. Musculoskeletal effects of these medications have a reported incidence of less than 1% and consist mainly of arthralgias and myalgias. Achilles tendon disorders are most common, including reports of sharp pain in the tendon a few hours after medication administration and reports of bilateral tendon ruptures. Investigators have studied the toxic effects of these medications. Tenocytes in the Achilles tendon demonstrated cellular degeneration. Pefloxacin administration demonstrated a decrease in proteoglycan production and oxidative damage of type I collagen in mouse Achilles tendons. In particular, there was a decrease in production of decorin, which is critical for tendon structural strength. Further studies are necessary to determine the exact nature of risk of these medications for tendon disorders.

Injury and Repair

Tendon injuries occur by one of three mechanisms. Direct trauma can result in transection of the tendon. Indirect injury is an avulsion of the tendon from its bony insertion. Indirect intrasubstance injury can result from intrinsic or extrinsic factors. Trauma frequently results in a direct injury to tendon (such as tendon lacerations in the hand). A bony avulsion can result from an overwhelming stress to the bony tendon unit (such as ring finger flexor digitorum profundus avulsion injuries). Repetitive submaximal overload or repetitive pressure against a bony surface, as seen by the supraspinatus beneath the acromion, can result in intrasubstance degeneration. Tendon healing following an injury mimics the wound repair response in other soft tissues. The four phases of healing (inflammation, proliferation, remodeling, and maturation) occur.

Rat and rabbit Achilles tendons have been used to study extrasynovial tendon healing. Following tendon injury, the gap fills with inflammatory products, blood cells, nuclear debris, and fibrin. Fibroblasts and capillary buds fill the gap between the tendon ends by proliferating from the paratenon. After 3 days, collagen synthesis can be detected. Type I collagen production is increased 15- to 22-fold. After 2 weeks, a fibrous bridge consisting of fibroblasts and collagen fibers fuses the tendon. Between 3 and 4 weeks, the collagen fibers begin to organize longitudinally in a process that continues for many months. The scar mass during the early stages of healing is much larger than the uninjured tendon, but gradually decreases in size during healing because of collagen reorganization and collagen fibril cross-linking. This process improves with appropriately applied stress.

Healing in tendons enclosed by a sheath has been a topic of research for many years. Early studies suggested that healing occurred by granulation tissue from the sheath. Recent investigations have demonstrated that tendon cells participate in the healing response. Pro-alpha-1 collagen mRNA has been demonstrated to be present in epitenon and endotenon cells in the healing flexor tendon. In healing flexor tendons, which undergo controlled passive motion, the intrinsic healing response of the epitenon is the predominant form of healing. In immobilized tendons, granulation tissue from the digital sheath and endotenon cellular proliferation dominate the healing response. During the intrinsic healing response collagen synthesis and vascular response are noted followed by collagen maturation and reorganization similar to the wound repair response seen in other tissues.

Factors Affecting Tendon Repair

Factors that affect tendon repair include suture repair type, continuous passive motion, gap formation, and load experienced by the healing tendon. Aggressive and early active motion and weight bearing have been demonstrated to increase the rate of tendon rupture and gap formation. On the other hand, early and controlled passive mobilization has been demonstrated to improve several factors involving tendon repair. Controlled passive motion improves the repair strength in the early period following repair and decreases adhesions. In the canine digital flexor tendon an eight-strand repair resulted in increased stiffness and load to failure of the repair at 3 and 6 weeks when compared with the Savage, Tajima, and Kessler types of repair. Gap formation (elongation) at the repair site of healing flexor tendons has been associated with adhesion formation and poor functional outcome. A study evaluating gap formation in the healing canine flexor tendon demonstrated a significant increase in ultimate force, repair site rigidity, and repair site strain in tendons with less than 3 mm of gap compared with tendons that have greater than 3 mm of gap. These differences were noted at both 10-day and 42-day time periods during mechanical testing and no difference was noted in the prevalence of adhesions.

Novel approaches to improve tendon healing are being studied. Cytokines such as PDGF, epidermal growth factor, and insulin-like growth factor-1 have been noted to improve tendon healing. Growth and differentiation factors 5 and 6 from the bone morpho-

genetic protein family used in a rat Achilles tendon healing model via collagen sponges at the injury site have demonstrated increased tensile strength of the healing tendon. The appropriate type and timing of cytokine delivery to facilitate the most rapid and quality repair has yet to be determined. Mesenchymal stem cells in a collagen matrix have been delivered to a rabbit Achilles tendon injury model (1-cm tendon gap) and structural and material properties were noted to be twice those of the control tissues.

Factors Affecting Tendon-to-Bone Healing

Tendon-to-bone healing is critical for success in numerous reconstructive surgical procedures. When tendon grafts heal within a bone tunnel, a fibrovascular interface forms between the bone and tendon. Bony ingrowth is noted in this interface with the eventual development of an indirect insertion in which tendon collagen fibers are continuous with bone. In rotator cuff repair, bone ingrowth also occurs in the interface between tendon and bone. Animal models show no advantage in repairing tendon to a cancellous bone trough versus repair directly to cortical bone. Studies have demonstrated that the strength of repair correlates directly with bone ingrowth into the fibrous interface.

In a human cadaver finger model, an eight-strand-suture technique resulted in a significant improvement in tendon-bone elongation when exposed to a 20-N force. The sutures were secured to a suture anchor or a dorsally placed button. The eight-strand repair secured to a dorsal button was stronger than the four- or eight-strand repair performed with a suture anchor. Bone morphogenetic protein-2 has been used to improve the tendon graft-to-bone tunnel healing in a canine model. Biomechanical testing of this model showed higher tendon pullout strength in the cytokine-treated tendons as compared with controls. Histologic and radiologic evaluation demonstrated more extensive bone formation around the tendon and closer bone tendon apposition.

Tendon Overuse Injury

Tendon overuse injuries result from repetitive microtrauma. The patient responds early with the inflammatory cell infiltration, tissue edema, and fibrin exudation. If the overload becomes chronic, the synovial cells and fibroblasts proliferate, capillaries form, and the paratenon thickens. The process of tendinosis involves alteration to cells, collagen fibers, and matrix components. A reparative and degenerative process affects the tendon. The tensile strength of the tendon decreases and microtears develop in the tendon. As tendon fibers fail, the resulting load on the rest of the tendon increases, which places it at risk for progressive failure. This process occurs at the lateral epicondyle in tennis elbow, at the inferior insertion or the patellar tendon due to patella tendinitis, and at the Achilles tendon insertion to calcaneus with Achilles tendinitis. With tendon failure, the typical wound repair response occurs in most tendons, but is limited in others, such as the rotator cuff.

Nerve

Structure and Function

A neuron consists of four distinct regions: the axon, dendrites, presynaptic terminal, and the cell body. The cell body only contains 10% of the volume of the neuron but is the metabolic center containing the nucleus and organelles for protein and RNA synthesis. The dendrites are branches from the cell body that receive signals from other nerve cells. Each cell body contains only one axon that is responsible for the conduction of information by propagating electrical signals. The action potential is an all-or-none phenomenon initiated from the axon hillock, the region where the axon originates. Proteins are synthesized in the cell body, assembled into the appropriate macromolecules, and sent down the axon using axoplasmic transport. Presynaptic terminals are specialized regions at the end of axons, which transmit information to dendrites or cell bodies. Axons insulated by a myelin sheath (produced by Schwann cells) conduct electrical impulses using less energy at a higher frequency and at a faster speed than noninsulated axons. Myelin consists of 30% protein and 70% lipid (mainly cholesterol and phospholipid).

The nerve fiber consists of the axon and its myelin sheath. Surrounding the nerve fiber is a basement membrane and connective tissue called the endoneurium. A collection of nerve fibers forms a fascicle. The perineurium is the connective tissue that surrounds the fascicle. Several fascicles together form the peripheral nerve, which is surrounded by a connective tissue layer called the epineurium that supplies a protective framework for the fascicles. The vascular supply of peripheral nerves relies on an intrinsic and extrinsic system. The intrinsic system is a vascular plexus in the epineurium, perineurium, and endoneurium. The extrinsic system consists of regional vessels, which enter the nerve trunk at various sites running in the connective tissue that surrounds the nerve trunk. Both systems are oriented longitudinally with anastomotic connections between them. The perineurial and endoneurial plexuses make up a defined vascular unit, which can remain intact when fascicles are separated. The endoneurial plexus consists of arterioles, venules, and capillaries, which form an anastomotic network along the fascicle. The capillaries are large, nearly twice the size of muscle capillaries with functional characteristics similar to those in the central nervous system. The blood-nerve barrier is similar to the blood-brain barrier protecting and maintaining an appropriate endoneurial environment.

Nerves have biomechanical properties and although testing is difficult, demonstrate a typical stress-strain relationship. A more linear region at higher stress follows a compliant, low-strained toe region. During normal physiologic function, nerves work in the toe region of the stress-strain curve. In repair situations, the nerves may be expected to operate under more stress when the ends of nerves are reopposed to span injury gaps. This is critical, for while nerves have demonstrated ultimate strain ranging from 20% to 60%, ischemic damage is noted at strain rates as low as 15%. In clinical situations, joints and extremities are frequently immobilized to protect nerve repairs.

Injury and Repair

Peripheral nerve injuries can be divided into two broad categories: those that result in no axon discontinuity and only temporary loss of nerve conduction, and those injuries where axons are damaged to a point where axonal degeneration occurs proximal and distal to the injury. Wallerian degeneration is a result of axon discontinuity. This process occurs within hours of the injury. The myelin surrounding the axon undergoes deterioration with loss of nerve conduction. This process extends proximally from the site of injury usually to the next node of Ranvier and distally to the target organ. Schwann cells of intact nerve fibers do not usually divide, but following injury these cells undergo mitosis with a cell proliferation peak at 3 days. The Schwann cells act in phagocytosis of myelin and axonal debris. The Schwann cells maintain cytoplasmic tubes called the bands of Büngner that run beneath the nerve fiber basal lamina. These Schwann cells assist the process of regeneration by synthesis of nerve growth factor. The nerve cell body also undergoes changes following peripheral nerve injury. The focus of the nerve cell body changes to synthesis of proteins necessary for axonal repair and growth instead of the previous production of neurotransmitters. At the tip of the regenerating axon is the growth cone, which accomplishes the process of axonal regeneration. In order for regeneration to occur, the zone of injury must be crossed by the growth cone to make contact with the endoneurial tubes of the distal nerve stump. The ability to complete this process is affected by several factors including amount of nerve damage, gap, and scar formation. Regeneration is accomplished at an average of 1 mm per day in adults but may be faster in children.

Classification systems exist for nerve injuries. Neurapraxia, usually secondary to compression, results in local myelin damage, but the axon remains in continuity. Axonotmesis by definition is a loss of continuity of the axon with some preservation of the nerve connective tissue. Neurotmesis results in physiologic discontinuity of the nerve, although the nerve may not be actually transsected. In Sunderland's classification system five types of nerve injury are described. Type 1 is equivalent to neurapraxia, types 2, 3, and 4 are equivalent to axonotmesis, and type 5 is equivalent to neurotmesis. Axonotmesis, type 2, is a loss of continuity of the axons with the endoneurium, perineurium, and epineurium intact. Axonotmesis, type 3, is loss of continuity of the axons and endoneurium with the perineurium and epineurium intact. Axonotmesis, type 4, is loss of continuity of the axons, endoneurium, and perineurium, with the epineurium intact.

Historically, it was believed that nerve repair should be delayed for 3 weeks to allow for completion of wallerian degeneration; however, more recent studies have demonstrated that immediate primary repair improves results. Primary repair requires adequate soft-tissue coverage, skeletal stability with low tension on the nerve repair, and a good vascular supply. Two types of nerve repair, grouped fascicular repair and simple epineurial repair, are possible. Theoretically, grouped fascicular repair is advantageous because axon realignment can be more accurate, although this may require additional dissection resulting in increased scarring and decreased vascular supply. Prospective studies comparing grouped fascicular repair with simple epineurial repair have not demonstrated an improvement with the fascicular repair. Researchers continue to try to identify factors that will improve nerve repair and nerve regeneration at the biologic level. Growth factors have been given systemically or locally with some promising results in animal models.

When primary repair is impossible, nerve grafting is required. Autogenous grafting remains the standard approach. The sural nerve or the medial and lateral antebrachial cutaneous nerve have commonly been used. For larger nerves, multiple segments of graft may be necessary. In this setting, a group fascicular repair is attempted. The direction of the nerve graft is reversed from proximal to distal, and a tension-free repair performed. In smaller nerves, a single segment of graft may be used. Investigations of larger nerve grafts in animal models have demonstrated slower revascularization compared with that of smaller multisegment nerve grafts. Allografts would be an excellent choice if the results were equivalent to autogenous grafts. Advantages of allografts include no donor nerve sacri-fice, faster surgical procedures, and the ability to store grafts in tissue banks. The main impediment to allograft use has been the immunogenic host response. A recent study demonstrated allograft repair results equivalent to autograft repair following a biologic detergent technique that removed the cellular components, which are immunogenic, without production of cell debris. Further work to improve allograft results and to develop other conduits for nerve regeneration will hopefully add other options in the future.

Annotated Bibliography

Meniscus

Stollsteimer GT, Shelton WR, Dukes A, Bomboy AL: Meniscal allograft transplantation: A 1- to 5-year follow-up of 22 patients. *Arthroscopy* 2000;16:343-347.

This article documents the technique of using cryopreserved meniscal allografts in 22 patients and 23 knees with an average follow-up of 40 months using the Internation Knee Documentation Committee, Lysholm, and Tegner scoring systems. The most significant finding was a clinical improvement in perioperative pain as measured by the Lysholm, and on follow-up MRI of a subset the average size of meniscus was 63% of normal. Other confounding variables or procedures performed during this study were not discussed.

Articular Cartilage

Browne JE, Branch TP: Surgical alternatives for treatment of articular cartilage lesions. *J Am Acad Orthop Surg* 2000;8:180-189.

This article provides a comprehensive review of treatment of articular cartilage lesions and a recommended approach. The authors state that currently there are no peer-reviewed prospective randomized controlled trials of surgical versus nonsurgical treatment for full-thickness articular cartilage defects.

Muscle

Terjung RL, Clarkson P, Eichner ER, et al: American College of Sports Medicine roundtable: The physiological and health effects of oral creatine supplementation. *Med Sci Sports Exerc* 2000;32:706-717.

This consensus statement by the American College of Sports Medicine summarizes the research on creatine supplementation to increase muscle strength during resistance training. Exercise performance during short periods of extremely powerful activity (for example, squats or bench press) can be enhanced, especially during repeated bouts of activity. However, creatine supplementation does not increase maximum isokinetic strength, the rate of maximal force generation, nor aerobic exercise performance. Although creatine supplementation exhibits small but significant physiologic and performance changes, these increases in performance are realized during very specific exercise conditions as outlined in the original research protocols. This suggests that the apparent high expectations for performance enhancement in sports evidenced by the extensive use of creatine supplements are inordinate.

Yan Z: Skeletal muscle adaptation and cell cycle regulation. *Exerc Sport Sci Rev* 2000;28:24-26.

This excellent review studies skeletal muscle adaptation to altered functional demands and its effect on the satellite cells as they are stimulated and differentiated into myofibrils. It is hypothesized that this process is of fundamental importance for adaptation of exercise because nuclei from satellite cells maintain a constant nuclear to cytoplasm ratio, and they also alter gene expression and thereby provide the mechanism by which skeletal muscle adapts to altered functional demands.

Ligament

Rodeo SA, Suzuki K, Deng XH, Wozney J, Warren RF: Use of recombinant human bone morphogenetic protein-2 to enhance tendon healing in a bone tunnel. *Am J Sports Med* 1999;27:476-488.

A study involving the canine long digital extensor tendon transplanted into a drill hole in the proximal tibia demonstrated that dogs treated with human bone morphogenetic protein-2 at the tendon-bone interface resulted in improved histologic and biomechanical healing.

Slauterbeck J, Clevenger C, Lundberg W, Burchfield DM: Estrogen level alters the failure load of the rabbit anterior cruciate ligament. *J Orthop Res* 1999;17:405-408.

In a study involving ovariectomized rabbits, estrogen supplementation resulted in a significant decrease in the ultimate load to failure of the ACL as compared with rabbits without estrogen supplementation.

Tendon

Gelberman RH, Boyer MI, Brodt MD, Winters SC, Silva MJ: The effect of gap formation at the repair site on the strength and excursion of intrasynovial flexor tendons: An experimental study on the early stages of tendon-healing in dogs. *J Bone Joint Surg Am* 1999;81:975-982.

Gap formation was studied at the repair site of dog intrasynovial flexor tendons. A gap of > 3 mm did not increase the prevalence of adhesions or decrease range of motion but did decrease the strength and stiffness of the repair.

Nerve

Best TJ, Mackinnon SE, Evans PJ, Hunter D, Midha R: Peripheral nerve revascularization: Histomorphometric study of small-and large-caliber grafts. *J Reconstr Microsurg* 1999;15:183-190.

Small-caliber and large-caliber nerve graft revascularization was studied, with a significantly improved and faster response noted in the small-caliber graphs at 7 and 40 days following repair.

Classic Bibliography

Arnoczky SP, Warren RF, Spivak JM: Meniscal repair using an exogenous fibrin clot: An experimental study in dogs. *J Bone Joint Surg Am* 1988;70:1209-1217.

Beiner JM, Jokl P, Cholewicki J, Panjabi MM: The effect of anabolic steroids and corticosteroids on healing of muscle contusion injury. *Am J Sports Med* 1999;27:2-9.

Best TM, Loitz-Ramage B, Corr DT, Vanderby R: Hyperbaric oxygen in the treatment of acute muscle stretch injuries: Results in an animal model. *Am J Sports Med* 1998;26:367-372.

Brittberg M, Lindahl A, Nilsson A, Ohlsson C, Isaksson O, Peterson L: Treatment of deep cartilage defects in the knee with autologous chondrocyte transplantation. *N Engl J Med* 1994;331:889-895.

Buckwalter JA, Mankin HJ. Articular cartilage: Degeneration and osteoarthritis, repair, regeneration, and transplantation. *Instr Course Lect* 1998;47:487-504.

Curl WW, Krome J, Gordon ES, Rushing J, Smith BP, Poehling GG: Cartilage injuries: A review of 31,516 knee arthroscopies. *Arthroscopy* 1997;13:456-460.

Fu FH, Harner CD, Johnson DL, Miller MD, Woo SL: Biomechanics of knee ligaments: Basic concepts and clinical application. *J Bone Joint Surg Am* 1993;75:1716-1727.

Gelberman RH, Manske PR, Akeson WH, Woo SL, Lundborg G, Amiel D: Flexor tendon repair. *J Orthop Res* 1986;4:119-128.

Hede A, Larsen E, Sandberg H: Partial versus total meniscectomy: A prospective, randomised study with long-term follow-up. *J Bone Joint Surg Br* 1992;74:118-121.

Jackson DW, McDevitt CA, Simon TM, Arnoczky SP, Atwell EA, Silvino NJ: Meniscal transplantation using fresh and cryopreserved allografts: An experimental study in goats. *Am J Sports Med* 1992;20:644-656.

Johnson DL, Urban WP, Caborn DN, Vanarthos WJ, Carlson CS: Articular cartilage changes seen with magnetic resonance imaging-detected bone bruises associated with acute anterior cruciate ligament rupture. *Am J Sports Med* 1998;26:409-414.

Loitz-Ramage BJ, Frank CB. Shrive NG: Injury size affects long-term strength of the rabbit medial collateral ligament. *Clin Orthop* 1997;337:272-280.

Mair SD, Seaber AV, Glisson RR, Garrett WE Jr: The role of fatigue in susceptibility to acute muscle strain injury. *Am J Sports Med* 1996;24:137-143.

Son YJ, Thompson WJ: Schwann cell processes guide regeneration of peripheral axons. *Neuron* 1995;14: 125-132.

Spindler KP, Clark SW, Nanney LB, Davidson JM: Expression of collagen and matrix metalloproteinases in ruptured human anterior cruciate ligament: An in situ hybridization study. *J Orthop Res* 1996;14:657-661.

Spindler KP, Schils JP, Bergfeld JA, et al: Prospective study of osseous, articular, and meniscal lesions in recent anterior cruciate ligament tears by magnetic resonance imaging and arthroscopy. *Am J Sports Med* 1993;21:551-557.

Taylor DC, Brooks DE, Ryan JB: Anabolic-androgenic steroid administration causes hypertrophy of immobilized and nonimmobilized skeletal muscle in a sedentary rabbit model. *Am J Sports Med* 1999;27:718-727.

Volek JS, Duncan ND, Mazzetti SA, et al: Performance and muscle fiber adaptations to creatine supplementation and heavy resistance training. *Med Sci Sports Exerc* 1999;31:1147-1156.

Watchmaker GP, Mackinnon SE: Advances in peripheral nerve repair. *Clin Plast Surg* 1997;24:63-73.

Chapter 2

Bone Healing and Grafting

Emil H. Schemitsch, MD, FRCSC

Mohit Bhandari, MD, MSc

Fracture Healing

Bone is unique in that it heals without a scar and generally is restored to its preinjury properties. Fracture healing can be divided into primary (osteonal) and secondary (callus) healing. Primary healing is associated with rigid fracture fixation (plate fixation). The progression of fracture healing requires stability of the fracture ends as well as a functional blood supply.

Stages of Healing

The majority of fractures heal through a combination of intramembranous and endochondral ossification (secondary healing). There are at least five stages of healing: (1) hematoma and inflammation; (2) angiogenesis and cartilage formation; (3) cartilage calcification and cartilage removal; (4) bone formation; and (5) bone remodeling. Immediately following a fracture, a hematoma develops that is believed to be a reservoir for important signaling molecules that have the capacity to initiate early events in fracture healing. Platelets in the clot release growth factors such as transforming growth factor-beta (TGF-β) and platelet-derived growth factor (PDGF), which play an important role in modulating cell proliferation and differentiation. Other growth factors (such as bone morphogenetic protein [BMP]) and cytokines (such as interleukin (IL) -1 and -6) are expressed during cartilage formation. By the first week, the periosteum undergoes an intramembranous bone formation response. At the same time, the fibrovascular stroma overlying the fracture site is infiltrated with chondrocytes and forms cartilage. By the second week, two distinct portions of the callus are visible by microscopy: hard callus (intramembranous ossification) and soft callus (endochondral ossification). Cartilage calcification proceeds in much the same manner as that in the growth plate. Chondrocytes hypertrophy and then calcify. The calcified cartilage becomes a prime target for vascular ingrowth, is removed by chondroclasts, and is replaced by new woven bone.

The woven bone is then remodeled over several months to form the lamellar structure of compact bone.

Recapitulation of Embryonic Skeletal Bone Formation

Bone formation and remodeling are continuous processes that begin during fetal development and continue throughout life. When injury to bone occurs, healing is affected by regeneration of new bone rather than scar tissue. In a recent study it has been demonstrated that Indian hedgehog (*ihh*) and core binding factor 1 (*cbf1*) influence both embryonic bone formation and fracture healing. In addition, vascular endothelial growth factor (VEGF) plays a critical role in cartilage hypertrophy during growth plate development and ossification associated with fracture healing.

Effects of Fracture Fixation on the Healing Response

Plate Fixation

Anatomic alignment and rigid fixation of the fracture with a plate alters normal fracture healing. Rigid plate fixation inhibits callus formation. In regions where there is direct cortical contact, primary healing occurs by direct haversian remodeling. Briefly, osteoclasts resorb bone and create a channel across the fracture ends (cutting cone), enabling blood vessels and osteoblasts to follow. This direct "osteonal" remodeling has three requirements: anatomic fracture reduction, rigid fixation, and intact blood supply. Motion at the fracture site will ultimately result in callus formation (secondary healing), and if excessive, will lead to plate failure and nonunion.

The decreased bone density at the site of a plated fracture within 8 weeks of plate fixation is direct evidence of haversian remodeling. Increases in cortical porosity, or "cancellization" of the cortical bone, remains a common finding beneath a plate. Limited contact dynamic compression plates have been designed to limit contact areas of the plate with the cortical surface of the bone to preserve blood flow and limit porosity. The relative advantage of this type of plate is based on its design properties and not its material composition (titanium versus stainless steel).

Intramedullary Nail Fixation

The popularity of intramedullary nail fixation for long bone fractures (especially femur and tibia) has led to important advances in the understanding of fracture healing after nail insertion. In contrast to the load-sparing effect of plates, intramedullary nails are load-sharing devices that promote secondary fracture healing. The use of reamed versus nonreamed intramedullary nails is a point of debate.

Research supporting use of reamed intramedullary nails has focused on the resultant increased blood flow to soft tissues and the reamed nail's superior biomechanical stability. In a sheep tibial fracture model, it was demonstrated that reaming prior to nail insertion significantly increases muscle and surrounding soft-tissue blood flow compared with nonreamed nails for up to 6 weeks. This increase in blood flow to soft tissues may enhance cortical revascularization and the biomechanical superiority of large diameter reamed versus smaller diameter nonreamed nails.

Advocates of nonreamed intramedullary nailing believe that this insertion technique optimally preserves the blood supply for fracture healing. The massive destruction of the endosteal blood supply (up to 70%) after intramedullary reaming has been reported in the literature. In a variety of animal models, limited reaming was noted to cause less devascularization of cortical bone than standard reaming and loose-fitting nonreamed intramedullary nails allowed for superior cortical revascularization at 11 weeks when compared with a tight-fitting nail.

In summary, experimental data suggest that reamed nails offer greater biomechanical stability (afforded by their larger size) and increased soft-tissue blood flow, while loose-fitting, nonreamed intramedullary nails preserve blood flow to cortical bone. Thus, the optimal implant would seem to be a loose-fitting intramedullary nail inserted with limited reaming.

External Fixation

Primary bone healing can also be observed with rigid external fixation. The rigidity of a frame is ultimately determined by many factors: increased pin diameter, increased pin number, decreased bone-rod distance, increased pin group separation, and half pins separated by 45°. The optimal condition for fracture healing with external fixation may actually involve controlled micromotion. Studies have shown that axial micromovement (30 min/day) starting 1 to 3 weeks after surgery in patients with externally fixed tibial shaft fractures significantly reduces time to independent weight bearing and overall delayed union rates. Axial displacements have been reported from 0.3 to 1.0 mm in patients with tibial shaft fractures treated with unilateral external fixation during weight-bearing gait.

Variables That Influence Healing

Previous clinical and experimental studies have reported a variety of prognostic factors for fracture healing, including fracture morphology (for example, comminuted and segmental fractures), distraction (fracture gaps), bone loss, high-energy mechanism of injury, high degree of soft-tissue injury, diabetes, alcohol consumption, smoking history, delay in surgical treatment, steroid use, anti-inflammatory drug use, anticonvulsant use, antibiotic use (ciprofloxacin), anticoagulant use, vasculopathy, increasing patient age, and gender. These studies have been limited by single-surgeon experiences, small study sample sizes, idiosyncratic choice of prognostic variables examined, lack of adjustment for multiple variables, and the use of outcomes measures that are subject to variable interpretations.

Blood Supply

The extent of soft-tissue damage is of paramount importance to fracture healing. Significant stripping of the soft tissues and periosteum in patients with high-energy fractures negatively impacts the local blood supply at the fracture ends. Moreover, the location of the fracture relative to the nutrient vessel is important because those fractures distal to the entry point of the vessel are at increased risk of healing complications. A compromised or lack of blood supply negatively impacts fracture healing. It has been reported that injury to one (or all three) of the vessels supplying the leg resulted in a threefold increase in the incidence of delayed union compared with that of fractures with intact vessels.

The role of blood supply in modulating fracture healing has shed light on the mechanism behind the observed clinical effects. Studies have confirmed the increase in blood flow and vascularity during fracture healing. Angiogenesis, or neovascularization, is a normal response to injury. Bone cells and chondrocytes can produce angiogenic factors in a regulated manner. There is increased expression of VEGF, a potent angiogenic factor, during fracture healing. In a study of patients with fresh fractures, high levels of endothelial-stimulating angiogenic factor were found, suggesting the importance of neovascularization signals during early healing.

Recently, the role of exogenous nitric oxide (NO) on the microcirculation of ischemic muscle has been investigated. NO is a potent vasodilator; rats treated with s-nitroso-N-acetylcysteine (100 nmol/100 g/min) showed a 7% to 23% increase in arteriole diameters resulting in an increase from 37% at baseline to 108% at 40 minutes of reperfusion blood flow. A control group only reached a maximum of 68% baseline at 90 minutes of reperfusion blood flow. The potential benefits of NO on rat femoral fracture healing have also been studied; the NO donor group had a 30% increase in callus size compared with controls.

Emphasis on the preservation of vascularity in fracture management also has led to important advances in implant insertion techniques, such as submuscular plate application. The use of such indirect reduction techniques has been shown to improve union rates without bone grafting.

Nonunion

Nonunion is defined as failure of a fracture to unite as evidenced by a lack of progression of healing on radiographs and clinical examination. A reproducible method for grading the stages of bony healing on plain radiographs after fracture or osteotomy has important clinical implications. Radiographic union frequently is used as a study end point and can be an invaluable index when findings on clinical examination are contradictory or unreliable. The assessment of fracture healing relies on serial radiographic examinations with clinical correlation. Successful fracture union should meet the following criteria: (1) the patient's ability to bear weight without pain; (2) the absence of clinically detectable motion at the fracture site; and (3) visible bridging callus across the fracture on plain radiographs. Other imaging techniques such as radionuclide imaging, CT, ultrasound, and resonant frequency analysis show potential in their ability to quantify healing in the experimental setting, but are significantly more costly and cumbersome in their application to clinical practice.

It has been suggested that the best single predictor of strength of a healing fracture is cortical continuity. The interrater reliability of a variety of radiographic parameters commonly used to assess fracture healing recently has been examined. The single most reliable parameter was the number of cortices bridged by fracture callus ($\kappa = 0.75$, 95% confidence interval, 0.61-0.89).

At the pathologic level, a nonunion is a fracture bridged with soft tissue. The gap tissue characteristics reflect the local mechanical and nutritional factors that predominate in the early weeks following the fracture. Nonunions are classified as hypervascular (hypertrophic) (Fig. 1) or avascular (atrophic) (Fig. 2) based on the capability to incite a biologic reaction. Hypertro-

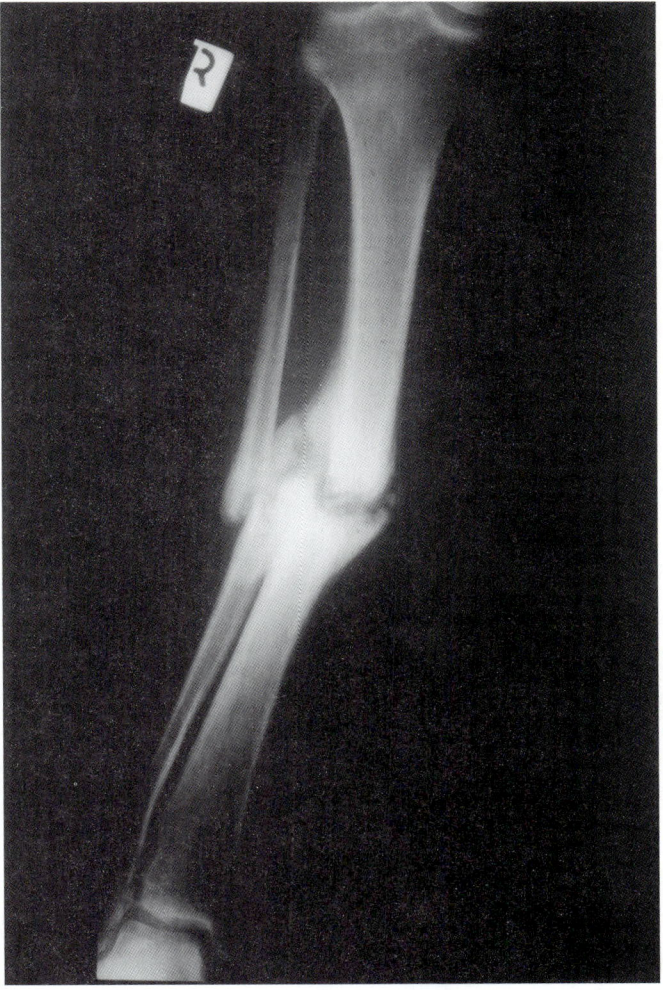

Figure 1 AP radiograph showing hypertrophic nonunion capable of biologic reaction with vascular bone ends and significant callus formation.

phic nonunions, with a predominance of fibrocartilage in the gap, can be effectively managed by stabilization alone. However, atrophic nonunions, with a fibrous tissue gap, often require bone grafting.

Biologic Enhancement of Fracture Healing
Bone Grafts

Bone grafts often serve a dual mechanical and biologic function. The overall success of a bone graft is based largely on its inherent biologic activity, its ability to activate surrounding tissues, and its ability to support ingrowth of host tissue. Osteogenesis refers to bone formation with no indication of cellular origin. When any graft is implanted, a consistent series of events occurs at the graft site: hemorrhage, inflammation, revascularization, substitution, and remodeling. Bone grafts can serve as a source of osteoinductive factors (promote bone formation) such as BMPs, TGF-β, insulin-like growth factors, acidic and basic fibroblast

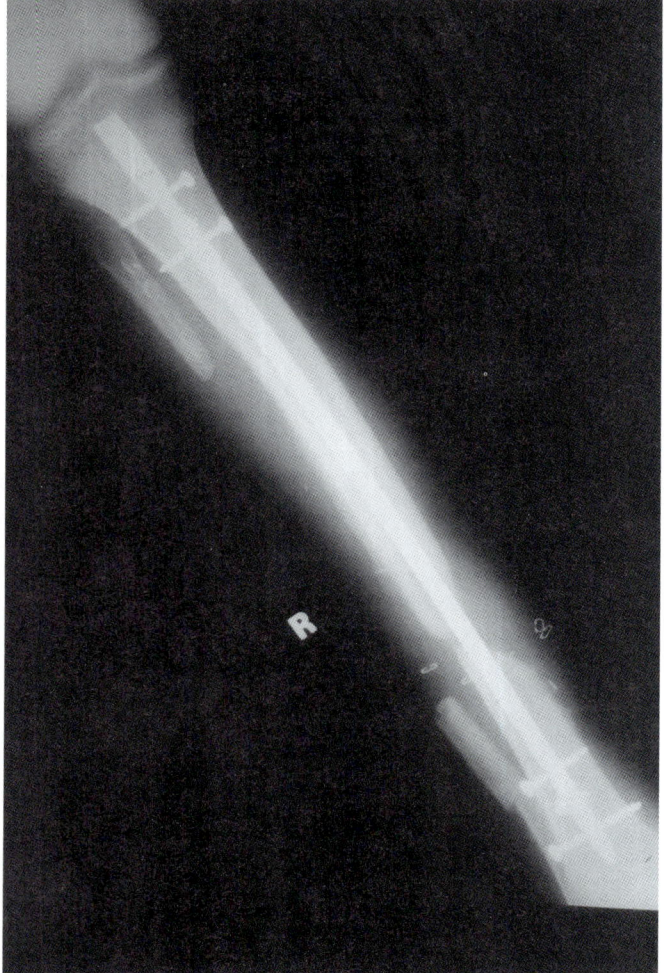

Figure 2 AP radiograph showing atrophic nonunion incapable of biologic reaction with avascular bone ends and lacking callus formation.

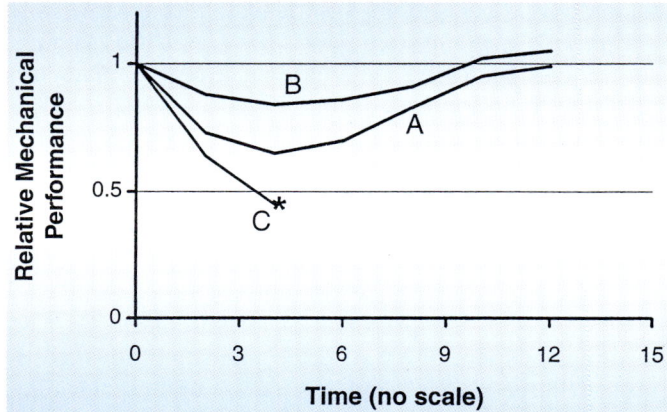

Figure 3 Temporal patterns of biomechanical property changes during cortical graft incorporation. Early resorption of the graft results in a decline in relative mechanical performance. However, strength returns as the bone formation processes eventually predominate. Various factors account for differences in resorption rates (A and B). Aggressive resorption can result in failure of the graft (C). *(Adapted with permission from Davy DT: Biomechanical issues in bone transplantation.* Orthop Clin North Am *1999;30:553-563.)*

growth factors (FGFs), PDGF, ILs, granulocyte colony-stimulating factors, and granulocyte-macrophage colony-stimulating factors. These factors (alone or in combination) can modulate the differentiation of mesenchymal stem cells into bone-forming cells. The health of the host bed is critical in bone graft success because new osteoprogenitor cells are recruited by induction of residual mesenchymal cells in the marrow, endosteum, periosteum, and connective tissue. In addition to osteoinductive effects, bone grafts can serve as a scaffold for the ingrowth of new host bone (osteoconduction).

Autogenous Bone Marrow

Autogenous bone marrow is composed of a rich supply of osteoprogenitor cells. Bone marrow can be aspirated from the iliac crest and injected into a fracture site or area of skeletal defect to stimulate osteogenesis. Favorable results have been reported with the use of bone marrow aspirates and appropriate stabilization in 100 patients with fractures. However, 20% of patients showed minimal bone forming response or no response at all to bone marrow grafting. A composite graft of autogenous bone marrow aspirate and demineralized bone matrix has been reported to produce similar radiographic and mechanical effects to open autogenous bone grafting in a canine nonunion model.

Autogenous Cancellous Bone Graft

Autogenous cancellous bone graft is osteogenic and is characterized by rapid revascularization and incorporation into the host site. Its increased surface area and rich source of osteoblasts and precursors compensate for its lack of structural support. After surgical cancellous bone implantation (usually obtained from the iliac crest), there is hemorrhage and inflammation at the graft site. Many of the osteocytes in the trabecular lacunae die, survived mostly by the surface osteoblasts that produce early new bone. The porous scaffold architecture of cancellous bone graft promotes facile infiltration of host tissues (blood vessels, osteoblasts, precursor cells) within 48 hours. Osteoclast precursors accompany the blood vessel ingrowth, and thus begin the process of graft resorption. Over time, osteoblasts surround "dead" trabeculae and lay down osteoid (unmineralized collagen type I). Ultimately, the bone graft is resorbed and replaced by new host bone. A period of bone remodeling ensues and may last up to several months.

Biomechanically, cancellous grafts have about 4% the strength of cortical bone grafts. The reason for the strength deficit is largely because cancellous grafts are 80% void fraction and 20% tissue fraction.

The relative advantages of autogenous cancellous bone grafts include their significant osteogenic potential, osteoconductive potential, and lack of immunogenicity. The relative disadvantages included a second surgical exposure to obtain the graft, donor site morbidity, and limited availability.

Cortical Bone Autografts (Nonvascularized)

In contrast to the rapid incorporation of blood vessels into cancellous bone grafts, cortical grafts must first rely on peripheral resorption by osteoclasts before revascularization, a process that can take months. Osteoclastic activity results in a significant weakening of the graft compared with host bone (Fig. 3). This graft weakness is most recognizable as a radiolucency of the cortical graft seen on radiographs (contrasted with the radiodensity of cancellous graft, which symbolizes new bone formation).

The healing of the graft-host interface to provide a stable union is similar to fracture healing (endochondral ossification). The relative advantages of cortical bone autografts include improved structural support and lack of immunogenicity. The relative disadvantages include a resistance to revascularization and remodeling.

Cortical Bone Autografts (Vascularized)

The addition of a functional blood supply to cortical bone grafts significantly reduces incorporation time. The majority of osteocytes survive the transplantation if ischemia time is limited. The stereotypic radiolucency of nonvascularized cortical grafts is not seen in vascularized grafts. Graft incorporation occurs quickly and significant weakening is not observed.

Allogeneic Bone Grafts

Allografts, or allogeneic grafts, are tissues transferred between two genetically different individuals of the same species. Modern processing of allogeneic bone grafts includes low-dose irradiation (< 20kGy) to destroy nonpathogenic surface bacteria (optional), physical débridement of all unwanted tissues, pulsatile water washes to remove cells and blood, ethanol to denature proteins and kill viruses/bacteria, and/or antibiotic soaks to kill remaining bacteria. Some bone also may be demineralized during this process. Allogeneic bone is typically stored between −20°C to −147°C, a temperature range that does not have an adverse effect on the bone material properties. For those tissues that have not been collected aseptically, gamma irradiation is used as a final sterilization step. Virucidal doses (30 kGy) will affect the mechanical properties of the graft; therefore, typical doses of irradiation fall under 20 kGy (Fig. 4).

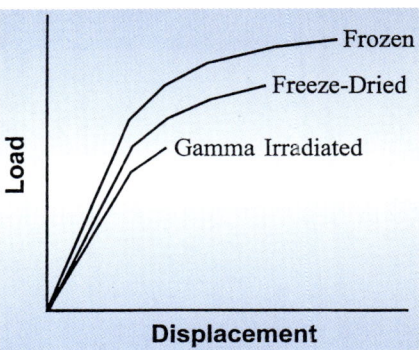

Figure 4 Treatment effects on the material behavior of allograft bone. *(Adapted with permission from Boyce T, Edwards J, Scarborough N: Allograft bone.* Orthop Clin North Am *1999;30:571-581.)*

The risk of viral transmission from an allogeneic bone graft is approximately 1 in 600,000. Most tissue banks have extensive screening protocols for allogeneic bone, including serologic tests for hepatitis B (surface antigen and core antibody), hepatitis C antibody, human immunodeficiency virus (HIV)-1 and -2 antibody, and HIV-P24 antigen. Some banks also conduct polymerase chain reaction testing for HIV.

Allogeneic graft incorporation occurs in much the same manner as with nonvascularized cortical autografts. Similar to the advantages of the cortical autografts, allogeneic grafts provide structural support. Additionally, allografts can be obtained in virtually unlimited quantities of various sizes for procedures where there is significant bone loss. The major disadvantage of allografts is immunogenicity and the potential risk of transmission of pathogens.

Bone Graft Extenders and Potential Substitutes

The term osteoconduction signifies a three-dimensional process that occurs after a porous material is implanted into adjacent bone and provides a scaffold for new bone formation. Blood vessels (perivascular mesenchymal tissues) and osteoprogenitor cells migrate into these porous spaces and incorporate the graft material with newly formed bone. Osteoinductive factors are those that have the capability of inducing osteoblast precursors to differentiate into mature bone-forming cells. Graft materials used in orthopaedic surgery are listed in Table 1.

Calcium Phosphates and Coraline Ceramics

The similarity of the exostructure of *Porites* and *Gonipora* (corals) to human cortical and cancellous bone has led to significant advances in the use of these materials as bone graft substitutes. The role of these ceramics as bone grafts is primarily osteoconduction. The major ceramics that are used clinically are calcium phosphates, hydroxyapatite, and tricalcium phosphates. Coraline

TABLE 1 | Grafting Materials Available for Orthopaedic Surgeons

Grafting Material	Osteo-conduction	Osteo-induction	Osteo-progenitor Cells	Mechanical Strength	Animal Studies	Human Studies
Cancellous autogenous bone graft	++++	++	++	−	Yes	Yes
Bone marrow	−	+/−	+++	−	Yes	Yes
Ceramics						
Pro-Osteon 200-500 (Interpore Cross International, Irvine, CA)	++++	−	−	+/−	Yes	Yes
Pro-Osteon 500 R (Interpore Cross International, Irvine, CA)	++++	−	−	+/−	Yes	No
Norian SRS (Norian Corporation, Cupertino, CA)	++++	−	−	+	Yes	Yes
α-BSM (Etex Corporation, Cambridge, MA)	++++	−	−	+	Yes	No
OsteoSet (Wright Medical Technology, Inc, Arlington, TN)	++++	−	−	+/−	Yes	Yes
Demineralized bone matrix	+	+++	−	−	Yes	Yes
Grafton allogeneic bone						
Matrix (Osteotech, Eatontown, NJ)						
Opteform (Regeneration Technologies, Inc, Alachua, FL)	+	?	−	+/−	NA	NA
Osteofil (Regeneration Technologies, Inc, Alachua, FL)	+	?	−	+/−	NA	NA
Dynagraft (GenSci Regeneration Laboratories, Inc, Irvine, CA)	+	?	−	+/−	NA	NA
Growth factors						
BMP-2	−	++++	−	−	Yes	Yes
rhBMP-7 (OP-1)	−	++++	−	−	Yes	Yes
Composites						
Collagraft (Zimmer, Warsaw, IN; and Collagen Corporation, Palo Alto, CA)	−	−	−	−	Yes	Yes

NA = Not available; OP-1 = osteogenic protein-1; + = produces effect; − = no effect
(Adapted with permission from Khan S, Tomin E, Lane J: Clinical applications of bone graft substitutes. Orthop Clin North Am 2000;31:389–398.)

hydroxyapatite (from genus *Gonipora*) is similar to cancellous bone with large pores (500-μm diameter) (Interpore 500, Interpore Cross International, Irvine, CA). A smaller pore size similar to cortical bone is derived from genus *Porites* (200-μm diameter) (Interpore 200).

The use of a coral-based hydroxyapatite bone graft substitute (Pro-Osteon; Interpore Cross International, Irvine, CA) for anterior cervical fusions has been reported to lead to significant rates of implant collapse but has revealed excellent biologic compatibility with good early creeping substitution for the implant with host bone. Overall, it has been shown that the mechanical strength of coraline implants is three times that

of normal cancellous bone 6 months after tibial metaphyseal grafting.

A biocompatible and resorbable calcium phosphate cement (composed of a combination of monocalcium phosphate, tricalcium phosphate, calcium carbonate, and a sodium phosphate solution), Norian Skeletal Repair System (SRS) (Norian Corporation, Cupertino, CA), is being used to augment fracture repair. Under physiologic conditions, it hardens within minutes into a carbonated hydroxyapatite in a nonexothermic reaction. When the reaction is complete (95% within 12 hours), its chemical composition is similar to the mineral phase of bone. Norian SRS undergoes the same in vivo remodeling as normal bone and has a final compressive strength of 55 mPa. It has shown favorable results in the augmentation of fixation in fractures of the hip, spine, and distal radius. However, there are concerns about the development of inflammation if the material migrates into a joint (that is, the radiocarpal joint). The use of Norian SRS has recently been expanded to the treatment of defects in complex calcaneal fractures. In a prospective study of 36 patients, earlier weight bearing (3 weeks) was achieved in the treatment group.

In an effort to more closely mimic the structure of natural bone, calcium orthophosphate cements have been developed (α-BSM; Etex Corporation, Cambridge, MA). These bone cements have favorable absorption characteristics and are easy to handle. The paste requires hours to harden at room temperature, but only 20 minutes at body temperature (37°C). The hardening reaction is endothermic and α-BSM is available in a variety of compressive strengths (5 to 40 mPa).

Calcium Sulfate

Calcium sulfate has long been used in its partially hydrated form of plaster of Paris. Newer forms of calcium sulfate are crystallized in highly controlled environments producing crystals of similar size and shape (OsteoSet; Wright Medical Technology, Inc, Arlington, TN). This material provides a void filler and is osteoconductive. Typically, OsteoSet is provided as pellets in two available sizes (4.8 × 3.3 mm or 3 × 2.5 mm). In vivo, the pellets dissolve in 2 months. In 26 patients with unicameral bone cysts treated with curettage and calcium sulfate pellets, the success rate was 92%. Antibiotics can also be added to the pellets to aid in the management of infected long bone defects.

With the increasing popularity of calcium sulfate as a defect filler, adverse events are now being reported. Three cases of severe inflammatory response in 15 patients treated with OsteoSet pellets for tumor defects have been reported. It was hypothesized that the rapid absorption of the pellets into a calcium-rich fluid stimulates inflammation.

Collagen Composites

Type I collagen is the most abundant protein in the extracellular matrix of bone. Collagen not only provides structural support to the matrix but also encourages the formation of hydroxyapatite crystals. Unfortunately, collagen alone functions poorly as a graft material. Collagraft (Zimmer; Warsaw, IN and Collagen Corporation, Palo Alto, CA), is a commercially synthesized composite of suspended bovine collagen, porous calcium phosphate ceramic, and autogenous bone marrow. It has been shown that Collagraft can augment grafts in anterior spinal fusions. Collagraft with autogenous marrow was compared with cancellous bone grafts in long bone fractures. There were no significant differences in fracture healing between groups.

Demineralized Bone Matrix

Acid extraction of bone removes the mineral phase of bone and leaves behind growth factors, noncollageneous proteins, and collagen. Demineralized bone matrix (DBM) is a potent stimulus for osteoinductive bone formation. Since the pioneering work of Urist in 1965, there have been many commercial applications for DBM alone and in combination with autogenous bone grafts or ceramics. DBM is commercially available in multiple forms, including gel (particulate), putty, and flex (sheet of fibers). It is possible that DBMs can be used as bone graft extenders, but not as substitutes for autogenous bone.

Bone Morphogenetic Proteins

BMPs comprise a family of at least 24 structurally-related growth factors from the TGF superfamily. These proteins have been shown to play an important role in the formation of bone by causing the differentiation of mesenchymal cells into chondroblasts and osteoblasts. With recent recombinant gene technology, BMPs have become available in sufficient quantities for clinical trials. BMP-2 and BMP-7 (osteogenic protein-1) have been shown to heal critical-sized defects in animal studies. A recent randomized controlled trial of 14 patients treated with lumbar interbody fusion cages (filled with either rh-BMP-2 or autogenous bone graft) revealed consistently higher fusion rates with rh-BMP-2. The use of BMP-7 (osteogenic protein-1) was evaluated in a placebo-controlled, randomized trial of 24 patients undergoing high tibial osteotomy and a critically-sized fibular defect. Nearly all patients in the BMP-7 group had new bone formation in the defect, whereas none of the placebo group had observable formation of new bone.

Peptide Signaling Molecules

Peptide signaling molecules stimulate chondroprogenitor and osteoprogenitor cells as well as differentiated chondrocytes and osteoblasts.

TGF-β acts as a key chemotactic mediator for fibroblasts and macrophages, enhances angiogenesis, and stimulates collagen synthesis and mesenchymal stem cell differentiation. The most concentrated isoform of TGF is TGF-β1; it is stored in platelets and is released in the fracture hematoma. Osteoblasts and chondrocytes synthesize TGF-β during endochondral ossification. In contrast to the dramatic effects of BMPs, TGF-β appears to augment fracture healing to a lesser extent. In a canine model, it was demonstrated that there were nonsignificant increases in the radiographic and histologic appearance of canine radii treated with TGF-β in a biodegradable polylactic acid/polyglycolic acid carrier as compared with carrier alone.

FGFs are involved in wound healing and repair. They act on stem cells, causing changes in migration, proliferation, differentiation, morphology, and function. Of the nine known members of the FGF family, acidic FGFs and basic FGFs are the most commonly studied. Experimental evidence suggests that basic FGF increases osteoblast, chondrocyte, and fibroblast mitogenesis and stimulates angiogenesis in a dose-response manner.

PDGF, synthesized by platelets, monocytes, and endothelial cells, has been shown to be a potent mitogen for all mesenchymal stem cells.

Physical Enhancement of Fracture Healing

Ultrasound

Fracture healing is dependent on an adequate blood supply to the cells. Ultrasound has been shown to increase the vascularity of the healing bone. As few as 10 days of ultrasound treatment have been shown to result in an increased bone blood flow that occurred immediately after removal of the ultrasonic wave stimulus. The relative effects of ultrasound are dependent on the intensity of the ultrasonic waves and the mode of exposure. In a study of a rat model of femoral fracture-healing, optimal parameters (intensity of 30 mW/cm^2 pulsed with 200 μs bursts of 1.5 MHz repeated at 1kHz for 20 min/day) were identified to augment fracture healing.

More than 168,000 studies have been published on the topic of ultrasound, of which 75 studies focus on its role in fracture healing. Of these, 23% (17 of 75) have been published since 1999. Six studies have specifically evaluated the efficacy of ultrasound by using a randomized trial design. A pooled analysis of these randomized trials suggests that in those patients (smokers and nonsmokers) with fractures of the tibia, scaphoid, or distal radius that are treated with casts, the addition of ultrasound treatments will reduce the time to fracture healing by approximately 3 weeks. However, ultrasound does not appear to have any additional benefit when tibial fractures are treated surgically with intramedullary nails with prior reaming.

The efficacy of ultrasound in the treatment of nonunions is limited. A recent nonrandomized observational study of 85 patients with nonunions treated with pulsed, low intensity ultrasound was reported. Results of 77 patients (90%) revealed, based on independent

radiographic and clinical assessments, that 67 (87%) of the fractures united. The mean time to healing from the initiation of ultrasound therapy was 5.5 $\pm$ 0.3 months. Despite promising results from observational studies, randomized trials are needed to prove the efficacy of ultrasound in nonunion management.

Pulsed Electromagnetic Fields

The use of electromagnetic fields to promote bone healing is based primarily on the theory that strain-generated electric potentials are signals for cellular processes during bone repair. It has been reported that electromagnetic fields stimulate growth factors important in modulating fracture healing.

For fracture healing (or nonunions), three types of electrical stimulation are available. (1) Direct current stimulation using electrodes; implantable or percutaneous electrodes deliver a constant current of 20 uA and 1.0 V to the fracture site. (2) Electromagnetic stimulation by inductive coupling; this system of external coils produces bursts with a repetition rate of 15 Hz, producing a current of 20 mV (10 uA/cm^2). (3) Capacitive coupling stimulation; noninvasive capacitive coupling; disk electrodes are coupled to the skin via a gel to produce a uniform field at the fracture site. The device produces a 60 KHz symmetric sine wave with a 5 V peak current and is used for 24 h/day.

The efficacy of pulsed electromagnetic fields on delayed tibial unions (16 to 32 weeks after casting) was examined in a placebo-controlled trial. Fifty-one patients were randomized to receive either pulsed electromagnetic fields (12 h/day for 12 weeks) or placebo. Forty-five patients (88%) complied with the study protocol. A greater proportion of patients in the treatment group achieved union (45% treatment versus 14% placebo, $P < 0.05$). The recent evidence from clinical studies for the use of pulsed electromagnetic fields is limited mainly to observational studies. A recent prospective study examined the use of low-intensity pulsed electromagnetic fields in 19 patients with nonunion of the long bones. The electric voltage pulse was 0.3 ms wide, repeating every 12 ms (frequency of about 80 Hz), peak magnetic fields were of the order of 0.01 to 0.1 m Tesla. Among the 13 patients who completed this treatment schedule (nonunions were present for a mean 41.3 weeks), 11 of them had successful bone healing (mean treatment period of 14 weeks). Two patients had bone gaps greater than 1 cm following removal of dead bone after infection.

Distraction Osteogenesis

Distraction osteogenesis has been applied to some of the most challenging conditions in orthopaedic surgery.

Indications for this technique include limb lengthening and the treatment of selected nonunions and deformities. In principle, distraction osteogenesis is a mechanical stretching of two vascularized bone surfaces at a predefined rate and rhythm to stimulate new bone formation in the expanding gap. It remains largely unknown how the mechanical force of distraction (or stretching) is translated into a biologic signal for new bone formation. A recent study showed increased expression of BMP-2, -4, and -7 in tibial distraction osteogenesis in New Zealand rabbits during the distraction phase; levels of these bone-inducing proteins declined when distraction was completed.

The technique of distraction osteogenesis involves placement of multiple transosseous wires or half pins through anatomic safe zones within the affected limb. Prior to beginning the distraction process, a latency period of approximately 5 to 21 days after osteotomy is recommended. The bone is then distracted at 1 mm/day at a rhythm of 0.25 mm every 6 hours. Simple lengthening can be achieved with monolateral fixators. Complex deformity correction usually requires ring fixators. Limb lengthening can be conducted over an intramedullary nail, especially in the case of femoral lengthening procedures. The use of an intramedullary nail allows earlier removal of the external fixator.

Despite the increasing popularity of circular external fixators for the treatment of fractures and nonunions, there are potential drawbacks of this technique. Pin tract infection remains a common problem—one of every ten pin sites will have a superficial infection (usually resolves with local pin site care and oral antibiotics). Most complications with distraction osteogenesis are proportionally related to the length of the distraction period and the experience of the surgeon. In experienced hands, distraction osteogenesis can produce significant improvements in physical function and quality of life.

Annotated Bibliography

Boden SD, Zdeblick TA, Sandhu HS, Heim SE: The use of rhBMP-2 in interbody fusion cages: Definitive evidence of osteoinduction in humans: A preliminary report. *Spine* 2000;25:376-381.
  Fusion was found to occur more reliably in patients treated with rhBMP-2 filled fusion cages than in controls treated with autogenous bone graft.

Connolly JF: Clinical use of marrow osteoprogenitor cells to stimulate osteogenesis. *Clin Orthop* 1998;355(suppl):S257-S266.
  Marrow osteoprogenitor cell use offers considerable improvement over standard open iliac crest grafting and is advantageous in stimulating osteogenesis in the management and prevention of nonunion.

Emami A, Petren-Mallmin M, Larsson S: No effect of low-intensity ultrasound on healing time of intramedullary fixed tibial fractures. *J Orthop Trauma* 1999;13:252-257.
  Thirty-two patients treated with reamed intramedullary nail insertion (range, 10 to 13 mm diameter nails) were randomly allocated to either ultrasound (n = 15) or placebo (n = 17). Independent, blinded assessment of radiographs revealed nonsignificant differences in healing rates between groups (155 days, ultrasound versus 125 days, placebo, $P < 0.05$). Healing was defined as radiologic bridging of three of four cortices.

Ferguson C, Alpern E, Miclau T, Helms JA: Does adult fracture repair recapitulate embryonic skeletal formation? *Mech Dev* 1999;87:57-66.
  Genetic mechanisms regulating fetal skeletogenesis also regulate adult skeletal regeneration. Key pathways include the Indian hedgehog and core binding factor 1 pathways.

Geesink RG, Hoefnagels NH, Bulstra SK: Osteogenic activity of OP-1 bone morphogenetic protein (BMP-7) in a human fibular defect. *J Bone Joint Surg Br* 1999;81:710-718.
  This article presents a randomized, double-blind study of 24 patients. All patients treated with osteogenic protein-1 and collagen carrier showed new bone formation in a fibular defect whereas no new bone was seen in collagen carrier alone.

Heckman JD, Ehler W, Brooks BP, et al: Bone morphogenetic protein but not transforming growth factor-beta enhances bone formation in canine diaphyseal nonunions implanted with a biodegradable composite polymer. *J Bone Joint Surg Am* 1999;81:1717-1729.
  Bone formation in a persistent osseous defect is increased when species-specific BMP incorporated into a polylactic acid-polyglycolic acid carrier is implanted at the site of the nonunion. TGF-ß1 at a dose of 10 ng per implant did not induce a similar degree of bone formation.

Hupel TM, Aksenov SA, Schemitsch EH: Cortical bone blood flow in loose and tight fitting locked unreamed intramedullary nailing: A canine segmental tibia fracture model. *J Orthop Trauma* 1998;12:127-135.
  These authors demonstrate that a loose-fitting nail spared cortical perfusion at the time of nail insertion more than a canal filling nail and allowed more complete cortical reperfusion 11 weeks after nailing.

Kenwright J, Gardner T: Mechanical influences on tibial fracture healing. *Clin Orthop* 1998;355(suppl):179-190.
  This study indicates that fracture mechanics should be controlled to provide amplitudes of movement in the first 4 to 6 weeks after fracture. The rigidity of fixation should be increased in the subsequent weeks until the fracture has healed and the frame is removed.

Mayr E, Rudzki MM, Rudzski M, Borchardt B, Hausser H, Ruter A: Does low intensity, pulsed ultrasound speed healing of scaphoid fractures? *Handchir Mikrochir Plast Chir* 2000;32:115-122.

Sixty patients with fresh scaphoid fractures were randomly allocated to ultrasound (n = 30) or placebo (n = 30). CT assessment of fracture healing revealed that significant reductions in the healing time with ultrasound (43 days versus 62 days, $P < 0.05$).

Rauch F, Lauzier D, Croteau S, Travers R, Glorieux FH, Hamdy R: Temporal and spatial expression of bone morphogenetic protein-2, 4, and 7 during distraction osteogenesis in rabbits. *Bone* 2000;27:453-459.

Immunohistochemical staining for BMP-2, -4, and -7 was evident within 7 days after a tibial fracture (prior to start of distraction) and localized to the mesenchymal cells and osteoblastic cells in the periosteal region. During distraction, cells resembling fibroblasts and chondrocytes exhibited intense staining.

Robinson D, Alk D, Sandbank J, Farber R, Halperin N: Inflammatory reactions associated with a calcium sulfate bone substitute. *Ann Transplant* 1999;4:91-97.

Fifteen implantations of OsteoSet were done after bone tumor resections. In three cases, a severe inflammatory reaction developed. In one case, serous drainage and an allergic reaction obligated graft removal.

Rubin C, Bolander M, Ryaby JP, Hadjiargyrou M: The use of low-intensity ultrasound to accelerate healing of fractures. *J Bone Joint Surg Am* 2001;83:229-270.

A review of the efficacy of low-intensity ultrasound in fracture management is presented.

Sarmiento A: On the behavior of closed tibial fractures: Clinical/radiological correlations. *J Orthop Trauma* 2000;14:199-205.

This article represents a comprehensive review of data obtained from 1,000 diaphyseal tibial fractures. There was a higher probability of delayed union in comminuted and segmental fractures. Maximal shortening of the fractures occurred at the time of injury, with no additional shortening experienced after weight bearing.

Schemitsch EH, Turchin DC, Kowalski MJ, Swiontkowski MF: Quantitative assessment of bone injury and repair after reamed and unreamed locked intramedullary nailing. *J Trauma* 1998;45:250-255.

This study demonstrates that greater injury or overall cortical porosity is associated with reamed nail insertion. There is no difference, however, between the amount of new bone formation after reamed and nonreamed nail insertion by 12 weeks after reaming.

Schildhauer T, Bauer TW, Josten C, Muhr G: Open reduction and augmentation of internal fixation with an injectable skeletal cement for the treatment of complex calcaneal fractures. *J Orthop Trauma* 2000;14:309-317.

Calcium phosphate cement augmentation of standard open reduction with internal fixation of joint depression type calcaneal fractures allows weight bearing as early as 3 weeks postoperatively.

Utvag SE, Grundnes O, Reikeras O: Effects of degrees of reaming on healing of segmental fractures in rats. *J Orthop Trauma* 1998;12:192-199.

Rats were divided into two groups: reaming to 1.6 mm with insertion of a 1.6 mm pin and reaming to 2.0 mm with insertion of a 2.0 mm pin. This study indicates that the degree of reaming does not significantly affect the healing pattern measured as restoration of mechanical characteristics.

Classic Bibliography

Bassett CA, Pawluk RJ, Pilla AA: Augmentation of bone repair by inductively coupled electromagnetic fields. *Science* 1974;184:575-577.

Brighton CT, Pollack SR: Treatment of recalcitrant nonunion with a capacitively coupled electrical field: A preliminary report. *J Bone Joint Surg Am* 1985;67:577-585.

Brighton CT, Shaman P, Heppenstall RB, Esterhai JL Jr, Pollack SR, Friedenberg ZB: Tibial nonunion treated with direct current, capacitive coupling, or bone graft. *Clin Orthop* 1995;321:223-234.

Cornell CN, Lane JM, Chapman M, et al: Multicenter trial of collagraft as bone graft substitute. *J Orthop Trauma* 1991;5:1-8.

Dickson K, Katzman S, Delgado E, Contreras D: Delayed unions and nonunions of open tibial fractures: Correlation with arteriography results. *Clin Orthop* 1994;302:189-193.

Grundnes O, Utvag SE, Reikeras O: Restoration of bone flow following fracture and reaming in rat femora. *Acta Orthop Scand* 1994;65:185-190.

Olerud S, Stromberg L: Intramedullary reaming and nailing: Its early effects on cortical bone vascularization. *Orthopedics* 1986;9:1204-1208.

Panjabi MM, Walter SD, Karuda M, White AA, Lawson JP: Correlations of radiographic analysis of healing fractures with strength: A statistical analysis of experimental osteotomies. *J Orthop Res* 1985;3:212-218.

Peltier LF, Jones RH: Treatment of unicameral bone cysts by curettage and packing with plaster-of-Paris pellets. *J Bone Joint Surg Am* 1978;60:820-822.

Rhinelander FW: Tibial blood supply in relation to fracture healing. *Clin Orthop* 1974;105:34-81.

Rhinelander FW: The vascular response of bone to internal fixation, in Browner BD, Edwards CC (eds): *The Science and Practice of Intramedullary Nailing.* Philadelphia, PA, Lea & Febiger, 1987, pp 25-59.

Sarmiento A, Sharpe FE, Ebramzadeh E, Normand P, Shankwiler J: Factors influencing the outcome of closed tibial fractures treated with functional bracing. *Clin Orthop* 1995;315:8-24.

Schemitsch EH, Kowalski MJ, Swiontkowski MF: Soft-tissue blood flow following reamed versus unreamed locked intramedullary nailing: A fractured sheep tibial model. *Ann Plast Surg* 1996;36:70-75.

Sharrard WJ: A double-blind trial of pulsed electromagnetic fields for delayed union of tibial fractures. *J Bone Joint Surg Br* 1990;72:347-355.

Urist MR: Bone: Formation by autoinduction. *Science* 1965;150:893-899.

Wang SJ, Lewallen DG, Bolander ME, Chao EY, Ilstrup DM, Greenleaf JF: Low intensity ultrasound treatment increases strength in rat femoral fracture model. *J Orthop Res* 1994;12:40-47.

Chapter 3

Biomechanics and Gait

Ann E. Barr, PhD, PT

Introduction

Instrumented gait analysis is becoming more influential in the development of new treatment approaches for musculoskeletal and neuromuscular disorders and the evaluation of their functional outcomes. To enhance the link segment models derived from video and force plate data, investigators now use either videofluoroscopic techniques in vivo to observe the movements of articular surfaces or instrumented prosthetic components to measure contact pressures and/or bending moments.

Components of Normal Gait

Stance phase occupies 60% of the gait cycle and consists of two periods of double limb support (initial and terminal), when the contralateral foot is in contact with the ground, and an intermediate period of single limb support, when the contralateral limb is engaged in swing phase. Stance consists of six periods: heel contact, foot flat, midstance, terminal stance, preswing, and toe-off. Swing phase occupies 40% of the gait cycle and consists of three periods: initial swing, midswing, and terminal swing.

Table 1 lists the time-distance parameters of normal gait. Stride time is the time it takes to perform a single stride. Stride length is the distance covered by a stride in the direction of locomotion. Step is defined as the action from initial ground contact on one foot until the initial ground contact of the opposite foot. Step length is the distance covered in the direction of locomotion. Step width is the distance covered perpendicular to the direction of locomotion. Two sequential steps comprise a stride. Cadence is the number of steps taken per unit time. Velocity is the distance covered in the direction of locomotion per unit time.

Normal angular kinematics and kinetics during gait are depicted in Figure 1. Ankle motion is bimodal with peak stance phase dorsiflexion (flexion) occurring late

in midstance and peak swing phase dorsiflexion occurring in terminal swing. Knee motion is bimodal with peak stance phase flexion occurring early in midstance, and peak swing phase flexion occurring at midswing. Hip motion is unimodal with peak flexion occurring during terminal swing. Moments cause a tendency for joint rotation. In this discussion, the term moment refers to the internal moment generated about the joint in question. A knee extensor moment, for example, is the internal moment of force that tends to rotate the knee joint in the direction of extension and occurs when the line of action of the tibiofemoral reaction force vector passes posteriorly to the axis of knee flexion-extension (that is, when the external moment tends to cause knee flexion). Activation by the knee extensors is required to counterbalance the tendency for knee flexion. Positive joint power values indicate concentric muscle contractions, whereas negative joint power values indicate eccentric muscle contractions. For example, during preswing, a high magnitude power generation peak by the concentrically contracting plantarflexors represents approximately two thirds of the total energy generated during walking and may contribute to propulsion. Alternatively, from heel contact to foot flat, power absorption by the eccentrically contracting quadriceps controls knee flexion during weight acceptance.

The following discussion highlights recent advances using technologically advanced gait analysis methods. The various common gait analysis methods and their respective strengths and limitations are listed in Table 2.

Hip Arthroplasty

Studies of in vivo acetabulofemoral pressures and femoral shaft bending moments in instrumented femoral prosthetic components have recently yielded provocative results pertinent to prosthetic wear, joint loads, and gait function. In one investigation using a device similar to the Austin-Moore femoral compo-

TABLE 1	Ranges of Normal Values for Time-Distance Parameters of Adult Gait at Free Walking Velocity
Stride or cycle time	1.0-1.2 strides/s*
Stride or cycle length	1.2-1.9 m†
Step length	0.65-1.1 m*
Step width	7.7-9.6 cm*
Cadence	90-140 steps/min†
Velocity	0.9-1.8 m/s†

*Values adapted from multiple sources as summarized in Craik RL, Oatis CA (eds): *Gait Analysis: Theory and Application*. St. Louis, MO, Mosby-Year Book, 1995.
†Values adapted from Whittle MW: *Gait Analysis: An Introduction*. Oxford, England, Butterworth-Heinemann, 1991.
(Reproduced with permission from Barr AE: Gait analysis, in Spivak JM, DiCesare PE, Feldman DS, Koval KJ, Rokito AS, Zuckerman JD (eds): *Orthopaedics: A Study Guide*. New York, NY, McGraw Hill, 1999, pp 209-216.)

nent, analysis of acetabular pressures, joint angular kinematics, ground reaction forces, and electromyography during free, fast, and slow ambulation and cane-aided ambulation suggested a greater role for the hip abductor musculature in producing peak contact pressures at the acetabulofemoral joint. Peak pressures occurred on the superoposterior aspect of the femoral head and preceded the peak ground reaction force and sagittal hip moment between midstance and terminal stance, suggesting that muscular contraction may be responsible for peak acetabular pressures. At slow gait velocity, peak acetabular pressures increased by approximately 20% even though ground reaction forces and hip moments are decreased at slow gait velocity. This counterintuitive finding shows that hip musculature can induce peak contact pressures during ambulation in excess of those estimated by conventional inverse dynamics techniques and, therefore, illustrates the limitations of such analyses. Presumably, greater muscular stabilization may be required at slower than normal gait velocities to control hip motion and is not necessarily compensated for by the velocity-mediated reduction in external joint loads. Clinical relevance from these findings includes patients with hip osteoarthritis who may adopt a slower gait velocity in response to joint pain and induce a paradoxical increase in hip joint forces.

Contralateral hand cane use at slow gait velocity reduced the peak acetabular pressures by as much as 40%, which coincides with a 45% reduction in gluteus medius activity. Cane use also further reduced ground reaction force magnitude, which may combine with the effect of decreased abductor activity to effectively reduce hip joint contact pressures.

Knee Arthroplasty

Controversy concerning posterior cruciate ligament (PCL)-retaining versus PCL-substituting prosthetic designs continues to be addressed in the literature. A recent study of 14 patients with a posterior stabilized design in one knee and a PCL-retaining design in the contralateral knee showed no effect of prosthetic design on knee motion, moments, or muscle activity during level walking, stair ascent, or stair descent. Cruciate-substituting designs have been reported to perform well in terms of wear and longevity in addition to their comparable performance in gait function.

Videofluoroscopic techniques that permit observation of prosthetic component surfaces in vivo have been used to evaluate both PCL-retaining and PCL-substituting prosthetic knee designs. Condylar lift-off occurs in all designs studied and seems to be related more to the abduction-adduction moments to which the knee is exposed during gait than to any design feature or surgical technique. Rotational motions, termed the screw home mechanism, also occur to some degree with total knee arthroplasty, and may even be reversed in some designs. These motions, when combined with a design that does not maintain high surface congruity while accommodating condylar lift-off and rotation, may prove detrimental to the tibial component. Flat-on-flat cruciate-retaining designs, therefore, perform worse in terms of wear than do low contact stress mobile-bearing designs. Finite element analyses tend to support the theory that the lower the conformity, the greater the susceptibility of the tibial surface to delamination.

Rotating-hinge total knee replacement designs play an important role in limb salvage procedures. Comparisons between normal knees and knees of patients with semiconstrained total knee arthroplasties showed age-related differences in gait and stair-stepping. Patients younger than age 50 years with a rotating hinge design performed in a manner similar to control subjects on time-distance as well as kinematic variables with few significant differences. The performance of patients older than age 50 years (range, 50 to 63 years) differed from that of controls and semiconstrained design recipients in that knee extension persisted in early to mid-stance, but they were still able to perform gait and stair activities at a high functional level.

Cerebral Palsy

Gait analysis has been useful for surgical planning in the treatment of patients with cerebral palsy. A recent prospective study of 97 patients with cerebral palsy

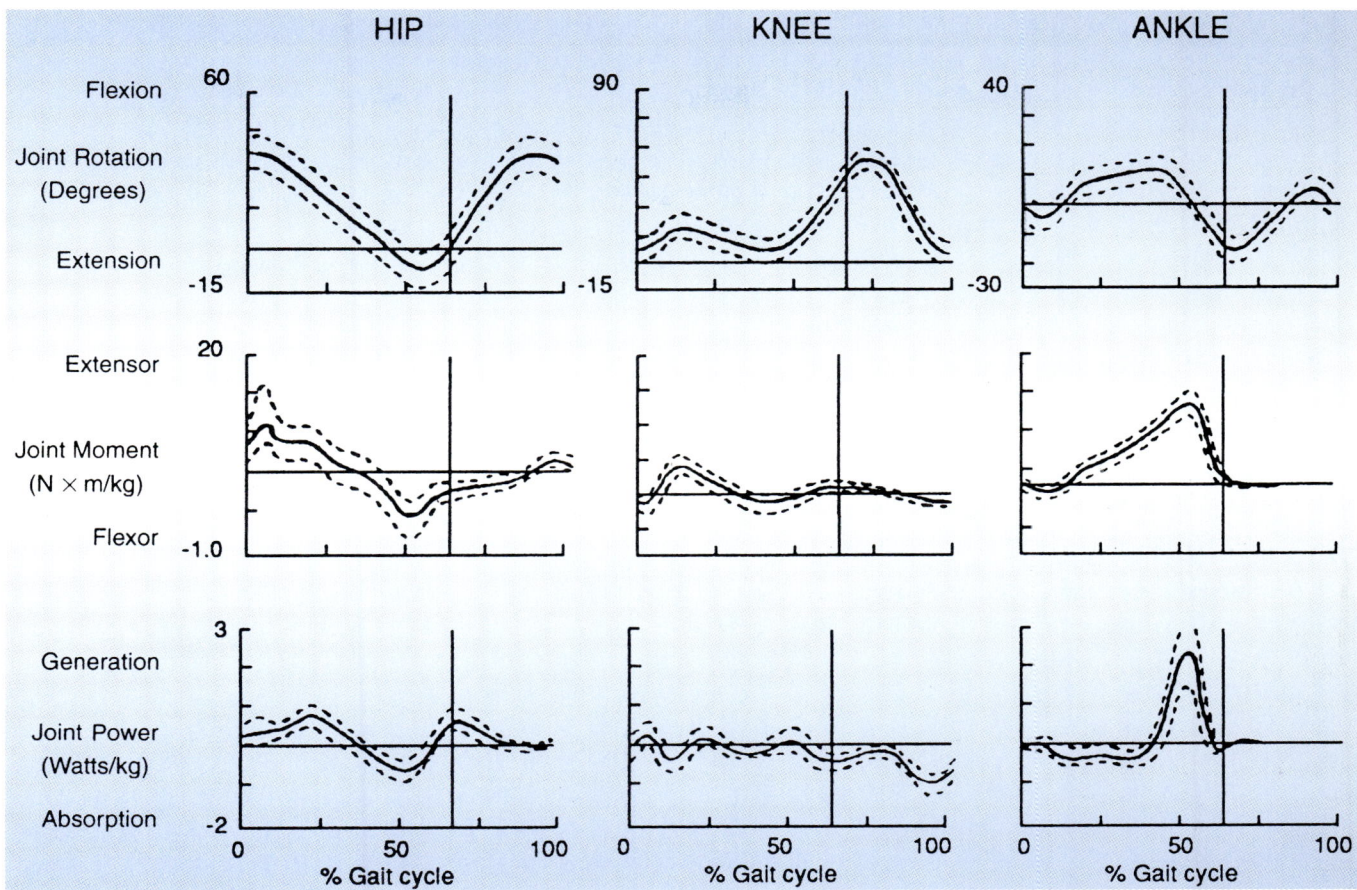

Figure 1   Graphic representation of the time histories of angular kinematics, internal joint moments, and joint powers about the sagittal plane (ie, flexion-extension motion axes) of the hip, knee, and ankle joints during the normal gait cycle as determined by combined angular kinematic and force plate analyses. Vertical lines indicate stance (from 0 to 60% of the gait cycle) and swing (from 60% to 100% of the gait cycle) phases. *(Reproduced with permission from Gage JR: Gait analysis in cerebral palsy. Clin Develop Med 1991;121:31.)*

showed that the addition of gait biomechanics data resulted in changes in surgical recommendations in more than half of the patients studied and was associated with a potential reduction in surgical cost.

Muscle-tendon lengthening procedures, sometimes in combination with tendon transfer procedures, can improve gait function in patients with spastic diplegia. It has been assumed that release of contracted tissues allows more normal positioning of the ankle and knee during gait. Although this is certainly the case, recent evidence suggests that muscle-tendon lengthening procedures also may have a limited but positive effect on ankle joint angular velocity. In patients with cerebral palsy, initial ground contact is frequently made with the toes rather than the heel. As a consequence, ankle angular velocity is reversed from the normal pattern of plantar flexion following heel strike to one of dorsiflexion following toe strike up to the middle of midstance as the heel is forced downward toward the floor. From the middle of midstance to terminal stance, patients with spastic diplegia will often undergo plantar flexion rather than the normal dorsiflexion that occurs as the

tibia advances over the stationary foot. This reversal of motion occurs because the velocity-dependent hyperactivity of the gastrocnemius-soleus complex is triggered when the tibia attempts to rotate forward over the stationary foot during ankle dorsiflexion and results in toe walking, which is characteristic of these patients. Nine months after muscle-tendon lengthening procedures, ankle dorsiflexion velocity was reduced at initial contact and dorsiflexion velocity was restored through midstance in patients with spastic diplegia. Lengthening of the gastrocnemius-soleus complex resulted in reduced activation of these muscles at initial contact and increased activation through midstance. Regardless of the specific muscle-tendon lengthening procedures and whether or not they were performed on multiple muscle-tendon units or in conjunction with tendon transfer, the greatest effect on angular velocity was at the ankle. These findings indicate that improved gait function is through restoration of more normal foot and ankle sensory feedback resulting from correction of sagittal plane joint contracture and is associated with increased stride length and gait velocity.

TABLE 2 | Strengths and Limitations of Gait Analysis Methods

Gait Analysis Method	Strengths	Limitations
Observational analysis	Widely available Can be enhanced by simple videotaping Allows classification of gross gait patterns Inexpensive	Subjective Not able to measure more subtle phenomena
Stride analysis	Provides quantitative information regarding time-distance parameters Easy and fast Low space requirements Relatively inexpensive	Does not permit angular kinematic and kinetic analysis Requires that patients have distinct swing phase in which floor contact is broken
Angular kinematic analysis	Permits precise measurement of joint angular excursions Objective and quantitative	Requires technically trained personnel for measurement and interpretation of results High space requirements Limited portability Costly
Force plate and pressure plate analyses	Permits precise measurement of external loads Permits inverse dynamics analyses Provides information regarding load patterns and distributions on stance limb	Limited usefulness in isolation May require permanent installation in "gait lab" Requires technically trained personnel for measurement and interpretation of results Costly
Electromyographic analysis	Provides measurement of motor performance and functional role of musculature Enhances interpretation of kinematic and kinetic parameters	Requires technical expertise for measurement and interpretation Subject to interference and artifact during sampling Invasiveness of intramuscular technique poses risk to patients Costly
Videofluoroscopic analysis	Permits direct observation of bones and implants during dynamic functional task Eliminates need for externally applied skin markers	Requires technical expertise for measurement and interpretation Costly

(Adapted with permission from Barr AE: Diagnostic testing: Gait analysis, in Spivak JM, Di Cesare PE, Feldman DS, Koval KJ, Rokito AS, Zuckerman JD (eds): Orthopaedics: A Study Guide. New York, NY, McGraw-Hill, 1999, p 381.)

One consequence of muscle spasticity on the developing skeleton is rotational deformities of the long bones; derotation osteotomies can improve gait. A recent retrospective study of a group of patients with tibial torsion deformities examined the effects of distal tibial and fibular derotation osteotomies on gait function 15 to 56 months (mean, 24.9 months) postoperatively. Kinematic improvements in foot progression angle and tibial rotation were statistically significant at both midstance and terminal stance for both internal rotation and external rotation osteotomies. A trend toward increased gait velocity was observed. In addition to the improvements in functional ambulation, this distal procedure is associated with a lower risk for peroneal nerve damage and may be preferable in patients for whom mediolateral tibial deformities do not need surgical correction.

As part of a comprehensive prospective clinical trial, the role of botulinum toxin A (BTX/A) in the management of dynamic gastrocnemius-soleus complex spasticity during gait in juvenile cerebral palsy was investigated. Twenty-five children were studied prior to and 3 weeks after treatment with BTX/A. In addition to expected improvements in sagittal plane kinematics, there also were improvements in ankle joint moment and power. In normal developing children, the internal ankle moment immediately following heel strike is dorsiflexor, meaning the ground reaction force vector of load bearing is posterior to the ankle joint (Fig. 1). From midstance to terminal stance, the normal ankle moment changes direction as the ground reaction force vector acts anterior to the ankle joint, producing an internal plantarflexor moment (Fig. 1). Ankle joint power in normal devel-

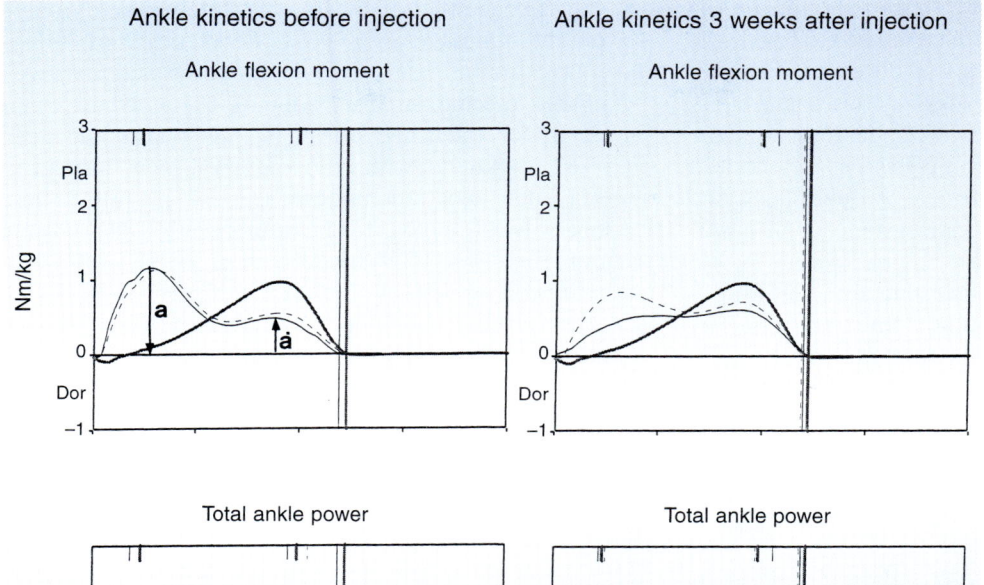

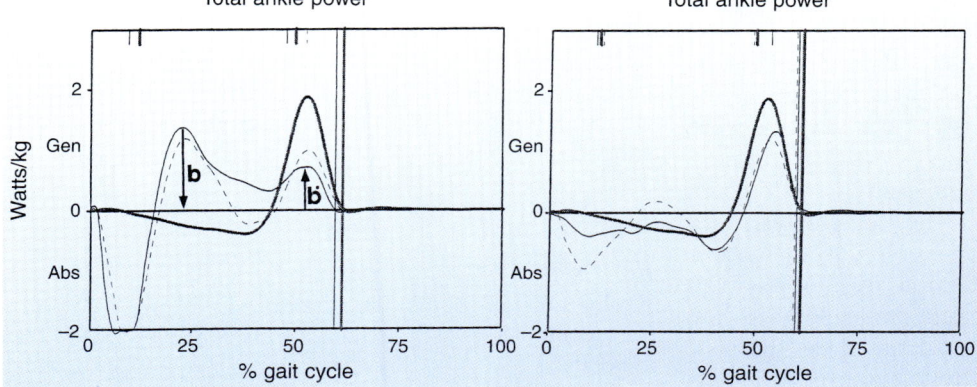

Figure 2 Effect of BTX/A injection to the gastrocnemius-soleus complex on ankle flexion moment and ankle power in a patient with spastic diplegia (light solid line, right limb; dashed line, left limb). Normal controls are shown (heavy solid line) for comparison. Locations of preinjection moment and power peaks are indicated by the letters a and b, respectively. *(Reproduced with permission from Boyd RN, Pliatsios V, Starr R, Wolfe R, Graham HK: Biomechanical transformation of the gastroc-soleus muscle with botulinum toxin A in children with cerebral palsy. Dev Med Child Neurol 2000;42:32-41.)*

oping children shows a power absorption phase from early to midstance, at which time the plantarflexors are lengthening to control the advancement of the tibia over the flat and stationary foot, followed by a power generation peak in late stance, which may correspond to a shortening contraction of the posterior calf musculature to assist in either toe-off or to control knee flexion in anticipation of the swing phase (Fig. 1). In children with spastic diplegia, a double-bump ankle moment curve is observed in which the earlier internal plantarflexor moment exceeds the latter. In Figure 2, the accompanying power profile shows a relatively high amplitude and foreshortened period of power absorption in early stance with an early transition to power generation for the remainder of stance in which two peaks are evident. Three weeks after BTX/A injection, gait analysis revealed a reduction of the first ankle plantarflexor moment peak with a resultant shift of the moment profile toward a more normal shape and marked decreases in the initial ankle power absorption peak and the early stance phase power generation peak (Fig. 2). These improvements persisted up to 24 weeks. These changes suggest that BTX/A can

help to reduce the abnormal response of a spastic muscle to the angular velocities typically present during gait. This treatment may be used alone or in conjunction with surgical correction of joint contracture and bony malalignment to further improve gait kinematics and kinetics.

Musculoskeletal Knee Injuries

Patients with anterior cruciate ligament (ACL) deficiency can develop a quadriceps avoidance gait pattern; investigators have attempted to characterize its development, the effects of reconstruction procedures on gait patterns, and the presence of additional patient strategies to control knee instability. Elimination or even reversal of the direction of the knee extensor moment normally present in early stance phase, or the quadriceps avoidance pattern, appears to develop slowly after ACL injury and may take years to emerge. Recent studies suggest that the prevalence of this pattern may be lower than originally estimated. Alternative patterns have been demonstrated with knee moment profiles within normal limits during early stance, but increases in knee extensor moments from midstance to terminal stance. In one investigation, an increase in knee flexion motion during early stance rather than the decrease associated with the quadriceps avoidance gait pattern was observed. The possible mechanism for the effectiveness of this gait adaptation is that increased knee flexion angle improves the efficiency of the hamstrings in compensating for the lack of ACL restraint. Increased periods of quadriceps and hamstrings activation observed duringstance phase corroborate this proposed mechanism.

One of the difficulties in observing and defining a typical ACL-deficient gait is that some patients may develop gait movement patterns that are more adaptive than those of other patients. One study attempted to examine this phenomenon by classifying patients with ACL deficiency according to their functional activity level prior to gait analysis. Patients who had returned to all preinjury activity without limitation and who rated knee function as 85% or higher compared to preinjury knee function were called copers. Patients who reported instability with activities of daily living and were scheduled for reconstructive surgery were called noncopers. Time from injury was shorter in noncopers than in copers, but laxity measurements did not differ between the two groups. Knee kinematics were within normal limits for the copers, but noncopers demonstrated reduced knee flexion of the involved side during loading response that persisted into late midstance. As might be expected from these findings, noncopers demonstrated lower knee extensor moments during stance phase. It is interesting to note that copers also demonstrated lower knee extensor moments on the involved side during stance phase despite their normal knee flexion motion. Examination of knee joint power profiles suggested different mechanisms for controlling the knee extensor moments for these two ACL-deficient groups. In noncopers, a power absorption peak for the plantarflexors coincided with peak knee flexion on the involved side, which indicates that the gastrocnemius muscle probably contributes to reduced knee extension and compensatory posterior tibial translation in the absence of the ACL. On the other hand, copers exhibited an attenuation of knee power absorption during the first 20% of stance phase, which suggests a transfer of power away from the potentially unstable knee joint. It would appear that the latter strategy imparts stability while maintaining essentially normal arthrokinematics, which may be crucial to the prevention of osteoarthritic changes following ACL injury and explains why copers had a higher functional level. It is also important to note that for both copers and noncopers, quadriceps strength as measured by isokinetic torque testing did not correlate with the altered knee kinematics or kinetics. This finding indicates that strength measurements alone may

not be sufficient indicators of functional dynamic movement adaptations in ACL deficiency and, therefore, have limited use for recommending activity level.

Another mechanism for reducing the knee extensor torque about the knee during stance phase has been observed in patients with patellofemoral pain. Instead of altering knee joint kinematics, the peak magnitude and loading rate of the vertical component of the ground reaction force vector is reduced in some subjects. This gait pattern is consistent with ACL-deficient patients who are copers in that muscular demands causing compression of the patellofemoral joint are reduced, but not at the expense of normal knee arthrokinematics.

Another possible contributing factor to the emergence of a quadriceps avoidance gait pattern is the presence of knee joint effusion, which has been shown to reduce knee extensor torque throughout stance phase in an incremental joint capsule injection model of effusion. The development of joint effusion in patients with chronic knee instability due to ACL deficiency cannot be ruled out as a contributing factor to gait adaptations.

Annotated Bibliography

Hip Arthroplasty

Krebs DE, Robbins CE, Lavine L, Mann RW: Hip biomechanics during gait. *J Orthop Sports Phys Ther* 1998;28:51-59.

A comprehensive report of simultaneously collected in vivo acetabular contact pressures, hip joint torques, and electromyographic activities of the hip musculature in an 85-year-old man showed the location and timing of peak hip contact pressures during gait at different speeds and with and without the use of a cane. Small areas of contact stress were observed and gait speed had an opposite effect than expected on the peak contact pressures.

Park S, Krebs DE, Mann RW: Hip muscle co-contraction: Evidence from concurrent in vivo pressure measurement and force estimation. *Gait Posture* 1999;10:211-222.

The extent of hip muscle co-contraction was studied by comparing in vivo endoprosthesis measurements on hip articular cartilage and force estimations from external kinematic and kinetic measurements. Internal direct measurements of hip contact pressure exceeded external estimates.

Knee Arthroplasty

Bolanos AA, Colizza WA, McCann PD, et al: A comparison of isokinetic strength testing and gait analysis in patients with posterior cruciate-retaining and substituting knee arthroplasties. *J Arthroplasty* 1998;13:906-915.

Fourteen patients underwent TKA with a posterior-stabilized design on one limb and a PCL-retaining design on the contralateral limb. No differences in objective measurements of knee joint kinematics and electromyographic activity were observed during gait on a level walkway and stairs.

Draganich LF, Whitehurst JB, Chou LS, Piotrowski GA, Pottenger LA, Finn HA: The effects of the rotating-hinge total knee replacement on gait and stair stepping. *J Arthroplasty* 1999;14:743-755.

Ten subjects with rotating-hinge TKA and 10 with semiconstrained TKA were compared with older normal controls during gait and stair-stepping. Younger TKA patients performed similarly to control patients, whereas older TKA patients showed some kinematic differences but were able to perform at a high functional level.

Stiehl JB, Dennis DA, Komistek RD, Crane HS: In vivo determination of condylar lift-off and screw-home in a mobile-bearing total knee arthroplasty. *J Arthroplasty* 1999;14:293-299.

Eighteen of 20 subjects (90%) with low-contact stress cruciate-sacrificing, mobile-bearing TKA observed with videofluoroscopy during gait showed both medial and lateral condylar lift-off. Screw home motion also was present and sometimes reversed.

Stiehl JB, Komistek RD, Dennis DA: Detrimental kinematics of a flat on flat total condylar knee arthroplasty. *Clin Orthop* 1999;365:139-148.

Fourteen subjects with flat-on-flat PCL-retaining TKA performed deep knee bends or level gait while being observed with videofluoroscopy. Tibiofemoral contact positions were posterior in all subjects throughout the gait cycle with lateral condylar lift-off, but with minimal screw home motion occurring in most subjects.

Cerebral Palsy

Boyd RN, Pliatsios V, Starr R, Wolfe R, Graham HK: Biomechanical transformation of the gastroc-soleus muscle with botulinum toxin A in children with cerebral palsy. *Dev Med Child Neurol* 2000;42:32-41.

Twenty-five children with cerebral palsy underwent gait analysis before and 3 to 24 weeks after BTX/A injection of the gastrocnemius-soleus muscles. Improvements in ankle moment and power following injection suggest a biomechanical transformation of muscle.

Granata KP, Abel MF, Damiano DL: Joint angular velocity in spastic gait and the influence of muscle-tendon lengthening. *J Bone Joint Surg Am* 2000;82:174-186.

Muscle-tendon lengthening procedures of the lower extremity in spastic diplegia were shown to have a positive influence on foot placement and ankle angular velocity during the stance phase of gait.

Kay RM, Dennis S, Rethlefsen S, et al: The effect of preoperative gait analysis on orthopedic decision making. *Clin Orthop* 2000;372:217-222.

Ninety-seven patients received preoperative gait analysis; 70 of them had specific treatment plans before gait analysis, and 62 of these plans were altered as a result of gait analysis. As a result, the average number of surgical procedures was reduced by 1.5 per patient.

Stefko RM, de Swart RJ, Dodgin DA, et al: Kinematic and kinetic analysis of distal derotational osteotomy of the leg in children with cerebral palsy. *J Pediatr Orthop* 1998;18:81-87.

A retrospective review of 10 ambulatory children with cerebral palsy who underwent distal tibial and fibular derotation osteotomies showed improved foot placement, tibial rotation, gait velocity, and ankle moments.

Musculoskeletal Knee Injuries

Powers CM, Heino JG, Rao S, Perry J: The influence of patellofemoral pain on lower limb loading during gait. *Clin Biomech* 1999;14:722-728.

Fifteen female subjects with patellofemoral pain showed slower gait velocity, decreased stance phase knee flexion, and decreased peak vertical ground reaction force loading rate. This results in reduced risk of additional injury caused by impulse loading.

Roberts CS, Rash GS, Honaker JT, Wachowiak MP, Shaw JC: A deficient anterior cruciate ligament does not lead to quadriceps avoidance gait. *Gait Posture* 1999;10:189-199.

Eighteen ACL-deficient subjects were studied and found to have both quadriceps activation and knee extensor moments during early and midstance. This pattern is not consistent with the quadriceps avoidance gait pattern and suggests other adaptations among these patients.

Rudolph KS, Eastlack ME, Axe MJ, Snyder-Mackler L: Movement patterns after anterior cruciate ligament injury: A comparison of patients who compensate well for the injury and those who require operative stabilization. *J Electromyogr Kinesiol* 1998;8:349-362.

Gait adaptations following ACL injury were studied in 16 patients classified as highly functional copers or reduced function noncopers. Copers transferred power away from the affected knee while maintaining normal arthrokinematics, whereas noncopers reduced knee extensor moments at the expense of normal knee arthrokinematics.

Torry MR, Decker MJ, Viola RW, O'Connor DD, Steadman JR: Intra-articular knee joint effusion induces quadriceps avoidance gait patterns. *Clin Biomech* 2000; 15:147-159.

In a joint effusion model, 14 healthy subjects underwent incremental injection of saline into the knee joint capsule. A quadriceps avoidance gait pattern progressively emerged, suggesting that this pattern may be associated with effusion as well as knee instability.

Chapter 4

Bearing Surfaces in Total Joint Arthroplasty

Michael D. Ries, MD

Current Issues

Ultra-high molecular weight polyethylene (UHMWPE) has been used as a bearing surface in total joint arthroplasty for over 30 years. Survivorship of both hip and knee arthroplasty is greater than 90% at 10 years and 80% at 20 years. Despite the favorable survivorship figures, young patients who require total joint arthroplasty can expect to undergo future revision surgery; therefore, efforts to further improve the in vivo behavior of UHMWPE as a bearing surface are warranted. Improvements in quality control have included better consolidation of UHMWPE resins to minimize fusion defects, elimination of impurities such as calcium stearate, and elimination of sterilization-induced oxidation.

Recent research has focused on the effects of sterilization on UHMWPE wear and mechanical properties. Gamma irradiation sterilization of UHMWPE causes polymer chain scission and oxidation, which adversely affect both wear and mechanical properties. However, gamma irradiation can also produce cross-linking of the polymer chains, which improves wear resistance. Enhanced polyethylenes or highly cross-linked polyethylenes have been developed to further improve the wear resistance of the material. Highly cross-linked polyethylenes demonstrate markedly improved wear behavior in hip simulator studies, but are associated with a decrease in mechanical properties (yield strength, ultimate tensile strength, and fatigue strength).

Previous efforts to improve the wear behavior of polyethylene, such as the addition of carbon fibers (carbon reinforced polyethylene), hot isostatic pressing (Hylamer), and heat pressing have not been associated with demonstrated improvements in wear resistance in vivo. Although current joint simulator studies may accurately predict in vivo behavior, clinical studies will be necessary to determine if highly cross-linked polyethylenes enhance the longevity of total joint arthroplasty.

Hard-on-hard bearing surfaces (metal-on-metal and ceramic-on-ceramic) have been used extensively in Europe, where improvements in manufacturing and design of the implants have been evaluated clinically with favorable results. However, concerns with hard-on-hard bearings include metal ion toxicity and ceramic wear and fracture.

UHMWPE Processing

UHMWPE implants are made from small powders that are formed by one of three methods. The powders are either compression molded into sheets and implants machined from the compression molded material, ram extruded into rods and then machined into implants, or molded directly into the final shape. With each method the powders are exposed to variable temperatures and pressures to consolidate the material. It may not be possible to directly mold some implants, such as those with complex geometries or modular locking mechanisms.

Clinical and implant retrieval studies of UHMWPE sterilized by gamma irradiation in air have demonstrated that wear behavior may be influenced by resin type, manufacturing method, or both. Directly molded Hi-fax 1900 total knee tibial components were found to have more surface wear (scratching and embedded metallic debris) and less fatigue wear (delamination) than similar components machined from ram extruded GUR 415 resin. The molded Hi-fax 1900 components also demonstrated less oxidation than the machined GUR 415 components. Both groups of implants were sterilized by gamma irradiation in air, suggesting that either the resin type or manufacturing method or both may influence resistance to oxidative degradation and associated wear behavior. However, most currently available UHMWPE implants have not been sterilized by gamma irradiation in air and it is not clear if wear behavior of these implants will be affected by resin type or manufacturing method.

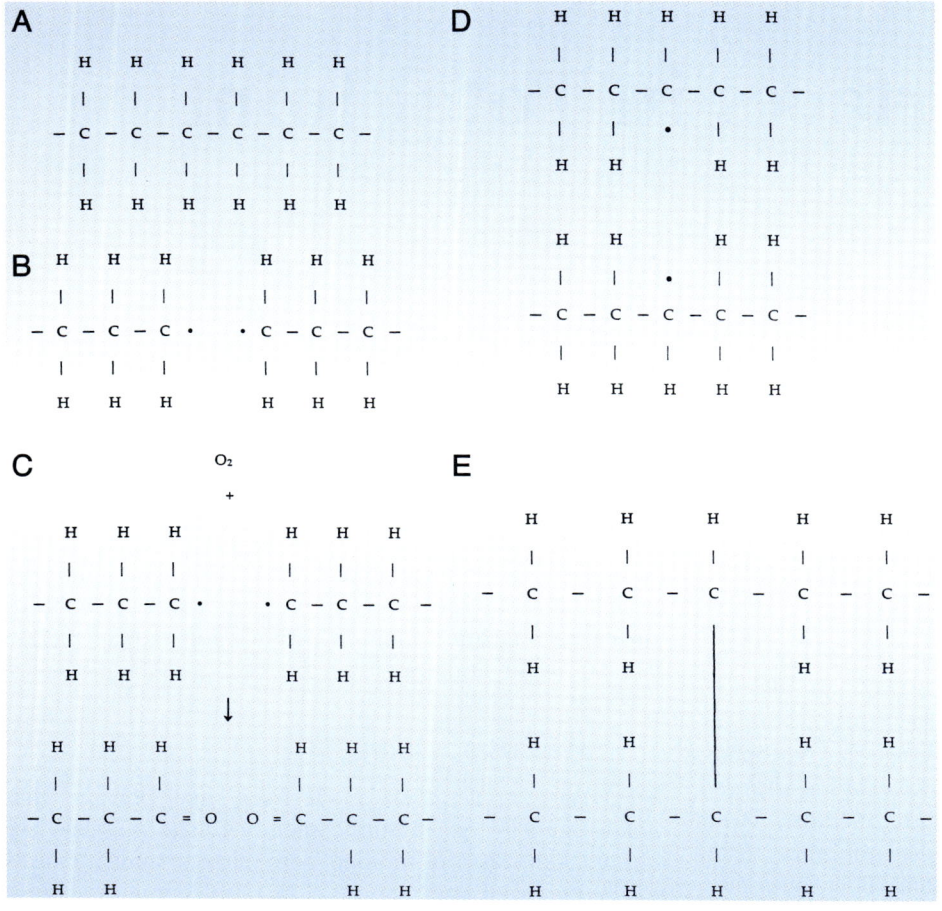

Figure 1 Molecular events by which gamma radiation cross-links two polymer chains. **A,** UHMWPE polymer chain. **B,** After gamma irradiation, UHMWPE polymer chain is split into smaller chains (scission). **C,** Oxygen forms terminal carbonyl groups. **D,** Two UHMWPE polymer chains with free radicals. **E,** Cross-link between two polymer chains.

UHMWPE Sterilization

The method of sterilization can affect UHMWPE wear and mechanical behavior. Gamma irradiation sterilization of UHMWPE causes polymer chain scission and cross-linking. UHMWPE consists of polymer chains with multiple carbon and hydrogen atoms connected by covalent bonds (Fig. 1, *A*). Each covalent bond consists of two shared electrons.

When UHMWPE is exposed to gamma irradiation sterilization, the radiation has sufficient energy to break a covalent bond in the polymer chain into two electrons or free radicals (Fig. 1, *B*). If oxygen is present, it can react with the free radicals to form a chemically stable carbonyl group. This process is oxidative degradation (Fig. 1, *C*).

The free radicals can exist for many years. As oxygen diffuses into the UHMWPE implant, such as during shelf storage, oxidative degradation continues to occur. The effect of gamma irradiation in air is to lower the molecular weight of UHMWPE. A decrease in molecular weight has an adverse effect on both wear resistance and mechanical properties. After gamma irradiation in air, UHMWPE wear resistance and fatigue strength are decreased.

Alternatively, UHMWPE implants can be sterilized by gamma irradiation in the absence of oxygen (in argon or nitrogen gas; or a vacuum). If oxygen is not present, a different chemical reaction (cross-linking) occurs. Free radicals are still produced by the gamma irradiation. The free radicals can combine to form a covalent bond or cross-link between two polymer chains (Fig. 1, *D* and *E*).

Cross-linking improves the wear behavior of UHMWPE. Hip simulator studies have demonstrated that less wear occurs with UHMWPE that is gamma irradiated in an inert atmosphere, compared with unsterilized or gas-sterilized UHMWPE. However, UHMWPE that is gamma irradiated in an inert atmosphere also undergoes some oxidation, probably because oxygen may be trapped within the material at the time of sterilization and oxygen also can diffuse into the component over time in vivo.

Gas sterilization with ethylene oxide or gas plasma is also used for sterilization of UHMWPE implants. The chemical structure of UHMWPE is not altered and its mechanical properties, including fatigue strength, are maintained. However, wear resistance is not improved because there is no cross-linking of the polymer surface.

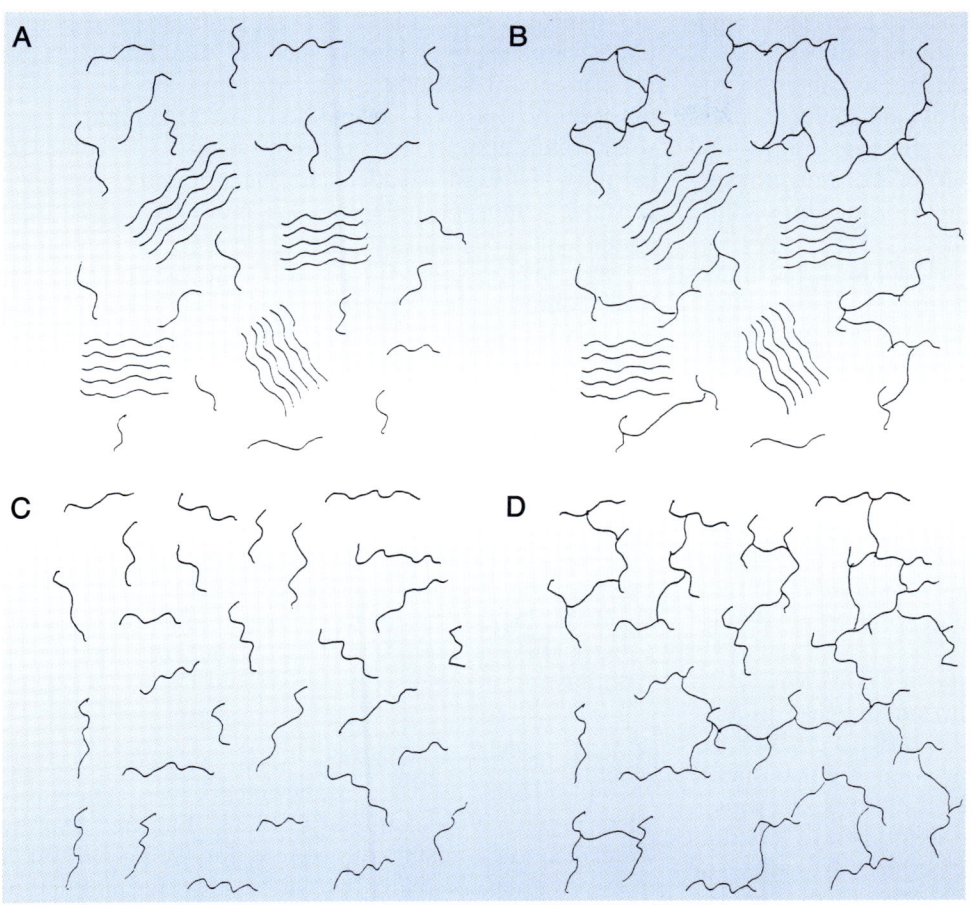

Figure 2   **A,** Schematic diagrams of semicrystalline structure of UHMWPE. Crystalline regions are shown in which the polymer chains are parallel and close to one another. Amorphous regions are shown in which the polymer chains are randomly oriented. **B,** When UHMWPE is irradiated at room temperature, cross-links develop in the amorphous but not the crystalline regions. **C,** When UHMWPE is heated above its melting point (135°C), polymer chains in the crystalline regions separate and the entire material becomes amorphous. **D,** UHMWPE that is irradiated above its melting point becomes very highly cross-linked because a large portion of the polymer chains are in the amorphous state during irradiation.

Currently, UHMWPE implants are sterilized by gamma irradiation in an inert atmosphere, ethylene oxide, or gas plasma. Each method minimizes the oxidative degradation that occurs in implants sterilized by gamma irradiation in air.

Highly Cross-Linked Polyethylenes

In an effort to improve the wear behavior of UHMWPE, highly cross-linked polyethylenes have been developed. UHMWPE can become highly cross-linked by exposure to electron beam or high-dose gamma irradiation, or by exposure to chemicals such as peroxide.

UHMWPE is a semicrystalline amorphous polymer. Portions of the material are in a crystalline phase in which the polymer chains are arranged in a parallel or lamellar fashion. Other areas are amorphous, and the polymer chains are randomly oriented (Fig. 2, *A*). When UHMWPE is irradiated at room temperature, cross-linking occurs in the amorphous but not the crystalline regions (Fig. 2, *B*). Free radicals that form in polymer chains within the crystalline region recombine because the polymer chains are nonmobile. The amount of cross-linking is dependent on the irradiation dose and processing temperature.

If UHMWPE is heated above its melting point (135°C), the polymer chains in the crystalline regions separate so that the entire material is in an amorphous state (Fig. 2, *C*). UHMWPE that is irradiated at high temperature above its melting point (melt-irradiated) becomes very highly cross-linked (Fig. 2, *D*). When the cross-linked, melt-irradiated material is cooled to room temperature, the crystallinity is less than that of conventional UHMWPE because polymer chains that were previously in a crystalline phase are cross-linked and cannot recrystallize.

Because irradiation produces free radicals, many free radicals are present in highly cross-linked polyethylene. In order to neutralize the free radicals and avoid oxidation, the material is annealed or heated. Melt-irradiated cross-linked polyethylene does not require subsequent annealing because the high temperature used neutralizes the free radicals. Highly cross-linked polyethylene irradiated at low temperature requires annealling after cross-linking.

Failure mechanisms of total hip and knee replacements are often different. The hip is more conforming than the knee; as a result, contact stresses in the knee are typically an order of magnitude greater than that of the hip.

UHMWPE wear mechanisms are affected by the magnitude of contact stress. At low contact stress such as occurs in the hip, surface wear mechanisms (abrasion and adhesion) predominate, whereas at high contact stress such as in the knee, fatigue wear mechanisms (pitting and delamination) typically occur. However, polyethylene material fatigue can also lead to liner dissociation failure of modular acetabular components.

Highly cross-linked polyethylenes demonstrate markedly improved wear behavior in hip simulator studies. However, cross-linking changes the amorphous or both the amorphous and crystalline regions of the polymer, which decreases its static mechanical and fatigue characteristics.

The static mechanical and fatigue strength are affected by the amount of cross-linking. Currently available highly cross-linked polyethylenes meet the minimum American Society for Testing and Materials mechanical standards. However, the minimum fatigue strength necessary for UHMWPE used in total joint replacements is not clear.

Cross-linking limits the mobility of UHMWPE polymer chains and is associated with an increase in stiffness and decrease in ductility. If a fatigue crack is initiated, growth of the crack is slowed by the ductile tearing of the polymer at the crack tip. However, highly cross-linked polyethylenes demonstrate less ductility and more rapid fatigue crack growth. The decrease in fatigue resistance is related to the amount of cross-linking. Very highly cross-linked UHMWPE may be more appropriate for use in total hip replacements than total knee replacement because of the greater fatigue strength requirements of total knee tibial components.

The cross-linked polyethylenes represent a class of materials with similar but not identical characteristics because of differences in processing methods. These differences include heating above or below the melt temperature, radiation source, radiation dose, and final method of sterilization (Fig. 3).

Counterface Material

Counterface materials used in total joint replacements include cobalt-chrome, ceramic (alumina or zirconia), stainless steel, and titanium. Titanium is a relatively soft metal that has been associated with cases of severe third-body abrasive wear and has been abandoned as a bearing surface. Either cobalt-chrome or ceramic (alumina or zirconia) can be safely applied to a modular cobalt-chrome or titanium total hip femoral component, whereas a stainless steel modular head coupled with a cobalt-chrome or titanium femoral component may lead to galvanic corrosion. Cobalt-chrome is therefore the preferred metallic bearing surface in total

hip arthroplasty. Ceramic bearing surfaces have potential advantages over metals such as increased abrasion resistance and wettability. In vitro and in vivo studies of ceramic femoral heads demonstrate slightly less wear than cobalt-chrome femoral heads. However, ceramic femoral heads can occasionally fracture. Ceramic femoral heads are also more expensive than cobalt chrome.

Scratches are often observed on the surfaces of femoral components retrieved from failed total knee arthroplasties. A single scratch can substantially increase the rate of UHMWPE wear. Modifications to the cobalt-chrome femoral component such as nitrogen ion bombardment or thermally-driven diffusion hardening may be helpful to improve scratch resistance and reduce UHMWPE wear in total knee arthroplasty. Alumina and zirconia ceramic total knee femoral components have also been used clinically. Concerns have been raised about the risk of fracture with these implants. An oxidized zirconium total knee femoral component has been approved by the Food and Drug Administration for use in the United States.

Metal-on-Metal Bearings

Metal-on-metal total hip replacements were commonly used in the 1960s and early 1970s. Failures usually occurred as a result of aseptic loosening although many of these implants provided long term function similar to metal-UHMWPE bearings.

Metal-on-metal bearings used in total hip arthroplasty are made of cobalt-chrome. The volume of wear generated from a metal-on-metal bearing is considerably less than that from a metal-UHMWPE bearing. Factors that may affect the metal-on-metal wear rates include the clearance (difference in radius between the femoral head and acetabular bearing surface), surface roughness, and carbon content of the cobalt chrome alloy. A small clearance provides more contact area between the two surfaces, which decreases contact stress, whereas a large clearance permits more fluid flow into the joint. If the clearance is too small and exceeds manufacturing tolerances, the joint articulation may become excessively tight and equatorial rather than polar contact occurs between the bearing surfaces, which can increase frictional torque and cause loosening. This effect on the joint has been implicated as a cause of failure of the McKee-Farrar metal-on-metal hip replacements. Increased wear is also associated with increased surface roughness, but the effect of other material variables such as use of cast versus forged cobalt-chrome and carbon content are less clear.

Early clinical results with modern metal-on-metal hip replacements are comparable to those of metal-UHMWPE bearings and demonstrate less aseptic loos-

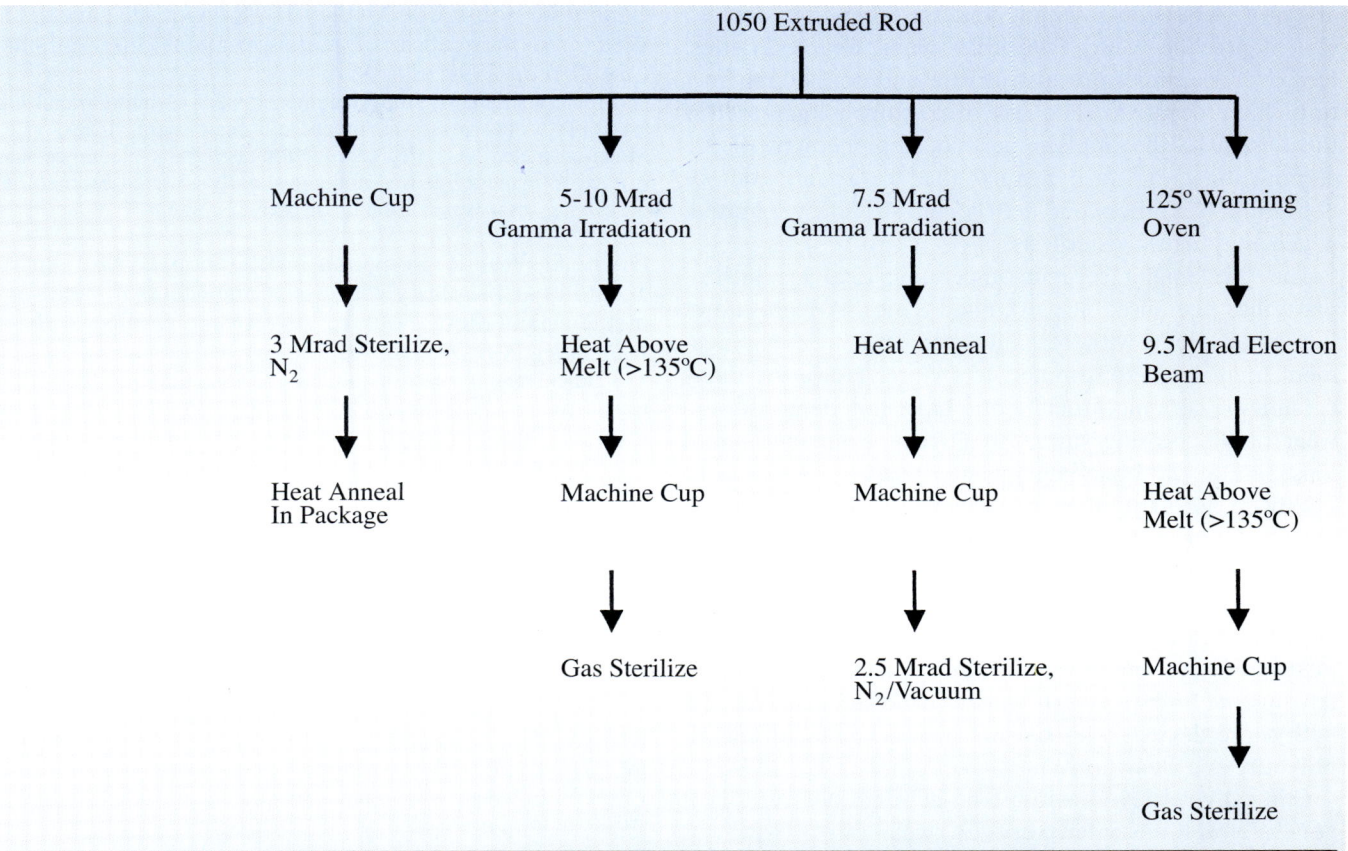

Process Name	Heat Stabilized	CISM (cold irradiated subsequent melt)	CIAN (cold irradiated annealed non-melt)	WIAM (warm irradiated adiabatic melt)
Product Name	Duration ™	(1) Marathan ™ (2) XLPE ™	Crossfire ™	(1) Durasul ™ (2) Longevity ™
Manufacturer	Stryker Howmedica Osteonics	(1) Depuy/J&J (2) Smith and Nephew	Stryker Howmedica Osteonics	(1) Sulzer (2) Zimmer

Figure 3 Current methods used to manufacture moderate to highly cross-linked polyethylenes.

ening than metal-on-metal designs used in the 1960s and 1970s. However, concerns with metal-on-metal hip replacements include the generation of metal particulate debris, which may travel to the distal sites as well as local osteolysis.

In patients with metal-polyethylene total joint replacements, metal as well as polyethylene particles can be found at distant sites. In a study of postmortem specimens from patients with metal-polyethylene total joint replacements, metallic wear particles were identified in the para-aortic lymph nodes in 68% and in the liver or spleen in 38% of the patients. The serum and urine levels of cobalt and chromium are elevated in patients with metal-on-metal articulations. Metals can travel to distant sites in ionic form and little is known about the long-term

clinical effects of elevated serum and urine metal levels. Cancer risk has not been shown to be increased in patients who have received metal-on-metal hip replacements. However, long-term studies with large numbers of patients are needed to accurately assess this risk.

Ceramic-on-Ceramic Bearings

Ceramic femoral heads that articulate against UHMWPE are made of alumina or zirconia. Zirconia has greater toughness than alumina; therefore, it is less likely to fracture. Alumina-on-alumina has more favorable wear characteristics than zirconia-on-zirconia. Ceramic-on-ceramic bearing surfaces made of alumina demonstrate extremely low volumetric wear rates. Ceramic surfaces are more abrasion-resistant and wettable than metals, which provide very favorable wear characteristics. However, ceramics are also brittle and occasional fractures have occurred. The risk of fracture is increased if the design of the implant permits impingement of the ceramic head or neck against the acetabular component rim. Ceramic wear debris can also be generated, which may cause osteolysis.

The Mittlemeier ceramic-on-ceramic total hip arthroplasty has been used in the United States. A high rate of loosening, along with ceramic head and neck impingement, may have contributed to failure. However, many ceramic-on-ceramic articulations have not demonstrated wear of the bearing surface but failed from mechanical loosening at the bone-implant interface.

Newer implant designs permit bony fixation to metallic femoral and acetabular components while using a modular ceramic acetabular liner and femoral head to provide the ceramic-on-ceramic bearing. The acetabular liners are not self-centering, and incorrect positioning of the liner during surgery may lead to fracture of the liner. However, early clinical reports with these devices demonstrate results similar to metal-polyethylene bearings.

Clinically retrieved ceramic-on-ceramic bearings have generally demonstrated very low wear rates. However, some cases of catastrophic wear have occurred. These cases have been attributed to alumina grains that pulled out from the ceramic surface, leading to increased roughness or third-body abrasives. Improvements in manufacturing have led to a decrease in the grain size and corresponding decrease in wear rates. In addition to grain size, wear rates have been correlated with patient weight, age, male gender, nonoptimal cup inclination, and component migration.

Annotated Bibliography

Baker DA, Hastings RS, Pruitt L: Study of fatigue resistance of chemical and radiation crosslinked medical grade ultrahigh molecular weight polyethylene. *J Biomed Mater Res* 1999;46:573-581.
    Resistance to fatigue crack propagation is decreased by cross-linking. Highly cross-linked polyethylenes may not be appropriate for use in high contact stress cyclic loading applications such as fixed bearing total knee replacements.

Chan FW, Bobyn JD, Medley JB, Krygier JJ, Tanzer M: Wear and lubrication of metal-on-metal hip implants. *Clin Orthop* 1999;369:10-24.
    In a hip simulator study volumetric wear of metal-metal hip arthroplasty bearings was much less than metal UHMWPE. Metal-on-metal wear decreased with decreasing clearance and surface roughness but was not significantly affected by material processing (cast versus forged) or carbon content.

Dorr LD, Wan Z, Longjohn DB, Dubois B, Murken R: Total hip arthroplasty with use of the Metasul metal-on-metal articulation: Four to seven-year results. *J Bone Joint Surg Am* 2000;82:789-798.
    Clinical results with a modern design metal-on-metal hip replacements are comparable to metal UHMWPE. Loosening rates are lower than the metal-on-metal hip replacements used in the 1960s and 1970s.

McKellop HA, Shen FW, Campbell P, Ota T: Effect of molecular weight, calcium stearate, and sterilization methods on the wear of ultra high molecular weight polyethylene acetabular cups in a hip joint simulator. *J Orthop Res* 1999;17:329-339.
    Calcium stearate is sometimes added to UHMWPE to facilitate processing. There was no difference in hip simulator wear between calcium stearate free UHMWPE and UHMWPE with calcium stearate. Volumetric wear was higher for UHMWPE sterilized by ethylene oxide compared to UHMWPE which was gamma irradiated presumably due to cross-linking produced by irradiation.

McKellop H, Shen FW, Lu B, Campbell P, Salovey R: Development of an extremely wear-resistant ultra high molecular weight polyethylene for total hip replacements. *J Orthop Res* 1999;17:157-167.
    Highly cross-linked polyethylenes can be produced by chemical or radiation cross-linking. Remelting after irradiation cross-linking extinguishes free radicals and resists oxidation. Highly cross-linked polyethylenes tested in hip simulators demonstrate dramatically reduced wear.

Prudhommeaux F, Hamadouche M, Nevelos J, Doyle C, Meunier A, Sedel L: Wear of alumina-on-alumina total hip arthroplasties at a mean 11-year follow-up. *Clin Orthop* 2000;379:113-122.
    Clinically retrieved alumina ceramic bearings demonstrated variable wear rates. Smaller grain size was associated with a decrease in wear rate.

Urban RM, Jacobs JJ, Tomlinson MJ, Gavrilovic J, Black J, Peoc'h M: Dissemination of wear particles to the liver, spleen, and abdominal lymph nodes of patients with hip or knee replacement. *J Bone Joint Surg Am* 2000;82:457-476.
    Postmortem specimens from 29 patients and biopsy specimens from 2 patients with metal-polyethylene total hip or knee replacements demonstrated both metal and polyethylene particles in the para-aortic lymph nodes in most of the patients. In 38% of the patients metal particles had disseminated to the liver or spleen and in 14% of the patients polyethylene particles had disseminated to the liver or spleen.

Won CH, Rohatgi S, Kraay MJ, Goldberg VM, Rimnac CM: Effect of resin type and manufacturing method on wear of polyethylene tibial components. *Clin Orthop* 2000;376:161-171.

Clinically retrieved molded Hi-fax 1900 Miller-Galante I components were compared with clinically retrieved machined GUR 415 Miller-Galante II components. Both implant groups were sterilized by gamma irradiation in air. The Miller-Galante I components demonstrated more scratching and embedded metallic debris but less oxidative degradation and delamination than the Miller-Galante II components.

Yoon TR, Rowe SM, Jung ST, Seon KJ, Maloney WJ: Osteolysis in association with a total hip arthroplasty with ceramic bearing surfaces. *J Bone Joint Surg Am* 1998;80:1459-1468.

Wear particles generated by a ceramic-on-ceramic hip replacement can stimulate a foreign body response and osteolysis.

Classic Bibliography

Davidson, JA: Characteristics of metal and ceramic total hip bearing surfaces and their effect on long-term ultra high molecular weight polyethylene wear. *Clin Orthop* 1993;294:361-378.

Fisher J, Chan KL, Hailey JL, Shaw D, Stone M: Preliminary study of the effect of aging following irradiation on the wear of ultrahigh-molecular-weight polyethylene. *J Arthroplasty* 1995;10:689-692.

Fritsch EW, Gleitz M: Ceramic femoral head fractures in total hip arthroplasty. *Clin Orthop* 1996;328:129-136.

Ivory JP, Kershaw CJ, Choudhry R, Parmar H, Stoyle TF: Autophor cementless total hip arthroplasty for osteoarthrosis secondary to congenital hip dysplasia. *J Arthroplasty* 1994;9:427-433.

Ries MD, Weaver K, Rose RM, Gunther J, Sauer W, Beals N: Fatigue strength of polyethylene after sterilization by gamma irradiation or ethylene oxide. *Clin Orthop* 333:87-95.

Rimnac CM, Klein RW, Betts F, Wright TM: Postirradiation aging of ultra-high molecular weight polyethylene. *J Bone Joint Surg Am* 1994;76:1052-1056.

Rose RM, Nusbaum HJ, Schneider H, et al: On the true wear rate of ultra high-molecular-weight polyethylene in the total hip prosthesis. *J Bone Joint Surg Am* 1980;62:537-549.

Sedel L, Kerboull L, Christel P, Meunier A, Witvoet J: Alumina-on-alumina hip replacement: Results and survivorship in young patients. *J Bone Joint Surg Br* 1990;72B:658-663.

Sutula LC, Collier JP, Saum KA, et al: Impact of gamma sterilization on clinical performance of polyethylene in the hip. *Clin Orthop* 1995;319:28-40.

Visuri T, Pukkala E, Paavolainen P, Pulkkinen P, Riska EB: Cancer risk after metal on metal and polyethylene on metal total hip arthroplasty. *Clin Orthop* 1996;329(suppl):280-289.

Chapter 5

Blood Transfusion

E. Michael Keating, MD

Introduction

Transfusion medicine is an integral component of the practice of orthopaedic surgery. Although the topic of transfusion medicine covers the administration of blood and its components, the major emphasis for the practicing orthopaedic surgeon is hemoglobin (Hb) management. Proper Hb management requires that the surgeon have knowledge of transfusion practices, advantages and disadvantages of various approaches to Hb management, and strategies to avoid the need for blood.

General Principles of Transfusion Therapy

Red Blood Cell Antigen Systems

Several hundred red blood cell (RBC) antigen systems have been identified, but fewer than 12 of them are responsible for the majority of alloimmune transfusion reactions. Although the clinical significance of the various RBC antigen systems has been recognized for more than 100 years, the functional significance of many of these systems has only recently been understood. For example, blood group antigen-bearing proteins are responsible for the structural integrity of and transport of substances across the RBC membrane, receptors for complement components, adhesive properties, and enzymatic activity. Pretransfusion testing now routinely assesses the presence or absence of the major blood group antigens and their antibodies.

ABO Antigens

Blood group A and B antigens are expressed at birth. The blood group O phenotype results from the absence of transferase activity, which adds an immunodominant acetylgalactosamine or galactose molecule to the abundantly expressed RBC antigens A and B, respectively. Following infancy, healthy individuals develop circulating isoagglutinins to the A or B antigens they lack. Expression of A and B antigens is the major factor governing RBC transfusion practices. Studies are in progress to evaluate the use of enzymatic activity to convert group B and group A blood to the more common group O phenotype.

Rh Antigens

The Rh system is the most complex and immunogenic of the various blood group antigen systems. It consists of almost 50 antigens, including major antigens D, C, c, E, and e. Antisera to the Rh D antigen agglutinates 85% of human erythrocytes. In the absence of immunization by transfusion or pregnancy, antibodies to the Rh system are not detected routinely; however, blood is routinely typed for the presence of the Rh D antigen because of its immunogenicity and its association with Rh hemolytic disease of the newborn. Although RBCs lacking Rh antigens (Rh_{null} phenotype) are stomatocytes, and Rh_{null} disease is associated with hemolytic anemia, the exact function of the Rh antigens is unclear.

Other Clinically Significant Antigen Systems

Other than the ABO and Rh systems, the most clinically significant RBC antigen systems are Kell, Duffy, Kidd, and MNSs. Antibodies to these antigens generally are produced following transfusion therapy or after a fetomaternal hemorrhage during pregnancy. Anti-Kell is relatively common. Antibodies to this antigen can accelerate the clearance of transfused erythrocytes. Duffy negativity [Fy(a-b-)] is common in blacks. Patients with this phenotype can produce alloantibodies that may cause a delayed hemolytic transfusion reaction. Antibodies to the Kidd antigens (anti-Jk^a and -Jk^b) may be difficult to detect during pretransfusion testing and can cause a delayed hemolytic transfusion reaction. Antibodies to the MNSs antigens can be associated with clinically significant hemolysis.

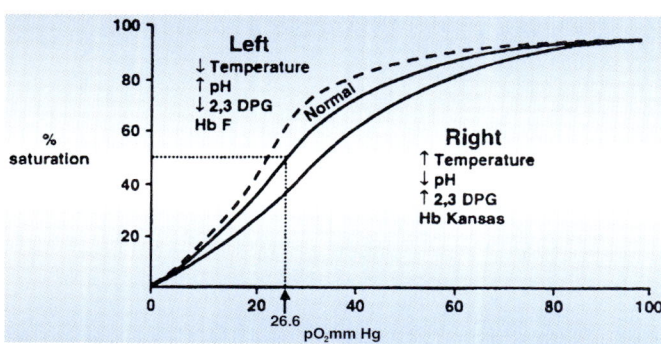

Figure 1 Mechanism of oxygenation. Oxygen dissociation curve for hemoglobin showing effects of temperature, pH, and 2,3-diphosphoglycerate content and hemoglobin type. *(Reproduced with permission from Goyette RG: Hematology: A Comprehensive Guide to the Diagnosis and Treatment of Blood Disorders. Los Angeles, CA, Practical Management Information Corporation, 1997, pp 333-354.)*

Red Blood Cell Transfusion Practices

Until the 1980s, the practice of blood transfusion was viewed as relatively risk-free. Consequently, transfusions were administered routinely before surgery to patients with Hb levels < 10 g/dL. With the recognition of human immunodeficiency virus (HIV) infection, and in light of the morbidity and mortality associated with other transfusion-related infection, such as hepatitis C virus (HCV), the advisability of routine transfusion based on a "trigger" Hb has been questioned. In treating a surgical patient with anemia, the potential immunomodulatory effects and not the risks of transfusion-related viral infections are of primary concern. In addition, the capacity of transfused RBCs to deliver oxygen is not optimal, especially when older units of RBCs are transfused. Therefore, blood management should be practiced, with the following guidelines: (1) patients should receive only the components necessary to correct a specific deficiency; and (2) therapy should be directed toward restoring functional levels of the missing component rather than guiding laboratory values back into the normal range.

RBCs are transfused to improve the blood's oxygen-carrying capacity (Fig. 1) rather than to correct hypovolemia. Studies have shown that patients with chronic anemia can function quite well with Hb levels in the 7 g/dL to 8 g/dL range because of a variety of compensatory mechanisms that exist to maintain tissue oxygenation in the face of anemia. These include alterations in tissue oxygen extraction and utilization as well as shifts in the oxygen dissociation curve caused by changes in erythrocyte 2,3-bisphosphoglycerate, pulmonary ventilation/perfusion, and cardiac output. This level of Hb is well tolerated in otherwise healthy patients with chronic anemia; however, Hb management is often necessary in the presence of acute anemia, cardiopulmonary disease, or other comorbidities.

A variety of RBC products are available from a hospital transfusion service, although whole blood is not always stocked by most blood banks. Packed RBCs are the component of choice to treat acute anemia. One unit of packed RBCs consists of the erythrocytes from one unit of whole blood minus most of the plasma. Leukocytes in one unit of blood can be responsible for a number of adverse events, including alloimmunization to HLA, transmission of cell-associated viruses (for example, cytomegalovirus, human T lymphotrophic virus [HTLV]-1 and -2), graft-versus-host disease, and immunomodulation. RBCs washed multiple times in saline may be transfused to patients with allergic reactions to plasma proteins (for example, immunoglobulin (Ig)E-mediated anti-IgA reactions). Finally, frozen RBCs can be deglycerolized and provide a source of rare blood types for patients without compatible units.

Red Blood Cell Substitutes

Ideas for RBC substitutes have existed for hundreds of years and yet none are available outside of clinical trials. Until the HIV epidemic, the ready availability of donated blood and the presence of hospital transfusion services, however, made artificial substitutes a low priority. Development of blood substitutes has revealed a number of potential problems that may limit their usefulness. For example, they have a short intravascular half-life, ≤ 2 days compared with the 120-day life span of a circulating RBC. In addition, absence of the RBC membrane allows oxygen to diffuse readily from the carrier molecule into the surrounding tissues, which causes imbalance of the microvasculature's autoregulatory mechanism. Consequently, as the second- and third-order arterioles constrict in an attempt to modulate the excess tissue oxygen levels, unwanted ischemia may develop. Hb molecules then readily scavenge nitric oxide. When this natural vasodilator is bound by large amounts of circulating free Hb, vasoconstriction develops and blood pressure can increase.

Hemoglobin Solutions

Hb is the RBC's natural oxygen carrier. Within the RBC, Hb molecules are protected from catabolism and survive the duration of the lifetime of the erythrocyte. However, free Hb rapidly dissociates into its subunits ($\alpha\beta$ dimers), which are oxidized and removed by the kidney. As seen in patients with crush injury, high concentrations of free plasma Hb can be nephrotoxic. In an attempt to prolong its intravascular half-life and decrease nephrotoxicity, the Hb molecule has been modified. These alterations include conjugating Hb with carrier molecules such as polyethylene glycol and dextran, creating intramolecular cross-links in individual Hb molecules to prevent them from dissociating into dimers, and polymerizing the molecule. An alternate approach that may avoid many of the problems of the solubilized Hb is to encapsulate the molecule with liposomal technology. The source of the Hb for these products has included outdated blood, bovine Hb, and recombinant human Hb, although these approaches have been associated with such issues as lack of supply, potential transmissible diseases (eg, bovine spongiform encephalopathy), and molecular and cost considerations, respectively.

Perfluorocarbon-Based Products

Perfluorocarbons are inert halogenated molecules that can carry large amounts of dissolved gases. For example, whereas normal human blood carries approximately 0.3 mL/dL of dissolved oxygen, 1 dL of a fluorocarbon solution can transport approximately 50 mL/dL. Although this property makes perfluorocarbons attractive RBC substitutes, they reside in the circulation for only a short time, require high concentrations of inspired oxygen, and blockade both the reticuloendothelial system and circulating granulocytes. Recipients may develop fever, a flulike syndrome, and dose-related thrombocytopenia. Initial studies in surgical patients with anemia were deemed ineffective, but recent evidence indicates that a second-generation fluorocarbon, perflubron, is more effective than autologous blood or colloid infusion in reversing physiologic transfusion triggers in orthopaedic surgery patients.

Adverse Effects of Transfusion Therapy

Infectious Complications

A number of infectious agents have been identified in the blood of humans. Although the risk of transfusion-associated disease with these agents is currently unknown, the potential for infection still exists. However, at the start of the 21st century, blood in the United States is safer than it has ever been.

Genomic Screening for Transfusion-Associated Pathogens

A variety of factors have contributed to the improved safety of the blood supply, such as extensive interviews to exclude high-risk donors, steps to inactivate lipid-enveloped viruses, surveillance to monitor for trends in infection, and testing for specific infectious agents. Screening procedures currently in place include those for the hepatitis B virus (HBV), HCV, HTLV-1 and -2, and HIV-1 and -2.

Screening has significantly reduced but not erased the risk for transfusion-associated viral infections. Viremia may occur during a window when antibodies may not be present or are present in such low concentrations that they are undetectable, and/or circulating antigen levels may be too low to be detected by conventional techniques. Therefore, a variety of techniques, including polymerase chain reaction (PCR), reverse transcriptase PCR, ligase-chain reaction, nucleic acid sequence-based amplification, and transcription-mediated amplification, have been used to detect silent infection in individuals.

Newly discovered transmissible pathogens may also be detected by nucleic acid amplification technology (NAT) testing, which can be used to separate patients with passive antibodies (for example, in neonatal HIV) from actively infected patients, differentiate strains, and detect asymptomatic infections. False negatives may occur when viral clearance is complete, subthreshold viremia is present, PCR primers are constructed from less conserved regions of the virus, or when blood is stored under conditions that promote degradation of the agent's genomic material. The sensitivity of NAT testing is on the level of 10^{-18} g nucleic acid. NAT is currently being used in both the United States and continental Europe to screen large plasma pools for infectious agents. Single-donor testing is attractive, but potentially costly.

Hepatitis

Despite screening procedures, posttransfusion HBV and HCV infections still occur. The risk of contracting HBV or HCV after a transfusion is estimated to be on the order of 1 in 30,000 to 250,000 and 1 in 30,000 to 150,000, respectively. Approximately 0.5% to 1.5% of healthy blood donors test positive for hepatitis, and this virus is a major cause of cirrhosis, hepatocellular carcinoma, and end-stage liver disease. Although the initial hepatitis infection is usually anicteric, infection becomes chronic in approximately 85% of patients. Infection by HCV has been reported from contaminated intravenous Ig preparations. Hepatitis A virus (HAV) is a nonenveloped RNA virus, predominantly transmitted by the enteric route. Transient HAV viremia does occur, however, and has produced cases of posttransfusion hepatitis A. The risk of HAV infection from a blood transfusion has been estimated to be 1 in 1,000,000. The transfusion-transmitted virus is a nonenveloped, circular, single-strand DNA virus that has a worldwide distribution, can be found in 1% to 40% of normal blood donors, appears to replicate in the liver, and has been identified in the serum of a patient with non-A-G posttransfusion hepatitis. The exact significance of transfusion-transmitted virus in human disease remains to be determined; it is possible that it may prove no more pathogenic than the hepatitis G virus.

Retroviruses

Blood is now screened for both HIV-1 and -2. The estimated risk of HIV infection from a single unit of blood ranges from 1 in 200,000 to 2 million. In March 1996, testing was instituted for the HIV-1 p24 antigen, which appears approximately 6 days before enzyme-linked immunosorbent assay (ELISA) tests for anti-HIV become positive. Despite the fact that the majority of HIV-1 infections are caused by the group M strain, outlier (group O) infections can also occur. Studies have found no evidence of significant group O infections in the United States, although the fact that existing HIV-ELISA tests must be modified to improve detection of this strain is an important factor. HIV-2 can lead to AIDS but has a low prevalence in the United States. HTLV-1 and 2 also are retroviruses. As a result of significant cross-reactivity, testing for HTLV-1 detects many cases of HTLV-2. Infection by HTLV-1 has been associated with tropical spastic paraparesis/myelopathy and adult T-cell lymphoma/leukemia. At this time, HTLV-2 has undetermined pathogenic significance other than rare reported cases of a mild myelopathy. Because both viruses are cell-associated, the risk of transfusion is greatest with cellular blood preparations such as RBCs or platelets. The risk of HTLV-1/2 infection from a single unit of blood is approximately 1 in 250,000 to 2 million.

Bacteria and Protozoa

Bacteria can contaminate a variety of blood products. It has been estimated that the chance for contamination of RBC units and platelet packs is approximately 1 in 500,000 and 1 in 12,000, respectively. Significant contamination is related to storage length and temperature. As a result, the prevalence of contaminated platelets is much higher than that of packed RBCs. In banked blood the most common organisms are cryophilic, gram-negative organisms such as *Yersinia enterocolitica*. Platelets are most often contaminated with gram-positive cocci such as Staphylococcus species. The possibility of bacterial contamination should be strongly considered when rigor and hypotension accompany transfusion.

Trypanosoma cruzi, the etiologic agent of Chagas' disease, is endemic in South and Central America and can survive storage for several weeks in a single unit of blood. Consequently, there is concern that this agent may enter the blood supply, particularly in areas with a high prevalence of Hispanic donors. Transfusion-associated malaria can be produced by all four human malarial species. Transmission results when an asymptomatic individual donates blood. *Babesia microti*, a protozoan parasite, can invade erythrocytes and produce a malaria-like illness. Following an acute infection, parasitemia can be lifelong and is particularly severe in the patient who has had splenectomy. Because there are no satisfactory serologic tests for either malaria or *Babesia microti*, the risk of transfusion can only be reduced by careful donor exclusion. There is no evidence that *Borrelia burgdorferi*, the spirochete that causes Lyme disease, can be transmitted by transfusion.

Human Herpesvirus 8

Human herpesvirus 8 (HHV-8) is associated with Kaposi's sarcoma and also is known as the Kaposi's sarcoma herpesvirus. Infection with HHV-8 has been associated with endemic and epidemic Kaposi's sarcoma, Castleman's disease, and body cavity-based malignant lymphomas. Although the primary mode of transmission appears to be sexual, the virus has been recovered from the blood of healthy blood donors, raising the possibility of transfusionassociated infection.

Immunomodulation

The significance of immunomodulation as a result of blood transfusion was first recognized in 1973 when transfusion prior to renal transplantation was noted to improve the survival of cadaveric renal allografts. Although controversy surrounds the significance of immunomodulation in the general surgical population, there is evidence that it can cause negative effects. Confounding variables complicate interpretation, but many retrospective studies of transfusion and postoperative infection conclude that transfusion is the single best predictor of postoperative infection. Orthopaedic-specific data document that transfusion is associated with an increased risk of bacterial infection and an extended hospital stay. Furthermore, the results of one recent retrospective study of almost 10,000 elderly hip fracture patients who underwent surgical repair concluded that blood transfusion was associated with a 52% greater risk of pneumonia. The basis for the immunomodulatory activity during transfusion therapy is not fully understood, but the effects are believed to be related to the presence of transfused leukocytes. For example, allogeneic lymphocytes continue to circulate for more than 1 year after transfusion in trauma patients. This may be associated with a mixed chimerism with the development of a state of relative immune tolerance. In addition, transfused mononuclear cells may incite an in vivo mixed lymphocyte culture reaction. Cytokines from this reaction include tumor necrosis factor, various interleukins, γ-interferon, and transforming growth factor-β, among others. Other potential reasons for the effect include the induction of anti-idiotypic antibodies, development of increased levels of suppressor lymphocytes, or the immunomodulatory effects of reactivation of a variety of latent viral infections by transfusion-related allogeneic stimulation. The potential for immunomodulation is a strong argument for administration of cellular blood products through a leukodepletion filter.

Transfusion Reactions

The incidence of hemolytic transfusion reactions is approximately 1 in 250,000 to 1 million. Approximately one half of the deaths are attributed to ABO incompatibility resulting from a clerical error. This most often occurs outside the laboratory and is the result of failure to match the blood to the patient. Delayed hemolytic transfusion reactions, which occur in approximately 1 in 1,000 units, present as shortened RBC survival and may masquerade as an immune hemolytic anemia. The incidence increases in heavily transfused patients. Febrile transfusion reactions are the most common type of adverse event associated with the administration of blood. These reactions may result from a reaction between recipient HLA antibodies and donor leukocytes or may be the consequence of elevated cytokine levels in an infused unit. Patients with a history of febrile reactions should receive units that have been leukodepleted prior to storage. Anaphylactic transfusion reactions are most often the result of IgE anti-IgA antibodies in IgA-deficient recipients. IgA deficiency is relatively common. To avoid these reactions, cellular blood products should undergo intensive washing. Transfusion-related lung injury may be caused by the presence of HLA or antineutrophil antibodies in the donor plasma. The severity of the reaction seems to depend on overall cardiopulmonary status.

Reducing the Risks of Blood Transfusion

Preoperative Autologous Donation

Preoperative autologous donation (PAD) offers several advantages, including absence of infectious and immunomodulatory complications, but the procedure is not without risks. The donation process can be associated with syncopal or ischemic events. In addition, reinfusion of autologous units can be accompanied by adverse events such as sepsis, volume overload, and hemolytic transfusion reactions, resulting from the same type of clerical errors that complicate allogeneic transfusions. Because healthy patients may require weeks to regenerate the blood lost during PAD, they typically have lower Hb levels right before surgery than before PAD. Perhaps the greatest shortcoming of the procedure is that many of these donated units are never used. Almost half of the autologous units donated in the total joint arthroplasty setting are not used. The labor-intensive nature of PAD may not be cost-efficient.

Epoetin Alfa

Erythropoietin has a central role in the regulation of erythropoiesis. The American Red Cross recommends that, if time permits, erythropoietin be administered to correct anemia instead of performing RBC transfusions. Epoetin alfa, the recombinant form of naturally-occurring erythropoietin, has been approved by the Food and Drug Administration for reduction of allogeneic blood transfusion in surgical patients. The greatest benefit is seen in patients with Hb levels in the range of 10 g/dL to 13 g/dL. Treatment with epoetin alfa significantly increases preoperative Hb levels and decreases the incidence of allogeneic blood transfusion in the orthopaedic population; in addition, epoetin alfa therapy is not associated with an increase in adverse events compared with placebo. It may be administered weekly (600 IU/kg), or approximately 40,000 units may be given subcutaneously 21, 14, and 7 days before surgery; a fourth dose is given on the day of the surgery. Compared with PAD, epoetin alfa treatment of total joint arthroplasty patients is accompanied by lower transfusions of allogeneic blood and higher postoperative Hb levels.

Acute Normovolemic Hemodilution

Acute normovolemic hemodilution limits the amount of RBCs lost during surgery. This technique is used infrequently during major orthopaedic procedures because it is logistically difficult to perform and requires a dedicated anesthesia team and careful monitoring to prevent surgical morbidity. Furthermore, acute normovolemic hemodilution can delay case turnaround times. It is not recommended for patients with significant preoperative anemia or organ system disease.

Blood Salvage Procedures

Although intraoperative blood salvage can recover approximately 60% of the RBCs lost during an orthopaedic procedure, a trained specialist usually is required to perform the procedure and, with the exception of major hip revisions, it may not be cost-effective in routine orthopaedic procedures performed outside of major teaching institutions. Blood can also be salvaged postoperatively from surgical drains and reinfused into the patient, but the product is hemodilute, partially hemolyzed, defibrinated, and may contain high concentrations of cytokines. This procedure is of limited usefulness in the general orthopaedic population and does not appear to be cost-effective.

An Approach to Hemoglobin Management in the Total Joint Arthroplasty Population

The outcomes of total joint arthroplasty and other major orthopaedic procedures are significantly influenced by the Hb management decisions made by the operating surgeon. The surgeon must weigh the risks, patient-specific considerations, and physiologic consequences before selecting a course of Hb management. Management decisions should be directed at reducing the risks of the transfusion of homologous blood, decreasing morbidity, shortening length of hospital stay, increasing vigor and strength, and improving quality of life. The initial state of the patient's Hb is an important variable when selecting among the various Hb management options. Patients with Hb levels ≥13 g/dL can be managed effectively with PAD. Those with Hb levels between 10 g/dL and 13 g/dL are prime candidates for Hb management with epoetin alfa. Although other Hb management options may be indicated clinically in some situations, they are often logistically difficult and do not provide clear advantages over either PAD or epoetin alfa.

Pharmacologic Agents

Fibrin Glue

Fibrin glue (sealant) can be used to improve hemostasis and decrease blood loss by providing a natural, flexible seal over suture lines. The material can be prepared from the patient's plasma or obtained commercially. The commercial preparations are virally inactivated. The fibrinogen and bovine thrombin are combined at the time of use in the presence of calcium to form the sealant. Some patients may form antibodies to factors V and II following exposure to the bovine thrombin.

Antifibrinolytics

Epsilon amino caproic acid and tranexamic acid inhibit plasminogen and plasmin binding to fibrin strands. When used prophylactically, they can reduce blood loss. In patients undergoing total knee replacement, a single dose of epsilon amino caproic acid, given before tourniquet release, resulted in a significant reduction in postoperative bleeding. Because of the risk of pathologic thrombosis, however, the use of these agents should be restricted to high-risk patients.

Aprotinin

Aprotinin is a serine protease with antifibrinolytic, antiplasmin antiactivated protein C, and antikallikrein activity that appears to preserve platelet function. It has been used to reduce blood loss and transfusion requirements in patients undergoing major orthopaedic surgery.

Annotated Bibliography

General

Keating EM: Hemoglobin management in hip arthroplasty. *Semin Arthopl* 2000;17:174-182.

This article discusses the advantages and disadvantages of a variety of approaches to Hb management in hip arthroplasty patients.

Adverse Effects of Transfusion Therapy

Bierbaum BE, Callaghan JJ, Galante JO, Rubash HE, Tooms RE, Welch RB: An analysis of blood management in patients having a total hip or knee arthroplasty. *J Bone Joint Surg Am* 1999;81:2-10.

This article describes the results of blood management practices in 9,482 total joint arthroplasty patients. The most important predictors of the transfusion of allogeneic blood were a low baseline Hb level and a lack of predonated autologous blood. Predonation of autologous blood is inefficient; 45% of units were not transfused. Transfusion of allogenic blood was associated with infection, fluid overload, and increased duration of hospitalization.

Carson JL, Altman DG, Duff A, et al: Risk of bacterial infection associated with allogeneic blood transfusion among patients undergoing hip fracture repair. *Transfusion* 1999;39:694-700.

Blood transfusion is associated with a 35% greater risk of serious bacterial infection and a 52% greater risk of pneumonia. These infections may be the most common life-threatening adverse effect of the transfusion of allogeneic blood.

Chamberland M, Khabbaz RF: Emerging issues in blood safety. *Infect Dis Clin North Am* 1998;12:217-229.

It is unlikely that the risk of transfusion-associated infection will ever be reduced to zero. Although the current blood supply in developed countries is safer than it has ever been, a number of challenges remain. These include variant HIV strains inconsistently detected by standard HIV tests, transmission of viruses through human preparations, and emerging agents (including prions).

Goodnough LT, Brecher ME, Kanter MH, AuBuchon JP: Transfusion medicine: First of two parts: Blood transfusion. *N Engl J Med* 1999;340:438-447.

Goodnough LT, Brecher ME, Kanter MH, AuBuchon JP: Transfusion medicine: Second of two parts: Blood conservation. *N Engl J Med* 1999;340:525-533.

This two-part series provides a general overview of blood transfusion medicine.

Reducing the Risks of Blood Transfusion

Allain JP: Genomic screening for blood-borne viruses in transfusion settings. *Clin Lab Haematol* 2000;22:1-10.

A number of techniques are available to detect blood-borne viruses during the window when antibody levels are low or nonexistent and antigen levels may be too low to be detected. A variety of molecular methods can be used. Although single donor testing is attractive, the cost is prohibitive. Therefore, nucleic acid amplification testing is only used to evaluate pooled plasma materials.

McFarland JG: Perioperative blood transfusions: Indications and options. *Chest* 1999;115(suppl 5):113S-121S.

The transfusion trigger has shifted from an empirical to a physiologic Hb level. A number of options can be used to reduce the patient's allogeneic blood needs. These include measures to increase the patient's Hb level (erythropoietin), decrease blood loss during surgery, and to substitute for intact RBCs. Pharmacologic agents that have the potential to reduce surgical blood loss include fibrin sealant, antifibrinolytics, and aprotinin.

Remy B, Deby-Dupont G, Lamy M: Red blood cell substitutes: Fluorocarbon emulsions and haemoglobin solutions. *Br Med Bull* 1999;55:277-298.

Hemoglobin solutions lack the antigenic characteristics of RBCs and do not require compatibility testing. Hemoglobin solutions are now undergoing phase III clinical trials. The perfluorocarbons are not blood substitutes; rather, they are a means to ensure tissue oxygenation during extreme hemodilution.

Spahn DR, van Brempt R, Theilmeier G, et al: Perflubron emulsion delays blood transfusions in orthopedic surgery. *Anesthesiology* 1999;5:1195-1208.

Perflubron emulsion is more effective than autologous blood or colloid infusion in reversing physiologic transfusion triggers.

Chapter 6

Coagulation and Thromboembolism in Orthopaedic Surgery

Jess H. Lonner, MD

Jay R. Lieberman, MD

Thromboembolic disease is common in patients who have had major lower extremity trauma, total hip and knee arthroplasty, and spinal cord injury. These injuries and surgical procedures are associated with venous stasis, endothelial trauma, and systemic initiation of the clotting cascade which all are risk factors for thrombosis. The risk of venous thromboembolism is compounded in the presence of hypercoagulable states classified as either primary (inherited) or secondary (Table 1). Inherited disorders involve deficiencies in one of the normal anticoagulant mechanisms, whereas secondary hypercoagulable states are clinical conditions that predispose to thromboembolic disease.

The likelihood of clot formation is compounded by reduction in levels of antithrombin III and impeded fibrinolysis that has been observed after total joint arthroplasty. Significant increases in fibrinopeptide A, thrombin-antithrombin complexes, and D-dimer were observed after tourniquet deflation after total knee arthroplasty (TKA) and with preparation of the femoral canal during total hip arthroplasty (THA). In one study, within 24 hours after surgery, 45% of limbs undergoing unilateral TKA had venographically proven deep vein thrombosis (DVT), 5% of which were popliteal thrombi. These results suggest that clot initiation and formation occur during surgery.

The Coagulation Cascade

The coagulation cascade consists of two pathways along which cofactors are variably activated, leading to fibrin clot formation. These pathways occur on or near phospholipid surfaces on platelets, endothelial cells, and white blood cells. The intrinsic and extrinsic pathways function independently until converging with the activation of factor X, which in turn activates prothrombin to form thrombin. The intrinsic pathway functions within components of blood, whereas the extrinsic pathway is activated by tissue lipoprotein. The formation of thrombin activates the conversion of fibrinogen to fibrin and is the essential component of the cascade necessary for thrombus formation. Prothrombin time (PT) measures the function of the extrinsic and common pathways, whereas partial thromboplastin time (PTT) measures the intrinsic and common pathways. Pharmacologic prophylaxis against clot formation will selectively intervene at different levels within the cascade.

Fibrinolysis acts to ensure blood vessel patency by removing fibrin deposits. Plasmin digests the fibrin and then activates other coagulation factors, including factors V and VIII, and fibrinogen. Finally, the clotting process is modulated, as well, by three natural anticoagulant pathways, including the heparin-antithrombin III pathway, the protein C-thrombomodulin-protein S pathway, and the tissue factor inhibitor pathway (Fig. 1).

Epidemiology of Venous Thromboembolic Disease

The risk of thromboembolic disease after THA and TKA, lower extremity and pelvis fractures, and spine surgery is variable, whether or not prophylaxis is used. DVT will likely occur in up to 58% of unprotected THA patients and 71% of unprotected TKA patients. These rates may be even higher for patients with hip or pelvic fractures. Proximal DVT may occur in as many as 31% of total joint arthroplasty patients and fatal pulmonary embolism in 0.1% to 0.5%. In general, most thrombi are small and have little clinical consequence. However, in proximal DVTs, particularly those of the pelvis, the risk of pulmonary embolism can be as high as 50%. The risk of chronic postthrombotic complications such as venous stasis ulcers, hyperpigmentation, and lower extremity pain as a result of DVT is lower than previously thought. Therefore, the primary goal of prophylaxis is to prevent symptomatic and fatal pulmonary embolism.

TABLE 1 | Risk Factors for Venous Thromboembolism

Primary hypercoagulable states

    Antithrombin III deficiency

    Protein C deficiency

    Protein S deficiency

    Activated protein C resistance

Secondary hypercoagulable states

    Bed rest or immobility longer than 5 days

    Malignancy

    Congestive heart failure

    Estrogen use or hormone replacement therapy

    Fractures of pelvis, hip, or leg

    History of myocardial infarction

    History of stroke

    Indwelling femoral vein catheter

    Inflammatory bowel disease

    Major surgery (particularly in operations involving abdomen, pelvis, and lower extremities)

    Multiple trauma

    Obesity

    Paralysis

    Prior venous thromboembolic disease

    Varicose veins

    History of smoking

Prevention

Thrombus formation begins intraoperatively. Consequently, thromboembolic prophylaxis should be initiated prior to or just after surgery and vigilance heightened within the first week or two after total joint arthroplasty and pelvis and hip fracture surgery.

Contemporary prophylactic interventions have contributed more to the declining incidence of fatal pulmonary embolism than of DVT. A combination of contemporary prophylaxis techniques, expeditious surgery, and early mobilization has reduced the risk of fatal pulmonary embolism after THA and TKA to between 0.05% to 0.4%. Considering the virtually uniform and consistent reduction in fatal pulmonary emboli with a variety of prophylactic measures, it is important to consider the inherent risks associated with the use of chemoprophylactic interventions. In light of these potential risks, it has been argued that routine chemoprophylaxis may not be warranted, citing a fatal pulmonary embolism rate of no higher than 0.4% without prophylaxis.

Pharmacologic options for DVT prophylaxis include warfarin, low molecular weight heparin (LMWH), and aspirin. Dextran and adjusted-dose heparin are no longer recommended. Mechanical approaches include early mobilization, pneumatic compression boots, and intermittent plantar compression. Short-course prophylactic therapy, used only until discharge from the hospital, is ineffective and in general is not recommended.

Influence of Anesthesia on Thromboembolic Disease

Epidural and spinal anesthesia may be more effective than general anesthesia for reducing the overall rate of DVT, proximal DVT, and pulmonary embolism in lower extremity arthroplasty. This increased effectiveness may be related to sympathetic blockade with subsequent vasodilatation and increased blood flow to the lower extremity observed with regional anesthesia. Additionally, with epidural anesthesia, depletion of antithrombin III is less likely than observed under general anesthesia, preserving a more normal clotting cascade. Hypotensive epidural anesthesia has been shown to further reduce the incidence of thrombosis after THA by limiting blood loss and augmenting blood flow to the lower extremity, which in turn reduces the likelihood of venous stasis.

Pharmacologic Thromboembolic Prophylaxis

Warfarin

Warfarin blocks transformation of vitamin K in the liver, thereby inhibiting the production of vitamin K-dependent clotting factors II, VII, IX, and X. In general, warfarin prophylaxis is given initially either the evening before or after surgery in a 5- or 10-mg dose. Previously, subsequent doses were determined by a sliding scale method, using PT, with a target PT level of 1.2 to 1.5 times the control value. However, interinstitutional variability in thromboplasm sensitivity has made standardization of PT difficult. The international normalized ratio (INR), which incorporates a correction factor, the internal sensitivity index, is used to determine appropriate levels of anticoagulation when using warfarin. The target INR generally should be maintained between 1.8 and 2.5. Clinically significant local and systemic bleeding complications have been reported with an incidence of between 1% to 5%.

With warfarin, the need for frequent monitoring of INR is inconvenient and expensive. Familiarity with the potential interactions with other medications is critical. Simultaneous use of nonsteroidal anti-inflammatory medications may increase the risk of peptic ulceration. It is not established whether the risk is diminished with cyclooxygenase-2 inhibitors. Other

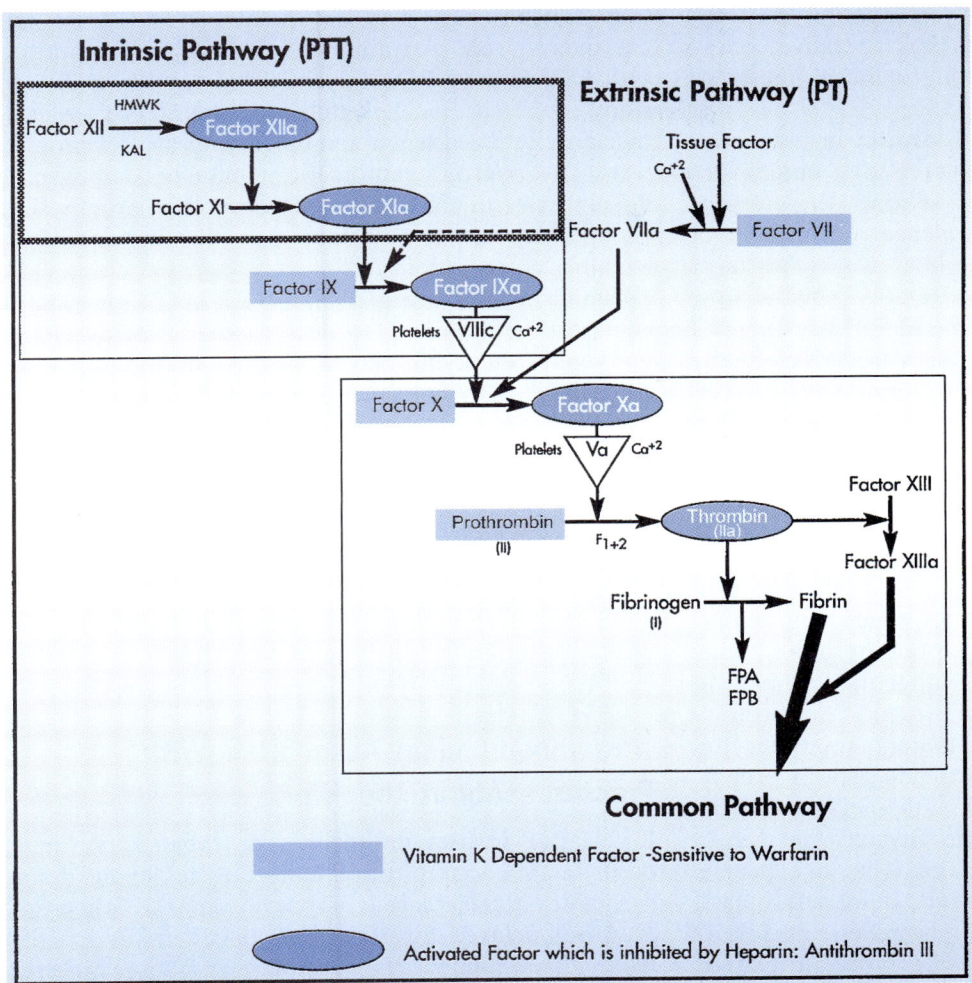

Figure 1 The coagulation pathways. Important features include the contact activation phase, vitamin K-dependent factors (affected by warfarin), and the activated serine proteases that are inhibited by heparin-antithrombin III. PT measures the function of the extrinsic and common pathways; the PTT measures the function of the intrinsic and common pathways. *(Adapted with permission from Stead RB: Regulation of hemostasis, in Goldhaber SZ (ed): Pulmonary Embolism and Deep Venous Thromboembolism. Philadelphia, PA, WB Saunders, 1985, p 32.)*

medications such as trimethoprim, cimetidine, phenytoin, and cefamandole may potentiate the anticoagulant effect of warfarin and increase the risk of bleeding complications. The delayed onset of action of warfarin leaves the patient relatively unprotected during the initial perioperative period, at which time the patient is at greatest risk for DVT. The major benefit of warfarin is not necessarily in the prevention of clot development, but more in limiting clot propagation. Except for one recent randomized prospective study of THA patients that showed that LMWH had a lower proximal DVT rate than warfarin, the incidence of proximal DVT with warfarin is generally not significantly different than with LMWH. In addition, there is no difference in the risk of fatal pulmonary embolism, which is generally considered less than 0.15%.

Low Molecular Weight Heparin

LMWH is created by depolymerization of standard unfractionated heparin. The molecular weight of these compounds ranges between 3,000 and 10,000 d, which allows these agents to function with different pharmacokinetics than standard unfractionated heparin (molecular weight between 12,000 and 15,000 d). LMWH has decreased ability to inactivate thrombin when compared with standard heparin because of its smaller size and prevents simultaneous binding of antithrombin and thrombin. LMWH has greater antithrombin-Xa activity than antithrombin-IIa activity. As a result of the limited effect on factor IIA, routine activated partial thromboplastin time (aPTT) monitoring is not required. LMWH has a bioavailability of 90% and prolonged half-life because of reduced binding of plasma proteins and therefore can be delivered once or twice daily. Dosages used for DVT prophylaxis do not increase either the PT or aPTT. Thrombocytopenia is less common with LMWHs than with unfractionated heparin. Potential limitations of LMWH include cost and need for parenteral administration, which makes compliance and administration of the drug more difficult after hospital discharge. Additionally, there may be an increased risk of bleeding complications observed, particularly if administered too soon after surgery. Use of LMWH is a relative contraindication to the use of indwelling epidural anesthetic agents.

LMWH is more effective than aspirin in preventing proximal DVT, but in direct comparative randomized trials, as well as in nonrandomized trials, there are no significant differences in the incidence of symptomatic or fatal pulmonary embolism compared with warfarin, aspirin, or mechanical pumps. Data show a dose response relationship with increased efficacy in DVT prevention at the expense of an increased risk of hemorrhagic events. Bleeding complications with LMWH have been observed in 2% to 12% of patients, but its efficacy, rapid onset, and short half-life make it a desirable option for total joint arthroplasty patients.

Aspirin

Aspirin prophylaxis has gained renewed interest in the United States because of evidence suggesting comparable rates of fatal pulmonary embolism and a better safety profile as compared with other medications. Its ease of administration, lack of a need for serologic monitoring of coagulation parameters, relatively low expense, and limited risks have made aspirin prophylaxis, alone or in combination with mechanical foot pumps, a desirable method of prophylaxis that can be easily used after patient discharge. The incidence of proximal DVT with aspirin after unilateral arthroplasty may be as high as 12% to 15%; however, the rate of fatal pulmonary embolism using aspirin antiplatelet prophylaxis has been no higher than 0.2% in a variety of studies.

In doses exceeding 100 mg per day, aspirin irreversibly binds and inactivates cyclooxygenase in both immature and circulating platelets, lasting the lifetime of the platelet (approximately 8 or 9 days). Aspirin inhibits thrombus plug formation by inhibiting platelet aggregation. The advantages of aspirin are its limited side effects, ease of administration, low cost, and the fact that no monitoring of blood clotting parameters is necessary. It may be easily continued after hospital discharge. The disadvantages of aspirin use are its higher overall incidence of DVT compared with other thromboprophylactic interventions. The risk of pulmonary embolism and fatal pulmonary embolism seems to be no higher than that of other methods. However, further randomized trials comparing aspirin with warfarin and LMWH are necessary to determine its role as a prophylactic agent in THA or TKA patients.

Mechanical Prophylaxis

External pneumatic compression boots are associated with a rate of proximal DVT that is slightly higher than that observed with warfarin in several series, but the overall risk of total DVT is lower, suggesting a shift in location of DVT from distal to proximal. One study observed that the rate of proximal DVT was significantly reduced when combined with aspirin prophylaxis. The risk of symptomatic pulmonary embolism is no higher than that observed with other prophylactic agents. Mechanical modalities have the lowest risk of bleeding complications.

The proposed mechanism of action of pneumatic compression devices is to decrease stasis by accelerating venous emptying and to increase fibrinolysis. Plantar compression boots work by mimicking the hemodynamic effect of plantar arch compression observed with ambulation. The advantage of mechanical compression devices is their limited risk of causing bleeding. Laboratory monitoring is unnecessary and side effects rare. However, patient compliance is a potential problem with these devices. Compression stockings alone do not decrease the risk of thromboembolic disease in total joint arthroplasty and should not be used alone.

Thromboembolism Associated With Fractures About the Hip

DVT after fracture of the hip has been reported to occur in 20% to 60% of patients. Several studies found a significantly increased risk of thrombosis when surgery was delayed for 2 days or longer, indicating that routine surveillance is necessary in these high-risk patients.

Thromboprophylaxis is standard in the care of a patient after hip fracture surgery. Recent studies have suggested significant reductions in the incidence of both proximal DVT and fatal pulmonary embolism when using mechanical or pharmacologic prophylactic measures, but careful monitoring of the elderly patient with hip fracture to watch for bleeding complications is essential. Further studies are required to optimize prophylaxis in this patient population.

DVT After Pelvic Fractures and Major Orthopaedic Trauma

The risk of asymptomatic thrombus formation may be as high as 34% after pelvis-acetabulum fractures. Pelvic thrombi are of particular concern because of a 50% risk of embolization. There may be an unexpectedly high risk of DVT in fractures distal to the hip, but whether routine prophylaxis is needed for all lower extremity fractures is uncertain.

LMWH has been shown to be effective at reducing the rate of proximal DVT after major orthopaedic trauma, but the overall rate of DVT may not change significantly. Mechanical plantar and calf vein compression may provide an excellent alternative to chemical prophylaxis, particularly in patients with increased bleeding risks. However, in a study of trauma patients in an intensive care unit setting and on a surgical ward, foot pumps were applied properly and functioning correctly only 59% of the time.

Spine Surgery

Although routine screening for lower extremity thrombi after major spinal surgery appears unwarranted, it may be appropriate in the presence of spinal cord injury. Mechanical prophylaxis with compression stockings and pneumatic boots may provide adequate anticoagulation for most posterior spinal fusions. The risk of bleeding complications may be elevated in those patients treated with chemoprophylaxis, but chemoprophylaxis may be an effective adjunct for patients with spinal cord injuries and for combined anterior and posterior spinal procedures.

Total Hip and Knee Arthroplasty

The risk of fatal pulmonary embolism without chemical or mechanical prophylaxis is approximately 0.4% after knee and hip arthroplasty. Routine prophylaxis has cut this rate in half. The risk of DVT continues to be between 15% to 25% after THA and 35% to 50% after TKA. The incidence of proximal thrombi, however, has been reduced to between 5% to 10% after THA and slightly lower after TKA.

Diagnosis of DVT

Clinical cues for diagnosing DVT after total joint arthroplasty, such as calf pain, swelling, palpable cords, or a positive Homans' sign, are not sensitive, specific, or reliable. Ascending contrast venography is accurate in diagnosing thrombi in both the proximal and distal veins, and it is less accurate above the inguinal ligament where many of the clinically significant emboli originate. Venography allows identification of nonocclusive thrombi, but is being used less frequently in many centers because it is invasive, painful, may induce anaphylactoid reaction and renal intolerance, and has been reported to precipitate thrombosis.

Ultrasonography is a popular and potentially effective technique for diagnosing DVT. Although accurate for detecting proximal thrombi, ultrasonography is less accurate in detecting small clots, thrombi of the calf, and those proximal to the inguinal ligament. The technique may be inaccurate for detecting fresh thrombi that are commonly soft and only partially compressible. Diagnostic yield may be enhanced by compression of veins that have nonechogenic, fresh clots. The sensitivity of the test is highly technician-dependent. Duplex ultrasonography, a combination of real-time ultrasonography and Doppler studies, creates audiologic and graphic depiction of venous flow that may increase the diagnostic accuracy.

Considering that approximately 50% of emboli that originate from thrombi are not visualized, it is likely that many clinically significant emboli arise from thrombi of the pelvic veins, which are particularly difficult to evaluate using ultrasonographs and standard ascending venography. Magnetic resonance venography (MRV) may emerge as an effective tool for diagnosing pelvic thromboses after total joint arthroplasty and major orthopaedic trauma. In one study, results showed a 39% incidence of pelvic thrombosis after hip arthroplasty, detected by MRV but not observed with either ascending venography or Doppler ultrasound. MRV may be an accurate test, but experience in interpretation and reduced costs will be necessary for this technique to become a common method for surveillance of thrombi.

Diagnosis of Pulmonary Embolism

Signs and symptoms common to pulmonary embolism, such as dyspnea, pleuritic chest pain, tachypnea, and tachycardia are nonspecific. Electrocardiogram may show nonspecific ST segment and T wave changes, but may be normal in up to 23% of patients with large pulmonary emboli. Arterial blood gas analysis may show hypoxemia and/or respiratory alkalosis, but a normal blood gas is not uncommon. The chest radiograph is more useful in excluding other diagnoses that may mimic pulmonary embolism and may aid in the interpretation of ventilation-perfusion scans.

Pulmonary angiogram, although highly accurate, is invasive, costly, and has a major complication rate of approximately 1%, which includes respiratory distress, renal failure, or hematoma requiring transfusion. The sensitivity, specificity, and accuracy of the ventilation-perfusion (V/Q) scan are low. A single V/Q scan may yield a falsely positive "high probability" result in as many as 15% of cases. This drawback is particularly dangerous considering the high rate of local and systemic bleeding that may result from intravenous heparinization. Diagnostic yield of the V/Q scan will be enhanced if used selectively, when clinical suspicion is high. Positive V/Q scans in asymptomatic patients and negative scans in symptomatic patients are both cause for concern and each may have negative impact erroneously on treatment. When a pulmonary embolism is suspected, a V/Q scan should be obtained initially. A "low probability" scan usually does not warrant further investigation unless clinical suspicion remains high.

Otherwise, a duplex ultrasound should be obtained to ensure the absence of a proximal clot that would require heparinization. A "high probability" V/Q scan generally should prompt treatment with intravenous heparin unless doubt still remains, in which case a confirmatory pulmonary angiogram is advisable. Approximately 75% of patients have V/Q scans of "intermediate probability," which often need to be confirmed with pulmonary angiograms.

Spiral CT may become a more routinely used method for detecting pulmonary emboli and has been shown to be more effective than V/Q scans in differentiating between emboli and other pulmonary disease.

Treatment of Established Thrombi

Clots proximal to the popliteal vessels should be treated because of an approximately 50% risk of embolization, but it remains controversial whether distal DVT of the calf should be treated because of conflicting data regarding risk of embolization. Calf thrombi are usually asymptomatic, typically resolve without treatment, have a low risk for embolization, and have little risk of contributing to postthrombotic syndrome. In one study, untreated calf DVT after THA was a precursor to proximal clot propagation in 17% to 23% of patients, but continued oral anticoagulant therapy or serial surveillance for this condition is reasonable. It is generally agreed that risk of embolization depends in part on clot size and location, although the "critical" size has not been established. The distribution of thrombi must be critically evaluated in planning treatment. If heparinization is withheld, close surveillance with serial duplex scans to detect proximal clot propagation may be advisable.

Traditionally, treatment of proximal DVT begins with intravenous heparin to prevent an extension of clots and recurrence of pulmonary embolism. LMWH has also been shown to be effective when using intravenous heparin. The goal is to prolong the aPTT to 2.0 times that of control. However, full heparinization within 5 days of joint replacement was accompanied by major bleeding events in more than one third of patients in one study, particularly if a bolus is given. Warfarin is instituted simultaneously with the heparin therapy and continued for 3 to 6 months; an INR of 2.0 to 3.0 is targeted. In one study, 6 months of warfarin therapy reduced the risk of late recurrence by 50% (9.5% versus 18.1%) compared with the conventional 6-week therapy, with an identical frequency of bleeding complications. Contraindications to the use of extended warfarin therapy include pregnancy, liver insufficiency, noncompliance, severe alcoholism, uncontrolled hypertension, active major hemorrhage, and inadequate follow-up. An inferior vena cava filter is generally reserved for those patients in whom full anticoagulation is absolutely contraindicated or in the event of recurrent pulmonary embolism despite intravenous heparin and a therapeutic aPTT.

Annotated Bibliography

Clagett GP, Anderson FA Jr, Geerts W, et al: Prevention of venous thromboembolism. *Chest* 1998;114(suppl 5):531S-560S.

This recent review article presents a discussion on the prevention of venous thromboembolism.

Colwell CW Jr, Collis DK, Paulson R, et al: Comparison of enoxaparin and warfarin for the prevention of venous thromboembolic disease after total hip arthroplasty: Evaluation during hospitalization and three months after discharge. *J Bone Joint Surg Am* 1999;81:932-940.

Venous thromboembolic disease occurred in less than 4% of 3,011 patients who received either enoxaparin or adjusted-dose warfarin during hospitalization. No thromboembolic prophylaxis was used after discharge, at a mean 7.5 days after surgery. There were no statistically significant differences between the two modalities in the incidence of DVT or mortality related to thromboembolic disease (0.13%). Ten percent of patients who received enoxaparin had bleeding complications, compared with 7.4% of those who received warfarin.

Cross JJ, Kemp PM, Walsh CG, Flower CD, Dixon AK: A randomized trial of spiral CT and ventilation perfusion scintigraphy for the diagnosis of pulmonary embolism. *Clin Radiol* 1998;53:177-182.

Spiral CT was significantly more accurate than V/Q scan for diagnosing pulmonary disorders (90% versus 51%, $P < 0.001$). There was no difference in the detection of pulmonary embolism, the condition was correctly diagnosed with spiral CT in 25% of patients in whom V/Q scans were nondiagnostic.

Dearborn JT, Hu SS, Tribus CB, Bradford DS: Thromboembolic complications after major thoracolumbar spine surgery. *Spine* 1999;24:1471-1476.

Seven cases of symptomatic pulmonary emboli occurred in a series of 318 major spinal procedures with prophylaxis that included thigh-length compression stockings and pneumatic compression leggings. Six percent of symptomatic pulmonary emboli cases occurred after anterior/posterior spinal fusions, whereas only 0.5% occurred after posterior decompression and fusion. The authors caution against relying on duplex ultrasound as a screening tool and question whether mechanical prophylaxis alone is adequate for combined anterior/posterior spinal fusions.

Freedman KB, Brookenthal KR, Fitzgerald RH Jr, Williams S, Lonner JH: A meta-analysis of thromboembolic prophylaxis following elective total hip arthroplasty. *J Bone Joint Surg Am* 2000;82:929-938.

A meta-analysis of all randomized controlled trials of prophylaxis after THA with follow-up bilateral venography found that warfarin and LMWH had the lowest rates of proximal DVT (6.3% and 7.7%, respectively). But there was no significant difference in the rate of fatal pulmonary embolism between warfarin, LMWH, aspirin, low-dose heparin, pneumatic compression, or placebo. LMWH had a significantly higher rate of wound bleeding complications (8.9%).

Ginsberg JS, Turkstra F, Buller HR, MacKinnon B, Magier D, Hirsh J: Postthrombotic syndrome after hip or knee arthroplasty: A cross-sectional study. *Arch Intern Med* 2000;160:669-672.

The incidence of postthrombotic syndrome was not significantly different in patients with either a distal or proximal DVT and those without DVT.

Hooker JA, Lachiewicz PF, Kelley SS: Efficacy of prophylaxis against thromboembolism with intermittent pneumatic compression after primary and revision total hip arthroplasty. *J Bone Joint Surg Am* 1999;81:690-696.

In a prospective study of 502 primary or revision THAs managed intraoperatively and postoperatively with thigh-high elastic compression stockings and thigh-high intermittent pneumatic compression sleeves, there was a 4% incidence of proximal DVT, a 0.6% incidence of symptomatic pulmonary embolism, and no fatalities from pulmonary embolism.

Hull RD, Pineo GF, Francis C, et al: Low-molecular-weight heparin prophylaxis using dalteparin in close proximity to surgery vs warfarin in hip arthroplasty patients: A double-blind, randomized comparison. The North American Fragmin Trial Investigators. *Arch Intern Med* 2000;160:2199-2207.

Dalteparin reduced the risk of proximal DVT to 0.8% compared to 3% with warfarin after total hip replacement. There was no difference in the rate of serious bleeding complications, but wound bleeding was increased when dalteparin was begun preoperatively.

Hull RD, Pineo GF, Francis C, et al: Low-molecular-weight heparin prophylaxis using dalteparin extended out-of-hospital vs in-hospital warfarin/out-of-hospital placebo in hip arthroplasty patients: A double-blind, randomized comparison. North American Fragmin Trial Investigators. *Arch Intern Med* 2000;160:2208-2215.

Extended dalteparin prophylaxis resulted in significantly lower frequencies of DVT compared with in-hospital warfarin therapy (3% compared to 9%).

Lotke PA: The role of aspirin for thromboembolic disease in total joint arthroplasty. *Am J Knee Surg* 1999;12:61-63.

In a consecutive series of 1,370 TKAs treated with 325 mg of aspirin twice daily for 6 weeks, the risk of fatal pulmonary embolism was 0.15%.

Pulmonary Embolism Prevention (PEP) Trial: Prevention of pulmonary embolism and deep vein thrombosis with low dose aspirin. *Lancet* 2000;355:1295-1302.

In this prospective randomized multicenter trial, there were 13,356 hip fracture patients and 4,088 elective total joint arthroplasty patients (50% received aspirin 160 mg daily for 35 days and 50% received placebo). The risk of fatal pulmonary embolism with aspirin therapy was 0.03% in the fracture group and 0.05% in the elective arthroplasty group.

Zahn HR, Skinner JA, Porteous MJ: The preoperative prevalence of deep vein thrombosis in patients with femoral neck fractures and delayed operation. *Injury* 1999;30:605-607.

Thirteen of 21 (62%) patients with femoral neck fractures had venographic evidence of DVT when surgical fixation was delayed more than 48 hours. This finding suggests that patients in whom surgical delay is necessary should be studied for the presence of DVT.

Classic Bibliography

Colwell CW Jr, Spiro TE, Trowbridge AA, et al: Use of enoxaparin, a low-molecular-weight heparin, and unfractionated heparin for the prevention of deep venous thrombosis after elective hip replacement: A clinical trial comparing efficacy and safety. Enoxaparin Clinical Trial Group. *J Bone Joint Surg Am* 1994;76:3-14.

Francis CW, Pellegrini VD Jr, Totterman S, et al: Prevention of deep-vein thrombosis after total hip arthroplasty: Comparison of warfarin and dalteparin. *J Bone Joint Surg Am* 1997;79:1365-1372.

Garino JP, Lotke PA, Kitziger KJ, Steinberg ME: Deep venous thrombosis after total joint arthroplasty: The role of compression ultrasonography and the importance of the experience of the technician. *J Bone Joint Surg Am* 1996;78:1359-1365.

Geerts WH, Code KI, Jay RM, Chen E, Szalai JP: A prospective study of venous thromboembolism after major trauma. *N Engl J Med* 1994;331:1601-1606.

Geerts WH, Jay RM, Code KI, et al: A comparison of low-dose heparin with low-molecular-weight heparin as prophylaxis against venous thromboembolism after major trauma. *N Engl J Med* 1996;335:701-707.

Leclerc JR, Geerts WH, Desjardins L, et al: Prevention of venous thromboembolism after knee arthroplasty: A randomized, double-blind trial comparing enoxaparin with warfarin. *Ann Intern Med* 1996;124:619-626.

Lieberman JR, Geerts WH: Prevention of venous thromboembolism after total hip and knee arthroplasty. *J Bone Joint Surg Am* 1994;76:1239-1250.

Lieberman JR, Wollaeger J, Dorey F, et al: The efficacy of prophylaxis with low-dose warfarin for prevention of plumonary embolism following total hip arthroplasty. *J Bone Joint Surg Am* 1997;79:319-325.

Millenson MM, Bauer KA: Pathogenesis of venous thromboembolism, in Hull R, Pineo GF (eds): *Disorders of Thrombosis*. Philadelphia, PA, WB Saunders, 1996, pp 175-190.

NIH Consensus Development Conference Statement: Prevention of venous thrombosis and pulmonary embolism. Bethesda, MD, U.S. Department of Health and Human Services, Office of Medical Applications of Research, 1986, vol 6, no 2.

Oishi CS, Grady-Benson JC, Otis SM, Colwell CW Jr, Walker RH: The clinical course of distal deep venous thrombosis after total hip and total knee arthroplasty, as determined with duplex ultrasonography. *J Bone Joint Surg Am* 1994;76:1658-1663.

Patterson BM, Marchand R, Ranawat C: Complications of heparin therapy after total joint arthroplasty. *J Bone Joint Surg Am* 1989;63:171-177.

Pellegrini VD Jr, Clement D, Lush-Ehmann C, Keller GS, Evarts CM: Natural history of thromboembolic disease after total hip arthroplasty. *Clin Orthop* 1996;333:27-40.

RD Heparin Arthroplasty Group: RD heparin compared with warfarin for prevention of venous thromboembolic disease following total hip or knee arthroplasty. *J Bone Joint Surg Am* 1994;76:1174-1185.

Robinson KS, Anderson DR, Gross M, et al: Ultrasonographic screening before hospital discharge for deep venous thrombosis after arthroplasty: The postarthroplasty screening study. A randomized controlled trial. *Ann Intern Med* 1997;127:439-445.

Warwick D, Williams MH, Bannister GC: Death and thromboembolic disease after total hip replacement: A series of 1,162 cases with no routine chemical prophylaxis. *J Bone Joint Surg Br* 1995;77:6-10.

Chapter 7

Selected Ethical Issues for Orthopaedic Surgeons

Charles H. Epps, Jr, MD

Introduction

The Hippocratic Oath has remained the cornerstone of medical ethics for more than 2,000 years. Even after several revisions the oath has remained true to its central theme: that the physician's first duty is to the patient. Current practice presents many challenges because there have been profound changes in society, national mores, and laws. Changes in the science and technology of the practice of medicine, the delivery of health care, the style/methods of practice by physicians, in the roles of other health care providers, and in the methods by which physicians are compensated are important factors as well. As a result, ethics for the physician has not escaped change. This chapter will review some of the practice situations orthopaedic surgeons currently face and cite some ethical considerations that may provide guidance for proper behavior.

Conflicts of Interest

Conflict of interest is perhaps the best concept with which to begin a discussion of medical ethics. One key element to answering other potential ethical dilemmas is uncovering any real or potential conflict of interest. Guidelines for conflicts of interest were issued by the Council on Ethical and Judicial Affairs (CEJA) of the American Medical Association (AMA) in 1986 and were revised in 1994. The opinion states, "Under no circumstances may physicians place their own financial interests above the welfare of their patients. The primary objective of the medical profession is to render service to humanity; reward or financial gain is a subordinate consideration. For a physician unnecessarily to hospitalize a patient, prescribe a drug, or conduct diagnostic tests for the physician's financial benefit is unethical. If a conflict develops between the physician's financial interest and the physician's responsibilities to the patient, the conflict must be resolved to the patient's benefit." The American Academy of Orthopaedic Surgeons® (AAOS) has adopted a similar statement on conflicts of interest: "The practice of medicine inherently presents conflicts of interest. Whenever a conflict of interest arises, it must be resolved in the best interest of the patient. The orthopaedic surgeon should exercise all reasonable alternatives to ensure that the most appropriate care is provided to the patient. If the conflict of interest cannot be resolved, the orthopaedic surgeon should notify the patient of his or her intention to withdraw from the relationship." These statements unequivocally establish the physician's primary obligation to the patient. It will also become apparent that conflict of interest is involved as a component of other ethical deviations.

Informed Consent

During the past 50 years, there has been a decided change in the manner in which surgeons and physicians obtain informed consent. In a paternalistic approach, physicians and surgeons told patients what was wrong and what was believed to be the appropriate treatment or procedure. After little or no information or choice, the patient was asked to sign the permit. Since the 1970s, the practice of true informed consent has evolved after several important court decisions defining this concept were handed down. Today, what constitutes informed consent accepts the premise that the patient's right of self-decision can be effectively exercised only if the patient possesses enough information to enable an intelligent choice and then makes that determination. The physician's obligation is to present the medical facts accurately to the patient or to the individual responsible for the patient's care and to make recommendations for management in accordance with good medical practice. Such information should include alternative modes of treatment, the objectives, risks, and possible complications of such treatment, and the complications and consequences of no treatment. Exceptions are permitted under certain circumstances: (1) where the patient is unconscious or otherwise incapable of consenting and harm from failure to treat is imminent; or (2) when risk disclosure poses such a serious psychological threat of detriment to the patient as to be medically contraindicated. The view that the physician may remain silent because divulgence might prompt the patient to forego needed therapy is considered paternalistic and is not acceptable.

Managed Care

The advent of managed care has brought a vastly different system that involves new mechanisms of health care delivery. The principal changes involve different reimbursement systems for providers and compiles referral restrictions and benefits. The managed care organization (MCO) endeavors to prevent unnecessary expenditure and at the same time ensure quality care. These conditions create a natural tension between the MCO and the provider, with the patient often caught in the middle. The AMA and the AAOS have attempted to provide guidelines for the practitioner. To summarize, in the MCO and any other health care delivery mechanism, the patient's interest is still the primary concern of the physician. If during the course of providing services, the orthopaedic surgeon learns that the MCO is limiting services, the surgeon has the ethical obligation to inform the patient of the diagnosis and the treatment options.

From an ethical standpoint, the orthopaedic surgeon can consider costs as one factor in determining appropriate care. In addition, the surgeon is obligated to practice within the scope of his/her personal education, training, and experience. When the relationship of the surgeon and the MCO is terminated, there is an ethical obligation to provide medically necessary care for the enrolled patient until appropriate referrals are arranged. In those instances where the orthopaedic surgeon unilaterally withdraws from participation in the MCO, adequate notice must be given directly to the patient indicating that the treating relationship will cease. Also, there is an ethical obligation for the surgeon to report recognized unethical activities of gatekeepers, specialists, and other professionals to the appropriate peer review authority. Because of the orthopaedic surgeon's special knowledge about the musculoskeletal system, there is an obligation to inform the officials and employees of MCOs, affiliated physicians, patients, and others when concerns regarding the quality of care arise.

Reporting Suspected Abuse or Neglect

Since the problem of child abuse first came to the forefront at least 25 years ago, its incidence has increased. Between 1986 and 1993, the number of abused and neglected children in the United States nearly doubled to 2.81 million. Other estimates place the number of children under the age of 18 years abused annually at 1.4 million. Teenagers are believed to be at twice the risk as children under the age of 3 years. As more has been learned about this problem, data indicate that spousal abuse, elder abuse, and maltreatment of disabled adults have reached alarming proportions.

As a result, the United States Child Abuse Prevention and Treatment Act of 1974 prompted nearly all states to adopt legislation requiring or permitting, without legal penalty, the reporting of elder and other abuse. In some cases, the victim and the suspected offender may plead with the orthopaedic surgeon to keep the matter confidential and not report it for investigation by public authorities. Some children, allegedly injured by their parents, may attempt to protect parents by saying that the injuries were caused by an accident. However, the orthopaedic surgeon has both a legal and an ethical obligation to comply with mandatory reporting statutes and state institutional policies requiring reporting of suspected cases of abuse or neglect.

Second Opinions

Under the conditions of current practice, patients may choose their physicians, request transfer of care, or terminate the patient-physician relationship at their discretion. In some circumstances, the choices may be somewhat limited by membership in a MCO.

Several circumstances may exist in the matter of a consultation or referral. If the consultation is initiated by the physician, it must be with the consent of the patient and may be temporary or permanent. If the aim is to transfer all care from one physician to another, the patient's consent is necessary. The patient may seek additional medical opinions or sever ties with the treating physician and seek care with another physician. When a physician wishes to transfer care to another physician, adequate notice should be given so that the patient can secure alternative care. Second opinions are sometimes required by the patient's insurance company prior to giving authorization to perform a procedure. In most MCOs the patient must comply and usually the choice of the provider to provide the additional opinion is at the discretion of the insurer. In some MCO plans, the patient may elect to give up a degree of free choice by accepting coverage.

In general, the second opinion physician is ethically obligated to return the patient to the treating physician. There is no breach of ethics if the patient chooses to terminate care with the original physician; however, it is not unethical for the second opinion physician to decline accepting responsibility for the patient's care under these circumstances. In most jurisdictions, obtaining copies of medical records or transferring them to another physician is within the patient's rights.

Sexual Harassment and Exploitation

While maintaining the patient's best interest as the primary concern, the orthopaedic surgeon is expected to provide competent and compassionate patient care and exercise appropriate respect for other health care professionals, colleagues, and society as a whole. Conduct that would constitute sexual harassment is unethical. Unwelcome sexual advances toward other members of the health care team caring for the patient may jeopardize patient care.

In the undergraduate and postgraduate environment, sexual harassment is considered to have occurred even if the relationship is consensual. The inherent inequality in the status and power that exists between medical supervisors and trainees produces the potential for sexual exploitation. The same power discrepancy is just as true in the relationship between the physician and patient.

Sexual Misconduct–Physician-Patient Relationship

The physician's primary interest is the welfare of the patient. Within the physician-patient relationship, the physician enjoys considerable knowledge, expertise, and status or power. The patient is vulnerable, both physically and emotionally, and sexual contact by the physician violates the patient's welfare. Therefore, all sexual contact and sexual relationships between physicians and their patients are considered unethical.

Legal penalties may be imposed and in some cases, civil action may be generated for malpractice. Criminal prosecution is pursued either under general sexual assault statutes or under recently enacted, more specific laws. In fact, Florida has a new statute that specifies that consent of the patient cannot be used as a defense by a physician against charges of misconduct.

In a situation when a physician and a patient become genuinely attracted to each other, at a minimum, the physician must terminate the professional relationship with the patient. Further, the physician is advised to consult with a colleague before initiating a relationship with the former patient because in great measure, the ethical propriety of a sexual relationship between a physician and a former patient depends on the nature and context of the former relationship. If the sexual contact occurred as a result of the use or exploitation of trust, knowledge, influence, or emotions derived from the former professional relationship, it is unethical. The AAOS and the AMA's CEJA both believe

that physicians have an obligation to report colleagues to the appropriate authorities when they become aware of alleged sexual misconduct. The one exception occurs when the physician learns of the sexual misconduct while treating the offending physician.

Sports Medicine

Because of training and experience, orthopaedic surgeons are often called upon to provide professional services to athletes. In these instances, as in all others, the patient's welfare is the primary concern. Athletes, especially professional athletes, who may have significant financial pressures to play in spite of injuries, present unique challenges. The pressure may come from the athlete, the coach, or the owner of a professional team. In the case of the scholastic athlete, the pressure may come from the athlete, the coach, or in some cases from the parent. Regardless of the circumstances, the patient athlete is best served when the orthopaedic surgeon remembers that the best interest of the patient is of primary concern.

Recently, the selection of team physicians by professional sports teams has involved questionable practices. Team physicians should be selected based on their level of competence, and it is unethical for them to be selected on the basis of fees paid by physicians or hospitals to the professional team. The care of professional athletes can have a significant impact on a physician's practice because of the publicity associated with these activities. However, these team physicians must be aware of the significant potential for conflict of interest, and keep in mind that their primary obligation is the care of the athlete.

Gender and Race

The physician, administrator, or educator must be conscious of and strive to avoid gender and racial discrimination. While the pool of female physicians has increased dramatically since the late 1970s, the number of underrepresented minorities has increased modestly and now appears headed for a decline. Men and women who do comparable work should be compensated equally. The academic setting should provide extension of tenure decisions through "stop the clock" programs and other mechanisms that facilitate the reentry of physicians who take time away from their careers to have a family. Physician managers in private practice and institutional administrators must consciously avoid policies and actions that would discriminate on the basis of gender and race. In academic institutions, special attention should be given to providing mentors and advisors who will encourage development and advancement of females and minorities.

TABLE 1	Qualifications for the Orthopaedic Surgeon as an Expert Witness

Current valid and unrestricted license to practice medicine in the state(s) in which he/she practices

Diplomate of or have satisfactorily completed the educational requirements of the American Board of Orthopaedic Surgery (or a specialty board recognized by the American Board of Medical Specialties), as well as qualified by clinical experiences, education or demonstrated competence in the subject of the case

Very familiar with the clinical practice, the applicable standard of care of orthopaedic surgery, and the relevant facts and history of the case at the time of the incident

TABLE 2	FTC Qualifications for Physician Advertisements

Table outlines four general rules, developed by the FTC, to determine if the physician advertisements are truthful and not false, deceptive, or misleading

Contain accurate information (explicit false claims or misrepresentation of material fact must be avoided)

No implied false claims or implied misrepresentations of material fact

No omissions of material fact

Material claims and personal representations made must be able to be substantiated

The fact that the number of underrepresented minorities has remained level or declined in recent years suggests that there is a need for a higher level of attention to these considerations.

Also, gender and race may play undesirable roles in medical decision making. Observations have confirmed disparities in health care and these may have resulted from treatment decisions, differences in income and education, sociocultural factors, prejudice, or failures by the medical profession. Physicians should examine their practices to ensure that their decisions are free of social or cultural biases that could be inadvertently affecting clinical judgment and thereby the delivery of medical care.

Orthopaedic Medical Testimony

The orthopaedic surgeon is often called upon to furnish medical evidence because patients may have third-party issues regarding personal injury, professional negligence, or workers' compensation issues. The medical witness must be impartial in any legal proceeding. The witness should prepare thoroughly and the testimony should be honest and truthful. The physician expert witness is entitled to fair monetary compensation for his/her time and expertise, but it is unethical to accept compensation that is contingent on the outcome of the litigation.

Conventional wisdom once held that there was a conspiracy of silence among physicians and that one physician would not testify against another. Such is hardly true today as it has been observed that testimony favorable to an issue can be literally purchased. There have been instances in which physicians have been allowed to testify about matters clearly outside the realm of their training and expertise. The orthopaedic community has accepted certain qualifications that the orthopaedic surgeon as expert witness should meet. These qualifications are outlined in Table 1.

Advertising

The orthopaedic surgeon has an ethical obligation not to use any medium or form of public communication in an untruthful, misleading, or deceptive manner for publicizing self or services. This principle of ethical conduct is founded in state and federal antitrust law and orders of the Federal Trade Commission (FTC). Because the patient is often relatively uninformed and assumes that the physician is revealing complete and accurate information, the patient is at risk for untruthful, misleading, or deceptive advertising and the use of false advertising destroys the trust relationship between physician and patient. Table 2 outlines four general rules, developed by the FTC, to determine if physician advertisements are truthful and not false, deceptive, or misleading.

Fee Unbundling and Other Billing Practices

The economic pressures of managed care, reduced fees, capitation, and the increasing numbers of underinsured and uninsured patients have resulted in significant reductions in physician income. As a result, some surgeons have resorted to fee unbundling and other measures to maintain income. Unbundling occurs when the charge for a specific procedure remains the same, but one or more components of the procedure is separated from the global service package and given a separate, additional fee. Physicians should not provide, prescribe, or seek compensation for services that they know are unnecessary. One area of abuse is in the treatment of personal injury litigants with so-called soft-tissue injuries. In some cases, the patients receive months and months of "physical therapy" including manipulations and injections and repeated diagnostic testing at great expense. Because there is no peer review in these cases, they in a sense can be considered the last frontier of unrestrained medical entrepre-

TABLE 3 | AAOS Recommendations/Guidelines for the Orthopaedic Surgeon Regarding the Acceptance of Gifts

Any gifts accepted by orthopaedic surgeons individually should primarily entail a benefit to patients and should not be of substantial value (eg, $100.00 or more). Accordingly, textbooks, modest meals and other gifts are appropriate if they serve a genuine educational function. Cash payments should not be accepted under any circumstances. For example, the attendance at Journal Clubs sponsored by orthopaedic manufacturers would be acceptable so long as there was no substantial financial benefit to the orthopaedist-in-training involved.

Individual gifts of minimal value are permissible as long as the gifts are related to the orthopaedic surgeon's work. For example, it is acceptable for an orthopaedic surgeon to accept small pharmaceutical samples or pens and notepads from orthopaedic manufacturers.

Subsidies to underwrite the costs of continuing medical education conferences or professional meetings can contribute to the improvement of patient care and, therefore, are acceptable. A subsidy given directly to an orthopaedic surgeon by a company's sales representative creates a relationship which could be perceived to influence the orthopaedic surgeon's use of the company's products and should be avoided. Any corporate subsidy should be received by the conference's sponsor, which in turn can use the money to reduce the conference's registration fee. This is appropriate and acceptable so long as the curriculum of the conference or meeting is determined solely by the organization sponsoring the educational course, not the orthopaedic manufacturer. Orthopaedic surgeons should not accept direct payments from a company to defray the cost of attending an educational conference.

Orthopaedic surgeons should not accept subsidies, directly or indirectly, from orthopaedic manufacturers to pay for or defray the costs of travel, lodging or other personal expenses of attending conferences of meetings, nor should they accept subsidies to compensate for their time. In addition, orthopaedic surgeons should not accept subsidies for hospitality outside of modest meals or social events held as part of a conference or meeting. It is appropriate for faculty at conferences or meetings to accept reasonable honoraria and to accept reimbursement for reasonable travel, lodging and meal expenses. It is also appropriate for consultants who provide genuine services to receive reasonable compensation and to accept reimbursement for reasonable travel, lodging, and meal expenses. Token consulting or advisory arrangements cannot be used to justify compensating orthopaedic surgeons for their time, travel, lodging, or other out-of-pocket expenses.

Scholarships or other special funds to permit orthopaedic surgeons in training to attend carefully selected educational conferences may be permissible as long as the selection of students, residents, or fellows who will receive the funds is made by the orthopaedist-in-training's institution or by the program sponsor.

Orthopaedic surgeons should not accept gifts with strings attached. For example, orthopaedic surgeons should not accept gifts if they are given in relation to a physician's surgical practice. In addition, when companies underwrite medical conferences or lectures other than their own, responsibility for and control over the selection of content, faculty, educational methods and materials should rest with the organizers of the conferences or lectures.

(Reproduced with permission from the American Academy of Orthopaedic Surgeons Committee on Ethics: Guide to the Ethical Practice of Orthopaedic Surgery, ed 3. Rosemont, IL, American Academy of Orthopaedic Surgeons, 1998, pp 38–39.)

neurship or medical exploitation in health care. Unbundling and unnecessary services are practices that are clearly unethical.

Gifts From Industry to Physicians

The matter of the relationship of physicians to the pharmaceutical and manufacturing industries has become the object of increased interest. Gifts from industry to the physician can serve as a marketing tool to promote the interests of industry. For years, pharmaceutical and industrial manufacturing representatives have provided information about their products and small gifts with the intent of promoting product name recognition and goodwill. Initially, these gifts were items such as pens, mugs, and note pads. Over the years, these gifts have become lavish and fre-

quently have involved paid vacations, free travel, expensive meals, and in some instances, actual cash. Studies have documented that even these small gifts clearly influence physician behavior.

Although most orthopaedic surgeons recognize these principles, many violations occur. In some instances, industry is now supporting direct subsidies for travel to Continuing Medical Education (CME) conferences, non-CME conferences, and housing expenses, sometimes even for the physician's family. In these instances, the physicians are clearly accepting something of value and it can be presumed that the manufacturers expect something in return. The manufacturer's incentive in providing expenses is profit-based and is to promote the manufacturer's product. It could be viewed that this practice constitutes a small step toward unrestricted collaboration between industry and the medical profession. Perhaps there are reasons for the breakdown, such as penetration of the market by MCOs, competition among industry representatives, and of course, reduced reimbursement to physicians. Orthopaedic surgeons are particularly susceptible because of the prevalence of technology associated with arthroscopy, total joint replacement, and fracture fixation systems. These circumstances do present serious conflicts of interest issues for the orthopaedic surgeon. At the same time, representatives of industry are using increasingly more aggressive marketing techniques. When Congress developed an interest in these practices and began investigations in the early 1990s, the AMA, through its CEJA, developed guidelines. The current AAOS guidelines regarding physician-industry relationships are outlined in Table 3.

Summary

Although this discussion of ethics for the practicing orthopaedic surgeon is not complete by any means, some of the most relevant concerns have been covered. Ethical codes, opinions, and ethical position statements are aspirations and at the same time, it is hoped that the orthopaedic surgeon will be inspired to a proper pattern of behavior toward patients, medical colleagues, and to society at large. The physician must always observe the law during practice, but there may be circumstances when ethical practice may dictate actions that actually exceed the legal requirements.

Annotated Bibliography

General Reference

American Academy of Orthopaedic Surgeons: *Guide to the Ethical Practice of Orthopaedic Surgery*, ed 3. Rosemont, IL, American Academy of Orthopaedic Surgeons, 1998, pp 1-70.

This is the third edition of this book that was first published in 1991. It provides standards of conduct and the essentials of ethical behavior for orthopaedic surgeons.

American Medical Association Council on Ethical and Judicial Affairs (eds): *Code of Medical Ethics: Current Opinions With Annotations*. Chicago, IL, American Medical Association, 2000.

This is the most comprehensive guide available to contemporary physicians. It has undergone regular revisions and includes the seven basic Principles of Medical Ethics and more than 180 ethical opinions of the AMA's Council on Ethical and Judicial Affairs on a wide spectrum of topics.

Lim EV, Aquino NJ: The orthopaedic surgeon and manufacturing industry relationship: Ethical guidelines. *Clin Orthop* 1999;368:279-286.

This article analyzes and reviews the relationship of orthopaedic surgeons to the orthopaedic implant industry in three areas of the relationship: (1) gifts from industry; (2) financial support of education and research; and (3) the relationship of industry to surgeon innovators.

Rothman DJ: Medical professionalism: Focusing on the real issues. *N Engl J Med* 2000;342:1284-1286.

Economic factors seem to assume primary importance among the factors currently affecting medical practice. This article explores the impact of these factors on professionalism, a concept that places the patient's interest above the physician's interest. Six strategies are suggested to promote and implement professionalism.

Wenger NS, Lieberman JR: An assessment of orthopaedic surgeons's knowledge of medical ethics. *J Bone Joint Surg Am* 1998;80:198-206.

This article describes the results of a survey instrument that evaluated knowledge of ethical issues among orthopaedic surgeons and their ability to handle ethical dilemmas.

Gifts

Pellegrino ED, Relman AS: Professional medical associations: Ethical and practical guidelines. *JAMA* 1999; 282:984-986.

The ethical challenges facing physicians and professional associations are discussed with special emphasis on the mission of associations.

Wazana A: Physicians and the pharmaceutical industry: Is a gift ever just a gift? *JAMA* 2000;283:373-380.

This article examines the extent and attitudes toward the relationship between physicians and the pharmaceutical industry and its representatives and its impact on the knowledge, attitudes, and behavior of physicians.

Managed Care

American Medical Association Council on Ethical and Judicial Affairs (eds): *Reports on Managed Care*. Chicago, IL, American Medical Association, 1998, pp 1-48.

This is a compilation of Council Reports from 1990-1998 concerning a variety of issues involving managed care.

Sullivan WM: What is left of professionalism after managed care? *Hastings Cent Rep* 1999;29:7-13.

This article examines the challenge of the "managed care revolution" which is requiring the medical profession to decide between a professionalism that is concerned with technical understanding and competence or playing a role in determining how to meet the collective health needs of US society.

Reporting Suspected Abuse or Neglect

Eisenstat SA, Bancroft L: Domestic violence. *N Engl J Med* 1999;341:886-893.

This is a review article that explores violence in the health care setting and principles of effective management.

White AA III (ed): Symposium: Issues of minorities in medicine and orthopaedics. *Clin Orthop* 1999;362:2-116.

This symposium emphasizing diversity, presents a spectrum of articles documenting the undergraduate, postgraduate, and practice experience of minorities with emphasis on orthopaedic surgery.

Rothman DJ: Medical professionalism: Focusing on the real issues. *N Engl J Med* 2000;342:1284-1286.

Economic factors seem to assuming prime importance among the factors currently affecting medical practice. This article explores the impact of these factors on professionalism, a concept that places patient's interest above the physician's interest. Six strategies are suggested to promote and implement professionalism.

Classic Bibliography

Emanuel EJ, Dubler NN: Preserving the physician-patient relationship in the era of managed care. *JAMA* 1995;273:323-329.

Epps CH Jr: Secondary gain as a factor in results of treatment, in Epps CH Jr (ed): *Complications in Orthopaedic Surgery*, ed 3. Philadelphia, PA, JB Lippincott, 1994, vol 1, pp 213-225.

Hillman BJ, Olson GT, Griffith PE, et al: Physicians's utilization and charges for outpatient diagnostic imaging in a medicare population. *JAMA* 1992;268:2050-2054.

Jonsen AR (ed): The nobility of medicine, in *The New Medicine and the Old Ethics*. Cambridge, MA, Harvard University Press, 1990, pp 61-79.

Katz J: Informed consent: Ethical and legal issues, in Arras J, Rhoden NK (eds): *Ethical Issues in Modern Medicine* ed 3. Mountain View, CA, Mayfield Publishing, 1989, pp 100-110.

Mitchell JM, Scott E: Physician ownership of physical therapy services: Effects on charges, utilization, profits, and service characteristics. *JAMA* 1992;268:2055-2059.

Pellegrino ED: Rationing health care: The ethics of medical gate keeping. *J Contemporary Health Law Policy* 1986;2:23-45.

Chapter 8

Imaging Beyond Conventional Radiology

Marie-Claude Miron, MD, FRCPC

Guy Grimard, MD, FRCSC

Raymond Lambert, MD, FRCPC, ABNM

Sophie Turpin, MD, FRCPC

Magnetic Resonance Imaging

Articular Cartilage

The accurate evaluation of articular cartilage remains problematic. The use of intra-articular gadolinium solution for evaluation of the cartilage is still controversial.

Two MRI techniques, which rely on alterations of the proteoglycan matrix in early osteoarthritis, have recently been described. First, the use of intra-articular or intravenous injection of gadolinium chelates has been advocated. This technique relies on diffusion of the contrast agent into altered regions of the proteoglycan matrix. Second, sodium MRI uses the attraction of positive sodium ions by the negative proteoglycan macromolecules; an increased sodium concentration in pathologic areas is measured. However, the resolution and signal-to-noise ratio of sodium MRI are low secondary to the low concentration of sodium ions in comparison with protons.

Ultimately, the goal of MRI of the articular cartilage is to detect biochemical abnormalities that precede morphologic changes, thereby assessing the biochemical properties of the cartilage rather than the surface morphology.

Tumors

The first step in the investigation of a suspected bone tumor is to obtain a plain radiograph, which most frequently yields a specific diagnosis. CT is effective in determining cortical destruction and in evaluating the calcified or ossified components of bone or soft-tissue lesions. MRI is the modality of choice for the staging of bone tumors because it detects skip lesions. MRI is also accurate in determining extracompartmental extension and invasion of cartilage such as the epiphysis and the growth plate, relatively common in osteosarcomas (80% detected on MRI compared to 60% suspected on plain films), and through the articular cartilage with involvement of the joint. However, in the latter situation, there may be a lack of specificity with false-positive results secondary to synovial inflammatory response to tumor. Perineoplastic edema is also difficult to distinguish from tumor invasion at MRI.

The use of contrast enhancement techniques to distinguish between benign and malignant tumors is controversial. In order to characterize more accurately the potential malignancy of a tumor, data have been published on quantitative estimation of enhancement as a function of time. Three parameters, the start, pattern, and progression of enhancement, have been studied. The study results are promising for the evaluation of soft-tissue masses with sensitivity and negative predictive value over 90% combining the three parameters. The results are less accurate for the evaluation of bone tumors, especially when attempting to distinguish low-grade malignant tumors from their benign counterparts.

Conventional MRI provides limited information about differentiating tumor necrosis from viable tumor. Clinically available contrast agents (gadolinium chelates) are of small molecular size and diffuse freely into the interstitial space, either into the necrotic tissue or the viable tumor. In recent studies on osteogenic sarcoma, a diffusion-weighted MRI technique was used to assess tumor necrosis. In tumor necrosis, there is increased membrane permeability and ultimately a breakdown of the cell membrane and the intracellular structures. Diffusion-weighted MRI is based on the random motion of the molecules that causes a phase dispersion of the spins, resulting in signal loss, and is the only noninvasive technique that measures differences between necrotic and viable tumor.

Pediatric Conditions

Gadolinium-enhanced MRI has shown the changing pattern of vascularization of the epiphysis and physis. When the ossification center is not yet visible in the epiphysis, the vascular canals are parallel, perpendicular to the plane of the epiphysis. With maturation they converge toward the center. In the evaluation of epiphyseal and transphyseal fractures, the weakest link is the zone of provisional calcification between bone and physeal cartilage. MRI not only allows visualization of the fracture line, but also reveals the associated vascular injury that may predispose to growth disturbances. Longitudinal fractures that cross the physis in the long axis of the bone are associated with the formation of a bony bridge in 75% of cases, whereas only 25% of patients develop a bony bridge when the fracture line is transverse, running along the physis.

On conventional MRI, bone in the early phases of Legg-Calvé-Perthes disease (LCPD) may not show signal abnormalities because the fatty marrow is mummified and as a result may present a normal fatty signal. The use of dynamic gadolinium-enhanced subtraction MRI has been successful in the diagnosis of early idiopathic necrosis of the femoral head, and visualization of early reperfusion. A recent study has shown reperfusion patterns in LCPD that appear to be related to prognosis. Sparing of the lateral pillar (or lateral column) of the femoral head by early reperfusion predicts a good prognosis. The necrosis and collapse of the lateral pillar result in deformity of the femoral head and insufficient acetabular coverage associated with poor prognosis. On gadolinium-enhanced subtraction MRI, reperfusion is characterized by an abnormally increased and persistent enhancement of the involved area compared with normal marrow (Fig. 1). The results are comparable to those with bone scintigraphy, but spatial resolution is better. Transphyseal reperfusion, occurring by neovascularization through the physis, is known to be a strong predictor of growth deformity and also is best seen on MRI. It is associated with a slow rate of reperfusion and a poor prognosis secondary to an early physeal closure.

Recently, gadolinium-enhanced MRI studies have also been performed to determine vascular abnormalities of the femoral head in pediatric patients treated with spica casting for reduction of dysplastic hips. A recent MRI study has shown that there is no vascular defect of the femoral head with hip abduction of less than 50°.

Computed Tomography

Volume-rendering spiral CT represents a significant advance in trauma imaging and patient management with changes in treatment decisions in up to 30% of pelvic fractures when compared with more conventional imaging. In anatomically complex areas such as ribs, pelvis, shoulder, and spine, a three-dimensional (3-D) reconstruction is especially valuable.

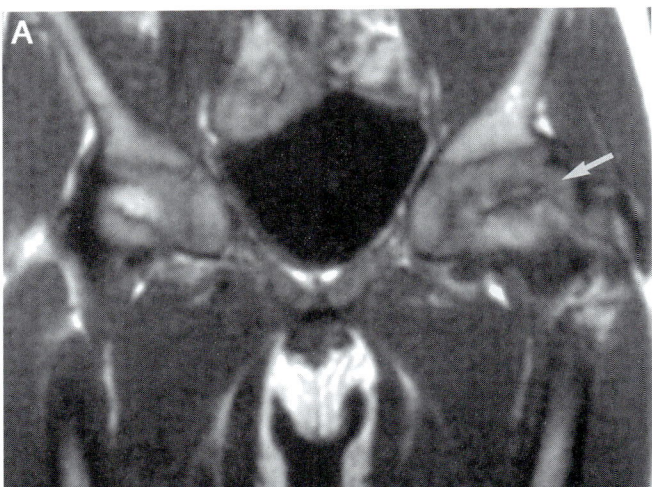

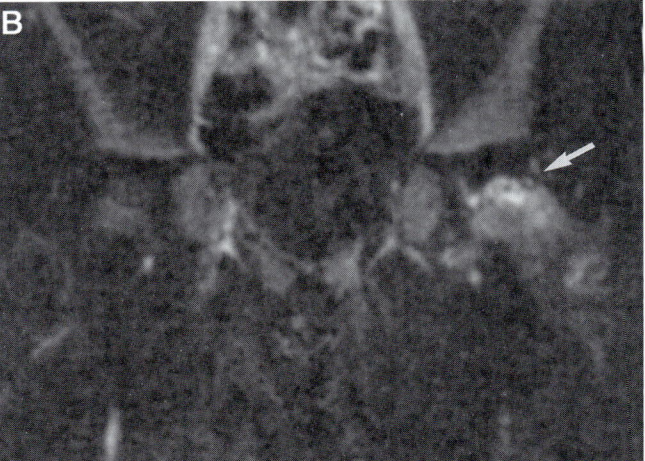

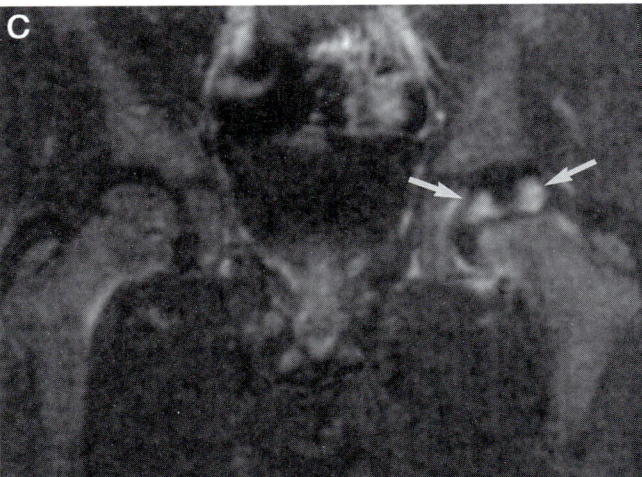

Figure 1 LCPD of the left femoral head. Evaluation of the proximal femur vascularization using dynamic gadolinium-enhanced subtraction MRI. **A,** A coronal precontrast image showing a normal right hip and abnormal signal of the left proximal femur (*arrow*). **B,** A 1-min gadolinium-enhanced subtracted image showing transphyseal reperfusion of the left proximal femur (*arrow*). **C,** A 2-min gadolinium-enhanced subtracted image showing reperfusion of the lateral and medial pillars of the left femoral head demonstrated as an abnormally increased and persistent enhancement of the revascularized areas (*arrows*) compared with normal marrow. (*Courtesy of Sebag et al, Hôpital Robert Debré, Paris, France.*)

The use of kinematic CT has been successful in the study of joint movements, especially for the diagnosis of tracking abnormalities of the patella.

MRI is the noninvasive modality of choice for meniscal imaging. Arthrographic CT (arthro-CT) with spiral CT also can be used for meniscal imaging secondary to recent technical improvements. However, the complex curvilinear morphology of the menisci remains difficult to assess by conventional arthro-CT. Recent studies have used dental CT software to optimize the evaluation of menisci by arthro-CT because the dental arches present the same curvilinear form as the menisci. This new technique offers high image quality with very fine details of meniscal and cartilage anatomy. This new technique demonstrated superficial cartilaginous lesions of the tibiofemoral cartilage not detected at conventional arthrography.

Ultrasonography

High-frequency transducers with increased spatial resolution, extended field-of-view technology offering an overview of regions up to 60 cm, 3-D ultrasonography and increased sensitivity of Doppler ultrasonography are the major technical improvements that have occurred in the past few years. Ultrasonography is particularly useful in the investigation of soft-tissue lesions.

There are significant advantages to this noninvasive, inexpensive technology. It produces dynamic images of soft tissues and joints, is unaffected by metal, and allows greater spatial resolution than MRI performed without surface coils.

Infection

Ultrasonography is useful in the early detection of osteomyelitis: the first ultrasonographic sign is deep soft-tissue edema followed by fluid collection adjacent to the infected bone. The diagnosis of osteomyelitis and septic arthritis may be difficult in neonates. Bone scan (technetium Tc 99m) sensitivity (reported to be 90% to 95% in osteomyelitis) decreases to 85% in neonates presenting with streptococcal infection (which can lead to bone lysis). Technetium Tc 99m is more sensitive to blastic reaction; the radionuclide uptake is less marked with bone lysis and a lesion needs to be at least 1.5 cm to be detected. Neonates and young children may present with superacute osteomyelitis with rapid formation of bone abscess. Therefore, a decrease in radionuclide uptake (cold spot) in these ischemic areas occurs, leading to misdiagnosis. Ultrasonography is therefore an important imaging modality for the early diagnosis of suspected osteomyelitis and septic arthritis.

Ultrasonography was used in a study of a cohort of neonates with osteomyelitis. Besides the soft-tissue lesions, there were changes in epiphyseal and metaphyseal echogenicity, which may lead to altered development of these structures and secondary growth disturbances. Intra-articular scarring was seen in the early stages of the disease and at 6 to 8 months after the onset of infection.

Trauma

In pediatrics, ultrasonography is particularly useful in the evaluation of the unossified epiphysis and is an easy and inexpensive method of locating displaced unossified fragments after trauma. Hemarthrosis, early callus, and displacement of the unossified epiphysis are readily seen.

Clubfoot

Ultrasonography has been used for the initial and follow-up evaluation of clubfoot. Evaluation of the navicular and of the relationship between the talus and the navicular is essential in order to understand this pathology. Because the navicular does not ossify before the patient reaches age 3 to 4 years, conventional radiographs are not accurate in evaluating the talonavicular relationship. An ultrasonographic technique recently has been described that outlines the talonavicular joint; medial subluxation or dislocation of the navicular described in clubfoot is well assessed using an ultrasonographic medial approach of the affected foot (Fig. 2). In addition, the equinus deformity of clubfoot has been studied using an ultrasonographic posterior approach. The parallelism of the talus and the calcaneus found in clubfoot is also well addressed with ultrasonography.

Hip

Hip ultrasonography has become the primary tool of investigation for developmental dysplasia of the hip (DDH). In a retrospective study of patients requiring surgical reduction for DDH, there was a significant decrease in osteonecrosis when the ossification center of the femoral head was present preoperatively at hip ultrasonography or on conventional radiographs, presumably secondary to the improved collateral circulation in older patients that replaces the end-vessel pattern found at birth.

Color and power Doppler ultrasonography have been used to map the vascularization of the femoral head in newborns and young infants. In patients treated for DDH, there is a correlation between increased hip abduction and reduction of femoral head blood flow; individual variations of the vascularization affect the patients' susceptibility to develop osteonecrosis when abduction is applied. When done periop-

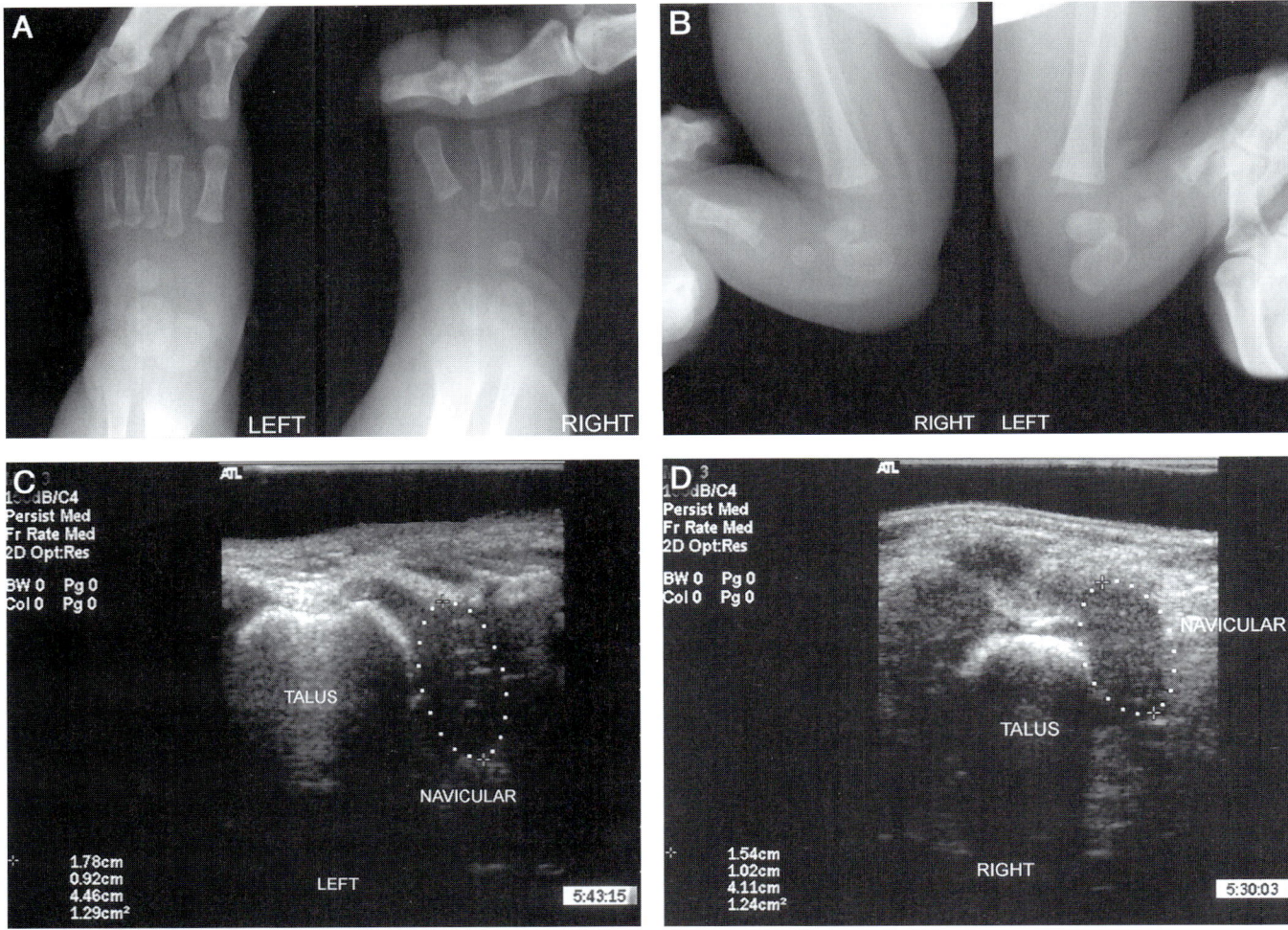

Figure 2 Radiographs taken from a 2-month-old patient with a right clubfoot. The left foot is normal. **A,** AP views of the feet. A decreased talocalcaneal angle and mild adduction of the forefoot are seen on the right side. **B,** Lateral views of the feet. The right foot shows rocker-bottom deformity, a decreased talocalcaneal angle, and an equinus deformity (decreased tibiocalcaneal angle). **C,** Medial ultrasonographic view of the left foot. Normal relationship between the talus and the navicular. The navicular is cartilaginous; the ossification center of the talus is present. **D,** Medial ultrasonographic view of the right foot. Medial subluxation of the navicular. Dysplastic and immature appearance of the talus compared with the normal opposite side.

eratively, Doppler ultrasonography of the hips defines the safe limits of hip abduction that permit adequate perfusion of the femoral heads.

Tumors

Gray-scale and Doppler ultrasonography are being used to characterize soft-tissue tumors and soft-tissue extension of bone tumors. On gray-scale imaging, malignant tumors tend to have irregular margins, heterogeneous echotexture, distortion of original tissue, and invasion rather than displacement of the adjacent structures. Doppler ultrasonography may add specificity in evaluating the neovascularity of a lesion. When studied with pulsed Doppler, the neovascularity of the lesion shows high systolic Doppler shifts, which represents high velocity flow, and high diastolic flow representing low impedance

flow because tumor vessels lack a normal muscularis. When studying the feeding arteries of the tumor, decreased vascular resistance of the affected limb is a criterion of metabolically active tumor.

The monitoring of the vascularity of a lesion and of the tumor-bearing limb may be helpful in the assessment of the effects of chemotherapy. Persistent or increased intratumoral blood flow are defined as poor response to therapy as when the resistive index of the feeding arteries of the affected limb remains low. However, other processes such as healing fracture or inflammation may affect blood flow.

Innovative Perspectives in Conventional Radiology

In order to decrease the radiation dose to the patient, a new imaging device has been designed to provide radiologic images of good quality. The originality of the device is its detector, a multiwire chamber. The device is based on the detection of x-rays in a gas (xenon and CO_2), conversion into electrons, and subsequent amplification. The major advantage of the detector is its great sensitivity to individual X photons, thus making it sensitive to low-dose exposures. Studies of a cohort of patients with scoliosis comparing conventional radiographs of the spine and pelvis and the new Charpak technique have shown similar diagnostic accuracy, with a substantial reduction in radiation dose. The mean ratio of the radiation dose between the two techniques is 13.1 for the spine x-rays and 18.8 for the pelvis x-rays.

A new system with the same features of low dosimetry with high resolution and fast acquisition time is currently under development. With this new system, a two-headed instrument, two perpendicular radiographs are taken simultaneously and then reconstructed with stereoradiographic algorithms. This new system provides images similar to those produced by 3-D CT using surface shaded rendering algorithm with very high morphometric precision. This system may in the future become an alternative to high radiation dose 3-D CT scanning in the evaluation of vertebral contours, especially in the evaluation of scoliotic patients.

Fluoroscopy plays a major role for real-time intraoperative localization of patient anatomy and positioning of surgical instruments. The greatest disadvantage of fluoroscopy is occupational radiation exposure, especially to the surgeon's hands. Spine surgeons are exposed to very high levels of radiation exposure: 10 to 12 times more than other musculoskeletal surgeons. The maximum level (cumulative total) of radiation exposure acceptable for the hands is 50 rem. This dose could be easily exceeded after as few as 120 spine surgeries if fluoroscopy is used on an average of 4 to 5 minutes per case. In a study in which 96 pedicle screws were placed in cadavers, it was noted that the dose rate to the torso is greater when the surgeon is placed on the same side as the x-ray source because of the scatter radiation (53.3 mrem/min versus 2.2 mrem/min when the surgeon is on the opposite side of the x-ray source). The results are similar for the radiation dose to the hands with an average of 58.2 mrem/min. The hand exposure doubled with surgery of cadavers weighing more than 150 lb.

Another disadvantage of fluoroscopy is that it provides one planar view at a time. Virtual fluoroscopy, by combining standard fluoroscopy with computer-aided surgical technology, counteracts the disadvantages of classic fluoroscopy. Virtual fluoroscopy allows acquired fluoroscopic images to be used for real-time surgical localization and instrument tracking. There is excellent correlation between the virtual fluoroscopic images and live fluoroscopy; mean probe tip error is 0.97 mm and mean trajectory angle difference is 2.7°. With this technique, the radiation exposure to the patient and the surgeon is significantly decreased.

Nuclear Medicine

New gamma cameras with higher resolution and capabilities of tomographic acquisition (single-photon emission CT) and new pharmaceuticals have led to new types of studies. Moreover, the recent clinical use of positron emission tomography (PET) has opened a new field of investigation with new metabolic tracers that produce high-resolution images and high diagnostic accuracy. PET scanning allows investigation in oncology, infection, and metabolic disease.

Bone and gallium scans have been used extensively for the detection of musculoskeletal infections. More recently, a labeled white blood cell (WBC) scan (with either indium In 111 or technetium Tc 99m) has become the method of choice for osteomyelitis diagnosis because it is highly sensitive and specific.

The multiphase bone scan (MBS) (flow phase, immediate static images, delayed phase images) is used to establish the diagnosis and differentiate osteomyelitis from other pathologies. On MBS, osteomyelitis demonstrates a pattern of increased regional perfusion during the flow and immediate phases, and a focal increased uptake on delayed phase. Soft-tissue infections cause a regional increased perfusion with no corresponding increased focal uptake on delayed images. In patients with osteomyelitis, combined MBS and gallium scan are more accurate than either scan alone. A labeled WBC scan (indium In 111 or technetium Tc 99m hexamethylpropyleneamine oxime [HMPAO]) combined with MBS are the most accurate studies for the diagnosis of bone infection. Studies have shown good diagnostic correlation between the two WBC labeled studies. Labeled WBC rarely accumulate at the site of noninfectious causes of bony remodeling; as a result, sensitivity and specificity is reportedly about 90% for the diagnosis of osteomyelitis. However, the use of labeled WBC scan is not recommended in the investigation of vertebral osteomyelitis because the scan may be normal or show reduced uptakes. The mechanism of gallium citrate Ga 67 uptake in inflammation is not completely understood. It is believed that the compound extravagates and binds to lactoferrin secreted by leukocytes and/or to the siderophores produced by bacteria in the infection site. New ways to detect inflammation and infection are currently under evaluation (polyclonal immunoglobulin [IgG], nanocolloids, avidin/biotin, streptavidin/biotin, polyethylene glycol-liposomes, and Tc 99m-ciprofloxacin).

PET using fluorine-18 fluorodeoxyglucose (18FDG-PET) has recently been reported to be useful for the investigation of osteomyelitis. 18FDG is an analog of glucose; it accumulates rapidly in infection because of the local increased glucose metabolism of activated inflammatory cells. In fractures and pseudarthroses, the FDG uptake is very low. 18FDG-PET can differentiate osteomyelitis from soft-tissue infection surrounding the bone because the 18FDG-PET has a very high resolution of a few millimeters. Unlike CT and MRI, metal implants do not affect imaging with 18FDG-PET. Recent reports in the literature have shown sensitivity for detecting bone infection (acute or chronic) greater than 95% and specificity between 70% to 90%. 18FDG-PET may also be used for treatment monitoring. Because the biodistribution is greatly influenced by glycemia, patients need to fast for at least 4 hours (diabetic patients must have tight control of their glycemia).

Annotated Bibliography

Magnetic Resonance Imaging

Baur A, Stäbler A, Brüning R, et al: Diffusion-weighted MR imaging of bone marrow: Differentiation of benign versus pathologic compression fractures. *Radiology* 1998;207:349-356.

Diffusion-weighted MRI was compared with conventional MRI in the evaluation of 30 patients with 39 vertebral compression fractures that were either benign or pathologic. Diffusion-weighted MRI of the bone marrow provided distinctive information to differentiate benign from pathologic fractures.

Jaramillo D, Villegas-Medina O, Laor T, Shapiro F, Millis MB: Gadolinium-enhanced MR imaging of pediatric patients after reduction of dysplastic hips: Assessment of femoral head position, factors impeding reduction, and femoral head ischemia. *AJR Am J Roentgenol* 1998;170:1633-1637.

In order to detect early osteonecrosis of the femoral head, an iatrogenic complication of dysplastic hip reduction, the authors evaluated the abnormalities of enhancement with MRI when abduction is applied to reduce dislocated hips. No abnormality has been described with abduction of less than 50°.

Sebag GH: Disorders of the hip. *Magn Reson Imaging Clin N Am* 1998;6:627-641.

Sebag G, Lamer S, Belarbi N, Hassan M: Advances in imaging of Legg-Calvé-Perthes disease, in Fonseca-Santos J, Aragao-Machado M, Santos C (eds): *Paediatric Radiology: The State of the Art in 2000*. Lisbon, Portugal, Springer, 2000, pp 61-64.

These two articles describe the results of the authors' work on MRI evaluation of LCPD and their innovative technique of investigation using dynamic gadolinium-enhanced subtraction for early diagnosis of LCPD and reperfusion pattern.

van der Woude HJ, Verstraete KL, Hogendoorn PC, Taminiau AH, Hermans J, Bloem JL: Musculoskeletal tumors: Does fast dynamic contrast-enhanced subtraction MR imaging contribute to the characterization? *Radiology* 1998;208:821-828.

The authors have performed dynamic contrast-enhanced subtraction MRI studies on 175 patients presenting with a musculoskeletal mass and have evaluated as a function of time the signal intensity of the tumors in order to characterize their malignant potential. This technique has proved to be useful to differentiate malignant from benign soft-tissue masses.

Computed Tomography

Coulier B: Use of dental CT software programs (Dentascan) for optimal arthroscopic CT of knee menisci. *JBR-BTR* 2000;83:303-308.

This new technique of imaging menisci by arthro-CT using dental CT software is an alternative to MRI of the menisci.

Pretorius ES, Fishman EK: Spiral CT and three-dimensional CT of musculoskeletal pathology: Emergency room applications. *Radiol Clin North Am* 1999; 37:953-974.

This article reviews the 3-D algorithms of reconstruction and the difference between volume rendering and surface shaded rendering; volume rendering is their preferred algorithm. Clinical applications of spiral CT and 3-D CT in the evaluation of musculoskeletal pathologies are also presented.

Innovative Perspectives in Conventional Radiology

Kalifa G, Charpak G, Maccia C, et al: Evaluation of a new low-dose digital x-ray device; First dosimetric and clinical results in children. *Pediatr Radiol* 1998;28:557-561.

Mitton D, Landry C, Veron S, Skalli W, Lavaste F, DeGuise JA: 3D reconstruction method from biplanar radiography using non-stereo corresponding points and elastic deformable meshes. *Med Biol Eng Comput* 2000;38:133-139.

These two articles review the innovative technique based on the work of Georges Charpak, winner of the Nobel Prize for Physics in 1992. This original technology significantly decreases the radiation dose to the patient as found in a study conducted on patients with scoliosis.

Nuclear Medicine

Elgazzar AH, Abdel-Dayem HM: Imaging skeletal infections: Evolving considerations, in Freeman LM (ed): *Nuclear Medicine Annual: 1999*. Philadelphia, PA, Lippincott-Raven, 1999, pp 157-191.

The role of nuclear medicine in the investigation of skeletal infection is reviewed. Classification and staging of osteomyelitis is well explained.

Kalicke T, Schmitz A, Risse JH, et al: Fluorine-18 fluorodeoxyglucose PET in infectious bone diseases: Results of histologically confirmed cases. *Eur J Nucl Med* 2000;27:524-528.

The histology of bone tissue in the context of bone infection is studied.

Stumpe KD, Dazzi H, Schaffner A, von Schulthess GK: Infection imaging using whole-body FDG-PET. *Eur J Nucl Med* 2000;27:822-832.

The authors have demonstrated that FDG-PET is a very sensitive tool in the investigation of infection (>95%).

Classic Bibliography

Bearcroft PW, Berman LH, Robinson AH, Butler GJ: Vascularity of the neonatal femoral head: In vivo demonstration with power Doppler US. *Radiology* 1996; 200:209-211.

Jaramillo D, Hoffer FA: Cartilaginous epiphysis and growth plate: Normal and abnormal MR imaging findings. *AJR Am J Roentgenol* 1992;158:1105-1110.

Midel A, Bieganski T, Bik K: Abstract: Neonatal septic arthritis and osteomyelitis: Value of ultrasound and conventional radiography. *34th Annual Congress European Society of Pediatric Radiology*. Lugano, Switzerland, European Society of Pediatric Radiology, 1997, p 53.

Sebag G, Ducou Le Pointe H, Klein I, et al: Dynamic gadolinium-enhanced subtraction MR imaging: A simple technique for the early diagnosis of Legg-Calvé-Perthes disease: Preliminary results. *Pediatr Radiol* 1997;27:216-220.

Treguier C, Darnault P, Chapuis M, Rambeau M, Bompais B, Bracq H: Abstract: Ultrasound evaluation of joint deformities in newborns with clubfoot. *34th Annual Congress European Society of Pediatric Radiology*. Lugano, Switzerland, European Society of Pediatric Radiology, 1997, p 63.

Chapter 9

Clinical Epidemiology

Charles T. Mehlman, DO, MPH

Measurement and Analysis

Epidemiologists measure and analyze data relative to disease and other health-related conditions. Disease frequency is most commonly discussed in terms of incidence and prevalence. The incidence (more precisely referred to as cumulative incidence) of a disease is the number of new cases identified during a specific period of time (follow-up), whereas prevalence is the total number of existing cases of a disease at one point in time. The two measures give two different types of information. Incidence indicates the rate at which new disease is developing. Prevalence reveals the total burden of disease for a given population and is intimately related to duration of the disease. Incidence may also be expressed in terms of the population's time spent at risk, and this is usually expressed in terms of person-years. An example is estimation of the risk of an automobile accident based upon time spent driving (in person-miles).

The key characteristics of a good instrument (such as a questionnaire, fracture classification system, or functional rating scale) are its reliability, validity, and responsiveness to change. Reliability assesses the ability of the instrument to reproducibly demonstrate the same result when used repeatedly under identical conditions. Validity relates to the instrument's ability to measure what it is intended to measure. One way of assessing an instrument's validity is by seeing how well it correlates with an existing gold standard. The level of agreement of the two instruments is then assessed using a correlation coefficient. The characteristic known as responsiveness to change measures an instrument's ability to detect clinically meaningful differences between subjects. What should be avoided are problematic ceiling or floor effects where all subjects score exceedingly high or low when the instrument is administered. An extreme example of a ceiling effect would be using a cerebral palsy functional assessment tool to measure physical performance of collegiate athletes.

Types of Studies

The core principles of information sharing found in epidemiology are dependent on useful information being generated through formal study. There are two broad categories of epidemiologic studies: interventional (also called experimental) and observational. In interventional studies the investigator actively intervenes to cause the subjects being studied to be exposed to a certain risk factor or treatment. The effect of this exposure (the outcome) is then analyzed and often compared with a control group. In observational studies the investigator does not intervene with respect to what happens to the study population, but does make detailed observations concerning exposures and outcomes. Because of logistic reasons, the period of follow-up is often shorter for interventional studies than observational studies. Interventional studies offer the highest level of scientific evidence for questions that lend themselves to the vigorous requirements of this study approach. Observational studies present fewer barriers but are more susceptible to design concerns that increase the likelihood of bias.

Epidemiologic studies may also be subdivided based on their structure. A randomized clinical trial is designed to provide information about how a particular treatment performs under ideal controlled circumstances. A group of patients with defined characteristics are admitted to the study and randomly divided in an effort to balance both known and unknown differences between the groups. A doctor or group of doctors with special expertise and/or training deliver the treatment in question to one group while the other group either receives placebo, no treatment, or standard treatment. Information is then collected as to the efficacy of the treatment in question. Randomized clinical trials are sometimes referred to as efficacy trials.

A cohort study is one in which a group of patients is followed and analyzed over a period of time regarding an outcome of interest. At times there may actually be a prospective nonrandomized study of two or more cohorts, and thus cohort studies may be interventional in nature. Orthopaedic cohort studies commonly involve one relatively large group of patients and are colloquially described as case series. Some cohort studies are purely descriptive, such as survival rates following treatment for osteosarcoma. Other cohorts may have an identifiable group of patients within it that were treated in a somewhat different fashion or were exposed to a different risk factor than the rest of the group. Such a group may serve as an internal control group for the study. An external control group may also be used and may consist of controls from a previous similar study, or it may be a second cohort of patients treated for the same problem via a different method than that of the first group of patients. This latter scenario may be designated as a double cohort study. The comparability of one cohort to another has major implications when it comes to the validity of control groups and generalizability to other populations. Because cohort studies frequently produce information about the incidence of disease, they are often referred to as incidence studies.

A case-control study is one in which all of its subjects are specifically chosen based on whether they have (cases) or do not have (controls) the disease or outcome of interest. By their very nature, case-control studies are retrospective in that they always look back to see how risk factors may differ between the two groups. The initial studies linking smoking and lung cancer, aspirin and Reye's syndrome, and asbestos and mesothelioma were all case-control studies. Such studies provide an estimate of the odds of developing a disease or outcome based on the analyzed risk factor or factors. An excellent example of an orthopaedic case-control study is that on passive smoking and Legg-Calvé-Perthes (LCP) disease. Ninety children with LCP (cases) were compared with 183 children without LCP (controls) regarding exposure to passive smoke. The odds were greater than five times higher for children with LCP being exposed to passive smoke than those without LCP. Case-control studies are considered to be the most efficient way to study very rare diseases as well as those that require long periods of follow-up. This efficiency of case-control studies does come at the price of heightened susceptibility to bias. Particular attention must be paid to case-control study design in order to minimize factors such as prevalence bias, information bias, selection bias, and misclassification bias.

Cross-sectional studies are structured so as to provide a broad view of the disease or condition that is being studied. The key aspect of a cross-sectional study is that it looks at a representative sample or an entire population of interest at one particular point in time. Because of this cross-sectional studies are sometimes referred to as survey studies or prevalence studies. Many important orthopaedic studies have been of a cross-sectional nature. These include classic studies on rotational alignment of the lower extremities in children as well as population-based studies on flatfeet. Cross-sectional studies offer little or no information concerning the cause and effect relationship of identified risk factors. The generalizability of a cross-sectional study may also be questioned if data were collected from subjects that are not representative of the larger true population.

Much emphasis has been placed on whether a study is prospective or retrospective in nature. An incorrect assumption is that the word prospective is synonymous with well planned and that any retrospective study is always some lesser species. This is clearly not the case. Prospective means that a research question was posed, a study protocol developed, and then data collected aimed at answering the research question all before the outcome of interest has occurred. Retrospective means that these same things all occurred after the appearance of the outcome of interest. All that is prospective is not profound, and all that is retrospective is not retarded. The merits of a study have much more to do with basic study design issues regarding patient selection, information collection, and methods for controlling bias, etc, rather than simply whether the study was prospective or retrospective.

One of the most common situations leading to confusion is when an author tries to identify a cohort study as a "prospective study" because the patients were seen and the information collected in a prospective fashion. This does little more than describe the mechanics of patient care whereby one sees patients, treats them, and records information in the patient's chart. A better definition of a prospective cohort study is one in which the relevant exposure (risk factor) may or may not have occurred at the time the study protocol is instituted and the outcome of interest certainly has not yet occurred. A retrospective cohort study is one in which all relevant events (exposures and outcomes) have already occurred by the time the study is initiated.

Threats to Validity

Validity may be considered to be the extent to which a study truly assesses what it proposes to assess. With respect to studies and study design, validity is discussed in terms of internal validity and external validity. Internal validity relates to how well a study answers the question it proposed to answer, whereas external validity relates to how well the question answered by the study applies to venues outside the study environment. Internal validity of a study may be viewed as a battle against confounding, bias, and chance. External validity addresses how applicable or generalizable a study's findings are to other patient populations.

The desire for a perfect study and the quest for useful information sometimes are conflicting goals. It is appropriate in most circumstances to focus on how valid a study is rather than how imperfect it is. A randomized clinical trial provides rather specific information about how the treatment in question works by minimizing the deleterious effects of bias and confounding and as such they have a high degree of internal validity. However, external validity may be compromised in randomized clinical trials because of their precisely defined patient populations. In other words, they may not be generalizable to a larger, more heterogenous patient populations.

Observational studies may offer a greater degree of generalizability than randomized clinical trials. Their ability to evaluate how effective specific treatments or interventions are in the "real world" has earned them the name "effectiveness studies". Observational studies are typically much less expensive than comparable interventional studies. The tradeoff is that observational studies may suffer from significant internal validity concerns. Although well controlled for in most randomized clinical trials, many significant concerns about bias exist for the typical observational study. If such study bias exists, it may prove to be detrimental to the study's validation. There are several different strategies aimed at overcoming such threats to internal validity in observational studies. Such strategies may be referred to as risk adjustment or as "controlling for other variables". One approach is to explicitly discuss known confounders and deal with them via stratified analysis, which is best when there are a small number of confounders. Multivariate analysis such as regression analysis may be required when there are multiple confounders. Linear regression is used when the outcome variable is continuous in nature, and logistic regression is appropriate when the outcome variable is discrete, such as success/failure, present/absent, etc. Logistic regression is the most commonly used multivariate technique in epidemiology to control for known confounders. None of these techniques can address unknown confounders.

TABLE 1 | Major Types of Bias

Selection Bias (BEND)	Information Bias (PRISM)
Berkson's	Prevalence
Exposure	Recall
Natural	Interviewer
Disease	Skewed follow-up
	Misclassification

Bias

Bias is any imperfection or systematic tendency that leads researchers to draw false conclusions from their study data. Clinical epidemiology studies may be influenced by two broad categories of bias: selection bias and information bias (also called observation bias). There are four types of selection bias and five types of information bias, identified by the acronyms BEND and PRISM, respectively, as outlined in Table 1 and discussed in the subsequent paragraphs; many other types of bias exist beyond those discussed here.

Selection bias is very dangerous because it strikes at the heart of any study: its subjects. Specifically, selection bias results in a study that attempts to compare noncomparable groups. Selection bias may take any of four major forms. The first of these is called Berkson's bias, which is when control subjects innocently chosen by researchers from certain settings (hospital inpatients for instance) may be significantly different from other study subjects. The second major type is exposure selection bias whereby subjects with a particular exposure history (or risk factor) are inappropriately included in a research study. Both types of bias are common concerns in case-control studies. The third type will be referred to here as natural selection bias. In the same way that Darwin's theory of natural selection teaches that the strong who survive are clearly different from the weak who die, natural selection bias teaches that those who volunteer for study participation are different from those who do not (that is, the general population). With disease selection bias, inappropriate inclusion of study subjects relative to their disease status (outcome status) may lead to significant bias concerns in cohort studies. An example of this would be the intellectually dishonest practice of including only patients with good outcomes in a study supporting a particular surgical procedure. Each of these different types of selection bias alone or in concert may be considered detrimental to a study's validity.

Information bias involves nonuniform data acquisition among study groups and may be grouped into five major forms. Prevalence bias may give rise to incorrect conclusions about a presumed relationship between a risk factor and a disease or outcome. In one such case, a particular blood test result was initially considered to indicate an increased risk of developing leukemia. It was later discovered that this same blood test result was found mainly in long-term survivors of the disease and was actually associated with a better overall prognosis. Recall bias describes instances where members of different study groups do not report events in a comparable manner. A good example of this would be asking the mother of a child with a congenital hand abnormality about problems during pregnancy versus asking the mother of a normal child. Interviewer bias describes the tendency for information to be collected or interpreted in a nonstandard fashion based on who is performing the task. A classic example of this would be a surgeon who rates the results of his or her own work or a surgeon who asks his or her own patients questions that lead them to respond according to the surgeon's own preconceptions. Skewed follow-up bias is a particularly common form of bias in orthopaedic clinical research that relates primarily to differential rates of patients lost to follow-up between study groups. Ideally, the patients lost should not differ significantly from those patients who remain, and the proportion who are lost should not be so great as to potentially change the study's conclusions if they were hypothetically found. Misclassification bias refers to errors in determining exposure (risk factors) and/or disease status (outcome) in study subjects. When misclassification occurs randomly it tends to bias a study toward the null hypothesis and lead to a type II error (failure to demonstrate a difference when one truly exists). When nonrandom misclassification occurs it can lead to either an overestimate or underestimate of the true relationship under study.

Association Versus Causality

Risk is a central concept in epidemiology. Classic epidemiologic jargon includes discussion of exposure, which leads to risk of developing disease. This same concept is often represented as risk factors that may result in certain outcomes The risk of developing a particular disease is linked in a probabilistic fashion to being exposed to a particular risk factor, provided that the case in question is not an extreme case in which everyone with the "risk factor" experiences the outcome of interest (for example, 100% of individuals exposed to the risk factor decapitation will develop the outcome called death).

Epidemiologists are focused on diseases, and in this context the word disease means any of a variety of health outcomes of interest. They wish to know what causes

TABLE 2	Bradford Hill Criteria
Strength—strong association of risk factor and disease
Consistency—replication in different populations
Specificity—risk factor leads to one particular disease
Temporality—cause precedes effect
Biologic Gradient—dose response relationship
Plausibility—existence of a biologic mechanism
Coherence—compatibility with existing knowledge
Experimental Evidence—replication in the lab
Analogy—similar risk factors show similar effects

them and what may be successfully used to treat or prevent them. What truly causes a disease is rarely completely understood and it is rare that 100% of those exposed develop disease. As a result, discussion is directed in terms of risk factors associated with the possible development of disease. What is perceived to be a risk factor may, in fact, be causally associated with the disease in question, the disease itself may actually be responsible for what is perceived to be a risk factor, or what is perceived to be a risk factor may in fact be no more than a red herring and the true cause of the disease is an unknown factor (confounder).

One approach to addressing the question of fallacious association versus true causation is to apply the Bradford Hill criteria (Table 2). These criteria serve as a useful framework for critical discussion of the likelihood of any particular risk factor being genuine. Even if all of Hill's criteria are satisfied it is still possible that the observed association is false. Other unknown and unmeasured factors may truly cause the disease. Confounding is considered to be present when the separate effects of two different variables cannot be distinguished. An example of this would be the effect that an unequal distribution of smokers has on the spinal fusion rates measured in two different adult study populations. Unequal distribution of confounders can lead to confusing findings from subgroup analysis, such as a treatment being shown to be effective in men and effective in women but ineffective for people in general (the two groups combined), a well-known phenomenon referred to as Simpson's paradox. One of the goals of randomization is to properly balance known and unknown confounders within different study groups.

An observed association may also be caused by systematic errors in selection of subjects and/or collection of information that led to false conclusions. One example of this is Berkson's bias, whereby control subjects are innocently drawn from a population (such as hospitalized patients) that is inherently different from the study group (perhaps subjects drawn from the general population). The final consideration relative to an observed association is that it may be caused by random variation found in the sample (chance). The likelihood of chance alone being the explanation for an observed association is evaluated via formal statistical analysis. Even if Hill's criteria were satisfied and the possibility of spurious results due to confounding, bias, and chance were ruled out, a final question concerning generalizability must be answered. Can the study results be applied to other patient populations or is the population that was studied so special and so different that the results may only apply to that population?

Annotated Bibliography

Abel U, Koch A: The role of randomization in clinical studies: Myths and beliefs. *J Clin Epidemiol* 1999;52: 487-497.
This article is an excellent review of several important myths and misconceptions regarding randomized clinical trials. The relative strengths and weaknesses of experimental and observational study designs are discussed.

Benson K, Hartz AJ: A comparison of observational studies and randomized, controlled trials. *N Engl J Med* 2000;342:1878-1886.
The authors discuss the concept of "treatment effect" and offer both surgical and nonsurgical examples that demonstrate that estimates of treatment effect from observational studies are neither consistently larger nor qualitatively different from randomized clinical trials addressing the same treatments.

Brunner HI, Giannini EH: Evidence-based medicine in pediatric rheumatology. *Clin Exp Rheumatol* 2000;18: 407-414.
This article is an excellent review that highlights both the roots and modern concepts of evidence-based medicine. The role of clinical epidemiology is strongly emphasized.

Freedman KB, Bernstein J: Sample size and statistical power in clinical orthopaedic research. *J Bone Joint Surg Am* 1999;81:1454-1460.
This article reviews the basic concepts of statistical sampling and hypothesis testing. The rationale behind power calculations as well as the commonly accepted standard of 80% power are discussed. Statistical significance versus clinical significance is also addressed.

Goodman SN: Toward evidence-based medical statistics: I. The P value fallacy. *Ann Intern Med* 1999;130: 995-1004.
The argument is made against unidimensional clinical study assessment based only on *P* values. The complementary information offered by confidence intervals is also discussed.

Goodman SN: Toward evidence-based medical statistics: II. The Bayes factor. *Ann Intern Med* 1999;130: 1005-1013.
This is an excellent summary of the basics of bayesian methodology and how it relates to clinical medicine. Concrete examples of this "consider the available evidence approach" include clinical decision making in the face of uncertainty and meta-analysis.

Hawker GA, Wright JG, Coyte PC, et al: Differences between men and women in the rate of use of hip and knee arthroplasty. *N Engl J Med* 2000;342:1016-1022.
A very large cross-sectional study demonstrated that the underuse of hip and knee arthroplasty is more than three times higher in women versus men. It is a strong example of an observational study design as well as the use of odds ratios and risk adjustment.

Kaska SC, Weinstein JN: Historical perspective: Ernest Amory Codman (1869-1940): A pioneer of evidence-based medicine: The end result idea. *Spine* 1998;23: 629-633.
This historic article provides valuable insight into one of the most prominent figures in orthopaedic outcomes research and epidemiology.

Kocher MS, Zurakowski D, Kasser JR: Differentiating between septic arthritis and transient synovitis of the hip in children: An evidence-based clinical prediction algorithm. *J Bone Joint Surg Am* 1999;81:1662-1670.
This article provides a strong example of how to develop and analyze a clinical prediction tool. This represents a significant conceptual step beyond aphorisms and "rules of thumb" to scientifically validated tools that may aid the clinical decision making process.

Marx RG, Bombardier C, Wright JG: What do we know about the reliability and validity of physical examination tests used to examine the upper extremity? *J Hand Surg Am* 1999;24:185-193.
According to this structured review of the literature, little information exists regarding the reliability and validity of common upper extremity physical examination maneuvers. Important terms such as impairment, reliability, validity, and accuracy are defined.

Mata SG, Aicua EA, Ovejero AH, Grande MM: Legg-Calve-Perthes disease and passive smoking. *J Pediatr Orthop* 2000;20:326-330.
The relationship of passive smoking with LCP disease is analyzed in a large orthopaedic case-control study. The odds of being exposed to the risk factor (passive smoking) were over five times higher for the LCP group than the control group.

Smith JS, Watts HG: Methods for locating missing patients for the purpose of long-term clinical studies. *J Bone Joint Surg Am* 1998;80:431-438.

The authors emphasize the importance of locating patients, because patients with bad outcomes tend to be more difficult to contact.

Szabo RM: Principles of epidemiology for the orthopaedic surgeon. *J Bone Joint Surg Am* 1998;80:111-120.

Basic epidemiologic principles as they relate to orthopaedic surgery are reviewed. A discussion of causal inference and the Bradford Hill criteria is presented.

Classic Bibliography

Bombardier C, Kerr MS, Shannon HS, Frank JW: A guide to interpreting epidemiologic studies on the etiology of back pain. *Spine* 1994;19(suppl 18):2047S-2056S.

Chang RW, Falconer J, Stulberg SD, Arnold WJ, Dyer AR: Prerandomization: An alternative to classic randomization: The effects on recruitment in a controlled trial of arthroscopy for osteoarthrosis of the knee. *J Bone Joint Surg Am* 1990;72:1451-1455.

Dorey F, Amstutz HC: Discrepancies in the orthopaedic literature: Why? A statistical explanation. *Instr Course Lect* 1993;42:555-564.

Dorey F, Nasser S, Amstutz H: The need for confidence intervals in the presentation of orthopaedic data. *J Bone Joint Surg Am* 1993;75:1844-1852.

Easterbrook PJ, Berlin JA, Gopalan R, Matthews DR: Publication bias in clinical research. *Lancet* 1991;337:867-872.

Ebramzadeh E, McKellop H, Dorey F, Sarmiento A: Challenging the validity of conclusions based on *P*-values alone: A critique of contemporary clinical research design and methods. *Instr Course Lect* 1994;43:587-600.

Hennekens CH, Buring JE, Mayrent SL (eds): *Epidemiology in Medicine*. Boston, MA, Little Brown & Company, 1987.

Hulley SB, Cummings SR, Browner WS (eds): *Designing Clinical Research: An Epidemiologic Approach*. Baltimore, MD, Williams & Wilkins, 1988.

Iezzoni LI: Risk and outcomes, in Iezzoni LI (ed): *Risk Adjustment for Measuring Health Care Outcomes*. Ann Arbor, MI, Health Administration Press, 1994.

Jefferys WH, Berger JO: Ockham's razor and Bayesian analysis. *Am Sci* 1992;80:64-72.

Morabia A: P.C.A. Louis and the birth of clinical epidemiology. *J Clin Epidemiol* 1996;49:1327-1333.

Rudicel S, Esdaile JE: The randomized clinical trial in orthopaedics: Obligation or option? *J Bone Joint Surg Am* 1985;67:1284-1293.

Chapter 10

The Physiology of Aging

Mathias P.G. Bostrom, MD

Joseph A. Buckwalter, MD

Neuromuscular Changes During Aging and the Effects on Mobility

Aging is a complex, natural phenomenon that often results in a decline in most physiologic systems of the body. The maintenance of some level of neuromuscular function is crucial for the elderly to maintain normal daily routines. Despite this necessity, the human aging process affects the neuromuscular system, resulting in an age-related decline in proprioception, decrease in lean muscle mass, and drastic alterations in balance that increase an individual's propensity for falling. It is important to understand the changes that are encountered throughout the aging process in an attempt to improve quality of life in the elderly patient.

Changes in Proprioception

Proprioception is a fundamental function required by all humans to perform their daily routines. Changes in proprioception that occur with advancing age affect the elderly by altering sense of balance and increasing the propensity for falls. Changes in proprioception include central nervous system (CNS) and peripheral nervous system (PNS) changes that affect coordination and musculoskeletal function by altering the neural control and stimuli of muscles, and affecting mobility in the elderly. Also, sight, hearing, and taste are affected with advancing age, resulting in changes in balance and equilibrium.

During aging, the CNS and PNS undergo several age-related changes. Cortical atrophy and a decline in neurotransmitter levels occur in the CNS. Between 45 and 85 years of age, the weight of the brain decreases by 20%. Cerebral blood flow steadily declines with advancing age, jeopardizing brain metabolism, and nerve conduction velocity slows 10% to 15%. These changes reduce reaction time and voluntary motor movement, resulting in reaction times of older adults

that are 20% longer than in young adults. The subsequent delay of motor and sensory function in the PNS is thought to be the major reason for the 35% to 40% increase in falls observed in adults age 60 years and older.

Accompanying old age are changes in the neural control and the stimuli of muscles. Single peripheral motor neurons innervate groups of skeletal muscle fibers forming a motor unit. Earlier studies have shown that with aging there is a marked loss of the total number of motor units in old muscles with remodeling of other motor units. More recently it has been shown that in aging skeletal muscle, the decrease in total motor units is actually a specific loss of fast motor units and an increase in slow motor units. This leads to the conclusion that there must be a reorganization of the motor unit pool during the aging of skeletal muscle, supporting the notion that with age some fast fibers may undergo denervation and others may be reinnervated by sprouting nerves from the slow motor units. These changes account for the reduction in reaction times and voluntary motor movements in the elderly.

The neuromuscular junction (NMJ) is the crucial link between the neural and muscular systems. Biochemical and functional changes at the NMJ affect the capability of the muscles to respond to neural stimuli. Alterations in the synaptic transmission across the NMJ greatly affect the magnitude to which individual muscle fibers are recruited for normal function. Studies show remodeling and fragmentation of the NMJ with age, suggesting a progressive degeneration of the NMJ. These changes affect the neuronal dependent muscular function of the elderly and impair their sense of balance and stability, intensifying the risk of falls.

Advancing age affects the senses in several ways. Cataracts, macular degeneration, and glaucoma are conditions commonly observed in the elderly. Hearing and vestibular function diminish with age, with approximately 90% of nursing home residents and 30% of the noninstitutionalized having significant hearing impairment. The loss of vestibular function leads to a loss of balance and also may contribute to the high rate of falls in the elderly.

Changes in Lean Muscle Mass

The most visible and profound changes that occur with advancing age are the alterations in the whole body composition. Throughout the life span there is a progressive decline in the lean muscle mass and a corresponding increase in fat mass. These changes begin beyond the fourth decade of life and continue well after the eighth decade. One of the tissues most affected is skeletal muscle, which undergoes considerable loss of both type I (slow) and type II (fast) fibers. There is also a decrease in fiber cross-sectional area that appears greater in the type II fibers. This decrease in excitable muscle mass leads to a concomitant prolongation of twitch contraction and a reduction in voluntary strength.

There is a decrease in the size of individual muscles with aging. Lean body mass decreases 15% to 30% by 80 years of age. Muscle strength and mass decrease between 30% and 50% from ages 30 to 80 years, with the loss of muscle mass accounting for most of the observed decrease in strength. The loss of muscle tissue is due to a decline in number of muscle fibers and atrophy of type II muscle fibers. A 26% reduction in the size of type II fibers from age 20 to 80 years is seen as being responsible for a large proportion of the age-related loss of muscle mass.

Age-related loss of muscle mass is contributed to by psychosocial factors that lead to decreased activity and result in disuse atrophy. There is a lack of predilection for physical activity as well as cultural factors that lead to less opportunity and lower expectations. Comorbidities including cardiovascular, pulmonary, and neurologic diseases compound these cultural factors. Overall there is a 40% decrease in muscle area and a 39% decline in the total number of fibers from age 20 to 80 years.

The loss of muscle mass is not a uniform occurrence; different muscles suffer atrophy to a different extent. This fact may relate to differences in their composition of fiber types. Furthermore, there is a greater loss of muscle mass in weight-bearing muscles compared to non–weight-bearing muscles. Loss of muscle mass also may be related to the age-associated decline in whole-body maximal oxygen consumption. However, the time course of the loss of muscle mass is very different from the decline in maximal oxygen consumption, which starts at the age of 25 years. The decrease in strength is related to a combination of changes in the intrinsic force-generating capacity of muscle, reduction in the number of muscle fibers, and reduction in the size of muscle fibers.

Changes in Balance and Increased Propensity for Falls

Functional dependence is one of the most serious health problems encountered by elderly people. While reduced muscle mass and strength are associated with increased frailty and risk of falling, changes in balance also contribute to falls in the elderly. The ability to maintain balance or postural stability is achieved by a complex interaction between the visual, vestibular, and proprioceptive systems. Body sway is the natural motion of the body when standing to counter the pulling down effects of gravity. Body sway has been shown to increase with age in both sexes, but females have demonstrated more sway than males. Thus, elderly individuals are less able to compensate for shifts in their center of gravity, have impaired ability to deal with environmental hazards, and are more likely to fall.

Balance is a complex activity requiring input from multiple sensory systems. Normal balance in humans changes with age. As aging occurs, balance function is lost through the loss of sensory elements, the ability to integrate information and issue motor commands, and musculoskeletal function. These changes compounded with other diseases common in aging populations further enhance the deterioration in balance function, leading to an increased predilection for falling.

The incidence of falls is known to increase with age, with up to a 35% to 40% increase in falls in people older than age 60 years, with even higher rates observed in females. In the US, falling is the leading cause of fatal injury in people older than 70 years. Among the community-residing populations, up to one quarter of persons aged 65 to 74 and one third or more of those aged 75 years or older fall annually. Fifty percent of these individuals experience multiple falls each year. Risk factors associated with falls include dementia, visual impairment, neurologic and musculoskeletal disabilities, medications, fear of falling, and environmental conditions. However, muscle weakness, changes in gait, and more importantly, changes in balance are the most significant risk factors associated with falling. The risk of falling increases linearly with the number of abnormalities. The risk factors for falling independently contribute to immobility and functional decline. The fear of falling adds to the decreased mobility and increased functional dependence.

The Effects of Aging on the Reparative Processes

Despite the intricate complexity of the human regenerative capacity for bone and soft tissues, there are alterations that occur with advancing age that decrease the efficiency of reparative and regenerative processes of bone and soft tissue. These alterations include decreases in the number of mesenchymal stem cells, which affect the efficacy and timing of fracture, ligament, and tendon healing in the geriatric population.

Mesenchymal Stem Cells

Mesenchymal stem cells (MSCs) reside in the bone marrow compartment with hematopoietic stem cells. In vitro MSCs appear to be multipotent for differentiating into osteoblasts, chondroblasts, adipocytes, fibroblasts, myoblasts and reticular cells. An age-related decrease in bone mass could reflect decreased osteoblasts secondary to an age-related loss of osteoprogenitors.

The decrease in skeletal mass with aging is associated with an age-related decrease in the number of osteoprogenitor cells. It has been postulated that the decrease in osteoprogenitor generation during aging results in a decrease in the number of osteoblasts and the age-related reduction in bone formation and alterations of the properties of bone in humans. Maintenence of the stem cell population might slow the age-associated loss of bone and improve reparative processes in bone.

Age-Related Changes in Articular Cartilage

Articular cartilage undergoes significant age-related changes in thickness, cell function and matrix tensile properties, composition and molecular organization. These changes precede and may contribute to degeneration of the tissue (fraying or fibrillation of the articular surface). In addition, like other collagenous tissues, articular cartilage develops a yellow-brown tinge with increasing age. This color change may result from posttranslational modification of the matrix proteins, but its significance remains unknown.

Basic investigations have identified significant alterations in cartilage that occur during skeletal maturation, and cross-sectional studies of human joints show that focal superficial fibrillation of articular surfaces first appears in many joints near skeletal maturity. These degenerative changes progressively increase in prevalence, extent, and severity with increasing age. The increasing prevalence of cartilage degeneration with age parallels the striking age-related increase in the prevalence of the clinical syndrome of osteoarthritis, that is, joint pain and stiffness associated with cartilage degeneration, increased subchondral bone

density, and the presence of osteophytes. These observations suggest that in some individuals, age-related superficial cartilage fibrillation progresses into deep clefts, fissures, fragmentation of the cartilage, and eventually large erosions that leave exposed subchondral bone and cause symptoms of osteoarthritis.

Despite the strong correlations between age, increased prevalence of cartilage degenerative changes, and increased prevalence of osteoarthritis, the relationship between the age-related tissue changes and the clinical syndrome of osteoarthritis remains poorly understood. The prevalence and severity of cartilage fibrillation varies among joints and among different regions of the same joint. Not all degenerative changes in articular cartilage are associated with joint pain and loss of motion and not all people with symptoms of osteoarthritis have radiographic evidence of osteoarthritis, nor do all degenerative changes progress with age, even in people with the clinical and radiographic diagnosis of osteoarthritis. Furthermore, age-related alterations in other tissue components of synovial joints including the synovium, subchondral bone, menisci, ligaments, and joint capsules may contribute to joint symptoms and musculoskeletal impairment.

The relationships between age changes in chondrocytes and degeneration of articular cartilage also remain unclear. Cell density declines sharply from birth until skeletal maturity, but most studies suggest that it remains relatively constant in adult life. However, cell morphology and synthetic function change with increasing age. The cells accumulate intracytoplasmic filaments and may lose some of their endoplasmic reticulum and their synthetic patterns change to produce different, more variable matrix proteoglycans. In addition, cells may become less responsive to anabolic growth factors, and a recent study has shown that human articular cartilage chondrocytes become senescent with increasing age. Age-related changes in chondrocytes may make the cells less effective in replacing degraded matrix macromolecules and in repairing the tissue following injury.

Studies of the mechanical properties of cartilage have not found age-related changes in compressive properties, but they have shown significant age-related decreases in tensile stiffness, fatigue resistance, and strength. The underlying matrix alterations responsible for the age-related changes in matrix tensile properties have not been identified, but water content generally decreases with age and both the proteoglycans and collagens that form the primary components of the articular cartilage matrix macromolecular framework undergo age-related changes.

The large aggregating matrix proteoglycans, aggrecan molecules, responsible for giving the tissue its stiffness

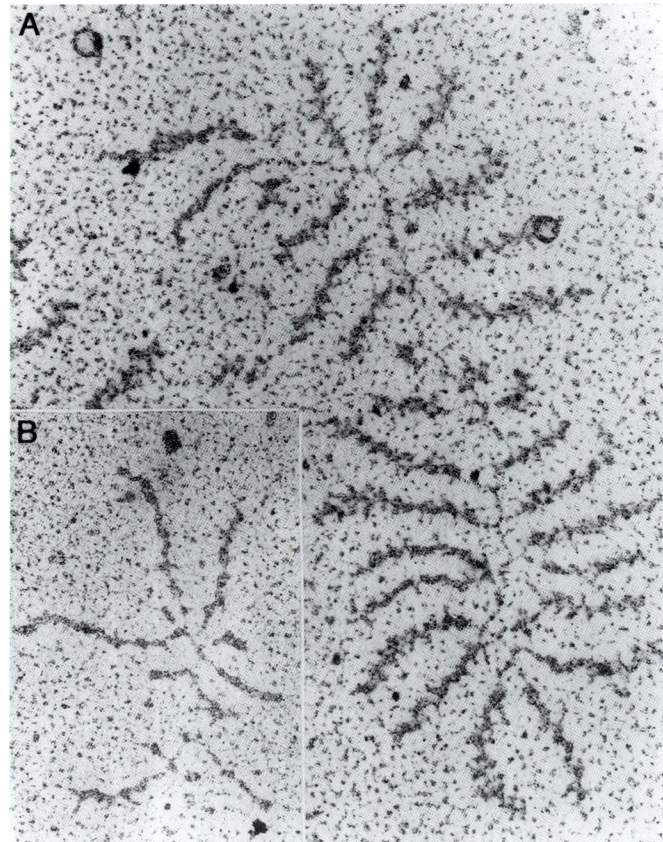

Figure 1 Electron micrographs of human articular cartilage proteoglycan aggregates consisting of central hyaluronan filaments and multiple attached aggrecan molecules. **A,** Proteoglycan aggregate from a newborn containing 30 aggrecan molecules. **B,** Proteoglycan aggregate from a 22-year-old containing 12 aggrecan molecules. Notice that the aggrecan molecules vary more in length than those from the younger person. (*Reproduced with permission from Buckwalter JA, Woo SL-Y, Goldberg VM, et al: Soft tissue aging and musculoskeletal function. J Bone Joint Surg Am 1993;75:1533-1548.*)

altered molecules accumulate in the matrix. Although the altered link proteins bind to hyaluronan and aggrecan, they may be less effective in stabilizing aggregates. Hyaluronan, the glycosaminoglycan that forms the central core molecules of proteoglycan aggregates, decreases in size and increases in concentration with increasing age. It is not certain if the increased concentration of hyaluronan results from increased synthesis or accumulation of degraded molecules. Because aggregation helps organize and stabilize proteoglycans within the matrix, the decline in aggregation and in aggregate size may alter the stability and mechanical properties of the matrix.

The cartilage matrix also contains nonaggregating proteoglycans such as decorin, biglycan, and fibromodulin. Decorin and fibromodulin interact with collagen fibrils and biglycan accumulates in the pericellular regions. The concentration of biglycan remains relatively constant while the concentration of decorin increases from about half the concentration of biglycan in newborns to twice the concentration of biglycan in adults. The functions of these proteoglycans have not been well defined, but they affect the formation, organization, and stability of the matrix and they can inhibit cell adhesion and migration. Thus, an increasing concentration of decorin may affect matrix turnover and inhibit repair.

The cartilage collagens also undergo age-related changes that may alter the tissue properties. During aging, cross-linking of collagen molecules may increase through nonenzymatic glycation reactions. The matrix collagen fibrils tend to increase in diameter with age, a change thought to be related at least in part to the decreased content of type XI collagen relative to type II collagen. Larger diameter collagen fibrils with a greater degree of cross-linking may be less flexible and make the cartilage matrix more rigid. The increased rigidity combined with decreased water content could limit the ability of the macromolecular framework to deform repetitively when loaded without damaging its structure. Increasing rigidity of the collagen framework and decreased water content might also interfere with the matrix turnover necessary to replace degraded molecules.

Maintaining articular cartilage function and synovial joint range of movement, even in the elderly, requires regular joint loading and motion. Marked decreased joint use decreases chondrocyte synthetic activity and adversely alters matrix composition and cartilage mechanical properties. It also decreases joint range of motion and may contribute to the age-related loss of muscle mass. However, repetitive high-intensity impact and torsional loading of joints may cause or accelerate joint degeneration. For these reasons, middle-age and older people, including those with mild joint degener-

in compression and resiliency undergo significant changes with skeletal maturation: they become much smaller and more variable in size (Fig. 1), their keratan sulfate content increases, their chondroitin sulfate content decreases, and the proportion of these molecules that form large aggregates declines, possibly because of an age-related decrease in aggregate stability. As these changes in aggrecan molecules occur, the size of proteoglycan aggregates decreases because of the decrease in aggrecan size and in the number of aggrecan molecules per aggregate.

The decline in aggregation and aggregate size probably results from several changes in the molecules and in the matrix. Proteolytic degradation leaves molecular fragments in the matrix that occupy space and that may bind to hyaluronan where they can inhibit aggregation of fully functional molecules. Link proteins, the protein molecules responsible for stabilizing and organizing large proteoglycan aggregates, also undergo increasing proteolytic modification with age and the

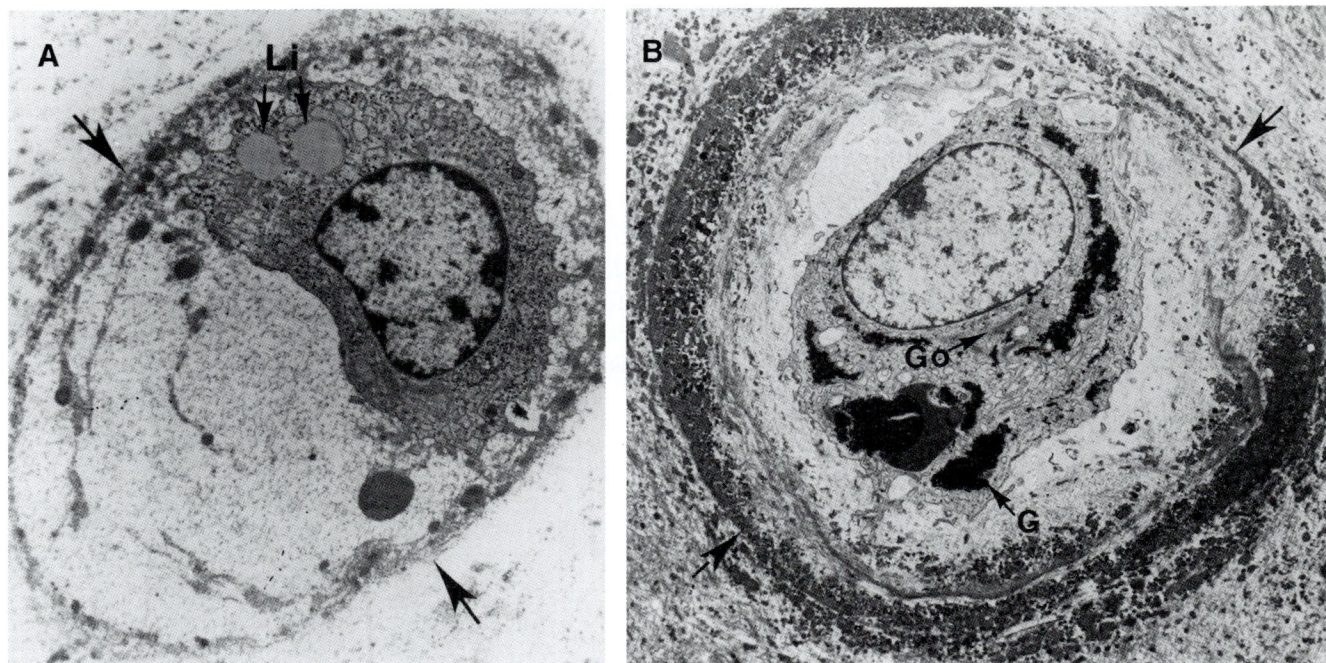

Figure 2 Electron micrographs of human nucleus pulposus cells. **A,** Electron micrograph of a cell from the central region of a child's nucleus pulposus. Li indicates lipid and the arrows mark the edge of the accumulation of electron dense matrix material. **B,** Electron micrograph of a cell from the central region of an elderly adult's nucleus pulposus. Go indicates Golgi membranes, G indicates glycogen, and the arrows mark the edge of the accumulation of dense matrix material. Notice the increased thickness of the rim of accumulated granular material surrounding this cell compared with the cell from the younger individual. *(Reproduced with permission from Buckwalter JA, Woo SL-Y, Goldberg VM, et al: Soft tissue aging and musculoskeletal function. J Bone Joint Surg Am 1993;75:1533-1548.)*

ation, should participate in regular physical activity that requires joint loading and motion and maintains joint range of motion. In general, activities that result in high-intensity impact and torsional loading of joints should be avoided.

Age-Related Changes in Intervertebral Disk

Back and neck stiffness and pain are among the most common complaints of middle-aged and older people. The relationship of these clinical problems to age-related changes in the soft tissues of the spine remain unknown, but no musculoskeletal tissue undergoes more dramatic age-related changes than the intervertebral disk. The most extensive changes occur in the central regions of the disk, the inner anulus fibrosus and nucleus pulposus. During skeletal growth and maturation the clear gelatinous nucleus pulposus of childhood becomes a firm, fibrous plate. In early adult life, fissures and cracks appear in the disk and then extend from the periphery to the central regions. These morphologic changes are accompanied by a decrease in proteoglycan and water concentration and an increase in noncollagenous protein concentration. Disk volume and shape also change, although these alterations have not been as well defined as the alterations in disk structure and composition. The age-related alterations in disk tissue appear to increase the probability of disk

herniation, and the age-related changes in the disk shape and volume can affect spine mobility and alter the alignment and loads applied to the facet joints, spinal ligaments, and paraspinous muscles. These alterations may contribute to age-related loss of spine mobility and strength, spinal stenosis, and degeneration of the facet joints.

Morphologic studies show that cell types and the number of viable cells change dramatically with age in the central regions of the disk. In infants, syncytial cords and clusters of notochordal cells occupy the central region of the nucleus pulposus, but by adolescence few of these cells remain. As the notochordal cells disappear, chondrocyte-like cells take their place. Following skeletal maturity, the number of viable cells in all regions of the disk declines sharply, but especially the central regions.

Electron microscopic studies of disk matrix show a progressive increase in mean collagen fibril diameter and in the variability of collagen fibril diameter with age. At the same time, dense granular filamentous osmophilic material accumulates throughout the matrix (Fig. 2). This material is concentrated in the regions immediately surrounding the cells of the central disk regions. Its composition has not been defined, but it may consist of degraded matrix molecules and noncollagenous proteins.

As the ultrastructure of the disk matrix changes and the proteoglycan concentration in the central regions of the disk declines, the proportion of proteoglycans that form aggregates and proteoglycan aggrecan size decrease. Proteoglycan aggregates from human infant intervertebral disk anulus fibrosus and vertebral cartilage end plate consist of a long central hyaluronan filament and multiple attached aggrecan molecules, a structure identical to the aggregates of hyaline cartilages. However, in human infants, only about one third of nucleus pulposus proteoglycan aggregates resemble these large aggregates; the other two thirds consist of monomer clusters that frequently lack a visible central hyaluronan filament. By adolescence, the proteoglycan population of the nucleus pulposus consists almost entirely of clusters of short aggrecan molecules and nonaggregated proteoglycans. A decline in the concentration of functional link protein may cause at least some of these change in proteoglycan aggregates.

The most critical variable responsible for the changes in central disk cells and their matrices appears to be declining nutrition. The disk cells rely on diffusion of nutrients through the disk matrix from blood vessels on the periphery of the anulus fibrous and within the vertebral bodies. The progressive age-related decline in the number of arteries supplying the region of the intervertebral disk presumably contributes to declining cell viability and biosynthetic function. At the same time, accumulation of degraded matrix macromolecules and decreasing matrix water content may interfere with diffusion through the matrix, further compromising cell nutrition. Factors that may accelerate the rate and increase the severity of age-related changes in intervertebral disk by altering the tissue or tissue nutrition include increased disk loading due to demanding physical activities, vibration or spinal deformity, and factors such as smoking, vascular disease, and diabetes that directly compromise the vascular supply.

Despite the apparent inevitability of age-related changes in the human intervertebral disk, regeneration of disk tissue may be possible. Experimental studies of the effects of enzymatic degradation of the normal central disk region extracellular matrix suggest that the cells can regenerate a matrix. Reexpansion of narrowed human disks after injection of enzymes has not occurred consistently, perhaps because of variability in the extent of disk degeneration, diffusion of the enzymes, the limited number of viable cells, or mechanical constraints that prevent reexpansion.

Age-Related Changes in Tendon, Ligament, and Joint Capsule

Middle-aged and older individuals can develop significant impairment as a result of alterations in tendons, ligaments, and joint capsules. Degenerative changes in dense fibrous tissues may result in spontaneous or low energy level ruptures of the shoulder rotator cuff, the long head of the biceps, tibialis posterior, patellar and the Achilles tendons, and sprains and ruptures of joint capsules and ligaments, including those of the spine and wrist. It is likely that at least some of the soreness following physical activity in middle-aged and older patients or chronic activity-related musculoskeletal pain results from injuries to the fibrous components of muscle tendon junctions or tendon, ligament, and joint capsule insertions into bone.

The tensile mechanical properties of at least some ligament-bone complexes deteriorate significantly with age. Investigation of the mechanical properties of the human anterior longitudinal ligament showed that the strength of the ligament-bone complex decreased approximately twofold from age 21 years to 79 years. A study of the mechanical properties of human femur-anterior cruciate ligament-tibia complexes from three age groups showed a progressive decline in tensile stiffness and ultimate load to failure with increasing age. The decrease in ultimate load to failure occurred most rapidly between the third decade of life (age 22 to 35 years) and middle age (40 to 50 years). Following middle age, ultimate load to failure continued to decrease; ligament-bone complexes from older individuals (60 to 97 years) failed at less than one third the ultimate load to failure of the younger ligament complexes. Another study of anterior cruciate ligament complexes found that the elastic modulus, ultimate tensile stress, and strain energy to failure were two to three times greater for complexes from young adults (age range 16 to 25 years) than for older people (age range 48 to 86 years). In older ligament-bone complexes, tensile failure occurred more frequently by rupture of the ligament substance than by avulsion from the bone, suggesting that the ligament substance may deteriorate more rapidly than the bone; however, this possibility warrants further study. Study of dog and rabbit medial collateral ligaments shows that their mechanical properties also deteriorate with increasing age following skeletal maturity, but the decline is more gradual than in the anterior cruciate ligament bone complexes. Therefore, the rate and extent of change in mechanical properties may vary among ligaments.

Detailed mechanical studies of the age-related changes in tendons and joint capsules have not been reported, but the similarities in structure, composition, and mechanical function between these tissues and ligaments, and the available evidence suggests that their mechanical properties also deteriorate with age. Furthermore, histologic degenerative changes in tendons appear more frequently with increasing age.

The tissue changes responsible for the age-related decline in the strength of dense fibrous tissues have not been clearly identified. In at least some locations, including the rotator cuff, the nutrition of dense fibrous tissue cells may decrease with age due to decreased vascular perfusion. The resulting decline in cell function may lead to tissue degeneration. Changes in the cell function, matrix composition, and organization of the matrix macromolecules that occur independently of alterations in nutrition may also contribute to the decline in mechanical properties.

Aging fibroblasts flatten and elongate, losing most of their rough endoplasmic reticulum and Golgi membranes. A study of tendon also showed that tissue from young animals had a high level of aerobic glycolysis, but the level of aerobic glycolysis declined with age to the point that it could not be detected in tissues from older animals. These changes may be associated with decreasing biosynthetic activity and possibly a decreased ability to participate in tissue turnover or respond to injury. Recent work also indicates that ligament cells are less able to respond to exercise in older animals.

Highly oriented fibrillar collagens form the bulk of the matrix in the dense fibrous tissues. Therefore, it seems reasonable to expect that the age-related decrease in tissue mechanical properties results from an alteration in the collagens. Although biochemical analyses have not shown dramatic age-related changes in tendon or ligament matrix composition, the collagen and water concentration of these tissues may decline slightly with age as the labile reducible collagen crosslinks decrease and the more stable nonreducible crosslinks increase. The properties of the tissues could also be affected by alterations in the organization and molecular structure of the collagens, and animal studies have suggested that the collagen fibril alignment and fiber bundle organization decrease with increasing age. Posttranslational modifications of the collagens may also contribute to the age-related decline in mechanical properties.

Given the magnitude of the age-related changes in the mechanical properties of knee ligaments, and probably in other dense fibrous tissues, and the known changes in the cells and matrices of these tissues, it is surprising that injuries to ligament, joint capsule, and tendon do not occur more frequently in older individuals. To some extent, decreasing levels of vigorous physical activity with increasing age may prevent injuries to these tissues.

Fracture Healing

During development, bone formation occurs through cartilage intermediaries (endochondral), within a collagen matrix without cartilage intermediaries (intramembranous), or by deposition of new bone on existing bone (appositional). All three types of bone formation occur throughout life and can contribute to the restoration of the skeleton after injury, disease, or the treatment of skeletal deformity. A decrease in the expression of growth factors may alter normal fracture healing and may contribute to the decline in fracture healing with age. Furthermore, the inductive potential of demineralized bone matrix from young animals is greater than that of the bone matrix from old animals, likely reflecting differences in the concentrations of osteoinductive growth factors.

The periosteum contains two layers, an inner and outer cambium layer. The cambium layer is responsible for appositional bone growth during development and comprises a large number of mesenchymal cells with osteogenic potential. However, the osteogenic potential of this tissue diminishes with aging. The periosteum is thinner in older individuals and the cellular contact dwindles, exposing the bone surface to physiochemical changes normally not under control of cells.

Most of the experiments done on fracture healing have been done in young or young adult animals and therefore, little data exist on fracture healing in older adult animals. Experiments performed to assess the effect of aging or fracture healing showed no differences in the biochemical parameters of fracture healing in young adult and older animals after 40 days of healing. Yet, after 80 days of healing, there was a marked delay in the fracture healing process in older animals as compared with that of the young adults. The healing fractures in young adult animals regained their mechanical properties after nearly 4 weeks of healing, whereas the strength and stiffness of femoral fractures in older adult rats neared intact values after 12 weeks. Thus, the mechanical properties of healing bone in young animals are much greater than in old animals, likely the result of a combination of factors.

Several mechanisms may explain the age-related decline in the rate of fracture healing. Aging is related to a general functional decline in the homeostatic mechanisms of skeletal tissues. The osteoprogenitor cell number is reduced with advancing age in both the bone marrow and periosteum. These cells are important targets and are the precursor cells necessary for osteoprogenitor cell proliferation. Another factor is a decline in the expression of osteoinductive cytokines and growth factors. One reason for this is a decline in the inflammatory response to injury. In addition, the bone inductive potential of demineralized bone matrix decreases with age. The inductive potential of bone matrix appears to be growth hormone-dependent, and growth hormone secretion decreases with age, reflecting the decreasing ability to repair fractures. Thus, a combination of factors result in decreased bone repair by endochondral, intermembranous, and appositional bone formation.

Exercise in the Elderly

The elderly population is increasing in both size and in proportion to the total population. The beneficial effects of exercise on both the physical and psychological aspects in the elderly are well documented. Exercise maintains mobility and independence in the elderly.

There are many effects of aging on the physiologic function of the body. The overall work capacity declines roughly 30% between the ages of 30 to 70 years. Muscle strength and mass decrease at the same degree. Similarly, cardiac output, maximum heart rate, and respiratory vital capacity show similar trends. Women lose 30% of their bone mass by age 70 years, and men lose half of that amount. Joint flexibility declines 25% to 30% and renal and liver function also decrease substantially. As much as 50% of this diminished function can be ascribed to disuse, and alternatively, this portion of the functional decline could be prevented by physical activity.

When prescribing exercise treatment in the elderly, special consideration must be given to the status of multiple organ systems, including cardiac, pulmonary, and musculoskeletal. The exercise regimen should be specifically catered to the patient's cardiovascular condition, musculoskeletal limitations, and personal goals. A substantial positive training effect can result from an exercise regimen that includes an appropriate warm-up and cool-down period in addition to walking, stretching, calisthenics, and other aerobic activities. A program similar to this can be effective if the proper intensity and duration is maintained.

In response to such a training schedule, elderly individuals experience increased stroke volume, maximum heart rate, and cardiac output. Maximal oxygen consumption is increased yet the change in respiratory function is negligible. As endurance and strength improve, fat will be replaced by lean muscle mass. Flexibility will be improved and bone demineralization will be reduced. Exercise has a soothing and calming effect on the elderly so that anxiety and depression may be prevented. The patient may experience an increase in self-respect as conditioning improves.

Lack of exercise is a common predictor of mobility decline, and mobility is related to increased risk of falling. Exercise training programs enhance the functional independence of the elderly through increased mobility. Elderly exercisers experience better motor control and coordination than elderly nonexercisers. Similarly,

elderly females who exercise display less postural sway than those who do not. Strength and balance training have been shown to be effective in improving balance and thus decrease the risk of falls. Furthermore, weight-bearing exercises have a beneficial effect on bone mass.

Perhaps the most obvious important research questions involve development of the most effective type of training for the elderly: a regimen that balances the risk of inactivity with the risk of exercise. A specific training program should consider the specific social needs of the subject, the goals and needs of the older population, and their reasons for participation, rather than using a training program already developed for a younger population. Moreover, it is essential to assess and compare the effects of various resistance programs and aerobic training on muscular endurance in the elderly. Modifying the intensity factors, duration, and frequency of training may play an essential role in the subject's compliance and adherence to the exercise program. The effect of training on functional activities such as balance, gait, muscle mass, and risk of falling are important.

An overly conservative attitude on the part of physicians, families, and elderly patients unfortunately has resulted in reduced activity, with an inevitable decrease in exercise tolerance and functional status. Elderly patients can maintain a reasonable level of exercise tolerance or can be rehabilitated to this level of activity with a proper physical program. The decline in overall function with age can be largely reduced.

Annotated Bibliography

Changes in Proprioception

Daley MJ, Spinks WL: Exercise, mobility, and aging. *Sports Med* 2000;29:1-12.

The elderly population is growing in both size and in proportion to the total population. The effects of exercise on mobility and aging are evaluated. Impaired balance and gait are the most significant risk factors for limited mobility and falls in the elderly.

Luff AR: Review: Age-associated changes in the innervation of muscle fibers and changes in the mechanical properties of motor units. *Ann NY Acad Sci* 1998;854:92-101.

In both humans and animals there is a progressive loss of muscle strength with age. Motoneurons are lost with age, and this occurrence is apparent in humans after the age of 60 years. The age-related loss of motoneurons and associated muscle fibers contributes to the reduced capacity of muscles with age.

Changes in Lean Muscle Mass

Martin PE, Grabiner MD: Aging, exercise, and the predisposition to falling. *J Appl Biomech* 1999;15:52-55.

Reduced muscular strength and muscle mass are associated with increased frailty and an increased risk of falls. With advancing age, there is a progressive decline in the lean muscle mass and a corresponding increase in fat mass.

Changes in Balance and Propensity for Falls

Konrad HR, Girardi M, Helfert R: Balance and aging. *Laryngoscope* 1999;109:1454-1460.

Normal balance changes with aging. As aging progresses, there is a loss of balance function through loss of sensory elements, and the ability to integrate information. These changes cause a marked increase in the risk of falling.

Mesenchymal Stem Cells

D'Ippolito G, Schiller PC, Ricordi C, Roos BA, Howard GA: Age-related osteogenic potential of mesenchymal stromal stem cells from human vertebral bone marrow. *J Bone Miner Res* 1999;14:1115-1122.

Mesenchymal stem cells reside in the bone marrow and are the progenitors for osteoblasts. There is an age-related decrease in bone mass due to a decreasing number of osteoblasts with aging. A decreasing number of mesenchymal stem cells may be responsible for the age-related reduction in the number of osteoblasts.

Aging and Osteoarthritis

Bank RA, Bayliss MT, Lafeber FP, Maroudas A, Tekoppele JM: Ageing and zonal variation in post-translational modification of collagen in normal human articular cartilage: The age-related increase in non-enzymic glycation affects biomechanical properties of cartilage. *Biochem J* 1998;330:345-351.

This article reports that age-related changes in human articular cartilage collagen can adversely affect the mechanical properties of the matrix and thereby increase the risk of cartilage degeneration.

Buckwalter JA, Martin JA, Mankin HJ: Synovial joint degeneration and the syndrome of osteoarthritis. *Instr Course Lect* 2000;49:481-489.

This article discusses the relationships between articular cartilage aging, joint degeneration, and osteoarthritis.

Exercise in the Elderly

Bemben MG: Age-related alterations in muscular endurance. *Sports Med* 1998;25:259-269.

The beneficial effects of exercise on both the physical and psychologic aspects in the elderly are well documented. There are many effects of aging on the physiologic function of the body. In prescribing exercise treatment in the elderly, special considerations must be taken into account.

Classic Bibliography

Andersson GBJ: Intervertebral disk: Clinical aspects, in Buckwalter JA, Goldberg VM, Woo SL-Y (eds): *Musculoskeletal Soft-Tissue Aging: Impact on Mobility.* Rosemont, IL, American Academy of Orthopaedic Surgeons, 1993, pp 331-347.

Buckwalter JA: Aging and degeneration of the human intervertebral disc. *Spine* 1995;20:1307-1314.

Buckwalter JA, Goldberg VM, Woo SL-Y (eds): *Musculoskeletal Soft-Tissue Aging: Impact on Mobility.* Rosemont, IL, American Academy of Orthopaedic Surgeons, 1993.

Buckwalter JA, Lane NE: Athletics and osteoarthritis. *Am J Sports Med* 1997;25:873-881.

Bak B, Andreassen TT: The effect of aging on fracture healing in the rat. *Calcif Tissue Int* 1989;45:292-297.

Carmeli E, Reznick AZ: Review: The physiology and biochemistry of skeletal muscle atrophy as a function of age. *Proc Soc Exp Biol Med* 1994;206:103-113.

Fielding RA: The role of progressive resistance training and nutrition in the preservation of lean body mass in the elderly. *J Am Coll Nutr* 1995;14:587-594.

Galea V: Changes in motor unit estimates with aging. *J Clin Neurophysiol* 1996;13:253-260.

Landin RJ, Linnemeier TJ, Rothbaum DA, Chappelear J, Noble RJ: Review: Exercise testing and training of the elderly patient. *Cardiovasc Clin* 1985;15:201-218.

Noyes FR, Grood ES: The strength of the anterior cruciate ligament in humans and Rhesus monkeys: Age-related and species-related changes. *J Bone Joint Surg Am* 1976;58:1074-1082.

Tideiksaar R (ed): *Falling in Old Age: Its Prevention and Treatment.* New York, NY, Springer Publishing, 1989, pp 1-9.

Tideiksaar R: *Falling in Old Age: Prevention and Management,* ed 2. New York, NY, Springer Publishing, 1997, pp 1-53.

Woo SL-Y, Hollis JM, Adams DJ, Lyon RM, Takai S: Tensile properties of the human femur-anterior cruciate ligament-tibia complex: The effects of specimen age and orientation. *Am J Sports Med* 1991;19:217-225.

Chapter 11

Outcomes Assessment and Evidence-Based Practice

Hans Kreder, MD

Introduction and Background

Outcomes research describes the notion of improving health outcomes by evaluating the end result of care. Apart from global health policies such as immunization, implementation of research findings to benefit a specific patient generally rests with individual health care providers. Ideally, relevant information from the literature should be considered when making decisions about patient care. The concept of integrating personal experience and knowledge with the best available scientific information is known as evidence-based practice. Strategies have been developed to make this process efficient and useful for the care of individual patients and groups of individuals.

Outcomes Research Strategies

The distinguishing features of outcomes research include (1) a focus on patient-based assessments; (2) evaluation of care involving the entire community or population; and (3) the hope that research findings will result in better health care, leading to a continuous loop of improvement in population health. Outcomes research encompasses many different research activities, including (1) innovative methods of forming large patient cohorts using administrative data and previously conducted research; (2) development, testing, and use of validated instruments to measure health from the patient's perspective; (3) incorporation of patient choice in decision analysis models; and (4) assessment of economic outcomes.

Traditional clinical trials involve the study of relatively small patient cohorts, usually from academic institutions. Outcomes research often involves innovative methods of establishing patient cohorts by using large administrative data sets or information from previous studies, or meta-analysis.

Meta-analysis involves a structured review and statistical collation of data from published and unpublished (if available) information. The intention is to boost statistical power by increasing sample size. The best information is obtained when high-quality randomized trials are included. Concerns regarding meta-analysis include publication bias (negative studies are less likely to be published, especially in the English language), and the questionable validity of combining data from trials of varying quality, with different interventions, populations, and time periods. Meta-analysis is not a substitute for a large, well-conducted, randomized trial. An evaluation of large, definitive, randomized trials completed after a prior meta-analysis found that meta-analysis correctly predicted a positive or negative treatment effect only two thirds of the time.

Administrative data have been used to evaluate new surgical procedures and to compare health delivery systems, specialist versus generalist care, and the performance of high versus low volume providers. Administrative data analysis is limited by the quality and type of information available in the data set. Studies often use claims data that were collected for the purpose of monitoring billings, and as such may not contain important information such as disease severity, patient function, or even the anatomic side being treated. As with all research, administrative data analysis must involve the definition of an appropriate inception cohort with well-defined inclusion and exclusion criteria (based on diagnostic and procedural codes). Predictor variables (variables affecting the outcome) and outcome variables must also be defined and validated. Finally, statistical adjustments must be made for patient characteristics such as age, sex, comorbid conditions, and length of follow-up.

Comprehensive clinical registries, such as total joint and cancer registries, have the potential to provide more clinically meaningful information than claims datasets. A registry should be set up with a clinical question or problem in mind to ensure that all relevant information is being collected and to avoid the expense of collecting unnecessary information. Future efforts

TABLE 1 | Overview of Components of ICIDH-2

	Body Function and Structure	Activities	Participation	Contextual Factors
Level of Functioning	Body (body parts)	Individual (person as a whole)	Society (life situations)	Environmental factors (external influence on functioning) plus personal factors (internal influence on functioning)
Characteristics	Body function Body structure	Performance of an individual's activities	Involvement in life situations	Features of the physical, social, and attitudinal world plus attributes of the person
Positive aspect (functioning)	Functional and structural integrity	Activity	Participation	Facilitators
Negative aspect (disability)	Impairment	Activity limitation	Participation restriction	Barriers/hindrances

(Reproduced with permission from Simeonsson RJ, Lollar D, Hollowell J, Adams M: Revision of the international classification of impairments, disabilities, and handicaps: Developmental issues. J Clin Epidemiol 2000;53:113-124.)

TABLE 2 | Nomenclature for Measuring Health

	Body	Individual	Society
Objective characteristics	Impairment	Performance (disability)	Involvement (handicap)
Subjective aspects	Somatic sensations	Perceived health	Domain-specific life satisfaction

(Reproduced with permission from Post MW, de Witte LP, Schrijvers AJ: Quality of life and the ICIDH: Towards an integrated conceptual model for rehabilitation outcomes research. Clin Rehabil 1999;13:5-15.)

should focus on (1) establishing comprehensive registries with national or international scope; (2) using technology to streamline the process of complete and accurate data collection; and (3) incorporating modularity and flexibility into the data collection process to allow for simple clinical studies through the registry data collection mechanism (such as deep vein thrombosis prophylaxis for total joint replacement).

Health Outcomes and Health Measurement

The goals of treatment are to prevent injury, disease, and death, to minimize disagreeable symptoms, and to maximize function and well-being. To compare the degree to which competing treatment strategies succeed in achieving these goals, health outcomes must be defined and measured in a consistent and valid manner.

The World Health Organization (WHO) concept of impairment, disability, and handicap has been refined in the new International Classification of Functioning and Disability (ICIDH-2). The concept put forward by the WHO provides a framework for understanding and measuring the positive and negative manifestations of

health conditions resulting from the interaction of an individual with the physical, social, and psychological environment (Table 1). These concepts have been developed into an operational definition pertinent to the discussion of instruments for health measurement (Table 2). It has been suggested that objective and subjective aspects should be considered within each of the three dimensions proposed by the WHO (body, individual, society). Objective measures focus on the performance of the body part, the individual alone, and the individual in a social context, whereas subjective measures seek to determine the individual's perception and reaction to this performance for each dimension. The components of this matrix-dimensional structure together represent the concept of well-being.

Objective determination of impairment at the body or organ level involves measures such as joint range of motion, muscle strength, and physical disfigurement. Subjectively, individuals might complain of pain, stiffness, or weakness caused by dysfunction at the organ level. Such organ dysfunction might disable that person from performing a particular task (such as reaching, running, or lifting). This disability is objectively measurable using questionnaires that ask about certain activities. The subjective consequences of the inability to perform a given activity may be quite varied. One individual may experience no sense of disability despite not being able to run, whereas this same physical difficulty might result in a perception of severe personal disability for another individual. Finally, a person may be unable to work, provide care, or otherwise participate in normal social activities because of a disability, with corresponding subjective consequences unique to that individual.

Historically, impairment measures comprised the mainstay of orthopaedic evaluations. With the advent of valid and consistent means of measuring health from the patient's perspective, the emphasis of evaluation has shifted toward subjective patient-based assessment. Health measurement instruments that sample broad aspects of mental and physical well-being are referred to as generic. These instruments can be used to compare the health effects of different diseases (such as renal failure versus arthritis), but they may not address all of the concerns that individuals with a specific condition might have. Disease-specific measurement instruments are intended to evaluate specific problems experienced by individuals with a particular health condition. Disease-specific instruments generally exhibit better evaluative properties than generic instruments, but they are less useful for comparing disparate health conditions. For a more complete picture of well-being, a generic questionnaire is often supplemented with a disease-specific instrument.

Evidence-Based Practice

Scientific evidence to support medical and surgical intervention lies at the core of modern medicine. The strength (or level) of evidence is a term meant to quantify the level of confidence that an observed result is indeed correct. The concept of evidence-based practice involves awareness by the practicing physician of the strength of evidence in support of the treatment that he or she is recommending to a particular patient in the clinical setting. Ideally, clinical decisions should be made considering relevant input from all sources, including the treating physician, the literature, and the patient. Evidence-based practice entails the application of defined strategies to facilitate the acquisition and integration of information from these sources into the clinical setting.

The steps involved in the application of evidence-based practice include (1) the identification of a specific question from clinical practice (that is, a problem related to diagnosis, treatment, etiology, or prognosis); (2) a focused search and retrieval of relevant external evidence (usually the literature); (3) critical appraisal

of the quality of the retrieved material; (4) distillation of the raw data from the retrieved literature into clinically relevant information; and (5) implementing a clinical decision by integrating the retrieved external information with internal information (personal experience, knowledge, and expertise), and patient expectations and preferences.

The literature search should aim to identify the best available evidence based on information in the abstract section. Once the full document is retrieved, a formal critical appraisal of the methods section must be performed before evaluating the results. Once the clinician has established the quality of an article, the next step involves determining the magnitude of the observed effect. Simple calculations are recommended to generate information from the raw data that has direct relevance to the clinical situation under consideration. For problems concerning a diagnostic test, the magnitude of a statistic known as the likelihood ratio allows the clinician to quantify the benefits derived from a diagnostic test. A large likelihood ratio (above 10 or below 0.1) corresponds to a test that provides useful information. The difference in outcome following different treatments can be quantified by odds ratios for categorical end points, and mean differences for continuous outcomes. Finally, it is important to consider whether the observed effect could be due to chance by computing confidence limits around the observed difference value. A precise outcome is one where the confidence limits are tightly clustered around the observed value.

Practicing evidence-based surgery involves regular literature review used to address specific questions arising from everyday clinical practice. This strategy of problem-based knowledge acquisition is more efficient than trying to stay abreast of the literature by regular reading, considering the time constraints of a busy clinical practice and the overwhelming amount of new information being published. Ongoing advances in technology will continue to facilitate this process as access to information is improved.

Annotated Bibliography

Freedman KB, Brookenthal KR, Fitzgerald RH Jr, Williams S, Lonner JH: A meta-analysis of thromboembolic prophylaxis following elective total hip arthroplasty. *J Bone Joint Surg Am* 2000;82:929-938.
This meta-analysis found that warfarin and low molecular weight heparin decreased the risk of proximal deep vein thrombosis and pulmonary embolism; however, low molecular weight heparin was associated with more bleeding complications.

Hawker GA, Wright JG, Coyte PC, et al: Differences between men and women in the rate of use of hip and knee arthroplasty. *N Engl J Med* 2000;342:1016-1022.

This study found that arthroplasty for severe arthritis was underutilized in both sexes, but the degree of underuse was more than three times as great in women as in men.

Kreder HJ: Evidence-based surgical practice: What is it and do we need it? *World J Surg* 1999;23:1232-1235.

This is an overview of the concept of evidence-based surgery.

Post MW, de Witte LP, Schrijvers AJ: Quality of life and the ICIDH: Towards an integrated conceptual model for rehabilitation outcomes research. *Clin Rehabil* 1999; 13:5-15.

This article proposes a framework for conceptualizing health measurement.

Simeonsson RJ, Lollar D, Hollowell J, Adams M: Revision of the international classification of impairments, disabilities, and handicaps: Developmental issues. *J Clin Epidemiol* 2000;53:113-124.

The new WHO concept of well-being is described.

Swiontkowski MF, Engelberg R, Martin DP, Agel J: Short musculoskeletal function assessment questionnaire: Validity, reliability, and responsiveness. *J Bone Joint Surg Am* 1999;81:1245-1260.

The development of a musculoskeletal outcomes assessment instrument is described.

User's Guide to Evidence Based Practice. Evidence Based Medicine Informatics Project. Available at http://www.cche.net/principles/content_all.asp. Accessed 1999.

This series provides detailed methodology for critically appraising the literature and quantifying the observed effects. The series also provides guidance in applying knowledge learned from the literature to everyday clinical practice.

Wright JG: Outcomes research: What to measure. *World J Surg* 1999;23:1224-1226.

This article provides an overview of health measurement.

Wright JG, Young NL, Waddell JP: The reliability and validity of the self-reported patient-specific index for total hip arthroplasty. *J Bone Joint Surg Am* 2000;82: 829-837.

This article reports on the validation of the self-reported version of a new type of outcome questionnaire that considers how individual patients weigh specific concerns in rating the outcome of total hip arthroplasty.

Classic Bibliography

Epstein AM: The outcomes movement: Will it get us where we want to go? *N Engl J Med* 1990;323:266-270.

Espehaug B, Engesaeter LB, Vollset SE, Havelin LI, Langeland N: Antibiotic prophylaxis in total hip arthroplasty: Review of 10,905 primary cemented total hip replacements reported to the Norwegian Arthroplasty register, 1987 to 1995. *J Bone Joint Surg Br* 1997;79:590-595.

Evidence-based medicine: A new approach to teaching the practice of medicine: Evidence-based medicine working group. *JAMA* 1992;268:2420-2425.

Gartland JJ: Orthopaedic clinical research: Deficiencies in experimental design and determinations of outcome. *J Bone Joint Surg Am* 1988;70:1357-1364.

Keller RB, Rudicel SA, Liang MH: Outcomes research in orthopaedics. *Instr Course Lect* 1994;43:599-611.

Kreder HJ, Deyo RA, Koepsell T, Swiontkowski MF, Kreuter W: Relationship between the volume of total hip replacements performed by providers and the rates of postoperative complications in the state of Washington. *J Bone Joint Surg Am* 1997;79:485-494.

LeLorier J, Gregoire G, Benhaddad A, Lapierre J, Derderian F: Discrepancies between meta-analyses and subsequent large randomized, controlled trials. *N Engl J Med* 1997;337:536-542.

Wennberg J, Gittelsohn A: Small area variations in health care delivery. *Science* 1973;182:1102-1108.

Chapter 12

Medical Care of Athletes

Eric C. McCarty, MD

Kurt P. Spindler, MD

Daniel C. Wascher, MD

Injury and Prevention

Fitness Profiles

Each sport has specific demands and requirements for participation and for prevention of injury. Attributes that may be important include cardiopulmonary fitness, strength, flexibility, body morphology, speed, agility, hand-eye coordination, and age. To identify athletes who may be at risk for injury, it is helpful to examine fitness profiles that are developed for each sport.

Gender-Specific Injuries

Types and rates of injuries are different in males and females. Basketball has been well studied with regard to gender differences. Females have a 25% greater risk of sustaining a grade I ankle sprain than do males, but there is no difference between genders in grade II or III sprains, fractures, or syndesmotic sprains. Female athletes have a significantly higher rate of knee injuries, including a three to eight times greater risk of anterior cruciate ligament (ACL) injuries than males. Various theories have suggested anatomic differences (including notch size and ACL size), joint laxity, hormones, proprioception, and training techniques. Women have greater knee laxity and less joint proprioception function than men. It is unclear which differences result in increased risk, but the role of hormonal fluctuations on the incidence of injury is an area of intense investigation.

Sport-Specific Injuries

Various sports are associated with particular injuries. In general, overhead sports such as tennis and baseball cause more problems with the shoulder and elbow than other sports. Contact sports that involve the head and neck (for example, football) are associated with a higher incidence of concussions and cervical spine injuries. Activities such as soccer, basketball, and football that involve pivoting and cutting maneuvers tend to produce more ACL injuries than other sports. Endurance participants such as long distance runners and cyclists tend to have overuse injuries of the lower extremity such as patellar tendinitis or iliotibial band tendinitis. Sports that involve gripping an object, such as racquet sports, often produce upper extremity tendinitis problems such as lateral epicondylitis. Ankle sprains occur in any sport that involves bipedal movement. The sports responsible for the greatest number of eye injuries are baseball, ice hockey, and racquet sports. Some injuries are almost always sport-specific (Table 1).

Age-Specific Issues

Regular participation in exercise and athletics has been shown to be beneficial for participants of all ages. In middle aged and older people, participation in some form of regular exercise has been shown to reduce age-related health declines and provide psychological benefits. A recent randomized controlled trial over a 10-year period demonstrated the benefits of a walking program in older women. Exercise prevented hip fractures from falls by increasing bone density, coordination, balance, and muscle strength.

Most studies suggest a positive role for organized sports participation in youth populations. Sports participation is associated with positive mental and physical health benefits, but also with an increased risk of injury. Most supervised sports training does not affect growth, maturation, or nutritional status during puberty. Over the past decade there has been an increased emphasis on one-sport specialization by children and adolescents. Adolescent burnout and parental fighting have sometimes resulted from the pressures placed on children to participate and to win. Young athletes who specialize in just one sport may be denied the benefits of varied activity while facing additional physical, physiologic, and psychologic demands from intense training and competition. Thus, children

TABLE 1 | Unique Sport-Specific Injuries

Sport	Injury
Ballet	Painful os trigonum
Baseball	Axillary artery thrombosis or aneurysm
Baseball/golf	Hamate fracture
Cycling	Ulnar neuropathy in Guyon's canal
Rock climbing	Annular pulley injury of proximal phalanx
Rowing	Stress fracture of rib
Volleyball	Suprascapular neuropathy
Wrestling	Auricular hematoma (cauliflower ear)

involved in sports should be encouraged to participate in a number of different activities to develop a wide range of skills.

Protective Equipment

The purpose of protective equipment is to prevent injury and protect injured areas from further injury. Basic characteristics of any type of protective device is that it conforms well to the body, does not or only minimally interferes with the athlete's performance, and does not present any danger to other participants. Custom-made mouth guards have been shown to be better than stock or mouth-formed (boil and bite) guards in the prevention of traumatic dental injuries. Soccer shin guards may provide protection against tibial fractures. Bicycle helmets reduce the risk of head and brain injury by 63% to 88% in cyclists of all ages and reduce the number of injuries to the upper and midfacial areas by approximately 66%. In hockey, the use of full-face shields instead of half-face shields significantly reduced the risk of sustaining facial and dental injuries without an increase in the risk of neck injuries, concussions, or other injuries. Most studies have demonstrated the effectiveness of wrist guards in limiting the severity of wrist injuries in sports such as inline skating or snowboarding; however, some studies do not show any biomechanical advantage. Proper eye and facial protection has been shown to minimize the risk of severe injury and potential vision loss in racquet and contact sports.

Shoewear

The type of shoewear needed varies and depends on the forces exerted on the foot. Soft-soled shoes have been found to be a factor in turf-toe injuries in football players. Football turf shoes need to have a firm sole to resist hyperextension of the first metatarsophalangeal joint. Removable metal forefoot inserts can provide the necessary firmness. Taping can help prevent great toe hyperextension. Shoewear may play an important role in the occurrence and treatment of stress fractures. High-top sneakers have been demonstrated to play a role in the prevention of inversion ankle injuries by significantly increasing the passive resistance to inversion already afforded by braces and tape.

Knee Braces

The use of knee braces in the prevention and rehabilitation of knee injuries may hold some advantages, but the overall effectiveness is inconclusive.

Prophylactic Braces

Prophylactic knee braces are used to decrease and potentially lessen the severity of knee injuries. In football, the most commonly injured ligament of the knee is the medial collateral ligament (MCL). Many braces have been designed to prevent valgus knee injury and subsequent MCL injury by providing a lateral strut over the joint.

Rehabilitation Braces

Rehabilitation braces are used primarily after ligamentous reconstruction of the knee to allow protected and controlled motion during healing. They are also used during rehabilitation of knee injuries treated nonsurgically. These braces may be helpful in multiligament knee reconstruction, but no demonstrable benefit has been shown on postoperative outcome after ACL reconstruction alone.

Functional Braces

Functional knee braces are designed to give stability and support during rotational, varus-valgus, and AP forces. They also can limit range of motion, especially extreme hyperextension and flexion. Knee control is gained by leverage from the brace and increased surface contact. Wearing a brace may enhance proprioception. Subjective improvement is reported with use of the functional brace after ACL reconstruction, but objective improvement is not evident when tested at physiologic stress levels. Current studies have not found any significant advantage in using a brace after ACL reconstruction. In fact, most braces appear to significantly slow hamstring muscle reaction times at the voluntary level. Energy expenditure and muscle fatigue have been shown to increase significantly with brace use. However, braces can be used to protect an MCL injury by limiting valgus forces or restricting extension or hyperextension after a posterior capsular strain.

Female Athlete Triad

The pressure of achieving or maintaining an unrealistically low body weight has led to the entity known as the female athlete triad. First used in 1992, this term encompasses three interrelated components: disordered eating, amenorrhea, and osteoporosis. The eating disorder may be anorexia nervosa, bulimia, or others. Amenorrhea usually occurs when the menstrual cycle ceases after menarche. Osteoporosis results from the menstrual dysfunction and lack of estrogen and can lead to bone fragility with increased fracture risk.

The prevalence of the female athlete triad is unknown and difficult to determine because of the underrecognition of the entity and the secretive nature of eating disorders. When an athlete is suspected of one component of the triad, she should be carefully screened for the other components. Screening includes an extensive medical, psychosocial, and nutritional history plus a comprehensive physical examination. Tests that may be helpful include bone densitometry, blood hormone levels, general blood chemistry, and urinalysis. When an eating disorder is suspected, the athlete needs to be evaluated by a multidisciplinary team of health care professionals trained in dealing with this problem. Once the diagnosis is made, intervention must involve nutritional and exercise counseling as well as psychotherapy. Hormone therapy may be beneficial. The prognosis is more favorable if the triad is detected early and treatment initiated.

The menstrual cycle can be affected by chronic exercise alone. However, secondary amenorrhea is unlikely without additional metabolic stressors. Prospective exercise studies have not shown that exercise causes secondary amenorrhea.

Preparticipation Examination

The primary objective of the preseason physical examination is to determine current medical status and identify any conditions that may predispose an athlete to injury or that may be potentially life-threatening. In approximately 1% of athletes screened at all levels, something found on the examination disqualifies them from competition, most often because of a musculoskeletal disorder. The second most common reason is a cardiac abnormality, although many cardiac abnormalities are not detected by routine preparticipation examination. The most common cardiac abnormalities causing disqualification from competition are valve problems (such as mitral valve prolapse) and rhythm and conduction irregularities, but the most serious cardiac problem in athletes is hypertrophic cardiomyopathy. This condition is the most common cause of sudden death in athletes age 12 to 32 years. Most athletes with this condition do not have any preceding symptoms to the event.

The key components to the preparticipation examination are the history, vital signs, general medical examination, and musculoskeletal examination. Other aspects such as fitness testing or body composition determination may be added. The routine use of ancillary tests (radiograph, electrocardiogram) is not recommended unless there is something in the history or physical examination that indicates a current or past problem. The current recommendation from the American Heart Association is that the routine use of a 12-lead electrocardiogram is not warranted in screening high school and collegiate athletes. Guidelines endorsed by the American Heart Association, the American Academy of Pediatrics, and the American College of Cardiology include a preparticipation physical examination on every athlete competing for the first time in high school and college. High school athletes need a repeat examination every 2 years, with an interim history taken in the alternating years. Collegiate athletes should have a comprehensive examination and history before competing in their first year, and each subsequent year an interim history and blood pressure measurement should be obtained. Any active problems are followed up every year.

Disqualification of an athlete depends on a number of criteria, such as the seriousness of the condition, whether the athlete is involved in a contact/collision, limited contact, or noncontact sport, the strenuousness of the activity, and whether other participants are at risk for injury. Contact and limited contact sports carry more contraindications for participation with medical conditions than noncontact sports because of the potentially harmful impact involved in the sports. These contraindications include various spine problems, heart conditions, internal organ disorders, and systemic dysfunction.

On-the-Field Evaluation

The evaluation of an injured athlete requires the ability to rapidly recognize and treat a multitude of problems. Access to emergency services should be readily available.

Equipment

The team physician's medical bag contains many of the medications and small equipment for proper initial treatment of an emergency on the sideline and for treating various ailments on the road (hotel, bus, plane) or in the training room. Typically, advanced cardiac life support medications are carried, as well as medications such as antibiotics, antihistamines, anti-inflammatory agents, gastrointestinal medications, local anesthestics (such as lidocaine), and an assortment of other medications. It is necessary to keep the bag well stocked and to restock it after every competition or trip. A list of possible contents is shown in Table 2.

In addition to the medical bag, some larger equipment may be helpful for the physician on the sideline or in a locker room on the road. These items may be necessary to treat a cardiac condition or splint an injured limb (Table 2).

Assessment and Treatment

Head and Neck Injuries

Head and neck injuries are common in contact sports. In football, head injuries are almost twice as frequent as neck injuries. The most common head injury in athletics is a concussion. An interassociation task force recently formulated some guidelines that are helpful in determining when to allow return to play for athletes with concussions (Table 3). To prevent potential cumulative brain damage and the second impact syndrome, any athlete still experiencing postconcussion symptoms (headache, dizziness, nausea, confusion, blurred vision) should not return to competition. After a concussion injury, brain cells are in an extremely vulnerable state because of metabolic dysfunction. The potentially devastating second impact syndrome (50% mortality rate) occurs from diffuse cerebral swelling with delayed catastrophic deterioration that occurs when an individual sustains a second, sometimes minor, trauma to the head before resolution of the symptoms of the first head trauma. Additionally, any athlete who sustains a prolonged loss of consciousness should be transported immediately to a hospital for further evaluation. It is important during the evaluation of an unconscious athlete to treat as though a cervical spine injury is present and to rule out any associated injuries.

Neuropsychological functions, such as memory, information processing, and the ability to plan, have been shown to be impaired in athletes who sustain concussions while participating in football or soccer. Neuropsychological testing is advocated as a sensitive means to assess cognitive impairment that occurs after a concussion. It could potentially provide objective measures for a physician in deciding when to allow the athlete to return to play.

Neck injuries include cervical sprains, fractures, spinal cord injury, transient quadriplegia, and stingers (burners). The most important goal of on-the-field assessment of an injured athlete with a suspected neck injury is to prevent any further injury. The head and neck must be immobilized with gentle longitudinal traction. In a football or hockey player, the helmet and chinstrap must remain in place until it can be deter-

TABLE 2 | Team Physician Equipment

The Medical Bag

Stethoscope	Vaseline and Xeroform gauze
Oral airway	Irrigation kit
Endotracheal tube	Telfa pads
Laryngoscope	Moleskin
Blood pressure cuff	Nail clippers
Angiocath needles (16 g and 18 g)	Packing (tampon)
Intravenous tubing	Forceps
Alcohol and Betadine swabs	Penlight
Betadine scrub	Otoscope/opthalmoscope
Hydrogen peroxide	Batteries
Sterile saline (small bottle)	Petroleum jelly
Cotton swabs	Tape (cloth, stretch)
Ace bandages	Reflex hammer
Plastic bandages (Band-aids)	Scalpels
Steri-strips	Fiberglass roll
Sterile gauze pads (2 × 2, 4 × 4)	Slings
Aluminum finger splints	Syringes
Gloves (nonsterile and sterile)	Needles
Thermometer	Scissors
Tongue depressors	Eye chart
Hemostats	Eye patch
Suture kit	Fluorescein strip
Suture	Ultraviolet penlight

Medications

Nonsteroidal anti-inflammatory drugs (variety)	Lidocaine, marcaine
Antibiotics (such as keflex, amoxicillin, zithromycin, ciprofloxacin, tetracycline, acetaminophen)	Antinausea medications (milk of magnesia)
	Bacitracin
	Albuterol inhaler
Analgesic (such as Tylenol with codeine)	Antifungal agent
Prednisone (medrol dose pack)	Sunscreen
Diphenhydramine	Cardiac medications (such as atropine, nitroglycerin, digoxin, verapamil, dopamine, beta-blocker)
Cough syrup	
Antihistamines (such as Claritin or Zyrtec)	
Muscle relaxant (such as Robaxin, Valium)	
Lomotil, loperamide	Eye drops
Epi-pen (injectable epinephrine)	

Sideline/Locker Room Equipment

Cardiac monitor/defibrillator	Fluids-D5 Ringer's lactate, normal saline
Crutches	
Stretcher	Oxygen tank with facemask
Spine board	Bolt cutter/screwdriver
Cervical collar (such as Philadelphia)	Cellular telephone
Slings	Splints (air and rigid)
	Blanket

mined in a controlled environment that no spine injury has occurred. Several studies have demonstrated that the maintenance of a neutral position of the neck and prevention of secondary injury to the cervical spine and spinal cord requires the shoulder pads to be left on until the helmet is taken off. If the airway needs to be accessed, the facemask can be removed. Any injury to the neck should be examined with radiographs and then further studies as deemed necessary.

The common stinger or burner occurs in 50% to 70% of college football players during a 4-year career. The injury typically results from a blow to the head or neck and presents as an intense sharp burning pain that radiates from the neck into the arm. It occurs as either a nerve root compression injury or a traction injury of the upper trunk of the brachial plexus (C5 and C6). Weakness and numbness sometimes occur. Symptoms and strength deficits typically improve rapidly, but it is not uncommon for deficits to be present for several days or weeks after the injury. A return to sports is not recommended until all symptoms have resolved and the neck and neurologic examinations are normal.

Transient quadriplegia is a temporary neurapraxia of the spinal cord that occurs without a fracture or dislocation. It is differentiated from a stinger in that both sides of the body are involved and complete paralysis can occur in both upper and lower extremities. The paralysis usually lasts no more than 10 minutes, and full recovery can be expected in most people. Athletes who have experienced transient quadriplegia usually have a narrowing of the anteroposterior diameter of the cervical canal with a ratio (Pavlov's ratio) of the canal to the vertebral body <0.8 as evident on lateral radiographs. However, narrowing of the spinal canal is evident in one third of asymptomatic football players and thus is not a contraindication in itself to participation in contact sports. There is no documented predisposition to permanent neurologic injury after an episode of transient quadriplegia, but more than one occurrence is a contraindication to further participation.

Eye Injuries

Ninety percent of eye injuries in athletes are preventable with proper eye protection. The sports in which eye injuries are most common are baseball (age 14 years or younger) and basketball (14 years and older). Testing for acuity and extraocular muscle function, inspection for lacerations, foreign bodies and abrasions of the cornea and sclerae, and examination of the anterior chamber for bleeding (hyphema) can all be easily done by the team physician. A patch should then be applied for more serious injuries (except for suspected globe rupture where an eye shield is more appropriate) and immediate referral to a specialist is recommended.

TABLE 3	Guidelines for Altered Consciousness/ Return to Play

After episode of altered consciousness, the athlete should be observed for a minimum of 15 minutes with serial neurologic evaluations

Athlete may return to play the same day if:

Signs and symptoms are cleared within 15 minutes or less at rest and exertion

Normal neurologic evaluation

No documented loss of consciousness

Athlete is excluded from same-day participation if:

Signs and symptoms do not clear within 15 minutes at rest or exertion

Documented loss of consciousness

Beware of vomiting after suspected head injury or new headaches in first 48 to 72 hours after a concussion (these conditions require further medical evaluation)

(Adapted with permission from Wojtys EM, Hovda D, Landry G, et al: Current concepts: Concussion in sports. *Am J Sports Med* 1999;27:676–687.)

Initial treatment for a hyphema is to keep the athlete supine with the head elevated 30° to 40°.

Thoracic Injuries

Thoracic injuries typically are caused by blunt trauma. The most common injury is a rib fracture, which can occur from direct impact or as a stress fracture, as often seen in rowers. The most serious injuries to the thoracic area are those to the heart and lungs. Although rare, low-energy impact to the chest (commotio cordis) can cause cardiac arrest and sudden death in a young athlete. Most of these incidents occur in youth baseball. The cause is hypothesized to be the timing of a chest blow during a narrow window within the repolarization phase of the cardiac cycle when the heart is electrically vulnerable. Resuscitative efforts sometimes are successful. There is inconclusive evidence that soft chest protectors or soft baseballs help prevent this injury. Other causes of sudden cardiac death in athletes are myocardial contusion, hypertrophic cardiomyopathy, cardiac disease (most common cause in older athletes), and electrical disturbances. Injuries to the lungs include pulmonary contusions and pneumothoraces. Tension pneumothorax in an athlete needs to be immediately recognized as absent breath sounds and treated with a 16-gauge needle placed in the second intercostal space at the midclavicular line.

Abdominal Injuries

Abdominal injuries in athletics usually occur from blunt trauma. The spleen is the most commonly affected organ; a ruptured spleen requires surgical intervention. Any athlete with an enlarged spleen should not be allowed to play a contact sport until it has been clinically resolved for at least 4 weeks. Hematuria in association with flank pain usually indicates trauma to the kidney(s). Kidney trauma is intracapsular 85% of the time and treatment is nonsurgical. Significant injury to the abdomen usually is present in athletes who have symptoms such as abdominal pain and tenderness, guarding, rigidity, hypotension, nausea, vomiting, and pallor. When in doubt, an abdominal CT should be obtained to rule out injury.

Heat and Cold Injuries

Heat injuries in athletes include a spectrum of ailments. Minor occurrences include heat edema (mild swelling), heat syncope (orthostatic hypotension of an athlete secondary to pooling of blood), and heat cramps. More significant heat injuries are heat exhaustion and heat stroke. Heat exhaustion, the most common heat-related illness, is characterized by signs of weakness, nausea, vomiting, confusion, headache, orthostasis, and the inability to continue in competition. The athlete's core temperature is less than 104°F. Heat stroke, the second leading cause of death in American professional football, is characterized by collapse accompanied by significant neurologic impairment (delirium, behavioral changes, coma), tachycardia, tachypnea, hypotension, and sometimes anhydrosis. The athlete's core temperature is greater than 105°F. The team physician must quickly assess the seriousness of heat illness and measure the core temperature with a rectal thermometer. It must be determined whether life support or emergency cooling measures must be instituted. A cooling tub can be used, or tepid water over the body with a fan blowing to promote evaporative cooling. Ice packs should be placed on the neck, groin, and axillae. In severe cases, rehydration should be instituted with intravenous fluids. Return to competition for the athlete with heat exhaustion is based on the severity and response to cooling, and it is mandatory that temperature and mental status are normal. With heat stroke, a return to competition can occur after complete recovery from any complications and the athlete has demonstrated the ability to acclimate to heat, a process that takes approximately 2 months to 1 year.

The team physician needs to take a lead role in the prevention of heat injuries. The athlete must acclimate to heat by exercising moderately in the heat. Avoidance of vigorous exercise is advised when the wet bulb-globe temperature is higher than 82°F. Hydration is another key component to prevention of heat illnesses. Hydration begins before the event or practice and continues throughout the period of exertion and afterward, with the goal that fluid intake should match sweat losses. During prolonged competition, water or preferably fluids that contain carbohydrates and electrolytes to assist water transport in the intestine and to improve palatability should be taken. Salt supplements with adequate fluid intake also have recently been found to be advantageous in preventing heat-related illnesses.

The team physician also may be faced with cold injuries such as chilblain, frostbite, and hypothermia. Chilblain is a localized superficial skin lesion caused by prolonged exposure to the cold that may blister and itch but is rarely a problem. Frostbite, which can be insidious in onset, is the destruction of exposed areas of skin that occurs by the freezing of the cells, leading to the formation of crystals within the cells with dehydration and ultimately cell death. Third-degree frostbite sometimes causes mummification and spontaneous amputation of the dead tissue. Treatment involves gentle rewarming in warm water (100°F to 104°F). There are varying degrees of hypothermia. Restoration of adequate core body temperature is the key in treatment of hypothermia. Proper layered clothing, staying dry, adequate fluids and food, and using common sense will prevent hypothermia.

Airway Injuries

Exercise-induced bronchospasm (EIB) is a transient airway constriction that occurs in both large and small airways after strenuous exertion. An athlete with EIB does not necessarily have a history of asthma. Symptoms include wheezing, coughing, or sometimes shortness of breath. Prevention is the primary goal in managing EIB. Measures include warming up before strenuous exercise, keeping the mouth and nose covered in cold weather, exercising in warm, humidified environments, and cooling down after exercise. Aerobic fitness and good control of baseline bronchial reactivity also help. Short- and long-acting inhaled $\beta2$-agonists are highly effective at reducing the magnitude of EIB and are the medications of choice in EIB prophylaxis.

Exercise-induced anaphylaxis is an uncommon yet potentially life-threatening condition. The symptoms are those seen in any anaphylactic reaction: wheezing, shortness of breath, rash, pruritus, erythema over the body, and potential vascular collapse. Exposure to certain allergens (foods, medications, environmental) near the start of exercise is thought to be the cause of this condition. Initial management is with epinephrine injection, an antihistamine, and transport to the nearest hospital. Prevention is predicated on identification of inciting allergens.

Muscle Injuries

Muscle injuries can be divided into muscle strains and muscle contusions. Muscle strains are indirect injuries caused by excessive eccentric loading of the muscle-tendon unit. Failure typically occurs at the myotendinous junction, although tendon avulsions from bone can occur. Risk factors for muscle strains include muscle weakness, decreased flexibility, inadequate warmup, muscle fatigue, and a history of previous injury. Muscle contusions are caused by direct compressive loads applied to the muscle.

Regardless of the injury type, muscle healing occurs in three distinct phases. The first phase is characterized by inflammation, necrosis of damaged muscle, and phagocytosis of necrotic debris. The second phase is characterized by activation of myogenic precursor cells, or satellite cells, and protein synthesis. These satellite cells proliferate and differentiate into myotubules and eventually into myofibers. The final phase is characterized by maturation or remodeling and gradual recovery of the functional properties of the muscle.

Traditionally muscle injuries have been initially treated with activity modification and modalites and occasionally brief immobilization, followed by a progressive stretching and exercise program. Nonsteroidal anti-inflammatory drugs (NSAIDs) are commonly used to limit pain and swelling after muscle injury. Experimental studies with NSAIDs in muscle injury have shown conflicting results, with some studies showing no effect on myofiber regeneration and others showing delayed muscle regeneration in the NSAID-treated group. Direct injection of corticosteroids into areas of muscle strain also has been advocated to promote healing. A recent review of 58 professional football players who received intramuscular corticosteroid injection for a severe, discrete hamstring strain showed a mean time to return to full activity of 7.6 days. No complications related to the injection were seen. However, using an animal muscle contusion model, investigators found that corticosteroid treatment caused irreversible disorganization of the healing muscle fiber structure and a marked decrease in force-generating capacity. Pulsed ultrasound also has been used to promote muscle healing in athletes. A recent study found that ultrasound promoted satellite cell proliferation but found no significant effect on overall muscle healing.

Overuse Injuries
Soft-Tissue Overuse Injuries

Overuse injuries are a frequent cause of morbidity and lost training time in military recruits. Between 25% to 30% of recruits undergoing basic training sustain overuse injuries, with approximately 75% of these in the lower extremity. The most common diagnoses are stress fracture, iliotibial band syndrome, patellar tendinitis, Achilles tendinitis, plantar fasciitis, and shin splints. Similar rates and distribution of injuries have also been found in civilian endurance runners. Anatomic risk factors for overuse injuries include decreased hamstring flexibility, dynamic pes planus, pes cavus, restricted ankle dorsiflexion, and increased hindfoot inversion. A recent study found that the addition of a hamstring stretching program in military basic trainees decreased lower extremity overuse injuries from 29% to 17%. Treatment of soft-tissue overuse injuries involves activity modification, NSAIDs, a stretching and strengthening program, and a gradual return to activity.

Stress Fractures

Repetitive exercise can cause strain within bone that exceeds its local strength and causes microdamage. A recent in vitro study showed high strains in the second metatarsal under normal walking conditions. Simulated muscle fatigue and plantar fascia release caused an increase in strain in the second metatarsal. Bone subjected to repetitive strain attempts to strengthen itself by remodeling, which first involves bone reabsorption, followed by new bone formation. If high strains continue during the reabsorption phase, the microdamage in the bone may progress to a stress fracture.

A stress fracture is characterized by pain during activity that is relieved by rest. On examination there is discrete tenderness over the area of the stress fracture. Plain radiographs often are negative initially. Bone scintigraphy shows increased uptake at the area of the stress fracture and remains the imaging study of choice. MRI is very accurate in diagnosing stress fractures and it is advantageous because it depicts the degree of bone involvement and helps to identify other injuries.

Risk factors for stress fractures include a rapid increase in exercise time or intensity, decreased lower extremity strength, low bone density, and a history of menstrual disturbances. Military recruits who played basketball regularly for at least 2 years before basic training had a significantly lower incidence of stress fractures than recruits who did not play basketball. Strategies to prevent stress fractures include gradually increasing physical activity, use of biomechanical shoe orthoses, and lower extremity strength training before beginning a high-intensity period of training.

Stress fractures in athletes are most common in the tibia, followed by the tarsal bones, metatarsals, femur, and fibula. Stress fractures also can occur in the trunk and upper extremity in weight lifters, overhead athletes, and rowers. Most stress fractures can be successfully treated by limiting activities, followed by a muscle strengthening program and a graduated return to activity. Some stress fractures have a poor prognosis for rapid healing with nonsurgical treatment, including the anterior tibia, fifth metatarsal metaphysis, navicular, and superior femoral neck. Early surgical intervention for fixation or bone grafting may be indicated for these areas.

Exertional Compartment Syndrome

Exertional or chronic compartment syndrome is thought to be caused by an exercise-induced increase in the intracompartmental pressure that is sufficient to impair local perfusion, leading to tissue ischemia, pain, and sometimes a temporary neurologic deficit. The most common locations are the anterior and deep posterior leg compartments. Patients present with exercise-induced pain in the affected compartment that improves quickly with rest. Physical examination at rest usually is normal. The definitive diagnosis is made on the basis of intracompartment pressure measurements. An elevated preexercise resting pressure and a prolongation of the time it takes for the pressure to return to normal after exercise are diagnostic of exertional compartment syndrome. Recent studies have shown that nuclear medicine imaging, MRI, and near-infrared spectroscopy may be useful noninvasive methods of diagnosing exertional compartment syndrome. If the condition does not improve with a period of rest followed by conditioning, fasciotomy of the involved compartment is performed. The results of fasciotomy for exertional posterior compartment syndrome are less favorable than for involvement of the anterior compartment.

Rehabilitation

Strengthening

Isometric exercise is contraction of a muscle against resistance with no change in its length. Isometric exercises are useful early in rehabilitation when injured or healing structures are being protected from motion. However, strength gains with isometric exercise are specific to the joint position used. Concentric exercise is contraction of a muscle against resistance with shortening of the muscle. Eccentric exercise is contraction of a muscle against resistance with lengthening of the

muscle. Eccentric activity is fundamental to most athletic endeavors. Eccentric training usually is begun during the later stages of rehabilitation because it generates large muscle forces that may cause joint pain and muscle soreness. Both concentric and eccentric exercises can be done as isotonic (against constant resistance) or isokinetic (at a constant velocity) exercises. Isotonic exercises can be done with free weights, machines, or manual resistance. The load placed on a muscle by the same weight at different points in the arc of motion may vary considerably. To overcome this variability, strength training machines have been designed with cam systems to increase loads at the range of motion where the muscle is able to generate larger forces. Isokinetic exercise can be done at slow (60°/s) or at high (300°/s) angular joint velocity. These machines are useful for assessing muscle strength and measuring a patient's rehabilitation progress. However, athletic activities involve much higher angular velocities than is possible with these devices. Open chain exercises are those in which a muscle group is exercising without any contraction from its antagonist group. An example is a leg extension exercise being performed by the quadriceps muscle group. Closed chain exercises are those in which there is cocontraction of opposing muscle groups. An example is a leg press exercise with contraction of both the quadriceps and the hamstring muscle groups. Closed chain exercises more closely simulate functional activities and minimize shear forces across the joints.

Flexibility

Flexibility training has not been conclusively proven to reduce athletic injuries but it is widely used in fitness regimens. Joint motion may be limited by capsular (static) structures or by muscular (active) tightness. When designing a rehabilitation program, it is important to recognize which structures are causing limitations of joint motion. Improvement in active flexibility occurs only when the joint is moved through a range of motion that places the surrounding muscles under tension. Three types of stretching exercises are widely used: static stretching, ballistic stretching, and proprioceptive neuromuscular facilitation (PNF). Static stretching places the muscle under a slow, gentle stretch that is maintained for 20 to 60 seconds. The steady stretch diminishes the muscle stretch reflex and allows gradual lengthening of the muscle-tendon unit. Ballistic stretching involves a forceful, quick movement to stretch the involved muscle. However, ballistic stretching can be counterproductive by activating the muscle stretch reflex and because of its forceful nature may cause muscle injury. PNF attempts to reduce muscle tone by stimulating Golgi tendon organs. The muscle is stretched by a partner and held at its end range for several seconds. A maximal isometric contraction is then performed and held for 5 to 10 seconds. This contraction provides maximum stimulation to the Golgi tendon organs, causing inhibition of the muscle under tension. The muscle is then relaxed and slowly stretched further by the partner. No specific technique is accepted as most effective; all three stretching methods have been shown to increase range of motion when performed on a regular basis.

Plyometrics

Plyometrics are resistance training exercises that involve the conversion from an eccentric muscle contraction to a concentric contraction to produce a forceful movement in a short period of time. An example of a plyometric exercise is jumping off of a box and on landing, immediately jumping back off the ground. Plyometrics have been shown to improve performance in activites that involve explosive muscular power, such as vertical leaping. Overly aggressive plyometric training can produce soft-tissue and joint overuse injuries.

Proprioception

Proprioception, defined as the sensation of joint movement and position, plays an important role in the neuromuscular control required for precision movements as well as for dynamic joint stability. Afferent feedback to the brain is provided by skin, muscle, joint, and ligament mechanoreceptors. Joint injury can cause a decrease in proprioception. Proprioceptive deficits after ACL injury are improved but not completely restored after ACL reconstruction. A recent study of ACL-deficient patients found that wearing a functional brace or a neoprene sleeve did not significantly improve proprioception. It has been postulated that proprioceptive deficits may predispose to further injury. Proprioceptive exercises such as joint repositioning and balance training should be incorporated early into rehabilitation programs.

Modalities

Cryotherapy can relieve pain, reduce muscle spasm, and cause vasoconstriction. The vasoconstriction effect is believed to decrease bleeding, inflammation, and edema formation after an acute injury. Extended application of ice can cause frostbite or neurapraxia of peripheral nerves. Contraindications to cryotherapy include rheumatologic conditions exacerbated by cold, such as Raynaud's phenomenon. Heat also is an effective analgesic and can relieve muscle spasm and joint stiffness by causing a relaxation and lengthening of connective tissue fibers. Heat also increases blood flow to tissue, which can promote lymphatic and venous drainage; however, after an acute injury, this increase in blood flow can exacerbate soft-tissue swelling or joint effusion. Prolonged application of heat can cause thermal injury. Ultrasound uses high-frequency sound waves to generate heat within deeper tissues; therapeutic effects include reduction in pain and muscle spasm. Ultrasound has been shown to enhance cellular proliferation and protein synthesis during the healing of skin wounds, muscle-tendon injuries, and fractures. Electrical stimulation also is widely used to decrease pain and promote healing of soft-tissue injuries. The electrical current can be applied by several techniques with variations in magnitude, polarity, waveform, and frequency.

Sport-Specific Conditioning

Periodization is a concept that involves varying the frequency, duration, and intensity of the workout during an athletic season that consists of five phases: active rest (with cross-training to give the athlete a mental and physical break); off-season phase (during which general athletic fitness is emphasized); preseason phase (high-intensity sport-specific workouts); early in-season phase (during which conditioning is high but not maximal); and late in-season or peaking phase (during which performance for intense competition is maximized).

Adjunctive Treatment

Local Steroid Use

Corticosteroids have been widely used, and abused, to decrease the pain and inflammation associated with athletic injuries. Corticosteroids inhibit phospholipase A_2 and thus both the cyclooxygenase and lipoxygenase pathways of the inflammatory cascade. Although corticosteroids relieve pain and may improve function, they have been shown to have a deleterious effect on the healing of acutely injured ligaments and tendons. Other complications associated with corticosteroids include systemic (such as poor glycemic control in diabetics) and local (fat atrophy, skin pigment changes, ligament and tendon rupture) effects. Corticosteroids should primarily be used in conjunction with rest and rehabilitation as part of a comprehensive program to treat chronic inflammatory conditions and should not be directly injected into tendons or ligaments.

Hyperbaric Oxygen

Hyperbaric oxygen has been shown to help healing of severe soft-tissue injuries, and recently has been promoted as a means to allow more rapid recovery after athletic exertion. A recent study showed no improvement in delayed-onset muscle soreness after hyperbaric oxygen therapy. Another investigation also found no improvement in muscle soreness but did find enhanced recovery of muscle torque in the treatment group.

Medical Issues

Ergogenic Supplements and Drugs

It has been well documented that anabolic steroids induce muscle hypertrophy and increase muscle strength. A recent animal study showed that muscle hypertrophy occurs even in sedentary populations. Widespread testing for anabolic steroids has appeared to decrease their use in collegiate and professional athletes, but not in recreational and high school athletes. A recent survey found that 3% of male and female middle-school students reported using anabolic steroids. Known side effects include endocrine, cardiac, hepatic, and psychological problems.

More recently, prohormones such as dehydroepiandrosterone (DHEA) and androstenedione have been used as anabolic agents. These compounds, which are available as so-called dietary supplements, are thought to be metabolized into anabolic steroids after ingestion. Although DHEA can increase testosterone levels in women, the changes are small and unlikely to have significant performance-enhancing effects. No increase in testosterone levels has been noted in men after ingestion of DHEA or androstenedione.

Several genetically engineered hormones are being used by athletes to improve performance. Human growth hormone and insulin growth factor-I increase muscle size and shorten muscle recovery time. Synthetic erythropoietin causes an increase in red blood cell production and increased aerobic endurance. Autologous transfusion, or blood-doping, can have a similar effect. The resulting polycythemia can cause stroke or myocardial infarction. Creatine is an amino acid dietary supplement that has also gained popularity among athletes. Creatine is converted to phosphocreatine, which can donate phosphorus to increase the formation of adenosine triphosphate, the energy source for skeletal muscle. Ingestion of 3 g/day causes small improvements in exercises involving short periods of high-intensity repetitive activity. Maximal isometric strength and aerobic performance are not affected. A weight gain is seen in the first few days of creatine use, probably because of water retention. Despite anecdotal reports, there is no definitive evidence of untoward side effects with creatine use. Hydroxymethylbutyrate (HMB) is another supplement purported to build muscle. Most studies have not shown an anabolic effect with the use of HMB.

Human Immunodeficiency Virus

The potential exists for human immunodeficiency virus, hepatitis, and other blood-borne pathogens to be trans-mitted during athletic contests. Athletes with active bleeding should be promptly removed from competition. Bleeding must be controlled and any wound properly covered before a player can return to competition.

Annotated Bibliography

Injury and Prevention

American Academy of Pediatrics: Committee on Sports Medicine and Fitness: Intensive training and sports specialization in young athletes. *Pediatrics* 2000;106: 154-157.

This statement reviews the potential risks of high-intensity training and sports specialization in young athletes.

Galloway M, Jokl P: Aging successfully: The importance of physical activity in maintaining health and function. *J Am Acad Orthop Surg* 2000;8:37-44.

This review article emphasizes the importance of regular physical activity for the older patient and reviews the requirements for exercise.

Lynch S, Renstrom P: Treatment of acute lateral ankle ligament rupture in the athlete: Conservative versus surgical treatment. *Sports Med* 1999;27:61-71.

A review of the assessment of the sprained ankle and the treatment options with the scientific basis behind conservative or surgical treatment is presented.

Messina D, Farney W, et al: The incidence of injury in Texas high school basketball: A prospective study among male and female athletes. *Am J Sports Med* 1999;27:294-299.

This prospective study examines the incidence of injury among high school basketball players and the differences in injury type, incidence, rate, and risk between male and female athletes.

Thacker S, Stroup D, et al: The prevention of ankle sprains in sports: A systematic review of the literature. *Am J Sports Med* 1999;27:753-760.

This article presents an extensive review of the published literature discussing the risk of ankle sprains in sports, methods to provide support, the effect of these interventions on performance, and comparison of prevention efforts.

Waninger K: On-field management of potential cervical spine injury in helmeted football players: Leave the helmet on! *Clin J Sport Med* 1998;8:124-129.

The author provides a critical review of the scientific evidence on cervical spine management in helmeted football players with suspected cervical spine injury.

Wing R: Physical activity in the treatment of the adulthood overweight and obesity: Current evidence and research issues. *Med Sci Sports Exerc* 1999;31(suppl 11):S547-S552.

This article reviews the randomized trials examining the role of physical activity in the treatment of adult overweight and obesity.

Knee Braces

Greene D, Hamson K, et al: Effects of protective knee bracing on speed and agility. *Am J Sports Med* 2000; 28:453-459.

This study demonstrated that the use of prophylactic knee braces on athletes does not significantly reduce speed or agility.

Risberg M, Holm I, et al: The effect of knee bracing after anterior cruciate ligament reconstruction: A prospective, randomized study with two years' follow-up. *Am J Sports Med* 1999;27:76-83.

This prospective randomized study evaluated the effect of rehabilitative and functional knee bracing after ACL reconstruction and found no significant difference for a majority of the parameters.

On-the-Field Injuries

Basilico F: Cardiovascular disease in athletes. *Am J Sports Med* 1999;27:108-121.

This article presents a review of cardiovascular diseases that may limit an athlete's participation in sports and potentially put an athlete at risk for sudden cardiac death. The cardiovascular preparticipation screening examination and guidelines for allowing athletes to play with heart conditions are discussed.

Latzka W, Montain S: Water and electrolyte requirements for exercise. *Clin Sports Med* 1999;18:513-524.

This article reviews the physiology and clinical applications for fluid and electrolyte maintenance during activity.

Matser E, Kessels A, et al: Neuropsychological impairment in amateur soccer players. *JAMA* 1999;282: 971-973.

This study demonstrated that participation in amateur soccer in general, and concussion specifically, are associated with impaired performance in memory and planning functions.

Wojtys E, Hovda D, et al: Current concepts: Concussion in sports. *Am J Sports Med* 1999;27:676-687.

A review of head injuries in sports, diagnosis, return to play, and other issues is presented.

Muscle Injuries

Beiner JM, Jokl P, Cholewicki J, et al: The effect of anabolic steroids and corticosteroids on healing of muscle contusion injury. *Am J Sports Med* 1999;27:2-9.

In a rat muscle contusion model, corticosteroids had a negative effect on muscle healing, whereas anabolic steroids improved the recovery of force generating capacity of injured muscle.

Donahue SW, Sharkey NA: Strains in the metatarsals during the stance phase of gait: Implications for stress fractures. *J Bone Joint Surg Am* 1999;81:1236-1244.

Strains were measured in cadaver second and fifth metatarsals after loading with a dynamic gait simulator. Strains in the second metatarsal were twice that of the fifth metatarsal. Simulated muscle fatigue and plantar fasciotomy increased peak strain in the second metatarsal.

Rehabilitation

Beynnon BD, Ryder SH, Konradsen L, et al: The effect of anterior cruciate ligament trauma and bracing on knee proprioception. *Am J Sports Med* 1999;27:150-155.

This study found the threshold to detection of passive knee motion was worse in knees with ACL deficiency. Wearing a functional knee brace or neoprene sleeve did not significantly improve proprioception in the ACL-deficient knee.

Staples JR, Clement DB, Taunton JE, et al: Effects of hyperbaric oxygen on a human model of injury. *Am J Sports Med* 1999;27:600-605.

This controlled, prospective, double-blind study found improvement in recovery of eccentric muscle torque with hyperbaric oxygen treatment but no effect on delayed onset muscle soreness.

Classic Bibliography

American Medical Society for Sports Medicine and the American Academy of Sports Medicine: Human immunodeficiency virus and other blood-borne pathogens in sports. *Am J Sports Med* 1995;23:510-514.

Arendt E, Dick R: Knee injury patterns among men and women in collegiate basketball and soccer: NCAA data and review of literature. *Am J Sports Med* 1995; 23:694-701.

Cantu RC: Guidelines for return to contact sports after a cerebral concussion. *Phys Sportsmed* 1986;14:75-83.

Fadale PD, Wiggins ME: Corticosteroid injections: Their use and abuse. *J Am Acad Orthop Surg* 1994;2: 133-140.

Garrett WE: Muscle strain injuries. *Am J Sports Med* 1996;24:S2-S8.

Kibler WB, Chandler TJ: Sport-specific conditioning. *Am J Sports Med* 1994;22:242-432.

Lephart SM, Pincivero DM, Giraldo JG, et al: The role of proprioception in the management and rehabilitation of athletic injuries. *Am J Sports Med* 1997;25: 130-137.

Maron BJ, Thompson PD, Puffer JC, et al: Cardiovascular preparticipation screening examination of competitive athletes. *Circulation* 1996;94:850-856.

Matheson GO, Clement DB, McKenzie DC, et al: Stress fractures in athletes: A study of 320 cases. *Am J Sports Med* 1987;15:46-58.

Otis C, Drinkwater B, et al: American College of Sports Medicine position stand: The Female Athlete Triad. *Med Sci Sports Exerc* 1997;29:1-9.

Schepsis AA, Martini D, Corbett M: Surgical management of exertional compartment syndrome of the lower leg: Long-term followup. *Am J Sports Med* 1993; 21:811-817.

Sitler M, Ryan J, Hopkinson W, et al: The efficacy of prophylactic knee brace to reduce knee injuries in football: A prospective, randomized study at West Point. *Am J Sports Med* 1990;18:310-315.

Torg JS, Pavlov H, Genuario SE, et al: Neurapraxia of the cervical spinal cord with transient quadriplegia. *J Bone Joint Surg Am* 1986;68:1354-1370.

Chapter 13

Multiply Injured Patients

Steven A. Olson, MD

David J. Hak, MD

Christopher G. Finkemeier, MD

H. David Moehring, MD

A 1998 consensus conference on the effectiveness of trauma centers in the United States reported that there is a 15% to 20% reduction in the risk of death as a result of a trauma center or system being in place. In the United States, the first de facto trauma centers were inner city hospitals, which for the most part provided emergency services to local populations. By contrast, within a modern trauma system, the hospital (trauma center) provides acute care for the severely injured patient, and is a key component of a system that encompasses all phases of care, from prehospital care through acute care and rehabilitation. This so-called "inclusive" trauma system was first described in the Centers for Disease Control and Prevention (CDC) position paper on trauma care systems, and was later redefined in the Model Trauma Care System Plan. The trauma center is a key component of this system, but the system recognizes the necessity of other health care facilities. The goal is to match a facility's resources with a patient's need so that optimal and cost-effective care can be achieved.

Once a trauma center is established, the care providers must triage the patients to determine which facility within the trauma system is most appropriate for that patient. Trauma scoring systems were initially created for the purpose of field triage. An effective field triage tool must be straightforward and user-friendly for prehospital personnel. The scoring system should accurately assess severity of injury—both anatomically and physiologically.

Trauma Scoring Systems

Revised Trauma Score

The revised trauma score (RTS) was developed as a system for field triage. The RTS comprises three parameters: the Glasgow coma score, respiratory rate, and systolic blood pressure. A value from 0 to 4 is assigned for each variable. An RTS score of 10 or less has been shown to accurately identify 97% of fatal injuries. The RTS is currently the most widely used prehospital field triage tool.

Injury Severity Score

The first significant scoring system to be based primarily on anatomic criteria was the injury severity score (ISS), which was created to define injury severity and was not intended to be a field triage system. The application of the ISS comes in providing researchers control of the variability of trauma severity for evaluating outcomes.

The ISS is based on the incorporation of anatomic indices and severity indices. The ISS uses injury severity developed in the abbreviated injury scale (AIS). The AIS was developed in 1971 by an American Medical Association Committee on Aspects for Automotive Safety and revised in 1990 (AIS-90). The ISS uses the highest AIS-90 score from the three most severely injured anatomic areas for any given patient. These AIS-90 values (1 to 5) are each squared, and then summed for a total ISS score. For example, a patient with a flail chest has an AIS-90 thorax of 4, a closed femur fracture AIS-90 skeletal system of 3, a ruptured spleen AIS-90 abdomen of 4; the ISS score for this patient would be 41. The ISS considers only the highest AIS-90 score from any single anatomic site. This decreases the ability of this score to predict injury severity in patients with multiple injuries within the same anatomic area. Nonetheless, the ISS has become an important predictor of injury severity and mortality and is one of the national standards for injury severity assessment. An ISS of 16 or more has been shown to be associated with a mortality of 10%.

New Injury Severity System

In response to the weakness of the ISS in predicting outcomes for a patient with severe injury to a single body area, the new injury severity system (NISS) was proposed. The NISS uses the AIS-90 injury severity

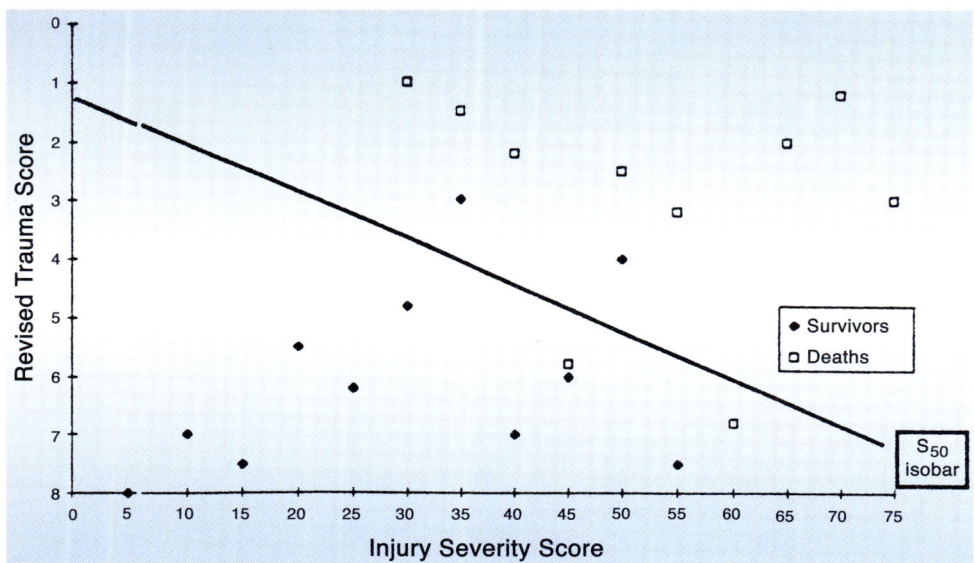

Figure 1 RTS plotted against ISS to predict mortality (the TRISS method). *(Reproduced with permission from Senkowski CK, McKenney MG: Trauma scoring system: A review. J Am Coll Surg 1999;189:491-503.)*

codes. The three highest AIS scores, regardless of anatomic area, are squared and summed to calculate the NISS score. Several reports have demonstrated that the NISS score provides a more accurate prediction of short-term mortality than the ISS scores in comparable populations.

The TRISS Method

The TRISS method for analyzing trauma data was developed by combining the anatomic criteria of the ISS with the physiologic criteria of the RTS. The TRISS method uses logistic regression analysis to correlate the RTS with the ISS to create a S_{50} isobar on which a 50% survival is predicted (Fig. 1). Patient probability of survival is plotted on the RTS versus ISS graph. The 50% survivor cutoff is arbitrary and only provides a method for isolating outlying patients in a particular patient population.

TRISS methodology can be used to compare trauma patient outcomes against a reference database (the Multiple Trauma Outcome Study, or MTOS). Using this method, any trauma service, regardless of size, can compare itself to the MTOS database for outcomes analysis. The TRISS method also can be used as a method of developing normative data for an individual trauma system's database as well.

Anatomic Profile

The anatomic profile is another trauma scoring system based on anatomic location. The anatomic profile is based on the AIS-90 scores with the important difference that the anatomic profile considers only four components. Component A includes head, brain, and spinal cord injuries; component B includes thoracic and anterior neck injuries; component C includes all other major injuries; and component D includes all minor injuries.

The ASCOT Method

The ASCOT (A Severity Characteristic of Trauma) method was developed in an attempt to improve TRISS methodology. The ASCOT system uses the anatomic profile (component scores A, B, and C) and the RTS in a method similar to TRISS methodology in an attempt to develop an S_{50} isobar to predict outcomes for both survival and death from traumatic injury.

The ICISS System

The idea to use ICD-9 (International Classification of Diseases) coded data to create an injury severity scoring system was in response to the amount of resources needed to implement an ISS based system. The resources needed to accurately classify patients by AIS, such as a designated trauma registry and staff to encode and enter the data, is substantial. Although many major urban trauma centers have dedicated staff to maintain trauma registries, smaller urban and rural centers often do not have these resources. These hospitals were previously unable to use the TRISS or ASCOT methodology for quality assurance.

The ICD system is an anatomically based nomenclature system. In 1996, the ICISS (International Classification of Diseases, 9th edition, Injury Severity Score) was created by calculating survival risk ratios using the North Carolina Trauma Registry data for each ICD-9 code. The ICISS system does hold promise as a tool for evaluating injury severity, particularly in those systems without an established trauma registry.

American College of Surgeons Guidelines

The American College of Surgeons (ACS) Committee on Trauma has recently updated "Optimal Resources for Optimal Care of the Injured Patient." This document identifies three distinct types of patients with musculoskeletal injury. The first group consists of patients with isolated closed musculoskeletal injury unassociated with any other fracture or injury potential. The second type of patient group comprises individuals who have multiple fractures of long bone or joint injuries with significant potential for life-threatening injuries. The third type of patient group consists of individuals who have multiple fractures of major long bones, the spinal column, and/or joints associated with additional injuries outside the musculoskeletal system. These patients usually require resources available at a Level 1 or Level 2 trauma center.

Closed Head Injury

Closed head injury is a term that describes a variety of conditions that affect the multiply injured patient with significant head trauma. Diffuse axonal injury occurs without mass lesion in about 25% of patients who die as a result of severe traumatic brain injury. This type of injury is one of the major causes of the persistent vegetative or severely disabled state resulting after traumatic brain injury. Ischemic brain injury is extremely common after severe head injury. It is estimated that 80% to 90% of patients who die of head injury show some elements of ischemia on histopathologic examination of brain tissue. The concept of delayed secondary brain damage is supported by the fact that 30% to 40% of patients who die after head injury experience a so-called lucid interval during which they were able to obey commands or speak. Trauma brain injury may be global or focal, with areas of hematoma or contusion. Recently, studies have shown that in regions of focal injury, what is called a flow-metabolism mismatch occurs, where cerebral blood flow may be significantly decreased and blood glucose utilization by brain tissue is increased.

Survival of the patient with a closed head injury is dependent on the maintenance of adequate cerebral blood flow. Cerebral blood flow is indirectly monitored by the calculation of the cerebral perfusion pressure (CPP), which is a difference between the mean arterial pressure (MAP) and the intracranial pressure (ICP); $CPP = MAP - ICP$. Normal ICP is 10 mm Hg or less. ICP greater than 20 mm Hg typically requires continuous monitoring and treatment. When ICP is increased

to the range of 30 to 35 mm Hg, venous drainage from the brain is impaired, further exacerbating cerebral edema. A minimum cerebral perfusion of > 18 mL/100 g of brain tissue/min is required for neural survival. Below 20 mL/100 g of brain tissue/min, the patient loses consciousness. As the ICP increases, CPPs fall and ischemia occurs. Brain death results when the cerebral perfusion is so severely compromised that oxygen and glucose delivery cease to meet the metabolic needs of the brain.

The classic approach to the management of the multiply injured patient with significant head trauma includes initial neurologic and serial examinations, as well as a rapid CT scan to define the extent of the brain injury. Surgical treatment is primarily directed at evacuation of significant hematomas. Nonsurgical management is designed to maintain adequate cerebral perfusion. It is often necessary to reduce the ICP in these patients using various methods, including hyperventilation, head elevation, and osmotic diuresis with mannitol. Multicenter studies have demonstrated that there is no significant improvement in outcome with the use of steroids for traumatic brain injury. Hypothermia has been proposed as a possible means of improving survival of patients with severe head injury. Treatment with moderate hypothermia to 33°C was shown to lead to hastened neurologic recovery in some patients. Unfortunately, coagulopathy, hypocalcemia, and arrhythmias are associated with this level of hypothermia. Correction and prevention of coagulation abnormalities, including prevention of hypothermia-induced coagulopathy, is also important. Newer progressive lesions on CT scans were reported to occur in 85% of patients with at least one abnormal clotting parameter at the time of admission.

Reports supporting the advantages of early fracture fixation in trauma patients have primarily focused on minimizing pulmonary complications. In patients with moderate to severe closed head injuries, concerns have been raised that early surgical fracture fixation may expose a vulnerable patient to the risk of secondary brain injury. The two most important determinants of secondary brain injury are hypotension and hypoxemia, conditions that may occur during extended orthopaedic surgical interventions. Early surgery for fracture fixation in the under-resuscitated patient has been reported to result in transient hypotension intraoperatively, which adversely affected neurologic outcomes. If surgery to stabilize orthopaedic injuries is undertaken in the initial hours after injury, the status of the patient's resuscitation must be carefully assessed. On occasion, invasive monitoring of hemodynamic parameters may be indicated in this setting.

Chest Trauma

In the multiply injured patient with thoracic injury, a major concern is lung damage with resulting progressive hypoxia. Pulmonary contusion, hemothorax, pneumothorax, and pulmonary laceration all are conditions that can result in significant hypoxia.

The respiratory management of the critically injured patient in the intensive care unit includes refinements of the ventilatory techniques, such as positive pressure support and permissive hypercapnia. These modifications lower energy expenditure by the patient and reduce the potential for barotrauma.

Controversy remains regarding the potential impact of intramedullary reaming in patients with severe pulmonary injuries. Embolization of marrow contents and bone fragments develops after fractures occur and may be exacerbated during intramedullary reaming. Embolized fat and fat-laden thrombi have been suggested to result in a mechanical blockage of the pulmonary microvasculature. It has been proposed that the inflammatory response to free fatty acids damages the pulmonary vascular endothelium, causing lung capillary leak and acute respiratory distress syndrome. Other authors have questioned whether intravascular fat embolization causes such an acute pathologic inflammatory response in the trauma patient. However, isolated embolization of marrow fat in a patient with a normal healthy physiologic state results in no clinically significant inflammation in the pulmonary vasculature. Adequate resuscitation and ventilatory support are the primary treatment modalities used for the resolution of shock in the trauma patient.

According to several recent clinical studies, the extent of the primary pulmonary injury is the major determinant in the development of pulmonary morbidity. A comparison of a large cohort of patients with femur fractures treated with reamed intramedullary nailing versus plating showed no difference in pulmonary morbidity based on skeletal fixation. The pulmonary complications correlated with the primary pulmonary injury.

Controversy exists regarding the best way to evaluate a patient with a suspected injury to the thoracic aorta. Several studies have confirmed aortography as the standard against which other methods should be compared. Recently, transesophageal echocardiography also has been used to evaluate potential traumatic aortic disruptions. The echocardiographic signs of aortic injury are complex and may be confined to a short section of the aorta. One study cautions that operator experience is necessary for echocardiography to be accurate. A patient with a mediastinal injury must be evaluated for possible aortic injury prior to repair of long bone injuries.

Abdomen

The FAST (Focused Assessment with Sonography for Trauma) is now routinely used in many trauma centers for the evaluation of blunt abdominal trauma. The study does not require transportation of the critically ill patient to other areas of the hospital, and can easily be repeated as a follow-up examination. The accuracy of the study, however, depends on the experience of the examiner, and injuries with little free fluid (such as a ruptured bowel) tend to be underestimated.

Although unstable patients with intra-abdominal injuries require immediate surgical intervention, stable patients with injuries of the spleen, liver, and kidneys are increasingly being managed conservatively with serial assessment using CT. The ACS provides definitions of the degree of hemorrhagic shock (Table 1).

Elevated intra-abdominal pressures may lead to a condition referred to as abdominal compartment syndrome, which may result in cardiac, pulmonary, renal, bowel abdominal wall/wound, and intracranial disturbances. Although the abdominal compartment syndrome may be caused by nontraumatic conditions, multiple trauma, massive hemorrhage, or protracted surgery with massive resuscitation are situations in which abdominal compartment syndrome is most frequently encountered. Fascial closure may be delayed following laparotomy in these patients until the intra-abdominal edema is resolved. In the interim, a 3-L sterile irrigation bag, also known as a Bogota bag, or other sterile flexible plastic barrier may be sewn to the fascia or stapled to the skin. Staged or damage-control laparotomy (rapid and focused control of major bleeding combined with packing and other salvage procedures (for example, stapled division of bowel injuries without resection, drainage of pancreaticoduodenal and biliary injuries) in order to avoid the vicious cycle caused by protracted surgical repairs, hypothermia, coagulopathy, and acidosis) also may be beneficial. The abdomen is temporarily closed as just described and the definitive intra-abdominal repairs are performed 24 to 36 hours later when physiologic abnormalities have been corrected.

Spine

There is significant difficulty in diagnosing fractures and dislocations of the cervical spine in unresponsive patients. It is often difficult to obtain adequate plain radiographs. CT scans may also fail to identify significant injuries. Recent reports have analyzed the use of dynamic fluoroscopy to rule out cervical spine injury in the comatose patient. This examination can only be done by an experienced physician. Flexion and extension of the patient's neck is done under live fluoros-

TABLE 1 | Estimated Fluid and Blood Losses Based on Patient's Initial Presentation

	Class I	Class II	Class III	Class IV
Blood loss (mL)	Up to 750	750–1500	1500–2000	> 2000
Blood loss (% blood volume)	Up to 15%	15%–30%	30%–40%	> 40%
Pulse rate	< 100	> 100	> 120	> 140
Blood pressure	Normal	Normal	Decreased	Decreased
Pulse pressure (mm Hg)	Normal or increased	Decreased	Decreased	Decreased
Respiratory rate	14–20	20–30	30–40	> 35
Urine output (mL/hr)	> 30	20–30	5–15	Negligible
Central nervous system/mental status	Slightly anxious	Mildly anxious	Anxious and confused	Confused and lethargic
Fluid replacement (3:1) rule	Crystalloid	Crystalloid	Crystalloid and blood	Crystalloid and blood

(Adapted with permission from *Advanced Trauma Life Support for Doctors, Student Course Manual*, ed 6. Chicago, IL, American College of Surgeons, 1997, p 98.)

copy, with the physician proceeding with further motion only if no abnormalities are seen. MRI also may be useful in this scenario in patients who are responsive, or who later become responsive and report neck pain, tenderness, or other neurologic symptoms referable to the spinal cord, and whose initial radiographs were normal. Active flexion and extension radiographs also may be useful in identifying ligamentous injuries causing instability.

Because of the consequences of a missed fracture of the thoracic and lumbar spine, screening radiographs are recommended for the trauma patient with the following history: multisystem blunt injuries, a fall from a height of 10 ft or more, ejection from a motor vehicle or motorcycle, a Glasgow coma scale score of 8 or less, a neurologic deficit, or back pain and tenderness on physical examination.

High-dose methylprednisolone is recommended for the treatment of acute spinal cord injury. Improvements in motor scores were seen in patients with incomplete spinal cord injuries if steroids were administered within 8 hours of injury. The recommended intravenous dose of methylprednisolone is 30 mg/kg body weight initially over 15 minutes, followed by an infusion of 5.4 mg/kg for 23 hours.

Pelvis/Lower Extremity

Retrograde intramedullary femoral nailing has gained popularity in the treatment of multiply injured patients with femoral shaft fractures. Advantages include simplified supine positioning, ability to perform simultaneous procedures, decreased surgery times, and decreased blood loss. In addition, independent fixation of associated femoral neck fractures is allowed, and violation of subsequent posterior sur-

gical approaches is avoided in patients with ipsilateral acetabular fractures. Concerns associated with retrograde femoral nailing include potentially lower union rates, violation of the knee joint, rotational and alignment errors, and creation of a stress riser at the proximal locking screw site, which could increase the risk of subtrochanteric fractures. Adequate canal fill is important in achieving union, and dynamization may be required at 6 to 12 weeks to minimize the risk of nonunion.

The risks and benefits of reaming in multiply injured trauma patients with long bone fractures are controversial. Reaming may be detrimental to patients with associated lung injuries. Intraoperative transesophageal echocardiography has confirmed that multiple embolic particles pass into the heart during intramedullary nailing. Embolization occurs during reaming, entry into the intramedullary canal, and during placement of nonreamed nails. The passage of particles into the left atrium and subsequently into the systemic circulation may occur in patients with patent foramen ovale (may be present in up to 20% of adults). Reamer design and technique have been shown to be important variables that impact intramedullary pressures during reaming. Reamers with deep cutting flutes and narrow drive shafts are preferred, whereas reamers with narrow flutes and thick drive shafts may increase the intramedullary pressure as the reamer is advanced. Intramedullary pressures also can be reduced by slow advancement of the reamer and intermittent irrigation of the intramedullary canal.

The rapid placement of temporary external fixation of long bone fractures has been proposed as an alternative to immediate intramedullary nailing. This method permits fracture stabilization while minimizing early secondary insults. Emergent external fixation of the femoral shaft can be achieved in 30 minutes or less. Conversion to definitive fixation is performed at a later time when the patient's condition has stabilized. A 97% union rate was achieved after secondary intramedullary nailing in a report of 54 severely injured patients with femoral fractures initially treated with emergent external fixation. A one-stage conversion from external fixator to intramedullary nailing was performed in patients with a relatively short duration of emergent external fixation (usually less than 2 weeks), no signs of systemic infection, no loosening of the external fixator pins, and no erythema or purulent pin tract drainage. The conversion to intramedullary nailing, when performed after a short period of external fixation, was found to be a safe treatment method for selected multiply injured patients, with an infection rate of 1.7%.

High-energy pelvic fractures may be associated with life-threatening bleeding. Emergent anterior external fixation has been shown to decrease mortality rates in these patients. Numerous biomechanical studies have shown that anterior pelvic external fixation alone fails to provide adequate stability of the posterior pelvis. Large pelvic clamps that compress the posterior pelvic ring have been designed; however, several iatrogenic injuries have been reported from the use of these devices, which require experience for proper placement on the deformed or displaced pelvis. Percutaneously placed iliosacral screws are being used for fixation of the posterior pelvic ring.

Vascular Trauma

The potential for possible vascular injuries should be suspected based on the mechanism of injury. Vascular injuries are known to occur with knee dislocations. There should be a high index of suspicion that a patient has had spontaneous reduction of a knee dislocation if there is evidence of injury to three or more ligaments of the knee, and evaluation for potential vascular injury should be considered. A pulse deficit (decreased or absent) in an injured extremity is an indication for an evaluation for vascular injury. When a pulse deficit is detected, all correctable causes should be addressed; these may include inadequate resuscitation and/or malalignment of fractures.

Several reports have investigated quantifying the pulse deficit with ankle/brachial index measurements. Ankle/brachial index measurements of more than 0.9 have been found to indicate no arterial injury on penetrating trauma.

Contrast arteriography remains the standard for evaluation of vascular injuries; however, in the multiply injured patient with an avascular limb the time required for formal angiography is rarely feasible. A single-shot angiogram on the operating room table or direct exploration in the region of injury is usually required. The management of life-threatening injuries in the multiply injured patient takes priority over limb salvage procedures. Immediate amputation may be required in the multiply injured patient with other serious injuries in addition to the vascular disruption.

Pathophysiology of the Multiply Injured Patient

In multiply injured patients, a systemic inflammatory response is developed as a result of injury to multiple organ systems and the products of resuscitation such as blood transfusions and surgically induced trauma. This initial inflammatory response is typically homeostatic and is orchestrated by macrophages, which release numerous cytokines (interleukin-1, tumor necrosis factor, etc) and is carried out by both macrophages and polymorphoneutrophils (PMNs). PMNs respond to both the systemic cytokines as well as local factors such as tissue complement and other chemoattractants. PMNs release superoxide anion (O_2) if they are restimulated as in the case of bacteremia, infection, additional injury, or surgery. Generally, the initial inflammatory response clinically lasts up to several days in trauma patients.

Many trauma patients experience a prolonged inflammatory response currently referred to as the systemic inflammatory response syndrome, which can lead to organ dysfunction such as the adult respiratory distress syndrome, and ultimately to multiple organ failure. Multiple organ failure after injury occurs in two time periods. Early multiple organ failure occurs without sepsis and is thought to result from the initial inflammatory response after injury. Late multiple organ failure occurs as a result of sepsis and is thought to be related to uncontrolled infection. Postinjury systemic inflammatory response syndrome can become activated as early as 6 to 12 hours after injury, and leads to multiple organ failure in one of two ways: the patient experiences a massive insult ("one-hit model") or sequential additive insults ("two-hit model"). Both models result in uncontrolled inflammation and diffuse autogenous tissue injury.

Data suggest that patients who underwent a major (3 hours or longer) surgical procedure on the third to fifth day following trauma had an increased risk of mortality. This observation suggested that a delayed second surgical procedure could act as a "second" hit, and exacerbate the patient's inflammatory system. Some investigators have tried to identify indicators of the inflammatory response that would predict which patients would be at risk for multiple organ failure if they were to undergo a second-hit surgical procedure. In one study, elevated C-reactive protein, decreased platelet count, and elevated neutrophil elastase were found to be significantly associated with patients developing multiple organ failure after delayed surgical procedures. Change in these parameters is a sensitive but nonspecific indicator of risk for an adverse consequence as the result of additional surgery.

Elderly Trauma Patients

The population-based accident mortality rate is higher for the elderly than for any other age group. Because of their increasingly active lifestyle, more elderly patients will be involved in injury mechanisms other than simple falls. Multiple studies have suggested that the ISS does not correlate with mortality in the elderly. One recent investigation that considered only high-energy trauma mechanisms for elderly patients demonstrated excellent correlation between ISS mortality in the elderly patient. In this patient population, an ISS of 18 or greater was correlated with a mortality rate of 37%. An ISS of 18 or less correlated with mortality of 4%. Early surgery for stabilizing fractures was not found to be an adverse risk factor for survival in the elderly population. The development of adult respiratory distress syndrome and sepsis was most highly correlated with mortality in this patient group. The elderly trauma patient has a greater incidence of significant comorbidities, and is more likely to have decreased physiologic reserve.

Prophylaxis Against Secondary Complications

Prophylactic therapy is indicated in the care of the multiply injured patient. The role of nutrition has become increasingly important. Current recommendations are to provide early enteral nutrition to patients who have a functional gastrointestinal tract. Several investigations have shown that lack of feeding the gut can lead to early sepsis with translocation of bacteria across the intestinal mucosa membrane. Early hypermetabolism is associated with injury and leads to protein calorie malnutrition. The appropriate caloric support for the multiply injured patient is important in this initial phase of treatment because secondary complications can be minimized.

Multiply injured patients can exhibit a stress response that includes the release of hormones that stimulate gastric acid production. When left unchecked, gastric ulcers can result in bleeding and, in rare cases, perforation. Agents that decrease acid secretion have played an important role in decreasing stress-induced bleeding. The use of histamine blockade

and/or mucosal barrier protection is required in any significantly multiply injured patient, and is especially indicated in those patients in whom oral intake is not possible.

Deep venous thrombosis and pulmonary embolism are major concerns in patients with multitrauma. Some form of prophylaxis or treatment is recommended. Some investigators argue that despite treatment to prevent deep venous thrombosis, the rate of death from pulmonary embolism remains unchanged, at about 1% in most series. The types of prophylaxis can be divided into pharmacologic (types of anticoagulation) and mechanical. Pharmacologic methods of prophylaxis that have been shown effective in decreasing the incidence of venous thrombosis in the trauma patient include administration of low molecular weight heparin, dose-adjusted unfractionated heparin, and vitamin K antagonists (warfarin). Mechanical methodologies of prophylaxis include early ambulation, segmental compression devices of the extremities, and foot pumps. Each of these methods of prophylaxis has been shown to decrease the incidence of venous embolism compared with no therapy. Pharmacologic methods uniformly report a greater reduction in the incidence of venous thrombosis as compared with mechanical methods; however, they are associated with a higher incidence of bleeding complications. In multiply injured patient populations with severe closed head injuries or acute spinal fractures, anticoagulation therapy is contraindicated because of the risk of intracranial bleeding. Unfortunately, the patient population with a lower extremity long bone fracture and closed head injury is at greatest risk for thromboembolism. The vena caval filters have been shown to be effective in the prevention of pulmonary embolism.

Multiply injured patients frequently have a severe soft-tissue injury associated with fractures. The use of antibiotics is indicated; recent data suggest that administration for more than 48 to 72 hours after definitive closure of the wound is unnecessary. Prolonged use of antibiotics may contribute to the development of antibiotic-resistant bacteria.

Compartment syndrome occurs most commonly in the calf but can occur in the thigh, foot, or upper extremity. Pain medication, multiple injuries, or bulky splints that prevent adequate examination are factors that may mask compartment syndrome. The classic findings of compartment syndrome are pain out of proportion to that expected with passive stretch, paresthesias, and a tense fascial compartment. In comatose, neurologically impaired, or multiply injured patients unable to cooperate with a physical examination, a delay in diagnosis may occur. Careful patient monitoring, palpation of the suspected compartment, and monitoring of compartment pressures is important in the early diagnosis of compartment syndrome. Recent investigations have reported that the perfusion gradient (diastolic blood pressure minus compartment pressure) is a critical factor. A perfusion gradient of 30 mm Hg or greater has been reported to be safe to observe. A perfusion gradient of 30 mm Hg or less is indicative of a fasciotomy. Occult compartment syndrome can occur in the multiply injured patient with prolonged hypotension. In this situation, compartment syndrome may develop even though the compartment is "soft" to clinical examination. Fasciotomy in severely traumatized extremities should be considered at the time of initial stabilization if there are elevated compartment pressures. With arterial injuries associated with prolonged ischemic time, prophylactic fasciotomy should be strongly considered, or the leg closely monitored for the development of postoperative compartment syndrome.

Mental Status

Confusion or disorientation (usually transient and nonprogressive) after surgery is common in the elderly and is often related to the trauma of injury, an unfamiliar environment, or the administration of multiple medications. However, a significant change in mental status or on a delayed basis should prompt suspicion for subdural or other intercranial hemorrhage, or brain injury. Prompt diagnosis is important because anticoagulants can be hazardous or fatal in this situation. A frequent source of agitation and confusion is delirium tremors associated with acute alcoholic withdrawal syndrome. Pharmacologic prophylaxis is recommended to prevent acute delirium tremors.

Secondary Survey: The Missed Injury

The rate of missed injuries has been reported as high as 10% in patients with closed head injuries, and 6% in patients without closed head injuries. Every multiply injured patient should undergo a thorough secondary survey once they are awake and alert following their initial resuscitation. Complaints of pain or stiffness in joints or extremities should be addressed with careful examination, and radiographic examination should be obtained when indicated.

Health Care Worker Risk

Blood-borne pathogen transmission occurs predominantly by percutaneous or mucosal exposure of workers to the blood or body fluids of infected patients. In a survey of over 3,000 participants, 87% of surgeons surveyed reported a blood/skin contact, and 39% reported a percutaneous blood exposure in the previous month. This type of exposure is particularly common in the care of the multiply injured patient with open wounds, with the potential for increased exposure to the health care worker. Precautions include handwashing after patient contact, the use of barrier precautions (gloves, gowns, and facial protection where indicated) to prevent contact, and minimal manual manipulation of sharp instruments and devices and prompt disposal of these items in puncture-resistant containers.

The three diseases of greatest concern for blood transmission are human immunodeficiency virus (HIV), hepatitis B, and hepatitis C. The estimated risk for HIV transmission after a percutaneous exposure to HIV-infected blood is approximately 0.3%, and that after mucous membrane exposure is approximately 0.09%. In vitro models have shown that increasing needle size and depth of penetration are associated with increased blood transfer volume, and that hollow-bore needles transfer greater volumes of blood than solid suture needles, and gloves reduced the amount of blood transferred upon a needlestick.

Recent studies have also shown that increasing viral load in the blood of the patient leads to an increased risk of seroconversion in the exposed health care worker. Once the health care worker has been exposed, postexposure prophylaxis may decrease the risk of seroconversion. A CDC retrospective case control study found that postexposure prophylaxis with zidovudine was associated with approximately an 80% decrease in risk for seroconversion among health care workers who had a percutaneous exposure to HIV-infected blood. The need for postexposure prophylaxis is determined by a combination of both the severity of exposure to the health care worker as well as the infectivity of the blood. For high-risk exposures, most authorities are recommending treatment with a nucleoside analogue reverse transcriptase inhibitor, such as zivovudine and lamivudine, as well as the addition of a protease inhibitor such as nelfinavir mesylate.

The risk of transmission of hepatitis B after a needlestick exposure to a nonimmune health care worker is at least 39% if the source patient is HBeAg+ (Hepatitis-B Antigen positive) and may be as low as 6% if the patient is HbeAg−. In a case review of hepatitis B-infected health care workers, fewer than 10% of workers recalled a specific percutaneous injury while approximately 30% recalled caring for a hepatitis B+ patient within 6 months prior to onset of their illness. The CDC recommends hepatitis B vaccination for all health care workers. If a nonimmune health care worker is exposed to hepatitis B virus, administration of the hepatitis B vaccine and hepatitis B immunoglobulin is highly effective in preventing infection after an exposure.

Hepatitis C virus can lead to chronic infection and severe liver dysfunction. Hepatitis C virus is typically transmitted by large exposures of blood, such as through a transfusion of packed blood cells or blood products. Overt percutaneous exposures to hepatitis C virus have also been documented as a means of hepatitis C transmission. The rates of seroconversion among health care workers who have inadvertent percutaneous exposures from hepatitis C-infected blood have ranged from 1.8% to 10%. There is currently no effective postexposure prophylaxis for the hepatitis C virus.

Annotated Bibliography

American College of Surgeons Committee on Trauma (editorial board): *Resources for Optimal Care of the Injured Patient, 1999.* Chicago, IL, American College of Surgeons, 1999.

Development, implementation, and quality assurance monitoring of trauma systems and trauma centers for ACS verification are reviewed.

Balogh Z, Offner PJ, Moore EE, Biffl WL: NISS predicts postinjury multiple organ failure better than the ISS. *J Trauma* 2000;48:624-628.

A comparison of NISS and ISS is done in a series of trauma patients. Results indicate a greater correlation of NISS scores and the development of posttraumatic multiple organ failure.

Bhandari M, Guyatt GH, Tong D, Adili A, Shaughnessy SG: Reamed versus nonreamed intramedullary nailing of lower extremity long bone fractures: A systematic overview and meta-analysis. *J Orthop Trauma* 2000;14:2-9.

The authors reviewed the literature and identified randomized clinical trials comparing reamed versus nonreamed intramedullary nailing for meta-analysis. Reaming intramedullary nailing reduced the absolute risk of nonunion by 7%.

Boulanger BR, McLellan BA, Brenneman FD, Ochoa J, Kirkpatrick AW: Prospective evidence of the superiority of a sonography-based algorithm in the assessment of blunt abdominal injury. *J Trauma* 1999;47:632-637.

The authors reviewed the use of FAST. They reviewed 706 patients with blunt trauma and in whom abdominal injury was suspected. The mean time for the diagnostic workup was 53 minutes with FAST, compared to 151 minutes with other methods.

Brumback RJ, Virkus WW: Intramedullary nailing of the femur: Reamed versus nonreamed. *J Amer Acad Orthop Surg* 2000;8:83-90.

The advantages and disadvantages of reamed and nonreamed intramedullary nailing of femoral shaft fractures are discussed.

Giannoudis PV, Smith RM, Bellamy MC, Morrison JF, Dickson RA, Guillou PJ: Stimulation of the inflammatory system by reamed and unreamed nailing of femoral fractures: An analysis of the second hit. *J Bone Joint Surg Br* 1999;81:356-361.

The authors report a prospective study of patients treated with reamed and nonreamed femoral nailing of femoral shaft fractures. Levels of serum interleukin-6 and neutrophilelastase rose significantly during the nailing procedure. However, there was no difference between reamed and nonreamed technique for femoral nailing.

Kushwaha VP, Garland DG: Extremity fractures in the patient with a traumatic brain injury. *J Am Acad Orthop Surg* 1998;6:298-307.

Fracture care in the patient with traumatic brain injury is discussed. Diagnosis, anesthetic risk, and review treatment of fractures by anatomic site are reviewed.

Mann NC, Mullins RJ, MacKenzie EJ, Jurkovich GJ, Mock CN: Systematic review of published evidence regarding trauma system effectiveness. *J Trauma* 1999; 47(suppl 3):S25-S33.

The authors review the literature of assessing the effect of trauma system/center implementation on patient outcomes. A 15% to 20% reduction in the risk of death after a trauma center/system has been implemented was reported.

Moed BR, Watson JT, Cramer KE, Karges DE, Teefey JS: Unreamed retrograde intramedullary nailing of fractures of the femoral shaft. *J Orthop Trauma* 1998;12:334-342.

In 35 femoral shaft fractures treated by retrograde intramedullary nailing, the rate of union was 94%. The importance of canal fill and early dynamization to minimize the risk of nonunion was emphasized in this study.

Nowotarski PJ, Turen CH, Brumback RJ, Scarboro JM: Conversion of external fixation to intramedullary nailing for fractures of the shaft of the femur in multiply injured patients. *J Bone Joint Surg Am* 2000;82:781-788.

In the emergent management of femur fractures in severely injured patients treated initially with temporary external fixation, direct conversion from external fixation to intramedullary nailing was performed. A 97% union rate was achieved with the planned secondary intramedullary nailing. Immediate external fixation followed by early intramedullary nailing is a safe treatment method for femoral shaft fractures in selected multiply injured patients.

Ogura H, Tanaka H, Koh T, et al: Priming, second-hit priming, and apoptosis in leukocytes from trauma patients. *J Trauma* 1999;46:774-783.

Serum from 24 severely injured patients was analyzed. Patients with increased priming of polymorphonuclear leukocytes had a significantly delayed incidence of apoptosis.

Prevention of pulmonary embolism and deep vein thrombosis with low dose aspirin: The Pulmonary Embolism Prevention (PEP) trial. *Lancet* 2000;355:1295-1302.

There were 13,356 patients undergoing surgery for hip fracture and 4,088 patients undergoing elective total joint arthroplasty enrolled in this prospective, randomized, double-blind trial comparing the daily administration of 160 mg aspirin with placebo. Patients were followed for 35 days and the incidence of mortality, in-hospital morbidity, and symptomatic pulmonary embolism and deep venous thrombosis analyzed. Aspirin reduced the risk of pulmonary embolism and deep venous thrombosis by at least a third.

Reinert MM, Bullock R: Clinical trials in head injury. *Neurol Res* 1999;21:330-338.

Relevant mechanisms of traumatic brain injury are reviewed, along with recent clinical trials of neuroprotective agents after traumatic brain injury.

Senkowski CK, McKenney MG: Trauma scoring systems: A review. *J Am Coll Surg* 1999;189:491-503.

The authors provide an excellent review of major trauma scoring systems currently in use today, along with an in-depth explanation of the origins of the systems and current applications.

Tornetta P III, Mostafavi H, Riina J, et al: Morbidity and mortality in elderly trauma patients. *J Trauma* 1999;46:702-706.

In patients with high-energy trauma mechanisms, strong correlation between injury severity score and mortality is reported. An ISS of 18 or greater was associated with a 37% mortality rate. The development of acute respiratory distress syndrome and sepsis was strongly correlated with mortality. Early fracture care in this population resulted in a slightly higher survivor rate, but it was not statistically significant.

Classic Bibliography

Bone LB, Johnson KD, Weigelt J, Scheinberg R: Early versus delayed stabilization of femoral fractures: A prospective randomized study. *J Bone Joint Surg Am* 1989;71:336-340.

Bosse MJ, Kellam JF: Orthopaedic management decisions in the multiple-trauma patient, in Browner BD, Jupiter JB, Levine AM, Trafton PG (eds): *Skeletal Trauma: Fractures, Dislocations, Ligamentous Injuries*, ed 2. Philadelphia, PA, WB Saunders, 1998, pp 151-164.

Botha AJ, Moore FA, Moore EE, Kim FJ, Banerjee A, Peterson VM: Postinjury neutrophil priming and activation: An early vulnerable window. *Surgery* 1995;118:358-365.

Davis JW, Parks SN, Detlefs CL, Williams GG, Williams JL, Smith RW: Clearing the cervical spine in obtunded patients: The use of dynamic fluoroscopy. *J Trauma* 1995;39:435-438.

Goarin JP, Catoire P, Jacquens Y, et al: Use of transesophageal echocardiography for diagnosis of traumatic aortic injury. *Chest* 1997;112:71-80.

Goris RJ, Gimbrere JS, van Niekerk JL, Schoots FJ, Booy LH: Early osteosynthesis and prophylactic mechanical ventilation in the multi-trauma patient. *J Trauma* 1982;22:895-903.

Knudson MM, Morabito D, Paiement GD, Shackleford S: Use of low molecular weight heparin in preventing thromboembolism in trauma patients. *J Trauma* 1996;41:446-459.

Moore FA, Sauaia A, Moore EE, Haenel JB, Burch JM, Lezotte DC: Postinjury multiple organ failure: A bimodal phenomenon. *J Trauma* 1996;40:501-512.

Stein SC, Young GS, Talucci RC, Greenbaum BH, Ross SE: Delayed brain injury after head trauma: Significance of coagulopathy. *Neurosurgery* 1992;30:160-165.

Waydhas C, Nast-Kolb D, Trupka A, et al: Posttraumatic inflammatory response, secondary operations, and late multiple organ failure. *J Trauma* 1996;40:624-631.

Chapter 14

Work-Related Illness, Cumulative Trauma, and Compensation

Peter C. Amadio, MD

Basic Definitions

The concepts of impairment, disability, and handicap have been codified by the World Health Organization, which has established an international classification of functioning and disability (ICIDH-2). An impairment is defined as a deviation or loss of body structure, or of physiological or psychological function. A disability is a limitation in the performance of an activity. It is possible to have impairment without disability, and vice versa. A handicap is a restriction in participation in life situations, such as at work, in school, or socially. In some instances, impairments and disabilities will produce handicaps, but not necessarily. Other factors, such as the physical, social, or attitudinal environment in which a person lives, or other personal factors not related to anatomic, physiological, or psychological impairments, often affect the nature and extent of handicaps. For example, the amputation of a finger is an impairment that might cause a disability in tying knots, but not necessarily in other activities. Whether such a person has a handicap would depend on their occupation and social milieu. In some cultures, for example, a finger amputation might result in social exclusion. Typically, workers' compensation systems ask the physician to determine permanent impairment at the conclusion of an episode of work-related injury or disease. Impairment assessment is the basis of the American Medical Association *Guides To The Evaluation of Permanent Impairment*, a guidebook currently in its fifth edition. The text converts all impairments into a percentage that indicates the degree of a person's impairment, so that dissimilar impairments may be compared and combined.

During an episode of work-related injury or illness, the physician is also asked to make determinations of disability, that is, whether the worker is able to perform any or all of their usual job duties. In some instances, a determination of permanent disability may also be requested, but this is a far more global issue than one of impairment. Impairment is based on (usually) clearly measured anatomic or physiologic losses. Permanent disability, as the term is commonly used medicolegally, actually only concerns work ability, and therefore also includes the concept of handicap, with its attendant assessment of the worker's job, the worker's social and educational status, and in some cases, the available job market. Thus, disability determinations are not simply physical in nature, and may require a multidisciplinary assessment.

Apportionment is a legal term that refers to the relative attribution of causes for a specific impairment, usually for the purpose of assigning legal responsibility. Thus, a worker who sustains an amputation of an index finger that had been previously injured would have the impairment apportioned between whatever impairment was present from the preexisting injury and that of the subsequent injury, by subtracting the percentage of initial impairment from that of the final impairment. In principle, this is a simple mathematical calculation, but in practice, unless the preexisting impairment was also the result of a work injury, the precise degree of preexisting impairment may be difficult or even impossible to determine. In such cases the rating physician is not obliged to guess at the preexisting impairment. Instead the physician is expected to adhere to a standard of "reasonable medical certainty or probability." This legal term is not precisely defined, but refers to what a reasonable person (in this case a physician) would conclude, usually based on a standard of more likely than not.

Maximum medical improvement is another legal term that refers to the point at which no further improvement is expected in a given condition. There is no set time for making this determination, which rests on the judgment of the physician.

Outcomes of Work-Related Illness and Injury

There is considerable literature that discusses the differences in outcome between occupational and non–work-related illness or injury. In most cases, in comparisons of patients with identical diagnoses who have different insurance coverage (with some being covered by workers' compensation and some by other forms of insurance), there are differences in the time off work after injury, and in satisfaction with outcome, both of which tend to be less than satisfactory for patients covered by workers' compensation. This is true across a broad spectrum of problems, from backache to knee arthritis or carpal tunnel syndrome (CTS). Those covered by workers' compensation are also more likely to return to a different job than those covered by other forms of insurance. More objective anatomic or physiologic results, for example, of range of motion or nerve conduction, tend to be similar for both work and non–work-related etiologies. Again, this observation has been repeated across a variety of conditions, from knee replacement or ligament reconstruction to carpal tunnel release or lumbar disk excision.

It is hypothesized that the differences in outcome for similar problems, based on insurance coverage, are a consequence of a flaw in the workers' compensation system, which often produces issues of possible secondary gain and may introduce an adversarial relationship between worker and employer. Ironically, the main goal of workers' compensation was to create a no-fault system—the worker sustains an injury in the workplace and is compensated, without having to show any fault on the part of the employer. When the compensable injuries were mostly of the obvious sort, such as a machine amputating a worker's hand, this system usually did function as designed. As those injuries became less common, a larger proportion of the claims became more subtle, arising from symptoms without a specific diagnosis. In such cases, a dispute might arise as to whether the problem was actually an "injury" or a "disease" as those terms are commonly interpreted, or simply a part of everyday life; or whether the problem, although a real malady, was indeed caused by work or instead arose outside the workplace. A worker, perhaps bereft of other forms of health or disability insurance, might try to associate more ills with work. On the other hand, an employer, in an attempt to limit insurance costs, might argue that symptoms noted in the workplace were not caused or aggravated by work, and either arose from activity outside the workplace, or simply reflected normal 'aches and pains' of everyday life.

In assessing whether a claim for workers' compensation coverage should be certified, the treating physician must consider whether the symptoms and signs fit any known pattern of disease or injury, whether the pattern is one that might be expected to arise from a worker's occupation, and whether there might be other, preexisting factors that contributed to the problem for which a claim is made. For example, an otherwise healthy factory worker who constantly lifts 40-lb boxes overhead might have a good claim for a work-related rotator cuff disorder, while an obese, diabetic secretary who types 2 or 3 hours per day might have a weak claim for work-related CTS.

In general, there is agreement between the work-related problem for which a claim is made and the job. For example, according to data compiled by the US Bureau of Labor Statistics, most claims for back injury arise in the trucking industry, a logical source because truckers not only must load and unload heavy cargoes, but are also subjected to vibration associated with long-distance driving. Both heavy lifting and vibration are known risk factors for back injury and lumbar arthritis. Claims for CTS come most commonly from factory jobs, where repetitive gripping in wrist flexion is a common task and a known risk factor for CTS. And although current thinking may suppose that there is an epidemic of work-related backache and CTS, a comparison of US Bureau of Labor Statistics and epidemiologic data suggests that a minority of the global burden of either backache or CTS are ever claimed as work-related, even when the symptoms are severe or chronic.

Pain Syndromes in the Workplace Setting

Pain is a common adjunct to many musculoskeletal disorders, whether work-related or not. In almost all instances, the pain is proportionate to the physically or physiologically definable pathology. In some instances, however, pain can be out of proportion to the known underlying pathology, either in severity or duration; a pain dysfunction syndrome may exist. Somatization is a psychiatric term that relates to syndromes of somatic pain. A somatization disorder exists when a patient has a multiyear history of multisystem somatic complaints, with no physical evidence of underlying disease. This disorder is most common in young females. There is little evidence that somatization disorder, as a specific psychiatric diagnosis, is prevalent in the working population, or that this diagnosis explains the complaints of very many individuals with workers' compensation claims.

A factitious injury is one that is self-inflicted. This may be associated with malingering, if the secondary gain is appropriate to the injury (for example, a soldier shooting a toe to avoid being sent to the front). A factitious disorder exists when no such secondary gain exists. The patients deliberately cause their own illness, often by manipulating a wound, applying tourniquets to create edema, or inoculating themselves with infectious agents. Factitious disorder is a severe psychiatric illness; fortunately it is extremely rare, both in general and in the workplace setting. A related condition describes patients who are Sad, Hostile, Angry, Frustrating, and Tenacious (the SHAFT syndrome), and who convince doctors to operate where no real pathology exists (factitious injury by proxy). With the SHAFT syndrome patient, it is wise for the physician to recall the Hippocratic admonition 'first, do no harm', and to eschew surgery when the only clear diagnosis is pain.

Malingering is the deliberate misrepresentation of symptoms to avoid a duty (such as to work). Its psychiatric counterpart is Munchausen syndrome, in which an individual feigns an illness in order to gain medical attention. Both of these conditions are rare in the workers' compensation population.

Social Aspects of Workplace Injury

The fact that few occupational injuries or illness are associated with overt psychopathology should not blind the treating physician to the social aspects of occupational injury, including workplace stress, conflicts with supervisors or coworkers, or other potentiators of symptoms such as depression or alcohol abuse. An accurate assessment for each of these factors should be a part of any evaluation of the disabled worker.

When return to work is problematic, professional case management may be helpful. A case worker is assigned to help coordinate rehabilitation and return-to-work issues. Case management may include worksite visits, on-the-job work hardening (exercise to build up endurance and strength after a period of disability), graduated return-to-work programs (slowly increasing hours and/or activity) and even job retraining. It is important in such circumstances that the management focus on, and serve, the interests of the injured worker, and not simply those of the employer or insurer.

Early return to work is almost always in the best interest of the worker, as it minimizes the sense of disability and lessens the effects of deconditioning, which inevitably accompanies a period of time away from work. There are two main exceptions when an early return to work can be detrimental: when no appropriate modified work exists (for example, a patient who works in a packing plant has a hand amputation that is successfully replanted, and the only available work is in a refrigerated room), or when a posttraumatic stress disorder is present. In workers with posttraumatic stress disorder, nightmares, flashbacks, and other fearful reactions may require a period of desensitization before return to work. Posttraumatic stress disorder is uncommon, but can develop after particularly severe injuries such as burns or amputations, especially when the expectation is that the worker will return to work at the same machine that caused the injury.

Ergonomics and Cumulative Trauma Disorders

Ergonomics is the science of fitting the job to the worker. Ergonomics takes into account the worker's physical capabilities and basic concepts of human anatomy and physiology to arrive at job and tool designs that are compatible with healthy physical function in the workplace. Annual reports of the US Bureau of Labor Statistics show that all causes of workplace injury have shown remarkable decreases in incidence over the past decade.

There has been much attention paid lately to the so-called cumulative trauma or repetitive trauma injuries. These conditions arise not from a single episode but as the accumulated result of repeated activity. A blister is a typical example of a cumulative or repetitive trauma injury; like the blister, most musculoskeletal cumulative trauma injuries are self-limited, provided that an initial period of rest from the inciting activity is provided. Moreover, most musculoskeletal cumulative trauma injuries become less frequent as the worker becomes conditioned to the specific activity. There are limits, of course; if rest is not provided or if the activity exceeds physiologic limits of force or duration, then no amount of conditioning will prevent inevitable tissue failure.

There is good evidence to suggest that many specific musculoskeletal disorders, including CTS, lumbar arthritis, and rotator cuff disease, can be the result of certain repetitive activities. Much of this evidence has been summarized in two documents, one released by the National Institutes of Occupational Safety and Health (NIOSH) and the other by the National Research Council (NRC). Both contain references to the numerous epidemiologic, clinical, and in many cases animal model studies that support the linkage of specific activities with specific conditions. When these conditions arise in the context of a job that includes risk factors for the condition, they are appropriately called work-related musculoskeletal disorders. This term also applies to any other musculoskeletal symptoms occurring in the workplace that meet certain criteria. Traditionally, these criteria have been described in the various state and federal workers' compensation statutes. Most recently, the US Department of Labor's Occupational Safety and Health Administration (OSHA) has promulgated additional workplace safety regulations, which incorporate much of the ergonomic data contained in the NIOSH and NRC reports. For the first time, US workplaces will have national standards for certain activities, such as lifting limits (50 lb is recommended as the upper limit for repetitive lifting without some sort of assistance) or keyboard use (4 hours per day is the recommended maximum). These rules, published in late 2000, will take effect in late 2002 and can be viewed at the OSHA web site, http://www.osha.gov.

Strategies for preventing workplace injuries can start with the OSHA guidelines and principles of ergonomics outlined above. Jobs should be designed to be within the physical capabilities of the average person wherever possible. Workplaces should be comfortable, and again where possible should be adjustable to varying sizes and shapes of workers. Workers must also practice workplace safety. Workers who are in poor physical condition or who do not use the safety equipment provided to them can undo the most carefully and safely designed job. Just as certain jobs can increase the risk of injury, so can certain worker attributes such as obesity and smoking. Both worker and workplace factors play a significant role in the etiology of certain workplace conditions, and both are potentially modifiable for the betterment of the worker.

Annotated Bibliography

Atlas SJ, Chang Y, Kammann E, Keller RB, Deyo RA, Singer DE: Long-term disability and return to work among patients who have a herniated lumbar disc: The effect of disability compensation. *J Bone Joint Surg Am* 2000;82:4-15.

Patients receiving compensation benefits were younger, more likely to be laborers, and reported more disability than those not receiving compensation benefits. Four years after diagnosis, compensation recipients were significantly more likely to be receiving disability benefits, and were less likely to have improved symptomatically with treatment. In both compensation and noncompensation patients, initial clinical findings and return to work rates were similar, and surgery significantly improved outcomes over no surgery.

Atroshi I, Gummesson C, Johnsson R, Ornstein E, Ranstam J, Rosén I: Prevalence of carpal tunnel syndrome in a general population. *JAMA* 1999;282:153-158.

This is probably the best epidemiological study on CTS available. Based on the population of Skane, in southern Sweden, a total of 2,000 subjects were not only questioned but

also examined clinically and with nerve conduction studies. Among the findings: CTS is present in roughly 2% to 3% of the population, although less than half of those have actually sought medical attention, and CTS is twice as prevalent in those with repetitive jobs as in those without.

Barsky AJ, Borus JF: Functional somatic syndromes. *Ann Intern Med* 1999;130:910-921.

This is an excellent review of the 'sick role' and the impact of litigation and compensation.

Bednar JM, Baesher-Griffith P, Osterman AL: Workers' compensation: Effect of state law on treatment cost and work status. *Clin Orthop* 1998;351:74-77.

This brief article reviews 275 injured workers and nonworkers from on metropolitan area crossing two states. The workers had more visits, therapy, and time off work than the nonworkers, and the workers in the state with more generous compensation benefits had more visits, therapy, and time off work than those in the less generous state.

Butterfield PG, Spencer PS, Redmond N, Feldstein A, Perrin N: Low back pain: Predictors of absenteeism, residual symptoms, functional impairment, and medical costs in Oregon workers' compensation recipients. *Am J Ind Med* 1998;34:559-567.

In this study of 340 compensation claimants, fitness was the strongest predictor of early return to work.

Carpenter JE, Flanagan CL, Thomopoulos S, Yian EH, Soslowsky LJ: The effects of overuse combined with intrinsic or extrinsic alterations in an animal model of rotator cuff tendinosis. *Am J Sports Med* 1998;26:801-807.

In this animal model, rotator cuff disease was simulated by repetitive use superimposed on a shoulder with an acromial osteotomy.

Hadler NM: *Occupational Musculoskeletal Disorders*, ed 2. Philadelphia, PA, Lippincott-Williams & Wilkins, 1999, p 433.

This text is required reading for anyone interested in the global issues surrounding the clinical problem of occupational injury. The problems arising from the medicalization of everyday 'predicaments' are clearly identified, and there is a strong argument against the current workers' compensation insurance system, which requires the patient, physician, employer, and health insurer to assign blame for rather than simply treating a given ill.

Hutton WC, Toribatake Y, Elmer WA, Ganey TM, Tomita K, Whitesides TE: The effect of compressive force applied to the intervertebral disc in vivo: A study of proteoglycans and collagen. *Spine* 1998;23:2524-2537.

An animal model confirms that spinal arthritis develops in response to repetitive loading.

Macfarlane GJ, Hunt IM, Silman AJ: Role of mechanical and psychosocial factors in the onset of forearm pain: Prospective population based study. *BMJ* 2000; 321:676-679.
  This article discusses the importance of mechanical and psychosocial factors.

National Research Council US: *Work-Related Musculoskeletal Disorders: Report, Workshop Summary, and Workshop Papers.* Washington, DC, National Academy Press, 1999.
  This well-referenced study is the latest word on the science behind cumulative trauma injuries and ergonomics, developed by a multidisciplinary panel commissioned by the National Academy of Science. The complete report is also available online at http://www.nap.edu/books/0309063973/html/index.html.

Classic Bibliography

Bellamy R: Compensation neurosis: Financial reward for illness as nocebo. *Clin Orthop* 1997;336:94-106.

Bernard BP, Putz-Anderson V (eds): *Musculoskeletal Disorders and Workplace Factors: A Critical Review of Epidemiological Evidence for Work-Related Musculoskeletal Disorders of the Neck, Upper Extremity and Low Back.* Atlanta, GA, US Department of Health and Human Services: DHHS no 97-141, 1997.

Gelberman RH, Hergenroeder PT, Hargens AR, Lundborg GN, Akeson WH: The carpal tunnel syndrome: A study of carpal canal pressures. *J Bone Joint Surg Am* 1981;63:380-383.

Grunert BK, Sanger JR, Matloub HS, Yousif NJ: Classification system for factitious syndromes in the hand with implications for treatment. *J Hand Surg Am* 1991; 16:1027-1030.

Hadler NM, Carey TS, Garrett J: The influence of indemnification by workers' compensation insurance on recovery from acute backache: North Carolina Back Pain Project. *Spine* 1995;20:2710-2715.

Mair SD, Seaber AV, Glisson RR, Garrett WE Jr: The role of fatigue in susceptibility to acute muscle strain injury. *Am J Sports Med* 1996;24:137-143.

Schoenmarklin RW, Marras WS, Leurgans SE: Industrial wrist motions and incidence of hand/wrist cumulative trauma disorders. *Ergonomics* 1994;37:1449-1459.

Chapter 15

Amputation and Prosthetics

Douglas R. Dirschl, MD

Paul Tornetta III, MD

Stephen H. Sims, MD

Introduction

Amputation of all or part of a limb may be performed as a result of trauma, peripheral vascular disease, tumor, infection, or congenital anomaly. Although advances in medical treatment and surgical techniques for salvage of traumatized or dysvascular limbs have resulted in a decrease in the incidence of major amputation, amputation rates in North America are still at approximately 5 to 10 per 100,000 population per year. There are more than 300,000 amputees in the United States alone. Diabetes mellitus has been associated with up to 70% of amputations. It has been suggested that amputation surgery should be considered reconstructive rather than ablative surgery, with amputation as the first step in the rehabilitation of a patient with a limb in which function cannot be restored. Recent emphasis has been on functional outcomes and patient satisfaction after amputation surgery, rather than the amount of tissue preserved or the residual limb length. In one report, 57% of patients rated their reintegration to work after amputation to be unsatisfactory. A multidisciplinary team approach is necessary for previous levels of function to be restored.

General Considerations

Metabolic Cost of Amputation

The metabolic cost of walking is inversely proportional to the length of the residual limb and the number of joints preserved. Self-selected walking speed decreases and oxygen consumption increases as the amputation level moves more proximal. In transfemoral amputees with severe peripheral vascular, cardiac, or other disease, the metabolic cost of walking can be so high that maximal energy is expended during normal walking. Although the metabolic requirements of ambulation after transtibial amputation are not significantly greater than those of nonamputees, transfemoral amputees expend 50% to 65% more energy walking than do nonamputees. Because these data were generated in gait laboratories and on treadmills, it is not unreasonable to suppose that the metabolic cost of walking distances or outdoors is even greater. This metabolic cost is probably one reason why elderly patients rarely achieve high levels of walking independence after transfemoral amputation. Results from one recent study indicated that only 40% of elderly patients undergoing transtibial amputation regained their preoperative functional status.

Weight Bearing (Load Transfer)

In order for an amputee to effectively bear weight using a prosthetic limb, the soft-tissue envelope of the residual limb must be an effective interface to accept and transfer the load from the prosthesis to the bone of the residual limb. In the ideal situation, the soft-tissue envelope should consist of a sufficient mass of mobile, nonadherent muscle and full-thickness skin, subcutaneous tissue, and fascia that can withstand the axial and shear stresses imparted to it when the residual limb pistons within the prosthetic socket. Because it is exceedingly rare for the prosthetic socket to achieve a perfect fit for the residual limb, a soft-tissue envelope that is not mobile and durable will eventually break down, resulting in ulceration.

Load transfer is accomplished either by direct or indirect means. Examples of direct load transfer are Syme's amputations or knee disarticulations. In these cases, the weight-bearing surface of the bone is broad and forces can be borne directly on the end of the residual limb. Prosthetic fit in this situation need not be intimate because the prosthesis is necessary only for suspension. Indirect load transfer occurs in amputations through the diaphyses of bones when the weight-bearing surface of the bone is too small to effectively dissipate end-bearing forces. Attempts at direct load transfer in these cases would result in rapid breakdown of the residual limb. The load in these situations is distributed by a prosthetic socket that achieves, as near as possible, total contact with the residual limb, thus distributing the load over a much greater surface area.

Wound Healing and Amputation Level

In determining the level of the amputation, functional considerations (preservation of residual limb length and functioning joints) must be balanced with the ability of the surgical wound to heal at those levels. Oxygenated blood in the soft-tissue envelope at the amputation level is a prerequisite for wound healing. A serum albumin level less than 3.5 g/dL generally indicates malnourishment and a total lymphocyte count less than 1,500/mm^3 generally indicates immune deficiency: either of these conditions is associated with a 40% to 50% incidence of poor wound healing and infection. Poor control of the serum glucose level in diabetic patients is also associated with a higher risk of poor wound healing and infection. If infection or gangrene makes urgent surgery necessary, open drainage of infection or open amputation can be done, followed by appropriate antibiotic therapy and/or metabolic support until wound healing potential can be optimized.

Several methods have been described to assist in assessing tissue oxygenation to predict if amputation is necessary or if the wound will heal at the proposed level of amputation. Physical examination may reveal a well-demarcated line of change in skin temperature, which may be a rough indicator of a healing level. Assessment of blood pressure also can be helpful in determining inflow of blood to the extremity. The ankle-brachial index, defined as the ratio of the systolic blood pressure measured at the brachial artery to that measured at the ankle, can be used in the lower extremity. An index of less than 0.45 indicates that incisions distal to the ankle will be unlikely to heal. Doppler indices also have been described. The Doppler pressure at the planned level of amputation divided by the Doppler pressure of the brachial artery can also be used for more proximal amputations. An index of ≥ 0.5 is considered indicative of minimal acceptable vascular inflow. Ankle pressure indices may be falsely elevated in the patient with peripheral vascular disease, however, because of vessel wall calcifications. Because digital vessels rarely calcify in peripheral vascular disease, toe pressures have been shown in some studies to be more reliable in these patients, with toe pressures of less than 30 mm Hg being highly predictive of the need for amputation. Measurements of skin perfusion pressure, a noninvasive study performed in the peripheral vascular laboratory, have indicated an 80% sensitivity in predicting limbs on which a surgical incision made at the location of the measurement will fail to heal.

Technetium-Tc 99m pyrophosphate scanning has been used to help predict the need for amputation. This test showed a demarcation between viable and nonviable muscle tissue in a series of patients with electrical burns and frostbite. The sensitivity and specificity of this test in determining viability were 94% and 100%, respectively.

Transcutaneous oxygen pressure measurements assess the partial pressure of oxygen diffusing through the skin. This noninvasive test, which has become the gold standard measurement of vascular inflow, can be performed at any location on an extremity that has intact overlying skin. Recent studies have documented 88% sensitivity and 84% specificity of the test. A threshold value of less than 20 mm Hg has been shown to yield high rates of wound healing complications. Transcutaneous oxygen pressure may be falsely low in patients who have a swollen extremity, cellulitis, or venous stasis changes.

Specific Conditions

The absolute indication for amputation as a result of trauma is an ischemic limb with nonreconstructable vascular injury. Some studies of high-grade open tibial fractures indicate that, unlike early amputation, limb salvage may be associated with a higher rate of sepsis, poorer functional results, and decreased potential for return to work. However, prospective studies have not confirmed these findings. Guidelines and scoring systems to assist in choosing immediate or early amputation of mangled limbs exist, but have been shown to be of little use when applied prospectively to an individual patient. These scoring systems are best used to provide general guidelines as to when salvage should be attempted, rather than as definitive decision-making tools. One specific indication often mentioned as an absolute indication for acute amputation in a mangled lower extremity is a lack of plantar sensation. It is believed that an insensate foot will provide poor function and be difficult to maintain without frequent skin breakdown. This belief has recently been disputed. One reason is that a lack of plantar sensation on presentation may represent a neurapraxia that can resolve rather than a permanent neurotmesis. A multicenter study examined patients with mangled extremities and a lack of plantar sensation. A difference in outcome between patients treated with acute amputation and those treated with limb salvage surgery could not be demonstrated with the sickness impact profile 2 years after injury. Only 14% of the attempted salvage group progressed to secondary amputation.

Peripheral vascular disease leads to more amputations than any other pathologic process. Diabetes mellitus is present in approximately 50% of patients with

TABLE 1 | Lower Extremity Amputations by Amputation Level and the Presence of Diabetes (National Hospital Discharge Survey Data 1989–1992)

Amputation Level	Diabetes		No Diabetes		Total	
	No.	%	No.	%	No.	%
Toe	21,671	40.3	12,427	24.1	34,098	32.3
Foot or ankle	7,773	14.5	2,967	5.8	10,740	10.2
Transtibial	13,484	25.1	11,048	21.4	24,527	23.3
Knee disarticulation	704	1.3	778	1.5	1,482	1.4
Transfemoral	8,612	16	20,028	38.8	28,640	27.2
Hip or pelvis	87	0.2	386	0.7	473	0.5
Not specified	1,378	2.6	3,971	7.7	5,349	5.1
Total	**53,709**	**100**	**51,605**	**100**	**105,309**	**100**

(Reproduced from Reiber GE, Boyko EJ, Smith DG: Lower extremity foot ulcers and amputation in diabetes, in Harris MI, Cowie CC, Stern MP, et al (eds): *Diabetes in America*, ed 2. Washington, DC, National Institutes of Health, Publication No. 95-1468, 1995, pp 409–428.)

peripheral vascular disease. The American Diabetes Association estimates that approximately 65,000 amputations of the lower extremity are performed annually in diabetic patients (Table 1). Amputation is performed in these patients for treatment of infection that cannot be controlled by other measures and in those patients with nonreconstructable peripheral vascular disease who have ongoing tissue loss or unrelenting pain with rest that is secondary to muscle ischemia.

The rehabilitation potential of the patient with peripheral vascular disease is much different than that of the trauma patient. Patients with peripheral vascular disease who require amputation are likely to have concomitant cardiovascular or cerebrovascular disease, poor nutrition, and a limited life expectancy, and a reasonable assessment of their projected functional independence after amputation is crucial. The biologic amputation level is the most distal functional amputation level that has a high probability of supporting wound healing and is determined by clinical examination and vascular studies. The rehabilitation amputation level is then determined by combining the biologic amputation level with the previously determined rehabilitation potential. The result will be the level of amputation that will maximize the potential functional independence of the patient while minimizing the risk for wound healing problems and infection. A recent trend, particularly in dysvascular patients, is the use of arterial bypass procedures to increase inflow in patients with critical limb ischemia. If the procedure is successful, the increased inflow can allow for a more distal amputation and better function.

Gas gangrene is a serious infection that frequently results in amputation. In clostridial myonecrosis, patients may have sepsis, pain, and delirium. There is a brownish discharge from the wound and crepitus of the soft tissues on palpation. To treat the infection, amputation must be above the level of tissue involvement and must be combined with appropriate adjunctive antibiotic therapy. Hyperbaric oxygen may also be of use in these difficult situations. Streptococcal myonecrosis is a tissue plane infection that is slower to develop than gas gangrene. Treatment requires excision of the involved muscle compartment, which can make preservation of function after an amputation challenging. Infection by anaerobic gas-forming gram-negative organisms is not uncommon in patients with diabetes. These infections often are polymicrobial, and treatment consists of wide débridement and broad-spectrum parenteral antibiotics. If systemic sepsis is present or local infection cannot be controlled, amputation may be indicated.

In patients with neoplasms in the extremities, amputations are rarely performed. Survival rates after limb salvage surgery are comparable in many cases with survival rates after amputation. Preoperative adjuvant therapy often will lead to tumor shrinkage and allow preservation of vital structures at the time of tumor excision. The goal of tumor surgery is to obtain clear margins and optimize survival. The decision for amputation versus limb salvage should be made after thoughtful individual consideration of the tumor type, location, prognosis, rate of local recurrence, expected functional outcome, and patient considerations.

Technical Considerations

Meticulous handling of the soft tissues is important to wound healing and ultimate functional outcome after amputation. The skin is often fragile as a result of impaired circulation or recent trauma. Flaps should be full thickness, avoiding lateral dissection between the skin, subcutaneous tissues, fascia, or muscle planes. The periosteum should not be stripped proximal to the level of bone transection so that regenerative bony overgrowth can be prevented. Bone edges should be round and smooth. Wounds present during amputation should not be closed under tension; even a small amount of soft-tissue tension during wound closure in a patient with diabetes or peripheral vascular disease may lead to wound breakdown and infection.

In general, muscles should be secured at their normal resting length, whether to bone (myodesis), periosteum, or antagonist muscle fascia (myoplasty). Restoring a stable muscle mass to the residual limb can improve function by preventing atrophy, improving muscular control of the residual limb, avoiding contracture, and establishing a stable soft-tissue envelope over the end of the bone for prosthetic load transfer.

All transected nerves form neuromas. To prevent these neuromas from being painful, nerves should be gently retracted distally and sharply transected as far proximally as possible with a fresh scalpel blade. The nerve should not be crushed with a clamp prior to transection because this can lead to postoperative phantom or limb pain that mimics reflex sympathetic dystrophy. Ligation, crushing, cauterization, capping, closure of the perineurium, and end loop anastomoses have not been shown to be more effective in preventing painful neuromas than simply burying the transected nerve end in local muscle. Perioperative continuous regional anesthesia should be a consideration to diminish long-term pain.

Split-thickness skin grafting is discouraged for amputation except in the presence of a mobile, resilient muscle mass and the skin grafting is essential to preserve a more functional distal amputation level. If functional concerns are paramount and grafted skin provides insufficient durability, reconstructive soft-tissue procedures, such as free tissue transfer or tissue expansion, may be considered. Complex soft-tissue reconstructive procedures are frequently unsuccessful in the patient with diabetes or peripheral vascular disease. The amputated portion of the limb should be considered as a possible source of skin for grafting or reconstruction.

Partial foot amputations are becoming more common. Preservation of the hindfoot can be an advantage in properly selected patients as limb length is maintained. Adequate vascular inflow must be present before a distal amputation can be considered. Revascularization can be considered if adequate flow is not present. When possible, great toe amputations should be distal to the proximal phalangeal base to preserve the sesamoids' insertion, or, if more proximal, the sesamoids should be excised. Second toe amputation proximal to the proximal phalangeal base may lead to hallux valgus and therefore is done as a ray resection rather than at the transmetatarsal level.

Complete transmetatarsal amputations are considered when the first ray or two other rays require amputation. The maximum metatarsal length should be maintained to aid in the terminal stance phase of gait. The amputation levels through each of the bones should mimic the natural shape of the metatarsals, being more proximal laterally than medially (each should be osteotomized 2 mm more proximal than the adjacent medial metatarsal). A minimum of 3 cm of the second metatarsal base should be maintained to preserve the Lisfranc ligament. The metatarsal osteotomies should be sloped from dorsal distal to plantar proximal. To offset the increased distal weight bearing seen in these patients, a percutaneous heel cord lengthening may be done. Full dorsiflexion of the foot should be possible with the knee extended.

Lisfranc amputations are done through all of the tarsometatarsal joints except the second, which should be osteotomized to preserve the stability of the medial cuneiform. Care should be taken to preserve the soft-tissue envelope around the fifth metatarsal base because the peroneus brevis and tertius and the plantar fascia are antagonists to the posterior tibial tendon medially. Loss of these structures may lead to inversion during gait. Likewise, the Achilles tendon insertion is relatively unopposed and should be transected or lengthened to avoid distal weight bearing on the stump and plantar flexion contracture. Amputation through Chopart's joint (calcaneocuboid and talonavicular) has similar risks of late plantar flexion contracture and in addition to release of the Achilles tendon; release of the posterior tibialis is suggested. The anterior process of the calcaneus should be beveled and the talus osteotomized at the level of the distal calcaneus so that there are no bony protrusions into the flap, which is based on the plantar surface proximally. Attaching the tibialis anterior to the toe extensor tendons through or under the plantar aspect of the talus allows for a stable neutral position of the hindfoot.

Transtibial amputation, the most common lower limb amputation, should be done 12 to 15 cm distal to the tibial plateau to allow adequate residual length for load transfer. The preferred surgical technique is use of a long, posterior myocutaneous flap to create a durable soft-tissue envelope for the residual limb.

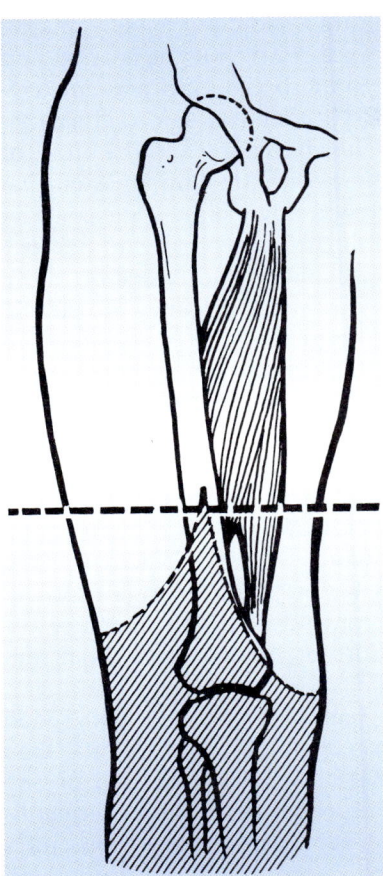

Figure 1 Diagram of skin flaps and bone resection for transfemoral amputation using elongated medial flap. *(Reproduced with permission from Gottschalk F: Transfemoral amputation, in Bowker JH, Michael JW (eds): Atlas of Limb Prosthetics: Surgical Prosthetic and Rehabilitation Principles, ed 2. St. Louis, MO, Mosby-Year Book, 1992, pp 501-507.)*

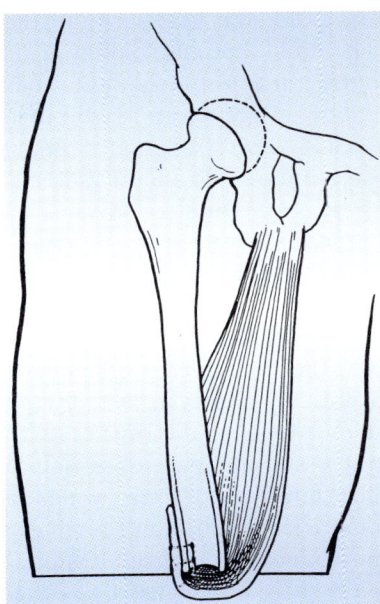

Figure 2 Technique of adductor myodesis. *(Reproduced with permission from Gottschalk F: Transfemoral amputation, in Bowker JH, Michael JW (eds): Atlas of Limb Prosthetics: Surgical Prosthetic and Rehabilitation Principles, ed 2. St. Louis, MO, Mosby-Year Book, 1992, pp 501-507.)*

When a posterior flap is not available, a posterolateral myocutaneous skew flap may be considered. A stable muscular envelope is created using myoplasty. Healing rates for transtibial amputations range from 30% to 92% as compared with approximately 90% in transfemoral amputations. If the popliteal pulse is palpable, the failure rate is only 10%. Overall, the revision amputation rate ranges from 5% to 30%.

Knee disarticulation may be advantageous as compared with transfemoral amputation and should be considered in patients with soft tissues that will support this level. The limb will be stable, end bearing, and suspension for the prosthesis is simpler because of the bulbous nature of the end of the residual limb. This amputation is now commonly done with a posterior flap similar to transtibial amputations. The patella ligament is attached to the cruciates, which are released from the tibia, and the gastrocnemius muscles are brought forward over the articular surface. This amputation level is also helpful to the nonambulator because it provides a long and stable lever arm for wheelchair transfers.

Because the metabolic cost of a transfemoral amputation is high, there is little room for error in providing an optimal stable and strong muscular envelope at this amputation level. Recent work has highlighted the need to maintain the femur in its normal alignment to provide the best control during gait. Ischial bearing containment prosthetic sockets are not capable of maintaining the normal biomechanical axis if the femur is aligned in abduction, and ambulation will be nearly impossible unless a strong muscular envelope allows the patient good control of the residual limb. An adductor myodesis is recommended. A medially based sagittal flap allows dissection of the adductor muscles from the femur. The femur is transected approximately 12 cm above the knee joint (Fig. 1). The adductor magnus is wrapped over the end of the cut residual femur and sutured to the lateral femoral cortex through drill holes (Fig. 2). The quadriceps mechanism, with its distal tendon intact, is then wrapped over the front of the residual femur and sutured to the posterior femoral cortex through drill holes. The residual femur is maintained in a neutral position throughout the procedure, to ensure the appropriate tension on the myodesis.

Postoperative Care and Complications

One goal of postoperative management of the residual limb is to avoid common complications such as swelling, edema, joint contracture, and postoperative pain. Residual limb care during the early postoperative period can enhance or detract from the ultimate functional outcome. If soft-tissue closure without tension is achieved and the vascular supply to the skin of the residual limb is good, a compression dressing (incorporating plaster of Paris, if desired) can help decrease swelling, edema, and postoperative pain. Excessive compression should be avoided if the vascularity of the soft-tissue envelope is less than optimal. Splinting is used to avoid joint contracture until the pain has decreased sufficiently to allow active and passive range of motion exercises. In patients with a good residual soft-tissue envelope, postoperative prosthetic limb fitting is initiated early, between 5 and 21 days after amputation. Immediate postoperative prosthetic fitting should be reserved for patients with stable, secure, highly vascular residual limbs, usually the young adult trauma patient.

Phantom limb sensation, the feeling that all or part of an amputated limb is present, occurs in virtually all adults after amputation and usually diminishes with time. Phantom limb pain is a burning, painful sensation in the distribution of the amputated limb, which a recent study indicates is more common than previously believed, occurring in more than 60% of adult amputees. Noninvasive therapies, such as increased prosthesis use, physical therapy modalities, intermittent compression, and transcutaneous electrical nerve stimulation, often will decrease the symptoms. If phantom limb pain is severe or persistent, active pain management with a proximal nerve block may be indicated. Persistent, localized residual limb pain is often related to an incompetent soft-tissue envelope, prominent underlying bony projections, or scarred deep tissue structures. In the amputee with peripheral vascular disease, ischemia of the residual limb can cause pain. Local nerve entrapment also can be a cause of persistent residual limb pain. One report demonstrated that only 9% of major amputees were completely pain free over a 4-week period of observation. Back pain was a significant cause of discomfort in this group.

Postoperative limb edema often occurs after amputation; this condition may cause pain and impede wound healing by increasing tissue and venous pressures. Rigid dressings, used judiciously, can help reduce soft-tissue edema. Soft dressings, combined with compression stump wrapping, can be helpful. Compression wraps, if too tight proximally, can produce bulbous distal swelling and a residual limb that is difficult to fit with a prosthetic socket. Late residual limb swelling can be produced by a prosthetic socket that is too tight proximally, causing congestion of the distal end of the residual limb. If this congestion is persistent it may lead to cellulitis and breakdown of the residual limb.

Joint contractures usually occur early after amputation, prior to prosthetic fitting. Contractures are best avoided by early range of motion, appropriate splinting, and early prosthetic fitting of the residual limb. The transfemoral amputee should be encouraged to lie prone after surgery to prevent hip flexion contracture,

and the transtibial amputee should not sit for long periods with the knee flexed. Early weight bearing and aggressive physical therapy also can help prevent contracture. Hip flexion or adduction contractures in transfemoral amputees can be caused at the time of surgery by myodesis done with the hip in excessive flexion or adduction. Preoperative static joint contractures must be corrected at the time of surgery because postoperative therapy will have little effect on these deformities, which may prevent optimal prosthetic fitting.

Wound breakdown after amputation is not uncommon, especially in patients with diabetes or peripheral vascular disease. Small areas of wound breakdown, if noninfected, can be treated open. Larger wounds can be managed with total contact plaster or plastic sockets and continued weight bearing, as long as there is no infection and the bone is not exposed. When the area of wound breakdown is larger, when bone is exposed, or when the soft-tissue envelope is tight, surgery for shortening and/or reclosure of the wound without tension may be indicated.

Many skin problems can be prevented with good hygiene, which includes keeping both the residual limb and the prosthetic socket clean, dry, and free of any residual soap or topical preparations. Contact dermatitis is often caused by residue from soaps or detergents and is best treated by ceasing use of the affecting chemical. Folliculitis or hydradenitis is common, and can be managed by meticulous hygiene, use of sweat-absorbing stump socks, and occasional use of oral antibiotics.

Prosthetic Considerations
Upper Extremity
The shoulder is the center of the functional sphere of the upper limb. The elbow acts to position the hand in space within this functional sphere, enabling the hand, or terminal device, to perform tasks. In the normal situation, multiple joint segments work concurrently to perform most upper limb tasks. Upper limb prostheses perform these same tasks sequentially; therefore, the length of the residual limb and the number of preserved joint segments correlate with functional outcome. Patients with upper limb amputations at or above the elbow are much less likely to wear their prosthesis than those with below-elbow amputation. Shoulder disarticulation and forequarter amputation provide only limited function.

Limb salvage is more critical in the upper limb than in the lower limb because intact sensibility is crucial to upper limb function. A partially functional upper limb is generally superior to an insensate, fully functional prosthesis. When upper limb amputation is necessary, prosthetic fitting should be initiated as soon as possible, perhaps even before solid wound healing has occurred. Prosthetic limb usage varies from 70% to 85% when prosthetic fitting is initiated within 30 days of amputation, as opposed to less than 50% when initiated at a later date.

Myoelectric prostheses continue to show improved function and are most useful in below-elbow amputations in patients without significant nerve injury proximally and with low physical demands. However, myoelectric prostheses are slow to perform tasks and are heavier and less durable than traditional mechanical prostheses.

Lower Extremity

Medicare designates amputees into five categories. K0 is a nonambulator, K1 a household ambulator, K2 a limited community ambulatory, K3 an unlimited community ambulatory, and K4 a high-functioning amputee who may be involved in sports. Prosthetic designs, especially feet, are reimbursed based on this classification. Two major recent advances in lower limb prosthetics are in the areas of socket and foot design. New plastics have allowed sockets to be lighter, more flexible, and more comfortable. The standard quadrilateral socket for transfemoral amputees is gradually being replaced by newer ischial containment socket designs, which more efficiently transfer load via increased contact with the residual limb. Silicone sleeves, used primarily in transtibial prostheses, improve comfort and suspension. Dynamic response feet now are available that provide spring and push-off during gait, decreasing the energy demands for walking and running and thus improving athletic ability and participation in recreational sports.

Foot Amputations

Toe amputations may lead to loss of some late stance phase stability, but patients function well with little disability and generally do not require prosthetic wear. An orthotic device with a filler may be helpful if multiple toes are amputated. Amputation of a peripheral ray (first or fifth) generally results in adequate function. An orthotic device may be required only to avoid metatarsal calluses, ulcers, or painful metatarsalgia secondary to weight transfer under the metatarsal heads. However, maintaining the first ray is important in push-off. In midfoot amputations including transmetatarsal, tarsometatarsal (Lisfranc), and Chopart, limb length is preserved. At each successive level the insertions of additional muscle units are lost. The use of an ankle-foot orthosis and forefoot filler for Lisfranc and Chopart amputations has yielded satisfactory results, offsetting the muscular imbalances of the flexors and extensors of the foot. Both a Syme's amputation (through-ankle amputation) and a modified Boyd

amputation (transcalcaneal) provide a durable, end-bearing residual limb that is rarely complicated by late ulceration or tissue breakdown. The amputation functions best if the articular surface of the tibial plafond is left intact and the malleolar flares are flattened. Prosthetic fitting can be challenging and is best done by an experienced prosthetist. Prosthetic use in 110 urban dwelling patients with partial foot amputations was reviewed in a recent report. Half of these patients used inserts in their shoes, 54% had special footwear, and none required a rocker bottom sole.

Transtibial Amputations

Patients with a below-knee amputation can be expected to have good return of function. It is important to maintain knee motion. The long posterior myocutaneous flap is standard, but good results have also been obtained with a posterolateral skew flap. Advances in prosthetic wear include flexible sockets, silicone liner suction for suspension, and dynamic response feet. The stationary ankle flexible endoskeleton is the most basic advance over the solid ankle cushioned heel foot. A small piece of wood is attached to the base of the keel, which is completed by a semirigid foam and belting materials that allow a smooth roll over the foot. The flexibility in the keel also allows for better accommodation to uneven surfaces by permitting small amounts of inversion and eversion. The stationary ankle flexible endoskeleton foot, however, does not provide enough stiffness or lever arm for push-off during higher level athletics, making a dynamic response foot necessary. In this design, the keel deforms under load, but its inherent memory allows for a return of energy upon removal of the load, similar to a spring. A split in the keel can allow inversion and eversion of the foot. The dynamic keel can be long or short and is fitted to each patient based on activity level, height, and weight. The most advanced type of foot is the articulated dynamic response foot. As opposed to the single keel design of the dynamic foot, the articulated dynamic foot has an articulation at the ankle with bumpers that permit specified amounts of motion. These feet are superior in accommodating uneven surfaces. The ideal foot prosthesis depends on the need for dynamic response versus the need to accommodate to uneven ground. For instance, running requires a greater dynamic response and golfing a greater need for inversion and eversion. The individual must be involved in the choice of feet. Some active individuals may wish to have several options for different activities.

Knee Disarticulations

Knee disarticulations are generally fitted with a polycentric knee, allowing for stable weight bearing. Results from a study of 80 consecutive knee disarti-

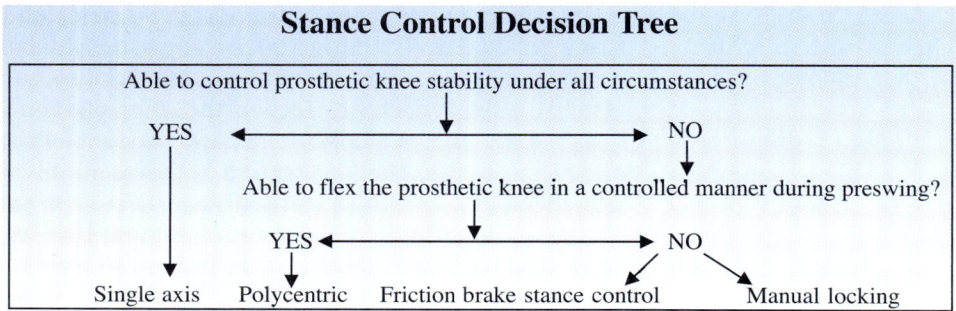

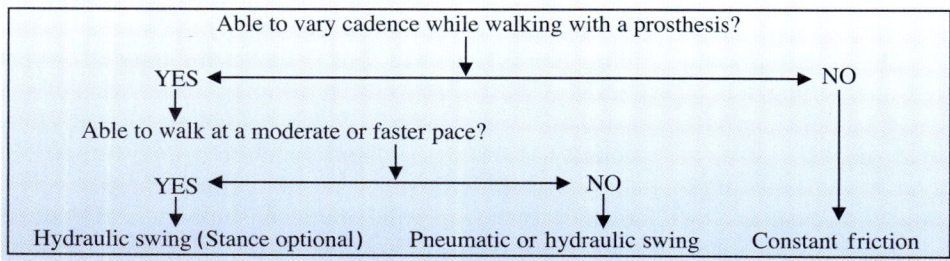

Figure 3 Stance control and swing control decision trees. *(Reproduced with permission from Michael J: Modern prosthetic knee mechanisms, in Gottschalk F, Brighton C (eds): Clinical Orthopaedics & Related Research Symposium: Amputation and New Prosthetic Devices. Philadelphia, PA, Lippincott-Williams & Wilkins, 1999, vol 361, pp 39-47.)*

culations demonstrated a 90% healing rate with the use of Doppler indices or transcutaneous oximetry. Twenty-five of the 27 patients who were independent ambulators before amputation were able to walk with their prosthesis.

Transfemoral Amputations

This level of amputation significantly increases the energy cost for walking. Transfemoral amputees with peripheral vascular disease or significant medical comorbidities are unlikely to be prosthetic ambulators. Suction suspension prostheses can work for the average to long stump and silicone liners similar to those used for below-knee amputations have also been used. Often, however, Silesian bandage or pelvic bands are required. A variety of options are available for the prosthetic knee joint; the type of knee used in a given situation must be fitted to the patient's needs. Recent work has been directed at the development of criteria for prosthetic prescription based on the patient's abilities in the stance and swing phases of gait as well as their desired activity level (Fig. 3).

Functional Outcome and Patient Satisfaction

Clearly documented functional outcomes after amputation have not been widely published in the literature. One reason may be because the majority of amputations done in the United States are in the elderly patient with peripheral vascular disease and other medical comorbidi-

ties; the fundamental treatment goal in these patients may be ablation of a dying, dead, or life-threatening limb, rather than an optimal functional outcome. Long-term follow-up is challenging in this group of patients; 1-year mortality rates can approach 20% after major surgery. One study reported a 40% 5-year mortality rate after lower limb amputation in the elderly. In patients age 80 years or older undergoing amputation, the 5-year survival rate was reported as 49% for nondiabetic patients as compared with only 19% in diabetic patients.

Only recently have data been available to help in understanding what factors might be most responsible for the variation in patients' perception of the result of lower limb amputations. In a study of 148 patients, an attempt was made to identify factors that correlate with the perceived result and should receive particular emphasis in the management of the lower limb amputee. The length of the residual limb did not correlate with the patients' perception of outcome, but other factors, including (1) condition of the contralateral limb; (2) comfort of the residual limb; (3) comfort, function, and appearance of the prosthesis; (4) social factors; and (5) the ability to participate in recreational exercise did; these areas might warrant more careful consideration in the rehabilitation of the lower limb amputee. Another study reported that patients who found a positive meaning in their amputation had favorable physical capacity and health. Anxiety, posttraumatic stress disorder, and changes in sexuality all are disorders that occur in amputees. The rate of alcohol abuse also is increased. Finally, 25% to 35% of amputees have symptoms that indicate depression, which warrants consultation with a mental health professional.

Annotated Bibliography

Bosse MJ, MacKenzie EJ, Kellam JF, et al: A prospective evaluation of the clinical utility of the lower-extremity injury-severity scores. *J Bone Joint Surg Am* 2001;83:3-14.

Five hundred fifty-six patients with high-energy open lower extremity injuries were prospectively studied. Sensitivity and specificity of the mangled extremity severity score, Limb Salvage Index, Predictive Salvage Index, the Nerve Injury, Ischemia, Soft-Tissue Injury, Skeletal Injury, Shock, and Age of Patient Score, and Hannover fracture scale for predicting amputation were determined. Sensitivity ranged from 0.33 to 0.51 and specificity from 0.84 to 0.98. Although specificity was relatively high, indicating that low scores may predict successful salvage, the sensitivity was very low, indicating that the scores are poor predictors of amputation.

Carter SA, Tate RB: The value of toe pulse waves in determination of risks for limb amputation and death in patients with peripheral arterial disease and skin ulcers or gangrene. *J Vasc Surg* 2001;33:708-714.

In this study, 309 patients (346 limbs) who presented with skin lesions and arterial disease were followed for an average of 5 years. The amplitude of toe pulse waves was measured. It was found that low pulse wave amplitude had a significant relationship to an increased risk for amputation or death in this patient group.

Dougherty PJ: Transtibial amputees from the Vietnam War: Twenty-eight year follow-up. *J Bone Joint Surg Am* 2001;83:383-389.

An excellent long-term report on the outcomes of young trauma patients is presented.

Dormandy J, Heeck L, Vig S: Major amputations: Clinical patterns and predictors. *Semin Vasc Surg* 1999;12:154-161.

This article examines outcomes of below-knee and above-knee amputations. In patients with below-knee amputations, full mobility was achieved two to three times more often when compared with patients who had above-knee amputations.

Dormandy J, Heeck L, Vig S: The fate of patients with critical leg ischemia. *Semin Vasc Surg* 1999;12:142-147.

This article examines amputation and mortality rates in patients with critical leg ischemia. A decline in major amputation rates is found in connection with an increase in revascularizations. The number of total amputations, however, appears to be increasing because of the aging of the population.

Early JS: Transmetatarsal and midfoot amputations. *Clin Orthop* 1999;361:85-90.

A detailed review of surgical techniques and indication for partial foot amputations is provided. Good surgical technique and the differences in muscle imbalance at each amputation level are important points.

Fergason J, Smith DG: Socket considerations for the patient with a transtibial amputation. *Clin Orthop* 1999;361:76-84.

A historic review of transtibial prosthetic socket designs is presented.

Fitzpatrick MC: The psychologic assessment and psychosocial recovery of the patient with an amputation. *Clin Orthop* 1999;361:98-107.

This article emphasizes the need for a preoperative assessment to determine the psychosocial needs of a patient who is facing amputation. A comprehensive plan to consider emotional response, possible complications, and psychosocial recovery should be part of the treatment program.

Frykberg RG, Arora S, Pomposelli FB Jr, LoGerfo F: Functional outcome in the elderly following lower extremity amputation. *J Foot Ankle Surg* 1998;37:181-185.

In 41 patients age 80 years or older who underwent major amputation, 40% had no change in function, 55% had diminished function. Residential status was worsened in 32%. The 5-year survival was 25% and worse for diabetic patients.

Gallagher P, MacLachlan M: Positive meaning in amputation and thoughts about the amputated limb. *Prosthet Orthot Int* 2000;24:196-204.

The Trinity Amputation and Prosthesis Experience scales and two open-ended questions were given to 104 amputees. Fifty six percent of the patients thought regularly about their amputated limb. Bilaterality and high amputation level predicted thinking about the limb. Forty-eight percent considered that something good had happened as a result of the amputation. Positive meaning correlated with higher physical capability and health scores, less athletic restriction, and higher levels of adjustment to limitations.

Goldberg T, Goldberg S, Pollak J: Postoperative management of lower extremity amputation. *Phys Med Rehabil Clin N Am* 2000;11:559-568.

This article presents a review of the initial management of the postoperative amputee focusing on appropriate splinting and physical therapy.

Gottschalk F: Transfemoral amputation: Biomechanics and surgery. *Clin Orthop* 1999;361:15-22.

An excellent review of the technique and outcome of transfemoral amputation. The relationship of the residual limb position to gait and ambulatory ability is reviewed highlighting the need to have an adducted limb.

Grady JF, Winters CL: The Boyd amputation as a treatment for osteomyelitis of the foot. *J Am Podiatr Med Assoc* 2000;90:234-239.

A review of the current technique and uses of the Boyd amputation for osteomyelitis is presented. This method allows for maintainance of the function of the heel pad as it preserves a portion of the calcaneus fused to the tibia.

Graham LA, Fyfe NC: Combined shock-absorbing shin and dynamic response. *Prosthet Orthot Int* 2000;24:246.

A discussion of shock absorption and dynamic response is presented.

Jensen TS, Nikolajsen L: Pre-emptive analgesia in postamputation pain: An update. *Prog Brain Res* 2000;129:493-503.

The role of preemptive analgesia in postamputation pain is discussed.

Kapp S: Suspension systems for prostheses. *Clin Orthop* 1999;361:55-62.

A review of the currently available suspensory systems for prostheses is presented with a chart of advantages and disadvantages.

Matsen SL, Malchow D, Matsen FA III: Correlations with patients' perspectives on the result of lower-extremity amputation. *J Bone Joint Surg Am* 2000;82:1089-1095.

A review of 148 patients determined the factors identified with quality of life, general satisfaction, infrequency of frustration. The findings demonstrated that factors other than the level of the amputation were most important to the patient perceived outcome.

Michael JW: Modern prosthetic knee mechanisms. *Clin Orthop* 1999;361:39-47.

A review of new technology and currently available prosthetic knee systems is presented in this article.

Misuri A, Lucertini G, Nanni A, Viacava A, Belardi P: Predictive value of transcutaneous oximetry for selection of the amputation level. *J Cardiovasc Surg* 2000;41:83-87.

Twenty patients who had amputations because of severe leg ischemia were studied with transcutaneous oximetry to select the correct amputation level. It was concluded that trancutaneous oximetry was an accurate method for selection of amputation level.

Pandian G, Kowalske K: Daily functioning of patients with an amputated lower extremity. *Clin Orthop* 1999; 361:91-97.

This article presents an examination of important considerations for amputation patients including preoperative assessment, education, postoperative follow-up, and rehabilitation.

Pinzur MS, Bowker JH, Smith DG, Gottschalk F: Amputation surgery in peripheral vascular disease. *Instr Course Lect* 1999;48:687-691.

An excellent review of the indications and techniques used in amputation surgery for peripheral vascular disease is presented.

Pinzur MS: Restoration of walking ability with Syme's ankle disarticulation. *Clin Orthop* 1999;361:71-75.

This article describes Syme's amputation and the use of dynamic response feet to regain ambulatory ability after amputation.

Pinzur MS, Labore A, Bednar M: Peripheral neuropathy in the hands of diabetic patients with lower extremity amputations. *Am J Orthop* 2001;30:121-124.

The remaining foot and right hand of 100 ambulating amputees were evaluated with Semmes-Weinstein monofilaments. There was a trend toward more severe insensitivity in the foot as compared with the hands in each of the groups evaluated, including insulin-dependent and noninsulin-dependent diabetic patients, and nondiabetic patients.

Pinzur MS, Bowker JH: Knee disarticulation. *Clin Orthop* 1999;361:23-28.

The authors recommend knee disarticulation when possible because the improved length is helpful for both ambulators and nonambulators. They reported that 25 of 27 (93%) of preoperative ambulators were able to use a prosthesis successfully. One patient required revision to a higher level, and one had only limited prosthetic use.

Rommers GM, Vos LD, Groothoff JW, Eisma WH: Mobility of people with lower limb amputations: Scales and questionnaires. A review. *Clin Rehabil* 2001;15: 92-102.

This article reviews the literature to present a comparison of mobility scales for patients with lower limb amputations.

Romo HD: Specialized prostheses for activities: An update. *Clin Orthop* 1999;361:63-70.

A review of the available categories of dynamic prosthetic feet is presented in this article.

Schuch CM, Pritham CH: Current transfemoral sockets. *Clin Orthop* 1999;361:48-54.

Prosthetic socket designs used for patients with transfemoral amputations are examined.

Smith DG, Fergason JR: Transtibial amputations. *Clin Orthop* 1999;361:108-115.

The long posterior flap technique and alternative techniques for transtibial amputations are discussed.

Smith DG: Principles of partial foot amputations in the diabetic. *Instr Course Lect* 1999;48:321-329.

An examination of the factors that influence the decisions-making process in amputation surgery for the patient with diabetic foot problems are presented.

Smith DG, Ehde DM, Legro MW, Reiber GE, del Aguila M, Boone DA: Phantom limb, residual limb, and back pain after lower extremity amputations. *Clin Orthop* 1999;361:29-38.

Ninety-two amputees were evaluated for type of pain and its intensity. All had Syme's or more proximal amputation with transtibial being the most common (63%). In this series, 66% were posttraumatic. Four types of pain were evaluated for frequency and intensity over a 4-week period: phantom limb pain, nonpainful phantom limb sensations, residual limb pain, and back pain. Nonpainful phantom limb sensations were present in 84%, phantom limb pain in 63%, residual limb pain in 76%, and back pain in 71%. For each type of pain, an average of 43% of the patients recorded the frequency of the pains to be more than half of the time. Of the types of pain, back pain was the most bothersome and most prevalent in patients with above-knee amputations and older patients. Sixty-three percent took no pain medication despite the pain and 36% of those who took pain medication used it daily. Nearly 50% of the patients recorded more than three types of pain during the 4-week period and only 9% recorded no pain.

Sobel E, Japour CJ, Giorgini RJ, Levitz SJ, Richardson HL: Use of prostheses and footwear in 110 inner-city partial-foot amputees. *J Am Podiatr Med Assoc* 2001; 91:34-49.

In this study, 110 patients with partial foot amputations were surveyed to determine the type of shoe insert or prosthesis that were being used. About one half of the patients wore a shoe-insert orthosis and 54% wore some form of footwear to protect the residual foot.

Webster JB, Levy CE, Bryant PR, Prusakowski PE: Sports and recreation for persons with limb deficiency. *Arch Phys Med Rehabil* 2001;82(suppl 1):S38-S44.

A review of the available sporting activities for amputees as well as some prosthetic considerations are presented.

Classic Bibliography

Chang BB, Bock DE, Jacobs RL, Darling RC III, Leather RP, Shah DM: Increased limb salvage by the use of unconventional foot amputations. *J Vasc Sirg* 1994;19:341-349.

Ewing JA: Detecting alcoholism: The CAGE questionnaire. *JAMA* 1984;252:1905-1907.

Lerner RK, Esterhai JL Jr, Polomano RC, Cheatle MD, Heppenstall RB: Quality of life assessment of patients with posttraumatic fracture nonunion, chronic refractory osteomyelitis, and lower-extremity amputation. *Clin Orthop* 1993;295:28-36.

Pinzur MS, Gold J, Schwartz D, Gross N: Energy demands for walking in dysvascular amputees as related to the level of amputation. *Orthopedics* 1992; 15:1033-1037.

Tornetta P III, Olson SA: Amputation versus limb salvage. *Instr Course Lect* 1997;46:511-518.

Wyss CR, Harrington RM, Burgess EM, Matsen FA III: Transcutaneous oxygen tension as a predictor of success after an amputation. *J Bone Joint Surg Am* 1988;70:203-207.

Yeager RA, Moneta GL, Edwards JM, Taylor LM Jr, McConnell DB, Porter JM: Deep vein thrombosis associated with lower extremity amputation. *J Vasc Surg* 1995;22:612-615.

Section 2

Systemic Disorders

Section Editors:
Paul E. DiCesare, MD
Regis J. O'Keefe, MD
James G. Wright, MD

Chapter 16

Bone Metabolism and Metabolic Bone Diseases

Randy N. Rosier, MD

Susan V. Bukata, MD

In the United States, one third of women older than age 65 years have osteoporosis, and with the aging of the population more men are also being affected. In 1995, $13 billion was spent for osteoporosis care. An estimated 300,000 hip fractures related to osteoporosis occur annually and the number is expected to increase threefold over the next 50 years.

Control of Bone Metabolism

Bone metabolism defines how bone functions as a part of the endocrine system. A metabolic bone disease or an abnormality in bone remodeling and repair occurs when there is an abnormality in hormonal control of bone function. Three different cell types, osteoblasts, osteocytes, and osteoclasts, control bone metabolism and are responsive to a variety of environmental signals. Osteoblasts are derived from a pluripotential mesenchymal stem cell and are the cells that synthesize organic bone matrix. These cells contain receptors for most of the hormonal factors involved in bone metabolism and they produce a variety of factors that influence the activity of other cells in bone. Osteoblasts also produce the enzyme alkaline phosphatase, which can be used to identify osteoblasts in histologic specimens, and can be measured in the serum as an indicator of bone formation.

Osteocytes are derived from osteoblasts that become encased in bone matrix and no longer form bone. Osteocytes connect with one another through long, thin cytoplasmic processes. Osteocytes have receptors for parathyroid hormone (PTH), and their rapid response to this hormone is produced by pumping calcium into the extracellular fluid, a process known as osteocytic osteolysis. The term osteocytic osteolysis is deceiving because osteocytes do not actually resorb bone but rather mobilize poorly crystallized calcium salts that surround them without affecting the organic matrix of the bone. Osteocytes also respond to mechanical signals in the bone and transmit these signals to other bone cells to increase bone remodeling in areas of maximal stress and strain.

Osteoclasts are derived from a hematopoietic monocyte cell precursor and are the cells responsible for bone resorption through enzymatic degradation. These giant multinucleated cells resorb bone by secreting proteins and lysosomal enzymes across their active ruffled membrane. The formation of active resorption cavities, known as Howship's lacunae, is the first stage in bone remodeling. Osteoclasts are responsive to a variety of factors produced by osteoblasts, including receptor activator of nuclear factor-κB ligand (RANKL), a recently recognized protein essential for the control of bone metabolism.

It was postulated that a signaling pathway exists between osteoblasts and osteoclasts that helped to regulate the balance between bone formation and resorption, and modulates the development and activity of osteoclasts. Recently, this signaling pathway was defined. A new member of the tumor necrosis factor superfamily, RANKL, has been identified as a part of this pathway as well as its signaling cell surface and soluble receptors, RANK and osteoprotegerin (OPG), and are described in detail in Table 1 and Figure 1.

Calcium

Calcium is an important regulator of many cellular functions including muscle contraction, blood coagulation, intracellular signal transduction, and control of cell membrane potentials. Homeostasis is maintained through interactions between the intestines, kidneys, and skeleton. Normal serum calcium concentrations range from 9 to 10.4 mg/dL with approximately half bound to proteins (primarily albumin), a small fraction bound to phosphate or citrate, and the remaining 50% in the free ionized form. Ionized calcium levels are carefully regulated within a very narrow limit and the skeleton is used as a reservoir for calcium when necessary.

TABLE 1 | RANK Signaling

	Bone-Related and Other Key Activities
RANKL	Expressed on cell surface of osteoblast/stromal cells
	Binds RANK on hematopoietic osteoclast precursor cells
	Stimulates osteoclast differentiation and osteoclast activity
	Inhibits osteoclast apoptosis
	Induces hypercalcemia when injected
	Loss of expression induces:
	osteopetrosis
	tooth eruption defects
	T and B cell differentiation defects
RANK	Receptor for RANKL
	Expressed on cell surface of hematopoietic osteoclast precursor cells and mature osteoclasts
OPG	Soluble decoy receptor for RANKL inhibits RANKL from binding to RANK
	Blocks osteoclast formation
	Increases bone mass
	Reduces hypercalcemia
	Overexpression induces osteopetrosis
	Loss of expression induces osteoporosis
	Prevents calcification of large arteries

(Reproduced with permission from Aubin JE, Bonnelye E: Osteoprotegerin and its ligand: A new paradigm for regulation of osteoclastogenesis and bone resorption. Medscape Women's Health 2000;5.)

All calcium is derived from the diet and its absorption from the intestines is regulated according to perceived body needs. Approximately 20% of calcium intake is absorbed through active transport in the duodenum by a calcium-binding protein, and through passive transport in the jejunum. Calcium is excreted in the kidney at a rate of approximately 150 to 200 mg per day, an amount that balances the calcium absorbed in the intestine. Most calcium is resorbed in the proximal tubule through a solvent gradient, although active transport occurs in the distal portions by a sodium-calcium exchange pump. Some calcium is also resorbed in the loop of Henle through an electrochemical gradient. Most regulation of calcium resorption occurs in the distal convoluted tubule where active calcium transport occurs. Calbindin, a vitamin-dependent, calcium-binding protein, assists in this transport against chemical and electrical gradients.

Dietary calcium requirements vary with age and efficiency of absorption. An increase in calcium intake is required during growth, pregnancy, and lactation. Calcium intake must be increased in older adults to counteract the effect of calcium loss caused by increased bone resorption (Table 2). Because the diets of most elderly people do not contain adequate calcium levels, supplementation is suggested, particularly for postmenopausal women.

Vitamin D

Vitamin D, a fat-soluble steroid hormone, plays an important role in the regulation of calcium metabolism and in stimulating and inhibiting genes that control the development of a variety of cells not associated with calcium metabolism. The two major sources of vitamin D are diet (in foods such as fatty fish, cod-liver oil, fortified cereals, bread, and milk) and from endogenous production in the skin during exposure to ultraviolet light. After exposure to sunlight, 7-dehydrocholesterol is converted into the biologically inert vitamin D_3 (cholecalciferol). A vitamin D binding protein then carries vitamin D_3 to the liver where it undergoes hydroxylation at its 25th carbon to become 25-hydroxyvitamin D_3 (calcifediol). This substance is catalyzed by two vitamin D 25-hydroxylases located in hepatic microsomes. Any agent (such as phenytoin) that affects hepatic function or induces P-450 microso-

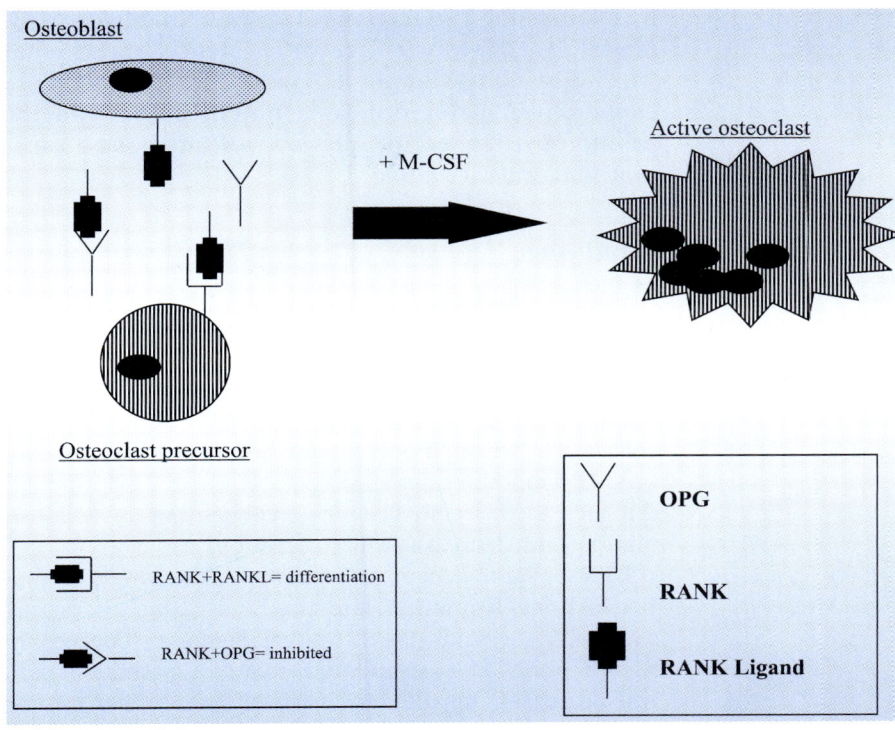

Osteoblast

+ M-CSF

Active osteoclast

Osteoclast precursor

RANK+RANKL= differentiation

RANK+OPG= inhibited

OPG

RANK

RANK Ligand

Figure 1 Diagrammatic representation of regulation of osteoclast development by RANKL/OPG/macrophage-colony stimulating factor (M-CSF). RANKL is produced by osteoblasts and stimulates osteoclast precursors to develop into mature osteoclasts through signaling events resulting from binding to the RANK receptor. Progression of osteoclastic differentiation also requires the action of M-CSF. OPG, which binds RANKL, acts as a soluble inhibitor and therefore modulates RANKL activity.

TABLE 2 | Recommended Calcium Intakes

Ages	Amount mg/day
Birth to 6 months	210
6 months to 1 year	270
1 to 3 years	500
4 to 8 years	800
9 to 13 years	1,300
14 to 18 years	1,300
19 to 30 years	1,000
31 to 50 years	1,000
51 to 70 years	1,200
71 or older	1,200
Pregnant and lactating	
14 to 18 years	1,300
19 to 50 years	1,000

Source: National Osteoporosis Foundation and the National Academy of Sciences

mal enzymes can alter production of 25-hydroxyvitamin D_3. Once produced in the liver, 25-hydroxyvitamin D_3 binds to α-globulin and becomes the principal circulating form of vitamin D. In the kidney, a second hydroxylation occurs at its first carbon by 1-α-hydroxylase to produce the biologically active form 1,25-dihydroxyvitamin D_3 This hydroxylation occurs in the mitochondria of proximal tubule cells and glomerulus. It is the rate limiting step in production of the biologically active form of vitamin D that is involved in calcium metabolism (Fig. 2). PTH controls 1-α-hydroxylase function, but levels of phosphate, calcium, and 1,25-dihydroxyvitamin D_3 also play a role in regulating hydroxylase activity.

A variety of factors can influence the production of vitamin D. In individuals with lighter skin tone, only 15 minutes of exposure of the hands and face to bright sunlight is needed daily to produce adequate amounts of vitamin D. In contrast, more sun exposure is needed to produce the same amount of vitamin D in those with darker skin tone and in those who wear sunscreen. Latitude, time of exposure, and season can have a dramatic effect on the amount of light exposure required. In adults, the recommended daily intake of vitamin D is 400 to 800 IU, an amount that should be increased if an individual does not have adequate sunlight exposure. The levels of circulating 25-hydroxyvitamin D_3 decrease with aging, and impaired renal function sometimes results in a reduction in 1,25-hydroxylase activity. These two factors can combine to affect vitamin D levels and calcium absorption in the elderly.

In the kidney, vitamin D increases resorption of phosphate in the proximal tubule. In the intestines, 1,25-dihydroxyvitamin D_3 regulates the production of the calcium-binding protein essential for calcium transport and absorption. Through this mechanism, exog-

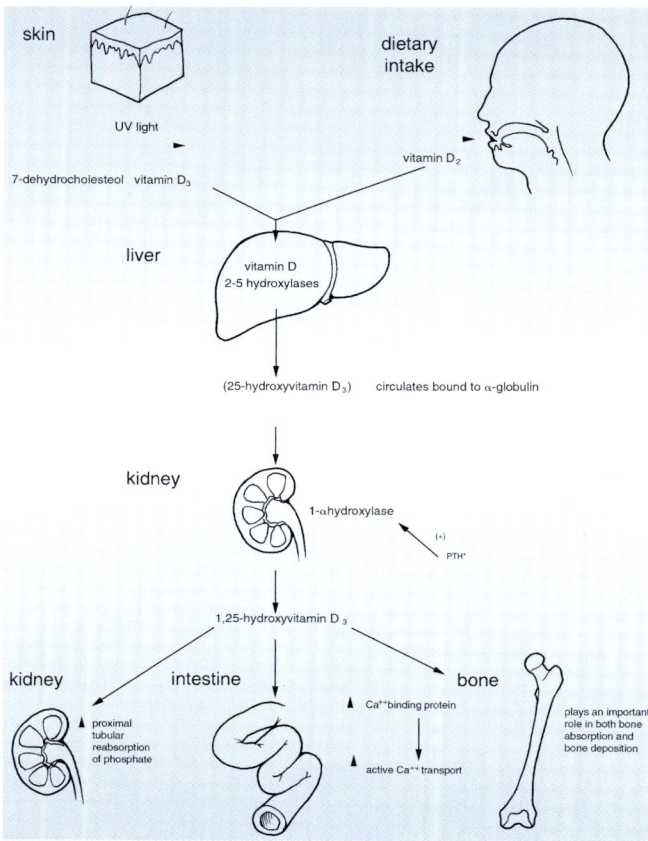

Figure 2 Vitamin D metabolism. *(Reproduced from Beaty JH (ed): Orthopaedic Knowledge Update 6. Rosemont, IL, American Academy of Orthopaedic Surgeons, 1999, pp 149-165.)*

enously administered vitamin D first works to increase calcium absorption and serum calcium levels. In bone, vitamin D enhances the mobilization of calcium stores in order to maintain serum calcium levels. 1,25-dihydroxyvitamin D_3 induces monocyte stem cells to differentiate into osteoclasts. Osteoblasts have receptors for 1,25-dihydroxyvitamin D_3 and produce a variety of cytokines and hormones that regulate osteoclast function in response to 1,25-dihydroxyvitamin D_3 and increase their resorptive activity. The production of RANKL by osteoblasts is regulated by 1,25-dihydroxyvitamin D_3. Osteoblasts also produce alkaline phosphatase, osteopontin, and osteocalcin in response to 1,25-dihydroxyvitamin D_3. There is no evidence that 1,25-dihydroxyvitamin D_3 actively influences bone mineralization except by maintaining normal extracellular levels of calcium and phosphorus. 1,25-dihydroxyvitamin D_3 is metabolized by its target tissues as well as the liver and kidneys.

25-hydroxyvitamin D_3 can also undergo hydroxylation at the 24 carbon to form 24,25-dihydroxyvitamin D_3. It was previously believed that 24,25-dihydroxyvitamin D_3 was biologically inactive and subsequently biodegraded, serving only as a mechanism for controlling production levels of 1,25-dihydroxyvitamin D_3. However, recent evidence shows that 24,25-dihydroxy-vitamin D_3 influences growth plate chondrocyte maturation as a potent mitogen in the proliferative zone, and plays a role in bone formation and fracture repair.

Parathyroid Hormone

The principal targets of PTH, the exclusive peptide produced by the four parathyroid glands, are the kidneys, intestines, and bone. PTH synthesis and release is related to low extracellular ionized calcium levels. A calcium sensing receptor on the surface of parathyroid cells works through a cyclic adenosine monophosphate (cAMP) modulated pathway to control PTH release. An increased serum calcium level inhibits cAMP formation and decreases PTH secretion.

PTH binds to receptors on osteoblasts, where it stimulates bone formation and the production of factors such as interleukin-6 (IL-6) that signal osteoclasts to resorb bone. PTH-stimulated osteoblasts secrete neutral proteases that degrade surface osteoid and initiate bone remodeling. Parathyroid hormone related protein (PTHrP) also increases osteoblast expression of RANKL and decreases production of osteoprotegerin in the development and progression of bone metastases in breast carcinoma. It is postulated that PTH has a similar effect on osteoblasts in normal bone metabolism. Osteoclasts do not have receptors for PTH. In addition to stimulating calcium release from bone, PTH decreases phosphorus reabsorption in the proximal tubule and increases distal tubule resorption of calcium in the kidney. PTH stimulates 1-α-hydroxylase activity in the kidney, increasing 1,25-dihydroxyvitamin D_3 production. This action in turn increases intestinal absorption of calcium through increases in calcium-binding protein expression, and provides the greatest effect on overall calcium quantities.

Calcitonin

Calcitonin, a hormone secreted by the parafollicular cells of the thyroid with low circulating levels, is not thought to be physiologically important in humans. In cell culture and animal models, calcitonin causes rapid dissolution of the ruffled cell membrane and inhibits osteoclastic bone resorption. Secretion of calcitonin is regulated acutely by calcium levels, increasing with high extracellular calcium levels and decreasing with lower levels. Calcitonin is active in the kidneys, intestines, and bone. Osteoclasts have receptors for calcitonin and exposure to the hormone causes rapid shrinkage of osteoclasts and decreased bone-resorbing activity. Calcitonin causes decreased reabsorption of calcium and phosphate in the kidneys, and increases secretion of sodium, potassium, chloride, and water and decreases the secretion of acid in the intestines.

Estrogens, Androgens, and Corticosteroids

There exists an association between decreased estrogen levels and increased rates of bone loss. Following oophorectomy or menopause, estrogen levels decrease by 80% and bone loss accelerates to a rate of 2% to 3% per year for 6 to 8 years before returning to the normal age-related rate of 0.3% to 0.5% per year. Estrogen receptors are found on both osteoblasts and osteoclasts, but the exact mechanism through which estrogen inhibits bone resorption is not known. However, it is likely that the effects are mediated by stromal cells found in the bone marrow. Estrogen deficiency results in an increase in IL-6 expression in these cells. In animal models, blocking IL-6 activity has ablated the bone loss associated with estrogen deficiency. Estrogen, in a dose-dependent manner, can suppress the pathway through which RANKL and macrophage-colony stimulating factor (M-CSF) induce monocyte precursors to develop into osteoclasts; however, this effect is independent of stromal cells. Obesity can protect against bone loss, probably because precursors of estrogen metabolites are stored in adipose tissue and higher levels circulate after loss of ovarian function.

The exact role of androgens in maintaining skeletal mass in men is not clearly defined, but they appear to play a role similar to that of estrogen. Men with idiopathic hypogonadotropic hypogonadism have reduced cortical and trabecular bone mass. Delayed puberty is also associated with osteopenia in men. Receptors for androgens are found on osteoblasts. Androgens prevent bone resorption and may stimulate increases in bone mass, but the exact mechanism through which they work is not known.

Corticosteroids decrease protein synthesis in general. They inhibit calcium absorption in the intestines, primarily by decreasing production of calcium-binding proteins. Corticosteroids increase calcium excretion in the kidneys, and very high doses inhibit both bone formation and bone resorption. They can indirectly stimulate secondary hyperparathyroidism through these mechanisms of action, leading to significant bone loss even with prednisone doses as low as 10 mg per day.

Thyroid Hormone

Thyroid hormones T4 (thyroxine) and T3 (3,5,3'-triiodothyronine) circulate bound to plasma proteins. They interact with specific cell receptors and bind to nuclear DNA. Increased levels of thyroid hormones stimulate both bone resorption and formation, but resorption occurs at a slightly greater rate and eventually results in net bone loss. Consequently, chronic hyperthyroidism or thyroid supplementation can contribute to osteoporosis. Women who receive thyroid hormone have lower bone mass in both axial and appendicular skeletons and have a higher risk for hip fracture.

Metabolic Bone Diseases

Metabolic bone disease results from a disruption in the balance between the normal processes of bone formation, mineralization, and bone remodeling. Diseases such as osteoporosis, osteomalacia, and hyperparathyroidism result in osteopenia and decreased bone density or quantity. Other conditions such as Paget's disease and osteopetrosis result in osteosclerosis and increased bone quantity or density.

Osteomalacia, Rickets, Renal Bone Disease, and Hyperparathyroidism

In osteomalacia, the total amount of bone is normal but there is inadequate mineralization of newly formed bone. Osteomalacia in children (rickets) is characterized by inadequate mineralization of the growth plate. Rickets and osteomalacia can occur from a variety of disorders, many of which affect calcium and phosphorus metabolism. Vitamin D deficiency and metabolism disorders, intestinal malabsorption, renal disorders, malignancy, and heavy metal intoxication with aluminum or iron all can cause osteomalacia. In the United States, rickets is now rare because of the fortification of foods with vitamin D.

Osteomalacia is still seen in the adult population, particularly in elderly individuals who are predisposed to bone disease by the mild malabsorption that often occurs with aging. Decreased renal function and liver diseases also affect vitamin D production in the elderly. It is estimated that 4% to 8% of hip fractures in the northern United States can be attributed to osteomalacia; many of those patients have vitamin D deficiency. Drugs such as phenytoin activate P-450 oxidases, which convert vitamin D precursors to inactive metabolites instead of 25-hydroxyvitamin D_3. Rickets and osteomalacia can occur from genetic disorders that affect vitamin D production or response. Type I vitamin D-dependent rickets results from a deficiency in 1-α-hydroxylase as a result of defective kidney development. Type II vitamin D-dependent rickets results from a defect in the vitamin D receptor complex.

A variety of renal diseases and complications associated with their treatment can lead to rickets and osteomalacia. In X-linked hypophosphatemic rickets, a renal tubular defect caused by a recently identified mutation in an endopeptidase gene called *PHEX* causes phosphate loss and results in an insufficient amount of phosphorus for bone mineralization. Unlike with other forms of rickets, bones appear characteristically radiodense due to a defect on osteoblast control of mineralization that also occurs. Chronic renal disease can result in renal osteodystrophy, a condition that is a combination of secondary hyperparathyroidism and osteomalacia. Hyperphosphatemia due to decreased renal function lowers serum calcium levels. Decreased 1-α-hydroxylase activity from renal disease results in reduced calcium absorption from the intestines. Lower calcium levels result in increased PTH secretion and bone resorption. Severe secondary hyperparathyroidism can develop in some patients, leading to formation of osteolytic lesions known as brown tumors. Although aluminum-containing phosphate-binding antacids are now rarely used to treat dialysis patients, many patients who received them in the past have developed aluminum bone toxicity. Aluminum deposited in the bone disrupts the formation of hydroxyapatite crystals and inhibits osteoblast function. Aluminum levels can be controlled by intermittent dosing of the chelator desferoxamine, and over several years the aluminum can be removed and normal bone turnover occurs.

Diagnosis of osteomalacia and rickets can be difficult. Radiographs often mimic other disorders and an iliac biopsy is often needed to confirm the diagnosis. Pseudofractures, or Looser's transformation zones, can sometimes be seen on the compression regions of long bones in patients with osteomalacia. These radiolucent lines result from multiple stress fractures that heal with unmineralized bone. Biochemical testing of patients with osteomalacia often shows elevated levels of alkaline phosphatase, and low levels of calcium, phosphorus, or vitamin D metabolites. Bone biopsy specimens show widened osteoid seams, and if tetracycline labeling was used the labels appear smudged together because of the slow rate of mineralization.

Treatment of osteomalacia depends on the etiology of the condition. All patients are given 1,500 mg of calcium daily. Table 3 shows additional treatments required.

Osteoporosis

Osteoporosis is a metabolic bone disease characterized by low bone mass and microarchitectural deterioration of bone tissue, leading to enhanced bone fragility and a consequent increase in fracture risk. Risk factors include low body weight (less than 85% ideal body weight or less than 120 lb), recent weight loss, a personal or family history of fragility fractures, and smoking. Genetics, including ethnicity (caucasian or Asian), play a role, and recent work has focused on identification of specific genetic loci that may be involved in osteoporosis. Environmental factors such as poor nutrition and low calcium intake, a sedentary lifestyle, and exposure to medications including steroids also play a role.

Osteoporosis is a silent and progressive disorder. Increased awareness of osteoporosis, especially in postmenopausal women, has led to increased screening. However, a large number of fragility fractures still occur in patients who have never been evaluated for osteoporosis. Standard radiographs often provide the first indication of bone loss, but osteopenia is not visible on plain radiographs until 30% to 50% of bone mineral is lost. Because prevention of fragility fractures is the mainstay of treatment, patients at risk need early evaluation and treatment.

Patient Evaluation
Any patient with osteopenia requires a thorough evaluation of medical history and risk factors in order to aid in the differential diagnosis of bone loss. Identifying a history of steroid use, alcoholism, or eating disorder is essential. Radiographic assessments and laboratory studies are needed to determine a diagnosis and disease stage for these patients.

Laboratory Studies
Secondary causes of bone loss must be ruled out. Serum measurements of calcium, phosphorus, vitamin D, basic electrolytes, thyroid function tests, and PTH should be obtained. A complete blood count and serum biochemical levels can identify any hematologic, mineral, or electrolyte disorders as well as reveal an unrecognized systemic disorder. Renal function is assessed by measuring blood urea nitrogen and creatinine levels. Liver function is assessed using the enzymes aspartate aminotransferase, alanine aminotransferase, alkaline phosphatase, and γ-glutamyl transpeptidase. Because alkaline phosphatase is produced by many tissues, including kidney, liver, intestines, and bone, fractionation may be helpful to identify the source if levels are elevated. For men, serum testosterone levels should also be measured.

To determine whether bone mass is decreasing, stable, or increasing, serum and urine can be tested for a variety of biochemical markers. Collagen cross-link products including N-telopeptide, pyridinoline, and deoxypyridinoline can be measured in urine and provide an approximation of the rate of bone resorption. A more specific marker for bone resorption was recently developed that measures carboxy terminal collagen cross-links, which are sometimes referred to as crosslaps, in serum. All of these products are excreted during bone resorption and provide a sensitive measurement for bone turnover rates, and can also be used

TABLE 3 | Treatment of Osteomalacia and Rickets

All patients	Calcium 1,500 mg/day
Vitamin D deficiency	Vitamin D$_2$ 50,000 IU 3 to 5 times per week
	After deficiency is overcome: 1,000 to 2,000 IL/day
Intestinal malabsorption	25-hydroxyvitamin D$_3$ 20 to 100 mg/day
Phenytoin-induced	25-hydroxyvitamin D$_3$ 20 to 100 mg/day
Type I vitamin D-dependent rickets	1,25-dihydroxyvitamin D$_3$ 2 to 3 μg/day until normal mineralization occurs
	0.5 to 1 μg/day with normal mineralization
Type II vitamin D-dependent rickets	1,25-dihydroxyvitamin D$_3$ 35 μg/day (variable success even with this massive dose)
X-linked hypophosphatemic rickets	1,25-dihydroxyvitamin D$_3$ 2 to 3 μg/day until normal mineralization occurs
	0.5 to 1 μg per day with normal mineralization
	Phosphorus 1 to 2 g/day
Renal osteomalacia	1,25-dihydroxyvitamin D$_3$ 1 to 2 μg/day
	Restrictions on dietary phosphate
	Partial or total parathyroidectomy if PTH levels cannot be controlled

to follow treatment effectiveness. Serum markers for alkaline phosphatase and osteocalcin (a bone-specific protein secreted by osteoblasts) are used to assess rates of bone formation and can also be used to follow treatment progress.

Occasionally a bone biopsy is needed to confirm a diagnosis of osteoporosis and differentiate bone loss from osteomalacia or occult malignancy. A transilial biopsy taken 3 cm posterior and 3 cm inferior to the anterior superior iliac spine can be assessed by light microscopy. A hematoxylin and eosin stain can help define the cellular components of the bone. Special stains such as von Kossa or trichrome readily distinguish mineralized and unmineralized matrix due to their different staining characteristics. Other special stains can be used to detect aluminum in bone, which can cause a mineralization defect in patients on renal dialysis. Tetracycline administered twice at a specified dose interval (for example, 250 mg oral tetracycline for 3 days, 12 days off, repeat for 3 days, biopsy 7 days after completion of second course) allows for the dynamic parameter of bone remodeling to be evaluated with fluorescence microscopy. The tetracycline accumulates in areas of active mineralization and the distance between labels allows determination of mineral apposition rate. Histomorphometry combines microscopy with a computer-assisted quantitative measurement that allows the extent of bone resorption and bone formation to be quantitated in a specimen. This technique allows additional parameters such as osteoblast and osteoclast number, trabecular area, and bone resorption sites to be determined.

Radiologic Assessment

Diagnosis of osteoporosis is made through measurement of bone density. Dual-energy x-ray absorptiometry (DEXA) is considered the gold standard. Radiation doses are very low (1 to 3 mrem compared with 25 to 50 mrem for an average chest radiograph) and scanning times are short, averaging 3 to 7 minutes per location scanned. Both axial and appendicular sites can be scanned using this technique. Quantitative CT (QCT) scanning is another method, but only can be used to measure densities in the lumbar spine. This technique compares bone measurements against measurements of a hydroxyapatite phantom embedded in plastic that is scanned simultaneously. QCT uses more radiation (100 to 200 mrem) and can be less precise; however, it is the only technique that can assess both trabecular and cortical areas separately.

Peripheral QCT (pQCT) uses the same principle as QCT to measure bone density but examines peripheral sites. Precision is comparable to that of DEXA in the measurement of bone density at the ultradistal radius, and unlike DEXA, pQCT can differentiate between cortical and trabecular bone, allowing for assessment of each component in response to therapies for osteoporosis. Quantitative ultrasound has attracted a lot of interest because it does not involve radiation and is relatively inexpensive. Attenuation of signal by overlying soft tissue affects measurements; thus, relatively superficial sites such as the calcaneus are the bones of choice for scanning. Using current equipment and techniques, calcaneal measurements only moderately correlate with hip and spine measurements obtained by

DEXA scanning and usefulness as a monitor for patients undergoing treatment has not been completely established. Quantitative ultrasound may prove useful as a screening technique for patients at risk for osteoporosis. Historically, single energy x-ray absorptiometry and radiographic absorptiometry had been used to assess bone density but have been supplanted by DEXA and QCT.

Diagnosis and Classification of Osteoporosis

The World Health Organization currently defines osteoporosis based on bone density measurements of the hips and spine, using the lowest measured level to define the stage of disease. Patients with bone densities 1 to 2.5 standard deviations (SD) below the mean peak bone mass measurements (the T-score) are considered to be osteopenic, with mild to moderate bone deficiency. Bone densities greater than 2.5 SD below the mean peak bone mass measurements are used to define osteoporosis, with a history of fragility fracture defining severe osteoporosis.

Once a diagnosis of osteoporosis is established, it should be classified as high turnover or low turnover. In high turnover osteoporosis, the activity of osteoclasts is enhanced and resorption lacunae are deeper and more numerous. Osteoblasts are unable to replace bone at the rates that osteoclasts are resorbing it, resulting in net bone loss. High levels of markers for both bone resorption and formation are detectable in the urine and serum. In low turnover osteoporosis, there is a failure of osteoblasts to form bone during normal bone turnover. Osteoclasts resorb bone at a normal or even slightly decreased rate, and collagen cross-link products are measured at levels similar to premenopausal levels. Serum tests for bone formation are at greatly decreased levels, indicating the deficiency in bone formation.

The primary form of osteoporosis that occurs at menopause has been categorized as type 1 osteoporosis. This form is six times more prevalent in women than men and is related to estrogen deficiency rather than calcium intake. This high turnover osteoporosis results in net bone loss at rates of 2% to 3% per year for a period of 6 to 10 years. Trabecular bone is most often affected, and there is an association with vertebral fractures. Type 2 osteoporosis occurs in individuals older than age 75 years in a 2:1 ratio of women to men. Both trabecular and cortical bone are affected and there is an association with hip fractures. Sometimes referred to as senile or involutional osteoporosis, it is generally a form of low turnover osteoporosis and is associated with a lifetime of calcium deficiency. Recently it has been noted that both high and low turnover osteoporosis can occur in any age range, which emphasizes the importance of determining the rate of bone loss. Osteoporosis due to secondary causes can occur at any age and depends on a secondary factor to disturb the balance between bone formation and bone resorption. Diseases (cancer, hormonal imbalances), drug use (steroids, chemotherapy, anticonvulsants), chronic renal failure, transplant medications, malnutrition, or immobilization can lead to secondary osteoporosis. The imbalance between bone formation and bone resorption can usually be reversed once the causative factor is removed. However, the loss in bone density often remains and leads to an increased risk of osteoporosis throughout life. Thus, patients with a remote history of childhood cancer or an eating disorder are at increased risk of osteoporosis.

Treatment

The principal goal of osteoporosis treatment is prevention. In the treatment of children, adolescents, and young adults, an emphasis on attaining maximal peak bone mass during age of 20 to 30 years must be stressed. Adequate nutrition, weight-bearing exercise, adequate calcium and vitamin D intake, and maintenance of normal menstrual cycles all are important components to achieving peak bone mass. Young female athletes who experience extended periods of amenorrhea and young men and women suffering from anorexia or malnutrition are at particular risk for developing osteoporosis. Once bone loss has begun to occur, therapeutic agents can be used to slow the rate of loss. Because of continued bone formation, antiresorptive therapies can actually increase bone mass. Some therapies designed for direct stimulation of bone formation are under development. Weight-bearing exercise also appears to play an important role in maintaining muscle mass and may stimulate osteoblasts for 24 to 48 hours following activity.

Multiple therapeutic agents are currently used to help slow the rate of bone loss in osteoporosis (Table 4). Calcium supplements are inexpensive and enhance the benefits of estrogen and antiresorptive agents. However, they cannot be used in isolation at menopause for prevention of bone loss. Few individuals are able to achieve recommended daily intakes of 1,500 mg of calcium per day through diet alone. Supplements are available in two forms, and absorption is best achieved in divided doses of 500 mg or less. Calcium carbonate supplements contain 40% elemental calcium but require normal stomach acidity for adequate absorption. Calcium carbonate absorption is reduced when ingested with meals high in fat or fiber, and this form of calcium supplementation can be associated with gas and constipation. Calcium citrate supplements are 21% elemental calcium and can be absorbed in the absence of acidity, an important factor given the high percentage of elderly individuals who are achlorhydric.

Calcium citrate supplements also tend to ameliorate constipation.

Vitamin D is critical for calcium absorption. Supplementation leads to enhanced bone mass in vitamin D-deficient individuals, but it is unclear if supplements provide any benefit to vitamin D-competent individuals. Recommended daily doses of vitamin D are 400 IU to 800 IU, with higher doses used to treat vitamin D-deficient individuals. Initially, vitamin D-deficient patients are treated with the active metabolite 1,25-dihydroxyvitamin D_3. However, 1,25-dihydroxyvitamin D_3 has a short half-life (4 hours) and is expensive, so supplementation is changed to the longer lasting and less expensive vitamin D_2 or vitamin D_3 (half life, 2 months) once the deficiency has been corrected.

The mainstay of bone loss prevention in postmenopausal osteoporosis is estrogen treatment. Estrogen is important in bone metabolism at many levels. Osteoblasts have estrogen receptors, but their exact role in bone metabolism is not clearly defined. Many other cell types also contain estrogen receptors including intestinal and renal cells. Estrogen can indirectly affect calcium homeostasis by modulating dietary calcium absorption and renal excretion of calcium. Estrogen therapy, considered the first line of defense for prevention of osteoporosis, also decreases osteoclast activity, again through unknown signaling pathways. Estrogen deficiency does not occur until menopause, when the rate of bone loss suddenly increases to 2% to 3% per year. Perimenopausal bone loss is prevented by estrogen therapy in 80% of women and bone density is maintained at the level that existed upon initiation of therapy. This prevention of bone mass loss is not maintained after the withdrawal of therapy, and rapid bone loss occurs such that after 7 to 10 years bone density approaches the levels of individuals who had never been treated with estrogen therapy. Thus, it is advantageous to begin estrogen therapy at the onset of menopause, as early as possible, and to maintain it for the remainder of an individual's life. However, bone loss that may have occurred during the perimenopausal period cannot be regained.

Daily doses of 0.625 mg of conjugated estrogen in combination with progestin are recommended for bone-sparing effects. Progestin is essential because unopposed estrogen clearly increases the risk of developing endometrial cancer. Individuals in early menopause may experience some breakthrough bleeding with this therapy. Estrogen therapy is available in both oral and transdermal forms and works best in combination with 1,000 mg daily calcium supplementation. Some studies have shown other nonosseous benefits, including decreased rates of coronary artery disease and lessening of menopausal symptoms. Other studies

TABLE 4 | Treatments for Osteoporosis

Treatment	Dosage
Estrogen/progestin combination	0.625 mg/day conjugated estrogen with progestin
	Both oral and transdermal forms
	Give with 1,000/mg per day calcium supplements
Selective estrogen receptor modulators	Raloxifene: 60/mg per day
Bisphosphonates	Alendronate: 10/mg per day or 70/mg per week
Calcitonin	200/IU per day, nasal spray
Calcium supplements	Total dietary intake goal of 1,500/mg per day
	Give supplements in divided doses of 500 mg or less
	Available as calcium carbonate or calcium citrate
Vitamin D	400 to 800/IU per day of vitamin D_2
	Higher doses per day vitamin D deficient
	May need 1,25-dihydroxyvitamin D_3 if severe deficiency

have shown no cardiovascular benefit of estrogen therapy in individuals without underlying cardiovascular disease. Estrogen therapy is particularly controversial with regard to breast cancer risk. Some studies showed an increased risk of breast cancer (14 per 100 compared to 11 per 100 in untreated individuals); however, overall mortality was still decreased in the treated group, a finding attributed to possible cardiovascular benefits of treatment. Other studies have shown no differences in breast cancer risk. Current recommendations suggest that estrogen therapy is contraindicated in individuals with a personal history of breast cancer or estrogen responsive tumor, with first degree relatives with breast cancer, with liver disease, with undiagnosed abnormal vaginal bleeding, and with a history of blood clot formation.

Advances in the understanding of estrogen receptors led to the identification of two estrogen receptors with varying distributions in different tissues. Some molecules may stimulate one receptor while inhibiting the other. Therefore, a new class of drugs, known as selective estrogen receptor modulators, have been developed. These drugs act as an estrogen antagonist in breast tissue, but as an agonist in bone. Tamoxifen is not used in osteoporosis treatment because it also stimulates endometrial tissues and can cause postmenopausal symptoms in up to 50% of patients. Raloxifene selectively stimulates estrogen receptors in bone, and therefore is not associated with such side effects. Raloxifene has also been shown to reduce the incidence of breast cancer by 50% when compared with standard estrogen replacement therapy. Although neither drug is as effective as estrogen, they both increase bone mass and prevent vertebral fractures.

Bisphosphonates represent the other major category of agents used for treating bone loss. These analogs of pyrophosphate bind to the surface of hydroxyapatite crystals and inhibit crystal resorption, although their exact mechanisms of action are not known. Amino-bisphosphonates act as a mechanism of bisphosphonate activity in osteoclasts; they interfere with the mevalonate metabolic pathways and may alter lipid modification of membrane proteins and intracellular signaling. Bisphosphonates reduce the production of proteins and lysosomal enzymes by osteoclasts and reduce the rates at which new bone remodeling units are formed. They may induce osteoclast apoptosis and interfere with the differentiation of precursor cells into mature osteoclasts. These drugs are not metabolized and are excreted intact in the urine. Their half life is approximately 10 years and cessation of treatment does not lead to rapid bone loss.

First-generation drugs such as etidronate inhibit both bone formation and resorption. Second- and third-generation drugs such as alendronate and risedronate inhibit bone resorption at rates 1,000 times greater than their effects on bone formation. Alendronate has been used for several years and produces a 50% decrease in fracture rates at the hip, spine, and wrist after 1 year of treatment. Small bone mass gains of 2% to 4% per year in vertebrae and 1% to 2% in the hip are seen in the first 4 years of treatment. Guidelines for pharmacologic therapies for osteoporosis have been proposed by the National Osteoporosis Foundation. Recommended dosing of alendronate is 10 mg daily for individuals with bone densities > 2 SD below peak bone mass and 5 mg daily for individuals with bone densities > 1.5 SD below peak bone mass, if other risk factors for osteoporosis are present. Because calcium, food, and beverages greatly affect absorption, the medication must be taken on an empty stomach with no food or beverage intake for an additional 30 minutes. Significant gastrointestinal side effects such as esophagitis and dyspepsia are seen in 10% to 15% of patients treated with alendronate; this rate is lower with risedronate (dosing 5 mg daily for all patients), which was recently approved by the Food and Drug Administration (FDA) for treatment of osteoporosis.

Calcitonin in doses of 200 IU daily given as a nasal spray has also been shown to be effective in stabilizing spinal bone mass and decreasing vertebral factors. It does not affect cortical bone and shows no influence on hip fracture rates. Interestingly, calcitonin has an analgesic effect with painful vertebral fractures, but does not change their rate of healing.

In addition to the standard techniques for treating long bone fractures resulting from osteoporosis, a new approach has been taken in the treatment of vertebral compression fractures. Augmentation of the vertebral bodies with a modified polymethylmethacrylate (PMMA) cement has been successful in relieving pain associated with these insufficiency fractures. This form of PMMA has a lower viscosity and longer working time than standard PMMA, allowing for injection into the vertebral body. Two techniques have been used. In vertebroplasty, PMMA is injected percutaneously into the vertebral body. In kyphoplasty, a balloon catheter is placed into the vertebral body to create a space for the PMMA. Once the balloon is expanded on the right and left side of the vertebral body, PMMA is injected into the cavity. Although these procedures appear promising, the long-term benefits and potential risks are still being determined.

Future Directions

Therapies currently under investigation focus on the development of agents that would increase bone mass and strength. Daily low dosing of PTH and PTHrP increased vertebral bone mass in both animal and human trials, but cortical bone mass gains were not present. These agents increased the life span of osteoblast by decreasing their apoptotic rate. Sodium fluoride is mitogenic for osteoblasts, increasing the recruitment and differentiation of precursors. High doses lead to the production of abnormal, undermineralized bone with decreased bending strength. Lower doses of slow-release sodium fluoride combined with calcium supplementation produced gains in bone density and decreased fracture rates. The recently described signaling pathway that includes RANK, RANKL and OPG offers new potential targets and agents for treatment of osteoporosis. The expression of several genes, including the vitamin D receptor, estrogen receptors, and type Ia collagen genes have been examined for a genetic role in the pathogenesis in osteoporosis. The individual influence of any of these genes is controversial, but each may increase susceptibility to the development of osteoporosis. However, other factors clearly play a role in the pathogenesis and progression of osteoporosis besides these individual genes.

In a patient with a high-risk fracture, the role that osteoporosis may have played should be considered. In order to help decrease the risk of another fracture caused by osteoporotic bone, these patients should undergo an evaluation for osteoporosis and begin appropriate pharmacologic therapy as necessary.

Osteoporosis in Men

Although osteoporosis is more common in women (lifetime risk of an osteoporosis-related fracture is 40% in women compared with 13% in men), it is estimated that 20% of the costs of osteoporosis in the United States are due to fractures in men. Studies of vertebral bone density measured by quantitative CT suggest that the rate of bone loss in men associated with aging is greater than previously estimated and equal to the age-related bone loss rate in women. Young men have a much greater peak bone mass on average than do young women, which may account in part for the lower rate of osteoporosis in men. Although hypogonadism is clearly associated with the development of osteoporosis in men, it is not clear whether declining androgen levels seen with aging contribute to bone loss in otherwise healthy men. Estrogen may also play a role in maintaining bone mass in men, but the exact role of estrogens has yet to be defined.

Men who have a low energy fracture, radiographic evidence of bone loss, or a medical condition that is considered an increase risk for bone loss should be evaluated for osteoporosis. The initial workup is the same for both men and women as described earlier in this chapter, with the exception of possibly adding a testosterone level measurement for men. Therapy for idiopathic and age-related osteoporosis should include adequate calcium and vitamin D and an antiresorptive drug. Bisphosphonates are as effective in men as they are in women. Calcitonin nasal spray also appears to reduce further bone loss. Hypogonadal patients also should receive treatment with testosterone; however, exact treatment regimens have yet to be established.

Osteopetrosis

Osteopetrosis (Albers-Schönberg disease or marble bone disease) defines a rare group of bone metabolism disorders in which there is decreased osteoclastic resorption of bone and cartilage, but normal bone formation. This condition results in increased bone density and marrow space obliteration. Histologically, the bone consists of cores of calcified cartilage surrounded by areas of new bone, usually immature woven bone. The disordered architecture of the bones makes them more fragile and susceptible to fractures. In some forms of the disease, osteoclasts can be present in large numbers, but are abnormal. They lack their functional ruffled borders and are not found in Howship's lacunae. In other forms of the disease osteoclasts are decreased in number or even absent.

Both the radiographic appearance and the clinical severity can be variable. Radiographs demonstrate a diffuse symmetric increase in bone density. Long bone metaphyses are widened with a characteristic pattern of transverse sclerotic bands alternating with lucent bands. Vertebrae develop sclerotic bands underlying the endplates, resulting in a "rugger jersey" appearance. At least nine forms of osteopetrosis exist as one of four phenotypes, each varying in severity. The majority of patients present with the mild, autosomal dominant form also known as the adult (tarda) form. Patients have a normal lifespan and may be asymptomatic or have mild anemia. Patients may also have a history of a few fractures. The congenital form (juvenile, infantile, malignant) is an autosomal recessive disorder and the most severe form of the disease. Patients die during childhood (younger than age 10 years) and present with severe anemia, thrombocytopenia, hepatosplenomegaly, and a compromised immune system. They can have cranial and optic nerve palsies. Patients often sustain multiple fractures and are prone to osteomyelitis. Another autosomal recessive form is characterized by intermediate severity between the adult and infantile forms. An additional rare form is associated with renal tubular acidosis and a mutation in the carbonic anhydrase II gene that results in lower than normal levels of this enzyme available for bone resorption. These patients also can have cerebral calcifications that often result in mental retardation.

The varying patterns of bone involvement seen between and within each subtype demonstrates the genetic heterogeneity of this disease. The molecular basis for most forms of the disease remains unknown. Besides the carbonic anhydrase II gene defects, defects in osteoblast function that limit their ability to synthesize M-CSF have been identified. This cytokine is essential for the recruitment and development of mature osteoclasts. The RANK/RANKL/OPG signalling pathway is also essential for osteoclast recruitment and development, and animal studies suggest that these genes may play a role in some forms of osteopetrosis.

Treatments for osteopetrosis vary with the form of the disease. Some patients with the severe infantile form improve after bone marrow transplantation from HLA-compatible donors. Early intervention appears important because severely narrowed marrow spaces are less likely to engraft with the transplanted bone marrow. Only about 40% of patients find appropriate matched donors, and the transplant is successful in only half of these patients. Of patients with successful bone marrow transplantation, half are cured of the disease. Some success has been reported using large doses of 1,25-dihydroxyvitamin D_3 and a diet low in calcium. The exact mechanism of action of 1,25-dihydroxyvitamin D_3 is unknown, but it appears to stimulate the formation of the ruffled border on osteoclasts and may increase the rate of fusion of osteoclast progenitor cells to form mature active osteoclasts. The only FDA-approved treatment for osteopetrosis is interferon γ-1b. It increases superoxide secretion by osteoclasts, resulting in increased bone resorption by the osteoclasts. This activity has influenced the supposition that some of the genetic defects in osteopetrosis may be correctable, although the genes involved have not been identified.

Paget's Disease

Paget's disease is second to osteoporosis as the most common metabolic bone disease. An ethnic and geographic prevalence of the disease is seen in addition to clustering in families. The disease is rare in Asia and more prevalent in Northern Europe, North America, Australia, and New Zealand. In these regions, up to 4% of Anglo-Saxon individuals older than age 55 years have Paget's disease, and many of these people are asymptomatic. The incidence of the disease increases with age and is rarely seen in patients younger than age 40 years. Although the etiology of Paget's disease remains unknown, two recent studies of large kindreds identified a possible gene that increases an individual's susceptibility to the disease. However, not all kindreds possessed this gene. No studies have conclusively demonstrated a link between Paget's disease and a specific HLA antigen. There is some evidence supporting a viral etiology. Viral inclusion bodies have been found in osteoclasts of involved bone in some patients with Paget's disease. These inclusion bodies resemble those of ribonucleic acid paramyxoviruses such as respiratory syncytial virus and measles. The focality of Paget's disease and the lack of new foci once the disease is established place the ideas of a systemic origin for the disease in question. Increased levels of IL-6 have been found in pagetic foci, suggesting that the bone microenvironments may influence the establishment and progression of the disease.

Three histologic phases of the disease are observed. There is a marked increase in bone resorption with an increase in the number and size of osteoclasts, sometimes referred to as the hot phase. Osteoclasts form irregular resorption cavities and bone marrow is replaced by fibrovascular tissue. Collagen breakdown products are detectable in urine during this phase. In the intermediate phase there is a rapid increase in osteoblast activity and new bone formation, with an increase in alkaline phosphatase activity. The new bone forms irregular, thick seams with widened lamellae and irregular cement lines, resulting in the mosaic pattern characteristic of pagetic bone. Woven bone is prominent, especially subperiosteal, and mineralization occurs at twice the normal rate. In the final or cold phase, both osteoclastic and osteoblastic activity decrease. Densely sclerotic, enlarged, deformed bones

with thickened trabeculae are characteristic. Patients with periarticular involvement may develop secondary osteoarthritis.

Because most patients are asymptomatic, Paget's disease is often diagnosed incidentally on routine radiographs in its final phase. Bone, joint, or low back pain are common symptoms. The entire progression of the disease evolves over many years and radiographic appearance depends on the phase of the disease at the time of diagnosis. Radiographs initially show radiolucency in affected bones. In long bones a wedge- or flame-shaped lucency begins in the metaphysis and points toward the diaphysis. The lucency then advances into the diaphysis at approximately 1 cm per year. This phase is followed by osteoblast activity during which the lucencies are converted to radiodense regions. In the polyostotic form of Paget's disease all of the lesions are at approximately the same stage, indicating that onset of disease was likely the same for all sites. The intense uptake seen on bone scan can often be helpful in identifying regions affected by Paget's disease, even before changes are evident on plain radiographs. Paget's disease in the spine often affects the lumbar vertebrae and radiographic changes from thickening of the end plates and subcortical bone can result in a "picture frame" appearance. Compression of the nerve root and cord can occur from enlargement of the vertebral body. Compression fractures of vertebrae can occur in the earlier osteolytic phase of Paget's disease.

Patients should be thoroughly evaluated and followed up using biochemical markers such as alkaline phosphatase and urinary bone resorption markers such as N-telopeptides. Those with active and symptomatic Paget's disease should be treated. Bisphosphonate therapy has become the standard of care. Initially, patients were treated with etidronate, but long-term therapy interfered with osteoid mineralization. Newer therapies, with second-generation bisphosphonates such as alendronate (40 mg daily), risedronate (30 mg daily), and tiludronate (400 mg daily) that do not inhibit mineralization have had better results. Calcitonin has been used because of its ability to directly inactivate osteoclasts. It is generally given in an injectable form because there is decreased bioavailability with the nasal spray and an optimal nasal spray dose is not known. However, patients with mild disease may improve with the 200 IU daily dose used for osteoporosis. Up to 60% of patients develop antibodies to the calcitonin, decreasing its effectiveness. Calcitonin may become the alternate therapy for individuals who do not tolerate bisphosphonates.

Pagetic lesions are well tolerated with the exception of those of the acetabulum, which cause osteoarthritis, and the spine, which cause neural compression. The bone, although radiodense, is brittle because of its disordered architecture. Fractures occur on the convex side of bones and can result in a bowing deformity. Paget's disease can precipitate high output cardiac failure because of the increased vascularity of the affected bones and the subsequent demand on the cardiovascular system. This condition alone is an indication for treatment, even in the absence of skeletal complaints.

High-grade sarcoma can develop in approximately 1% of patients with Paget's disease, more commonly in patients with polyostotic lesions than in those with solitary lesions. Sixteen percent of Paget's sarcomas are multifocal. Osteosarcoma, often the telangectatic variant, is most common but fibrosarcomas and chondrosarcomas can also be seen. Because of the increased vascularity of pagetic bone, carcinomas sometimes metastasize to these regions, emphasizing the importance of radiographic follow-up and possibly biopsy in aggressive or evolving lesions in pagetic bone.

Annotated Bibliography

General Texts

Colditz GA: Relationship between estrogen levels, use of hormone replacement therapy, and breast cancer. *J Natl Cancer Inst* 1998;90:814-823.

A comprehensive review of the biology relating hormones to breast cancer is presented. The article reviews all English language studies relating estrogen replacement therapy to increased risk of breast cancer.

Cosman F, Lindsay R: Selective estrogen receptor modulators: Clinical spectrum. *Endocr Rev* 1999;20:418-434.

This article presents a review of the effects of selective estrogen receptor modulators and their possible clinical applications.

Favus MJ (ed): *Primer on the Metabolic Bone Diseases and Disorders of Mineral Metabolism,* ed 4. Philadelphia, PA, Lippincott-Williams & Wilkins, 1999.

This comprehensive text addresses all aspects of bone metabolism and the diseases that result from abnormal bone metabolism. Physiology, genetics, clinical disease presentations, basic science, and treatments for metabolic bone disorders are discussed.

Hofbauer LC: Osteoprotegerin ligand and osteoprotegerin: Novel implications for osteoclast biology and bone metabolism. *Eur J Endocrinol* 1999;141:195-210.

This article reviews the newly recognized proteins RANK, RANKL (RANK ligand or osteoprotegerin ligand), and osteoprotegerin and their correlation to bone metabolism. Implications for basic science as well as clinical applications addressed.

McCarthy EF, Frassica FJ (eds): *Pathology of Bone and Joint Disorders With Clinical and Radiographic Correlation.* Philadelphia, PA, WB Saunders Company, 1998.

This comprehensive text on bone histology and pathology has several chapters addressing normal physiology of bone, bone metabolism, metabolic bone diseases, and Paget's disease with corresponding representative radiographs and histology plates.

Osteoporosis

Avioli LV: The role of calcitonin in the prevention of osteoporosis. *Endocrinol Metab Clin North Am* 1998;27:411-418.

This article describes the role of calcitonin in the treatment of osteoporosis and discusses dosing regimens and possible mechanisms of action.

Cummings SR, Black DM, Thompson DE, et al: Effect of alendronate on risk of fracture in women with low bone density but without vertebral fractures: Results from the Fracture Intervention Trial. *JAMA* 1998;280:2077-2082.

A prospective trial with the bisphosphonate alendronate demonstrates a reduction of vertebral fractures among women with osteoporosis as an adjunct to the previous FIT trial that demonstrated a similar reduction in hip and wrist fractures.

Ettinger B, Black DM, Mitlak BH, et al: Reduction of vertebral fracture risk in postmenopausal women with osteoporosis treated with raloxifene: Results from a 3-year randomized clinical trial: Multiple Outcomes of Raloxifene Evaluation (MORE) Investigators. *JAMA* 1999;282:637-645.

A prospective trial with the selective estrogen receptor modulator, raloxifene, demonstrates increased bone mineral density in the hip and spine and a reduction in vertebral fractures in postmenopausal women.

Lane JM, Russell L, Khan SN: Osteoporosis. *Clin Orthop* 2000;372:139-150.

This article presents a comprehensive review of the basic science of osteoporosis. The latest diagnostic and therapeutic strategies are presented.

Mirsky EC, Einhorn TA: Bone densitometry in orthopaedic practice. *J Bone Joint Surg Am* 1998;80:1687-1698.

The tools currently used for determination of bone density, clinical indications for their use, and interpretation of results are discussed.

Physician's Guide to Prevention and Treatment of Osteoporosis. Washington, DC, National Osteoporosis Foundation, 1998.

A concise summary of the diagnosis and treatment of osteoporosis including current dosing recommendations for all pharmacologic treatments is presented.

Reginster J, Minne HW, Sorensen OH, et al: Randomized trial of the effects of risedronate on vertebral fractures in women with established postmenopausal osteoporosis: Vertebral Efficacy with Risedronate Therapy (VERT) Study Group. *Osteoporos Int* 2000;11:83-91.

Important prospective evaluation of fracture risk reduction of the new bisphosphonate approved by the FDA are discussed, along with a review of some of the gastrointestinal side effects of bisphosphonate therapy.

Paget's Disease

Siris ES: Paget's disease of bone. *J Bone Miner Res* 1998;13:1061-1065.

This article provides a thorough review of pathology, pathophysiology, and treatment for Paget's disease.

Classic Bibliography

Chapuy MC, Arlot ME, Duboeuf F, et al: Vitamin D3 and calcium to prevent hip fractures in the elderly woman. *N Engl J Med* 1992;327:1637-1642.

Dawson-Hughes B, Dallal GE, Krall EA, Sadowski L, Sahyoun N, Tannenbaum S: A controlled trial of the effect of calcium supplementation on bone density in postmenopausal women. *N Engl J Med* 1990;323:878-883.

Delmas PD, Bjarnason NH, Mitlak BH, et al: Effects of raloxifene on bone mineral density, serum cholesterol concentrations, and uterine endometrium in postmenopausal women. *N Engl J Med* 1997;337:1641-1647.

Delmas PD, Meunier PJ: The management of Paget's disease of bone. *N Engl J Med* 1997;336:558-566.

Eyre DR: Bone biomarkers as tools in osteoporosis management. *Spine* 1997;22(suppl 24):17S-24S.

Felson DT, Zhang Y, Hannan MT, Kiel DP, Wilson PW, Anderson JJ: The effect of postmenopausal estrogen therapy on bone density in elderly women. *N Engl J Med* 1993;329:1141-1146.

Finkelstein JS, Neer RM, Biller BM, Crawford JD, Klibanski A: Osteopenia in men with a history of delayed puberty. *N Engl J Med* 1992;326:600-604.

Grampp S, Genant HK, Mathur A, et al: Comparisons of noninvasive bone mineral measurements in assessing age-related loss, fracture discrimination, and diagnostic classification. *J Bone Miner Res* 1997;12:697-711.

Grodstein F, Stampfer MJ, Colditz GA, et al: Postmenopausal hormone therapy and mortality. *N Engl J Med* 1997;336:1769-1775.

Jilka RL, Hangoc G, Girasole G, et al: Increased osteoclast development after estrogen loss: Mediation by interleukin-6. *Science* 1992;257:88-91.

Kaplan FS, August CS, Fallon MD, Dalinka M, Axel L, Haddad JG: Successful treatment of infantile malignant osteopetrosis by bone-marrow transplantation: A case report. *J Bone Joint Surg Am* 1988;70:617-623.

Key LL Jr, Rodriguiz RM, Willi SM, et al: Long-term treatment of osteopetrosis with recombinant human interferon gamma. *N Engl J Med* 1995;332:1594-1599.

Kiel DP, Felson DT, Anderson JJ, Wilson PW, Moskowitz MA: Hip fracture and the use of estrogens in postmenopausal women: The Framingham Study. *N Engl J Med* 1987;317:1169-1174.

Mankin HJ: Metabolic bone disease. *Instr Course Lect* 1995;44:3-29.

Prince RL, Smith M, Dick IM, et al: Prevention of postmenopausal osteoporosis: A comparative study of exercise, calcium supplementation, and hormone-replacement therapy. *N Engl J Med* 1991;325:1189-1195.

Schneider DL, Barrett-Connor EL, Morton DJ: Thyroid hormone use and bone mineral density in elderly women: Effects of estrogen. *JAMA* 1994;271:1245-1249.

Shapiro F: Osteopetrosis: Current clinical considerations. *Clin Orthop* 1993;294:34-44.

Stewart AF: PTHrP(1-36) as a skeletal anabolic agent for the treatment of osteoporosis. *Bone* 1996;19:303-306.

Chapter 17

Musculoskeletal Oncology

H. Thomas Temple, MD

Denis R. Clohisy, MD

Evaluation

Age, gender, types of symptoms, duration and location of tumor, antecedent trauma, and constitutional complaints are very important factors in the clinical history of a patient with a bone tumor. Knowing when a tumor occurs, its location, and its size and extent provides valuable information about a disease and narrows the differential diagnosis. Certain tumors are age-specific. For example, metastatic neuroblastoma would not be expected in a patient older than age 10 years. Conversely, myeloma is a disease that rarely occurs before the fourth or fifth decades. For many tumors of bone, there is a clear male predominance. However, giant cell tumor and low-grade surface (parosteal) osteosarcomas are more common in women.

Tumor location can help to predict the histologic diagnosis based on the particular bone and the tumor's location in the bone (Fig. 1). The majority of adamantinomas and ossifying fibromas are found in the tibial diaphysis, osteoblastomas of the spine occur in the dorsal elements, and osteosarcomas usually occur in the metaphyseal ends of rapidly growing bones such as the distal femur, proximal tibia, and proximal humerus. Chondroblastomas are almost always found in the epiphyses of long bones. Large tumors are more likely than small tumors to be malignant and tumors in multiple sites in young individuals are more often benign, whereas multiple synchronous tumors in older adults are usually malignant (metastatic).

Most patients with malignant tumors of bone have pain and discomfort. Pain that is present with both activity and rest, especially night pain, is worrisome and demands further attention. Many patients with benign tumors are completely asymptomatic and seek medical attention because of an unrelated problem, and radiographic studies reveal an unexpected abnormality. Weight loss, fever, malaise, sweats, and chills can occur with certain tumors, usually small round blue cell tumors such as Ewing's sarcoma, lymphoma, and eosinophilic granuloma. Alcohol, tobacco use, and a family history of cancer should be determined. Environmental and occupational exposure to cancer-causing agents is difficult to elicit but important to establish.

Physical examination should include a general survey of all organ systems. It is important to document the location and size of the lesion, the presence or absence of deformity, overlying skin changes, swelling, joint motion, crepitus, auscultation (especially if a vascular tumor is suspected), palpation of regional lymph nodes, and a careful neurologic and vascular assessment.

Generally, laboratory data is nonspecific and of limited value in the diagnosis of most bone tumors. Certain tests, however, can help to differentiate between tumors and tumor-like conditions of bone. For example, a complete blood count and erythrocyte sedimentation rate can be useful in differentiating tumor from infection. Serum chemistries, particularly calcium, phosphorus, alkaline and acid phosphate, and lactate dehydrogenase are very useful. Hypercalcemia as well as abnormalities of alkaline and acid phosphatase can be associated with metastatic diseases as well as metabolic bone diseases. Specific tumor markers such as prostate specific antigen and serum immune electrophoresis can be helpful in the diagnosis of metastatic prostate cancer and multiple myeloma, respectively. These and other tumor markers are valuable in the evaluation of patients for disease recurrence and response to treatment.

Imaging Studies

Radiographs

All patients with a suspected bone tumor should have biplanar radiographs that include the joints above and below the lesion. The biology of the lesion can be assessed by evaluating the margin, the fundamental relationship of the tumor to the bone, the internal matrix that identifies the general type of tumor (bone,

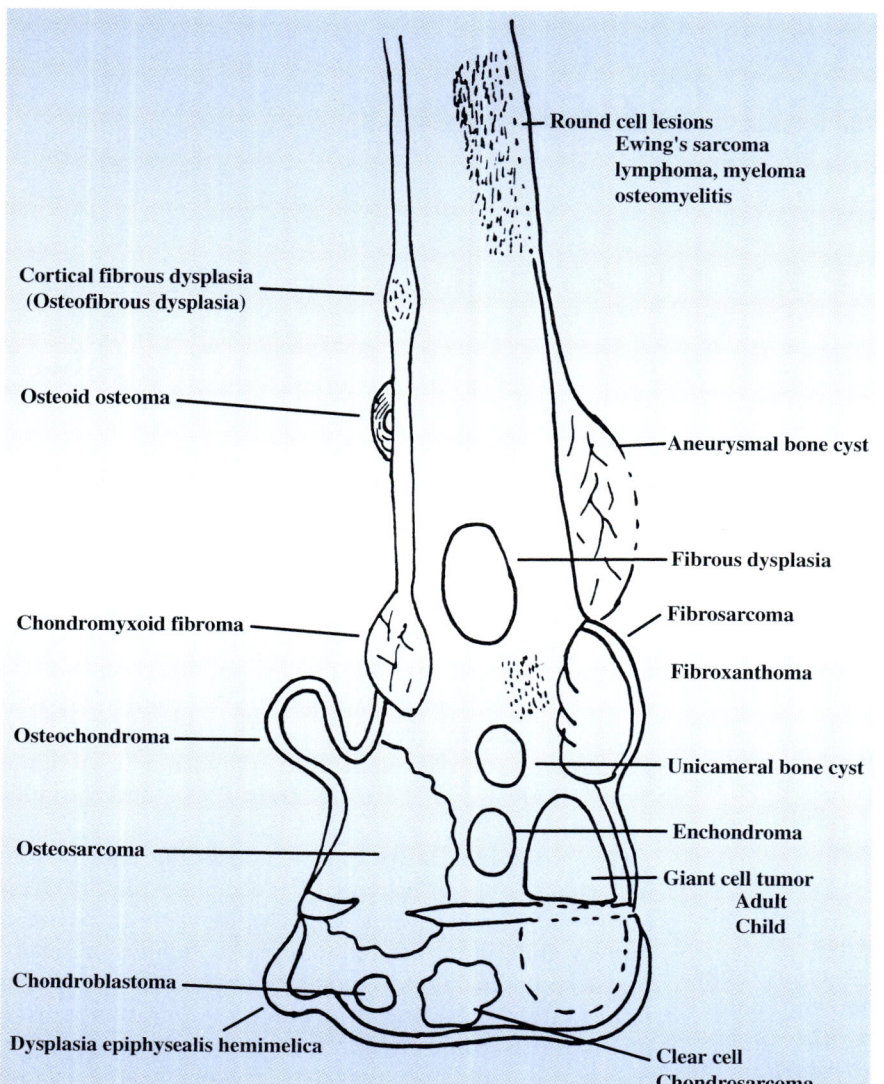

Round cell lesions
Ewing's sarcoma
lymphoma, myeloma
osteomyelitis

Cortical fibrous dysplasia
(Osteofibrous dysplasia)

Osteoid osteoma

Aneurysmal bone cyst

Fibrous dysplasia

Fibrosarcoma

Chondromyxoid fibroma

Fibroxanthoma

Osteochondroma

Unicameral bone cyst

Osteosarcoma

Enchondroma

Giant cell tumor
Adult
Child

Chondroblastoma

Dysplasia epiphysealis hemimelica

Clear cell
Chondrosarcoma

Figure 1 Diagram showing tumor location. *(Reproduced with permission from Madewell JE, Ragsdale BD, Sweet DE: Radiologic and pathologic analysis of solitary bone lesions: Part I. Internal margins. Radiol Clin North Am 1981;19:715-748.)*

cartilage, or fibrous) and periosteal reaction, the bone's response to tumor destruction. A narrow zone of transition between the lesion and normal bone or a geographic margin suggest a benign disease process, whereas a wider zone of transition and permeative or moth-eaten patterns of destruction suggest a more aggressive benign or malignant tumor. Tumors of osseous origin such as osteoid osteoma, osteoblastoma, or osteosarcoma produce a characteristic internal matrix pattern that has a cloud-like appearance whereas cartilage tumors such as enchondroma or chondrosarcoma have mineralization patterns reminiscent of arcs and rings, stippled calcifications, and flocculations. Fibrous tumors generally have an immature or woven bone matrix whose appearance is described radiographically as ground glass. Periosteal reactions around benign tumors or tumor-like conditions are generally smooth or laminated whereas aggressive tumors cause onion

skin or star-burst patterns of periosteal new bone formation.

Bone Scintigraphy

Bone scintigraphy can identify other skeletal sites of tumor, either skip metastases within the same bone or distant sites. Whole body technetium Tc 99m-methylene diphosphate scintigraphy is commonly used for staging and surveillance purposes, and tumor response to chemotherapy can be assessed as well. Diminished radiotracer uptake has been shown to occur in tumors with a favorable response to chemotherapy. In some tumors of bone, particularly cartilage lesions, the intensity and uniformity of uptake may be helpful in distinguishing benign from malignant tumors. Thallium 201 has also been used to assess tumor response to chemotherapeutic intervention, particularly in patients with osteosarcoma. For patients in whom myeloma is suspected, a skeletal survey is necessary to determine other sites of disease because of the high false-negative results associated with bone scintigraphy.

Computed Tomography

CT best demonstrates cortical and endosteal destruction as well as subtle matrix production. It is useful in localizing small lesions in complex bones, especially those in the spine, pelvis, and hindfoot. Soft-tissue extension of tumor and its relationship to nerves and blood vessels are adequately visualized on CT for the purpose of image-directed biopsy procedures. CT of the chest is necessary in all patients with malignant primary tumors of bone because metastatic disease spread is most common in the lungs. Spiral CT has been reported to be a more sensitive modality to detect early lung metastases. A novel use of CT has been to assess the local host response in bone after chemotherapeutic intervention to predict the amount of tumor necrosis or chemosensitivity of osteosarcoma.

Angiography

Diminished tumor vascularity after chemotherapy has been shown to correlate with improved survival for patients with osteosarcoma. Otherwise, this modality is not particularly useful in staging musculoskeletal tumors and has been replaced by MRI. Therapeutically, angiography is chiefly used preoperatively for chemoembolization or mechanical embolization of malignant tumors.

Magnetic Resonance Imaging

For surgical planning, MRI is perhaps the most important radiographic study because it provides anatomic details of the tumor's relationship to muscle compartments, adjacent joints, and neurovascular structures. Dynamic contrast MRI has been used to identify the most viable or vascular areas of a tumor. This technique can assess tumor response to chemotherapy before surgery, and can demonstrate early disease recurrence after surgery.

Biopsy

Although the biopsy is technically a minor procedure, major adverse consequences can occur if it is done incorrectly. Unlike carcinomas, sarcomas are highly implantable in soft tissue. For this reason, biopsy tracks are considered contaminated and must be excised during tumor resection. Biopsy tracks should traverse only one compartment and be placed along the planned course of resection; nerves, vascular structures, and joints should be avoided. In addition, hemostasis must be meticulous because hematoma contami-

nates adjacent normal tissue, which too must be resected. The leading edge of the soft-tissue component of tumor should be targeted, and needle or open biopsy directly into bone should be avoided or minimized to avoid stress risers and hemorrhage. The site and direction of needle placement is very important for future reconstruction because contaminated tissues must be removed at the time of resection.

At most cancer centers, needle biopsies are now performed when technically feasible. The clear advantages of needle biopsy are lower cost (at most institutions), decreased risk of hematoma, accurate image guidance, and avoidance of regional or general anesthesia. However, needle biopsy has a higher risk of sampling error and special studies such as flow cytometry, gene rearrangement, electron microscopy, and immunohistochemical staining are sometimes not possible due to small tissue quantities. Open biopsy provides more tissue for both diagnostic and research purposes, but is associated with increased morbidity and requires removal of more tissue at the time of tumor resection.

Studies show that biopsy errors increase the need for amputation and decrease survival. Two studies have shown that biopsy errors are more frequent in community or referring hospitals and urge that biopsies be performed in the institution at which definitive treatment is planned.

Staging

Staging is the process of identifying a tumor and determining its extent. Because treatment and prognosis depend on the tumor stage, the staging process must be organized and efficient and should be done at a center dedicated to the diagnosis and treatment of musculoskeletal tumors. A multidisciplinary team approach is necessary to arrive at the correct diagnosis and for optimal treatment. Staging is an ongoing process before, throughout, and after treatment because tumor surveillance continues for many years after completion of therapy.

The most common staging classification used by orthopaedic oncologists is the Enneking staging system that has been adopted by the Musculoskeletal Tumor Society (Table 1). This system is designed to guide treatment of malignant musculoskeletal tumors of bone and soft tissue. Patients with malignant bone tumors are stratified into three groups based on tumor grade (high or low), location within or outside a compartment, and the presence or absence of metastases (lymph nodes, distant organs, or skip metastases).

An alternative staging system is the American Joint Committee on Cancer, which considers whether the tumor is confined to bone (T1) or extends beyond bone (T2), grade (G1-4), nodal involvement (N) and

TABLE 1	Musculoskeletal Tumor Society Staging System

Stage	Histologic Grade	Compartment	Metastatic
IA	Low	Within	No
IB	Low	Outside	No
IIA	High	Within	No
IIB	High	Outside	No
III	Any	Any	Yes

(Reproduced from Mizel MS, Miller RA, Scioli MW (eds): Orthopaedic Knowledge Update: Foot and Ankle 2. Rosemont, IL, American Academy of Orthopaedic Surgeons, 1998, pp 11-26.)

distant tumor spread (M). This information was previously summarized in a Table appearing in *OKU 6*.

Molecular Biology of Neoplasia

During neoplasia, the genes that regulate cell proliferation are dysregulated and the net result is excessive DNA synthesis and cell division. Genes that lead to neoplasia are called oncogenes and their discovery has rapidly accelerated the understanding of how selected proteins are required for normal cellular homeostasis and how these proteins can encourage tumor cell survival, growth, and spread.

Proteins are the building blocks that assemble cells and maintain and monitor their performance and function. They are involved in motility, phagocytosis, membrane receptor processing, intracellular signaling, cell adhesion, and exocytosis. Proteins also make up the molecules within the cell nucleus that bind to DNA regulation sites and influence gene expression. Examples of this group of molecules are the cyclins, a family of proteins that guide the cell through cell division and the transcription factor E2F. Enzymes are another form of protein that have critical nuclear and cytoplasmic functions. Enzymes that function inside the nucleus transcribe DNA, process RNA, and activate critical molecules involved in gene regulation. One example is a family of enzymes called cyclin-dependent kinases (CDKs).

Enzymes that function or are located in cytoplasmic organelles play critical roles within and outside the cell. These enzymes catalyze cytoplasmic biochemical reactions required for cell function and homeostasis, and they perform vital extracellular functions after secretion from the cell. These functions include extracellular matrix degradation and activation of extracellular growth factors and cytokines. Finally, growth factors and cytokines are proteins. These molecules are often responsible for cell-to-cell or extracellular matrix-cell communication and they influence an inexhaustible number of cellular events.

Knowing how important proteins are for cell performance and function, it follows that abnormalities in their quantity or construction would be expected to result in disease and would be expected to be at the origin of neoplasia. For this reason, tremendous energy and resources have focused on identifying the genes that encode for vital proteins and on understanding how expression of these genes is regulated.

Genes are composed of coding and noncoding regions. The coding regions provide a DNA sequence that can be transcribed into messenger RNA (mRNA) and ultimately translated into chains of amino acids, which form proteins. The noncoding regions (promoter regions) provide binding sites for nuclear enzymes and signaling proteins, called transcription factors, that influence gene expression, or transcription. For example, mRNA polymerase, the enzyme that transcribes DNA into RNA, binds to the noncoding region of genes before they can be transcribed. Additional DNA binding sites are present for transcription factors. These proteins can encourage (enhancers) or discourage (repressors) gene expression.

The transcription factor E2F is important in musculoskeletal tumors. This protein acts as an enhancer and is responsible for transcription of a set of genes that initiate DNA synthesis and cell division. An example of how altered gene expression can cause or can be associated with musculoskeletal neoplasia is illustrated by the protein encoded by the retinoblastoma gene, pRb (Fig. 2). This protein binds to and inactivates the transcription factor E2F. During the initial phase of normal cell division, pRb is phosphorylated by a cyclin/CDK holoenzyme. This phosphorylation inactivates pRb and frees E2F, allowing E2F to bind to the promoter region of various genes involved in DNA synthesis. This action results in a stimulus for cell division. Because the active (unphosphorylated) form of pRb blocks transcriptional activation of DNA synthesis genes, pRb is called a tumor suppressor gene.

Two tumor suppressor genes have been closely associated with bone sarcomas, the *RB* gene (*pRb*) and the *TB53* (*p53*) gene. The *RB* gene has been found to be absent or expressed at low levels in osteosarcoma and other cancers, permitting higher levels of activation of E2F. Similarly, the *TB53* gene has been found to be absent or expressed at low levels in rhabdomyosarcoma and osteosarcoma. Identification of the association between absent or greatly diminished expression of these genes and sarcomas provides direction for current research on the cause and cure for these devastating cancers.

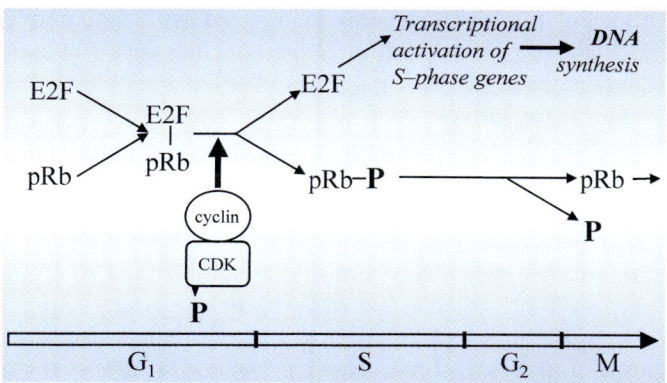

Figure 2 Interaction between the retinoblastoma protein and cyclin/CDK complexes. pRb = active retinoblastoma protein; pRb-P-inactive (phosphorylated) retinoblastoma protein; E2F = transcriptional factors. *(Reproduced from Clohisy DR: Growth and metastasis of musculoskeletal tumors, in Buckwalter JA, Einhorn TA, Simon SR (eds): Orthopaedic Basic Science: Biology and Biomechanics of the Musculoskeletal System, ed 2. Rosemont, IL, American Academy of Orthopaedic Surgeons, 2000, pp 428-441.)*

The molecular process that ultimately results in neoplasia in most cases will prove to be complex and, from a molecular biology standpoint, multifactorial. One contributing element can be modified gene expression, as illustrated by the tumor suppressor genes *RB* and *TB53*. A second type of molecular alteration that can contribute to neoplasia is chromosomal or gene abnormalities.

One type of chromosomal alteration associated with bone and soft-tissue sarcomas is gene translocation. A gene translocation occurs when two chromosomes exchange pieces, forming a chimeric gene. Chromosomal translocations are the most common gene rearrangement associated with neoplasia. As might be expected, the most common chromosomal translocations in cancer cells involve genes that encode transcription factors. After the translocation event, novel proteins (fusion proteins) can result from the positioning of coding sequences from two genes that are normally located on different chromosomes in continuous sequence. Fusion proteins can be responsible for the malignant phenotype and are tumor type-specific.

Ewing's sarcoma and some soft-tissue sarcomas have been shown to have distinct gene translocations. Unique and specific gene translocations have been identified for several soft-tissue sarcomas, including myxoid liposarcoma (chromosomes 12:16), synovial sarcoma (X:18), and rhabdomyosarcoma (2:13). Ewing's sarcoma (11:22) is the only bone sarcoma distinguished by a specific gene translocation thus far. The chimeric genes in each of these malignancies are suspected to encode for fusion proteins that act as transcription factors. For example, the 11:22 fusion gene associated with Ewing's sarcoma encodes for a transcription factor that contains the transactivating domain encoded by the *EWS* gene and the DNA binding domain encoded by the *FLI-1* gene.

Identification of chromosomal abnormalities in musculoskeletal cancers will benefit the diagnosis of these tumors in the future and may benefit their treatment as well. Accuracy of diagnosis is enhanced, as modern molecular diagnostic techniques can identify specific gene rearrangements in cancer cells. Potential new treatments are provided by the opportunity to invent immune-based treatments targeting the fusion proteins.

Tumors of Bone
Osseous Tumors of Bone
Enostosis
An enostosis or bone island is a hamartoma—normal tissue in an abnormal location. In this case, there is normal cortical bone in the medullary canal. These lesions are asymptomatic, are generally found incidentally, and are most common in the cranial sinuses, cranial vault, and mandible as well as the ilium and the proximal femur. They are generally smaller than 2 cm and are radiodense with spiculated borders that blend with the surrounding cancellous bone. Generally there is no radiotracer uptake on bone scan but in giant enostoses (those exceeding 2 cm), uptake can be seen in up to 30% of lesions. Enostoses can be multiple and this condition is termed osteopoikilosis, a rare autosomal dominant condition.

Treatment is observation unless the diagnosis is in doubt, especially for patients with giant enostoses in unusual locations. In these cases, biopsy may be necessary to establish the correct diagnosis.

Osteoid Osteoma
This is a common and painful vascular lesion of uncertain etiology most often affecting individuals during the first and second decades of life. Pain at night is characteristic and is typically relieved with salicylates. Although the disease is self-limiting, clonal chromosomal changes have been demonstrated, suggesting that osteoid osteoma, like osteoblastoma, may be neoplastic. Osteoid osteoma is most often located in the cortex of long bones but can be periosteally and (rarely) medullary-based. CT is most effective in identifying this lesion. Focal intense radiotracer uptake is seen on bone scintigraphy. The nidus is radiolucent, generally measuring less than 1.5 cm, and there is an abundance of surrounding reactive and sclerotic bone. In the spine, like osteoblastoma, osteoid osteoma typically occurs in the posterior elements and may cause scoliosis. Microscopically, osteoid osteoma consists of fibrovascular stroma with woven bone formation, similar to osteoblastoma.

Most patients complain of pain, and initial treatment is with nonsteroidal anti-inflammatory drugs (NSAIDs). In those patients in whom NSAIDs are contraindicated or who develop complications related to their use, or in those whose symptoms are refractory to chronic NSAID use, surgery is a reasonable alternative. The efficacy of the COX-2 inhibitor family of NSAIDs has not been studied in patients with osteoid osteoma but may offer a safer method of long-term treatment of this disease.

En bloc excision was the favored surgical treatment in the past but the current trend is toward simple excision and curetting of the nidus. Less invasive techniques such as radiofrequency ablation and CT-guided percutaneous core needle excision have been effective; reported recurrences are low with minimal treatment complications.

Osteoblastoma

Osteoblastoma accounts for less than 1% of all bone neoplasms and is most often seen in the metaphyseal area of long bones, the posterior elements of the spine, and the collective bones of the foot. The condition is predominant in males during the second and third decades of life. Osteoblastoma may be indolent and appear more like an osteoid osteoma, or it can be aggressive and confused with osteosarcoma.

Osteoblastoma is composed of trabeculae of woven bone in a rich fibrovascular stroma. There may be some osteoblastic mitotic activity but no atypia. Secondary aneurysmal changes have been reported in up to 10% of cases. Osteoblastoma can be distinguished from osteosarcoma by osteoblastic rimming of newly formed bone and by the absence of permeation and entrapment of host bone. Aggressive osteoblastomas are distinct in that the osteoblasts are quite large and epithelioid in appearance. Sheet-like osteoid production and stromal hemorrhage can also be seen. Metastases have been reported to occur in patients with osteoblastoma but are very rare; local disease recurrence is far more common. Thorough curetting is adequate for most osteoid–osteoma-like osteoblastomas, but wide local excision is necessary for aggressive lesions.

Osteosarcoma

Although a number of variants exist, osteosarcoma is a malignant tumor of bone that makes bone, and can occur either within bone or on its surface. Conventional osteosarcoma is medullary-based, high-grade, and has a bimodal frequency. The majority of tumors occur in adolescent patients, males more often than females, and a small number occur in older patients who received radiotherapy in the past or in patients with Paget's disease. Despite being the most common primary malignancy of bone, osteosarcoma is rare compared with carcinomas such as lung, breast, and prostate, affecting approximately 2,000 patients in the United States annually.

Since the advent of multiagent chemotherapy, patient survival has improved dramatically. High-dose methotrexate in conjunction with adriamycin, and *cis*-platinum, are the principal drugs currently used to treat osteosarcoma. Typically, patients receive chemotherapy preoperatively, are restaged, and then undergo surgery for local disease control. In the past, amputation was the standard of care but with successful chemotherapeutic intervention, advanced surgical techniques, and better imaging modalities, limb salvage is possible in up to 90% of patients.

Local recurrence correlates with the adequacy of the tumor resection and tumor response to chemotherapy. In a study of 540 patients with nonmetastatic osteosarcoma, there were 31 patients with local recurrence (6%). Interestingly, only 1 patient with a local recurrence was free of disease at 15 months, 3 were alive with uncontrolled disease, and 27 died of disease. The authors concluded that patients with inadequate surgical margins should undergo immediate amputation, especially patients with a poor response to chemotherapy.

There are several different histologic subtypes of high-grade intraosseous osteosarcoma: osteoblastic, chondroblastic, fibroblastic, telangiectatic, and small cell. Although the histologic pattern is diverse, there is ostensibly no difference in treatment for these different subtypes and the common histologic thread that runs between these tumors is the presence of malignant mesenchymal cells that make osteoid. No statistically significant difference in outcome (survival) has been shown based on histologic subtype.

It is clear that survival in osteosarcoma and other high-grade malignant tumors of bone, such as Ewing's sarcoma, is dependent on tumor location. For example, survival is greater for patients with tumors arising in the appendicular skeleton whereas patients with tumors of the pelvis and spine have much worse outcomes. The 5-year survival in patients with pelvic osteosarcoma has been reported to be between 26% to 34% in two recent studies. Tumor stage at the time of presentation is also prognostically significant. Osteosarcoma commonly metastasizes to lung parenchyma and patients presenting with stage III disease have a far worse disease outcome than patients without metastases. These patients are generally treated with high-dose chemotherapy and simultaneous resection of the primary tumor as well as the lung nodules. In one study, the combination of surgery (pulmonary metastastectomy) and chemotherapy improved survival while in another, the prognosis was poor with overall 5-year

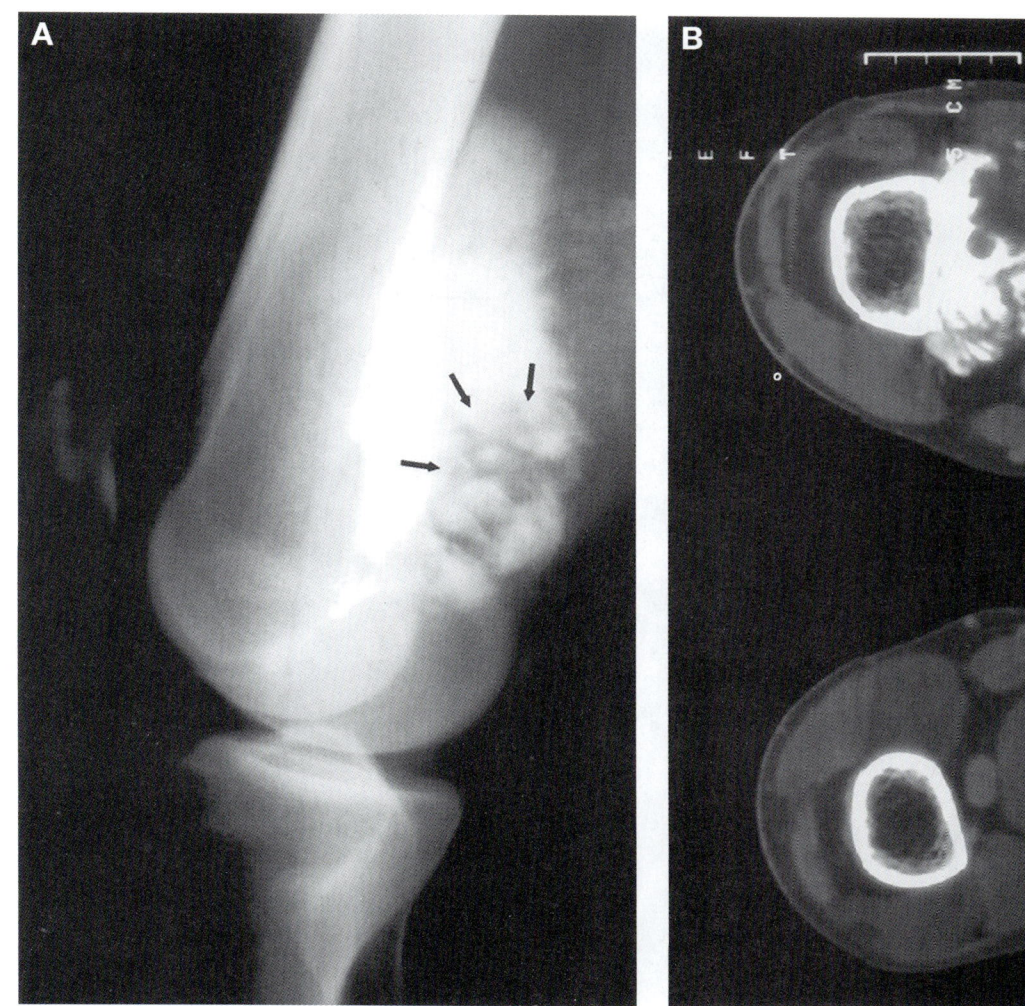
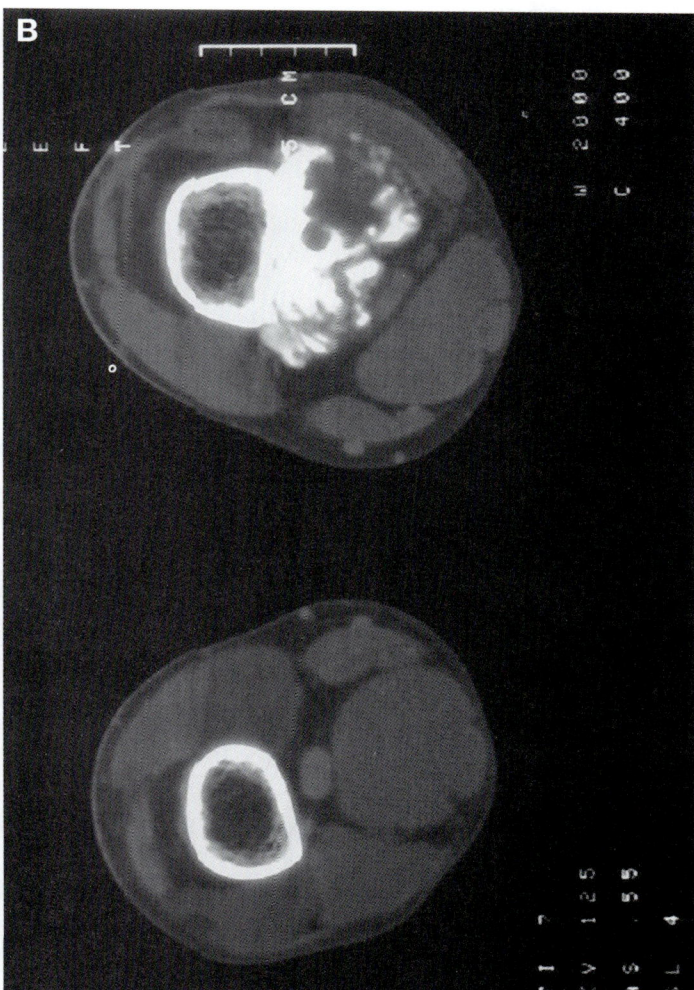

Figure 3 **A,** Lateral radiograph demonstrating lucency within a surface osteosarcoma (parosteal osteosarcoma) indicated by the arrows. This region proved to be a focus of high-grade osteosarcoma (dedifferentiated osteosarcoma). **B,** CT scan showing a low-attenuation area corresponding to the lucency seen on the lateral radiograph.

survival of 17% for patients with synchronous lung metastases versus 79% for patients with localized disease. Patients with other concomitant metastases to sites such as lymph nodes and bone have a very poor prognosis.

Other prognostic factors that adversely affect survival are expression of P-glycoprotein, high alkaline phosphatase, high lactic dehydrogenase, vascular invasion, large tumor size, no alteration in DNA ploidy after chemotherapy, and the absence of antiheat shock protein 90 antibodies after chemotherapy. P-glycoprotein is a product of the multidrug resistance gene complex and DNA ploidy studies represent the relative proportion of cells in the various stages of DNA replication.

Surface or parosteal osteosarcomas generally occur around the third and fourth decades of life and unlike conventional osteosarcoma are more common in women. Parosteal osteosarcoma is usually found on the posteromedial aspect of the knee and is closely apposed to the cortex. In one study, the cortex was invaded by tumor in more than 70% of patients and in 44% of patients, tumor was found extending into the medullary cavity. Parosteal osteosarcoma is typically a low-grade malignant tumor but may harbor foci of higher-grade tumor, especially when they recur, and are usually identified as radiolucent areas on radiographs or low attenuation areas on CT (Fig. 3). The differential diagnosis includes osteochondroma and myositis ossificans. Parosteal osteosarcoma is distinguished from osteochondroma in that it lacks corticomedullary trabecular continuity—a radiographic feature present in all osteochondromas. The pattern of zonation seen radiographically and histologically is different in myositis ossificans where the periphery of the tumor appears more mature than the central portion. This pattern of maturation is reversed in patients with osteosarcoma (Fig. 4). Treatment is complete excision, and adjuvant chemotherapy is not necessary unless high-grade areas are found histologically.

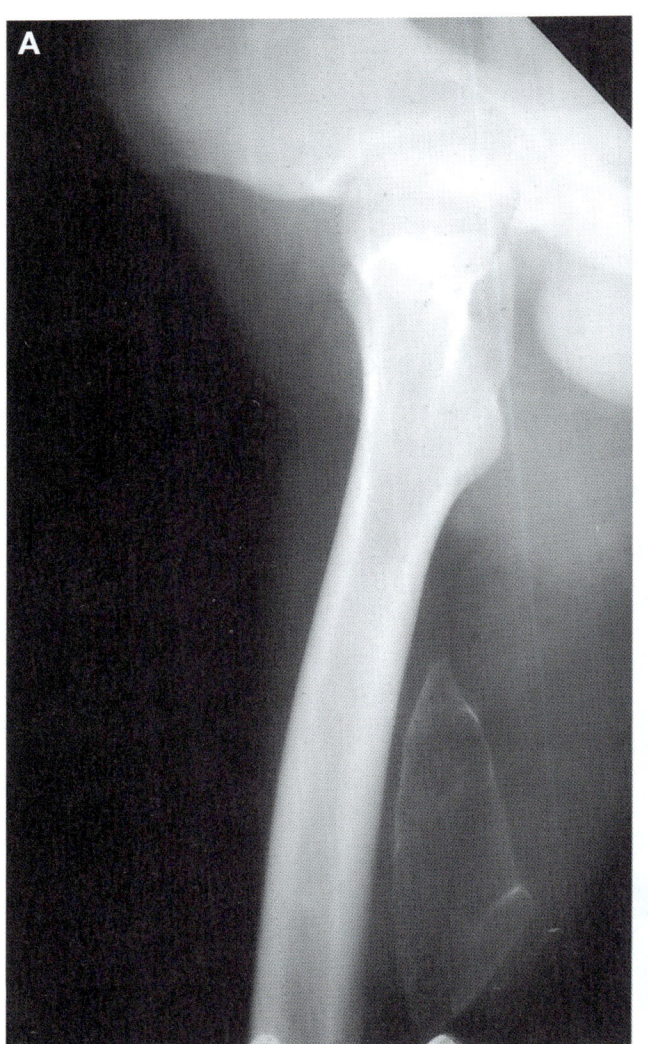
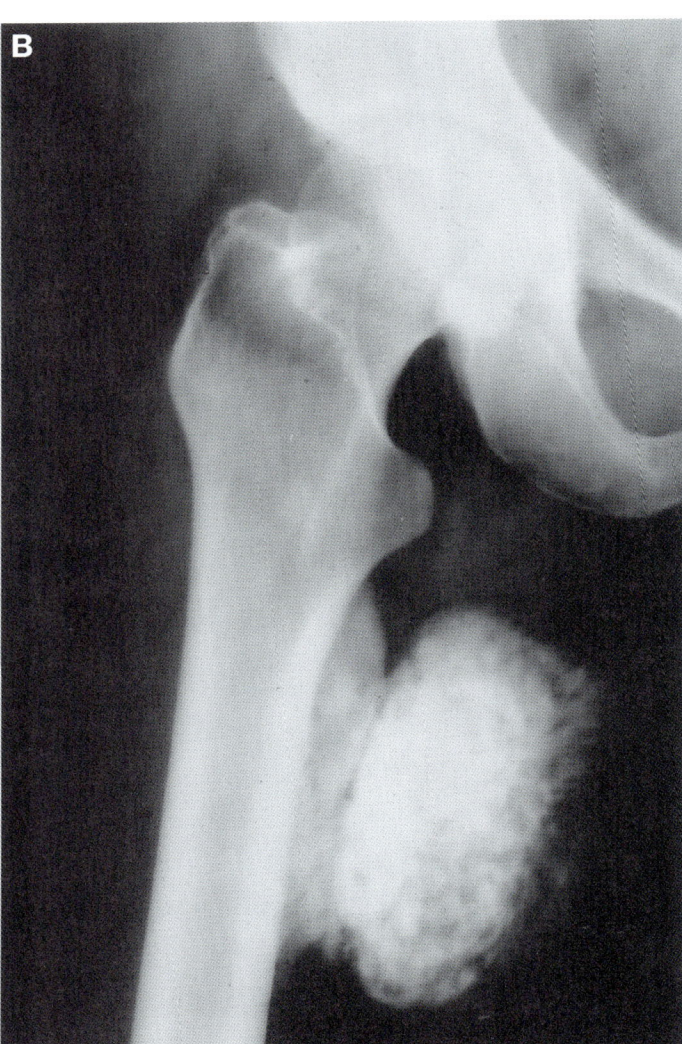

Figure 4 **A,** Lateral radiograph of the proximal femur revealing a juxtacortical osseous mass with smooth, well-defined borders representing myositis ossificans. **B,** AP radiograph of the proximal femur showing a juxtacortical mass with ill-defined peripheral borders and a more mature-appearing pattern of mineralization centrally that is typical of parosteal osteosarcoma.

Periosteal osteosarcoma is intermediate grade with predominant chondroid differentiation. Unlike parosteal osteosarcoma, it rarely grows into the medullary space. Treatment is wide local resection and chemotherapy is generally given. High-grade surface osteosarcoma represents 8% of all osteosarcomas and is often found in the diaphysis of long bones, especially the femur. Like conventional osteosarcoma, it is treated with chemotherapy and wide local resection.

Low-grade central osteosarcoma is a very rare tumor that generally occurs in an older age group and can be confused with benign conditions, especially fibrous dysplasia. Metastases are uncommon. Unlike fibrous dysplasia, low-grade central osteosarcoma produces dense osseous matrix that is better demonstrated on CT. Histologically, the stroma is more cellular than that seen in fibrous dysplasia and osteoid production is apparent. Treatment is wide local excision.

Tumors of Cartilage

Osteochondroma

Solitary osteochondromas occur sporadically and are thought to arise from a defect in the perichondral ring. They are attached to the surface of the bone by an osseous stalk. The unifying feature of all osteochondromas is the presence of osseous trabecular continuity between the stalk and medullary canal. Generally, patients complain of a painless mass; however, pain may be present for a variety of reasons that include tendinitis, bursitis, and neural compression, fracture through the base of the stalk, osteonecrosis of the cartilage cap, and malignant transformation. Vascular pseudoaneurysms have been reported.

Malignant transformation is rare, especially for patients with solitary tumors, and it does not occur before skeletal maturity. Osteochondromas in proximal appendicular

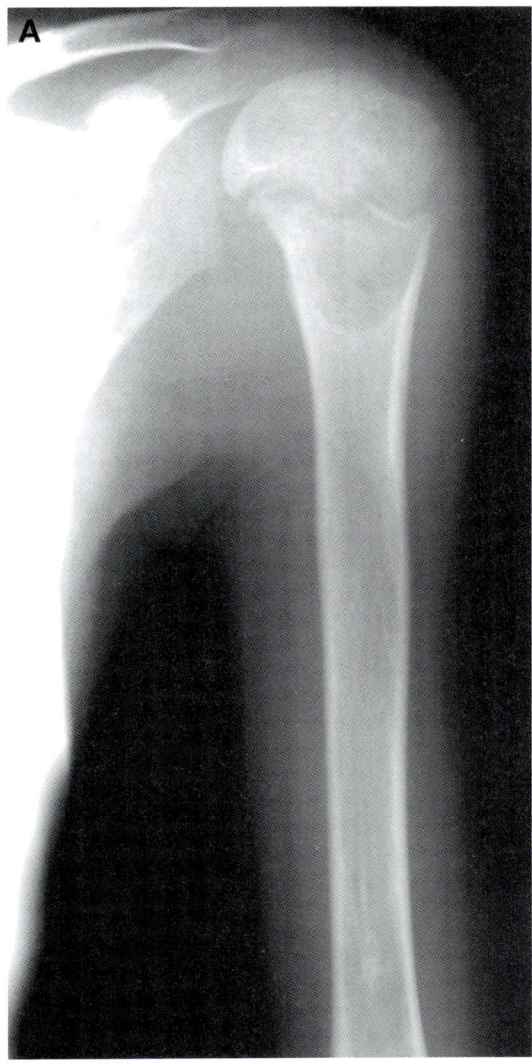

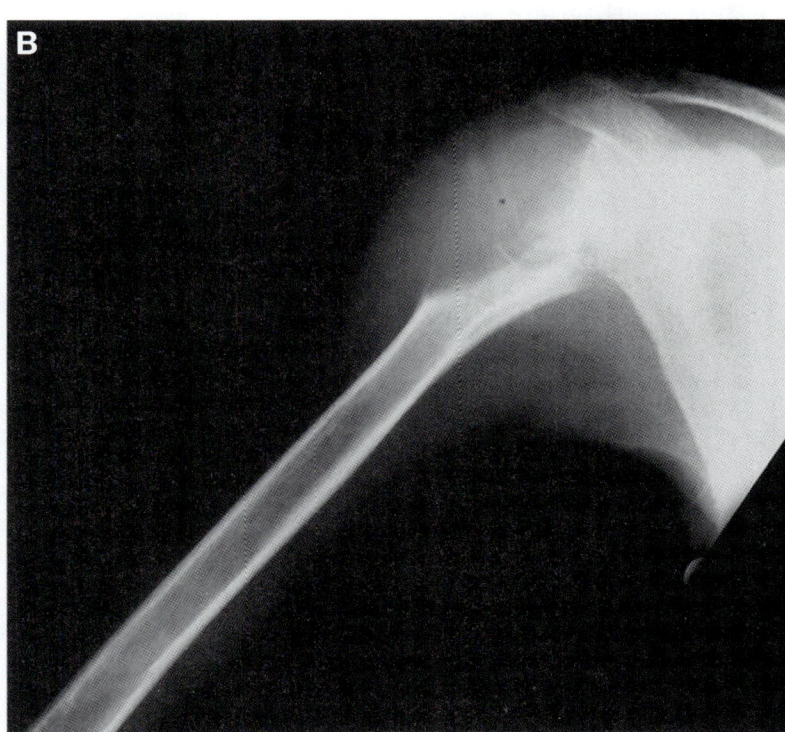

Figure 5 **A** and **B,** AP and lateral radiographs of a 9-year-old boy with an aggressive chondroblastoma of the proximal humerus. Note that the lesion crosses the physis and involves both the epiphysis and metaphysis.

sites and axial locations seem to be at greater risk than more distal appendicular lesions. Malignant transformation is more often seen in patients with multiple hereditary osteochondromatosis, an autosomal dominant condition that is genetically heterogenic and associated with mutations of gene loci *EXT1* and *EXT2*, two putative tumor suppressor genes. Radiographic features in patients with malignant transformation of osteochondromas include: thickening of the cartilage cap often accompanied by dystrophic mineralization, lysis of a portion of the stalk, and underlying bone and intramedullary invasion that has been observed in 33% of patients in one study.

Treatment is observation for asymptomatic tumors. For painful lesions, excision of the osteochondral excrescence including the stalk, cartilage cap, and overlying bursa may be necessary. In children the lesions are typically adjacent to the growth plate and excision should be delayed until the cessation of growth if possible.

Chondroblastoma

Chondroblastoma is a rare, epiphyseal-based tumor that is most commonly diagnosed in the first two decades of life. This tumor is associated with genetic abnormalities in chromosomes 5 and 8. Chondroblastoma can be locally aggressive and, on rare occasions, metastasize to the lung (Fig. 5). It is most often seen in the ends of long bones as well as the collective bones of the foot and ankle. In the foot, the talus is most frequently involved and in up to 50% of cases, cystic changes occur and are confused with a simple bone cyst. In the foot and ankle, the lesion always effaces subchondral bone in contrast with a simple cyst, which occurs in the anterior aspect of the calcaneus but does not extend into subchondral bone. Chondroblastomas are often painful and because of their epiphyseal location, frequently cause effusions.

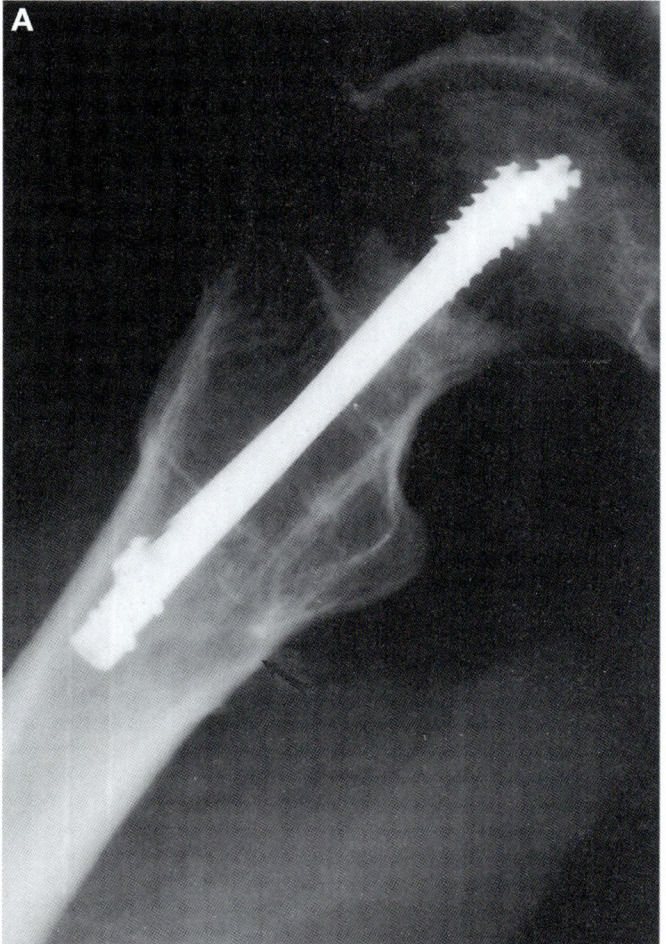

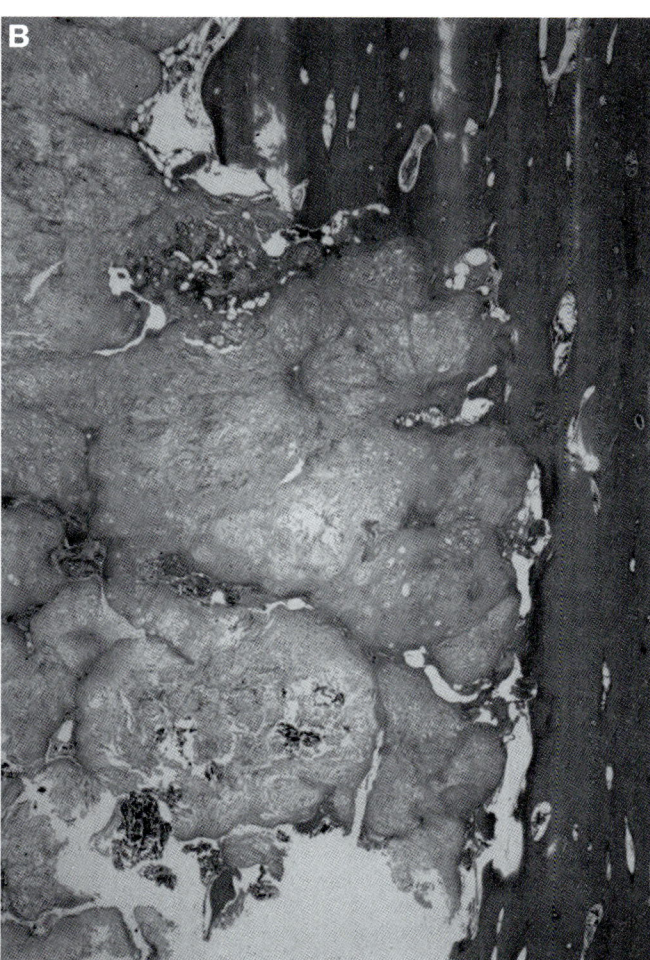

Figure 6 **A,** Lateral radiograph of a 49-year-old woman who sustained a nondisplaced femoral neck fracture 4 years prior to presentation with a radiolucent abnormality in the subtrochanteric region of the femur with deep endosteal scallops (*arrow*). **B,** A biopsy reveals a low-grade chondrosarcoma growing in a lobular pattern and scalloping the endosteal surface of cortical bone.

Radiographically, chondroblastomas are generally radiolucent with rare mineralization and a sclerotic border. Chondroblastomas may be destructive and have poorly circumscribed margins. The lesion is composed of polygonal stromal cells and occasional giant cells. The cell nuclei have a characteristic indentation or cleavage. Occasionally the cells involute and the cell membranes mineralize, giving the microscopic appearance of chicken-wire calcification.

Most chondroblastomas are treated by curetting and burring and have been reported to recur in 15% and 25% of cases in two large series of patients. Some authors advocate the use of phenol as an adjunct; however, because of the proximity of these lesions to the growth plate and articular surface, it should be used with caution.

Chondromyxoid Fibroma

Chondromyxoid fibroma is a rare benign tumor found in the metaphyseal ends of long bones, short

tubular bones of the foot, and less commonly in the hand. The tumor occurs during the third and fourth decades of life. This neoplasm has a characteristic rearrangement on chromosome 6 at position q13 (6q13). However, the role that this genetic alteration plays in the development and pathogenesis of this tumor is still unknown.

Pain is the typical presenting complaint. The tumor is eccentric and radiolucent with internal septations and a markedly thinned cortex. Matrix production is subtle and is seen in 34% of patients. A mixed pattern of cellularity is seen microscopically with hypercellular spindled areas juxtaposed to hypocellular loose fibromyxoid stroma. Treatment is aggressive curetting and bone grafting.

Enchondroma

Enchondromas develop when physeal cartilage does not undergo ossification, becomes entrapped in bone, and ultimately resides in the metaphysis or diaphysis.

Anomalies that occur peripherally in the physis become periosteal or cortical chondromas whereas those that occur centrally are termed enchondromas. Multiple enchondromas are seen in patients with Ollier's disease. The presence of hemangiomata with multiple enchondromas occurs in patients with Maffucci's syndrome. Malignant transformation is rare in patients with a solitary enchondroma, but occurs in 25% of patients with Ollier's disease and Maffucci's syndrome.

Enchondromas are mixed radiolucent and radiodense abnormalities with mineralizations that appear as arcs and rings or flocculations. Most enchondromas have increased radiotracer uptake on bone scan. Active enchondromas can be difficult to distinguish from low-grade chondrosarcomas. Endosteal scalloping appreciated on radiographs or CT that exceeds two thirds of the cortex is highly suspicious for malignant transformation (Fig. 6). This finding, along with pain and radiotracer uptake that exceeds the intensity of uptake in the ipsilateral iliac spine with a heterogeneous uptake pattern, is strongly suggestive of malignant change. Location is also very important. Cartilage tumors located in the proximal appendicular skeleton or in axial locations, scapula, and pelvis are more worrisome than lesions in the small tubular bones of the hands and feet. Pathologists will accept hypercellularity and a moderate degree of atypia in lesions of the small tubular bones before making a malignant diagnosis. Similar microscopic changes in tumors in more proximal appendicular or axial sites would immediately evoke a malignant diagnosis. More than with any other tumor, correlation between the clinical, radiographic, and microscopic findings is essential in making the correct diagnosis.

Treatment for a solitary enchondroma is observation. Treatment of low-grade chondrosarcoma is controversial and there is increasing evidence that extended curetting and adjunct thermal (methylmethacrylate) or chemical cautery may be adequate. Wide local excision is also an acceptable treatment but is now less commonly used for low-grade tumors.

Chondrosarcoma

Chondrosarcoma may occur as a primary lesion or secondarily in preexisting benign antecedent tumors such as osteochondroma, enchondroma, or in previously irradiated tissue. It is common in the pelvis and the ends of long bones in the appendicular skeleton. This tumor is most common after the fourth decade and affects men more often than women. Aside from primary and secondary lesions, chondrosarcoma varies histologically by grade, histologic subtype (conventional, mesenchymal, clear cell, dedifferentiated), tumor grade, and location (intraosseous or juxtacortical).

Chondrosarcomas are resistant to chemotherapy and radiotherapy; thus, surgery alone is the treatment of choice for all chondrosarcomas except the dedifferentiated subtype. The use of chemotherapy in high-grade conventional chondrosarcoma is controversial. High levels of P-glycoprotein expression may render chondrosarcoma resistant to chemotherapy.

Dedifferentiated chondrosarcoma is a high-grade poorly differentiated sarcoma that arises in an antecedent low-grade chondrosarcoma. There is evidence that there is a common monoclonal origin of this tumor and given the substantial number of genetic alterations between the high- and low-grade components, early separation from the common precursor clone is likely. This tumor has a poor prognosis despite aggressive chemotherapy and resection.

Survival for patients with chondrosarcoma depends on tumor size, grade, location, and adequacy of surgical resection. Exciting developments in basic science that may have therapeutic consequences for patients with chondrosarcoma involve metalloproteinase inhibitors and effects of fluoroquinolones on chondroid matrix resulting in tumor growth arrest.

Fibrous Tumors of Bone
Unicameral Bone Cysts

Unicameral bone cysts are developmental anomalies of the physis where there is a transient failure of ossification of physical cartilage and cyst formation. They occur in patients during the first and second decades of life and are usually found incidentally or after a fracture. Unicameral bone cysts spontaneously resolve in late adolescence and rarely persist into adulthood. The most common location is the proximal humerus, followed by the proximal femur. In older adolescent patients and young adults, the anterior aspect of the calcaneus is a frequent site. On radiographs, unicameral bone cysts are well marginated, radiolucent lesions that are centrally located and that expand and thin the cortex. The fallen fragment sign (a comminuted fracture fragment within the cyst) is often observed in patients with pathologic fractures. The cyst is filled with thin, yellowish fluid that is often blood-tinged. The cyst wall is composed of fibrovascular tissue with giant cells and reactive bone. In long-standing and traumatized lesions, cholesterol clefts and macrophages with hemosiderin deposition are seen.

There are active and latent cysts; active cysts are juxtaposed to the physis and latent cysts are located away from the physis. Treatment is controversial and ranges from observation to aspiration and injection of steroids or bone and collagen products, to curetting and bone grafting, and even subtotal diaphysectomy. Despite treatment, recurrence is common, especially in active cysts. Most surgeons recommend treatment consisting of aspiration and injection for large and active lesions. Bone grafts may be optimal in patients with a large lesion in the proximal femur where pathologic fracture has increased morbidity.

Fibrous Dysplasia

In fibrous dysplasia, fibrous tissue with metaplastic bone replaces normal lamellar bone, resulting in structural weakening of the bone and increased risk of pathologic fracture. Progressive deformities can occur due to microscopic fractures. The disease is most commonly solitary but may also be multifocal. The degree of skeletal involvement in patients with polyostotic disease is highly variable. Albright's syndrome is a combination of polyostotic fibrous dysplasia, café-au-lait spots, and endocrinopathies.

The femur and humerus are most frequently involved. On radiographs, fibrous dysplasia is characterized by deep endosteal scallops and a prominent ground glass matrix. The proximal femur may develop a shepherd's crook deformity, so named because the upper end of the femoral shaft resembles a shepherd's crook, from multiple recurrent microfractures. Fractures occur on the tension side of affected bones. Microscopically, fibrous dysplasia consists of thin osseous trabeculae that is without a prominent osteoblastic lining and fibrous stroma. The arrangement of the osseous trabeculae is reminiscent of Chinese letter characters.

The orthopaedist's role in treating patients with fibrous dysplasia is to prevent deformity and treat pathologic fractures. If bone graft is used, cortical allograft is a reasonable choice because it provides structural support and is resorbed less readily than autograft or cancellous allograft. Internal fixation is a useful adjunct to bone grafting in the proximal femur and other locations where there is a risk of pathologic fracture. Tumor progression has been observed in pregnant women and in women taking birth control pills, underlining the functional importance of estrogen receptors in this tumor.

Fibroxanthoma

Fibroxanthoma is probably the most common musculoskeletal tumor occurring in up to 30% of children. The tumor is recognized during the first two decades of life and is generally self-limiting. It occurs in all long bones but most prominently in the femur, tibia, and humerus. In one series, fibroxanthomas were multiple in 8% of patients. Multiple lesions are commonly seen in patients with neurofibromatosis. Fibroxanthoma is also known as nonossifying fibroma but because the natural tendency for this lesion is to involute and ossify, this description is confusing. Other names include fibrous cortical defect and metaphyseal cortical defect.

Treatment is observation unless the lesion presents a risk for pathologic fracture. In a Mayo Clinic study, two variables were identified to be associated with increased pathologic fracture risk. These variables were tumor size exceeding 50% of the diameter of bone and longitudinal extension greater than 22 mm. These criteria, however, do not take into consideration tumor site or the degree to which the lesion had already ossified at the time of diagnosis. For pathologic fractures, immobilization and reassessment of the tumor after fracture healing is indicated.

Ossifying Fibroma/Adamantinoma

Ossifying fibroma is generally diagnosed during the first and second decades of life as an incidental finding unless there is associated deformity and/or a fracture. Radiographically the abnormality is radiolucent and there is a strong predilection for the anterior cortex of the tibia. Anterior tibial bowing may be present. Fractures and pseudofractures are not uncommon. On microscopic examination, the lesion is strikingly similar to fibrous dysplasia except that the osseous trabeculae have prominent osteoblastic rimming. Immunohistochemical studies have revealed the presence of cytokeratin in most examined specimens. Adamantinoma is similar but contains nests of epithelioid cells.

Observation is prudent with serial radiographs to document the presence or absence of disease progression. Bracing is recommended for young patients with bowing deformities. For older patients (adolescents and adults) with progressive symptomatic disease or impending pathologic fracture, complete surgical excision is indicated with bone grafting and internal fixation. For young patients with dramatic bowing deformities in whom bracing is difficult, impending pathologic fractures or fracture nonunions, resection, and Ilizarov application and bone transport may be indicated. There remains controversy as to whether ossifying fibroma represents a precursor of adamantinoma or is on a continuum with this malignant process. Adamantinoma is a low-grade malignancy treated by wide surgical excision.

Malignant Fibrous Histiocytoma

Malignant fibrous histiocytoma of bone is a relatively rare high-grade malignant tumor that occurs in

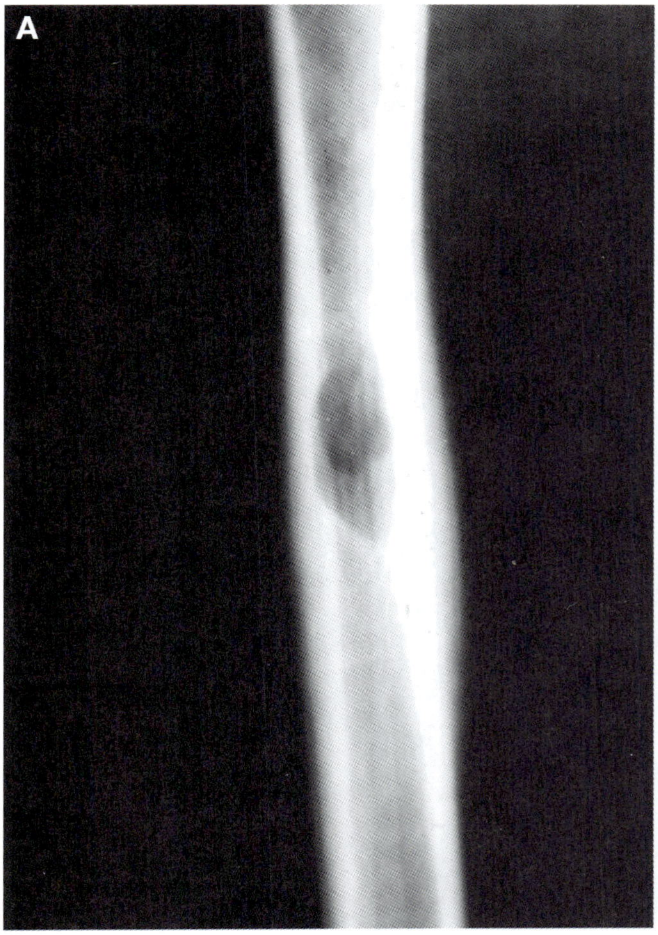

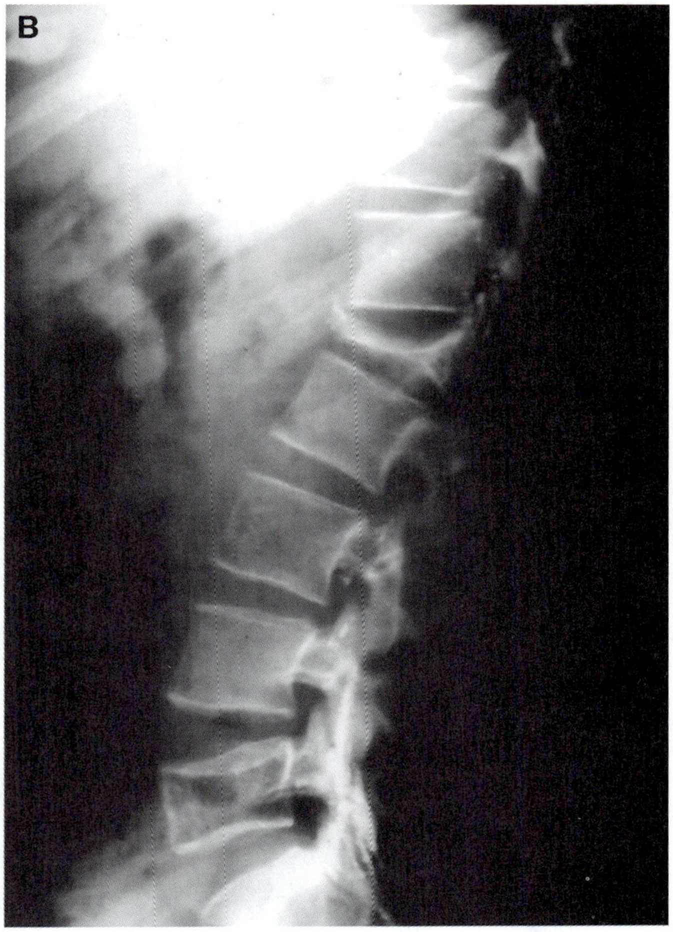

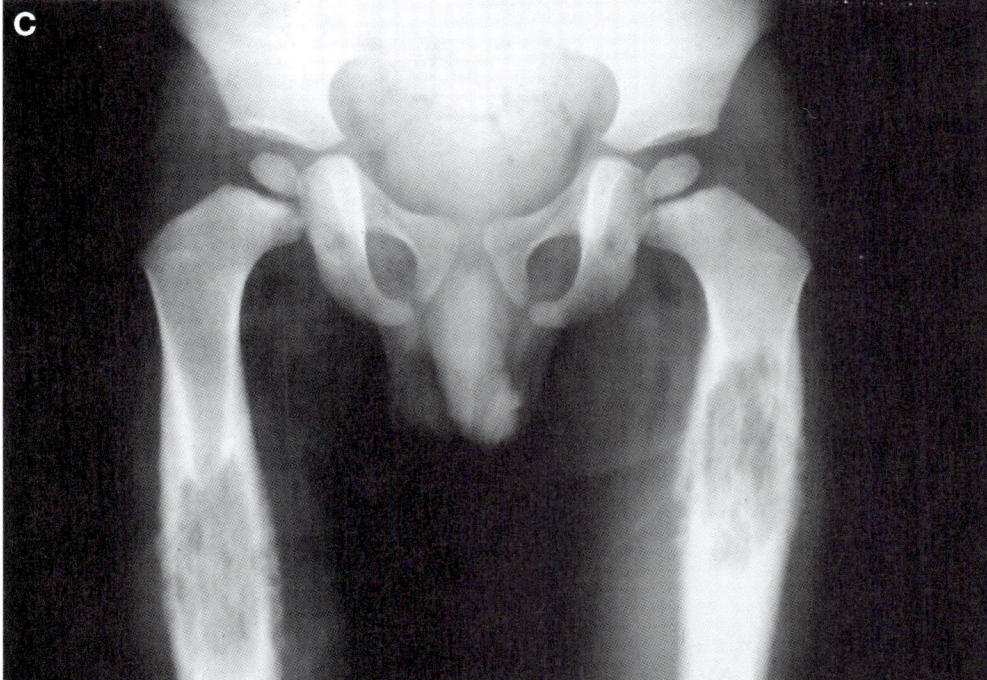

Figure 7 **A,** Radiograph of a 14-year-old boy with solitary Langerhans cell histiocytosis of the mid femoral diaphysis. This is a radiolucent lesion with a beveled inferior edge. **B,** Radiograph of a 12-year-old girl with back pain and no neurologic symptoms with prominent vertebra plana of L1. **C,** Radiograph of a 3-year-old boy with polyostotic involvement of the skeleton with two aggressive appearing lesions in the mid-proximal one third of the femora with permeative areas of lysis and aggressive periosteal reactions.

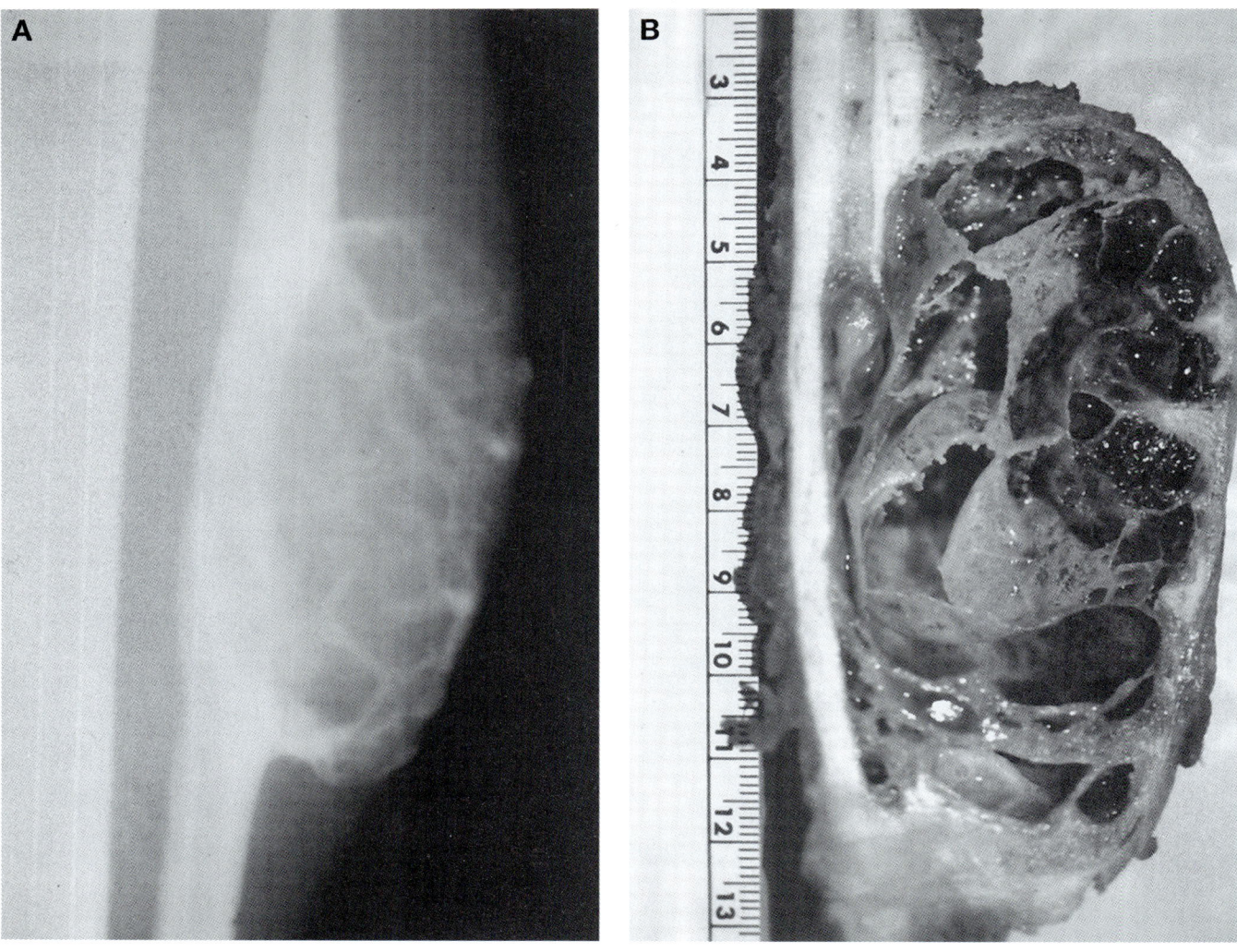

Figure 8 **A,** AP radiograph of the fibula showing an aneurysmal bone cyst that is large and cortically based with prominent septations. **B,** Coronally cut gross specimen shows the blood-filled septations.

patients after the fourth or fifth decades of life. It may occur as a primary tumor or secondarily in a benign antecedent such as a bone infarct or osteomyelitis. The tumor is metaphyseal, most commonly found around the knee, and is highly destructive. Treatment is similar to that of osteosarcoma with multiagent chemotherapy and surgical resection. Survival for patients with this disease ranges from 0 to 70%. Survival is dramatically improved for patients who are healthy enough to undergo chemotherapy. Lung metastases are common.

Small Round Blue Cell Tumors

Langerhans Cell Histiocytosis

Langerhans cell histiocytosis, also known as eosinophilic granuloma, is a tumor that most often affects children during the first and second decades of life. Langerhans cell histiocytosis ostensibly is a spectrum

of diseases that primarily affect the skeleton but can also affect the reticuloendothelial system and visceral organs. In its simplest form, it involves the skeleton either as a solitary lesion or in a polyostotic fashion. Hand-Schüller-Christian disease is a constellation of findings that includes multiple osseous lesions, exophthalmos, and diabetes insipidus. The most extreme form of the disease, Letterer-Siwe, occurs in infants and is a combination of polyostotic lesions and multiple organ involvement. This rare disease is fatal in most cases and requires bone marrow transplantation.

Patients with Langerhans cell histiocytosis usually present with bone pain but may also have constitutional symptoms such as fever and malaise with elevated white blood cell counts and erythrocyte sedimentation rates. A wide spectrum of osseous changes are seen radiographically, ranging from well delineated margins (Fig. 7, *A*) to permeative lesions with areas of osseous destruction and soft-tissue masses (Fig. 7, *C*). Vertebral body collapse can be observed (vertebra plana) (Fig. 7, *B*) and is usually managed nonsurgically with bracing. For patients with vertebra plana and progressive neurologic deficits, decompression, bone grafting, and instrumentation are necessary.

The histologic hallmark of Langerhans cell histiocytosis is the presence of histiocytes in a background of mixed chronic inflammatory cells including eosinophils. The defining histologic characteristic is the Langerhans histiocyte with a large central nuclear cleft and Birbeck bodies seen on electron microscopy.

When the diagnosis is certain, observation is the treatment of choice for most nonaggressive solitary lesions because this disease is self-limiting and resolves spontaneously. If the diagnosis is in question, needle biopsy and injection with methylprednisolone has been advocated by one center. Curetting and bone grafting for larger lesions and in older patients is necessary. For young patients with polyostotic disease, especially with visceral involvement, low-dose chemotherapeutic regimens have been used. Low-dose irradiation has also been used for treatment of multiple local lesions that are progressive.

Ewing's Sarcoma

Ewing's sarcoma peaks between the ages of 10 and 30 years and is most common in the metadiaphysis of long bones. Radiographically, Ewing's sarcoma is lytic with permeative bone destruction, an onion-skinned periosteal reaction, and a large circumferential soft-tissue mass. Cytogenetic studies have consistently found a translocation of chromosomes 11 and 22 resulting in the formation of a fusion protein, EWS-FLI 1, that forms at the chromosomal junction.

Treatment consists of multiagent chemotherapy before and after surgery. Surgery for local disease control seems to confer a survival benefit in most studies. Radiotherapy, however, is very effective in achieving local disease control as well, and should be combined with surgery when tumor margins are close or positive.

Important prognostic factors are tumor stage, site (worst in the spine and pelvis), size of the tumor at presentation (patients with tumors > 100 cm^3 have a worse prognosis than patients with smaller tumors), response to chemotherapy (necrosis observed in more than 90% of the specimen is favorable), and lactic dehydrogenase (LDH) levels (increased LDH is associated with worse outcomes). Overall, the survival rate in patients with Ewing's sarcoma who receive intensive combined treatment is 60%. In one study of 975 patients, the 5-year survival rate for patients with nonmetastatic Ewing's sarcoma was 55% versus 22% for patients presenting with metastases.

Aneurysmal Bone Cyst

Aneurysmal bone cyst is a term used to describe expansile, blood-filled, intramedullary lesions (Fig. 8). Although the etiology of the aneurysmal bone cyst remains unclear, many medullary-based lesions are secondary to other benign antecedent tumors such as chondromyxoid fibroma, fibroxanthoma, or osteoblastoma. Trauma may be an etiologic factor in surface aneurysmal bone cysts.

Radiographs show that this tumor is eccentric and cortically based, with marked expansion of the periosteum. There is often a honeycombed internal architecture caused by osseous septations. A well-defined margin is usually present but, in spine tumors especially, the margin can be poorly defined. Prominent fluid-fluid levels are present on MRI and CT.

Treatment is excision for cortically based or surface tumors and curetting, burring, and thermal or chemical adjuncts for central lesions. Recurrence of medullary lesions has been reported to be 25%. Spontaneous regression can occur. Tumor recurrences in spine locations are very common. The role of radiation therapy in the primary or adjunct treatment of this disease is not well studied.

Other Tumors
Chordoma

Chordoma is a rare tumor that arises from notochord remnants and is most often encountered in older adults. The sacrum is the most common site of disease, followed by the sphenoccipital and cervical spine, but the tumor may occur anywhere in the midline neural axis. Constipation is an early symptom, followed by difficulty sitting. Much later in the course of disease, bowel and bladder control are lost. Unfortunately, diagnosis is almost always delayed.

Lumbosacral radiographs are difficult to interpret because of overlying bowel gas that obscures osseous detail. A lateral radiograph may show a large soft-tissue density. CT shows osseous destruction and a low attenuation soft-tissue mass that often displaces the rectum anteriorly. The mass is uniformly hyperintense on T2 pulse-weighted MRI sequences with an intensity approaching a fluid signal. The characteristic cell is the multivacuolated physaliferous cell in a bluish myxoid background.

Treatment is surgical and despite wide margins on gross and microscopic examination, local recurrence is common. External beam radiotherapy is often administered after resection or repeat resection for recurrent tumors. Postoperative surveillance is important for monitoring local recurrence and to a lesser extent, distant metastases to the lungs primarily and the liver occasionally. Chordomas are typically low grade and metastases generally occur later or after multiple local recurrences.

Soft-Tissue Tumors

With the common use of MRI to image the appendicular skeleton, benign soft-tissue tumors are being detected with greater frequency now than ever before. As a result, orthopaedic surgeons are often involved in the initial assessment of extremity soft-tissue tumors. There are two questions that must ultimately be addressed while evaluating a patient with a soft-tissue tumor: can a diagnosis be established without a biopsy, and is a biopsy necessary?

Management of soft-tissue tumors begins with the medical history, proceeds to physical examination, may involve imaging, and may require tissue diagnosis via biopsy. Most patients who are evaluated for soft-tissue tumors report the presence of a soft-tissue mass. It should be determined if the mass has increased in size and if so, how rapidly; whether there is a history of trauma; if there is one or more than one mass; and whether the patient has a syndrome that is characterized by soft-tissue tumors. Enlargement of a mass is worrisome and suggests a malignancy. A history of trauma or intense physical activity supports but does not prove the presence of a muscle injury or myositis ossificans. Finally, the presence of neurofibromatosis type I suggests that the mass may be a neurofibroma.

Physical examination should evaluate adenopathy in the region of the mass, exclude the presence of neurofibromatosis type I, and then focus on the physical characteristics and location of the tumor. The presence of adenopathy is supportive of an infection but can be seen with some sarcomas, such as rhabdomyosarcoma and synovial sarcoma. Clinical features of neurofibromatosis type I include café-au-lait macules, two or more soft-tissue tumors, axillary freckling, tibial bowing, and scoliosis. Physical examination of soft-tissue tumors should estimate the size of the tumor, determine if the lesion is superficial to or deep to the superficial fascia, and should establish if the tumor is soft and malleable or firm. The consistency of the mass is important because common benign tumors such as lipomas and hemangiomas typically are soft and malleable and malignancies usually are firm.

After completion of the history and physical examination, imaging and/or biopsy usually is necessary to establish a diagnosis. Patients with tumors that cannot be diagnosed as benign on physical examination need further evaluation. The objective of additional evaluation is to establish a diagnosis. Occasionally this can be accomplished through imaging studies alone, but a biopsy usually is necessary. MRI is the preferred imaging study because it will provide detailed information about the size and location of the mass and with selected benign soft-tissue tumors, it will provide a definitive diagnosis. Soft-tissue tumors that sometimes can be diagnosed with MRI include lipomas, hemangiomas, angiolipomas, myxomas, tumors resulting from muscle injuries, and synovial cysts. If there is any question about the diagnosis, then a biopsy should be performed.

Principles of performing a biopsy must prioritize oncologic consideration and must follow guidelines outlined earlier in this chapter. The location and size of the tumor will determine if an excisional biopsy, needle biopsy, or incisional biopsy should be performed. Excisional biopsy may be performed on subcutaneous, small, and easily excised lesions with a peripheral margin of normal tissue. Needle biopsy may be performed on large, easily palpable, firm masses that are not adjacent to vital neurovascular structures, and incisional biopsy should be performed when neither excisional biopsy or needle biopsy seems appropriate.

Broad categories of soft-tissue tumors are benign, locally aggressive, and malignant. The number of possible benign tumors is large. Typically resection of benign lesions is through a marginal excision, although complete intralesional excision may be adequate in some cases. The most common locally aggressive tumor is fibromatosis, also referred to as extra-abdominal desmoid tumor. Fibromatosis is locally invasive and a high rate of local recurrence should be expected. A wide margin containing a cuff of normal tissue is desired. Malignant soft-tissue tumors, independent of histologic grade, should be treated with either a radical surgical margin and no radiation, or a marginal or wide surgical margin plus radiation therapy. The radiation can be delivered to the tumor bed by implantable radioactive beads or external beam irradiation. External beam irradiation may be performed before or after surgery. When preoperative radiation is used, that is, radiation treatment after the biopsy but before the tumor resection, a higher incidence of major wound complications will occur following definitive tumor resection when compared with definitive tumor resection followed by postoperative radiation. The majority of limb salvage procedures involve marginal resections (particularly adjacent to neurovascular structures) and radiation therapy.

All patients with soft-tissue sarcomas should be staged with a chest CT scan and a bone scan of the entire skeleton. Patients with pulmonary metastases at the time of diagnosis should be treated initially with chemotherapy. Following induction chemotherapy, treatment should focus on local control using surgical resection of the primary tumor, followed by radiation if indicated based on the surgical margin. Chemotherapy is typically resumed following surgical resection of the primary tumor.

The role of chemotherapy in treating patients with soft-tissue sarcomas who at the time of diagnosis do not have pulmonary metastasis remains controversial. Numerous randomized clinical trials have drawn different conclusions regarding the impact on disease-free interval and overall survival. Data suggest, however, that if chemotherapy is beneficial for these patients, it will be helpful for those patients with large, high-grade sarcomas. This theory is based on known risk factors for tumor metastasis: size larger than 5 cm, high histologic grade, and location deep to the superficial fascia.

At the completion of treatment all patients with soft-tissue sarcomas must be followed diligently for a relapse of the cancer. This follow-up should include clinical evaluation for any new symptomatology that could represent a tumor recurrence or metastasis, physical examination for tumor recurrence at the site of primary tumor, and scheduled imaging of the previous tumor bed and lungs. The Musculoskeletal Tumor Society and other cooperative cancer study groups do not have consensus recommendations on the schedule or means for surveillance tests to detect local or distant sarcoma relapse; however, several salient factors should be included in all follow-up protocols. Patients should be followed for at least 10 years; follow-up should be every 3 to 4 months for at least 2 years, and each follow-up should involve assessment for both local and distant relapse. Exact schedules vary from center to center and the means of evaluation vary. As a minimum, interval assessments should involve obtaining a review of systems, physical examination of the previous tumor bed, and a chest radiograph. As a maximum, such assessments may involve MRI of the previous tumor bed, chest CT scan, and a bone scan of the entire skeleton.

The estimated survival of patients with soft-tissue sarcomas depends predominantly on their oncologic stage at the time of diagnosis and the histologic grade, size, and location of the sarcoma. Patients who have pulmonary metastases at the time of diagnosis have the lowest chance of survival and with current treatment, their median survival is less than 12 months. The chance of long-term survival is significantly better in patients who do not have pulmonary metastases at the time of diagnosis. This group of patients has an overall 5-year survival of approximately 75%. However, within this group of patients, the probability of survival decreases with increased histologic grade, increased tumor size, and deep location.

Limb Salvage

For limb salvage surgery to be widely accepted, when compared with amputation, survival rates must be similar and function must be equivalent or better. In one large multi-institutional study of patients with osteosarcoma of the distal femur treated with adjuvant chemotherapy, there was a slightly higher risk of local recurrence in the limb salvage group and overall survival was similar in patients treated with either amputation or limb salvage. However, this study was not randomized and there are more recent data to suggest that local recurrence may have an adverse effect on survival. In another study that compared energy expenditures for patients who had limb salvage surgery versus distal transfemoral amputation, it was shown that the difference in energy expended was far greater in patients with amputations than patients who retained their limb independent of knee fusion. This difference between groups was even more pronounced as gait velocity increased.

There are no absolute contraindications to limb salvage but several clinical situations exist that make limb salvage less attractive than amputation. Pathologic fracture causes tumor contamination of the adjacent soft tissues and leads to an increased risk of disease recurrence with limb salvage. Recent studies have demonstrated a decrease in survival in osteosarcoma patients with a pathologic fracture. Young patients in whom large limb length differences are anticipated after tumor resection may be better treated with amputation or with a rotation or turn-up plasty. Patients with distant disease, especially extrapleural disease and skip metastases, may be better served by amputation to control local disease and restore function quickly because expected survival is short. Neurovascular involvement is another relative contraindication for limb salvage surgery. Arteries and veins can be resected en bloc with the tumor; however, the functional deficits left by the loss of major nerves, particularly the sciatic nerve, may be so great that amputation would be more appropriate. Typically, limb salvage is more aggressively pursued in the upper extremity where nerve grafting and tendon transfers compensate for loss of major motor nerves.

The choice of reconstruction after tumor resection should depend on the type and extent of the defect, anticipated function, and the surgeon's familiarity with certain techniques. Allografts have long been used to reconstruct large defects and joints after tumor resection. The advantages of allografts are that they are biologic and can incorporate into host bone over time. They have ligamentous attachments so that joint function and stability can be reconstructed; this is useful after proximal tibial resections in restoring the extensor mechanism. Complications of allografts are high, and include fracture in up to 20% of patients and infection occurring in 8% to 12%. Joint degeneration is common in osteoarticular grafts because of impaired chondrocyte viability and joint instability. Allografts are not always readily available and have the potential for disease transmission.

Metal reconstruction of large segment and joint defects has improved with modularity, replacement of a straight uniaxial hinge with a rotating hinge, better methods of soft-tissue attachment, and improved cement techniques. Prosthetic breakage is relatively rare with metal components and periprosthetic infection is less frequent than with allograft reconstruction. Soft-tissue attachment to metal remains problematic but more importantly, aseptic loosening is the major cause of failure of implants and increases over time.

For small intercalary defects, especially around the ankle and distal radius, vascularized autografts have been used with success. Vascularized fibulae are used most often, followed by vascularized iliac crest grafts. The fibula hypertrophies over time and healing is predictable at the osteosynthesis sites. Vascularized fibulae have also been used with allografts to improve the rate and quality of healing at allograft host junction sites. This technique is probably better suited for nonunion repairs at allograft host junctions.

Bone transport has gained popularity for intercalary defects following tumor resection of diaphyseal lesions, especially low-grade tumors such as adamantinomas that do not require adjuvant chemotherapy. Good results with this technique usually occur over a long period of time, but this can be emotionally difficult for some patients. Pin tract infections, nerve and arterial injuries, nonunions, and fractures are common.

Despite its popularity and frequency, limb salvage surgery for malignant musculoskeletal tumors remains imperfect and complicated. The length of surgery and concomitant blood loss, extent of resection, especially of adjacent soft tissues, patient immunosuppression due to the cancer and chemotherapy, and adjuvant use of radiotherapy are factors that affect the outcome. Better surgical techniques and liberal use of rotational and free flap coverage, improved prosthetic designs and modularity, standardized and regulated guidelines for allograft retrieval and processing, better means of fixation of grafts to bone, and most important, patient selection have all contributed to limb salvage success. Improvement in fixation of prostheses and biologic grafts to bone, application of growth factors, and improved knowledge of tumor biology will undoubtedly enhance the functional quality and long-term success of limb salvage surgery.

Mechanism of Metastasis

The process by which cancer cells spread throughout the body is complex and comprises several distinct and necessary steps. In broad terms, each of these steps is an interaction between cancer cells and the surrounding local environment. The local environment consists of noncancerous normal host cells and the extracellular matrix, and surrounding tissues. The three generic steps unique to cancer cell behavior are: (1) degradation of extracellular matrix; (2) attachment to and detachment from extracellular matrix; and (3) movement through the extracellular matrix.

To understand the cellular and molecular basis of the interactions between cancer cells and the local environment around these cells, it is important to be familiar with the general concepts of extracellular matrix degradation and cell adhesion. Extracellular matrix degradation plays a critical pathologic role in cancer cell invasion of normal tissue, and cancer cell spread and growth; it facilitates entry of cancer cells into adjacent cancer-free tissues. Extracellular matrix degradation provides chemotactic factors and extracellular scaffolding that guide cancer cell motility, and it can provide matrix-residing factors that stimulate cancer growth.

Extracellular matrix degradation is performed by enzymes, and the family of enzymes that is distinguished as a major contributor to the pathophysiology of cancer metastasis is matrix metalloproteinases (MMPs). MMPs have been associated with the metastatic phenotype of essentially all types of cancers, and it is clear that these enzymes have an effect on tumor cell invasion, adhesion, and migration. There are at least 16 MMP family enzymes. MMPs are zinc-dependent enzymes that present in diverse species such as plants, birds, and mammals. They are a component of many pathologic processes, including normal wound healing, bone remodeling, angiogenesis, and inflammation. MMPs are secreted by normal cells as well as by cancer cells, and their enzymatic activity reflects the net result of a tightly regulated biochemical system. Two regulatory steps influence the overall enzymatic activity of MMP family enzymes: activation of secreted MMPs and levels of inhibitors of MMPs. MMPs are secreted in an inactive proform. Activation of proform enzymes is a critical and necessary step in determining the amount of degradative activity. Naturally-occurring inhibitors of MMPs, tissue inhibitors of metalloproteinases, are prevalent in healthy and diseased tissues and the tissue level of these molecules is a major determinant of the cumulative activity of MMPs.

Cell adhesion is central to the ability of any cell, whether normal or malignant, to migrate locally in any tissue or to recognize (home to) target tissues that will permit a nurturing environment for survival and growth. Adhesive interactions occur between similar cells, dissimilar cells, and between cells and the extracellular matrix. Metastasis involves detachment from the local site and adhesion to the site of metastasis. Adhesion or detachment is initiated through cell surface proteins that recognize specialized binding sites on neighboring cells or in the extracellular matrix. The two most widely studied groups of these cell surface proteins or protein assemblies are integrins and cell adhesion molecules. Integrins are heterodimeric transmembrane cell surface receptors, composed of α and β subunits, and these molecules bind a three amino acid sequence composed of RGD that is found on a number of extracellular matrix proteins. The matrix molecules recognized by integrin receptors include laminin, fibronectin, vitronectin, and different types of collagen. Two cell surface adhesion molecules involved in normal tissue homeostasis and in disease are vascular cell adhesion molecule (VCAM) and intercellular cell adhesion molecule (ICAM).

To manifest the malignant phenotype, cancer cells must degrade extracellular matrix, attach and detach from the matrix, and move through the matrix. These cellular events must occur at both ends of the metastatic process: tumor invasion through and exodus from tissue of origin and tumor attachment and invasion of a distant tissue. At the site of primary tumor (breast or prostate, for example), tumor cells produce MMPs that degrade extracellular matrix and provide access through the primary tissue's basement membrane and into the systemic circulation. MMP-2, gelatinase (gelatinase B) and MMP-9 are suspected to play a pathologic role in this initial step in metastasis. Migration of these cancer cells through the extracellular matrix, basement membrane, and vessel wall is under the direction of integrin receptor and cell adhesion molecules such as VCAM.

After entering the bloodstream, tumor cells form small cell aggregates and travel throughout perfused tissues until a region for tumor cell binding is identified. The initial site of binding in target tissue such as bone is the endothelial wall. After invasion through the endothelium, cancer cells bind to bone-matrix proteins and other components of the bone marrow microenvironment. Cell-to-cell aggregation can be performed by ICAM and homing to bone as a distant target, can be mediated by tumor cell expression of integrins such as $\alpha_v\beta_3$ and/or $\alpha_4\beta_1$. $\alpha_v\beta_3$ is an integrin complex used by osteoclasts to bind bone matrix proteins such as osteopontin and bone sialoprotein (BSP). Interestingly, it is suspected that $\alpha_v\beta_3$ integrin expression on human breast and prostate cancer cells facilitates anchoring of these cells to the bone microenvi-

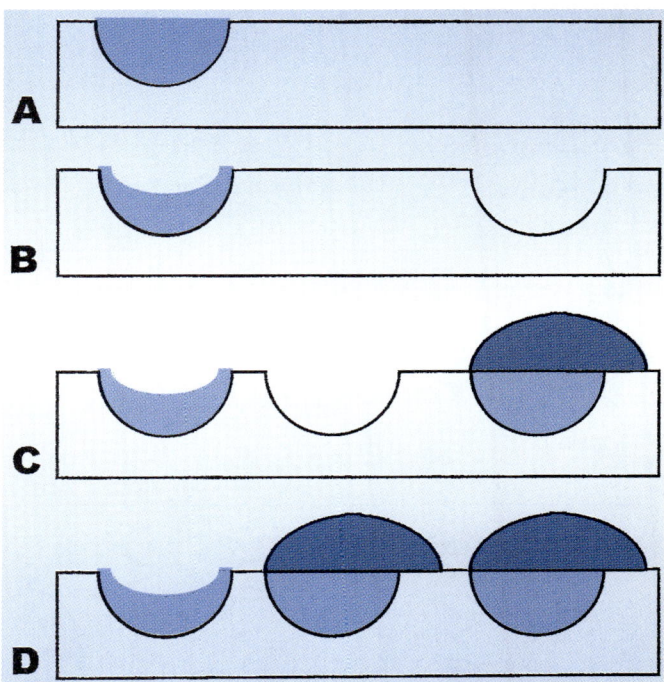

Figure 9 Summary of the effects of cancer on bone. **A,** Normal bone with a remodeling unit and no net loss or gain in bone mass. Crescent-shaped bone surface represents site of previous osteoclastic bone resorption and half-moon shaped light grey region represents subsequent osteoblastic bone formation. **B,** The net bone response to tumor that induces a purely radiolucent lesion on radiograph is depicted. Osteoclastic bone resorption exceeds osteoblastic bone formation and attempts to fill sites of osteoclastic bone resorption are incomplete. **C,** The net bone response to tumor that induces a mixed (radiolucent and radiodense) lesion on radiograph is depicted. Osteoclastic bone resorption exceeds osteoblastic bone formation in some areas while tumor-induced bone formation (dark grey) exceeds resorption in other areas. **D,** The net bone response to tumor that induces a purely radiodense tumor on radiograph is depicted. Tumor-induced, osteoblastic bone formation exceeds osteoclastic bone resorption.

ronment, and it has been shown that these cells secrete BSP, a ligand for $\alpha_v\beta_3$. This establishes the theoretical paradigm where roaming osteotrophic cancer cells enter the bone microenvironment expressing $\alpha_v\beta_3$ and secreting BSP. Upon contacting the bone matrix, tumor-secreted BSP anchors to bone matrix hydroxyapatite crystals and provides an RGD binding site for breast cancer $\alpha_v\beta_3$ integrin. The integrin-BSP binding interaction then attaches the breast cancer to bone matrix, establishing a microscopic focus of metastatic bone cancer. Another potential means for establishing microscopic cancer foci in bone is through binding of tumor-expressed $\alpha_4\beta_1$ with VCAM expressed by bone marrow-residing vascular endothelium.

After the microscopic aggregate of bone cancer cells has taken residence in bone, it will lay dormant and therefore clinically irrelevant until it can invade the skeletal tissue. Bone cancers invade bone by stimulating normal host osteoclasts to destroy bone. This tumor-induced, osteoclast-mediated osteolysis initiates the development of almost all clinically evident skeletal cancers, whether these cancers appear on radio-

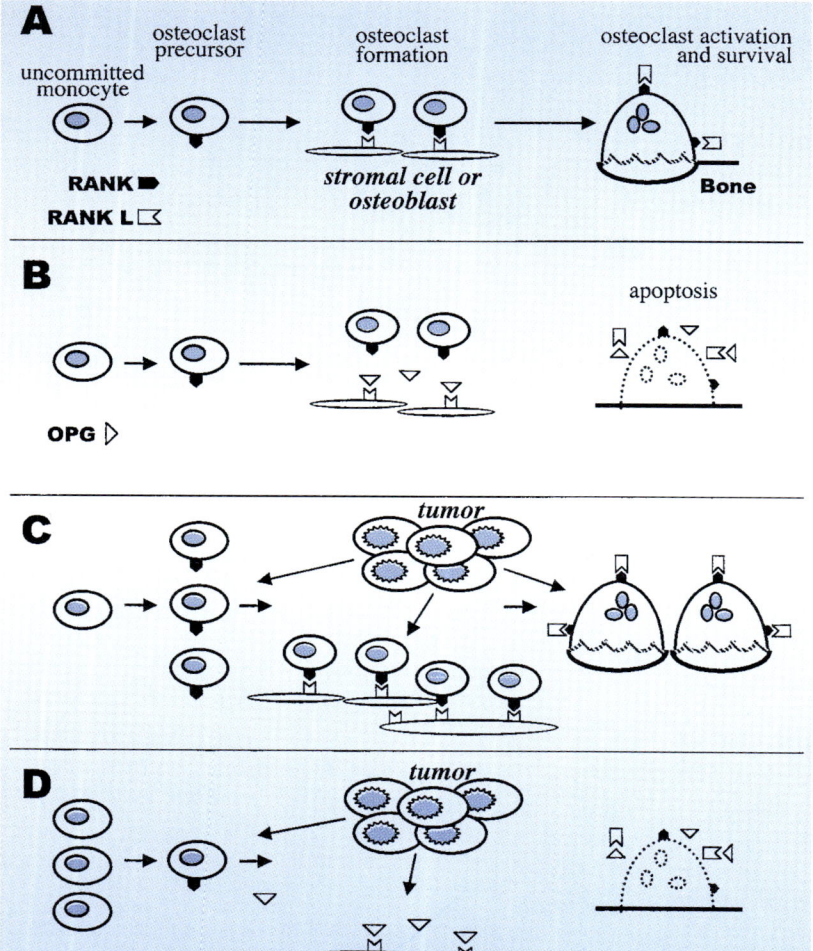

Figure 10 Osteoprotegerin blocks cancer-induced bone loss and osteoclastogenesis. **A,** Cell-to-cell contact between RANK (on osteoclast precursor cells) and RANKL (on stromal cells or osteoblasts) is required for physiologic osteoclast formation. **B,** OPG binds to RANKL. This interaction blocks osteoclast formation and induces osteoclast death (apoptosis). **C,** Osteolytic cancers increase the number of osteoclast precursors, increase expression of OPG ligand, and increase the number of osteoclasts. **D,** OPG treatment has important influences at sites of tumor, including decreases in the number of osteoclast precursors, decreased expression of OPG ligand, and decreased number of osteoclasts.

graphs to be radiolucent, radiodense, or both. The molecular mechanisms through which cancers interact with bone are not entirely clear. These processes involve regulation of osteoclast formation and activity through the osteoprotegerin-receptor activator of nuclear factor-κβ ligand (OPG-RANKL) signaling pathway, which will be described later.

The mechanisms through which bone cancers stimulate an osteoblastic reaction are unknown, but are being intensely investigated. Cancer-induced bone formation is undoubtedly performed by osteoblasts and osteoblastic cancers probably secrete molecules that directly or indirectly stimulate intramembranous bone formation. This bone formation most likely involves the recruitment, differentiation, and stimulation of osteoblasts to form bone. The search for prostate cancer-secreted molecules that may stimulate bone formation has determined that the potent vasoconstrictor endothelin 1 is produced by many of these cancers and is capable of inducing osteoblastic bone formation. Other proposed osteoblastogenic tumor-secreted fac-

tors include transforming growth factor-beta, fibroblast growth factor, and the bone morphogenetic proteins.

Influence of Cancer on Bone Cells

Recently, the means through which osteoblastic bone formation and osteoclastic bone resorption maintain the delicate balance required for a healthy skeleton has been determined. Historically, diseases of bone mass have been described as representing an uncoupling of bone formation and bone resorption. In the past 5 years, the mystery of coupling has been solved by the discovery of a system of molecules called OPG and RANKL. Recent investigation of the role of this regulatory system in bone cancer has provided new insight into understanding how bone cancers interact with normal bone cells and result in pathologic bone loss.

Cancer influences the skeleton by perturbing normal skeletal remodeling. There are four distinct phases that comprise physiologic skeletal remodeling: a resting phase, a bone resorption phase, a reversal phase, and a bone formation phase. When the cumulative activity of all four phases is totaled over time, the net change in bone mass is zero. Skeletal remodeling proceeds systematically through each phase, beginning and ending with the resting phase. The bone resorption phase involves osteoclastic bone removal. This process must always precede the reversal and formation phases. Bone formation is always initiated by osteoblasts through production of collagen and is completed through deposition of crystals within the newly produced bone matrix.

Cancer can disrupt the extent, but not the sequence, of each phase of bone remodeling (Fig. 9). Tumors such as lung cancer that are purely radiolucent on radiographs induce exaggerated activity in the bone resorption phase and deficient response in the bone formation phase (Fig. 9, *B*). Tumors such as breast cancer that are mixed on radiographs induce exaggerated activity in the bone resorption phase, and in some regions during the formation phase (Fig. 9, *C*). Radiodense tumors such as prostate cancer stimulate an overactive bone resorption phase and a markedly exaggerated bone formation phase (Fig. 9, *D*). The important concepts to be understood are that the bone resorption phase is active in all bone cancers independent of their radiographic appearance, and that tumors themselves (other than osteosarcomas) do not make bone or destroy bone, but influence normal bone cells to perform these tasks. These general concepts underscore the importance of defining the mechanism through which bone cancers induce osteoclast-mediated bone loss. Discovery and characterization of the OPG-RANKL system as the pivotal regulator of osteoclast formation and performance has provided opportunity to determine if OPG, RANKL and/or RANK-expressing cells play a role in cancer-induced, osteoclast-mediated osteolysis.

RANKL is a recently discovered molecule that promotes and is required for osteoclast formation and survival. RANKL is a member of the tumor necrosis factor (TNF) ligand family. It is a transmembrane protein that functions as a ligand. This ligand is made by stromal cells and osteoblasts and recognizes two TNF-receptor family molecules, RANK and OPG. Binding of RANKL to RANK manifests its biologic activity, while binding to OPG inactivates or sequesters RANKL, blocking its biologic activity. RANKL stimulates osteoclast formation and function at all steps in the osteoclast life cycle and is required for each step to occur (Fig. 10, *A*). RANKL affects mononuclear osteoclast precursor cells by directing their differentiation and commitment to the osteoclastic lineage. It exerts its effects by binding to its receptor RANK, which

is located on the surface of osteoclasts and their precursors.

In contrast, OPG is a potent inhibitor of osteoclastic bone resorption. Unlike other TNF-receptor family members, it lacks transmembrane and cytoplasmic domains and is secreted as a soluble protein. (Fig. 10, *B*). OPG affects mononuclear osteoclast precursor cells by blocking their ability to differentiate along the osteoclast lineage. The molecular action of OPG is quite straightforward. OPG simply acts as a soluble secreted decoy receptor for a cell surface or secreted RANKL.

Murine models of bone cancer show that the OPG-RANKL system is involved in cancer-induced bone loss. Specifically, osteolytic cancer has been shown to increase expression of RANKL at sites of tumor in bone, and to increase the number of RANK-expressing osteoclast precursor cells at sites of tumor (Fig. 10, *C*). As expected, treatment of tumor-bearing mice with OPG eliminates osteoclasts and their precursors from sites of tumor and blocks cancer-induced osteolysis (Fig. 10, *D*). The mechanism through which tumors stimulate local production of RANKL in vivo have not been definitively established. Research currently supports two mechanisms for local production of RANKL in vivo at sites of tumor. One is tumor cell production of RANKL and the second is tumor cell production of factors that induce RANKL, such as parathyroid hormone-related protein, prostaglandin E_2, and interleukin-1.

Because the majority of bone cancers are bone metastases, and because patients with skeletal metastases generally have incurable cancer, the focus of clinical care is palliation from the complications of bone cancer. These complications include pain, immobility, pathologic skeletal fracture, and hypercalcemia of malignancy. With an understanding of bone remodeling and cancer's effect on bone as previously discussed, it follows that the osteoclast plays a major role in the development of the clinical complications of bone cancer. Specifically, excessive osteoclastic bone resorption causes pain and immobility, leads to skeletal weakening and fracture, and causes hypercalcemia. It is with this knowledge that osteoclast-targeted therapies have been studied over the past 5 years as a means for decreasing the frequency of skeletal complications related to bone cancer. These studies have shown that bisphosphonate therapy decreases the number of skeletal complications in patients with advanced cancer. It is hoped that therapies may advance further if OPG or a related molecule becomes available for use in humans.

The OPG-RANKL system has provided insight into the pathophysiology of giant cell tumors of bone as well as in cancer-induced osteolysis. As giant cell tumors of bone are composed of multinucleated osteoclast-like cells, investigators have recently explored the possibility that molecules that regulate osteoclastogenesis may contribute to the pathophysiology of giant cell tumors. Analysis of gene expression in giant cell tumors has shown that RANKL expression is high in spindle-shaped, stromal-like cells, RANK-expressing mononuclear cells are present, and OPG expression is not increased. These new and exciting findings suggest that RANKL is involved in the tumor cell-induced osteoclast-like cell formation in giant cell tumors and they suggest that the ratio of RANKL/OPG among tumor cells may contribute to the degree of osteoclastogenesis and bone resorption in these tumors.

Current Management of Skeletal Metastasis

Cancer is the second leading cause of death in the United States, with 1.5 million new cases diagnosed in the year 2000. Among this staggering number of new cases, nearly half of these patients will have cancers that commonly spread to bone, specifically, cancers of the prostate, breast, lung, and kidney. These malignancies will spread to bone in at least 50% of all affected patients and in up to 90% of patients with advanced disease, resulting in hundreds of thousands of patients annually with new skeletal metastases.

The impact of bone metastases on quality of life and overall morbidity of malignant diseases is substantial. Quality of life and morbidity are negatively impacted by cancer-related skeletal events. These events include pain, decreased mobility, hypercalcemia, skeletal fracture, spinal cord or nerve root compression, and bone marrow dysfunction secondary to tumor infiltration. Cancer-related skeletal events occur, on average, two to four times per year in patients with advanced bone-seeking cancers such as breast cancer and myeloma. Caring for patients with skeletal complications of cancer is challenging and can be fraught with problems. These patients are extremely ill and benefit greatly from the expert care and skill that orthopaedic surgeons can provide.

Evaluation of Bone Metastasis

Despite advances in the medical management of patients with skeletal metastases, the orthopaedic surgeon remains an irreplaceable participant in the care of these patients. Effective evaluation and thoughtful treatment recommendations require broad clinical skills, familiarity with skeletal imaging modalities, knowledge of nonsurgical means for treating bone metastases, and surgical skill.

Evaluation of patients with skeletal metastases begins with clinical evaluation that includes evaluation of the patient's coagulation status and potential for hypercalcemia and will include elements of the patient's medical history and laboratory studies. In most circumstances, medical and oncologic consultation is beneficial.

Imaging studies are required to evaluate the area(s) of known skeletal metastases and to assess the overall extent of skeletal involvement. In a patient who is known to have metastatic disease, plain radiographs are often sufficient to make all clinical decisions. Occasionally, when surgical stabilization is indicated, it is helpful to obtain axial imaging via MRI or CT scan. Both imaging modalities will give precise information regarding the extent of skeletal destruction, and as a result, may direct the surgeon's choice of internal fixation. In addition to imaging the area of known skeletal disease, it can be important to assess the overall extent of skeletal involvement. Under most circumstances this is best accomplished with a bone scan. In selected circumstances, radiographic skeletal surveys are superior to bone scans. Those circumstances include when the primary tumor is myeloma or where a site of known skeletal disease does not manifest increased isotope activity on bone scan. Identification of any new skeletal lesions by bone scan should be followed by evaluation with biplanar radiographs to determine the risk of pathologic fracture.

Treatment of Bone Metastasis

As several options for treatment of skeletal metastases are available and can be used to treat a single disease site, coordinating care with a multidisciplinary team of physicians is important. The modalities that must be considered include traditional narcotic and anti-inflammatory medications, intravenous bisphosphonates, chemotherapy, radiation, surgical stabilization of affected bones, and/or surgical decompression of neural tissue.

The most critical determinant in coordinating the management of bone metastases is pain. As a general rule, patients with no or minimal pain should be treated with chemotherapy (if it is part of their ongoing treatment) as well as with intravenous bisphosphonates and analgesic medications. The administration of analgesics is often best in sustained-release oral tablets, or dermal patches. In patients with constant pain and/or pain aggravated by limb use, a more aggressive treatment plan is indicated. Specifically, in addition to analgesic medication and bisphosphonates, these patients should have external beam irradiation to the involved skeletal site and the site may need surgical stabilization either before or after radiation.

Some patients with skeletal metastases who are being considered possible candidates for surgery may have limited survival. As a result, both the patient and the treating orthopaedic surgeon(s) must have a clear understanding of the indications for and goals of surgical treatment. There are three indications for surgical treatment of skeletal metastases and there are two goals of treatment. The first indication is to stabilize a pathologic fracture. The second is to strengthen a bone at high risk for pathologic fracture. The third indication is to treat bone metastases sites that are painful despite radiation therapy. The goals of surgical treatment are twofold. From the patient's perspective, the goal is to decrease pain and to optimize mobility and function. From the surgical technique perspective, the goal of surgical treatment is to provide immediate and permanent skeletal stabilization. Radiation of painful skeletal metastases is excellent treatment when administered to sites that are not at high risk for fracture. Ninety percent of patients treated with radiation will receive some pain relief and more than half will experience complete relief of pain. In patients who experience pain relief, the majority experience it within 2 weeks of receiving radiation treatments. In general, therefore, patients who need radiation to control pain from skeletal metastases and do not have radiographic evidence of impending skeletal fractures should have surgical stabilization of the affected bone only if their pain persists despite radiation or if their pain recurs following an initial response to radiation. Response rates to radiation will vary with the type of primary tumor. Myeloma and metastatic breast and prostate cancers will respond the best, and other types of cancers, such as lung cancer, will not respond as well.

Planning for surgical stabilization of bones affected by skeletal metastases should focus on providing immediate and permanent stabilization. Achieving immediate stabilization acknowledges that osseous union is unlikely to occur and is not necessary for successful treatment. Achieving immediate stabilization eliminates the need for external immobilization devices after surgery and facilitates postoperative mobility and rehabilitation. Permanent skeletal stabilization is important because of the possibility of extended patient survival. Although survival can be weeks or months in some patients, others may survive for years, reflecting the wide range of median survivals noted in patients with advanced cancers. Patients with advanced lung cancer have a median survival of less than 6 months, in contrast to the median survival in patients with advanced prostate (40 months) or breast cancer (24 months).

The site of skeletal metastases often plays a major role in the method of surgical reconstruction. The three anatomic osseous locations that lead to alternative means of reconstruction are the axial skeleton, the metaphyseal and diaphyseal region of long bones, and epiphyseal regions of long bones. Lesions involving the axial skeleton (spine, pelvis, and scapula) that require surgical treatment are almost always best managed with intralesional removal of tumor and replacement of the resultant skeletal deficiency with bone cement or allogeneic cortical bone graft. In most instances, internal fixation spanning the defect can be used to enhance the reconstruction. When reconstructing lesions of the spine, typically located in one or more vertebral bodies, preoperative evaluation should address the possibility of spinal cord compression. If this condition is noted, then surgical decompression should be performed at the time of tumor excision and surgical stabilization. When stabilizing vertebral body defects, internal fixation must extend to uninvolved bone at both ends of the defect. Internal fixation devices can be located anteriorly or posteriorly and should follow general principles applied to each region of the spinal column.

Surgical reconstruction of metastatic tumors involving the pelvis can be divided broadly into two groups: lesions that involve the subchondral bone of the acetabulum, and lesions that do not. Among lesions not involving the subchondral region of the acetabulum, those involving the ilium and supra-acetabular region require surgical treatment most often. Lesions contained by bone require simple intralesional tumor excision and cementation of the resultant defect. Tumor deposits resulting in extensive cortical bone loss, particularly medially, should be reconstructed with pelvic reconstruction plates or Steinmann pins as well as bone cement. Selected internal fixation devices should span the defects and when possible, should engage normal bone at the proximal and distal sites of the osseous defect.

When surgically treating lesions involving the subchondral region of the acetabulum, pelvic reconstruction and total hip arthroplasty is usually necessary. Such treatment will involve intralesional tumor removal followed by reconstruction. The femoral side of the hip is managed with a standard femoral prosthesis and the acetabular reconstruction usually requires reconstruction of the pelvic defect prior to placement of the acetabular cup. Cavitary, contained pelvic defects may require no acetabular augmentation, or may require augmentation using either a portion of the resected femoral head and/or bone cement. A standard acetabular cup is appropriate. Pelvic defects with an intact acetabular rim and disruption of the medial wall will require augmentation with the resected head and/or cement, and may require medial wire mesh to contain the cement. A standard cup or a protusio ring cup are both appropriate. Defects of the lateral and superior acetabulum should be filled with cement, and continuity between the reconstructed region and uninvolved bone should be established through placement of large Steinmann pins into the superior ilium or across the sacral iliac joint. Wire mesh may be necessary to contain the cement. A protrusio ring cup or roof-ring support with a cemented acetabular cup is optimal. A high rate of hip dislocation has been reported in several series (up to 10%) and use of a constrained acetabular cup is appropriate in some cases.

Stabilization of long bones with diaphyseal and/or metaphyseal metastases is best performed by achieving rigid internal fixation above and below the tumor. Fixation can be accomplished with intramedullary devices or plates. Where possible, gross tumor should be removed (intralesional) and bone cement should be used liberally to enhance fixation and stability.

Stabilization of long bones with epiphyseal metastases can be performed with either arthroplasty or internal fixation augmented with bone cement. The type of arthroplasty performed will depend on the anatomic location. The need for arthroplasty reconstruction is most common with tumors of the proximal femur. Such lesions are best treated by hemiarthroplasty. Hemiarthroplasty also provides the best reconstruction for lesions involving the proximal humerus, while a rotating hinged total knee arthroplasty is the optimal reconstruction for lesions of the distal femur and proximal tibia. Contiguous metaphyseal and diaphyseal bone loss sometimes require segmental replacement with a massive prosthesis.

Deciding whether a patient should undergo prophylactic surgical stabilization of a bone containing a metastasis can be challenging and the definition of an impending pathologic fracture is controversial. This situation is most often encountered in lesions of long bones. Four variables should influence the decision for or against surgery: osseous location of the lesion, type of pain, the tumor's influence on the bone, and size of the lesion. Regarding location, the peritrochanteric femoral neck region is at highest risk. The type of pain most suggestive of an impending fracture is functional pain, that is, pain related to movement. Purely radiolucent (lytic) lesions are at the highest risk of fracture, followed by mixed and then radiodense (blastic) lesions. Lesions encompassing two thirds of the bone diameter or 50% of the cortex have a high risk. Overall size has also been considered an important variable. Lesions larger than 2.5 cm in the proximal femur have been considered at increased risk. However, considerations of size are dependent on the particular bone, as well as the other clinical and radiographic features. A radiolucent lesion in the femoral neck or intertrochanteric region that is painful with limb movement and involves a region two thirds the diameter of the bone requires prophylactic fixation. With long bone lesions that are less risky, each factor should be weighed in making a recommendation for or against surgery. The upper extremities should be carefully evaluated in patients undergoing lower limb reconstruction, because they will likely become weight bearing during postoperative rehabilitation.

Several special considerations that must be addressed when treating patients with skeletal metastases include the patient's general medical condition, the potential for disease at multiple skeletal sites, and identification of richly vascular tumors. Consideration of coagulation status and risk of treatment-associated deep venous thrombosis is required. Coagulation system deficiencies generally can be identified in the medical history and review of systems, but platelet number and coagulation indices should be determined. The majority of patients undergoing surgical treatment for skeletal metastases have several risk factors for developing deep venous thrombosis. These include cancer-induced coagulation abnormalities, prolonged bed rest and inactivity, and pelvic or lower extremity surgery. When one or more of these risk factors is present, pharmacologic prophylaxis for deep venous thrombosis is recommended postoperatively.

Some skeletal metastases can induce a rich vascular supply to the tumor. Extremely vascular tumors are most commonly renal and thyroid cancer metastases. Failure to address the potential for massive bleeding from such tumors preoperatively may result in uncontrolled, life-threatening hemorrhage during surgery. Assessing the potential for highly vascular tumors should begin with a preoperative arteriogram and, if indicated, embolization of the sites of arterial inflow to the tumor. This type of evaluation is recommended for tumors that are present in anatomic locations where tourniquet control of surgical bleeding is not feasible. These locations include the spine, scapula, proximal humerus, pelvis, and proximal femur.

Bisphosphonates and Bone Metastasis

With an understanding of the pivotal role of osteoclasts in the pathophysiology of all bone metastases, the role of osteoclast-inhibiting bisphosphonates has been examined in patients with skeletal metastases. Findings have revealed that bisphosphonates, particularly the intravenous agent pamidronate, have a dramatic effect on cancer-related skeletal events. Pamidronate decreases skeletal pain in up to 50% of patients with skeletal tumors from myeloma, breast cancer, or prostate cancer. Pamidronate also decreases the need for radiation treatment to bone, pathologic skeletal fracture, surgery to bone, and hypercalcemia in women with advanced breast cancer as well as in patients with advanced myeloma.

Bisphosphonates provide an exciting advancement in the treatment of cancer patients with skeletal metastases. Several points must be mentioned, however: proper treatment is 90 mg of pamidronate given intravenously as a single monthly dose; duration of treatment is at least 9 months; pamidronate treatment has no effect on survival; and a significant proportion of patients still have skeletal complications despite treatment (breast cancer, 51% and myeloma, 24%). Thus, the osteoclast has clearly been defined as a target for potential new agents to inhibit metastases-induced bone loss.

Annotated Bibliography

Imaging Studies

Geirnaerdt MJ, Hogendoorn PC, Bloem JL, Taminiau AH, van der Woude HJ: Cartilaginous tumors: Fast contrast-enhanced MR imaging. *Radiology* 2000;214: 539-546.

The purpose of this study was to distinguish benign from malignant cartilage tumor using fast-contrast MRI in 37 patients. Early enhancement was seen in chondrosarcoma but not in patients with enchondroma. Differentiation of benign from malignant based on enhancement was possible with a sensitivity of 61%, specificity 95%, positive predictive value 92%, and negative predictive value 72%.

Biopsy

Dupuy DE, Rosenberg AE, Punyaratabandhu T, Tan MH, Mankin HJ: Accuracy of CT-guided needle biopsy of musculoskeletal neoplasms. *AJR Am J Roentgenol* 1998;171:759-762.

Over a three-year period, the authors performed 176 core needle biopsies and 45 fine needle aspirations for musculoskeletal neoplasms. The accuracy for needle biopsy was 93% and 80% for fine needle aspiration. The complication rate for both techniques was < 1%. The authors conclude that CT directed biopsy is safe and effective but warn that clinical, radiographic and pathologic correlation is necessary in all cases.

Tumors of Bone

Bacci G, Ferrari S, Mercuri M, et al: Predictive factors for local recurrence in osteosarcoma: 540 patients with extremity tumors followed for minimum 2.5 years after neoadjuvant chemotherapy. *Acta Orthop Scand* 1998;69: 230-236.

At a mean follow-up of 7.5 years (range: 2.5 to 15 years) local recurrence was seen in 31 patients (6%) and correlated with negative surgical margins and response to chemotherapy. Only 1 of 31 patients with local recurrence was disease-free 15 months after the last treatment. The authors concluded that an immediate amputation should be considered in tumors removed with inadequate margins especially if the histologic response to preoperative chemotherapy was poor.

Rosenthal DI, Hornicek FJ, Wolfe MW, Jennings LC, Gebhardt MC, Mankin HJ: Percutaneous radiofrequency coagulation of osteoid osteoma compared with operative treatment. *J Bone Joint Surg Am* 1998;80:815-821.

The rates of recurrence and persistent symptoms were compared in a consecutive series of 87 patients managed with surgical excision and 38 patients with percutaneous ablation with radiofrequency. Recurrence in patients treated surgically and with radioablation was 9% and 12%, respectively.

Temple HT, Scully SP, O'Keefe RJ, Katapurum S, Mankin HJ: Clinical outcome of 38 patients with juxtacortical osteosarcoma. *Clin Orthop* 2000;373:208-217.

All 38 patients who presented with previously untreated low-grade juxtacortical osteosarcoma were alive at 6.7 years follow-up. Intramedullary extension was seen in 17 patients (45%) and tumor violated the adjacent cortex in 71% of patients. Close but negative margins were adequate in achieving local disease control and preventing metastases in these patients. Intramedullary extension did not increase the risk of metastatic disease.

Tumors of Cartilage

Berend KR, Toth AP, Harrelson JM, Layfield LJ, Hey LA, Scully SP: Association between ratio of matrix metalloproteinase-1 to tissue inhibitor of metalloproteinase-1 and local recurrence, metastasis, and survival in human chondrosarcoma. *J Bone Joint Surg Am* 1998;80:11–17.

Chondrosarcoma recurrence was associated with a higher ratio of matrix metalloproteinase-1 to tissue inhibitor of metalloproteinase-1 and was a moderately significant independent predictor of a poor outcome.

Lee FY, Mankin HJ, Fondren G, et al: Chondrosarcoma of bone: An assessment of outcome. *J Bone Joint Surg Am* 1999;81:326-338.

Two hundred twenty-seven patients with chondrosarcoma were reviewed. Patients with high-grade lesions were older and more commonly had pathologic fracture, metastases, local recurrence and death. Predictors of metastases and death in patients with high-grade tumors were local recurrence, pelvic tumors, tumors larger than 100 cm^3, ploidy abnormalities (aneuploidy and high mean DNA index), histologic grade 3 tumor, and dedifferentiated histology.

Murphey MD, Flemming DJ, Boyea SR, Bojescul JA, Sweet DE, Temple HT: Enchondroma versus chondrosarcoma in the appendicular skeleton: Differentiating features. *Radiographics* 1998;18:1213-1237.

The authors analyzed 187 patients with enchondroma (n = 92) and chondrosarcoma (n = 95). Radiographic factors that were important in distinguishing enchondroma from chondrosarcoma were deep endosteal scalloping (greater than two thirds of the cortex), cortical destruction and the presence of a soft-tissue mass, periosteal reaction, and marked and heterogeneous uptake on bone scintigraphy.

Ramappa AJ, Lee FY, Tang P, Carlson JR, Gebhardt MC, Mankin HJ: Chondroblastoma of bone. *J Bone Joint Surg Am* 2000;82:1140-1145.

Of 47 patients on which adequate information was obtained, tumors were typically located in the epiphyses or apophyses of long bones and were associated with pain and limited range of motion. Most patients had excellent functional outcomes although three developed osteoarthritis. Tumor recurrence occurred in seven patients (15%), most commonly in lesions arising around the hip. Three patients had a second recurrence and one had a third recurrence. Two patients developed metastases, one patient died, and another was alive after metastatectomy.

Wu CT, Inwards CY, O'Laughlin S, Rock MG, Beabout JW, Unni KK: Chondromyxoid fibroma of bone: A clinicopathologic review of 278 cases. *Hum Pathol* 1998;29:438-446.

Two hundred seventy-eight cases of chondromyxoid fibroma were studied and the clinical, radiologic, and pathologic features reviewed. Intralesional excision was recommended with a recurrence rate of 25%.

Fibrous Tumors of Bone

Qureshi AA, Shott S, Mallin BA, Gitelis S: Current trends in the management of adamantinoma of long bones: An international study. *J Bone Joint Surg Am* 2000;82:1122-1131.

This is a retrospective study from 23 different institutions for 70 patients with biopsy-proven adamantinoma. Limb salvage was attempted in 64 patients (91%) and limb retention was 84%. An intercalary allograft was most commonly used and reconstructive complications overall were 48%. Local recurrence was seen in 8.6% of patients at 5 years and 18.6% at ten years; metastases were documented in 2 patients before surgery and occurred in 7 patients (10%) after surgery. Wide resection margins were associated a lower rate of local recurrence than marginal or intralesional resection.

Wilkins RM: Unicameral bone cysts. *J Am Acad Orthop Surg* 2000;8:217-224.

Etiology, diagnosis, and contemporary treatment are reviewed in this excellent article.

Small Round Blue Cell Tumors

Bacci G, Ferrari S, Bertoni F, et al: Prognostic factors in nonmetastatic Ewing's sarcoma of bone treated with adjuvant chemotherapy: Analysis of 359 patients at the Istituto Ortopedico Rizzoli. *J Clin Oncol* 2000;18:4-11.

The authors studied 359 patients with nonmetastatic Ewing's sarcoma of bone. On multivariate analysis they found a number of prognostic factors associated with poor outcomes that included: male sex ($P < 0.02$), age older than 12 years ($P < 0.006$), fever ($P < 0.001$), anemia ($P < 0.0025$), high LDH ($P < 0.001$), axial location ($P < 0.04$), radiation therapy only for local disease control ($P < 0.009$), and type of chemotherapy regimen ($P < 0.0003$). They concluded that in surgically treated patients, the most important prognostic factor was the preoperative tumor response to chemotherapy.

Yasko AW, Fanning CV, Ayala AG, Carrasco CH, Murray JA: Percutaneous techniques for the diagnosis and treatment of localized Langerhans-cell histiocytosis (eosinophilic granuloma of bone). *J Bone Joint Surg Am* 1998;80:219-228.

Thirty-four of the 35 lesions diagnosed by needle biopsy and injected with methylprednisolone healed. There were no local recurrences at a mean follow-up of 90 months. There were no complications associated with this procedure.

Current Management of Skeletal Metastasis

Clohisy DR, Ramnaraine ML, Scully S, et al: Osteoprotegerin inhibits tumor-induced osteoclastogenesis and bone tumor growth in osteopetrotic mice. *J Orthop Res* 2000;18:967-976.

In vivo findings provide insight into the mechanism through which tumors induce osteoclastogenesis and osteolysis, by demonstrating that tumors increase RANKL expression and the number of RANK-expressing cells at sites of tumor, effects which are blocked by OPG treatment.

Huang L, Xu J, Wood DJ, Zheng MH: Gene expression of osteoprotegerin ligand, osteoprotegerin, and receptor activator of NF-$\kappa\beta$ in giant cell tumor of bone: Possible involvement in tumor cell-induced osteoclast-like cell formation. *Am J Pathol* 2000;156:761-767.

By using semiquantitative reverse transcriptase polymerase chain reaction, findings suggest that OPG ligand is involved in osteoclast-like cell formation in giant cell tumors. It is speculated that the ratio of OPG ligand/OPG by tumor cells may contribute to osteoclastogenesis in giant cell tumor.

Classic Bibliography

Enneking WF, Spanier SS, Goodman MA: A system for the surgical staging of musculoskeletal sarcoma. *Clin Orthop* 1980;153:106-120.

Harrington KD, Sim FH, Enis JE, Johnston JO, Diok HM, Gristina AG: Methylmethacrylate as an adjunct in internal fixation of pathological fractures: Experience with three hundred and seventy-five cases. *J Bone Joint Surg Am* 1976;58:1047-1055.

Hortobagyi GN, Theriault RL, Porter L, et al: Efficacy of pamidronate in reducing skeletal complications in patients with breast cancer and lytic bone metastases: Protocol 19 Aredia Breast Cancer Study Group. *N Engl J Med* 1996;335:1785-1791.

Imbriaco M, Yeh SD, Yeung H, et al: Thallium-201 scintigraphy for the evaluation of tumor response to preoperative chemotherapy in patients with osteosarcoma. *Cancer* 1997;80:1507-1512.

Madewell JE, Ragsdale BD, Sweet DE: Radiologic and pathologic analysis of solitary bone lesions: Part I. Internal margins. *Radiol Clin North Am* 1981;19:715-748.

Pisters PW, Leung DH, Woodruff J, Shi W, Brennan MF: Analysis of prognostic factors in 1,041 patients with localized soft tissue sarcomas of the extremities. *J Clin Oncol* 1996;14:1679-1689.

Ragsdale BD, Madewell JE, Sweet DE: Radiologic and pathologic analysis of solitary bone lesions: Part II. Periosteal reactions. *Radiol Clin North Am* 1981;19:749-783.

Rosier RN, O'Keefe RJ, Teot LA, et al: P-glycoprotein expression in cartilaginous tumors. *J Surg Oncol* 1997;65:95-105.

Rougraff BT, Simon MA, Kneisl JS, Greenberg DB, Mankin HJ: Limb salvage compared with amputation for osteosarcoma of the distal end of the femur: A long-term oncological, functional, and quality-of-life study. *J Bone Joint Surg Am* 1994;76:649-656.

Scully SP, Temple HT, O'Keefe RJ, Mankin HJ, Gebhardt M: The surgical treatment of patients with osteosarcoma who sustain a pathologic fracture. *Clin Orthop* 1996;324:227-232.

Simonet WS, Lacey DL, Dunstan CR, et al: Osteoprotegerin: A novel secreted protein involved in the regulation of bone density. *Cell* 1997;89:309-319.

Sweet DE, Madewell JE, Ragsdale BD: Radiologic and pathologic analysis of solitary bone lesions: Part III. Matrix patterns. *Radiol Clin North Am* 1981;19:785-814.

Tong D, Gillick L, Hendrickson FR: The palliation of symptomatic osseous metastases: Final results of the Study by the Radiation Therapy Oncology Group. *Cancer* 1982;50:893-899.

Unwin PS, Cannon SR, Grimer RJ, Kemp HB, Sneath RS, Walker PS: Aseptic loosening in cemented custom-made prosthetic replacements for bone tumours of the lower limb. *J Bone Joint Surg Br* 1996;78:5-13.

Chapter 18

Infection

David M. Scher, MD

Brent Wise, MD

Antibiotic Resistance

Antibiotic resistance emerged soon after the introduction of antibiotics. Bacterial resistance can now be demonstrated against all available classes of antibiotics.

The prevalence of drug-resistant *Streptococcus pneumoniae* has increased with penicillin-intermediate resistance rates as high as 51%. Unfortunately, multidrug resistance among pneumococci increases as penicillin and cephalosporin minimal inhibitory concentrations increase. Almost all drugs have been affected, including the fluoroquinolones and carbepenems. Fortunately, vancomycin has remained effective against all pneumococcal strains.

Methicillin-resistant strains of *Staphylococcus aureus* (MRSA) are now endemic in some hospitals and long-term care facilities. The prevalence of MRSA in the United States has increased from 2% to 39.7% during the past 2 decades. An altered penicillin-binding protein mediates methicillin resistance. Strains of MRSA are resistant to all beta-lactam antibiotics. Resistance to non–beta-lactam antibiotics such as clindamycin, tetracycline, trimethoprim-sulfamethoxazole, and ciprofloxacin has increased disproportionately compared with MRSA. Vancomycin intermediate-resistant strains of *S. aureus* have been reported.

The enterococci have gradually become a major cause of nosocomial infections, accounting for 10% to 12%. Vancomycin-resistant enterococci (VRE) has been found in as many as 52% of samples. Ampicillin resistance has been reported to be as high as 83%. Most of the VRE outbreaks have involved clonal dissemination, leading to the enactment of strict isolation precautions in hospitals.

Factors leading to the emergence of resistance include the widespread, inappropriate use of broad-spectrum antibiotics, use of antibiotics in animal husbandry and in fisheries, increase in the number of immunocompromised patients, and prolonged survival of debilitated patients. Resistance develops by either direct genetic exchange or spontaneous mutation. Direct genetic exchange usually involves small, independently-reproducing strains of DNA called plasmids. The mechanisms of resistance include enzymatic inhibition, alteration of porin channels, outer or inner membrane permeability, target proteins, or metabolic pathways, and antibiotic efflux.

New agents are being developed to combat the problem of drug resistance. Linezolid, the first antibiotic of a new class of antibiotics called oxazolidinones, has been approved for use in countering MRSA and VRE. The streptogramin quinupristin-dalfopristin has also been recently approved for use in dealing with VRE infections. However, the use of narrow-spectrum antibiotics based on culture and sensitivity is imperative to diminish the risk of antibiotic resistance. Proper hand washing by physicians and allied health care workers is the most important means of controlling nosocomial transmission.

Osteomyelitis in Adults

The etiologies and management of osteomyelitis are different in children and adults. Osteomyelitis in the adult may have a hematogenous source, typically the result of intravenous drug abuse. The more common causes of adult osteomyelitis are trauma (primarily open fractures and severe soft-tissue injury), vascular insufficiency, diabetes, and surgical wound infections. When the signs and symptoms have developed within 10 days of the initial etiology, the infection is considered to be acute. However, with infections that have been present for more than 10 days, necrotic bone is likely to develop, reflecting chronic osteomyelitis. The progression of chronic disease may occur over months or years.

Radiographic and laboratory studies (white blood cell count [WBC], erythrocyte sedimentation rate [ESR], and C-reactive protein [CRP]) may be used as part of the diagnostic investigation. Radiographs may show periosteal elevation or bone resorption. If plain radiographs are nondiagnostic and the physical examination is nonspecific, additional studies may be useful. Technetium Tc 99m scanning can demonstrate areas of increased metabolic activity. MRI is the most sensitive diagnostic method for identifying subtle findings, such as edema resulting from early inflammation. CT may be helpful to delineate subtle bone destruction, to characterize the extent of the disease, and to guide biopsies or assist in surgical planning.

Recent studies have focused on establishing cost-effective treatment regimens that minimize recurrence. After identifying the infecting organism and determining bacterial sensitivities, treatment for acute osteomyelitis without bone necrosis and devascularization is parenteral antibiotic therapy alone (a 4- to 6-week course). Outpatient parenteral therapy has been shown to be successful and cost effective. The role of oral antibiotics in the treatment of osteomyelitis continues to be clarified. After aggressive single-stage surgical débridement, a short course of parenteral antibiotics may be followed by oral treatment for 6 weeks, with a cure rate equaling that resulting from parenteral treatment. Oral treatment with quinolones has been shown to be effective for some gram-negative infections, but their efficacy for most gram-positive infections, including staphylococcal osteomyelitis, remains controversial.

Local antibiotic delivery systems are under investigation as both adjuvant and alternative treatments. Antibiotic-laden polymethylmethacrylate beads are commercially available with gentamicin (not available in the United States) or can be easily made using vancomycin or tobramycin powder. Their use typically involves surgical débridement followed by implantation of beads to fill resultant dead space. High local concentrations of antibiotic can be obtained with minimal systemic absorption. A second surgical procedure is frequently necessary for bead removal followed by either bone grafting and/or soft-tissue transfer.

Cases of chronic, draining osteomyelitis that are recalcitrant to treatment and accompanied by vascular or immune deficiency may be best managed with amputation. There is an association between squamous cell carcinoma and chronic osteomyelitis with a draining sinus (between 0.2% and 1.7%).

Septic Arthritis in Adults

In adults the etiology of septic arthritis may be one of hematogenous spread or direct inoculation by contiguous spread, or infection from a surgical wound. The most common risk factors in adults are intravenous drug abuse, hemoglobinopathy, immune suppression following organ transplantation, and rheumatoid arthritis. The early pathogenesis involves joint inoculation followed by infiltration of polymorphonuclear leukocytes (PMNLs). The low oxygen tension of this environment impedes the bactericidal activity of the PMNLs. Bacterial toxins can cause cell death and result in the release of proteolytic enzymes that degrade cartilage. It has been postulated that a delayed immune response may then develop, stimulated by bacterial antigens and exotoxins, which results in the influx of T lymphocytes. These T lymphocytes may play a role in the development of postinfectious arthritis.

Neisseria gonorrhoeae, from a hematogenous source, is the most common infecting organism in adult septic arthritis. Joint sepsis develops in approximately 1% to 3% of patients with gonococcal infection. The organism is more common in women and recent menstruation or pregnancy predisposes to dissemination of local infection. Systemic signs such as migratory polyarthralgias, fever, dermatitis, and tenosynovitis are indicative of the bacteremic form, whereas the suppurative form is characterized primarily by monoarticular septic arthritis with a large, purulent effusion. The second most common causative organism in adult septic arthritis is *S. aureus*. Bacterial surface collagen receptors (more likely to be present on *Staphylococcus sp.* that cause joint infections than those involved in other infections) of *S. aureus* have recently been identified. Consequently, this virulence factor gives *S. aureus* a particular affinity for articular cartilage. *S. epidermidis*, an occasional causative organism in septic arthritis, is seen almost exclusively as a postoperative infection. The presence of both of these organisms have recently been reported following arthroscopic procedures. Cannulated instruments have been implicated as a potential source of contamination in these cases; consequently, special sterilization procedures have been suggested. *Salmonella* joint sepsis occurs following septicemia as a result of gastrointestinal infection. These patients typically have an underlying hemoglobinopathy, such as sickle cell disease, or a depressed immune system, frequently as a result of systemic lupus erythematosus.

Patients with septic arthritis usually present with localized joint pain, increased warmth, and restricted motion. Laboratory studies (WBC count, ESR, and CRP) are usually elevated. Radiographs should be obtained to assess bone involvement and joint erosion. The most important diagnostic study is joint aspiration. Cell counts greater than 50,000 cells/mL, composed predominately of PMNLs, indicate joint sepsis. Debate continues over the relative effectiveness of serial aspirations versus arthroscopic or open irrigation and débridement; surgical irrigation and débridement should be done within 72 hours if the patient does not demonstrate marked improvement from serial aspirations. Antibiotic therapy based on the results of the

Gram stain and patient risk factors should be initiated after cultures have been obtained. In most adult patients, initial treatment is administration of an antibiotic such as ceftriaxone, to cover *S. aureus* and *N. gonorrhoeae*. Patients with immunosuppression or hemoglobinopathy must have antibiotic coverage for *Salmonella* and MRSA. It is also essential that the joint fluid be examined for the presence of crystals because crystalline arthropathy can mimic joint sepsis. Parenteral antibiotics are continued for 4 to 6 weeks along with range of motion exercises. A recent study using polymerase chain reaction to detect bacterial DNA in septic joints has demonstrated the persistence of bacterial DNA 3 weeks after initiation of treatment, despite sterile cultures after 3 days.

Soft-Tissue Infections in Adults

Soft-tissue infections range from local cellulitis requiring a short course of narrow-spectrum antibiotics to life-threatening fasciitis. It is imperative to distinguish the early presentation of necrotizing fasciitis from cellulitis, erysipelas, or other superficial and more benign infections. The most important elements in establishing this diagnosis are failure to respond to appropriate antibiotics, rapid enlargement of the involved area, and systemic signs (including tachycardia, hypotension, acidosis, hyperthermia, or hypothermia). Patients at risk are those who are immunocompromised, and those with underlying medical conditions (such as diabetes, liver disease, or alcohol-related conditions) and local tissue hypoxia resulting from surgical wounds, radiation therapy, or cutaneous scars. Physical findings include erythema and tenderness with occasional subcutaneous crepitus. Radiographs may reveal the presence of subcutaneous air, but usually are not diagnostic. MRI may be useful to distinguish cellulitis from necrotizing fasciitis in early stages.

Necrotizing fasciitis is frequently a polymicrobial infection caused by anaerobic, aerobic, gram-positive, and/or gram-negative organisms. Group A streptococci, which have surface receptors and exotoxins that contribute to their virulence, are frequently the causative organism along with staphylococci. Treatment involves management of systemic symptoms. Complete surgical débridement must be initiated early. Multiple débridements are typically necessary and mortality has been reported to be between 9% and 26%.

Musculoskeletal Infections in Children

Microbiology

S. aureus remains the most common causative organism for both osteomyelitis and septic arthritis, followed by *Streptococcus*. A recent comprehensive, multicenter, prospective study identified *S. pneumoniae* as the cause of 4% of cases of osteomyelitis and 20% of cases of joint sepsis. Children with sequelae of the infection (contractures and joint destruction) were younger than those with no sequelae (mean age of 6.4 months versus 18.6 months). The recent introduction of pneumococcal vaccines will likely have a dramatic effect on the incidence of these infections, as has been the case with *Haemophilus influenzae*.

Previously *H. influenzae* type B was the next most common cause of osteomyelitis and was the most common cause of septic arthritis in children 2 years of age or younger. Since the introduction of the *H. influenzae* type B vaccine, which is now administered at 2 months of age, influenza essentially has been eliminated as a cause of osteomyelitis or septic arthritis. Another infectious organism with which children may become infected is *Pseudomonas aeruginosa*, typically as a result of foot puncture wounds.

Acute Hematogenous Osteomyelitis

The initial signs and symptoms of osteomyelitis in children are pain, fever, and a limp. Frequently there is also a concomitant history of minor trauma that may play a role in the development of bacteremia and in creating a nidus for infection. In addition to the physical examination, the diagnosis is established with the aid of laboratory studies (WBC, ESR, CRP) and radiologic studies (radiographs, technetium bone scan, ultrasound) (Figs. 1 and 2). Aspiration is essential for isolation of the infecting organism as well as identification of a possible abscess requiring surgical drainage. Septic joints have been shown to occur adjacent to the infected bone in 33% of patients. Septic arthritis adjacent to osteomyelitis typically occurs most commonly in the knee, followed closely by the hip, ankle, and shoulder. An antibiotic effective against gram-positive organisms (cefazolin 100 mg/kg/day) should be administered parenterally once blood and bone cultures are obtained. Blood cultures are typically positive 40% to 50% of the time. The patient should be switched to oral antibiotics for 6 weeks once fever has abated, and there should be minimal or no discomfort and the CRP returned to normal levels. Follow-up assessment of CRP should also be done at approximately 1 week following initiation of oral antibiotics and at the termination of treatment to ensure efficacy. A recent long-term follow-up study of osteomyelitis and septic arthritis has demonstrated the effectiveness of a similar regimen involving early conversion to oral antibiotics with almost no sequelae.

Some uncommon variants of osteomyelitis have recently been reported. Hematogenous calcaneal osteomyelitis accounts for about 4% of all osteomyelitis

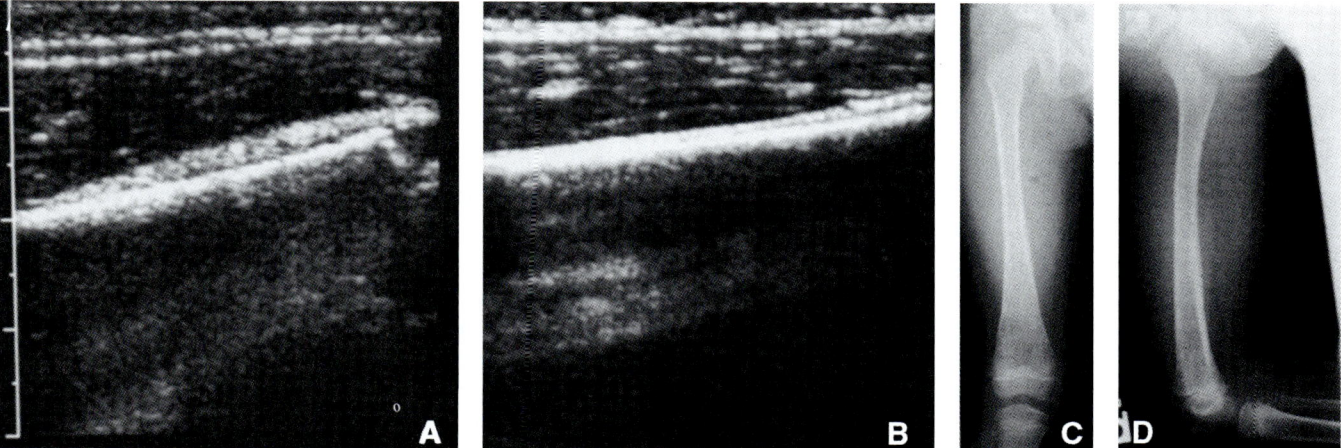

Figure 1 Radiographs of the femur of a 4-year-old girl with right distal femoral osteomyelitis. Sagittal ultrasound views of the right (**A**) and the normal left (**B**) distal femurs. Periosteal elevation is demonstrated in **A,** suggesting a subperiosteal abscess. The patient underwent irrigation and débridement with decompression of the abscess and drilling of the distal femoral cortex. **C** and **D,** AP and lateral views, respectively, of the femur 6 months after surgery. Radiodense areas of the distal femur consistent with the prior infection are apparent, but the physis remains open.

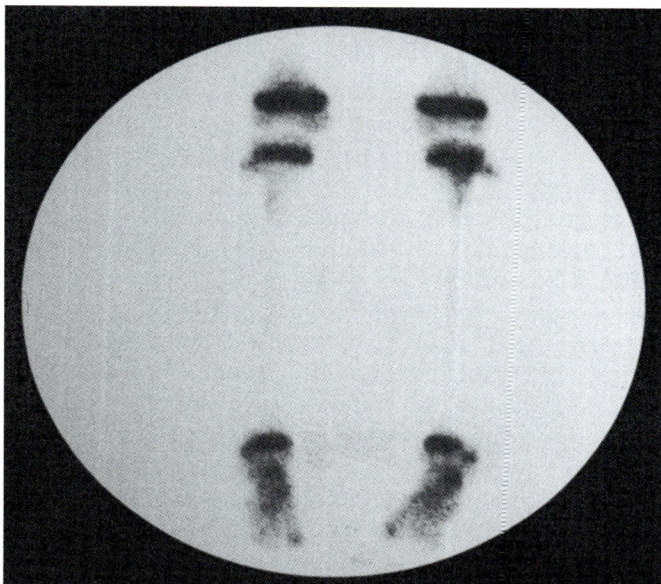

Figure 2 Bone scan of the left proximal tibia of a 5-year-old girl with osteomyelitis, demonstrating increased uptake.

cases; however, when it does occur the diagnosis can be difficult to confirm. Children may present with low-grade or no fever and the WBC and CRP may not be elevated; the ESR typically is elevated. Bone scans are essential in the absence of radiographic abnormalities and, once the diagnosis has been established, this infection can be successfully managed in the same manner as in other bones. Another rare association with hematogenous osteomyelitis is epiphyseal separation that can occur in neonates. This condition must be recognized and treated with surgical fixation and immobilization, in addition to the appropriate surgical and medical treatments for osteomyelitis.

Septic Arthritis

Septic arthritis in children is most common at age 2 years or younger. Affected patients typically present with pain, fever, and the inability to walk (in cases involving lower extremity joints). In young children, the distinction between transient synovitis and septic arthritis of the hip can be difficult; however, four easily obtainable predictors (fever, inability to bear weight, ESR greater than or equal to 40 mm/h, and serum WBC greater than or equal to 12,000/mm^3) can be used to establish the probability of septic arthritis. If none of these predictors are present, the probability of septic arthritis is less than 0.2%. If one, two, three, or four predictors are present, the probabilities are 3%, 40%, 93.1%, and 99.6%, respectively.

The diagnosis is confirmed by joint aspiration, which demonstrates WBCs (predominantly PMNLs) greater than 50,000/mm^3. Gram stain and cultures and sensitivities are obtained and irrigation and débridement done with placement of a deep drain. Blood cultures are positive in 40% to 50% of cases and joint cultures may be positive in 30% to 82% of cases. Parenteral antibiotics are administered after cultures have been obtained and are continued until there has been clinical improvement as evidenced by no fever, decreased pain, increased hip motion, and ambulation. CRP may also be monitored to determine the patient's response to therapy. Early conversion to oral antibiotics, following approximately 1 week of therapy, is safe and effective in patients with community-acquired, gram-positive septic arthritis.

Uncommon Infections

Diskitis, vertebral osteomyelitis, pyomyositis, and pyogenic sacroiliitis all should be considered when evaluating a child with a limp, inability to walk, and signs of infection. Children with diskitis and vertebral osteomyelitis will have back pain and tenderness. Children with diskitis usually are younger (the condition is uncommon in children older than age 8 years) than those with vertebral osteomyelitis and may have nonspecific laboratory findings. Children with vertebral osteomyelitis are more likely to be febrile and appear ill; this diagnosis is rare in children age 3 years or younger. MRI will establish either diagnosis, and management should consist of blood cultures followed by antibiotic therapy.

Pyomyositis is a rare condition that results from the combination of bacteremia and pathophysiologic alterations in the local muscle environment. Skeletal muscle typically is resistant to bacterial seeding, even in the presence of bacteremia. However, muscle that has been subjected to minor trauma or subclinical infection with bacteria, viruses, or parasites may be predisposed to pyomyositis. There are three described phases of this infection: the initial invasive phase, the suppurative phase, and the late phase (includes fluctuance and more severe systemic manifestations). Most patients present during the suppurative phase because of increasing symptoms. The diagnosis is best confirmed using MRI with gadolinium contrast; however, this test is so sensitive that it may suggest bone involvement as well. The treatment of pyomyositis involves antibiotics against the infecting organism (usually *S. aureus*), and surgical débridement for patients in the late and suppurative stages.

Pyogenic sacroiliitis usually occurs in older children or young adolescents, although it can present at almost any age. It is characterized by complaints of low back and hip pain as well as fever, which is frequently low grade, and a limp or the inability to walk. A technetium bone scan will confirm the diagnosis, but MRI may be necessary to diagnose an abscess. Treatment is usually with antibiotics alone, but in patients who are unresponsive to antibiotics alone, open débridement may be necessary to identify an organism and drain abscesses.

Lyme Disease

Lyme disease is the multisystem disease caused by infection with *Borrelia burgdorferi*, spread by ticks of the *Ixodes ricinus* complex (*I. scapularis* in the northeast, northern, Midwest, and southern United States; *I. pacificus* in the Pacific Coast states; *I. ricinus* in Europe; and *I. persulcatus* in Asia). These ticks carry the gram-negative spirochete between humans and its reservoir: the white-footed deer mouse. The deer is not a source of infection. The immunopathogenesis of the disease is probably related to the immunologic and inflammatory changes induced by *B. burgdorferi*. Lyme disease is divided into three clinical stages: early localized, early disseminated, and late.

Early localized Lyme disease is characterized by erythema migrans, the pathognomonic skin lesion that occurs approximately 1 week after the tick bite (range, 1 to 30 days). Early disseminated Lyme disease occurs within 6 to 9 months of the onset of infection and can be manifested by atrioventricular nodal block and mild pericarditis. Early neurologic symptoms, including lymphocytic meningitis, radiculoneuritis, and cranial neuritis, may also be present.

The musculoskeletal features of untreated Lyme disease include arthralgia and intermittent episodes of monoarthritis. The arthritis, which may mimic acute septic arthritis, can occur within days to months of the onset of infection. The synovial fluid is inflammatory, with a WBC count of 10,000 to 25,000 mm^3, and always with a predominance of neutrophils. Additionally, the fluid often reaccumulates rapidly after aspiration. Chronic inflammatory arthritis is the dominant feature of late Lyme disease. The involved joint, most frequently the knee, is usually swollen but not very painful. Small joint inflammation is not common and its presence should suggest a different diagnosis. Although the inflammatory synovitis typically dissipates after months to years, the arthritis may become chronic. Persistent arthritis despite antibiotic therapy is associated with HLA-DR4 and serum immunoglobulin G that is reactive with *B. burgdorferi*'s outer surface protein A.

Studies have shown that oral antibiotics are usually effective in treating Lyme arthritis. Current practice is to give a 3- to 6-week course of oral amoxicillin as initial therapy, with intravenous therapy reserved for refractory cases or arthritis associated with central nervous system disease. Refractory cases may be characterized by a reinflammation of the affected joint, inflammation of a second joint, or evidence of new extra-articular infection. A vaccine for Lyme disease is available and is recommended for patients in endemic areas, but its role in patients who already have Lyme arthritis remains unclear.

Reactive Arthritis

Reactive arthritis was originally defined as synovitis developing after a distant infection, and it was distinguished from postinfectious arthritis because of the absence of bacterial components in the joint tissue. Studies have focused on the arthritides triggered by infections with *Enterobacteriaceae* and *Chlamydia* in the patient with the HLA-B27 haplotype. However, non-HLA-B27 associated arthritides have been well described and reactive arthritis is now considered to occur in two forms: HLA-B27 associated and

TABLE 1 | Bacteria Triggering Reactive Arthritis—Manifestations at the Entry Site

Site of Entry	Clinical Manifestations	Bacteria
Gastrointestinal tract	Diarrhea	*Yersinia enterocolitica**
	Gastroenteritis	*Salmonella typhimurium**
	Enterocolitis	*Shigella flexneri**
	Oligo- and asymptomatic infection	*Campylobacter jejuni/fetus**
		*Clostridium difficile**
		Brucella abortus/mellitensis
Urogenital tract	Urethritis, cystitis	*Chlamydia trachomatis**
	Cervicitis	*Ureaplasma urealyticum*
	Prostatitis, epididymitis	*Mycoplasma hominis*†
	Salpingitis, endometritis	*Neisseria gonorrhoeae*
	Often asymptomatic infections	Bacille Calmette-Guérin
		Gardnerella vaginalis
Bronchopulmonary	Bronchitis, pnuemonia, sinusitis	*Chlamydia pneumoniae*
	Angina tonsillaris	β-hemolytic streptococci
	Tuberculosis	*Mycobacterium tuberculosis*
Skin/mucosa	Erythema chronicum migrans	*Borrelia burgdorferi*
	Acrodermatitis chronica atrophicans	*Staphylococcus aureus*
	Skin infections joint infections	
	Cat-scratch disease	*Bartonella*
	Brucellosis	*Brucella abortus/mellitensis*
	Leptospirosis	*Leptospira*

*Reactive arthritis triggering bacteria associated with HLA-B27
†Association is uncertain
(Reproduced with permission from Kuipers JG, Kohler L, Zeidler H: Reactive or infectious arthritis. Ann Rheum Dis 1999;58:661-664.)

nonassociated. The infection preceding reactive arthritis can be urogenic, enterogenic, respiratory tract-associated, or idiopathic, and the arthritis is believed to develop as a T cell-mediated reaction. Table 1 summarizes the site of entry, clinical manifestation, and causative bacteria.

Enteric causes of reactive arthritis are often treated with nonsteroidal anti-inflammatory drugs (NSAIDs) alone, usually until the CBC and ESR have normalized. Viable Chlamydia species may persist in the joints of patients with reactive arthritis and antibiotic treatment of the initial infection as well of the subsequent arthritis can be beneficial. The use of both antibiotics and NSAIDs is justified.

In addition, many transient arthritides are caused by viral infections. Rubella infection of both the wild type and after immunization is a common cause of arthralgias or arthritis in adolescents, but is rare in young children. Parvovirus B19 is also a common cause of acute arthritis in children and young adults. As viral arthritides are self-limiting, the treatment is NSAIDs combined with symptomatic measures.

Musculoskeletal Manifestations of Retroviral Infection

Musculoskeletal infections constitute an unusual clinical manifestation in patients with human immunodeficiency virus (HIV) infection (0.3% to 3.5%). Septic arthritis is the most commonly reported infection of the musculoskeletal system. *S. aureus* is the most commonly isolated agent, in approximately one third of cases. Osteomyelitis is a more serious infection and half the reported cases were caused by atypical mycobacteria. The mortality rate has been reported as high as 20%.

A wide range of HIV-associated rheumatologic manifestations have been described, including Reiter's syndrome or reactive arthritis, psoriatic arthritis, arthralgias, painful articular syndrome, and undifferentiated spondyloarthopathies. Unlike infections, these complaints are relatively common (54.8%) and tend to be more frequent during the late stages of HIV infection. Several worldwide studies appear to indicate an association between HIV and seronegative spondyloarthopathies. HIV-associated arthritis is generally self-limited and most patients respond to conventional first- and second-line anti-inflammatory medications.

Osteonecrosis is becoming a more reported finding in HIV disease. A recent MRI-based survey of 339 asymptomatic HIV-positive patients showed 15 (4.4%) to have osteonecrosis. The etiology of osteonecrosis in the HIV-positive patient is unclear, but either previous or concomitant steroid use or the hyperlipidemia induced by the current protease inhibitors may be causative factors.

Human T lymphotropic virus type I (HTLV-1), is another retrovirus that is present in widely scattered, apparently unrelated populations in the world. The two best-studied areas are the islands of southwestern Japan, where approximately 20% of adults are seropositive, and the Caribbean basin, where 2% to 5% of black adults are seropositive. HTLV-1 associated myelopathy, also know as tropical spastic paresis, is a chronic, progressive, demyelinating disease that affects the spinal cord and white matter. The lifetime incidence of HTLV-1 associated myelopathy in HTLV-1 carriers is estimated to be 5%. Gait disturbances and weakness and stiffness of the lower limbs are common. Lower extremities are affected to a greater degree than upper extremities. Spasticity may be moderate to severe and low back pain is common. HTLV-1 has also been implicated in arthropathy with HTLV-1 proviral DNA demonstrable in synovial tissue and synovial fluid lymphocytes. Patients in endemic areas with these symptoms should be screened for HTLV.

Annotated Bibliography

Antibiotic Resistance

Sieradzki K, Roberts RB, Haber SW, Tomasz A: The development of vancomycin resistance in a patient with methicillin-resistant Staphylococcus aureus infection. *N Engl J Med* 1999;340:517-523.

The authors investigated the microbiologic properties of a MRSA strain that was resistant to vancomycin as well. The bacteria were shown to be susceptible to vancomycin when combined with a β-lactam antibiotic.

Smith TL, Pearson ML, Wilcox KR, et al: Emergence of vancomycin resistance in Staphylococcus aureus: Glycopeptide-intermediate Staphylococcus aureus working group. *N Engl J Med* 1999;340:493-501.

This study reports the first two infections in the United States caused by MRSA that had intermediate resistance to vancomycin. The Centers for Disease Control and Prevention guidelines for preventing the spread of vancomycin resistance are reviewed along with the situations in which vancomycin use should be discouraged.

Virk A, Steckelberg JM: Clinical aspects of antimicrobial resistance. *Mayo Clin Proc* 2000;75:200-214.

The epidemiology of the major resistant organisms, the factors that have led to the development of resistance, and current solutions for treating many of these infections are discussed. Several newly Food and Drug Administration-approved antibiotics are also discussed.

Osteomyelitis in Adults

Swiontkowski MF, Hanel DP, Vedder NB, Schwappach JR: A comparison of short- and long-term intravenous antibiotic therapy in the postoperative management of adult osteomyelitis. *J Bone Joint Surg Br* 1999;81:1046-1050.

Single-stage, aggressive surgical debridement, with the assistance of laser Doppler flowmetry to assess bone viability and soft-tissue coverage, followed by 5 to 7 days of parenteral antibiotics and 6 weeks of oral antibiotics, effectively eradicated chronic osteomyelitis in 91% of patients. The use of long-term intravenous antibiotics with these adjuvants was shown to be unnecessary.

Septic Arthritis in Adults

Blevins FT, Salgado J, Wascher DC, Koster F: Septic arthritis following arthroscopic meniscus repair: A cluster of three cases. *Arthroscopy* 1999;15:35-40.

Three cases of septic arthritis of the knee following arthroscopic meniscal repair are reported. The authors attribute these infections to inadequate cleansing of the cannulas used in the repair.

van der Heijden IM, Wilbrink B, Vije AE, Schouls LM, Breedveld FC, Tak PP: Detection of bacterial DNA in serial synovial samples obtained during antibiotic treatment from patients with septic arthritis. *Arthritis Rheum* 1999;42:2198-2203.

The authors used polymerase chain reaction to detect bacterial DNA in synovial fluid samples from six adult patients being treated for septic arthritis. Bacterial DNA was still present in two patients after 21 and 22 days of treatment, respectively, and was absent in another at 26 days. Polymerase chain reaction may become a useful tool in the diagnosis and management of joint infections.

Verdrengh M, Erlandsson-Harris H, Tarkowski A: Role of selectins in experimental Staphylococcus aureus-induced arthritis. *Eur J Immunol* 2000;30:1606-1613.

A murine model of *S. aureus* septic arthritis was used to elucidate the contribution of selectin adhesion molecules to leukocyte infiltration. They found that when the selectin molecules were blocked by a variety of mechanisms, the severity of early arthritis was less but the subsequent clearance of bacteria from the body was also diminished.

Musculoskeletal Manifestations of Retroviral Infection

Berman A, Cahn P, Perez H, et al: Human immunodeficiency virus infection associated arthritis: Clinical characteristics. *J Rheum* 1999;26:1158-1162.

This prospective study of patients with HIV infection demonstrated that 7.8% of these patients had arthritis, which was not due to any other inflammatory arthritis. In those studied, rheumatoid factor and HLA-B27 were negative. The authors conclude that HIV-associated arthritis, like that in other viral disorders, is acute in onset, or short duration and not associated with erosive changes.

Soft-Tissue Infections in Adults

Fontes RA, Ogilvie CM, Miclau T: Necrotizing soft-tissue infections. *J Am Acad Orthop Surg* 2000;8:151-158.

This review article covers the clinical characteristics of severe soft-tissue infections with respect to the diagnosis, microbiology, and treatment.

Musculoskeletal Infections in Children

Bradley JS, Kaplan SL, Tan TQ, et al: Pediatric pneumococcal bone and joint infections: The Pediatric Multicenter Pneumococcal Surveillance Study Group (PMPSSG). *Pediatrics* 1998;102:1376-1382.

This multicenter study reports the characteristics of bone and joint infections caused by penicillin-susceptible and penicillin-nonsusceptible strains. The response to therapy of the two groups is similar. The age of children who had seqelae from the infection were younger than those who did not.

Christiansen P, Frederiksen B, Glazowski J, Scavenius M, Knudsen FU: Epidemiologic, bacteriologic, and long-term follow-up data of children with acute hematogenous osteomyelitis and septic arthritis: A ten-year review. *J Pediatr Orthop* 1999;8:302-305.

This study is a retrospective review of 69 children with acute hematogenous osteomyelitis and 48 children with septic arthritis at median 10-year follow-up. The outcome was favorable, with only 3% having major sequelae and 2% having minor sequelae. The major sequelae were a moderate femoral head deformity following septic arthritis, vertebral wedging and loss of disk space height, and osteonecrosis of the femoral head.

Fernandez M, Carrol CL, Baker CJ: Discitis and vertebral osteomyelitis in children: An 18-year review. *Pediatrics* 2000;105:1299-1304.

This retrospective review compares the clinical characteristics and radiographic findings of 57 children with either diskitis or vertebral osteomyelitis. Children with diskitis were younger than those with vertebral osteomyelitis and the duration of symptoms was shorter. Radiographs were usually diagnostic in the patients with diskitis, but not with vertebral osteomyelitis. The authors conclude that patient age and clinical presentation frequently distinguish the two diagnoses and recommend MRI for definitive diagnosis.

Howard AW, Viskontas D, Sabbagh C: Reduction in osteomyelitis and septic arthritis related to Haemophilus influenzae type B vaccination. *J Pediatr Orthop* 1999;19:705-709.

This retrospective study compares patient cohorts with septic arthritis and osteomyelitis before and after the introduction of the Haemophilus influenza type B vaccine in Ontario, Canada. The vaccination has succeeded in eliminating *H. fluenzae* as an infective organism in pediatric septic arthritis and osteomyelitis. The authors recommend that empiric antimicrobial therapy may cover only gram-positive organisms in vaccinated children.

Jaakkola J, Kehl D: Hematogenous calcaneal osteomyelitis in children. *J Pediatr Orthop* 1999;19:699-704.

Twenty-one patients with hematogenous calcaneal osteomyelitis were studied. The average patient age was 2.9 years. Local tenderness, swelling, and erythema were the most common findings. The authors recommend maintaining high suspicion for the diagnosis of hematogenous calcaneal osteomyelitis in the limping child to avoid potential treatment delays, which would result in persistent symptoms and growth disturbance.

Kim HK, Alman B, Cole WG: A shortened course of parenteral antibiotic therapy in the management of acute septic arthritis of the hip. *J Pediatr Orthop* 2000;20:44-47.

This article presents a retrospective review of 20 patients with culture-positive septic arthritis treated with surgical débridement and parenteral antibiotics, followed by early conversion to oral antibiotics. Patients were switched to oral antibiotics when they demonstrated clinical improvement, characterized by the absence of fevers, decreased pain, increased hip motion, and increased ambulation. The authors conclude that community-acquired, gram-positive septic arthritis may be safely treated with early conversion to oral antibiotics following surgical drainage and initial parenteral antibiotics, once the patients demonstrate an adequate clinical response.

Kocher MS, Zurakowski D, Kasser JR: Differentiating between septic arthritis and transient synovitis of the hip in children: An evidence-based clinical prediction algorithm. *J Bone Joint Surg Am* 1999;81:1662-1670.

Data from all 282 patients were collected and an algorithm developed to differentiate between those with septic arthritis and toxic synovitis. The authors were able to identify four independent multivariate clinical predictors: history of fever, inability to bear weight, ESR greater than or equal to 40 mm/h, and serum WBC count greater than 12,000/mm^3. The probability of septic arthritis was determined to be < 0.2% for zero predictors, 3% for one predictor, 40% for two predictors, 93% for three predictors, and 99.6% for four predictors. The authors recommend using the predicted risk of septic arthritis, based on the number of predictors present, to assist in guiding the diagnostic workup.

Lyon RM, Evanich JD: Culture-negative septic arthritis in children. *J Pediatr Orthop* 1999;19:655-659.

In this retrospective study, the records of 67 patients with septic arthritis were reviewed. A causative organism was identified in only 30% of patients. All were treated by surgical drainage and antibiotic therapy. The authors suggest that the incidence of culture-negative septic arthritis has been underestimated and that the same management be applied regardless of culture results in children who are otherwise suspected of having joint sepsis.

Perlman MH, Patzakis MJ, Kumar PJ, Holtom P: The incidence of joint involvement with adjacent osteomyelitis in pediatric patients. *J Pediatr Orthop* 2000;20:40-43.

A retrospective review of 66 patients with osteomyelitis determined that 33% had sepsis of the adjacent joint and that the most commonly involved joint was the knee. The authors recommend careful evaluation of the adjacent joint in children with osteomyelitis.

Spiegel DA, Meyer JS, Dormans JP, Flynn JM, Drummond DS: Pyomyositis in children and adolescents: Report of 12 cases and review of the literature. *J Pediatr Orthop* 1999;19:143-150.

Twelve cases of pyomyositis are described with regard to the clinical findings, diagnosis, and treatment. Three stages of the disease are described reflecting the pathophysiology of the infection. MRI is the optimal diagnostic tool, although its sensitivity makes distinguishing local edema from osteomyelitis difficult. Treatment depends on the stage, but is typically managed by surgical débridement and antibiotics.

Classic Bibliography

Culp RW, Eichenfield AH, Davidson RS, Drummond DS, Christofersen MR, Goldsmith DP: Lyme arthritis in children: An orthopaedic perspective. *J Bone Joint Surg Am* 1987;69:96-99.

Lew DP, Waldvogel FA: Osteomyelitis. *N Engl J Med* 1997;336:999-1007.

Morrissy RT, Haynes DW: Acute hematogenous osteomyelitis: A model with trauma as an etiology. *J Pediatr Orthop* 1989;9:447-456.

Nelson JD: The bacterial etiology and antibiotic management of septic arthritis in infants and children. *Pediatrics* 1972;50:437-440.

Ring D, Johnston CE II, Wenger DR: Pyogenic infectious spondylitis in children: The convergence of discitis and vertebral osteomyelitis. *J Pediatr Orthop* 1995;15:652-660.

Szer IS, Taylor E, Steere AC: The long-term course of Lyme arthritis in children. *N Engl J Med* 1991;325:159-163.

Waldvogel FA, Medoff G, Swartz MN: Osteomyelitis: A review of clinical features, therapeutic considerations and unusual aspects: Osteomyelitis associated with vascular insufficiency. *N Engl J Med* 1970;282:316-322.

Chapter 19

Arthritis

Cathy S. Carlson, DVM, PhD

Osteoarthritis

Osteoarthritis (OA) is the most common form of arthritis, affecting approximately 40 million people in the United States, and is a leading cause of physical disability, increased need for health care, and impaired quality of life. By the year 2020, this disease is expected to affect nearly 60 million people in the US. Despite its prevalence, there is relatively little known regarding the etiology, pathogenesis, and progression of this disease. This lack of knowledge is due in part to confounding factors in human epidemiologic studies, including individual variations in physical activity, diet, and medical history; the poor correlation between symptoms of OA and radiographic lesions; and the inability to detect early disease. In addition, morphologic, cell culture, and biomechanical studies of human tissues are limited because the only joint tissues that usually are available are those obtained at surgery from patients with severe OA. Also, for many years OA was regarded as a simple, age-related, degenerative, wear and tear phenomenon and even as an inevitable consequence of aging, views that led to negative approaches to both research and treatment.

OA is a noninflammatory degenerative joint disease that is characterized by articular cartilage degradation, subchondral sclerosis, osteophyte formation, and changes in the soft tissues including the synovial membrane, joint capsule, ligaments, and muscle (Fig. 1). Synovial inflammation can also be present. Although the pathologic changes in OA are fairly well defined, particularly in the late stages of the disease, defining the clinical disease is much more difficult because pathologic changes in the knee joints visualized in vivo by routine radiographic techniques and by clinical MRI techniques correlate poorly with clinical symptoms. It appears that OA may actually be a group of overlapping disorders, probably not of the same etiology but gradually converging on the same end point with similar morphologic and clinical outcomes. Systemic factors, genetics, and local factors (such as biomechanically- or biochemically-mediated events) may control the site and severity of disease.

Until recently, the study of articular cartilage lesions was the main focus of OA research. Articular cartilage consists of relatively low numbers of chondrocytes that are separated by an extracellular matrix of collagens (90% to 95% type II), other proteins, and proteoglycans. Because of the large negative charge of the component proteoglycans, water is held within the cartilage, providing it with the tensile strength needed to absorb high load forces. Adult articular cartilage contains neither a vascular supply nor innervation and, thus, has a poor ability to heal. Experimentally-induced partial-thickness defects may remain virtually unchanged morphologically for at least 6 months and probably longer. Areas of damaged articular cartilage are an important pathologic feature of OA (Fig. 2). The fundamental event resulting in the destruction of articular cartilage in OA appears to result from an imbalance between anabolic and catabolic processes. The extracellular matrix of cartilage is degraded by matrix metalloproteinases that are induced by cytokines. Cytokines also blunt chondrocyte compensatory synthesis pathways required to restore the integrity of the degraded extracellular matrix. Mechanical factors also undoubtedly play a role in cartilage destruction.

Although articular cartilage damage has historically been an area in which research into treatments for OA has been concentrated, OA is increasingly appreciated to be a disorder of the entire synovial joint and not simply of articular cartilage. There is emerging evidence, for example, that an increased thickness of subchondral bone (sclerosis), a feature that is commonly appreciated in late-stage human disease, may be an important early feature in the pathogenesis of this disease, possibly preceding morphologic changes in articular cartilage. Recent evidence also demonstrates specific architectural changes in the subchondral tra-

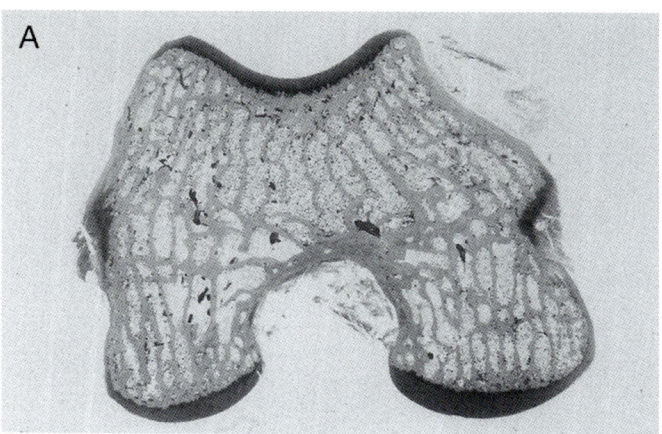
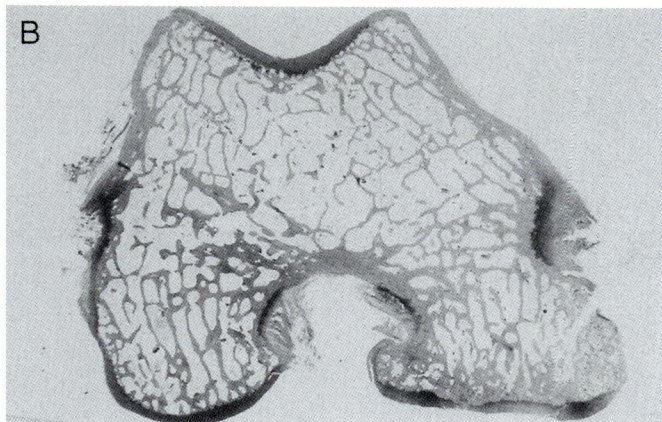

Figure 1 Photomicrograph of a coronal histologic section from a normal femur **(A)** and a femur exhibiting changes of severe OA **(B)**. In addition to loss of articular cartilage in OA, there are marked changes in subchondral and periarticular bone leading to changes in condylar shape, particularly of the medial femoral condyle (right side in both photos).

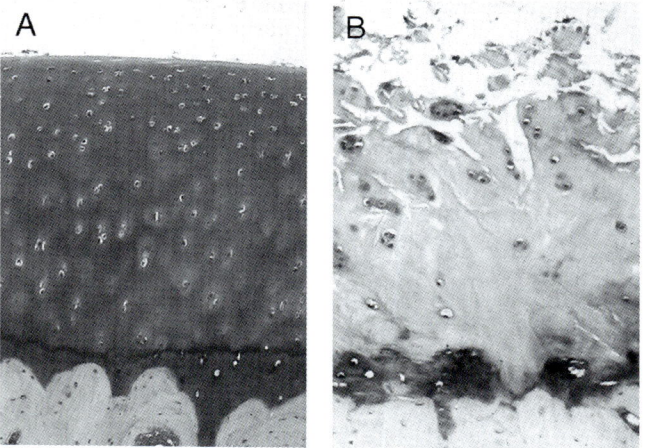

Figure 2 Photomicrograph of normal adult articular cartilage **(A)** compared with severely osteoarthritic articular cartilage **(B)**, in which there is marked fibrillation and loss of matrix staining.

becular bone in OA that are consistent with an acceleration of bone turnover, which appears to be a part of the pathophysiologic process in the progression of the disease.

Risk Factors

Risk factors for OA include age, gender, genetic predisposition, mechanical stress and/or joint trauma, and obesity. The disease is uncommon in adults younger than age 40 years, but is the most common chronic disease in later life, with more than 80% of those age 75 years and older being affected. The prevalence of OA increases progressively with age at all joint sites. The mechanisms for the association of OA with age, however, have not been clearly defined, although data is emerging from studies in other tissues showing that cellular responses to growth factors can decrease with age. A significant age-related decline in chondrocyte response to insulin-like growth factor-1 (IGF-1), which stimulates the production of proteoglycans and collagen and also stimulates production of integrins (cell receptors that bind extracellular matrix proteins and are important for tissue repair), recently has been demonstrated.

Overall, women are about twice as likely as men to have OA. The pattern of joint involvement also differs with gender, with women having a greater number of joints involved and more frequent complaints of morning stiffness, joint swelling, and nocturnal pain. Before age 45 years, however, the disease prevalence is lower in women than in men, with a marked increase in prevalence occurring after 55 years of age, particularly in the knee. These gender differences in OA incidence were first recognized over 150 years ago and were thought to be linked to postmenopausal estrogen deficiency. In support of this theory, several recent epidemiologic studies have found that estrogen replacement therapy is associated with a lower than expected risk of knee and hip OA in postmenopausal women. In addition, functional estrogen receptors recently have been demonstrated in adult articular cartilage, suggesting the potential for estrogen regulation in chondrocytes.

OA also appears to have a genetic component. There is a significantly higher concordance of OA in all joint areas among monozygotic twins than among dizygotic twins. Segregation analysis of population data suggests that OA is a polygenic disorder but the identity of the genes involved remains unknown. Studies of a rare familial form of OA suggest that an autosomal dominant mutation in type II collagen may be an important factor.

Another important risk factor, particularly for OA of the knee and, to a lesser extent, the hip, is obesity. Increased force across the weight-bearing joints probably explains most of the risk, although metabolic factors may also play a role. Weight loss appears to lower the risks of radiographic and symptomatic knee OA and recent clinical trial data suggest that weight loss may ameliorate symptoms. Although the majority of the evidence is from studies in women, greater body mass index in young men also has been shown to be associated with an increased risk of subsequent knee, but not hip, OA. Heavy physical activity also is an important risk factor for the development of knee OA, particularly in elderly obese individuals. Light and moderate activities, however, do not appear to increase risk and, in fact, appear to be beneficial.

Nonsurgical Management

No nonsurgical management has been documented to affect the progression of OA. Pharmacologic therapy for OA is presently only palliative and is based on the use of analgesic or nonsteroidal anti-inflammatory agents (NSAIDs). NSAIDs are the most commonly prescribed agents for alleviating the pain associated with this disorder, but can cause serious adverse effects, such as gastrointestinal tract and kidney disorders and disorders in hemostasis, particularly in the elderly population. Although the cyclooxygenase-2 inhibitors are associated with a lower rate of complications than conventional NSAIDs, there is an urgent need for finding pharmacologic therapies for OA that are both effective and relatively safe.

The use of the nutraceuticals glucosamine sulfate and chondroitin sulfate (recommended dose: 1,500 mg glucosamine and 1,200 mg chondroitin sulfate) for the treatment of OA recently has attracted substantial attention in the literature. Glucosamine, a hexosamine sugar that is a basic building block for the biosynthesis of glycosaminoglycans and proteoglycans, and chondroitin, a glycosaminoglycan that is found in the proteoglycans of articular cartilage, are both derived from animal products, administered orally, and are to some degree absorbed from the gastrointestinal tract. Cell culture data indicate that these compounds are capable of increasing proteoglycan synthesis in chondrocytes from articular cartilage. A recent study evaluated the benefit of glucosamine and chondroitin preparations for OA symptoms using a meta-analysis combined with systematic quality assessment of clinical trials of these preparations in knee and/or hip OA. The main finding was that both glucosamine and chondroitin are likely to be effective therapies for the symptomatic management of OA. Overall, it appears that these compounds are safe; however, their efficacy in the treatment of OA requires further study.

Intra-articular Injections

Intra-articular injections fall into three categories: corticosteroids, hyaluronic acid, and cytokines. It has been suggested that corticosteroids can improve symptoms, but they also are reported to impair the physiology of normal cartilage and induce arthropathy. Intra-articular viscosupplementation using cross-linked hyaluronan (hyaluronic acid) is classified as a device rather than a drug. Hyaluronic acid compound injection has been associated with functional improvement in up to 77% of patients. This therapeutic approach is based on the observation that synovial fluid in OA knees has decreased viscosity and elasticity, and its native hyaluronan has a lower molecular weight than that found in normal healthy knees. The best response is seen in patients with mild OA changes on radiographs, but even patients with severe changes demonstrate some response to treatment. There have been no reported systemic reactions with hyaluronic acid injections, but local reactions consisting of transient pain and swelling may occur. Experimentally, cytokines and growth factors (transforming growth factor-beta 1, IGF-1, and bone morphogenetic proteins) have been shown to improve cartilage metabolism in vitro and are currently being studied in animal models. In the future these agents may be delivered by injection or through local implantation into a defect in the joint surface with use of a carrier matrix.

Surgical Treatment

Biologic healing and regeneration of cartilage recently have generated a great deal of interest. Two new intra-articular procedures, autogenous osteochondral grafting (mosaicplasty) and autologous chondrocyte implantation (ACI), have shown promise in some patients with knee articular cartilage defects. To date, only lesions on the femoral condyles and trochlear groove have been effectively treated. The two procedures improved knee function in 2- to 5-year follow-up studies in carefully selected patients. Patients most likely to benefit are those with normal knee alignment, no evidence of ligamentous instability, no evidence of arthritis on the corresponding tibial surface, and radiographically normal or near-normal knee joints. For grade III or IV defects less than 2 cm^2 (size limit due to concerns about donor site morbidity), mosaicplasty is used. Autologous grafts of cylindrical osteochondral plugs (10- to 15-mm deep grafts containing articular cartilage and cancellous bone) are taken from non–weight-bearing articular surfaces, preferably the intercondylar notch or the anterior femoral condyle. The osteochondral plugs are press-fitted into matching holes drilled into the bony base of the chondral defect. Difficulties with this procedure include limited harvest-

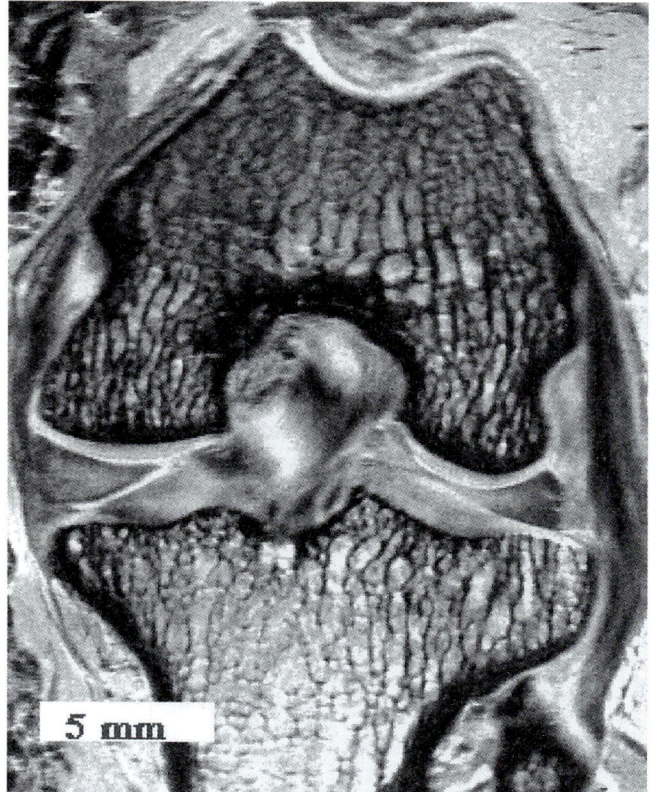

Figure 3 Micro MRI study of a monkey knee joint. The micro MRI technique is currently applicable only for small specimens and produces images of near-histologic quality. (Courtesy of Dr. Farshid Guilak, Duke University Medical Center.)

ing areas, varying cartilage thicknesses, establishing contour and congruence, physical damage from fracture, and possible poor plug fixation. An additional and potentially serious concern is development of OA at the donor sites.

For chondral defects greater than 2 cm² (up to 15 cm²), ACI may be used. A biopsy of healthy osteochondral tissue weighing approximately 200 to 300 mg is obtained from the intercondylar notch or another non–weight-bearing surface area. This tissue is sent to a commercial facility where it is cultured for approximately 3 weeks to produce 10 to 12 million times the number of live autologous chondrocytes. An arthrotomy is performed approximately 3 to 4 weeks after the arthroscopic biopsy to implant autologous chondrocytes. A periosteal cover is sutured to the edges of the defects and the cultured cells are then injected under the flap. Two-year outcome studies in the US have revealed significant improvement in patient function and symptoms compared with baseline conditions. Second-look arthroscopies and biopsy specimens reveal a repair tissue of hyaline-like cartilage in 74% of patients. Longer follow-up and double-blind comparisons with other techniques are necessary to determine the long-term efficacy of ACI in treating focal articular cartilage defects of the knee.

There is currently interest in the enzymatic digestion and exposure of the edges of cartilage defects to promote incorporation of neocartilage produced by whatever method is used for the regeneration of cartilage. This is because even when there is excellent regeneration of cartilage, there is incomplete remodeling at the junction between the neocartilage and the adjacent cartilage. The approach of enzymatic digestion may improve the bonding of such regenerated tissue to the defect edges.

Radiofrequency energy probes recently have been introduced to surgically remove or smooth roughened articular cartilage. Although published reports indicate that the response is favorable, unpublished data demonstrates that chondrocyte necrosis can occur with this technique. The lowest voltage setting possible should be used, because articular cartilage necrosis may not be apparent grossly and may be a clinically silent lesion for a prolonged period of time.

Future Challenges

Tissue engineering approaches have the potential to improve the management of patients with articular defects. Appropriate scaffolds and adhesives as well as methods for the local and temporal delivery of cytokines are needed. Adaptation of these techniques so that they can be performed arthroscopically would be ideal. Biologic challenges include the variable quality and quantity of the cartilage that is produced, decreasing responsiveness with age, bonding to the adjacent cartilage, and restoration of the subchondral bone. Most importantly, it will be necessary to clarify the process of chondrogenesis and its regulation at the cellular and molecular levels so that it can be intelligently controlled and optimized. Evaluation of future therapeutic techniques will require high resolution and volumetric MRI studies for accurate identification of focal articular cartilage defects and generalized cartilage loss. Currently it is possible to achieve results that approach histologic resolution in animal studies, in which the area to be imaged is relatively small (Fig. 3); however, this is not yet possible in humans.

Rheumatoid Arthritis

Definition and Prevalence

Rheumatoid arthritis (RA) is a chronic inflammatory disease characterized by hyperplasia of the synovial lining cells, angiogenesis, and infiltration of mononuclear cells resulting in pannus formation, cartilage erosion, and ultimately joint destruction. It affects 0.5% to 1% of the population worldwide, with women being affected almost three times as often as men. The prevalence increases with advancing age. RA results in a high degree of disability, as well as shortening of life expectancy that is equivalent to that of patients with Hodgkin's disease, diabetes, and stroke. Despite intensive study, the cause of RA remains unknown, and the disease is defined using a set of empirically derived clinical criteria. Major features of active disease include symmetrical polyarthritis with joint swelling and tenderness, and morning stiffness lasting for 1 hour or longer. Additional characteristics of RA include subcutaneous nodules, presence of rheumatoid factor (in about 80% of patients with RA), and radiographically evident erosions or juxta-articular osteoporosis in or adjacent to the involved joints. RA can affect any joint, but it is usually found in metacarpophalangeal, proximal interphalangeal, and metatarsophalangeal joints, as well as in the wrist and knee. Estrogen and pregnancy mitigate disease development of RA. The symptoms of RA are improved by pregnancy in about 75% of pregnant patients, but relapses within 6 months postpartum occur in 90% of cases.

Pathogenesis

RA typically has been viewed as an autoimmune disease; however, although humoral and cellular immune responses to autoantigens (such as production of rheumatoid factor) occur in RA, none of these autoreactive phenomena are specific to RA, present in all patients, or clearly linked to the destruction of cartilage and bone, which frequently is the ultimate consequence of long-term rheumatoid synovitis. The role of T cells in RA also is currently a matter of debate. Although T cells are abundant in the inflamed joint, critically involved in animal models of RA, and implicated in human RA by the association of class II major histocompatibility complex (MHC) alleles with RA, a T cell-centered view of the disease has not yet led to clearer insight into the etiology of RA or to breakthroughs in its treatment. In addition, T cell-derived lymphokines are not the most abundant cytokines in synovial tissue or fluid, and attempts to treat RA using novel T cell-depleting biologic therapeutic agents such as monoclonal antibodies have not been effective. Viral etiologies also have been hypothesized, both in dogs (in which the disease occurs naturally) and in humans. Finally, the results of twin and family studies clearly implicate an important role for genetic factors in the etiology of RA. However, the complex nature of this disease has hampered progress in defining the genetic determinants.

The synovium contains two principal cell populations. Type A synoviocytes belong to the monocyte-macrophage family and have potent phagocytic ability

and the capacity to secrete large quantities of proinflammatory cytokines. Type B synoviocytes are specialized fibroblasts that produce hyaluronic acid and collagen and, in an inflammatory milieu, also can secrete cytokines, proteases, and other inflammatory mediators. Type A and B synoviocytes are present in greatly increased numbers in RA synovium, along with other functionally important cell populations. In addition, neutrophils in synovial fluid and chondrocytes in adjacent articular cartilage are important contributors to inflammatory pathways in the RA joint.

Most investigators would agree that the natural history of RA involves exposure, in genetically susceptible individuals, to an unknown environmental agent that triggers an autoimmune response leading to the production of mediators, particularly cytokines. These agents drive the pathophysiologic processes that lead to the clinical manifestations of RA. Therapeutic intervention in this chain of events is possible at a number of sites. However, most efforts have been concentrated on modulating either T-lymphocyte responses or the activities of various arthritogenic cytokines.

Pharmacologic Treatment

Presently, less than 5% of patients with seropositive RA remain in long-term disease-free remission. In addition, virtually all patients with RA have or develop osteoporosis as a complication of the disease or its treatment. Radiographic damage is seen in more than 70% of patients with RA within the first 2 years of disease, and radiographic progression is seen in almost all patients. In most patients, the consequences of RA seem to be considerably more severe than the side effects of contemporary disease-modifying antirheumatic drugs.

Currently, a preventive strategy is evolving in which early aggressive control of inflammation with disease-modifying antirheumatic drugs is used, seeking to minimize long-term joint damage. Glucocorticoids are the most potent suppressors of inflammation and may be needed to control severe polyarticular disease until disease-modifying antirheumatic drugs have been added and take effect. At that point, the glucocorticoids should be tapered and discontinued. Second-line therapy should be instituted at the time of diagnosis and continued as long as any evidence suggests ongoing active disease. Methotrexate is the drug most commonly used in combination therapy because of its favorable efficacy and toxicity profile. Evidence from randomized, controlled clinical trials and observational studies have indicated increased efficacy and acceptable (and often lower) toxicity for combinations of methotrexate and one or more other disease-modifying antirheumatic drugs. Much interest also has been expressed in the "step-down" approach in which RA is treated aggressively very early in its course and, after clinical control is achieved, some drugs are withdrawn and therapy continued with the least toxic drugs. Treatment should focus on suppressing inflammation and pannus development and limiting erosive disease in the first year or two.

Many of the more recently developed pharmaceutical agents for the treatment of RA are directed against cytokines that are disease mediators. The most important candidate appears to be tumor necrosis factor (TNF). TNF is made primarily by mononuclear cells and binds to cell-surface receptors on lymphocytes, monocytes, polymorphonuclear leukocytes, and endothelial cells. TNF triggers several of the most central and critical events in the acute and chronic synovial inflammation and ultimate tissue destruction characteristic of RA, including induction of multiple additional cytokines and chemokines (such as interleukin [IL]-1, IL-6, and IL-8), expression of adhesion molecules and increased levels of class I MHC determinants, synthesis and release of proteases and prostaglandin E_2 by synovial fibroblasts (which is important in erosion of cartilage and bone), and synovial neoangiogenesis. It is present at biologically significant levels in RA synovial tissue and fluid.

Etanercept and infliximab are two TNF-α antagonists recently approved by the Food and Drug Administration that have powerful anti-inflammatory effects in patients with RA. Etanercept is a recombinant genetically engineered fusion protein composed of the Fc portion of IgG fused to the extracellular domain of the p75 human TNF-α receptor. The fusion protein results in a soluble receptor that binds to TNF, prevents its interaction with cell surface receptors, and renders it biologically inactive. Treatment with etanercept (subcutaneous injections twice a week) is reported to result in substantial improvement in the extent of joint inflammation in human patients, and this improvement is enhanced by combination with methotrexate. Adverse effects of etanercept are influenza-like symptoms and reactions at the injection site, which usually abate after the first few injections. Infliximab is a monoclonal antibody that binds TNF-α and is given intravenously once every 8 weeks. Potential long-term risks of these TNF-α antagonists have not been established. To date, neither drug has an increased risk of malignancy, autoimmune disease, or infection. TNF-α blockers have substantial activity in patients with RA who are recalcitrant to other disease-modifying antirheumatic drugs.

IL-1 receptor antagonist, a naturally-occurring specific inhibitor, blocks the binding of IL-1 to its cell surface receptors but does not possess agonist activity. Trials of IL-1 receptor antagonist show a relatively modest anti-inflammatory effect and a possible retardation of joint damage. Other approaches to inhibiting the proinflammatory activities of TNF and IL-1 are currently under investigation and include treatment with recombinant IL-4, -10, or -11. IL-4 and -10 both inhibit the release and function of IL-1, TNF-α, and other proinflammatory cytokines (IL-6 and -8); inhibit the production of matrix metalloproteinases; and increase the secretion of natural inhibitors of cytokines, such as IL-1 receptor antagonist and soluble TNF receptor. IL-11 is an anti-inflammatory cytokine that can reduce production of TNF-α; IL-1, -12, and -6; and nitric oxide. Clinical trials evaluating recombinant IL-4, -10, and -11 in the treatment of RA are now in progress.

Leflunomide, a pyrimidine synthesis inhibitor with clinical efficacy generally equivalent to methotrexate, also has recently been approved for the treatment of RA patients. Leflunomide appears to be as effective as methotrexate but, unlike that drug, does not necessitate monitoring for bone marrow toxicity. Adverse effects reported include rash, alopecia, allergy, weight loss, thrombocytopenia, and diarrhea.

Annotated Bibliography

Centers for Disease Control and Prevention: Impact of arthritis and other rheumatic conditions on the health-care system: United States, 1997. *JAMA* 1999;281: 2177-2178.
    This article provides figures on the impact of arthritis on the health-care system in the United States.

Fox DA: Cytokine blockade as a new strategy to treat rheumatoid arthritis: Inhibition of tumor necrosis factor. *Arch Intern Med* 2000;160:437-444.
    A detailed summary of TNF and methods of neutralizing this cytokine in patients with RA is presented.

Herndon JH, Robbins PD, Evans CH: Arthritis: Is the cure in your genes? *J Bone Joint Surg Am* 1999;81: 152-157.
    This article reviews the background and techniques of using gene therapy to treat RA. Studies in animal models and a brief description of a human clinical trial are included.

LaPrade RF, Swiontkowski MF: New horizons in the treatment of osteoarthritis of the knee. *JAMA* 1999;281: 876-878.
    This article reviews the techniques of autogenous cartilage implantation, autogenous osteochondral grafting, and hyaluronic acid injection.

Matteson EL: Current treatment strategies for rheumatoid arthritis. *Mayo Clin Proc* 2000;75:69-74.

This is a concise review of current clinical treatments for RA. NSAIDs and disease-modifying antirheumatic drugs are the primary focus of discussion.

McAlindon TE, LaValley MP, Gulin JP, Felson DT: Glucosamine and chondroitin for treatment of osteoarthritis: A systematic quality assessment and metaanalysis. *JAMA* 2000;283:1469-1475.

This article discusses meta-analysis of double-blind, randomized, placebo-controlled trials of 4 or more weeks' duration that tested glucosamine or chondroitin for knee or hip OA and reported extractable data on the effect of treatment on symptoms. The results suggest that some degree of efficacy appears probable for these preparations.

O'Driscoll SW: The healing and regeneration of articular cartilage. *J Bone Joint Surg Am* 1998;80:1795-1812.

This article presents a comprehensive review of current concepts and data, both biologic and clinical, related to the healing and regeneration of articular cartilage.

Pincus T, O'Dell JR, Kremer JM: Combination therapy with multiple disease-modifying antirheumatic drugs in rheumatoid arthritis: A preventive strategy. *Ann Intern Med* 1999;131:768-774.

This article presents a summary of combination therapies for RA and includes results from multiple human clinical trials.

Wright KE, Maurer SG, DiCesare PE: Viscosupplementation for osteoarthritis. *Am J Orthop* 2000;29:80-89.

A detailed assessment of viscosupplementation in the management of OA is presented, along with summaries of studies in animals and humans.

Chapter 20

Connective Tissue Disorders

Nancy Hadley Miller, MD

Introduction

Heritable connective tissue disorders are those that are capable of being inherited, or, in any one individual, that may occur by a new mutation. Typically a single unifying defect involving the extracellular matrix is the underlying cause of these disorders. Significant advances within the field of molecular genetics and in the understanding of heritable connective tissue disorders have led to the identification of the basic genetic defect for multiple disorders.

Ehlers-Danlos Syndrome

Ehlers-Danlos syndrome (EDS) is a heterogeneous group of heritable connective tissue disorders characterized by skin extensibility, articular hypermobility, and tissue fragility. The clinical variability and genetic heterogeneity of these disorders has long been recognized. The traditional classification system developed in 1988 delineated 11 types of EDS on the basis of clinical manifestations and mode of inheritance. Although valid, this approach relies significantly on the subjective interpretation of clinical signs. However, the recent identification of the molecular and biochemical basis of EDS now allow for a modification of the current classification to include this information in the diagnostic criteria of the EDS type.

The classification defines six major types of EDS, each with a clearly defined or potentially defined molecular basis (Table 1). The clinical traits used for diagnostic criteria are skin hyperextensibility, joint hypermobility (as assessed using the Brighton scale), easy bruising, tissue fragility, mitral valve prolapse and proximal aortic dilatation, chronic joint and limb pain, kyphoscoliosis, arthrochalasis, and dermatosparaxis. Major criteria are characterized by high diagnostic specificity and their presence is either essential for clinical diagnosis or highly indicative and laboratory confirmation is warranted whenever possible. Minor criteria have low diagnostic specificity, and the presence of one or more minor criteria contributes to the diagnosis of a specific type of EDS. In the absence of major criteria, the diagnosis cannot be established. The presence of minor criteria is suggestive of an EDS-like condition, the nature or molecular etiology of which is unknown.

Under the new classification system, the former EDS types I and II are grouped together as the classical type of EDS, and have a common genetic etiology of mutations in the *COL5A1* or *COL5A2* genes. The earlier differentiation of EDS types I and II was based on the severity of skin manifestations, which can now be attributed to genotype/phenotype interaction.

The hypermobility type of EDS (formerly type III EDS) is characterized by multiple joint dislocations and is distinct from other EDS types. Developmental milestones may be delayed due to joint instability and hypermobility. Scoliosis occurs in 50% of patients with hypermobility EDS, and these patients should be treated in the same manner as those with idiopathic scoliosis. The potential need for more aggressive surgical treatment due to increased progression secondary to joint flexibility may be considered.

The vascular (formerly type IV) form of EDS is caused by mutations within the *COL3A1* gene. Complications related to this disorder are rare in childhood. Twenty-five percent of individuals will have had a complication by age 20 years, and more than 80% by age 40 years. Median age of survival is approximately 48 years. The primary cause of death is arterial rupture; however, significant morbidity is associated with visceral rupture and uterine rupture during pregnancy.

The kyphoscoliosis form of EDS corresponds to the former type VI or ocular-scoliotic type. The common etiology of this group is a deficiency of lysyl hydroxylase, a collagen-modifying enzyme. There is marked scoliosis and significant muscular hypotonia. The condition should be considered in the initial diagnostic

TABLE 1 | Ehlers-Danlos Syndrome

| | | | Clinical Findings |
New	Former	Transmission*	Major
Classical	Type I (Gravis)	AD	Skin hyperextensibility Widened atrophic scars (manifestation of tissue fragility)
	Type II (Mitis)	AD	Joint hypermobility
Hypermobility	Type III (hypermobile)	AD	Skin involvement (hyperextensibility and/or smooth and velvety skin) Generalized joint hypermobility
Vascular	Type IV (vascular)	AR (rare) or AD	Thin, translucent skin Arterial/intestinal/uterine fragility or rupture Extensive bruising
Kyphoscoliosis	Type VI (ocular-scoliotic)	AR	Generalized joint laxity Severe muscle hypotonia at birth Scoliosis at birth, progressive Scleral fragility and rupture of the ocular globe
Arthrochalasia	Type VIIA and VIIB	AD	Severe generalized joint hypermobility Congenital bilateral hip dislocation
Dermatosparaxis	Type VIIC	AR	Severe skin fragility Sagging, redundant skin
Other forms	Type V	X-linked	Similar to classical
	Type VIII (periodonitis type)	AD	Similar to classical with periodontal friability
	Type X (fibronectin-deficient)	AD	Mild, similar to classical Poor clotting

*AD = autosomal dominant; AR = autosomal recessive
(Adapted from Beaty JH (ed): Orthopaedic Knowledge Update 6. Rosemont, IL, American Academy of Orthopaedic Surgeons, 1999, pp 217-223.)

TABLE 1 | Ehlers-Danlos Syndrome, continued

Clinical Findings	
Minor	**Minor**
Smooth, velvety skin Spheroids	*COL5A1* mutations
Complications of joint hypermobility Muscle hypotonia, delayed gross motor development Easy bruising Tissue extensibility and fragility (for example, hiatal hernia, anal prolapse in childhood, cervical insufficiency) Positive family history	
Recurring joint dislocations Chronic joint dislocations Positive family history	Unknown
Hypermobility of small joints Tendon muscle rupture Talipes equinovarus (clubfoot) Early-onset varicose veins Arteriovenous, carotid-cavernous sinus fistula Pneumothorax/pneumohemothorax Positive family history, sudden death in close relatives	*COL3A1* mutations
Tissue fragility, including atrophic scars Easy bruising Arterial rupture Marfanoid habitus Microcornea Radiologic osteopenia Family history	Deficiency of lysylhydroxylase, a collagen modifying enzyme
Skin hyperextensibility Tissue fragility, including atrophic scars Easy bruising Muscle hypotonia Kyphoscoliosis Radiologically mild osteopenia	Deficient processing of amino-terminal end of prox 1(I) or prox 2(I) chains of collagen type I
Soft, doughy skin texture Easy bruising Premature rupture of fetal membranes Large hernias	Deficiency of procollagen 1 N-terminal peptidase
	Unknown; described in single family
	Unknown; existence as autonomous entity uncertain
	Unknown; described in single family

work-up of a floppy infant, and may also be confused with the severe neonatal form of Marfan syndrome.

The former types VIIA and VIIB EDS comprise the arthrochalasia group of EDS. Patients with this condition have mutations that lead to a deficiency in processing the amino-terminal end of proalpha-1 or proalpha-2 collagen type I chains due to mutations involving the substrate sites within the procollagen type I chain. The condition can be detected biochemically through the extraction of these molecules and mutational analysis. Congenital bilateral hip dislocation has always been present in biochemically proven individuals.

The dermatosparaxis type of EDS, formerly known as type VIIC EDS, is primarily characterized by skin fragility and bruising. The underlying cause is a deficiency of procollagen 1 N-terminal peptidase, and can be detected biochemically.

The remainder of the EDS types (V, VIII, IX, X, and XI) have not been included in the revised classification to date for a variety of reasons. Types V and X have each been described in a single family and potentially do not represent a subset of EDS. EDS type VIII is similar to the classical type except that the condition also presents with periodontal friability. The existence of this syndrome as a separate entity is uncertain. EDS type IX has been redefined as an X-linked recessive condition allelic to Menkes' syndrome. Former EDS type XI, also known as familial joint hypermobility syndrome, was removed from the EDS classification due to its lack of specific diagnostic criteria, and may be redefined as its relationship to EDS becomes more clear.

Functional orthopaedic manifestations of the most common types of EDS (classical, hypermobility, and vascular types) have recently been assessed. There are no significant differences in history of joint dislocation, swelling, or types of orthopaedic surgical procedures experienced among these types. Joint pain is more frequently reported in patients with hypermobile EDS. Ambulation and upper extremity function and strength are impaired significantly in these patients. Back or neck pain is commonly reported (67%) among all patients, but did not correlate with the presence or absence of spinal deformity. Regarding musculoskeletal function, hypermobile EDS is considered the most debilitating form of the disease.

Osteogenesis Imperfecta

Osteogenesis imperfecta (OI), or 'brittle-bone disease,' is a group of heritable disorders characterized by either a reduction in the production of normal type I collagen, or the synthesis of abnormal collagen as a result of mutations in the type I collagen genes, with varying clinical severity. Major clinical characteristics are osteopenia, variable degree of short stature, and progressive skeletal deformities. Blue sclera, joint laxity, late-onset deafness, and dentinogenesis imperfecta may also be observed.

The Sillence classification of OI has long been useful in categorizing the clinical varieties based on clinical, genetic, and radiologic criteria (Table 2). Although this clinical outline provides a framework for classification, not all patients fit the specified criteria for a particular type. In addition, affected members of a particular family with the same genetic defect may present with varying phenotypes, or unrelated individuals with the same phenotype may have differing genetic defects. Long-term prognosis, however, strongly correlates with the Sillence type.

Impairment parameters in OI have been shown not always to predict functional limitation and disability. Many patients with OI compensate for their condition with the use of braces, ambulatory devices, and other aids, and lead functional and productive lives. Nonsurgical treatment strategies have primarily focused on the improvement of functional ability and the adoption of compensatory mechanisms to improve function, as opposed to improving range of motion and muscular strength. The developmental framework for children with OI, especially in the most severe types, differs from that of healthy children.

An alternative therapeutic strategy is directed toward improving the osteopenia and bone fragility, which are a result of the structural abnormalities in bone tissue and reduced rate of osteogenesis. A variety of agents including anabolic steroids, sodium fluoride, magnesium oxide, and calcitonin have been used in an attempt to reduce the risk of fracture, but none have resulted in sustained improvement. Bisphosphonate compounds, potent inhibitors of bone resorption, are now being used in children with severe OI. Following the cyclic administration of intravenous pamidronate (7.0 mg/kg body weight/yr given at 4- to 6-month intervals for 1.3 to 5.0 years), an increase in bone density, a reduction in bone resorption, and a decrease in the incidence of radiologic confirmed fractures have been reported.

Marfan Syndrome

Marfan syndrome is an autosomal dominant condition for which diagnosis is made primarily through clinical criteria. The molecular etiology of this disorder is a mutation within the *FBN1* (fibrillin 15) gene localized at 15q21. Molecular diagnosis has a limited role within this disorder because of the inability to detect sporadic mutations in a very large gene, and because mutations in the same gene cause other conditions, especially

TABLE 2 | Osteogenesis Imperfecta

Type	Transmission*	Main Biochemical Defect	Orthopaedic	Miscellaneous
IA	AD	Decreased production of type I collagen	Mild to moderate bone fragility, osteoporosis, normal stature	Blue sclerae, hearing loss, easy bruising, dentinogenesis imperfecta absent
B	AD		Short stature	More severe than IA with dentinogenesis imperfecta
II	AD, AR, and mosaic	Substitutions of glycyl residue in X1 or X2 chains in triple helix	Multiple intrauterine fractures, extreme bone fragility	Usually lethal in perinatal period, delayed ossification of skull, intrauterine growth retardation
A			Long bones broad, crumpled; ribs broad with continuous beading	
B			Long bones broad, crumpled; ribs discontinuous or no beading	
C			Long bones thin, fractured; ribs thin, beaded	
D			Severely osteopenic with generally well-formed skeleton; normal-shaped vertebrae and pelvis	
III	AD and AR (rare)	Abnormal type I collagen	Progressive deforming phenotype, severe bone fragility with fractures. At birth, scoliosis, severe osteoporosis, extreme short stature	Hearing loss, short stature, blue sclerae becoming less blue with age, shortened life expectancy, dentinogenesis imperfecta, relative macrocephaly with triangular facies
IVA	AD	Shortened proalpha (I) chains	Mild to moderate bone fragility, osteoporosis, bowing of long bones, scoliosis	Light sclerae, normal hearing, normal dentition, dentinogenesis imperfecta absent
B	AD			Dentinogenesis imperfecta present

*AD = autosomal dominant; AR = autosomal recessive
(Adapted from Beaty JH (ed): Orthopaedic Knowledge Update 6. Rosemont, IL, American Academy of Orthopaedic Surgeons, 1999, pp 217-223.)

those in the same phenotypic continuum as the Marfan syndrome.

Marfan syndrome is pleiotropic, exhibiting diverse manifestations within multiple organ systems, many of which appear in middle and late adulthood. Diagnostic criteria have primarily focused on the three organ systems prominently involved—musculoskeletal, ocular, and cardiovascular (Table 3). However, skin, lungs, adipose tissue, and the central nervous system are often included. Currently, the diagnosis in an index case, in which family history is not contributory, relies on major criteria in at least two organ systems and the involvement of a third organ system. For an individual who has a family member with Marfan syndrome, the presence of a major criterion in the family history, and one major criterion in an organ system, and involvement of a second organ system are essential for diagnosis.

Cardiovascular abnormalities of Marfan syndrome are the primary factors contributing to increased morbidity and mortality. Beta-adrenergic blockades are currently used therapeutically in an effort to protect the aorta from both dilatation and dissection. Although this philosophy originated 30 years ago, it has yet to be conclusively proven. Multiple studies have confirmed the reduction in inotropy and chronotropy in individuals with Marfan syndrome. While some studies suggest the slowing and actual prevention of aortic dilatation, others suggest that a select number of patients, for unknown reasons, are responsive to beta-adrenergic blockage, while others are not. Current studies are

TABLE 3 | Marfan Syndrome

System	Major Criteria	Minor Criteria
Musculoskeletal*	Pectus carinatum; pectus excavatum requiring surgery; dolichostenomelia; wrist and thumb signs; scoliosis > 20° or spondylolisthesis; reduced elbow extension; pes planus; protrusio acetabuli	Moderately severe pes excavatum; joint hypermobility; highly arched palate with crowding of teeth; facies (dolichocephaly, malar hypoplasia, enophthalmos, retognathia, down-slanting palebral fissures)
Ocular†	Ectopia lentis	Abnormally flat cornea; increased axial length of globe; hypoplastic iris or hypoplastic ciliary muscle causing decreased miosis
Cardiovascular‡	Dilatation of ascending aorta ± aortic regurgitation, involving sinuses of Valsalva; or dissection of ascending aorta	Mitral valve prolapse ± regurgitation; dilatation of main pulmonary artery without valvular or peripheral pulmonic stenosis or obvious cause below 40 years; calcification of mitral anulus below 40 years; or dilation or dissection of descending aorta below 50 years
Family/genetic history§	Parent, child, or sibling meets diagnostic criteria; mutation in *FBN1* known to cause Marfan syndrome; or inherited haplotype around *FBN1* associated with Marfan syndrome in family	None
Skin and integument‖	None	Stretch marks not associated with pregnancy, weight gain, or repetitive stress; or recurrent or incisional hernias
Dura§	Lumbosacral dural ectasia	None
Pulmonary‖	None	Spontaneous pneumothorax or apical blebs

*Two or more major or one major + two minor criteria required for involvement
†At least two minor criteria required for involvement
‡One major or minor criterion required for involvement
§One major criterion required for involvement
‖One minor criterion required for involvement
(Reproduced from Beaty JH (ed): Orthopaedic Knowledge Update 6. Rosemont, IL, American Academy of Orthopaedic Surgeons, 1999, pp 217-223.)

attempting to confirm a beneficial effect of beta-adrenergic blockade and to study the usefulness of alternative agents such as verapamil.

The MASS Phenotype

The MASS phenotype is a condition characterized by mitral valve involvement, mild aortic dilatation, striae atrophicae, and skeletal involvement. The MASS phenotype came to clinical attention in the study of patients suspected of having Marfan syndrome, but who had little or no aortic enlargement or dissection, no ectopia lentis, and no family history of Marfan syndrome. Inheritance of this phenotype appears to be autosomal dominant in nature; however, both conditions can occur in the same family. Some individuals with MASS phenotype have a mutation in *FBN1*, usually of a type that eliminates most or all of the expression of a defective protein from the mutant allele. Thus, the resultant microfibrils within the extracellular matrix are fewer in number, but more functional. It is important to distinguish MASS phenotype from Marfan syndrome so that patients with MASS phenotype are not labeled with a more serious disease and treated inappropriately. Patients with MASS phenotype have mitral valve prolapse that necessitates regular echocardiographic and clinical follow-up, and endocarditis prophylaxis. Mitral valve regurgitation can develop with age, especially in men.

Homocystinuria

Homocystinuria is an autosomal recessive disorder of sulfur amino acid metabolism that is caused by a mutation within the gene encoding for the enzyme cystathionine beta synthase. This enzyme controls the rate-limiting step of the transsulfuration pathway and requires pyridoxal phosphate. A deficiency of cystathionine beta synthase activity results in elevated levels of homocysteine as well as methionine in plasma and urine and decreased levels of cystathionine and cysteine. The major clinical symptoms include ectopia lentis, vascular disease with life-threatening thromboembolisms, skeletal deformities, osteoporosis, and mental retardation. Because of its phenotypic similarities to the MFS, the recognition of homocystinuria is essential so that the condition can be treated effectively. The wide spectrum of mutations are primarily missense mutations and are unique from one family to another. However, despite the consistency of a mutation within a sibship, the clinical phenotype often varies within the sibship. Despite heterogenous mutations, many specific mutations will respond to vitamin B6 (pyridoxine) therapy. The daily administration of pyridoxine appears to enhance the activity of the deficient enzyme, resulting in a normalization of plasma and urine levels of sulfur amino acids.

Annotated Bibliography

Beighton P, De Paepe A, Steinmann B, Tsipouras P, Wenstrup RJ: Ehlers-Danlos syndromes: Revised Nosology: Ehlers-Danlos National Foundation (USA) and Ehlers-Danlos Support Group (UK), Villefranche, 1997. *Am J Med Genet* 1998;77:31-37.

This article discusses proposed revision of the classification of Ehlers-Danlos syndrome based primarily on the molecular basis of each type with the definition of major and minor diagnostic criteria.

Glorieux FH, Bishop NJ, Plotkin H, Chabot G, Lanoue G, Travers R: Cyclic administration of pamidronate in children with severe osteogenesis imperfecta. *N Engl J Med* 1998;339:947-952.

A study designed to assess the effect of bisphosphonate on bone resorption in patients with OI is presented. Cyclic administration of the drug improved clinical outcome, reduced bone resorption, and increased bone density.

Kraus JP, Janosik M, KozichV, et al: Cystathionine beta-synthase mutations in homocystinuria. *Hum Mutat* 1999;13:362-375.

This article presents an excellent review of the different mutations resulting in homocystinuria with the most frequently encountered mutations reported.

Pepin M, Schwarze U, Superti-Furga A, Byers PH: Clinical and genetic features of Ehlers-Danlos syndrome type IV: The vascular type. *N Engl J Med* 2000;342:673-680.

This article presents the largest review of EDS IV patients and the natural history of the disorder.

Pyeritz RE: The Marfan syndrome. *Annu Rev Med* 2000;51:481-510.

The most recent and thorough review of the Marfan syndrome and its phenotypic continuum is presented.

Stanitski DF, Nadjarian R, Stanitski CL, Bawle E, Tsipouras P: Orthopaedic manifestations of Ehlers-Danlos syndrome. *Clin Orthop* 2000;376:213-221.

A comprehensive review of a large population of EDS patients and their orthopaedic problems is presented. The most debilitating findings within each condition are reviewed.

Classic Bibliography

Ainsworth SR, Aulicino PL: A survey of patients with Ehlers-Danlos syndrome. *Clin Orthop* 1993;286:250-256.

Beighton P, Solomon L, Soskolne CL: Articular mobility in an African population. *Ann Rheum Dis* 1973;32:413-418.

Boers GH, Polder TW, Cruysberg JR, et al: Homocystinuria versus Marfan's syndrome: The therapeutic relevance of the differential diagnosis. *Neth J Med* 1984;27:206-212.

Cole WG: The molecular pathology of osteogenesis imperfecta. *Clin Orthop* 1997;343:235-248.

De Paepe A, Devereux RB, Dietz HC, Hennekam RC, Pyeritz RE: Revised diagnostic criteria for the Marfan syndrome. *Am J Med Genet* 1996;62:417-426.

Dietz FR, Mathews KD: Update on the genetic bases of disorders with orthopaedic manifestations. *J Bone Joint Surg Am* 1996;78:1583-1598.

Hanscom DA, Winter RB, Lutter L, Lonstein JE, Bloom BA, Bradford DS: Osteogenesis imperfecta: Radiographic classification, natural history, and treatment of spinal deformities. *J Bone Joint Surg Am* 1992;74:598-616.

Joseph KN, Kane HA, Milner RS, Steg NL, Williamson MB Jr, Bowen JR: Orthopaedic aspects of the Marfan phenotype. *Clin Orthop* 1992;277:251-261.

Raff ML, Byers PH: Joint hypermobility syndromes. *Curr Opin Rheumatol* 1996;8:459-466.

Silence DO, Senn A, Danks DM: Genetic heterogeneity in osteogenesis imperfecta. *J Med Genet* 1979;16:101-116.

Chapter 21

Genetic Disorders and Skeletal Dysplasias

Benjamin A. Alman, MD, PhD

Disorders Caused by Chromosome Abnormalities

Down Syndrome: Trisomy 21

Down syndrome, the most common chromosomal disorder, occurs in about 1 in every 5,000 births to women age 30 years or younger, and once in every 250 births to women age 35 years or older. Complete trisomies account for 95% of cases, and mosaicism (when only some cells contain the trisomy) or translocations comprise the remainder of cases. There is a five-megabase region on the long arm of chromosome 21 that when duplicated causes the classic Down phenotype. A combination of ultrasound features (short bone length), and maternal laboratory tests (human chorionic gonadotropin and alpha-fetoprotein levels) can aid in the prenatal diagnosis.

The clinical findings in Down syndrome are short stature and a characteristic facies, with upward slanting eyes, epicanthal folds, and a flattened profile. The hands show a single transverse flexion, often called a simian crease. Although mental retardation is present, there is a wide variation in IQ. Congenital heart disease, duodenal atresia, and hearing loss can occur. About 1% of affected individuals develop leukemia. There is a high incidence of endocrinopathy, in particular hypothyroidism. Infections are common, although the reason for this is unclear. Individuals exhibit premature aging and an early development of mental deterioration similar to that in Alzheimer's disease. With appropriate management for the cardiac, endocrine, and gastrointestinal abnormalities, most affected individuals live to adulthood.

Orthopaedic Manifestations

One out of every five individuals with Down syndrome has a musculoskeletal condition, related primarily to joint instability. Although this instability is attributed to ligamentous laxity, other factors, such as changes in the shape of the joints and changes in the site of ligament insertions, may also contribute. The outcome of surgical intervention for joint instability is not as good as for individuals without Down syndrome, a finding that probably is related to multiple factors including abnormal cell behavior caused by trisomy 21, abnormal joint shapes, and laxity of the soft tissues. Ten percent of affected individuals develop an increased atlantoaxial distance on cervical spine films. In most cases the increased interval is not associated with symptoms. Although the natural history of the cervical spine in individuals with an increased atlantoaxial distance is not completely known, studies of asymptomatic patients have not identified any acute episodes of spinal cord compromise. Furthermore, the reported complication rate for atlantoaxial arthrodesis in Down syndrome is high, although recent reports on fusion of the occiput to C2 or C3 show much better results. For these reasons, the surgical management for the atlantoaxial articulation focuses on symptoms rather than on radiographic findings. Symptoms, however, can be difficult to identify because patients may have subtle findings, such as a change in gait pattern. Measurement of the atlantoaxial interval has a poor reproducibility in patients with Down syndrome, questioning the true incidence of this radiographic finding. In addition, there are a broad range of other cervical malformations, including laminar defects, odontoid hypoplasia, and spondylolisthesis that can occur, often complicating interpretation of the cervical spine films. Surgery is reserved for patients with identified myelopathy. Because treatment is based on symptoms rather than on radiographic findings, the practice of obtaining routine cervical spine radiograph has been questioned by such organizations as the American Academy of Pediatrics' Committee on Sports Medicine and Fitness. Scoliosis and spondylolisthesis can occur in Down syndrome, probably at a higher incidence than in the unaffected population. Management, however, is the same as for individuals without Down syndrome.

Progressive hip dysplasia can occur during the first decade of life. Often these children have unstable joints. Although it is suggested that hip instability leads to functional problems later in life, it is unclear if surgical intervention improves outcome. Hip surgery in these patients has a high failure rate, especially in those with habitual dislocation. If undertaken, surgery must correct all deformity of the soft tissue and bone. Successful total joint replacement in adult patients has been reported. Brace treatment for children younger than age 6 years has been advocated, although only small numbers of children have been studied. Slipped capital femoral epiphysis occurs, may be bilateral, and is associated with a high incidence of osteonecrosis. Patellar dislocations are often asymptomatic. Surgical treatment has a high failure rate, and if undertaken in the symptomatic individual, correction of all the bone and soft-tissue deformity should be done. Planovalgus deformity with a hallux valgus deformity can develop, with the weight of the patient as a possible factor in the development of foot problems. Modification of shoe wear will be effective in most cases. Symptoms that mimic rheumatoid arthritis can develop.

Turner's Syndrome

This syndrome is caused by a single X chromosome and occurs only in girls, with an incidence of 1 in 2,500 births. In two thirds of cases all of the cells are XO, while in most of the rest the chromosome abnormality is mosaic (some cells are XO, while others are XX). Affected girls have a webbed neck, low hairline, short stature, and sexual infantilism. Because of a lack of sex steroid hormones, puberty does not occur and secondary sex characteristics do not develop. Most children are now treated with exogenous estrogen. More recently, growth hormone has also been administered, resulting in an increase in height of about 8 cm. However, because of the modest increase in height, the use of growth hormone supplementation remains controversial. Scoliosis is common, and is managed similar to idiopathic scoliosis, although patients must be monitored frequently if using growth hormones. Varus of the elbow is common, but it rarely causes disability. Most individuals have low bone density, believed to be related to the lack of sex steroid hormone. Intelligence and life expectancy are normal. There is a higher than expected incidence of juvenile rheumatoid arthritis. Girls with only one X chromosome are susceptible to X-linked recessive disorders, such as Duchenne muscular dystrophy.

TABLE 1 | Diagnostic Criteria for NF1

Six or more café-au-lait spots whose greatest diameter is 5 mm in prepubertal and 15 mm in postpubertal patients

Two or more neurofibromas of any type, or one plexiform neurofibroma

Axillary freckling

Optic glioma

Two or more Lish nodules (iris hamartomas)

A distinctive osseous lesion

A first-degree relative with NF1

Disorders Caused by Abnormalities in Tumor-Related Genes

Neurofibromatosis

Neurofibromatosis type 1 (NF1) is the most common disorder known to be caused by a mutation in a single gene, occurring in about 1 in 3,000 newborns. Although there are several forms of neurofibromatosis, musculoskeletal problems occur primarily in NF1. There are a variety of clinical findings that can occur in NF1, such as café-au-lait spots, neurofibromas, axillary freckles, Lisch nodules (retinal hamartomas), and bone deformity, most of which are absent in the newborn, but develop over time. NF1 is an autosomal dominant disorder, the diagnosis of which can be made based on clinical findings (Table 1). The condition is caused by a mutation in the gene that encodes for the protein neurofibrillin. This protein plays a role regulating a cell signaling pathway called Ras, and mutations in NF1 result in an increase in Ras signaling, leading to abnormal cell growth. Because it is an autosomal dominant disorder, only one of the two copies of the gene is mutated. However, in tumors in patients with NF1, the normal copy becomes lost or mutated, further dysregulating Ras signaling, leading to uncontrolled cell growth and neoplasia. Affected individuals can have a normal life span, but have a higher incidence of malignancy and hypertension because of renal artery stenosis.

Scoliosis is common, and occurs in two patterns. Most curves resemble an idiopathic pattern, and can be managed in a manner identical to curves in idiopathic scoliosis (see chapter 48). However, some curves have a dystrophic pattern, involving a short segment (four to six levels), with distortion of the vertebrae and ribs. In children younger than age 7 years, curves have an up to 80% chance of becoming dystrophic. The presence of rib penciling is a telltale sign that curves will become dystrophic. Dystrophic curves are refractory to brace treatment, relentlessly progressive, and, especially in cases associated with kyphosis, can lead to paralysis. They are best managed with early anterior and posterior surgical stabilization. Dystrophic curves in advanced stages are difficult to stabilize, sometimes requiring preoperative traction, anterior strut grafts, or vascularized grafts. Dural ectasia (an outpouching of the dura) and intraspinal neurofibromas can occur in these patients, and preoperative MRI of the spinal cord is necessary to plan surgery.

Pseudarthrosis of long bones is typical, with the tibia being the most common location. Ulnar, clavicular, radial, and femoral locations are also reported. An anterolateral bow in the tibia is a precursor to a pseudarthrosis. This prepseudarthrosis deformity should be managed with a total contact orthosis to prevent fracture. Intramedullary fixation works well as the initial treatment for the established pseudarthrosis. Salvage procedures include vascularized bone grafting and distraction osteogenesis techniques. Despite the success of surgical techniques to preserve the limb in tibial pseudarthrosis, gait analysis shows that the gait pattern with limb salvage is not always as good as with a below-knee amputation, especially in children treated at a young age for the pseudarthrosis.

A variety of neoplastic processes, most of which are benign and do not require surgical intervention, can occur in neurofibromatosis. Plexiform neurofibromas are difficult to manage because of their vascularity and infiltrative nature. It is difficult to distinguish neurofibromas from neurofibrosarcomas, and early reports suggesting a different enhancement pattern on CT scan have not been substantiated. Lesions that rapidly change in size or become symptomatic should be managed as a potential sarcoma. Children with neurofibromatosis have a propensity to develop other malignancies such as Wilms' tumor and rhabdomyosarcoma.

Multiple Hereditary Exostosis

Multiple hereditary exostosis is characterized by multiple osteochondromas. The condition is inherited in an autosomal dominant manner and is caused by a mutation in one of the three *EXT* genes. These genes code for a protein that regulates the way Indian hedgehog diffuses through the extracellular matrix. Indian hedgehog regulates the development of chondrocytes in the growth plate. When the *EXT* genes are mutated there is a maldistribution of Indian hedgehog, with too much present in some locations, and not enough in other locations. This discrepancy results in growth plate chondrocytes growing in the wrong direction, resulting in an osteochondroma. It can also cause angulation of the growing bone. Five potential clinical problems related to this disorder are the osteochodroma itself,

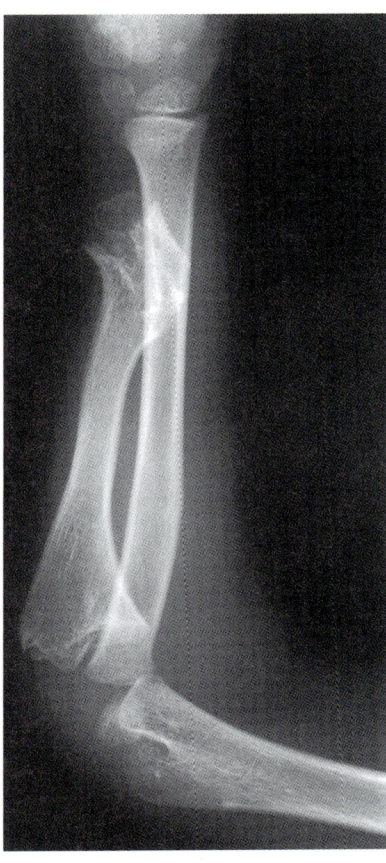

Figure 1 Severe forearm deformity in a child with multiple exostoses. Despite the radiographic deformity, this child was asymptomatic.

limb-length inequality, angular deformity of the bone, subluxation or dislocation of a joint secondary to an osteochondroma, and malignant degeneration. Only symptomatic osteochondromas require excision. Care must be taken to avoid damage to the adjacent growth plate and to remove the entire cartilaginous portion if surgery is undertaken. Limb inequality can be managed with epiphysiodesis, stapling, shortening, or distraction osteogenesis. Angular deformity can be managed with osteotomy, hemiepiphysiodesis, or stapling when symptomatic. Many deformities of the upper extremity do not cause symptoms (Fig. 1). Dislocation of the radial head can be treated with excision at skeletal maturity. Malignant degeneration is a relatively rare occurrence, and should be suspected in lesions that grow or become symptomatic after skeletal maturity.

Enchondromatosis

A genetic cause for enchondromatosis, also called Ollier's disease, has not been identified. However, it is often discussed with osteochondromatosis because both conditions are associated with cartilaginous lesions in bone. Enchondromatosis is characterized by multiple enchondromas in the metaphyseal portions of the bones, with streak-like lucencies on radiographs (Fig.

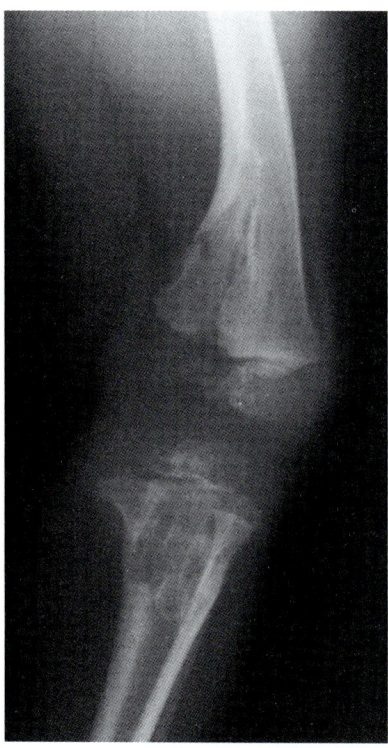

Figure 2 Characteristic streaking lucencies of multiple enchondromatosis. The lesions start at the growth plate and progress toward the diaphysis of the bone.

2). The lesions can result in a short or deformed limb. The limb deformity is managed similar to the deformities in multiple osteochondromatosis. Malignant degeneration is more common than in osteochodromatosis, and should be considered in any lesions that grow or become symptomatic after skeletal maturity. Maffucci's syndrome is multiple enchondromatosis associated with soft-tissue hemangiomas, and is associated with a very high rate of malignancy (exceeding 50%).

Disorders Caused by Abnormalities in Genes Important in Normal Skeletal Development
Cleidocranial Dyplasia

Cleidocranial dyplasia, also called cleidocranial dysotosis, is caused by a mutation in the *CBFA1* gene, which regulates the expression of genes in cells destined to become osteoblasts. Mutations in *CBFA1* cause abnormalities in structures formed directly from osteoblast cells. Patients have abnormalities in the development of anterior midline bone structures. The most characteristic clinical finding is a lack of development of clavicles, so that patients can adduct their shoulder girdles far enough to allow the shoulders to touch in front of their body. Midline skull defects and persistent fontanels are present, as well as midline anterior pelvic defects (lack of development of the pubic bones). A recent radiographic study suggests that the typical

appearance of the femoral head is similar to a chef's hat, suggesting a generalized abnormality in the development of the proximal femoral chondroepiphysis. Coxa vara can develop, and should be treated with an osteotomy.

Nail-Patella Syndrome

There are four musculoskeletal findings in nail-patella syndrome: nail dysplasia, patellar hypoplasia, elbow dysplasia, and iliac horns. This syndrome is caused by a mutation in the *LMX1B* gene, which plays a role in regulating expression of genes during normal skeletal and renal development. A restricted range of motion and contractures of the joints are additional findings. Knee deformity is variable and surgical intervention may be required to allow for more normal patellar tracking. Bone and soft-tissue abnormalities both need to be corrected to maintain proper patellar alignment. Quadricepsplasty may be required for a contracted quadriceps, but more commonly, knee flexion deformity requires hamstring release and posterior capsulotomy. Residual deformity is managed by osteotomy. Dislocated radial heads do not require treatment unless symptomatic, in which case excision is indicated. The nephropathy associated with nail-patella syndrome causes significant morbidity and mortality. Patients should be referred to a nephrologist early in the course of the disease for appropriate management.

Disorders Caused by Abnormalities in Genes That Play a Role in the Processing of Proteins
Diastrophic Dysplasia

In diastrophic dysplasia, multiple cartilaginous structures are involved, including the trachea, ear, and ligaments. The condition is caused by a defect in the *DTD* gene, which encodes for a sulfate transporter, the impaired function of which leads to undersulfation of proteoglycans in cartilage matrix and abnormalities in the hydraulic properties of cartilage. Affected individuals are of short stature, a condition that becomes progressively more apparent with growth. The pinnae of the ears have a characteristic swelling referred to as a cauliflower ear. Neonates can develop tracheomalacia, a condition that can be fatal. An abducted hitchhiker thumb and symphalangia may be present.

Kyphosis in the cervical spine occurs early in life, but often resolves. Persistent cases can become more symptomatic as degenerative changes develop later in life, and should be managed with arthrodesis. Scoliosis is often associated with kyphosis. The progression can be rapid, especially in younger children; early anterior

TABLE 2 | Types of Mucopolysaccharidoses

Type	Name	Inheritance Pattern*	Stored Substance and Enzyme Defect†
I	Hurler/Scheie	AR	HS + DS; alpha-L-idurinidase
II	Hunter	XLR	HS + DS; iduronidase-2-sulfatase
III	Sanfilippo	AR	HS; four subtypes with different enzymes
IV	Morquio	AR	KS, CS; three subtypes with type A caused by *N*-acetylgalactosamine-6-sulfatase, type B caused by β-D-galactosidase, and type C of unknown cause
V This designation no longer used (previously called Scheie)			
VI	Moroteux-Lamy	AR	DS + CS, Arylsulfatase B, *N*-acetylgalactosamine-4-sulfatase
VII	Sly	AR	CS + HS + DS, *N*-β-D-glucuronidase
VIII		AR	CS + HS, glucuronate-2-sulphatase

*AR = autosomal recessive; XLR = X-linked recessive
†CS = chondroitin sulfate; DS = dermatan sulfate; HS = heparan sulfate; KS = keratan sulfate

and posterior fusion can provide good outcomes. The condition of the hips is initially normal, but a flexion contracture may develop with time. Limitation of motion is associated with the onset of arthritic changes later in life. The knees have flexion deformities, valgus alignment, and patellar subluxation. In some patients the knees are completely unstable. The feet have a rigid equinovarus deformity, which requires extensive soft-tissue surgery, and possibly a talectomy. Recurrences of the foot deformity are common and these are treated with salvage procedures.

Mucopolysaccharidoses

This group of disorders is caused by abnormal function of a specific lysosomal enzyme that degrades a sulfonated glycosaminoglycan. The incomplete degradation product accumulates in the lysosomes themselves. There are a variety of subtypes, most inherited in an autosomal recessive manner (Table 2). Features common to these disorders include corneal clouding, visceromegaly, epiphyseal deformation, contractures, cardiac disease, and deafness. The diagnosis can be made using urine analysis for the specific glycosaminoglycan. Hurler's syndrome is the most common disorder, and is quite severe, with patients living only up to the second decade. Hunter's syndrome is less severe, with patients having a normal life span. Affected individuals have upper cervical instability, kyphosis of any region of the spine, hip deformity, and malalignment of the lower limbs. Bone marrow transplant has been used in severe cases to arrest progression.

Disorders in Which Causative Genetic Abnormality is Not Yet Known

Larsen's Syndrome

Autosomal dominant and autosomal recessive forms of this syndrome are reported, although most cases are sporadic in occurrence. Current research points to a gene abnormality located on the third chromosome, but the exact gene has not been identified. In children born with multiple dislocations of large joints, especially the knees, Larsen's syndrome should be considered as the diagnosis. The condition is characterized by a flat face with a broad forehead and hypertelorism. The cervical spine may develop kyphosis associated with hypoplastic vertebral bodies. The cervical spine deformity may occur more frequently than previously appreciated, and is best managed with early posterior spine fusion, even within the first 18 months of life. In the lower extremities, knee dislocations have traditionally been managed before other deformities. Stable knees are a necessity for ambulation, and open reductions are required if the knees are dislocated, but a lack of stabilizing ligamentous structures, such as the anterior cruciate ligament, can still result in an unstable joint requiring bracing. Cast manipulation can result in a fracture of the bones, and is rarely, if ever, successful in stabilizing the knee. Because the knees are usually hyperextended, stabilization of the knee relaxes the hamstrings, making simultaneous open reductions of the hip and knee possible. Dislocated hips also almost always require open techniques to achieve reduction. However, a high failure rate is associated with surgery to relocate the dislocated hips, leading some physicians to advocate leaving the hips dislocated (especially in bilateral cases) or delaying surgical treatment until after the child is old enough to combine open reduction with pelvic and femoral osteotomies. The most common foot deformity is a clubfoot. Circumferential releases usually are performed after the knee and hip are stabilized. Complications related to anesthesia can occur because of the mobile infolding arytenoid cartilage and tracheomalacia, conditions that are especially problematic in the newborn and sometimes require a delay in surgical management.

Distal Arthrogryposis

The term arthrogryposis refers to a physical finding (stiff joints with a lack of skin creases). Distal arthrogryposis primarily involves the hands and feet, as opposed to the generalized form of arthrogryposis (arthrogryposis congenita multiplex or amyoplasia), which involves the large joints as well. Unlike the generalized form of arthrogryposis, which is not an inherited condition, the distal forms are inherited in either an autosomal dominant or autosomal recessive manner. Distal arthrogryposis can be classified into type I, with isolated hand and foot deformity, and type II (also called Freeman-Sheldon syndrome), which also involves the face. In type I, studies suggest a causative gene mutation on the first chromosome. In both forms, the hand has a cuplike palm, with a single palmar crease and ulnar deviation of the metacarpophalangeal joints. Despite the deformity, the hands are usually quite functional and surgical intervention usually is not required. The feet are stiff with either clubfoot deformity or congenital vertical talus, and surgical treatment for the foot deformities is almost always required. Patients with distal arthrogryposis type II have a higher than expected incidence of scoliosis, which can be managed similar to idiopathic scoliosis. Complications from anesthesia are related to laryngeal cartilage abnormalities.

Skeletal Dysplasias

Skeletal dysplasias are a group of disorders usually associated with short stature. Traditionally they are classified by the part of the bone that is abnormal. Recent studies have uncovered the molecular genetic cause of many of these disorders. Although there are a variety of clinical differences between the various skeletal dysplasias, many have in common instability of the cervical spine, a condition that should be assessed.

Spondyloepiphyseal Dysplasia

Spondyloepiphyseal dysplasia is characterized by a short trunk and limb dwarfism with abnormalities of the physes and spine. The condition can be classified into congenita and tarda forms. The congenita form is present at birth, and is caused by mutations in type II collagen inherited in an autosomal dominant manner. The tarda form is milder, with most patients developing manifestations at about 4 years of age until adolescence. The tarda form is an X-linked condition caused by a mutation in the *SEDL* gene, which plays a role in regulating intracellular protein trafficking. The exact mechanism by which the *SEDL* gene mutation causes abnormal chondroepiphyseal formation has yet to be determined.

The congenita form is accompanied by coxa vara, valgus alignment at the knees, scoliosis, kyphosis, and increased lumbar lordosis. The hands have a normal appearance. Severe myopia, retinal detachments, and sensorineural hearing loss can be present. The skeletal deformities may give affected individuals a waddling gait pattern with increased lumbar lordosis and a protuberant abdomen. The tarda form is associated with hip pain or stiffness (generally in the second decade), flattened vertebrae (platyspondyly), and in many cases, scoliosis. There is failure or delay of ossification of the proximal femoral epiphysis, os pubis, distal femoral epiphysisis, talus, and calcaneus. Coxa valga is apparent. In the tarda form, the involvement is less severe, with the hips showing radiographic changes similar to Legg-Calvé-Perthes disease (except for bilateral, fairly symmetric involvement), and the spine showing platyspondyly.

Odontoid hypoplasia can predispose to upper cervical instability and cause myelopathy. More severely involved individuals are at higher risk for cervical instability. Lower extremity malalignment may be treated with osteotomies. The delay in proximal femoral ossification should not be mistaken for dislocation of the hips. Pain caused by degeneration of the articular cartilage of the hips can be treated with osteotomies, but total joint replacement may be required. Scoliosis and kyphosis are treated using the usual treatment principles for these spinal deformities. Most individuals with lower extremity deformity will not require surgery; however, if contemplated, surgery should be done for realignment of the lower extremities, rather than concentrating on a single joint.

Multiple Epiphyseal Dysplasia

This autosomal dominant disorder causes short stature and premature arthritis because of a defect in the epiphyses of bones. There is some similarity in presentation to the tarda form of spondyloepiphyseal dysplasia, but there is minimal spinal involvement, if any. The disorder has varying degrees of severity, and there can be variability of severity within a single family. It can be caused by a mutation in cartilage oligomeric protein (whose function in cartilage is not yet completely understood) or by a mutation in type IX collagen, which plays a role in the organization of collagen in the chondroepiphysis. Interestingly, mutations in cartilage oligomeric protein are also responsible for pseudoachondroplasia. Occasionally there is osteonecrosis of the epiphyses, seen most commonly at the proximal femur.

The hips are often most severely involved, and the proximal femoral epiphyses appear late, and are irregular in shape and fragmented. This appearance is quite similar to that seen in Legg-Calvé-Perthes disease, although multiple sites are involved, which all have a similar radiographic appearance. Unlike in Legg-Calvé-Perthes disease, the hips do not experience typical changes in radiographic appearance with time. Most patients present with hip symptoms. More severe involvement early in life is a predictor of a worse outcome. In patients younger than age 8 years, containment of the femoral head has been advocated, although femoral osteotomy is usually not performed because of underlying coxa vara. There are no comparative studies, however, showing an advantage to containment surgery. Older patients may have hinge abduction, or incongruity of the lateral portion of the femoral head that may be improved by proximal femur osteotomy. Knee deformity may be treated with osteotomy, although malalignment in younger individuals may recur with growth. Osteochondritis dissecans can occur, and is treated using the usual treatment principles. Because there is an intrinsic abnormality of the articular cartilage, osteotomies are at best temporizing procedures, and many individuals ultimately undergo total joint arthroplasty.

Achondroplasia

Achondroplasia is an autosomal dominant disorder caused by a mutation in the fibroblast growth factor receptor type 3. Most cases, however, are caused by new mutations, with increased paternal age as a risk factor. Fibroblast growth factor regulates chondrocytes early in their development, and the causative mutations interfere with the normal progression of chondrocyte maturation. The entire chondroepiphysis develops abnormally, with a greater effect in regions of greatest endochondral growth, giving rise to the characteristic rhizomelic shortening (there is worse shortening of the proximal bone). Children are identified at birth by the characteristic face (frontal bossing and midface hypoplasia), and short humerus and femur (Fig. 3). Infants are usually hypotonic. Some have foramen magnum stenosis; however, the use of screening tests to evaluate for this condition, and its surgical management are

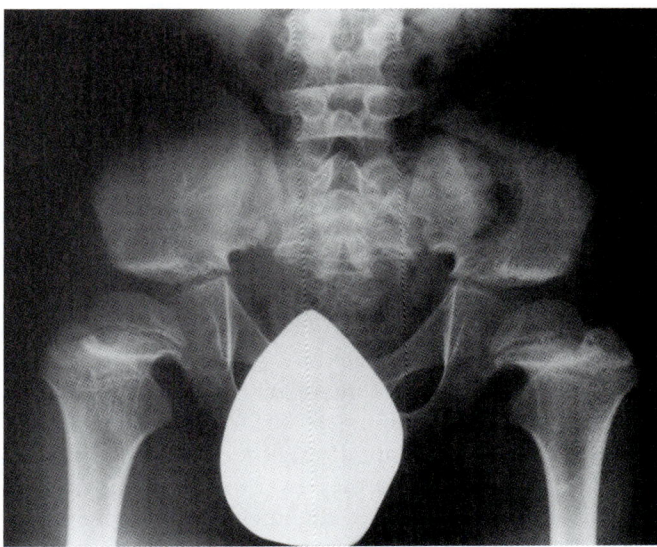

Figure 3 A pelvic radiograph of a child with achondroplasia. Flared iliac wings, short femoral necks, and a narrow interpedicular distance to the lower lumber vertebrae are shown.

controversial topics. Although the majority of affected individuals do not require surgery to correct the foramen magnum stenosis, this diagnosis should be considered in infants with an unusual neurologic picture.

The most severe problems are related to the spine. Unlike other forms of skeletal dysplasias, cervical instability is unusual. Kyphosis of the lumbar spine develops in infants, but usually spontaneously resolves in early childhood, when better trunk control develops. Protocols involving delayed sitting and bracing for the kyphosis are advocated; the rare progressive case that persists past young childhood requires surgery (anterior and posterior arthrodesis). Instrumentation into the spinal canal (for example, with hooks) is hazardous because a congenital spinal stenosis associated with a narrow space between pedicles is present. In the lumbar spine, the distance between the pedicles narrows, rather than increases, in a caudal direction. Patients may become more symptomatic later in life when degenerative changes are superimposed on the congenital stenosis. Decompression of the spine is performed in symptomatic cases. Genu varum occurs, and osteotomies can be performed in the patient with severe deformity and symptoms. Distraction osteogensis and the use of growth hormones to increase stature are controversial treatments for these individuals. Although growth hormone will increase growth velocity, there is patient-to-patient variability in the effect, and it is unknown how much the patient's final height is improved. Distraction osteogenesis is associated with lengthy treatment. Most children with achondroplasia are not treated for short stature. Although studies show that teenagers with achondroplasia have issues about body image, analysis of adults show that function and self image are similar to that of unaffected adults.

Pseudoachondroplasia

This disorder resembles achondroplasia, because of the rhizomelia, but is caused by a mutation in the gene encoding for cartilage oligomeric matrix protein. Hip changes develop that are similar to multiple epihyseal dysplasia. Osteoarthritis is a significant problem in adulthood. Radiographs of the spine show platyspondyly and anterior beaking in children, characteristics that can aid in confirming the diagnosis. Affected individuals can develop genu valgum, genu varum, or a windswept alignment to the lower extremities, with valgus of one leg and varus alignment to the other. Surgery is indicated to realign the lower extremities when the deformity is severe. As in multiple ephiphyseal dysplasia, there are no studies to indicate if hip surgery alters the outcome.

Metaphyseal Chondrodysplasias

This condition is characterized by abnormalities in the metaphyseal portion of the bone, often resulting in bowing of the lower limbs. There are many types of metaphyseal dysplasia. The Schmidt type is autosomal dominant and is caused by a type X collagen gene mutation. The Schmidt type is a relatively mild form, often not diagnosed until the child is 2 or 3 years of age. It needs to be considered in the differential diagnosis of a toddler with bowed legs. The Jansen type, also autosomal dominant, is caused by a mutation in the parathyroid hormone-related protein receptor, which regulates the differentiation of growth plate chondrocytes. Involvement is more severe in the Jansen than in the Schmidt type, and hypercalcemia may be present. The McKusick type is also called cartilage-hair hypoplasia, and is associated with systemic problems including lymphadema, neutropenia, immunodeficiency, and malabsorption. This is a rare disorder identified primarily in the Amish population. Surgical intervention in metaphyseal chondrodysplasia is indicated for children with progressive bowing of the lower limbs.

Annotated Bibliography

Down Syndrome

Greene WB: Closed treatment of hip dislocation in Down syndrome. *J Pediatr Orthop* 1998;18:643-647.

According to this study, long-term bracing (6 to 8 months) will result in stable, reduced hips in children age 6 years or younger with dislocated hips and Down syndrome.

Kioschos M, Shaw ED, Beals RK: Total hip arthroplasty in patients with Down's syndrome. *J Bone Joint Surg Br* 1999;81:436-439.

The hip can become quite symptomatic in adult patients. Despite concerns about performing arthroplasty in this patient population, these authors found that total hip replacement can be successful in the adult patient with Down syndrome.

Merrick J, Ezra E, Josef B, Hendel D, Steinberg DM, Wientroub S: Musculoskeletal problems in Down Syndrome European Paediatric Orthopaedic Society Survey: The Israeli Sample. *J Pediatr Orthop Br* 2000;9:185-192.

This article presents a review of the variety of musculoskeletal deformities that can occur in Down syndrome.

Wellborn CC, Sturm PF, Hatch RS, Bomze SR, Jablonski K: Intraobserver reproducibility and interobserver reliability of cervical spine measurements. *J Pediatr Orthop* 2000;20:66-70.

This study is one of several series showing poor intraobserver reproducibility to cervical spine measurements in Down syndrome.

Turner's Syndrome

Wihlborg CE, Babyn PS, Schneider R: The association between Turner's syndrome and juvenile rheumatoid arthritis. *Pediatr Radiol* 1999;29:676-681.

Patients with Turner's syndrome have a higher than expected incidence of juvenile rheumatoid arthritis.

Neurofibromatosis

Crawford AH, Schorry EK: Neurofibromatosis in children: The role of the orthopaedist. *J Am Acad Orthop Surg* 1999;7:217-230.

This article presents a comprehensive review of the orthopaedic manifestations of neurofibromatosis.

Durrani AA, Crawford AH, Chouhdry SN, Saifuddin A, Morley TR: Modulation of spinal deformities in patients with neurofibromatosis type I. *Spine* 2000;25:69-75.

Patients presenting with scoliosis at age 6 years or younger have a high chance of developing a dysplastic curve. Rib penciling is a sign that the curve will become dysplastic.

Karol LA, Haideri NF, Halliday SE, Smitherman TB, Johnston CE II: Gait analysis and muscle strength in children with congenital pseudarthrosis of the tibia: The effect of treatment. *J Pediatr Orthop* 1998;18:381-386.

Gait analysis of patients treated with limb salvage procedures for tibial pseudarthrosis shows a disturbed gait pattern, especially in individuals with an early onset of neurofibromatosis, compared with patients who eventually underwent an amputation.

Parisini P, Di Silvestre M, Greggi T, Paderni S, Cervellati S, Savini R: Surgical correction of dystrophic spinal curves in neurofibromatosis: A review of 56 patients. *Spine* 1999;24:2247-2253.

This retrospective study strongly suggests that anterior and posterior fusion is required for dystrophic curves.

Multiple Hereditary Exostosis

Carroll KL, Yandow SM, Ward K, Carey JC: Clinical correlation to genetic variations of hereditary multiple exostosis. *J Pediatr Orthop* 1999;19:785-791.

This article presents an attempt to correlate the genotype with the phenotype in multiple exostosis. A review of the implications of the various types and locations of osteochondromas is provided.

Enchondromatosis

Chew DK, Menelaus MB, Richardson MD: Ollier's disease: Varus angulation at the lower femur and its management. *J Pediatr Orthop* 1998;18:202-208.

The variety of treatments available for lower extremity deformity in multiple enchondromatosis and their outcomes are reviewed.

Cleidocranial Dysplasia

Aktas S, Wheeler D, Sussman MD: The 'chef's hat' appearance of the femoral head in cleidocranial dysplasia. *J Bone Joint Surg Br* 2000;82:404-408.

A typical appearance of the femoral head, similar in shape to a chef's hat, is present in the early stages of disease. This suggests that there is a disorder in the development of the proximal femoral chondroepiphysis in cleidocranial dysostosis.

Nail-Patella Syndrome

Dreyer SD, Zhou G, Baldini A, et al: Mutations in LMX1B cause abnormal skeletal patterning and renal dysplasia in nail patella syndrome. *Nat Genet* 1998;19:47-50.

Mutation in the *LMX1B* gene causes nail-patella syndrome.

Diastrophic Dysplasia

Baitner AC, Maurer SG, Gruen MB, DiCesare PE: The genetic basis of the osteochondrodysplasias. *J Pediatr Orthop* 2000;20:594-605.

This article reviews the underlying genetic defect responsible for inherited disorders of the growth or remodeling of cartilage.

Crockett MM, Carten MF, Hurko O, Sponseller PD: Motor milestones in children with diastrophic dysplasia. *J Pediatr Orthop* 2000;20:437-441.

Motor milestones are slightly delayed in individuals with diastrophic dysplasia.

Matsuyama Y, Winter RB, Lonstein JE: The spine in diastrophic dysplasia: The surgical arthrodesis of thoracic and lumbar deformities in 21 patients. *Spine* 1999;24:2325-2331.

Scoliosis is often associated with kyphosis, and deformity in younger children can be rapidly progressive. Early anterior and posterior arthrodesis is advocated.

Peltonen J, Vaara P, Marttinen E, Ryoppy S, Poussa M: The knee joint in diastrophic dysplasia: A clinical and radiological study. *J Bone Joint Surg Br* 1999;81:625-631.

The knee can be very unstable in individuals with diastrophic dysplasia.

Remes V, Tervahartiala P, Poussa M, Peltonen J: Cervical spine in diastrophic dysplasia: An MRI analysis. *J Pediatr Orthop* 2000;20:48-53.

Remes V, Marttinen E, Poussa M, Kaitila I, Peltonen J: Cervical kyphosis in diastrophic dysplasia. *Spine* 1999;24:1990-1995.

These two studies show that cervical kyphosis is common at birth, but usually resolves. Later in life, degenerative changes can cause these kyphotic deformities to be more symptomatic.

Vaara P, Peltonen J, Poussa M, et al: Development of the hip in diastrophic dysplasia. *J Bone Joint Surg Br* 1998;80:315-320.

The hip is normal at birth, after which flexion contratures develop. Limited motion is associated with the development of osteoarthritis.

Larsen's Syndrome

Babat LB, Ehrlich MG: A paradigm for the age-related treatment of knee dislocations in Larsen's syndrome. *J Pediatr Orthop* 2000;20:396-401.

This case series describes the different treatments available for the dislocated knee in Larsen's syndrome in individuals of various ages.

Skeletal Dysplasias

Gedeon AK, Colley A, Jamieson R, et al: Identification of the gene (SEDL) causing X-linked spondyloepiphyseal dysplasia tarda. *Nat Genet* 1999;22:400-404.

The Sedlin gene is identified as mutated in the X-linked tarda form of spondyloepiphyseal dysplasia.

Keiper GL Jr, Koch B, Crone KR: Achondroplasia and cervicomedullary compression: Prospective evaluation and surgical treatment. *Pediatr Neurosurg* 1999;31:78-83.

This article presents a review of the clinical presentation and surgical treatment of foramen magnum stenosis in achondroplasia.

Mahomed NN, Spellmann M, Goldberg MJ: Functional health status of adults with achondroplasia. *Am J Med Genet* 1998;78:30-35.

This study of adults with achondroplasia shows that individuals have an overall good outcome as measured using the SF-36 instrument.

Classic Bibliography

Arms DM, Strecker WB, Manske PR, Schoenecker PL: Management of forearm deformity in multiple hereditary osteochondromatosis. *J Pediatr Orthop* 1997;17:450-454.

Doyle JS, Lauerman WC, Wood KB, Krause DR: Complications and long-term outcome of upper cervical spine arthrodesis in patients with Down syndrome. *Spine* 1996;21:1223-1231.

Francomano CA, McIntosh I, Wilkin DJ: Bone dysplasias in man: Molecular insights. *Curr Opin Genet Dev* 1996;6:301-308.

Johnston CE II, Birch JG, Daniels JL: Cervical kyphosis in patients who have Larsen syndrome. *J Bone Joint Surg Am* 1996;78:538-545.

McKeand J, Rotta J, Hecht JT: Natural history study of pseudoachondroplasia. *Am J Med Genet* 1996;63:406-410.

Mundlos S, Otto F, Mundlos C, et al: Mutations involving the transcription factor CBFA1 cause cleidocranial dysplasia. *Cell* 1997;89:773-779.

Pauli RM, Breed A, Horton VK, Glinski LP, Reiser CA: Prevention of fixed, angular kyphosis in achondroplasia. *J Pediatr Orthop* 1997;17:726-733.

Chapter 22

Neuromuscular Disorders

Mark F. Abel, MD

John S. Blanco, MD

Diane L. Damiano, PhD, PT

Stephen R. Skinner, MD

R. Tracy Ballock, MD

Cerebral Palsy

Epidemiology and Etiology

Cerebral palsy (CP) is a heterogeneous condition that results from a static brain lesion occurring prior to or for a variable time after birth. The brain lesion is permanent and has deleterious effects on subsequent growth and development. The incidence of CP is 1 to 3 cases per 1,000 live births, making it the most prevalent childhood physical disability. Premature infants, especially those born at less than 32 weeks' gestation, are at increased risk for developing CP. The etiologies of CP include embolic, hemorrhagic, and hypoxic brain injuries as well as insults caused by brain malformations and infections. Excluded from this group are patients with genetic syndromes, metabolic derangements (enzyme deficiencies), and progressive neuromuscular conditions as well as those with acquired brain injury occurring beyond childhood. Other risk factors identified include maternal chorioamnionitis, placental bleeding, multiple pregnancies, hypotension, hypoventilation, hypoxia, and pulmonary insufficiency. In general, 50% to 60% of patients have evidence of prenatal or perinatal causes and 5% have postnatal causes, leaving approximately 35% of patients without obvious etiology. Functional prognosis in CP is related to the associated comorbid conditions. As the extent of brain injury increases, patients are more likely to have seizures (30%), mental retardation (40%), visual impairments (16%), hydrocephalus (14%), malnutrition (15%), and complex movement disorders (20%).

All treatments for CP are palliative and many have similar indications. Unfortunately, the majority of studies on treatments for CP are retrospective, uncontrolled cohort studies for which impact on function and disability has not been measured.

Classification

The classification of CP is based on the type of movement abnormality (physiologic classifications) and the body region affected (anatomic classification) (Table 1).

The physiologic classification is based on the manifested muscle tone and movement disorder and groups patients into those with spasticity and those with extrapyramidal or dystonic movements. Spasticity is characterized by hyperreflexia, clonus, and velocity-dependent resistance to joint motion. Writhing or jerking movements of the extremity, termed athetosis, chorea, and ballismus, are indicative of extrapyramidal motor damage, such as to the basal ganglia. Ataxia or impaired balance suggests injury to the cerebellum. Hypotonia or low muscle tone is another form of motor dysfunction. In general, spasticity responds best to current interventions, such as rhizotomy, muscle-tendon surgery, and benzodiazepines, whereas the extrapyramidal movement patterns are less predictably controlled.

In the anatomic classification, hemiplegia refers to involvement of one side of the body, diplegia to involvement of the legs primarily with relative sparing of the upper extremities, and quadriplegia to four-extremity involvement. Patients with quadriplegic involvement are totally dependent because they lack selective movement of all extremities and have truncal imbalance.

The physiologic and anatomic classifications emphasize the positive clinical signs (spasticity) associated with CP, and do not focus on so-called negative clinical signs such as weakness and impaired balance (Table 2), which are poorly measured and also relatively neglected by most treatment regimens.

Diagnosis and Evaluation

Patient history and physical examination, using such methods as three-dimensional motion analysis (for

TABLE 1 | Classification of CP

Type	Prevalence
Physiologic	
Spastic	80%
Extrapyramidal (Dystonic)	20%
Athetosis	
Chorea, ballismus	
Ataxia	
Hypotonia	
Anatomic	
Diplegia	50%
Hemiplegia	30%
Quadriplegia (total body involved)	20%

Treatment Options

Treatments for CP alter limb posture and/or muscle tone with the intent of improving function. Ankle-foot orthoses (AFOs) and walkers are prescribed to control posture and enhance balance. Neurotoxins, particularly botulinum toxin, are used to temporarily weaken selected muscles directly or by chemical neurolysis (with alcohol and phenol). Oral medications, intrathecal baclofen, and selective dorsal rhizotomy help reduce muscle tone and spasticity. Physical therapy helps maintain joint mobility and enhance function. Orthopaedic interventions, including muscle-tendon surgery, osteotomy, and arthrodesis, are used to alleviate the effects of contractures, stabilize joints, and optimize limb alignment for walking. Gait analysis, done with the help of cameras linked to computers, in-floor force plates, and dynamic electromyography (EMG), has become a fundamental part of assessing the movement complexities associated with CP. Through preintervention and postintervention assessments, the indications for and effects of a number of orthopaedic, neurosurgical, and orthotic procedures have been refined. For muscle-tendon surgery in particular, the gait data are used in conjunction with physical assessments to determine which specific procedure(s) will provide appropriate balance of muscle activity, not only across a joint, but also between adjacent joints.

detailed assessment of dynamic movement), radiographs (for assessing the skeleton), and brain imaging modalities, are fundamental to the diagnosis and assessment of CP. The diagnosis of CP must be confirmed by establishing that the deficits are not progressive and are the result of a brain injury.

The age for achieving motor milestones has prognostic implications. Prognosis for independent ambulation is guarded if sitting balance is not achieved by 2 years of age. Retained primitive reflexes including the Moro reflex, the extensor thrust, the tonic neck reflexes, and failure to develop the stepping response or the protective parachute responses beyond 24 months of age portend poorly for ambulation. Hand dominance before 18 months of age suggests contralateral brain injury. Combat crawling or lack of reciprocal lower extremity movements is often seen in patients with diplegia. According to several studies, acquisition of major gross motor skills, such as the ability to walk, plateau around 7 years of age.

For patients with spastic diplegia, enhancing walking ability is usually of primary concern. Treatment methods for spastic hemiplegia are focused on enhancing walking and improving upper extremity function, although these patients compensate well with the other side to overcome deficits on the affected side. Quadriplegic patients are dependent on others for their daily needs and have little capacity for functional improvement. The orthopaedic objectives are to improve trunk and limb position for seating, prevent painful joint dislocations, and prevent contractures from interfering with hygiene.

TABLE 2 | Clinical Signs

Clinical Signs in CP	Treatment Options
Positive Signs	
Hypertonicity (spasticity)	Selective dorsal rhizotomy, muscle-tendon surgery, intrathecal baclofen, botulinum toxin, bracing
Static contractures	Muscle-tendon surgery
Torsional deformities/joint deformity	Osteotomies, arthrodesis
Negative Signs	
Weakness	Physical therapy
Poor balance	Walking aids, bracing

Casting, Bracing, and Seating Systems

Casts are used for postoperative protection, to stretch muscle-tendon units, and reverse contractures. In young patients (age 4 years or younger), cast treatment may be effective and once completed allows bracing with an AFO. However, in the absence of additional treatment, recurrent contractures are common after stress casting. Botulinum toxin-A (BTX-A) injection may be useful as an adjunct to casting.

The goals of AFOs are to correct or control limb alignment, enhance stability, and to prevent contracture development. For patients with pronounced equinus, weakness, and crouch, and for midfoot collapse, bracing should be offered if not precluded by static contractures. AFOs also are used in nonambulatory patients to support the foot and prevent deformities that may preclude shoe wear.

For quadriplegic patients, seating systems play an integral role in providing trunk support, thus allowing mobility, and therefore have a favorable impact on quality of life. A variety of components, including cushioning, molded seats, propulsion controls, and supports for the head, trunk, and upper extremities, are currently available.

Botulinum Toxin

The neurotoxin produced by the *Clostridium botulinum* species has achieved widespread acceptance over the last decade in its ability to selectively weaken spastic muscles in CP. BTX-A, marketed under the name Botox in the United States, has largely replaced phenol and alcohol as a chemodenervating agent because its effects are more predictable and adverse effects are infrequent.

The mechanism of action for and recovery from BTX-A are still being studied. When injected into the muscle, BTX-A enters the nerve terminal to block release of acetylcholine. With time, new nerve terminals sprout and reattach to the muscle end plate to reverse weakening effects. The weakness is evident within 24 to 72 hours and lasts from 2 to 6 months. Systemic spread of BTX-A after local injection does occur but thus far total body doses of 10 to 12 units/kg do not seem to have significant deleterious effects in the short term. Because of dosing limitations and its short duration of action, BTX-A is most commonly used for localized treatment of a few muscles and in young children before significant muscle-tendon contractures have developed. BTX-A may be useful as an adjunct to serial casting by reducing the stretch response and eliminating some tonic muscle activity.

Transient pain from the injection is the most frequent complaint; however, serious adverse reactions are rare. However, clinical series include cases of bladder incontinence, seizures, constipation, and difficulty with swallowing and breathing. In addition, safe administration of the injection in patients with conditions of muscle weakness such as myasthenia gravis or muscular dystrophy is less certain. Aminoglycosides such as gentamicin may potentiate the neuromuscular blockade and should not be used concomitantly. Because the possible formation of antibodies can reduce effectiveness of subsequent injections, they should not be repeated at less than 3-month intervals. Finally, long-term effects and chronic usage have not been adequately studied, so multiple repeat injections must be performed cautiously and when alternative, safer methods fail.

Oral Medications

Gamma-amino butyric acid (GABA) is an inhibitory neurotransmitter that acts both peripherally and centrally. Baclofen mimics and diazepam potentiates GABA's action and produces sedation in conjunction with reduction of peripheral spasticity. These muscle relaxants are commonly used to ameliorate diffuse spasticity but adverse side effects have tended to restrict their use to the severely spastic patients with total body involvement or in the postoperative setting to treat spasms associated with healing. Baclofen and diazepam are the most frequently used oral medications in treating CP. Cessation after prolonged use of either drug can produce adverse effects including seizures, muscle irritability, and hallucinations.

Intrathecal Baclofen

Oral baclofen does not readily pass through the blood-brain barrier; consequently, high blood concentrations are often required before spasticity is reduced and with these concentrations, sedation is frequently problematic. Intrathecal baclofen administration has drastically reduced dose requirements to affect lower extremity spasticity so that central sedation is much less problematic. A reservoir and programmable pump has been designed to deliver baclofen at a rate commensurate with the desired spasticity reduction. The pump is placed subcutaneously over the abdomen and a catheter leading from the pump is positioned at the thoracolumbar junction for reduction of lower extremity muscle tone, and at a higher level if a more diffuse effect is desired. The drug diffuses into the spinal cord and variable distances cephalad as a function of the concentration. Thus higher infusion rates are more likely to reduce trunk tone, exacerbate weakness, and produce sedation.

The standard pump is approximately the size of a hockey puck; a thinner pediatric version also exists. However, bulkiness of the pumps precludes implantation in small subjects. Adjusting the dose takes several months and refills are required approximately every 3 months. Complications requiring surgery or pump removal have been reported in 10% to 20% of patients. These include catheter and pump malfunctions, untoward drug reactions including respiratory depression, and infections. Furthermore, drug tolerance and withdrawal reactions are significant concerns.

Selective Dorsal Rhizotomy

Over the past 15 years, selective dorsal rhizotomy has been used in the United States for management of spasticity in patients with diplegia. Although selective dorsal rhizotomy also has been used in nonambulatory patients, experience is less extensive and outcome less well documented. Technical aspects of the procedure and patient selection criteria vary; consequently, conclusions regarding effectiveness are still being debated.

Selective dorsal rhizotomy is based on the belief that, in spastic diplegia, heightened responses to afferent impulses, whether from the muscle spindle or skin, spread to adjacent levels and interfere with function. In fact, after selective dorsal rhizotomy, reflexes and resistance to passive limb movement generally are reduced in the lower extremities but the functional gains are variable. Thus, the relationship between spasticity reduction and functional gains are still debatable. Complications are rare but can include bowel and bladder incontinence if sacral rootlets are not properly identified, lower extremity dysesthesia, and dural leaks. Furthermore, musculoskeletal deformities, including spinal deformities, hip subluxation, midfoot subluxation, and muscle-tendon contractures, still can develop after selective dorsal rhizotomy.

Physical Therapy

For decades, physical therapy has been a mainstay of nonsurgical management of motor dysfunction in CP, as a stand-alone intervention or as a supplement to other treatments. Recent trends in physical therapy have begun to specifically address muscle weakness, and studies suggest that strength and endurance training can have pronounced positive effects on gait and motor function. Finally, a greater focus on functional goals in physical therapy, rather than merely addressing movement quality or developmental milestones, has been shown to produce measurable positive outcomes. The goals of physical therapy differ in nonambulatory or quadriplegic patients and tend to focus on prevention of secondary musculoskeletal deformities that could interfere with optimal positioning, patient comfort, or ease of care.

Muscle-Tendon Procedures

Muscle-tendon procedures, including lengthening, releases, or transfers, are done in patients with CP to alter agonist-antagonist balance, overcome static contractures, and enhance dynamic limb alignment when function, hygiene, or joint stability is believed to be compromised. Muscle-tendon procedures are recommended when less invasive methods such as casting and bracing are ineffective. The rationale for use of muscle-tendon procedures in spastic diplegia is based on the belief that shortening of the muscle-tendon units and restriction of joint motion will produce postural abnormalities that in turn lead to abnormal joint loading and ultimately to premature degenerative arthritis.

To achieve functional gains after muscle-tendon procedures, iatrogenic deformities caused by weakness and by unmasking spastic antagonists must be avoided. Overlengthening of the hamstrings can precipitate knee hyperextension, excessive pelvic flexion in stance, and/or poor knee flexion in swing, hampering foot clearance (stiff knee gait). With Achilles tendon overlengthening, push-off is reduced and excessive knee crouch can develop. Muscle units with a broad, fibrous aponeurotic expanse at their muscle-tendon junction can be lengthened by transection of this aponeurosis (recession), followed by manual stretching until the desired joint position is achieved. Muscle-tendon units conducive to aponeurotic lengthening include the semimembranosus, biceps femoris, gastrocnemius-soleus complex, and iliopsoas muscles. The muscle-tendon unit may be released from its origin or insertion (tenotomy), virtually eliminating its function at the joint spanned. Tenotomy tends to be performed for smaller muscles (such as the semitendinosus, the adductor longus, and gracilis muscles) within a group that span a joint. Tendon Z-lengthening, as opposed to release, is frequently done but the "right" length at which to reconnect must be determined. If too much slack is introduced, weakness and new deformities will ensue. Excessive muscle-tendon lengthening is virtually impossible to reverse.

Muscle-tendon procedures are the only techniques available to overcome static shortening of the tendinous portion of the muscle-tendon unit; however, specific indications and outcomes have yet to be ascertained through clinical trials. Consequently, the role of specific muscle-tendon procedures such as iliopsoas lengthening and rectus femoris surgery (transfers or releases) is uncertain.

Osteotomies and Arthrodesis

Rotational osteotomies are done to ameliorate severe in-toeing or out-toeing gait. The skeleton functions as a series of levers over which the muscles work; theoretically, the torsional deformities commonly seen in CP reduce muscle efficiency and function so that rotational osteotomies and subtalar correction are done to restore alignment and enhance muscle function.

Osteotomies are often combined with muscle tendon procedures to correct the accompanying contractures.

Arthrodesis in people with CP is reserved for treatment of pain associated with end-stage joint deterioration where ligamentous and muscle constraints cannot be reconstructed and/or when articular cartilage is severely damaged. Common sites for arthrodesis include the subtalar and midfoot joints for planovalgus foot deformity, the first metatarsophalangeal joint for dorsal bunions or hallux valgus, the wrist for severe flexion deformities, and the thumb interphalangeal joint or metacarpophalangeal joint.

Management of Specific Anatomic Regions

Spine

In patients with CP, the majority with severe scoliosis tend to be totally dependent for all needs, and many are mentally retarded, have seizures, impaired swallowing, and a propensity for respiratory infections. These associated comorbid conditions and the rigidity of the curves increase the risks and expense of correction. The goals of surgical treatment are to stop curve progression and obtain correction to enhance sitting posture, pulmonary function, and digestion, thus easing the care burden. Infection rates have been reported to be as high as 15% after surgery, and other complications, which include pneumonia, ileus, pseudarthrosis or neurologic injury, bring the overall complication rate to approximately 20%.

Hip

The incidence of subluxation in spastic quadriparesis ranges from 25% to 50% and perhaps a third to one half of these patients will experience hip pain. Furthermore, the adduction and other contractures that accompany hip subluxation make sitting and perineal hygiene difficult. Treatment in the form of orthopaedic procedures or with tone reduction techniques are used in hopes of altering the adverse consequences of hip subluxation.

Hip subluxation in CP results from chronic muscle hypertonicity, especially in the adductor group. Radiographic dysplasia with subluxation may become apparent between 2 to 4 years of age; without intervention, complete dislocation is often evident by approximately 7 years of age. The acetabulae become globally deficient and the femurs have increased neck-shaft angles along with excessive anteversion. In chronic cases, not only does the acetabular roof become eroded, but the femoral head becomes steeple-shaped from the combined pressure of the acetabulum medially and the labrum and gluteal muscles laterally. Subluxation in CP is typically measured using the Reimers migration index.

Muscle releases traditionally are performed in children younger than 4 years of age with restricted hip motion, hypertonicity, and minimal bony pathology (migration index 30%). A common approach has been to release muscles of the adductor group. Although anterior branch obturator neurectomy is detrimental to ambulatory function, in nonambulatory patients with hip subluxation, the benefits of neurectomy as an adjunct to muscle releases are unclear. Other muscles that are often released to manage hip subluxation include the iliopsoas and the proximal hamstrings. Early soft-tissue releases may prevent progressive subluxation in approximately 60% of cases but chronic hypertonicity, pelvic obliquity, and scoliosis combine to produce recurrent subluxation in the remaining 40%. Long-term, postoperative hip abduction bracing has been suggested to lower the incidence of recurrent subluxation.

Osteotomies, either acetabular, femoral, or both, are done for later stages of subluxation. In the absence of controlled studies, indications and success rates vary considerably. As a general guideline, for children between 4 to 8 years of age with a migration index between 30% to 50%, soft-tissue releases should be combined with femoral varus, shortening osteotomies, or acetabular osteotomies. On the acetabular side, equivalent results have been reported with a variety of osteotomies including hinging acetabuloplasties, rotational acetabular osteotomies, and augmentation acetabuloplasties. External rotation of the femoral shaft is often done in conjunction with varus and shortening to lower the femoral anteversion. Combined acetabular and femoral osteotomies are recommended for patients older than 8 years of age and with a migration index greater than 50%.

Using these guidelines, success as determined by radiographic measures of migration percentage can be achieved in 70% to 80% of cases. Patients with severe spasticity, especially those with asymmetric hypertonicity, are at high risk for resubluxation. In addition, the poor baseline health of many patients increases the rate of complications such as hip stiffness, hypersensitivity, skin breakdown, recurrent subluxation, and other perioperative complications such as pneumonia, urinary infections, and ileus. The high rate of adverse outcomes is especially prevalent in patients with severe spasticity and has been the impetus behind approaches to address the hypertonicity, either as preventive or as adjunctive treatments, with intrathecal baclofen or oral antispasmodic medications. Once muscle tone has been reduced, then contractures and bony pathology are addressed.

Salvage operations for older patients with chronically subluxated or dislocated and painful hips include proximal femoral resection and/or valgus osteotomies. Proximal femoral resections have been reported in retrospective analysis to improve pain in 70% of cases. Valgus procedures are done to realign the adducted femur when this position adversely affects pelvic alignment and sitting. Total hip replacement for spastic CP has been described but experience and follow-up are limited.

Knee

Chronic knee flexion deformities are common in spastic CP and often are addressed differently for ambulatory and nonambulatory patients. For ambulators, stance phase knee crouch increases the load on the patella, resulting in patella alta, fragmentation of the inferior patellar pole, and patellofemoral arthritis. Early in the course of treatment, quadriceps strengthening may be used for patients with sufficient motor control. Bracing, such as with floor-reaction AFOs, can be used to restrain anterior tibial translation. Hamstring lengthening is commonly used to overcome contractures and promote knee extension during stance. However, if swing phase spasticity of the quadriceps is not recognized, the resultant stiff knee may impede foot clearance. Consequently, hamstring lengthening is often combined with posterior transfer of the rectus femoris to the hamstrings.

Lengthening of the hamstrings in nonambulatory patients can be done distally if knee flexion deformities interfere with sitting or dressing. Alternatively, proximal release of the hamstring will increase hip flexion and abduction as well as knee extension if hip and knee deformities both impede sitting.

Foot

Foot deformities are extremely common in spastic CP and, like hip and knee deformities, they may produce functional deficits or interfere with shoe wear. In addition to equinus, other related deformities include pes planovalgus (spastic flatfoot), equinovarus, hallux valgus, and dorsal bunions.

Pes planovalgus is prevalent in patients who ambulate while crouched and who have contractures of the posterior calf muscles. Braces may stabilize the leg and foot to delay or prevent development. Surgical management often entails lengthening of the posterior calf musculature, particularly the gastrocnemius-soleus complex and possibly the peroneus brevis, followed by subtalar realignment procedures including extra-articular fusions and, more recently, lateral calcaneal lengthening osteotomies.

In addition to the crouch posture and associated calf contractures, the pes planovalgus deformity is commonly associated with hallux valgus, external tibial torsion, and femoral adduction and internal rotation. The dynamic relationships between limb segments should be considered if surgical treatment is planned at any

one segment. If not, recurrent deformities are likely. Adjunctive procedures include dorsiflexion osteotomies of the first metatarsal or rotational osteotomies of the tibia and/or the femur.

Hallux valgus or dorsal bunions are common in patients with spastic CP. Techniques for surgical management typically involve metatarsal osteotomies and soft-tissue realignments. Metatarsophalangeal fusion is another technique that can be used for severe and chronic metatarsophalangeal subluxation, although it may hamper crawling and walking in some cases.

Upper Extremity

Upper extremity deformities include thumb-in-palm contractures, wrist and finger flexion and elbow flexion contractures, forearm pronation deformities, and shoulder rotational and abduction deformities. Some of these deformities create difficulties performing activities of daily living and can create functional deficits from impaired grasp, release, and reach. However, functional gains from various treatments including BTX-A injections, bracing, and surgery have been difficult to quantify and it has been suggested that surgery to improve limb position for hygiene purposes or to make the arm more effective in performing tasks is a more achievable goal.

Myelomeningocele

Spina bifida is a term describing a variety of neural tube birth defects. Spina bifida occulta describes failure of fusion of the posterior vertebral elements and occurs in 10% of the general population. It is not associated with neurologic impairment. Other forms of spinal dysraphism include diastematomyelia and lipomeningocele. Spina bifida cystica refers to a group of disorders including meningocele, myelomeningocele, and myelocele. These conditions involve cystic distention of the meninges in addition to the bifid posterior spinal elements, with varying degrees of spinal cord and nerve root protrusion and neurologic injury (Fig. 1). These congenital malformations occur during the first month of fetal development.

Current figures for the prevalence of myelomeningocele in the United States are between 0.41 to 1.43 cases per 1,000 live births, which translates into 6,000 to 11,000 newborns with myelomeningocele in the United States each year. Factors that have led to a decrease in the number of children born with spina bifida include prenatal diagnosis via alpha-fetoprotein levels, ultrasound screening (allowing elective termination of pregnancy), and increased dietary intake of folic acid before pregnancy. Current recommendations are for women of childbearing age to take a vitamin supplement containing 0.4 mg of folic acid daily. The

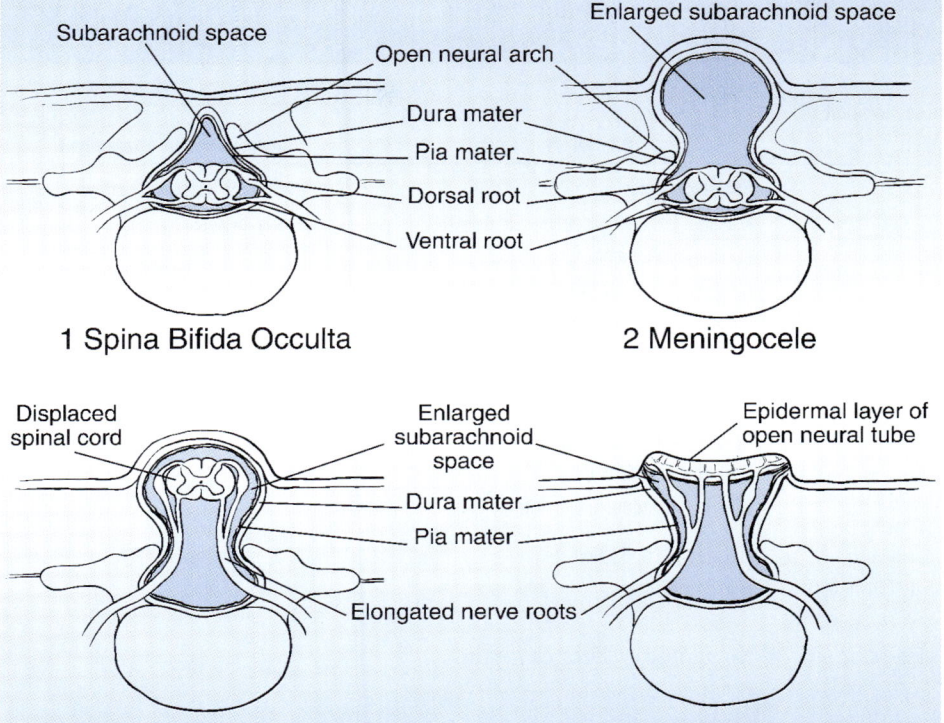

1 Spina Bifida Occulta

2 Meningocele

3 Myelomeningocele

4 Myelocele

Figure 1 Diagrams of spina bifida. *(Adapted with permission from Broughton NS, Menelaus MB (eds): Menelaus' Orthopaedic Management of Spina Bifida Cystica, ed 3. London, England, WB Saunders, 1998, p 3.)*

average recurrence risk of neural tube defects for parents with one affected child is approximately 5%. In addition to the effect of folic acid levels on the incidence of neural tube defects, myelomeningocele can be caused by teratogens such as alcohol and anticonvulsants. The role of cesarean section delivery in decreasing the risk of infection and neurologic injury as a result of birth trauma is controversial but is considered in certain situations, such as significant sac protrusion on ultrasound. Fetal surgery is currently in the investigational stage of development.

The main causes of death in this population have been hydrocephalus, central nervous system infection, and renal failure. Improvements in neurosurgical and urologic care are expected to improve the life expectancy of these patients. Intellectual function is almost always impaired to some degree, although 65% of these patients have intelligence in the normal range. Those with poorly treated hydrocephalus and those who require shunts have, on the average, lower intellectual function. As in all neuromuscular conditions, maximizing independence, communication skills, and mobility are the goals of management. Ambulation skills are not the sole defining component of a successful treatment plan. Neurologic level at L4 or distal is probably the most important factor in determining ambulation ability. A multidisciplinary approach is crucial in preventing fragmented treatment and suboptimal results.

Orthopaedic Considerations

Documented serial orthopaedic and neurologic examinations are a key component in avoiding deterioration of function because of progressive neurologic loss. Common causes of progressive spasticity and/or functional loss include cord tethering, syringomyelia, hydrocephalus, malfunctioning shunt, and posterior fossa compression secondary to Arnold-Chiari malformation. Any patient exhibiting worsening spasticity, progressive extremity deformities, rapidly increasing scoliosis, back pain, or radiculopathy should be suspected of having an evolving intraspinal or intracranial process. Patients with myelomeningocele will often have asymmetric neurologic levels as well as a variance in the function of muscles distal to the level of cord injury.

In addition to closely monitoring any changes in neurologic function, other goals include maintaining flexible joints with functional ranges of motion, monitoring skin integrity, and maintaining a stable and balanced axial skeleton. The use of orthotic devices based on neurologic level is a mainstay in maximizing function in the face of weakness, flaccidity, or spasticity (Table 3). Lengthening or releasing contracted soft tissues is often necessary to achieve a braceable joint.

Spinal Deformities

Spinal deformities include congenital scoliosis, kyphosis, and lordosis plus paralytic and/or developmental

| TABLE 3 | Function, Clinical Problems, and Common Brace Alternatives for Different Motor Levels in Myelomeningocele | | |

Myelomeningocele Level*	Probable Adolescent/Adult Function†	Clinical Problems	Common Brace Alternatives†
Thoracic	Sitter	Spinal deformity Hip subluxation/dislocation (acquired) Congenital clubfoot Congenital vertical talus	Parapodium or swivel walker Seating devices Mobility devices
L1-L2	Independent sitter, hands free; possible household ambulation with RGO braces	Spinal deformity Hip flexion deformity Hip subluxation/dislocation (acquired) Congenital clubfoot Congenital vertical talus Hip flexion, adduction deformity	RGO seating devices Mobility devices
L3	Household, community ambulator with KAFO or AFO braces (presence of strong quadriceps makes possible)	Hip flexion, adduction deformity Higher incidence of hip subluxation or dislocation Hip subluxation/dislocation (acquired) Congenital clubfoot Congenital vertical talus	KAFO, occasionally AFO
L4-L5	Community ambulator with AFO braces	Acquired calcaneus foot deformities Foot ulcerations (insensitivity and high level of activity) Hip subluxation/dislocation (acquired) Congenital clubfoot Congenital vertical talus	KAFO initially, then AFO
Sacral	Community ambulator or normal with or without AFOs	Acquired cavus feet, claw toes, ulcers Hip subluxation/dislocation (acquired) Congenital clubfoot Congenital vertical talus Major urologic problems common	AFO, UCBL, or none

*Functional level is defined as distal level with grade III-V strength. Changes in function, such as disabling spasticity, loss of function or strength, or scoliosis may be a result of associated hydrocephalus. Chiari II malformation, or tethered cord syndrome. Factors affecting ambulation as adolescent or adult include motor level, central nervous system deficits, obesity, scoliosis, lower extremity contractures, motivation, and intelligence.
†RGO, reciprocating gait orthosis; AFO, ankle-foot orthosis; KAFO, knee-ankle-foot orthosis; UCBL, University of California Berkeley Laboratory orthosis
(Reproduced from Beaty JH (ed): Orthopaedic Knowledge Update 6. Rosemont, IL, American Academy of Orthopaedic Surgeons, 1999, p 238.)

deformities. Scoliosis in patients with myelomeningocele is discussed in chapter 48.

Lumbar kyphosis, a challenging spinal deformity to treat, is most frequent in the patient with thoracic level disease and may have deleterious effects on pulmonary function, sitting ability, and abdominal volume. The lumbar kyphosis is frequently associated with thoracic lordosis and will exacerbate preexisting pulmonary compromise. Nonsurgical management does not prevent progression; skin ulcerations, related to the prominent gibbus and the poor soft-tissue coverage in the region, add to the challenge. Surgical treatment may require soft-tissue expanders to improve skin coverage prior to instrumentation. Vertebral decancellation procedures in younger patients and formal kyphectomy in older patients, usually accompanied by transection of the spinal cord remnant, are followed by segmental instrumentation to the sacrum.

Hip Deformities

Management of hip subluxation is controversial but there is consensus that the primary goal is to maintain hip mobility and a level pelvis by treating soft-tissue contractures. The etiology of hip deformities is multifactorial with muscle imbalance, contractures, positioning, and spinal alignment as contributing factors. Thoracic level patients generally have flaccid hips; however, many in this group develop progressive hip subluxation and dislocation. Hip instability may also occur in patients with midlumbar level paralysis with functioning hip adductors and flexors but with paralyzed hip abductors and extensors. Because restoration of normal muscle balance and function cannot be achieved, prophylactic hip surgery to prevent hip dislocation seems ill advised. In general, hip dislocations are not painful and probably do not affect ambulation, seating, or bracing requirements. Furthermore, supple pain-free dislocated hips are better than located hips rendered stiff as a result of multiple surgeries and scarring. However, if unilateral subluxation and muscle contractures are creating pelvic imbalance in ambulatory children with good quadriceps function, surgery aimed at establishing hip concentricity sometimes with the additional goal of muscle rebalancing may be warranted.

Knee Contractures and Torsional Deformities

Knee flexion contractures are the most common problem encountered at the knee. A multicenter study of patients with myelomeningocele documented a 10° flexion contracture at birth, which eventually increased to 17° in the thoracic and upper lumbar level patients. Many of these patients often will have hip flexion contractures and calcaneus deformities at the ankle as well. If an increasing flexion deformity at the knee restricts ambulation and/or makes bracing difficult, surgical release can be performed. In some cases hamstring release alone is insufficient and a posterior capsulotomy of the knee may be needed. Full knee extension should be possible intraoperatively. In the patient nearing skeletal maturity, a distal femoral extension osteotomy or anterior distal femoral physeal stapling may be performed. Osteotomies done in younger patients often result in recurrence with further growth.

Torsional deformities can impede walking and mandate bulky orthotic devices to ameliorate the resulting gait disturbance. In neurologically normal children, torsional deformities remodel with time; those in the myelomeningocele population generally do not. Rotational osteotomies are effective treatment and should be performed when functional difficulties are present. External tibial torsion in combination with ankle valgus and a planovalgus foot deformity can make brace wear difficult and result in excessive valgus forces across the knee. This combined deformity is difficult to manage with orthotic devices and can result in ulcer-

ation over the prominent medial malleolus. Tibial osteotomies done in the supramalleolar region can correct the rotational deformity as well as any valgus inclination of the distal tibia seen on a standing radiograph of the ankle.

Foot Deformities

The goal of treatment is to achieve a plantigrade foot that can be braced or placed in shoes. Because many patients with myelomeningocele have varying degrees of insensate plantar skin, preserving flexibility is important. Nonsurgical treatment of clubfoot deformities is rarely successful, but a preliminary period of casting to stretch contracted skin and allow for growth of the foot prior to surgery is helpful. At the time of comprehensive release, nonfunctioning tendons can be released or resected rather than lengthened to decrease the significant recurrence rate in these patients. Long-term use of an AFO is required to maintain a corrected position. Recurrences can be salvaged with talectomy.

Calcaneus deformities caused by unopposed anterior tibialis function can lead to plantar ulceration. Treatment consisting of anterior release or, in patients younger than 4 years of age, transfer of the anterior tibialis posteriorly to the calcaneus may be performed. The transfer should be done in those patients with full strength in the transferred tendon and no spasticity should be present. Equinus deformity can result in some cases, but tendon transfer may decrease orthotic requirements.

Valgus deformities are common and can occur at the level of the ankle joint as well as at the subtalar joint. Standing radiographs can help to determine the site of pathology. Whenever possible, soft-tissue releases and osteotomies should be performed rather than arthrodesis to avoid a stiff foot that is prone to ulceration, increased stresses at adjacent joints, and arthritis.

Fractures

Pathologic fractures as a result of osteopenia are common in patients with myelomeningocele and can occur after minimal trauma. Weight-bearing activities facilitated by standing tables, parapodiums, and orthotic devices have been shown to decrease the fracture incidence. Patients with fractures frequently have erythema, warmth, swelling, low-grade fever, and elevated white blood cell count. Radiographs may reveal periosteal elevation. These signs and symptoms combined with reduced pain perception and no clear history of trauma can suggest infection as the underlying diagnosis. Patients with this clinical picture should be presumed to have a fracture until proven otherwise. Limited cast or splint immobilization, often less than 1 month in duration, combined with weight bearing as soon as feasible is the preferred treatment. Chronic physeal fractures with delayed healing may require prolonged immobilization and occasionally internal fixation to promote healing.

Nonorthopaedic Considerations

Latex allergy or sensitivity is common in patients with myelomeningocele, affecting 20% to 70% in various series. Up to 20% of patients will have a history of a latex reaction. Multiple surgical exposures are thought to be a major etiologic factor so that the incidence increases with age and surgical exposures. The reactions can range from urticaria to severe anaphylaxis. Given the prevalence of latex reaction, routine universal precautions to limit latex exposure in all patients with myelomeningocele is advised.

Neurodegenerative Conditions

Neurodegenerative disorders have in common progressive functional decline secondary to muscle or neurologic degeneration. With muscular dystrophies, the primary defect is in the muscle; for the hereditary motor-sensory neuropathies (Charcot-Marie-Tooth polyneuropathies), the peripheral nervous system is the primary site of disease; for the spinal muscular atrophy syndromes, anterior horn cell function is defective; and for Friedreich's ataxia, degeneration is primarily in the spinocerebellar system. Progress in modern molecular genetics has enhanced understanding of the etiology of neurodegenerative diseases and changed previous classifications (Table 4).

The initial evaluation should include the neonatal history and recollections of intrauterine fetal movements, the timing of gross motor milestones, and the family history. The key point is to distinguish whether the child's disability is static or progressive. Physical examination must include assessment of gait, neurologic examination including manual muscle testing, assessment of sensation, balance and reflexes. The posture of the limbs, motion of the joints, and status of the spine should be noted. Facial features and other organ system pathology may help confirm the diagnosis.

Laboratory testing frequently includes measurements of serum creatine phosphokinase (CPK) and aldolase enzymes, which often are elevated in dystrophic muscle diseases. Other molecular and genetic testing should be performed based on clinical suspicion.

EMGs and nerve conduction velocity tests can often distinguish between primary disease of muscle (myopathy) and primary disease of nerve (neuropathy). In cases of myopathy, EMGs show low amplitude, often polyphasic potentials with decreased duration of response. Nerve conduction velocity should be normal in myopathy but decreased in demyelinating neuropathies. Axonal diseases are characterized by decreased compound muscle action potentials. In neuropathy, the EMGs show increases in the amplitude and duration of the action potentials in chronic disease, although fibrillation potentials of low amplitude can be seen early in the disease.

Biopsy of muscle and nerve is commonly required in the diagnostic work-up and this should be coordinated with the pathologist to enhance diagnostic value. Weak muscles should be biopsied, but they should not be so atrophic that the muscle tissue has been replaced by fibrous tissue and fat. The vastus lateralis and tibialis anterior are often selected in the lower extremity, whereas the triceps and biceps are commonly chosen in the upper extremity. Nerve biopsy is almost always performed using the sural nerve behind the distal fibula.

Malignant hyperthermia has been associated with anesthetic agents including halogenated inhalational agents or succinylcholine in patients with primary muscle diseases, particularly central core disease. Malignant hyperthermia is potentially lethal and can be associated with rhabdomyolysis and myogloginuria. Cardiac abnormalities and pulmonary disease are other common problems that must be evaluated prior to surgical intervention. A vital capacity of less than 30% to 40% of predicted volumes is associated with serious anesthetic risk, including the need for prolonged ventilatory support and possible tracheostomy. Weakness of pharyngeal muscles can lead to aspiration.

Because of the permanent and progressive nature of the disease process, musculoskeletal deformities occurring in patients with neurodegenerative diseases tend to worsen over time, and these deformities often are rigid. Casting and bracing may help prevent progression of deformity or partially compensate for muscle weakness, but surgery often is required for amelioration of hip, spine, and other extremity deformities.

Progressive spine deformities are best treated with segmental instrumentation and posterior fusion when pulmonary function is relatively preserved. Outcomes are compromised when anterior fusion is required, pulmonary function is severely impaired, or the curves are so large and stiff that a balanced spine cannot be achieved. The goal of the instrumentation is to obtain curve correction without the need for postoperative orthotic support.

TABLE 4 | Neurodegenerative Disorders

Muscle Disease	Inheritance	Molecular Defect	Common Phenotype
Duchenne muscular dystrophy	XR	Dystrophin (frame shift mutation)	Male, severe proximal and axial weakness, progressive (dystrophic absent), later contractures and spinal deformity, some MR
Becker muscular dystrophy	XR	Dystrophin (in-frame deletion)	Male, less severe than DMD, proximal weakness (dystrophin deficient)
Limb girdle muscular dystrophy 1A	AD	5q22-34 region	Poorly described
Limb girdle muscular dystrophy 1B	AD	Calveolin-3	Poorly described
Limb girdle muscular dystrophy 2A	AD	Calpain 3	Usually leads to early wheelchair dependence
Limb girdle muscular dystrophy 2B	AD	Dysferlin	Adolescent or early adult onset
Limb girdle muscular dystrophy 2C-F	AR	Subunits of sarcoglycan (complex defective)	Both genders, mild to severe muscle weakness, similar to DMD and Becker muscular dystrophy
Congenital muscular dystrophy (Merosin-deficient form)	AR	Laminin-$\alpha2$	Onset in infancy, variably progressive, diffuse weakness, contractures feet, hands, arthrogryptotic, facial muscles, weak peripheral neuropathy occasionally, cerebral hypomyelination
Congenital muscular dystrophy (Fukuyama form)	AR	Fukutin (heart, muscle, brain, pancreas)	Onset in infancy, MR, ocular deficits, diffuse weakness, seizures, most die by age 20 years, orthopaedic problems similar to merosin-deficient form
Fascioscapulohumeral muscular dystrophy	AD	4q35 region (deletion of tandem repeats)	Weakness proximal to distal, difficulty whistling, closing eyes, winged scapula, some with hand, leg, and axial weakness
Myotonic dystrophy	AD	Protein kinase (repeat in 3' CTG)	Most common adult onset but also more severe congenital form; associated with mild MR, frontal baldness, weakness of throat muscles, persistent contraction, distal weakness first, then proximal; cardiac conduction and other organ abnormalities
Emery-Dreifuss muscular dystrophy	XR	Emerin	Fibrosis common of elbows, Achilles tendon and posterior cervical muscle; cardiac abnormalities common
Congenital myopathy	AD-central core, nemaline core XR-Myotubular	Ryanodine receptor for central core, other gene products unknown	Hypotonic infants, weakness leads to developmental delay; reports of malignant hyperthermia; long faces, high-pitched voices, scapular winging, arachnodactyly, joint contractures, clubfeet dislocated hips
Polyneuropathies (hereditary motor sensory neuropathy)			
Type I and III hypertrophic type	Most AD, some recessive varieties (more severe)	Deficient peripheral myelin protein, myelin protein zero	Sensory defects and distal weakness of clawing hands and feet, equinovarus, scoliosis, hip dysplasia; decreased reflexes; weakness usually slowly progressive, with onset in childhood except Dejerine-Sottas (III) variety has infantile onset
Type II axonopathy	AD and XR	Not known	Rarer, with normal reflexes, neuronal loss, leading to sensory and motor defects Severity variable
Others (IV-VII)	Variable	Not known	Includes cases associated with phytanic acid excess, familial spastic paresis, optic atrophy and retinitis pigmentosa
Motor neuron disease: spinal muscular atrophy	AD	Survival motor neuron gene defect leads to early death of anterior horn and brain neurons (linked to 5q)	Werdnig-Hoffman (I): onset birth to 6 months, with severe and diffuse weakness, early death Type II: intermediate Kugelberg-Welandeg: onset in childhood with normal life expectancy Osteopenia with fractures, contractures and scoliosis
Freidreich's ataxia (spinocerebellar degeneration)	AR	Frataxin: unstable GAA trinucleotide repeat at 9q21	Onset in adolescents with ataxia, dysarthria, and progressive loss of motor function, decreased reflexes, scoliosis, cardiomyopathy

XR = X-linked recessive; AD = autosomal dominant; AR = autosomal recessive; DMD = Duchenne muscular dystrophy; MR = mental retardation
See reference Younger and Gordon 1996 for other metabolic myopathies and myasthenic syndromes

Muscular Dystrophies and Myopathies

The discovery of mutations in genes encoding key sarcolemmal membrane proteins, including dystrophin and the sarcoglycans, that link the actin cytoskeleton to the surrounding extracellular matrix has resulted in a unifying hypothesis of muscle membrane instability as the cause of many forms of muscular dystrophy. Absence of these key proteins leads to membrane instability with muscle contractions and then fiber damage with increases in serum CPK and aldolase. Repair is aborted and muscles are replaced with fibrous tissue and fat.

The Dystrophinopathies

Duchenne and Becker muscular dystrophies are both caused by mutations in the gene encoding dystrophin; therefore, these two disorders are collectively referred to as dystrophinopathies. The gene encoding for dystrophin is the largest cloned mammalian gene, carrying 2.5 million base pairs. Defects in this gene account for 70% of males with muscular dystrophy.

Duchenne muscular dystrophy (DMD) is a fatal X-linked recessive condition resulting in the absence of dystrophin and progressive axial and appendicular muscle weakness. DMD is the most common inherited muscle disease, affecting 1 in 3,500 boys, and is caused by a frameshift mutation in the dystrophin gene located on the short arm of the X chromosome (Xp21.2). This gene mutation results in the synthesis of an unstable protein that is rapidly degraded. In the absence of dystrophin, the sarcolemma is no longer protected from acute injury during a forceful muscle contraction, resulting in muscle fiber necrosis, inflammation, and replacement by fat and fibrous tissue. The serum CPK level may be elevated over 100 times its normal level in DMD.

Boys with DMD develop progressive proximal muscle weakness, contractures of the joints of the upper and lower extremities, and eventually become wheelchair-dependent. The clinical features of DMD often become apparent between 3 and 6 years of age. Patients may exhibit a delay in independent ambulation, toe walking, frequent episodes of tripping and falling, or difficulty with running or climbing stairs. With time, gluteal weakness leads to excessive lumbar lordosis and a circumducting gait to compensate for weak hip flexors. Weakness in the pelvic girdle and proximal thigh muscles makes it difficult for patients with DMD to arise from a sitting position on the floor without using their upper extremities to force the knees and hips into extension (Gower's sign). Pseudohypertrophy of the calf muscles is common in the ambulatory phase. Cardiac muscle is involved in most patients, resulting in sinus tachycardia and right ventricular hypertrophy. Mild mental retardation is common. Most patients stop walking by age 12 years and often die of pulmonary insufficiency by age 20 years if ventilatory support is not provided.

Although prednisone may be of short-term benefit in preventing progressive weakness, the lack of a specific medical treatment has caused therapeutic efforts to focus on myoblast transplantation and gene therapy. To date, however, these new genetic manipulations have not been successful clinically.

Orthopaedic treatment consists primarily of physical therapy and bracing to prevent contractures, surgery to release the contractures that have occurred in spite of therapy, and spinal fusion for the scoliosis that develops once the patient has become wheelchair-bound. Treatment of scoliosis is addressed in chapter 48. The contractures are primarily manifested as flexion and abduction contractures of the hips, knee flexion contractures and equinus or equinovarus contractures of the ankles. If multilevel tenotomies are offered to preserve upright walking posture, tendon surgery includes the tensor fascia lata, iliotibial band and gastrocnemius tendon with concomitant release, transfer, or lengthening of the posterior tibial tendon.

Myotonic Dystrophy

Myotonic dystrophy is the most common form of adult onset muscular dystrophy, with a frequency of 1 in 8,000 live births, but there is a more severe congenital form that is associated with delayed motor development and mental retardation. Despite the autosomal dominant inheritance pattern, the congenital form is nearly always inherited from an affected mother. The disease is caused by a marked expansion in the number of triplet cytosine-thymine-guanine (CTG) repeats in the untranslated region of the gene encoding a protein kinase that appears to be involved in phosphorylation of muscle-specific sodium channels. The disease affects skeletal muscle, smooth muscle, myocardium, the brain, and the eyes.

The age of onset is proportional to the length of the CTG repeat, but most cases become evident in adolescence. The adult-onset patients develop myotonia (inability to relax skeletal muscle), gonadal atrophy, cataracts, frontal baldness, heart disease, diabetes mellitus, and dementia. Wasting of the temporalis and masseter muscles results in the characteristic long, narrow face. In the congenital form, hypotonia, feeding difficulties caused by pharyngeal weakness, respiratory failure, and facial weakness are more prominent. Approximately 25% of infants with myotonic dystrophy die because of failure to develop adequate respiratory function. Muscle function often improves after the neonatal period in those who survive. Myotonia is absent at birth but usually develops by age 10 years. Mild or moderate mental retardation affects 75% of children. Muscle biopsy reveals fiber atrophy with central nuclei rather than myopathic changes.

Unlike many muscle diseases, in myotonic dystrophy weakness of distal muscles of the hands and feet is apparent first. Equinovarus foot deformites may be seen at birth and are difficult to treat, often requiring talectomy. Contractures of the wrist and elbows are common, along with hip dislocation in infants and children. Spine deformity is more common in patients with positive family histories (and, correspondingly, long CTG repeats).

Hereditary Motor-Sensory Neuropathy

The features of a polyneuropathy causing weakness and wasting of the legs and feet initially and subsequent wasting of the hands (Charcot-Marie-Tooth) is presently referred to as hereditary motor-sensory neuropathies (HMSN). This most common form of polyneuropathy occurs with a frequency of 1 in 2,500 individuals. There are at least seven types of hereditary motor-sensory neuropathy and the most common variety has an autosomal dominant pattern of inheritance but recessive and X-linked varieties also exist. Two broad categories or HMSN are recognized, the hypertrophic, demyelinating (types I and III), and the rarer, axonal (neuronal) type II. The genetics of these disorders is being established but it is recognized that they are caused by either DNA duplications or point mutation defects in genes controlling myelination (peripheral myelin protein and myelin protein zero). An X-linked dominant disorder has been associated with defects in the gene for connexin, a connecting protein involved with myelination.

HMSN typically occurs in childhood but the Dejerine-Sottas variety (HMSN III) first occurs in infants. Although sensory neuropathy does occur, motor neuropathy characterizes the HMSN. For the demyelinating, hypertrophic form, nerve conduction velocities are uniformly decreased (Table 4), with nerve biopsy showing the "onion bulb" hypertrophy of the myelin sheath. For the neuronal form, the nerve conduction velocities may be only slightly slowed but the compound muscle action potential is decreased. Demyelination also is seen. Muscle biopsy shows atrophy of fiber groups.

Common clinical findings include weakness of distal muscles, more so in the lower than the upper extremity. The intrinsic muscles of the foot are affected first, then the peroneals. Deep tendon reflexes are diminished or absent in demyelinating forms, especially at the ankles. Sensory function (for example, vibration sense, light touch and position sense) often are impaired distally. In some varieties, patients have tremors, ataxia, spastic paraparesis, deafness, optic atrophy, and retinitis pigmentosa.

Musculoskeletal deformities usually begin with the foot. Intrinsic muscle weakness results in claw toes, plantar flexion of the first metatarsal head, and pes cavus. Toe deformities can be treated by flexor to extensor tendon transfers, transfer of the long extensor to the metatarsal head, and interphangeal fusions. Flexible cavus can be treated with plantar release or plantar and medial release. In an effort to balance muscle force across the foot, tendon transfers such as centralization of the tibialis anterior or transfer of the tibialis posterior to the dorsum of the foot has been useful. Heel cord lengthening is rarely required. Usually the appearance of equinus is at the forefoot rather than the ankle. Fixed bony varus or cavus deformity can be managed with osteotomy of the os calcis or midtarsal bones. Triple arthrodesis should be reserved as a salvage procedure. The Coleman block test is used to differentiate fixed from flexible deformities by having the patient stand with the lateral border of the foot on a 1-cm block. If the heel tilts out of varus, then this is evidence of a flexible hindfoot deformity that can be treated with primarily forefoot surgery.

Hip dysplasia occurs in 6% to 8% of patients with HMSN. Pain is present in patients age 5 to 15 years and osteotomy of the pelvis or upper femur may be required.

Hand problems are essentially those of intrinsic muscle weakness. Transfers such as the flexor digitorum subliminis to the adductor pollicis brevis may be useful to enhance pinch grasp. Nerve compression neuropathy can be improved by surgical releases.

Scoliosis may occur in as few as 10% of patients or in as many as 50%, depending on the population studied and the criteria used to make the diagnosis. Scoliosis is more common in females and there is general agreement that the curves resemble idiopathic scoliosis.

Friedreich's Ataxia

Friedreich's ataxia is an autosomal recessive disorder caused by an unstable trinucleotide repeat (GAA) at the *9q21* gene locus and producing spinocerebellar degeneration. The incidence is 1 in 50,000 live births. The gene codes for a protein called frataxin. As with myotonic muscular dystrophy, in which there is also an unstable repeat of a trinucleotide group, the severity of the symptoms is proportional to the length of the repeat.

In general, symptoms begin before age 20 years. Progressive ataxia and difficulty with gait are the most common presenting symptoms. Dysarthria is common. Physical examination will usually demonstrate absent deep tendon reflexes in both the upper and lower extremities. However, upper motor neuron signs, such as the Babinski, are often positive. Decreases in vibration and position sense may be observed. Muscle weakness is common. The first muscles to weaken are the limb girdle muscles of the lower extremity, particularly the hip extensors and abductors. Cardiomyopathy is often present and can be identified by electrocardiography. All patients develop scoliosis. The CPK level is normal. Electromyograms demonstrate loss of motor units in a neurogenic pattern. The nerve conduction velocities are slowed. Fewer than half the patients will have optic atrophy, nystagmus, distal muscle weakness, deafness, or diabetes mellitus.

Most individuals with Friedreich's ataxia start using a wheelchair at least part-time during the second decade of life. The ataxia and poor balance, rather than the muscle weakness, cause these patients to stop walking. Most patients die of cardiomyopathy or pneumonia in the fourth or fifth decade of life.

The most common foot deformity in Friedreich's ataxia is pes cavovarus. Tenotomy, lengthening, or transfer of tibialis anterior and/or posterior tendons have been used to maintain plantargrade foot position. Triple arthrodesis is a salvage procedure.

All patients will develop scoliosis and the curve patterns are similar to those observed in idiopathic scoliosis. Approximately two thirds also have kyphosis. If the disease onset is early in life, curve progression is likely. Spinal orthoses may slow the rate of curve progression, but the device may make ambulation more difficult. Some individuals with later onset of disease symptoms may never reach 40° and the curve may not progress after skeletal maturity. In curves greater than 40°, posterior spine fusion is recommended whereas combined anterior and posterior fusion may be required for particularly large and rigid curves.

Spinal Muscular Atrophy

The spinal muscular atrophies occur at a rate of 1 in 20,000 live births. All are autosomal recessive disorders involving a mutation at the *5q13* locus, the site of the survival motor neuron gene. The disease process involves degeneration of anterior horn cells and brainstem motor nuclei. The loss of anterior horn cells is acute and nonprogressive, but progressive weakness can occur as growth progresses beyond muscle reserve. Antenatal diagnosis is available through the survival motor neuron gene deletion test.

The spinal muscular atrophies are generally divided into three types depending on the natural history and severity of symptoms. Spinal muscular atrophy type I, Werdnig-Hoffman disease, is the most severe type with onset at birth to 6 months of age. These children are profoundly hypotonic, weak, never sit without support, and generally die before age 2 years. Type II is intermediate, with signs and symptoms apparent before 18 months. These children can sit but do not stand, and life expectancy is into the fourth and fifth decades of life. Type III is the mild form also known as Kugelberg-Welander disease with onset after 18 months of age. Patients do walk and have a normal life expectancy.

Hip subluxations and dislocations are not unusual in the face of proximal muscle imbalance. If subluxation is identified early, adductor tenotomy and iliopsoas recession may prevent dislocation. Later, upper femoral varus osteotomy, open reduction, or pelvic osteotomy may be considered. Posterior acetabular coverage of the femoral head is poor in spinal muscular atrophy, and this fact will affect the selection of pelvic osteotomy.

Patients who survive into adolescence will develop progressive scoliosis because of muscle weakness. About one third of the patients will have associated kyphosis that progresses as well. Bracing can help provide sitting balance and may slow the rate of curve progression in both ambulatory and nonambulatory patients, but the spinal orthoses can interfere with activities of daily living. If scoliosis measures more than 40° and the forced vital capacity is more than 30% to 40% of predicted, full-length, posterior spine fusion with segmental fixation is considered. Fixation to the pelvis is recommended to address pelvic obliquity. Complications are common and include hemorrhage, pulmonary problems, loss of fixation, infection, pseudarthrosis, and death. Postoperative bracing is not well tolerated. In patients with marginal ambulatory abilities, walking may be impossible after long spinal fusions because the patients can no longer balance by trunk posturing.

Annotated Bibliography

Cerebral Palsy

Abel MF, Damiano DL, Pannunzio M, Bush J: Muscle-tendon surgery in diplegic cerebral palsy: Functional and mechanical changes. *J Pediatr Orthop* 1999;19: 366-375.
  The effects of muscle-tendon surgery done as isolated procedures in patients with spastic diplegia are prospectively reviewed.

Auff E, Poewe W: The clinical applications of botulinum toxin type A. *Eur J Neurol* 1999;6(suppl 4):1-125.
  This supplement is devoted to reports on the use of botulinum toxin.

Badawi N, Watson L, Petterson B, et al: What constitutes cerebral palsy? *Dev Med Child Neurol* 1998;40:520-527.

The types of CP and etiologic relationships are described.

Cabanela ME, Weber M: Total hip arthroplasty in patients with neuromuscular disease. *J Bone Joint Surg Am* 2000;82:426-432.

This article presents the Mayo Clinic experience in treating spastic patients with total hip arthroplasty. Hip replacements were performed on 15 ambulatory patients with good results. Pain relief seemed to be the greatest benefit rather than functional increases. There was a relatively high number of complications.

Damiano DL, Abel MF: Functional outcomes of strength training in spastic cerebral palsy. *Arch Phys Med Rehabil* 1998;79:119-125.

The functional impact of a rigorously defined program of isotonic strengthening on patients with spastic CP is described.

McLaughlin JF, Bjornson KF, Astley SJ, et al: Selective dorsal rhizotomy: Efficacy and safety in an investigator-masked randomized clinical trial. *Dev Med Child Neurol* 1998;40:220-232.

This article presents results from one of three randomized, single institutional trials evaluating the functional impact of rhizotomy. Findings show that selective dorsal rhizotomy is safe and reduces spasticity in children with spastic diplegia. However, physical therapy alone resulted in independent mobility at 24 months, as did physical therapy plus rhizotomy.

McNerney NP, Mubarak SJ, Wenger DR: One-stage correction of the dysplastic hip in cerebral palsy with the San Diego acetabuloplasty: Results and complications in 104 hips. *J Pediatr Orthop* 2000;20:93-103.

This article presents a retrospective review of 92 patients with CP undergoing extensive hip reconstruction with acetabular and femoral osteotomies, soft-tissue release, and in some cases, capsulorrhaphies. Details of the acetabuloplasty are illustrated. This series shows that high complication rates can be expected but ultimately a high percentage of radiographic success in terms of stable positions can be achieved. Effects on pain reduction and seating are less obvious. Guidelines for reconstructions of chronic deformities are provided.

Myelomeningocele

Banta J: Neuromuscular scoliosis. *Spine* 2000;1:219-232.

A review of the management of neuromuscular scoliosis, including the myelomeningocele population, is presented.

Broughton NS, Menelaus MB (eds): *Menelaus' Orthopaedic Management of Spina Bifida Cystica*, ed 3. London, England, WB Saunders, 1998.

All relevant topics regarding spina bifida cystica are covered including embryology, epidemiology, orthotics, deformities and their treatment, and rehabilitation strategies.

Drennan JC: Current concepts in myelomeningocele. *Instr Course Lect* 1999;48:543-550.

This article presents a discussion of foot deformities and their treatment as well as a review of latex allergy and sensitivity in the myelomeningocele population.

Greene WB: Treatment of hip and knee problems in myelomeningocele. *Instr Course Lect* 1999;48:563-574.

A discussion of the various deformities at the hip and knee including surgical and nonsurgical care is presented.

McLone DG: Care of the neonate with a myelomeningocele. *Neurosurg Clin North Am* 1998;9:111-120.

This article presents an excellent review of the neurosurgical treatment of the newborn with myelomeningocele.

Selber P, Dias L: Sacral-level myelomeningocele: Long-term outcome in adults. *J Pediatr Orthop* 1998;18:423-427.

Forty-six adults with sacral level myelomeningocele were studied. At final follow-up, 41 of 46 were community ambulators. Aggressive management of neurosurgical problems such as tethered cord, correction of musculoskeletal deformities, and avoidance of foot fusions were thought to result in better outcomes.

Neurodegenerative Disorders

Birch JG: Orthopedic management of neuromuscular disorders in children. *Semin Pediatr Neurol* 1998;5:78-91.

This article presents a discussion of the principles, rationales, and treatment strategies for musculoskeletal deformities associated with Duchenne muscular dystrophy, spinal muscular atrophy, fascioscapulohumeral dystrophy, and Charcot-Marie-Tooth disease.

Hart DA, McDonald CM: Spinal deformity in progressive neuromuscular disease: Natural history and management. *Phys Med Rehabil Clin North Am* 1998;9:213-232.

The prevalence, natural history, and treatment of spine deformity in the muscular dystrophies, spinal muscular atrophy, and Friedreich's ataxia are discussed.

McDonald CM: Neuromuscular diseases, in Molnar GE, Alexander MA (eds): *Pediatric Rehabilitation*, ed 3. Philadelphia, PA, Hanley & Belfus, 1999, pp 289-330.

This article gives a comprehensive description of childhood neuromuscular diseases with an extensive bibliography.

Tsao CY, Mendell JR: The childhood muscular dystrophies: Making order out of chaos. *Semin Neurol* 1999;19:9-23.

How the transition from the premolecular to molecular era of myology has transformed the diagnosis and categorization of childhood muscular dystrophies is discussed.

Classic Bibliography

Beauchamp M, Labelle H, Duhaime M, Joncas J: Natural history of muscle weakness in Friedreich's ataxia and its relation to loss of ambulation. *Clin Orthop* 1995;311:270-275.

Blair E, Stanley FJ: Issues in the classification and epidemiology of cerebral palsy. *Mental Retard Dev Disab Res Rev* 1997;3:184-193.

Bleck EE (ed): *Orthopaedic Management in Cerebral Palsy*. London, England, MacKeith Press, 1987.

Brin MF: Botulinum toxin: Chemistry, pharmacology, toxicity, and immunology. *Muscle Nerve* 1997;6(suppl): S146-S168.

Broughton NS, Menelaus MB, Cole WG, Shurtleff DB: The natural history of hip deformity in myelomeningocele. *J Bone Joint Surg Br* 1993;75:760-763.

Cambridge W, Drennan JC: Scoliosis associated with Duchenne muscular dystrophy. *J Pediatr Orthop* 1987; 7:436-440.

Carter GT, Abresch RT, Fowler WM Jr, Johnson ER, Kilmer DD, McDonald CM: Profiles of neuromuscular diseases: Hereditary motor and sensory neuropathy, types I and II. *Am J Phys Med Rehabil* 1995;74(suppl 5):S140-S149.

Carter GT, Abresch RT, Fowler WM Jr, Johnson ER, Kilmer DD, McDonald CM: Profiles in neuromuscular diseases: Spinal muscular atrophy. *Am J Phys Med Rehabil* 1995;74(suppl 5):S150-S159.

Dietz FR, Mathews KD: Update on the genetic bases of disorders with orthopaedic manifestations. *J Bone Joint Surg Am* 1996:78:1583-1598.

Gage JR, DeLuca PA, Renshaw TS: Gait analysis: Principles and applications with emphasis on its use in cerebral palsy. *J Bone Joint Surg Am* 1995;77: 1607-1623.

Johnson ER, Abresch RT, Carter GT, et al: Profiles of neuromuscular diseases: Myotonic dystrophy. *Am J Phys Med Rehabil* 1995;74(suppl 5):S104-S116.

Kurz LT, Mubarak SJ, Schultz P, Park SM, Leach J: Correlation of scoliosis and pulmonary function in Duchenne muscular dystrophy. *J Pediatr Orthop* 1983; 3:347-353.

Miller F, Bagg MR: Age and migration percentage as risk factors for progression in spastic hip disease. *Dev Med Child Neurol* 1995;37:449-455.

Rideau Y, Duport G, Delaubier A, Guillou C, Renardel-Irani A, Bach JR: Early treatment to preserve quality of locomotion for children with Duchenne muscular dystrophy. *Semin Neurol* 1995;15:9-17.

Vignos PJ, Wagner MB, Karlinchak B, Katirji B: Evaluation of a program for long-term treatment of Duchenne muscular dystrophy: Experience at the University Hospitals of Cleveland. *J Bone Joint Surg Am* 1996;78: 1844-1852.

Worton R: Muscular dystrophies: Diseases of the dystrophin-glycoprotein complex. *Science* 1995;270:755-756.

Younger DS, Gordon PH: Diagnosis in neuromuscular diseases. *Neurol Clin* 1996;14:135-168.

Chapter 23

Pediatric Hematologic and Related Conditions

Norman Y. Otsuka, MD, FRCSC

Hemophilia

Hemophilia is a bleeding disorder resulting from a deficiency in either plasma factor VIII (hemophilia A) or factor IX (hemophilia B). Both hemophilia A (classic) and hemophilia B (Christmas) are X chromosome-linked recessive disorders and are indistinguishable clinically. Hemophilia A occurs in 1 per 5,000 live male births and is approximately six times more common than hemophilia B. More than 370 different mutations have been identified in the gene for factor VIII. Prenatal diagnosis is possible by linkage studies or direct gene analysis, but more than one third of hemophilia cases are the result of spontaneous mutations. Postnatal diagnosis is made by direct assay of plasma factor VIII or IX activity levels. Hemophilia is classified as mild when factor levels are 5% to 30% of normal, moderate when factor levels are 1% to 5%, and severe when less than 1%. Most children with hemophilia have the severe form, with bleeding manifestations beginning around 1 year of age.

Hemarthrosis is the most frequent bleeding complication in children with hemophilia. The knee is the most commonly affected joint, followed by the elbow and then the ankle. Other acute musculoskeletal complications include soft-tissue hematomas, compartment syndrome, carpal tunnel syndrome, and femoral neurapraxia. In patients with hemophilia, the first-line therapy for each of these complications is factor replacement. The deficient factor can be replaced continuously or with intermittent boluses. Several forms of factor VIII and IX are available. Most pediatric patients are now treated with high purity plasma-derived or recombinant factor concentrates that are substantially more costly than less pure products. In general, the plasma activity level will increase 2% for every unit/kg of factor VIII given and 1% for every unit/kg of factor IX given. To treat most bleeding episodes in muscles and joints, circulating levels of the deficient factor must reach 40% to 50% of normal. Surgical procedures require replacement to 100%.

With repeated exposure to blood, the synovium of a joint hypertrophies and becomes hypervascular, leading to a progressive cycle of synovitis and more bleeding. The precise pathophysiology of chronic synovitis is unknown, but iron deposition (from breakdown of hemoglobin) stimulates synoviocyte proliferation and the release of inflammatory cytokines and inhibits chondrocyte activity. Chronic synovitis can be treated surgically with either open or arthroscopic synovectomy. Bleeding episodes are reduced in 80% of patients after synovectomy.

Chronic synovitis has several other deleterious effects on joint function in addition to destroying articular cartilage. Flexion contractures often develop because of chronic swelling and pain in the joint. The hyperemia of synovitis may cause asymmetric physeal growth, leading to significant angular deformities. At the end stages of hemophilic arthropathy, young patients may face severe disabilities with few treatment options. Total joint arthroplasty can be useful in adults with hemophilic arthropathy but has been associated with high rates of loosening and infection, especially in patients seropositive for human immunodeficiency virus (HIV).

Patients who have factor levels greater than 1% rarely develop significant hemophilic arthropathy. As a result, there has been growing interest over the past decade in prophylaxis for patients with severe hemophilia. Primary prophylaxis involves the maintenance of factor levels between 1% to 5%, starting at age 1 to 2 years, before significant joint hemorrhage occurs. Patients treated with primary prophylaxis required four times as much factor concentrate as "on-demand" treated patients (factor given when bleeding occurs), but had less than one hemarthrosis per year and had clinically and radiographically normal joints at 10-year follow-up. Secondary prophylaxis involves patients who are treated after an established pattern of bleeding but before frequent joint bleeding occurs. Secondary prophylaxis did decrease the episodes of hemarthrosis but the joints continued to deteriorate.

Up to one third of patients with severe hemophilia A develop inhibitors (antibodies) that neutralize factor VIII's coagulant activity. Inhibitor formation is rare (incidence of <4%) in patients with hemophilia B. Persistent inhibitor formation is one of the most serious treatment complications of hemophilia because it renders the patient resistant to factor replacement and significantly alters the morbidity and mortality of hemophilia. It is not yet possible to predict which patients will form inhibitors. Patients with genetic mutations (such as deletion) that eliminate endogenous factor production appear to be at greater risk of reacting to exogenous factor. If inhibitor titers are low, higher doses of factor replacement may be used to treat hemorrhage. In patients with high titers, an activated prothrombin complex concentrate can be used to bypass the deficient clotting factor. The best long-term treatment option requires daily factor infusion to render the patient immunologically tolerant to the clotting factor. Before 1985, more than 50% of patients with hemophilia who were treated with plasma-derived factor concentrates were infected with HIV. HIV transmission from clotting factor concentrate has not been documented since 1986 because of improved testing and purification methods.

Sickle Cell Disease

Sickle cell disease is a hereditary disorder of hemoglobin that distorts red blood cell architecture, leading to hemolytic anemia and microvascular occlusion. About 1 in 600 African-Americans are homozygous for the abnormal hemoglobin S gene (sickle cell anemia). Sickle cell anemia also can occur if hemoglobin S is inherited with other abnormal β-globulins. Eight percent of African-Americans carry a hemoglobin S gene and a normal β-globulin gene (sickle cell trait). These individuals normally do not have anemia or other significant clinical manifestations.

Pneumococcal sepsis is the leading cause of death among infants with sickle cell disease, and preventive treatment is with penicillin prophylaxis and vaccination. Although sickle cell disease can affect splenic, hepatic, renal, and neurologic function, musculoskeletal symptoms account for 80% of all hospital admissions. Musculoskeletal complications include bone infarction (sickle cell crisis), osteomyelitis, and osteonecrosis. Dactylitis, tenderness and swelling of the digits on the hands and feet, is the earliest manifestation of bone infarctions that affect up to 73% of patients age 6 months to 4 years. Children who have an episode of

dactylitis before the age of 1 year are at higher risk of having severe sickle cell disease later in life. Painful bone and joint crises occur most frequently between age 3 years and skeletal maturity. Symptoms can include swelling, tenderness, fever (usually less than 39°C) and leukocytosis, making severe sickle cell disease difficult to distinguish from infection. Most vaso-occlusive crises respond to analgesics, oxygen, and hydration in 3 to 7 days. Recent studies have demonstrated a significant reduction in the frequency of sickle cell crisis with long-term administration of hydroxyurea. This chemotherapeutic agent increases fetal hemoglobin concentrations, which improves red blood cell function.

Infections are common in patients with sickle cell disease, but compared with the frequency of sickle cell crisis, the incidence of osteomyelitis remains low (< 1% per year). Differentiating acute bone infarction from osteomyelitis is often difficult because of significant overlap in symptoms, laboratory values, and radiographic findings. Routine workup should include blood cultures and when infection is suspected, bone aspiration. Causative organisms include *Staphylococcus aureus*, *Salmonella*, and *Streptococcus pneumoniae*. MRI and bone scans have been used to identify cases of osteomyelitis, but ultrasonography may be equally effective and less expensive. Septic arthritis and sterile reactive arthritis have been reported but are relatively rare. All cases of subperiosteal abscess, osteomyelitis, and septic arthritis require surgical drainage.

Osteonecrosis of the femoral head is common in sickle cell disease, with a prevalence of 4.6% after age 10 years, and increasing to 32.5% in the fourth decade. The prognosis worsens with increasing age of onset. Total joint replacement is rarely indicated in young adults with sickle cell disease and when done in these patients increases the risk of infection and loosening.

Thalassemia

The thalassemia syndromes are a heterogeneous group of hemolytic anemias that result from absent or deficient synthesis of either α- or β-globulin chains. Thalassemia major (Cooley's anemia or β-thalassemia) is the severe form of the disease, usually accompanied by jaundice, hepatosplenomegaly, and transfusion-dependent anemia in the first year of life. In patients with thalassemia intermedia, disease presentation is variable, but these patients usually are not transfusion-dependent. Thalassemia minor patients have few symptoms and a normal life span.

Skeletal consequences of sporadically treated β-thalassemia include growth retardation, pathologic fractures, slipped capital femoral epiphysis, and premature osteoarthrosis. These problems stem from both

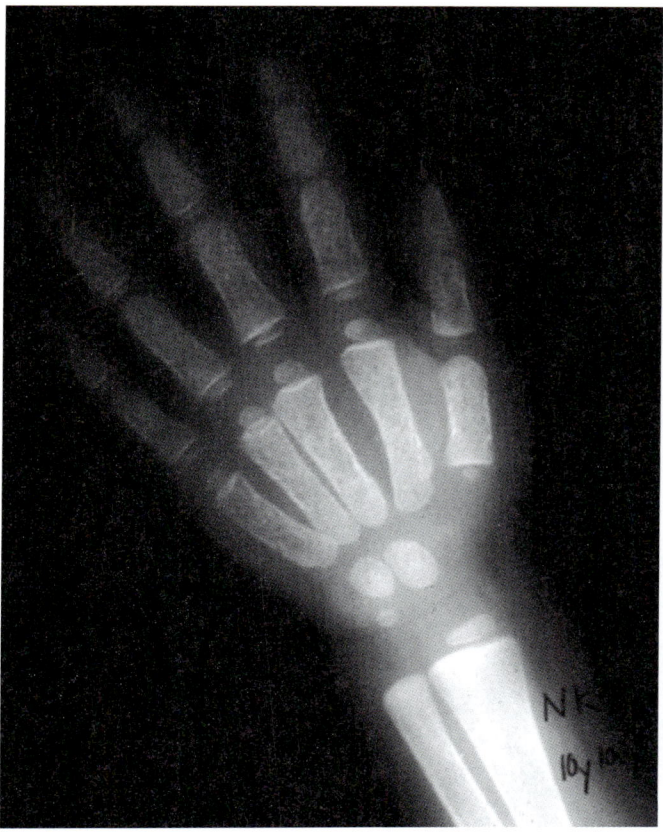

Figure 1 Radiograph of the hand of a 10-year-old child with thalassemia. Widened marrow spaces, thin cortices, and severe osteopenia are apparent. *(Courtesy of Beverly P. Wood, MD, Shriners Hospitals for Children, Los Angeles, CA).*

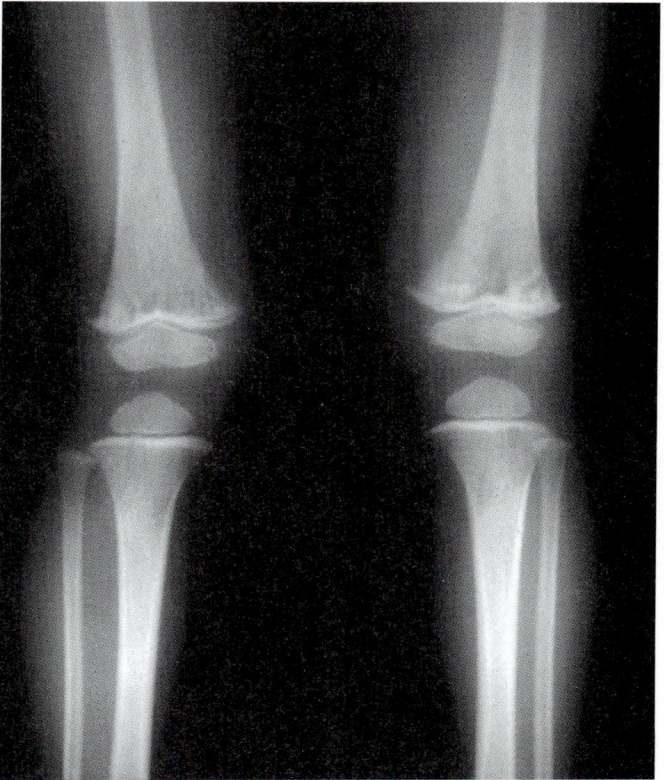

Figure 2 Radiograph of the lower extremities of a child with leukemia. Osteopenia, radiolucent metaphyseal bands, and periosteal changes are apparent. *(Courtesy of Beverly P. Wood, MD, Shriners Hospitals for Children, Los Angeles, CA).*

extreme bone marrow expansion and endocrinopathies (hypogonadism, hypothyroidism, growth hormone resistance). Radiographs may demonstrate widened marrow spaces, thin cortices, severe osteopenia (Fig. 1), and a "hair-on-end" appearance of the skull. Extramedullary hematopoiesis can also cause paraparesis by compression of the spinal cord. Early transfusion therapy (maintaining Hg > 9 g/dL) significantly reduces skeletal complications and when combined with iron chelation extends the life span of β-thalassemia patients into the fourth and fifth decade. Bone marrow transplantation and new supportive treatments reduce the morbidity associated with thalassemia. Recent advances in carrier screening and prenatal diagnosis have reduced the number of affected homozygotes in some at-risk Mediterranean populations.

Leukemia

Leukemia accounts for approximately one third of all childhood malignancies. Eighty percent of children with leukemia have acute lymphoblastic leukemia. The peak incidence occurs around 4 years of age. Common signs and symptoms of leukemia include lethargy, pallor, purpura, fever, lymphadenopathy, hepatospleno-

megaly, and bleeding. Up to 59% of children with acute leukemia have musculoskeletal symptoms. Extremity pain is most often localized to the metaphyseal region and described as intermittent, severe, and nonresponsive to salicylates. Children can present with back pain or a pathologic vertebral fracture.

Anemia, thrombocytopenia, and neutropenia are common laboratory findings in the early stages of disease, but peripheral blood counts are normal in 10% of patients. Identification of abnormal cells on a peripheral blood smear is diagnostic of leukemia. Three fourths of patients develop radiographic abnormalities. Severe radiographic changes can be asymptomatic, whereas symptomatic regions can have normal-appearing radiographs. Common manifestations include diffuse osteopenia and lytic lesions. Cortical lysis and periosteal new bone formation may mimic osteomyelitis. Radiolucent metaphyseal bands (called leukemia lines) are often associated with leukemia but occur in other chronic childhood diseases as a result of metabolic dysfunction (Fig. 2).

Bone pain associated with leukemia typically responds rapidly to chemotherapy. New chemotherapy regimens have increased the 5-year survival rate of acute lymphoblastic leukemia to more than 80%. Treatment with radiation and bone marrow transplant has also improved the prognosis. Radiation has been associated with mild scoliosis, slipped capital femoral epiphysis, and sarcomas. One of the most common complications of leukemia therapy, with a prevalence as high as 18%, is osteonecrosis of the femoral head. Osteonecrosis in these patients tends to affect multiple joints, often symmetrically. Treatment options include protected weight bearing, anti-inflammatory agents, core decompression, osteotomies, and total hip replacement.

Gaucher's Disease

Glucocerebroside is a primary component of cell membranes. Gaucher's disease, which is caused by a deficiency in the enzyme glucocerebrosidase, is characterized by accumulation of glucocerebroside in the lysosomes of macrophages attempting to handle normal cell turnover. Transmission is autosomal recessive and clinical severity is variable, even among patients of the same genotype. The disease is classified into three clinical types. Type I (chronic, nonneuropathic) is the most common (occuring in more than 90% of affected patients) and presents at any age with variable visceral and osseous involvement. It is particularly prevalent among Ashkenazi Jews. Type II (acute, neuropathic, infantile) is characterized by severe neural involvement and is usually fatal in infancy. Type III (subacute, neuropathic, juvenile) begins in childhood with gradually progressive neurologic dysfunction.

Splenomegaly is a hallmark feature of Gaucher's disease. Hypersplenism and marrow replacement result in anemia, leukopenia, and thrombocytopenia. The skeletal manifestations include abnormal widening of the metaphysis, pathologic fractures, bone crises, osteonecrosis, and eventually arthrosis. Pathologic fractures most commonly involve the spine and proximal femur. Many cases can be managed nonsurgically. Assessment for spinal deformity should be done routinely. Multiple compression fractures may result in significant thoracic kyphosis that has progressed to neurologic compromise in some patients (Fig. 3). Prognosis for children with osteonecrosis of the femoral head and Gaucher's disease is guarded; these patients are best managed initially with bed rest, analgesics, and activity modification. Splenectomized patients have improved cell counts but are at greater risk of pathologic fractures of the spine, osteonecrosis of the femoral head, and infection. Surgical treatment for fractures, osteonecrosis, or arthrosis is associated with increased rates of bleeding, infection, and prosthetic loosening with Gaucher's disease.

A Gaucher's disease crisis is characterized by acute, severe, localized bone pain that usually lasts several days. This disease is often difficult to differentiate from

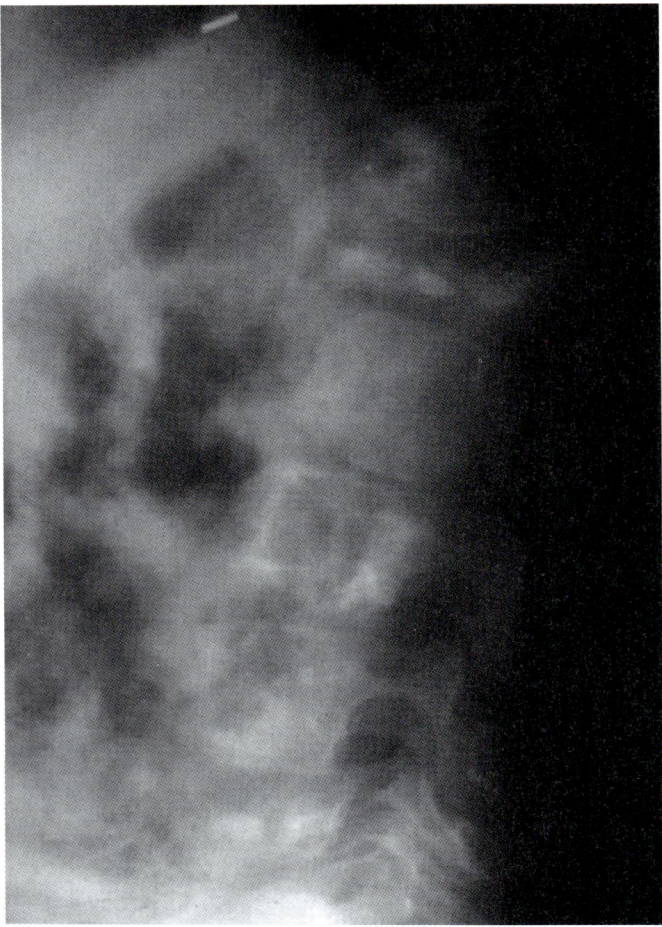

Figure 3 Gaucher's disease. Multiple compression fractures of the spine are seen. *(Courtesy of Beverly P. Wood, MD, Shriners Hospitals for Children, Los Angeles, CA).*

osteomyelitis because findings at presentation may include fever, an elevated white blood cell count, and an elevated erythrocyte sedimentation rate. Radiographic findings in the diseases are often similar as well, but unlike in osteomyelitis, increased uptake on a technetium Tc 99m scan is often not seen.

Enzyme replacement therapy (with alglucerase) is now available for patients with moderate to severe symptoms. Visceral changes can respond rapidly to enzyme replacement. With long-term replacement therapy, some skeletal manifestations of Gaucher's disease have been reversed.

Fanconi's Anemia

Fanconi's anemia is an autosomal recessive disease characterized by multiple congenital abnormalities, progressive bone marrow failure, and a predisposition to malignancy. Mutations in proteins that affect DNA repair cause the disease. Early diagnosis is critical to surgical planning, genetic counseling, and medical treatment. Carrier and prenatal testing is now available. A high variability in the phenotype and considerable overlap with other syndromes (vertebral, anal, cardiac, tracheal, esophageal, renal, and limb; Baller-Gerold syndrome; Bloom syndrome) make the diagnosis of Fanconi's anemia on clinical manifestations difficult. It is frequently associated with short stature, café-au-lait spots, microcephaly, and micrognathia. The most common skeletal anomaly is a radial deficiency of the hand or forearm. Anomalies extend from distal to proximal (thumb is abnormal if radius is abnormal). Lower extremity anomalies, such as hip and knee dysplasia, can occur but are less common. Ninety percent of patients develop aplastic anemia and 10% develop leukemia. The mean age of onset of anemia is 8 years and the mean survival is 16 years. In addition to transfusions, treatment of the anemia is with corticosteroids (to minimize growth and arrest) and androgens (oxymetholone). Bone marrow transplants and transplants of placental stem cells have been effective in some cases.

Thrombocytopenia With Absent Radii

Thrombocytopenia with absent radii syndrome is a rare autosomal recessive disorder characterized by congenital extremity anomalies and problems with hemostasis in infancy. It is distinguished from other radial deficiency syndromes by bilateral involvement and intact thumbs. Management of upper extremity anomalies includes adaptive devices for activities of daily living and centralization procedures in patients with good elbow and shoulder function. Lower extremity anomalies occur in up to 80% of patients and often require surgical intervention. Common deformities include genu varum associated with flexion contractures, tibial torsion, and talipes equinovarus. Occult hip dysplasia is common enough to warrant screening radiographs once a child reaches walking age. Hematologic findings are hypomegakaryocytic thrombocytopenia, periodic leukemoid reactions, and eosinophilia. Episodes of thrombocytopenia occur most frequently before the age of 2 years with morbidity and mortality secondary to intracranial hemorrhage. Prenatal diagnosis and in utero platelet transfusion are possible. If the patient survives beyond 2 years of age, thrombocytopenia typically resolves and a normal life span can be expected. Cardiac abnormalities (tetralogy of Fallot and atrial septal defect) and allergy to cow's milk are other common clinical features of thrombocytopenia with absent radii.

Annotated Bibliography

Hemophilia

Cohen I, Heim M, Martinowitz U, Chechick A: Orthopaedic outcome of total knee replacement in haemophilia A. *Haemophilia* 2000;6:104-109.
    Twenty-one consecutive total knee replacements were done in 16 patients with hemophilia. Knee scores were improved at follow-up of 5.6 years. Complications included three infections, two cases of arthrofibrosis, and no cases of loosening.

Kay MA, High K: Gene therapy for the hemophilias. *Proc Natl Acad Sci U S A* 1999;96:9973-9975.
    This article covers the recent advances and continuing challenges of gene therapy for hemophilia.

Penner JA: Management of haemophilia in patients with high-titre inhibitors: Focus on the evolution of activated prothrombin complex concentrate AUTO-PLEX T. *Haemophilia* 1999;5(suppl 3):1-9.
    Treatment with inhibitors for patients with hemophilia is discussed.

Roosendaal G, Vianen ME, Wenting MJ, et al: Iron deposits and catabolic properties of synovial tissue from patients with haemophilia. *J Bone Joint Surg Br* 1998;80:540-545.
    This article presents an in vitro analysis implicating iron deposition in synovitis. Hemosiderin-stained synovial tissue had increased production of inflammatory cytokines and catabolic effects on chondrocytes.

Rodriguez-Merchan EC: Management of the orthopaedic complications of haemophilia. *J Bone Joint Surg Br* 1998;80:191-196.
    A recent review of common orthopaedic manifestations of hemophilia and their treatment is presented.

Sickle Cell Disease

Miller ST, Sleeper LA, Pegelow CH, et al: Prediction of adverse outcomes in children with sickle cell disease. *N Engl J Med* 2000;342:83-89.
    The clinical course of 392 children with sickle cell disease was followed for an average of 10 years. The presence of dactylitis, severe anemia, and leukocytosis before 2 years of age were associated with more severe forms of sickle cell disease later in life.

Mukisi-Mukaza M, Elbaz A, Samuel-Leborgne Y, et al: Prevalence, clinical features, and risk factors of osteonecrosis of the femoral head among adults with sickle cell disease. *Orthopedics* 2000;23:357-363.
    Radiographic screening of symptomatic osteonecrosis of the femoral head revealed a prevalence of osteonecrosis as high as 37%.

Steinberg MH: Management of sickle cell disease. *N Engl J Med* 1999;340:1021-1030.

An excellent review of the current medical therapy for sickle cell disease is presented.

Thalassemia

Rund D, Rachmilewitz E: New trends in the treatment of beta-thalassemia. *Crit Rev Oncol Hematol* 2000;33: 105-118.

This review covers existing and potential therapeutic modalities for supportive and curative treatment of thalassemia.

Wonke B: Bone disease in beta-thalassaemia major. *Br J Haematol* 1998;103:897-901.

The skeletal manifestations of thalassemia are reviewed.

Leukemia

Kayser R, Mahlfeld K, Nebelung W, Grasshoff H: Vertebral collapse and normal peripheral blood cell count at the onset of acute lymphatic leukemia in childhood. *J Pediatr Orthop B* 2000;9:55-57.

Although infrequent, childhood leukemia can present with vertebral collapse and a normal peripheral blood count.

Wei SY, Esmail AN, Bunin N, Dormans JP: Avascular necrosis in children with acute lymphoblastic leukemia. *J Pediatr Orthop* 2000;20:331-335.

In an institutional review of 222 patients with acute lymphoblastic leukemia, 4% had symptomatic avascular necrosis, which typically involved multiple joints when present.

Gaucher's Disease

Kocher MS, Hall JE: Surgical management of spinal involvement in children and adolescents with Gaucher's disease. *J Pediatr Orthop* 2000;20:383-388.

In a study of four patients with kyphosis secondary to Gaucher's disease, three of the four patients had the rare type 3 form. Neurologic compromise from severe kyphosis developed in two patients.

Rodrigue SW, Rosenthal DI, Barton NW, Zurakowski D, Mankin HJ: Risk factors for osteonecrosis in patients with Type 1 Gaucher's disease. *Clin Orthop* 1999;362: 201-207.

In a series of 51 patients with Gaucher's disease, 15 had osteonecrosis. Male gender and splenectomy were independent risk factors for the presence of osteonecrosis.

Fanconi's Anemia

Garcia-Higuera I, Kuang Y, D'Andrea AD: The molecular and cellular biology of Fanconi's anemia. *Curr Opin Hematol* 1999;6:83-88.

The authors describe the structure and function of the Fanconi's anemia genes and the role of the encoded Fanconi's anemia proteins in controlling chromosome stability.

Thrombocytopenia With Absent Radii

Christensen CP, Ferguson RL: Lower extremity deformities associated with thrombocytopenia and absent radius syndrome. *Clin Orthop* 2000;375:202-206.

Of the 11 patients studied with thrombocytopenia with absent radii syndrome, 8 had lower extremity deformities. These deformities frequently required surgical correction.

McLaurin TM, Bukrey CD, Lovett RJ, Mochel DM: Management of thrombocytopenia-absent radius (TAR) syndrome. *J Pediatr Orthop* 1999;19:289-296.

The clinical course and surgical management of 23 patients with thrombocytopenia with absent radii syndrome were studied. The authors concluded that the greatest gains in independence come from simple adaptive devices and wheelchairs.

Classic Bibliography

Alter BP: Arm anomalies and bone marrow failure may go hand in hand. *J Hand Surg Am* 1992;17:566-571.

Gallagher DJ, Phillips DJ, Heinrich SD: Orthopedic manifestations of acute pediatric leukemia. *Orthop Clin North Am* 1996;27:635-644.

Nilsson IM, Berntorp E, Lofqvist T, Pettersson H: Twenty-five years' experience of prophylactic treatment in severe haemophilia A and B. *J Intern Med* 1992;232:25-32.

Smith JA: Bone disorders in sickle cell disease. *Hematol Oncol Clin North Am* 1996;10:1345-1356.

Section 3

Upper Extremity

Section Editors:
Frederick M. Azar, MD
Paul Tornetta III, MD
Arnold-Peter Weiss, MD
Michael A. Wirth, MD

Chapter 24

Shoulder and Arm: Pediatric Aspects

Bruce L. Gillingham, MD

Congenital Anomalies and Acquired Disorders

Glenoid Hypoplasia

Hypoplasia of the glenoid has become increasingly recognized as both a primary condition and as a constituent of skeletal dysplasias, mucopolysaccharidoses, and other conditions including Holt-Oram, Apert's, and de Lange's syndromes. The rim of the normal glenoid arises from two ossification centers that develop between age 9 to 16 years. Glenoid hypoplasia results when the inferior apophysis fails to ossify. The primary contribution of this ossification center is to raise the rim of the glenoid and convert the convex glenoid of the child to the gentle concave fossa of the adult. Glenoid hypoplasia is usually bilateral and symmetric. Symptoms are generally present by the second or third decade and typically are associated with an increase in physical activity. Physical examination often demonstrates limited forward flexion. Multidirectional instability is frequently present. Plain radiographs reveal decreased ossification of the lower two thirds of the glenoid and adjacent scapular neck. The surface of the abnormal bony glenoid is either smooth or indented (dentate glenoid) (Fig. 1). Associated radiographic findings include prominence of the coracoid, a large and elongated acromion, varus alignment of the proximal humerus, and flattening of the humeral head. Thickening of the inferior aspect of the labrum is seen on CT arthrography. MRI demonstrates persistence of the cartilaginous inferior glenoid anlage. Symptomatic patients respond well to a rehabilitation program that focuses or the rotator cuff, deltoid, and scapular stabilizers. It is unclear at present if glenoid hypoplasia predisposes to degenerative arthritis of the shoulder.

Congenital Pseudarthrosis of the Clavicle

Congenital pseudarthrosis of the clavicle is a rare anomaly distinct from fracture at birth, neurofibromatosis, and cleidocranial dysplasia. Unilateral, right-sided involvement is most common, but bilateral cases occur in 10% of affected individuals. Pseudarthrosis of the clavicle is primarily of cosmetic concern. There is little functional disability in children and adolescents. Although familial cases have been reported, no definite genetic pattern has been established. Several etiologies have been proposed, including failure of the two primary clavicular ossification centers to coalesce. Interference of fetal clavicular development caused by the close proximity of the vascular pulsations of the subclavian artery has also been postulated. The more cephalad position of the right subclavian artery as it passes over the first rib posterior to the midclavicle is central to this hypothesis. Cervical and highly placed first ribs accentuate this anatomic relationship. A vascular etiology is supported by left-sided involvement in dextrocardia and the presence of thoracic outlet syndrome according to the results of one study. Compression of the subclavian artery by the medial end of the lateral clavicular fragment was demonstrated on arteriogram in this case.

A painless, palpable prominence in the middle third of the clavicle is generally recognized in infancy. Radiographically, an obvious midclavicular separation is seen with the middle segment elevated and displaced forward and the lateral segment depressed and posterior. Callus and periosteal reaction are not present. Absence of cranial sutural and fontanelle defects and pubic diastasis distinguish this condition from cleidocranial dysplasia. Spontaneous union does not occur. Surgical intervention is indicated for the rare patient with pain or significant cosmetic deformity. Infants and younger children between 7 months and 6 years of age have been successfully treated without bone grafting or internal fixation. Resection of the fibrous pseudarthrosis and sclerotic bone ends with preservation of the periosteal sleeve and approximation of the medial and lateral clavicular segments using absorbable suture is performed. Children older than age 6 years may

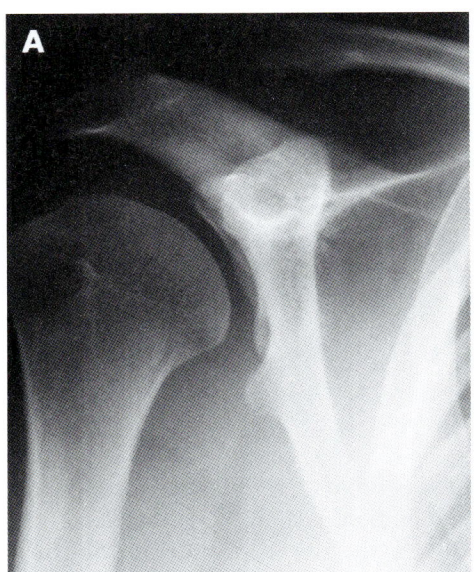
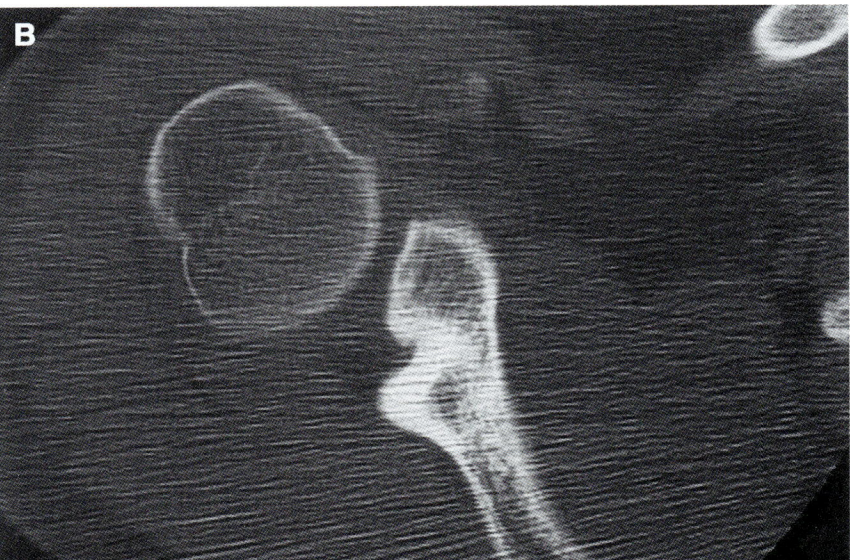

Figure 1 **A,** AP shoulder radiograph of an adult male with glenoid hypoplasia. Note dentate appearance of the inferior glenoid and associated flattening of the humeral head. **B,** Axial CT scan of the glenohumeral joint. Insufficiency of the posteroinferior glenoid is present with accompanying indentation of the articular surface.

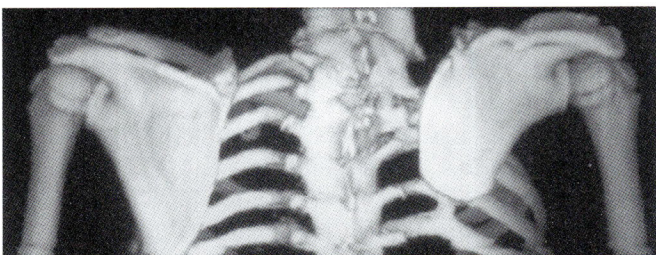

Figure 2 Three-dimensional CT reconstruction of bilateral shoulder girdle in a child with congenital undescended scapula. Elevation, malrotation, and hypoplasia of the scapula are present on the right side. Associated upper thoracic scoliosis is also present.

require autogenous bone grafting and compression plating following resection of the pseudarthrosis.

Congenital Undescended Scapula (Sprengel's Deformity)

The scapula lies at the level of C4 and C5 at the fifth week of gestation and migrates caudally below T3 by 12 weeks. Failure of descent results in a high, small, and wide scapula that is malrotated in comparison with to the opposite side (Fig. 2). Scapulothoracic motion is limited. The primary functional deficit is limitation of shoulder abduction to 90° to 100°. Associated anomalies are present in two thirds of patients and include scoliosis, hemivertebrae, rib synostosis, clavicular abnormalities, renal anomalies, and hypoplasia of the shoulder girdle musculature. In up to 50% of the patients, a fibrous band, cartilaginous bar, or omovertebral bone extends from the vertebral border of the superior scapular angle to a posterior element of the fourth to seventh cervical vertebrae. Improvement of

neck pain and cosmetic appearance can be accomplished with excision of the supraspinous portion of the scapula and omovertebral bone. Good results have been reported in adults using this technique. In cases of severe deformity and impairment, relocation of the scapula in a more physiologic position by muscle resection and reimplantation may be required. The Green procedure has been modified by avoiding dissection of the serratus anterior muscle and repositioning the scapula by rotation rather than caudad translation. Immediate postoperative mobilization is allowed and there is marked improvement in shoulder abduction. The average improvement in abduction after the procedure was 75° (range, 55° to 90°).

Congenital Brachial Plexus Palsy

Congenital brachial plexus palsy remains a challenging clinical problem and an area of active clinical interest and debate. The risk of congenital brachial plexus palsy increases in proportion to birth weight, with a median incidence of 0.9 cases per 1,000 live births in newborns weighing less than 4,000 g, 1.8 in newborns weighing 4,000 to 4,500 g, and 2.6 in newborns weighing more than 4,500 g.

Traction on the brachial plexus and forced lateral flexion of the head and neck during delivery are implicated as causative factors, along with shoulder dystocia, fetal malposition, cephalopelvic disproportion, high birth weight (as in maternal diabetes), and forceps delivery. Multiparity, prolonged second stage of labor, and breech position have also been reported as causative factors. Perinatal risk factors are absent in 30% of cases. Impaction of the posterior shoulder against

TABLE 1 | Classification of Congenital Brachial Plexus Palsy

Type	Relative Incidence (%)	Nerve Roots Involved	Clinical Appearance	Risk Factor
I Upper plexus (Erb-Duchenne)	80	C5, C6, +/−C7	Adducted, internally rotated shoulder	Macrosomia
II Panplexus	19	C5-T1	Flail, insensate arm	Macrosomia
III Lower (Klumpke's)	1	C8, T1	Paralyzed hand, intact shoulder and elbow; Horner's syndrome	Breech delivery

the sacral promontory and increased intrauterine pressure caused by uterine anomalies have been implicated in patients without shoulder dystocia.

The clinical pattern observed reflects the nerve roots involved (Table 1). Type 1, involving the upper plexus at C5, C6, and variably, C7 is four times more common than the other two types combined. It is important to identify whether the lesion is preganglionic or postganglionic. Preganglionic lesions, which generally involve the lower plexus (type 3), are avulsions from the spinal cord and motor function will not be recovered. Preganglionic lesions are suggested by the presence of Horner's syndrome (unilateral myosis, ptosis, enopthalmos, and anhydrosis of the ipsilateral face and neck), elevated hemidiaphragm, winged scapula, or the absence of rhomboid, rotator cuff, and latissimus dorsi function.

Physical examination is the most reliable method of assessing the severity of neural injury. Spontaneous motion of the shoulder, elbow, wrist, and finger should be observed. An intact Moro reflex is indicative of pseudoparalysis from clavicle or humeral birth fracture, septic arthritis of the shoulder, or other nonneurologic etiology. The presence of Horner's syndrome indicates a poorer prognosis. Serial examinations are necessary as the rate and extent of spontaneous recovery of elbow flexion, shoulder abduction, and extension of the wrist, fingers, and thumb help predict outcome. Imaging studies, including high-resolution MRI and CT myelogram, are commonly used to assess the status of the brachial plexus. MRI using phased array surface coils allows direct visualization of the plexus. Neuromas and root avulsions can sometimes be identified. CT myelogram is better in detecting pseudomeningoceles associated with root avulsion from the spinal cord. Electromyographic and nerve conduction velocity studies have not been shown to be consistently predictive of specific root damage and are best used to establish a preoperative baseline. The presence of sensory action potentials in paralyzed muscle groups is indicative of root avulsion because the sensory root ganglion is located outside the spinal cord.

More than 90% of children with congenital brachial plexus palsy spontaneously recover. Treatment in this group focuses on the prevention of contractures, par-

ticularly about the shoulder, by passive range of motion exercises performed while stabilizing the scapulothoracic joint. In general, excellent hand function is regained with variable return of shoulder function. Significant effort has been focused on identifying and treating the minority of patients in whom spontaneous recovery does not ultimately occur. Absence of biceps and deltoid function as well as wrist, thumb, and finger extension at age 2 to 3 months is considered pathognomonic of this group, although recovery at up to 9 months of age has been reported. Complete neurologic recovery is rare in infants who experience recovery of biceps function after the age of 3 months. A central question is whether microsurgical intervention in infancy improves outcome compared with natural history. The results of microsurgical repair at age 6 months were significantly better than for patients who had spontaneous recovery of biceps function at age 5 months in one recent series. Microsurgical repair is indicated in infants with total plexopathy, Horner's syndrome, or in those who have no evidence of biceps recovery within the first 6 months of life (Fig. 3). Neuroma resection and sural nerve grafting for neuromas in continuity or nerve transfer in the case of root avulsions is performed. Current techniques can improve, but not normalize, function. Secondary procedures are usually successful in improving the common residual deficits of strength and motion. Improvement of at least one functional grade, as assessed by the Mallet classification, have been reported.

Treatment for patients with chronic plexopathy must address muscle contracture and secondary bony deformity. Chronic muscle imbalance leads not only to internal rotation and adduction contracture of the shoulder but progressive glenoid retroversion and posterior subluxation of the humeral head. Evaluation of glenohumeral architecture is an essential component of preoperative planning. Subperiosteal release of the subscapularis origin is indicated by 1 year of age if less than 30° of external rotation is present in adduction. Transfer of the latissimus dorsi and teres major to the rotator cuff accompanied by pectoralis major release is indicated for significant internal rotation contracture and external rotation weakness in children between 2

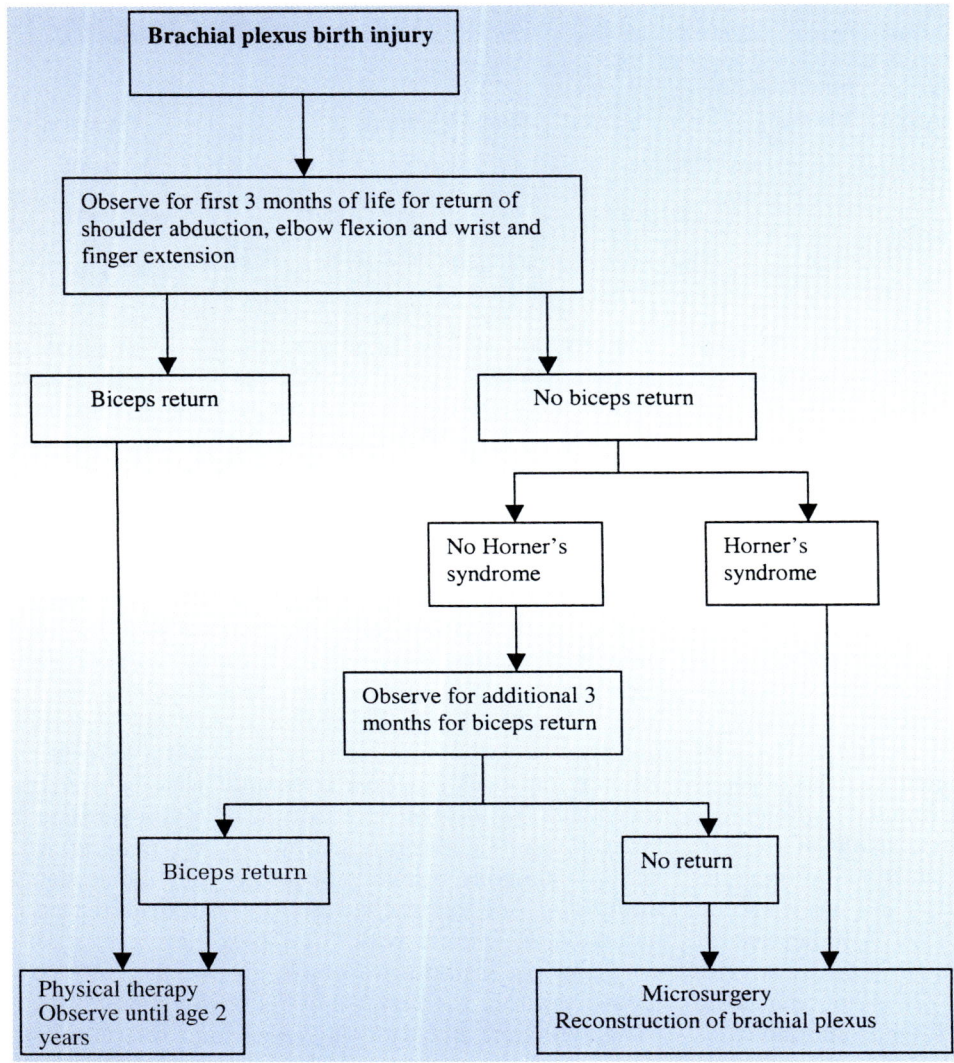

Figure 3 Algorithm for treatment of infants with incomplete recovery of neural function. *(Reproduced from Waters PM: Obsterical brachial plexus injuries: Evaluation and management.* J Am Acad Orthop Surg *1997;5:205-214.)*

and 7 years of age with minimal glenohumeral deformity. Closed reduction after contracture release is usually possible in the patient younger than age 4 years with concomitant posterior shoulder dislocation. Humeral external rotational osteotomy is the treatment of choice when severe flattening of the glenoid and humeral head is present. Active pronation can be improved in patients with supination contracture caused by C7-T1 involvement by biceps rerouting. If passive pronation is not possible, forearm osteotomy is required. Transfer of the triceps, pectoralis major, or latissimus dorsi can be used to augment weak elbow flexion. Shoulder fusion is reserved for skeletally mature patients with paralysis of the deltoid and rotator cuff but who have good hand function.

Septic Arthritis of the Shoulder

The shoulder is an uncommon site for septic arthritis. Less than 5% of the cases of septic arthritis in children involve the shoulder. Antecedent trauma, previous or concurrent infection, and the presence of indwelling catheters have been cited as risk factors. Delay in diagnosis is common, particularly in infants, who often remain afebrile. A whole body technetium bone scan should be obtained early in the evaluation of the neonate with suspected musculoskeletal sepsis because multifocal osteomyelitis is common. Pseudoparalysis of the affected limb caused by shoulder inflammation is frequently observed in patients with a septic shoulder. True paralysis caused by impingement of the swollen shoulder capsule on the brachial plexus can occur and resolves with resolution of the infection. Radiographs often demonstrate joint space widening. The presence of humeral metaphysis within the shoulder capsule increases the likelihood that concomitant osteomyelitis may be present. Although serial aspirations have been recommended for the treatment of shoulder sepsis, arthrotomy obviates the need for multiple invasive procedures in a young child and allows for a more thorough débridement. Loculated purulence may be found in the biceps sheath. Arthroscopic irrigation and débridement is also an option. A small joint arthroscope may be required in infants and toddlers. In neonates diagnosed 2 days or more after the onset of symptoms, damage to the physis and secondary ossification centers of the proximal humerus results in shortening of the arm and deformity of the humeral head, but loss of function is negligible.

Traumatic Injuries

Clavicular Birth Fractures

The clavicle is the most frequently fractured bone in the neonate during childbirth, with an incidence of between 0.2% to 4.4%. Fetal macrosomia (birth weight greater than 4,000 g) and shoulder dystocia leading to excessive pressure on the shoulder by the symphysis pubis have been implicated as the most common risk factors. Antenatal prediction is difficult, however, because the majority of cases occur in otherwise healthy infants after normal labor and delivery. Concomitant brachial plexus palsy is present in a small percentage of patients. Palpable crepitus and pseudoparalysis of the affected limb are usually present. Occasionally a late diagnosis is made on recognition of a palpable midclavicular prominence. In contrast to congenital pseudarthrosis of the clavicle, abundant callus will be present on radiographs. Simple immobilization for comfort for 10 to 14 days the only treatment that is required. Healing and remodeling is rapid and reliable.

Clavicle Shaft Fractures

The clavicle is the only osseous connection between the arm and trunk and is subjected to medially directed forces from the upper limb. The double curve shape and ligamentous and muscular insertions of the clavicle predispose the middle third of the structure to injury. More than 90% of clavicle fractures occur at the junction between the middle and distal third of the clavicular shaft. Closed treatment with a sling or figure-of-8 strap is effective. Distraction of the fracture by overtightening of the figure-of-8 strap should be avoided. Anticipatory guidance of the patient and parents regarding the natural history of the expected callus prominence and its subsequent remodeling over the first year after injury is essential. Open reduction and internal fixation with a low profile plate is reserved for open fractures; severely displaced, irreducible fractures; those that have buttonholed through the fascia or trapezius, tenting the skin; and the uncommon circumstance in which neurovascular compromise of the

mediastinal structures is present. Complications after midshaft clavicle fracture are rare.

Proximal Humeral Fractures

Proximal humeral physeal fractures are uncommon, comprising between 3% and 6% of all physeal injuries. Salter-Harris type I fractures occur in infants and children younger than age 5 years due to the transverse orientation of the physeal plate. Metaphyseal fractures are most common between age 5 and 11 years. In adolescence, when the physis has assumed a more conical shape, Salter-Harris II fractures predominate. Salter-Harris III and IV fractures of the proximal humerus are extremely rare. Closed treatment remains the standard of care for most of these injuries. The proximal humeral physis contributes 80% of the longitudinal growth of the humerus, providing tremendous remodeling potential for displaced and angulated fractures. In addition, little functional impairment results despite residual humeral shortening or imperfect remodeling at skeletal maturity. Up to 70° of angulation and 100% displacement is allowable in children under age 5 years, decreasing to 40° of angulation and 50% displacement as the patient nears physeal maturity. Closed reduction followed by percutaneous pinning is reserved for adolescents with completely displaced or unacceptably angulated fractures. Open reduction may be necessary in the rare circumstance of muscular or tendinous interposition.

Humeral Shaft Fractures

Humeral shaft fractures constitute only 3% of fractures in children younger than age 16 years. Transverse or short oblique fractures are the result of direct trauma. Spiral or long oblique fractures are caused indirectly by violent twisting. Fracture resulting from minor trauma may be caused by an occult unicameral bone cyst or other benign lesion. Stress fractures progressing to complete shaft fractures have been reported in skeletally immature throwing and overhead athletes; prodromal symptoms were present in each case.

Isolated closed injuries are best managed by closed methods, including hanging arm cast, coaptation splint, or collar and cuff bandage with early transition to fracture bracing. Humeral overgrowth will compensate for overriding of 1 to 2 cm. The amount of angulation that will correct with growth and remodeling decreases as the location of the fracture moves farther away from the proximal humeral physis. Angulation of 25° is allowable in proximal diaphyseal fractures, whereas only 15° or less should be accepted distally. Malrotation, which will not remodel, should be avoided. Surgical treatment is indicated to stabilize a so-called "floating elbow" (ipsilateral humeral and forearm fractures), multiple trauma in which the patient must remain recumbent, and head-injured patients in whom angulation and excessive shortening cannot be controlled due to spasticity. The emerging use of flexible intramedullary nails may decrease iatrogenic injury to the radial nerve and soft tissues compared with plating techniques, because of the minimal dissection required for their insertion. The risk of refracture can be minimized by leaving the nails in place until mature callus is present. Dynamic compression plates remain the treatment of choice for unstable fractures that require open treatment. External fixation should be reserved for fractures associated with significant soft-tissue involvement.

Annotated Bibliography

Bellemans M, Lamoureux J: Results of surgical treatment of Sprengel deformity by a modified Green's procedure. *J Pediatr Orthop* 1999;8:194-196.

In seven patients with congenital undescended scapula, treatment included a modification of the Green procedure that avoided dissection of the serratus anterior muscle and allowed for immediate postoperative mobilization. The scapula was repositioned by rotation rather than caudad translation, obviating the need for clavicular surgery. Patients gained an average of 75° of abduction and were subjectively satisfied.

Bennek J: The use of upper limb external fixation in paediatric trauma. *Injury* 2000;31(suppl 1):21-26.

External fixation yielded good results in five humeral shaft fractures associated with considerable soft-tissue damage. The external fixator was left in place for an average of 44 days. No nonunions or refractures occurred, and final alignment was satisfactory in all patients.

Beringer DC, Weiner DS, Noble JS, Bell RH: Severely displaced proximal humeral epiphyseal fractures: A follow-up study. *J Pediatr Orthop* 1998 18:31-37.

Persistent malposition following closed treatment did not result in functional impairment in 48 patients with severely displaced proximal humeral physeal fractures. Complications occurred in one third of patients treated with surgery but in none of the patients treated by closed methods.

Bos CF, Mol LJ, Obermann WR, Tjin a Ton ER: Late sequelae of neonatal septic arthritis of the shoulder. *J Bone Joint Surg Br* 1998;80:645-650.

Eight children were followed for a mean of 14 years after neonatal shoulder sepsis. Delay in diagnosis resulted in severe radiographic deformities but negligible functional loss.

Currarino G, Sheffield E, Twickler D: Congenital glenoid dysplasia. *Pediatr Radiol* 1998;28:30-37.

This radiologic study classifies glenoid dysplasia into five etiologic groups. Failure of ossification of the inferior glenoid apophysis is emphasized as the underlying etiology of this condition.

Doita M, Iio H, Mizuno K: Surgical management of Sprengel's deformity in adults: A report of two cases. *Clin Orthop* 2000;371:119-124.

Resection of the omovertebral bone and superomedial border of the scapula reduced neck pain and improved cosmetic appearance in two adults with Sprengel's deformity. Shoulder motion improved in only one patient.

Hoffer MM, Phipps GJ: Closed reduction and tendon transfer for treatment of dislocation of the glenohumeral joint secondary to brachial plexus birth palsy. *J Bone Joint Surg Am* 1998;80:997-1001.

Eight children were treated for shoulder dislocation caused by brachial plexus birth palsy with a combination of tendon releases followed by closed reduction and transfer of the latissimus dorsi and teres major to the rotator cuff. This method resulted in increased shoulder strength and active range of motion with improvement in activities of daily living.

Kaplan B, Rabinerson D, Avrech OM, Carmi N, Steinberg DM, Merlob P: Fracture of the clavicle in the newborn following normal labor and delivery. *Int J Gynaecol Obstet* 1998;63:15-20.

In this series of over 27,000 births, neonatal clavicle fracture occurred in 1.65% of vaginal deliveries and 0.2% of cesarean deliveries. The majority of fractures occurred in otherwise healthy newborns during normal labor and delivery.

Sales de Gauzy J, Baunin C, Puget C, Fajadet P, Cahuzac JP: Congenital pseudarthrosis of the clavicle and thoracic outlet syndrome in adolescence. *J Pediatr Orthop* 1999;8:299-301.

This interesting case report of thoracic outlet syndrome in an adolescent female in association with congenital pseudarthrosis of the clavicle offers indirect support for the vascular hypothesis for this condition.

Waters PM: Comparison of the natural history, the outcome of microsurgical repair, and the outcome of operative reconstruction in brachial plexus birth palsy. *J Bone Joint Surg Am* 1999;81:649-659.

Infants who had recovery of biceps function during the third through sixth month of life had significantly worse function than those who had recovery during the first 3 months. The clinical results for six patients who had microsurgical repair 6 months after birth were significantly better than those of the 15 patients who experienced recovery of biceps function at age 5 months.

Waters PM, Smith GR, Jaramillo D: Glenohumeral deformity secondary to brachial plexus birth palsy. *J Bone Joint Surg Am* 1998;80:668-677.

CT and MRI studies of 42 patients with residual brachial plexus birth palsy demonstrated excessive glenoid retroversion (mean glenoscapular angle of −25.7° compared with −5.5° on the unaffected side). Posterior glenohumeral subluxation was present in 62%. Progressive deformity was found with increasing age.

Classic Bibliography

Clarke HM, Curtis CG: An approach to obstetrical brachial plexus injuries. *Hand Clin* 1995;11:563-581.

Grogan DP, Love SM, Guidera KJ, Ogden JA: Operative treatment of congenital pseudarthrosis of the clavicle. *J Pediatr Orthop* 1991;11:176-180.

L'Episcopo JB: Tendon transplantation in obstetrical paralysis. *Am J Surg* 1934;25:122-125.

Lloyd-Roberts GC, Apley AG, Owen R: Reflections upon the aetiology of congenital pseudarthrosis of the clavicle: With a note on cranio-cleido dysostosis. *J Bone Joint Surg Br* 1975;57:24-29.

Peleg D, Hasnin J, Shalev E: Fractured clavicle and Erb's palsy unrelated to birth trauma. *Am J Obstet Gynecol* 1997;177:1038-1040.

Samilson RL: Congenital and developmental anomalies of the shoulder girdle. *Orthop Clin North Am* 1980;11: 219-231.

Wirth MA, Lyons FR, Rockwood CA: Hypoplasia of the glenoid: A review of sixteen patients. *J Bone Joint Surg Am* 1993;75:1175-1184.

Chapter 25

Shoulder and Elbow Injuries in the Throwing Athlete

Frederick M. Azar, MD

Steve Bernstein, MD

Ronald Scott Kvitne, MD

George A. Paletta, Jr, MD

Rotator Cuff Tears

Throughout the throwing motion, the shoulder is subjected to extremes of angular velocity and translation and distraction forces. Anterior glenohumeral translation forces of up to 40% of body weight are generated during the late cocking phase. Angular velocities of up to 7,000° per second are generated during the acceleration phase. Glenohumeral distraction forces of 1 to 1.5 times the body weight are generated during the release and follow-through phases. The bony geometry of the glenohumeral joint offers little inherent stability. As the primary dynamic stabilizer of the glenohumeral joint, the rotator cuff functions primarily through eccentric action to stabilize the humeral head in the glenoid, while muscles with larger lever arms (deltoid, latissimus, pectoralis major, teres major) propel the humerus relative to the scapula. The rotator cuff also resists superior translation of the humeral head. The scapulothoracic musculature and the long head of the biceps also play important roles in the dynamic stability of the shoulder. Shoulder pathology in throwing athletes occurs primarily as a result of the repetitive stresses that occur during the throwing cycle.

Rotator Cuff Lesions

The rotator cuff in throwing athletes is repeatedly subjected to abnormally high tensile and compressive forces, which frequently result in shoulder disability caused by a complex pattern of pathologic involvement that includes tendon inflammation, tendon fatigue and weakening, degeneration, tendinopathy, and, ultimately, failure with partial- or full-thickness tearing. The etiology of rotator cuff pathology in this patient population is multifactorial and includes both intrinsic and extrinsic factors. Common intrinsic factors include age-related tendon degeneration, alterations in tendon vascularity, impaired healing responses, and altered tendon matrix composition. Extrinsic factors include compression (subacromial or glenoid rim), tensile over-

load, and repetitive stress. Rotator cuff abnormalities may be the result of primary cuff failure or secondary to underlying conditions such as glenohumeral instability. The rotator cuff of a throwing athlete may fail because of primary impingement, secondary impingement, primary tensile failure, secondary tensile failure, or internal impingement. The articular side of the cuff is at particular risk because of the relative weakness of the articular side tendon fibers at their insertion site compared with fibers inserting on the bursal side. The key to successful treatment of rotator cuff pathology in a throwing athlete is recognition of underlying contributing factors such as instability.

In athletes with primary impingement, the rotator cuff is injured by compressive contact with the coracoacromial arch, undersurface of the acromion, or even an os acromiale. This classic impingement syndrome as originally described by Neer is uncommon in athletes younger than 35 years of age, but may be the pathophysiology of rotator cuff injury in an older throwing athlete in the later stages of the pitching career.

In athletes with primary tensile failure of the rotator cuff, the cuff typically fails as a result of repetitive tensile forces that occur during the release and follow-through phases of throwing, with no underlying pathology contributing to the development of cuff lesions. Early in the season, athletes susceptible to primary tensile failure may have acute tendinitis, whereas late in the season chronic overload cuff failure may occur.

Glenohumeral instability may contribute to rotator cuff disease in throwing athletes. Many throwers have some increased laxity of the dominant shoulder. Although the etiology of this increased laxity is unclear, it may be caused, in part, by capsular stretching as a result of repetitive stress. Elite throwers also often have some degree of posterior capsular contracture that can result in increased anterior translation forces on the humeral head during certain phases of throwing. Such instability can result in higher tensile demands on the rotator cuff as it works to limit increased anterior or posterior humeral head translation and may play a critical role in secondary tensile failure or impingement of the rotator cuff. The presence of underlying instability must be considered in the evaluation of a thrower's shoulder with rotator cuff pathology.

Internal impingement also may be the cause of rotator cuff pathology in throwing ahtletes. It is defined as impingement of the posterior–superior rotator cuff between the humerus and posterior–superior glenoid rim. In throwers, this impingement is thought to occur in the late cocking phase when the humeral head is abducted and maximally externally rotated. Such internal impingement is believed to be physiologic. A recent arthroscopic study demonstrated that 85% of 105 consecutive patients undergoing shoulder arthroscopy for a variety of diagnoses exhibited internal impingement at an average of 95° of abduction and 74° of external rotation. Consequently, it has been suggested that throwers develop symptomatic internal impingement as a result of the frequency and magnitude with which impingement occurs during late cocking.

The role of glenohumeral instability in the development of internal impingement has been debated. One theory suggests that anterior glenohumeral capsular laxity with an associated posterior capsular contracture is the essential lesion in the development of symptomatic internal impingement. Advocates of this theory recommend correction of the underlying preexisting anteroinferior instability as the primary treatment. In addition, they cite the fact that not all throwers with internal impingment have associated superior labral anterior and posterior (SLAP) tears. Another theory proposes that the essential lesion is a posterosuperior type II SLAP lesion with resultant anterior pseudolaxity and a posteroinferior capsular contraction predisposing the posterosuperior labrum to peelback forces in the abducted and external rotated position. In support of this theory, advocates cite as support an extremely high rate of return to throwing with surgical SLAP repair in conjunction with a focused postoperative posterior capsular stretching program.

Clinical Evaluation

A careful history and physical examination are essential in determining the cause of a thrower's pain. The athlete's age; onset, duration, and location of pain; and the phase of throwing during which pain occurs are all critical factors. Younger athletes often have problems with instability and secondary impingement, whereas older athletes are more likely to experience degenerative processes associated with primary impingement. Rotator cuff pain is typically anterior shoulder pain,

but can present in any distribution or during any phase of throwing. Attention should also be directed toward loss of velocity or control, because these can be subtle early symptoms of rotator cuff disease.

Physical examination must assess for abnormalities in range of motion, strength, and stability and incorporate specific tests for conditions such as labral lesions, SLAP lesions, acromioclavicular joint pathology, classic impingement, internal impingement, and biceps lesions. It is essential to compare the throwing shoulder to the contralateral shoulder. Normal adaptive changes in an elite thrower's shoulder include muscle hypertrophy and asymmetry, inferior scapular displacement, and increased external rotation and decreased internal rotation that produce an overall arc of motion similar to that of the opposite side.

Inspection of the supraspinatus and infraspinatus is important to rule out significant atrophy that may be suggestive of suprascapular neuropathy. Active and passive range of motion should be assessed with attention to glenohumeral-scapulothoracic rhythm. Weakness is the hallmark of rotator cuff pathology and although specific, is not very sensitive. Manual resistance testing of all components of the cuff must be done. It is important to differentiate true cuff weakness from weakness secondary to pain. Athletes with cuff tendinitis or subacromial bursitis may have pain that manifests as weakness during resisted motion. Subacromial injection of lidocaine can be used to help in diagnosis. Residual cuff weakness that persists after complete pain relief following subacromial injection is most likely indicative of rotator cuff pathology. The Neer and Hawkins impingement signs are used to evaluate for impingement. Tests for biceps and SLAP lesions should include palpation of the biceps and the Speed, O'Brien active compression, crank, Kibler anterior slide, and Jobe relocation tests. Instability is assessed using the load and shift test for glenohumeral translation, the sulcus sign, apprehension test, and Jobe relocation test. Internal impingement may be suggested by reproduction of the athletes' pain in abduction and maximal external rotation or by a positive posterior impingement sign.

Diagnostic Imaging

Standard radiographs should include four views: true AP in internal and external rotation, axillary, and supraspinatus outlet. Common abnormal findings in the thrower's shoulder include subchondral cysts or sclerosis of the greater tuberosity, which are best seen on the AP views. The AP view is also useful in assessing superior humeral head migration, calcific tendinitis, tuberosity avulsions, or acromioclavicular joint arthritis. The axillary view is best for evaluating the anterior and posterior glenoid margins. The supraspinatus outlet view is helpful in demonstrating acromial morphology and spurs. Specialized views that may be required include West Point axillary and Stryker notch views. CT arthrography is best for detecting bony and chondral lesions and osteochondritis dissecans lesions of the glenoid.

MRI remains the diagnostic test of choice for evaluation of rotator cuff and labral pathology. The location and extent of involvement of cuff pathology and the degree of cuff retraction are clearly delineated with MRI. Associated intra-articular pathology, such as a Bankart lesion, labral tear, or SLAP lesion also can be identified. Magnetic resonance arthrography can improve the detection of partial-thickness rotator cuff pathology and labral lesions. Abduction-external rotation positioning and traction views also can improve detection of internal impingement lesions.

Ultrasound has been reported as 84% accurate in diagnosing full-thickness rotator cuff tears. Its usefulness in the detection of partial-thickness tears is still uncertain. The use of ultrasound in detecting cuff pathology, although promising, is a relatively new concept and is heavily operator-dependent, and therefore should be limited to experienced physicians.

Ancillary Diagnostic Tests

Electromyography and nerve conduction velocity studies are indicated to rule out suprascapular neuropathy but are used only in instances of clinical suspicion. Isokinetic testing of the rotator cuff may also be helpful in identifying significant strength deficits.

Treatment

The treatment of rotator cuff pathology in a throwing athlete depends on an accurate diagnosis of the cuff disease and identification of any underlying contributing factors. Nonsurgical treatment is almost always the initial recommendation for throwing athletes with rotator cuff pathology other than a full-thickness tear. Such treatment must focus on the elimination of pain and inflammation as well as comprehensive rehabilitation of the entire upper extremity kinetic chain. Treatment begins with cessation of throwing, enforced active rest, modalities including ice, and a therapeutic course of nonsteroidal anti-inflammatory drugs. Once pain-free full motion has been achieved, a period of strengthening is initiated that focuses primarily on the rotator cuff and scapular stabilizers, and a progressive throwing program (Thrower's Ten program) is begun (Table 1). Resisted exercises with the arm in the functional position of abduction and external rotation should not begin until the athlete is pain-free in that position. The

TABLE 1	The Thrower's Ten Program

Dumbbell exercises for strengthening deltoid and supraspinatus musculature

Prone horizontal shoulder abduction

Prone shoulder extension

Internal rotation strengthening at 90° shoulder abduction using tubing

External rotation strengthening at 90° shoulder abduction using tubing

Elbow flexion/extension strengthening exercises using tubing

Serratus anterior strengthening (progressive push-ups)

Diagonal "2" shoulder flexion/extension pattern strengthening using tubing

Press-ups

Dumbbell wrist flexion/extension and pronation/supination

late strengthening phase should include eccentric cuff strengthening exercises and plyometrics. With strength restored, the athlete can begin functional reconditioning of the rotator cuff with attention to proper throwing mechanics and a progressive interval throwing program. When full functional strength, range of motion, and normal throwing mechanics have been achieved, the athlete may begin a return to full activity. Subacromial cortisone injection for therapeutic purposes should be used cautiously.

If an extended 3-month course of comprehensive nonsurgical treatment fails to return the athlete to preinjury participation level, surgical intervention may need to be considered. The surgical treatment of choice and the likelihood of its success are dependent on accurate identification of the etiology of the cuff disease and the extent of cuff involvement.

Athletes with true primary compressive rotator cuff disease (a small subset of older throwing athletes) should be treated with arthroscopic subacromial decompression and débridement of the site of cuff tear. The use of arthroscopic subacromial decompression in throwing athletes younger than age 35 years generally should be avoided, because the prognosis for return to preinjury level of participation is poor. In a recent report of young athletes treated with arthroscopic decompression and débridement, only 66% had satisfactory results, with only 45% returning to preinjury participation level. In an effort to improve results in these patients, some authors have recommended subacromial débridement with preservation of the coracoacromial ligament.

The surgical treatment of primary tensile cuff disease that has failed extensive rehabilitation is arthroscopic débridement of the rotator cuff tear undersurface if less than 50% to 75% of the cuff thickness is involved.

Surgical treatment must be followed by an extended postoperative rehabilitation program that ultimately emphasizes eccentric functioning of the posterosuperior cuff.

A difficult therapeutic dilemma is the high-grade partial-thickness rotator cuff tear involving more than 50% to 75% of the cuff thickness. If more than 50% of the cuff thickness is involved, takedown and repair of the cuff tear should be considered.

Secondary compressive or secondary tensile cuff pathology is caused by underlying primary glenohumeral instability, which must be corrected. Failure to treat the underlying glenohumeral instability is equal to a failure to treat the underlying essential lesion. Open or arthroscopic capsulolabral reconstruction or, more recently, thermal capsulorrhaphy is required in addition to treatment of the cuff pathology.

A full-thickness rotator cuff tear in a young throwing athlete requires early surgical intervention and carries a poor prognosis. Few elite throwing athletes have successfully returned to competition after full-thickness cuff tears. Open anterior acromioplasty and repair of the full-thickness cuff tear has a reported 88% good or excellent result in the general population; no reliable results in throwing athletes have been published. Results of this techique are related to the preoperative tear size, quality of tendon tissue, difficulty of tendon mobilization, and associated tear in the long head of the biceps. Massive, irreparable rotator cuff tears usually are not seen in competitive overhead athletes.

Arthroscopic decompression and mini-open repair of full-thickness cuff tears has advantages over open repair, including preservation of the deltoid origin, better diagnosis and treatment of associated intra-articular pathology, and the opportunity for more aggressive, early rehabilitation. The mini-open repair has produced results similar to those of open repair and is the treatment of choice for small, unretracted tears.

An all-arthroscopic repair technique for full-thickness tears is being used more frequently. One study reported 49 good or excellent results in 53 patients at 2- to 3-year follow-up using this technique. However, the patients in this study were not a group of throwing athletes. Longer follow-up is required to assess the efficacy of this technique. Open or mini-open repairs remain the gold standard for surgical treatment of the full-thickness tear in the throwing athlete.

Surgical Treatment of Internal Impingement

The diagnosis of internal impingment can be difficult. The athlete often complains of posterior shoulder pain, especially during the late cocking phase, and may also complain of pain in the follow-through phase. Physical examination findings may include a positive crank test or posterior shoulder pain with abduction and external rotation. Pain may then be reduced or eliminated with application of a posteriorly directed force on the humeral head. A diagnostic intra-articular lidocaine injection may be helpful in differentiating internal impingement from primary impingement or other extra-articular causes of pain. Plain radiographs usually are normal. Magnetic resonance arthrography, with traction and abduction-external rotation views, is the most helpful imaging study because it often demonstrates blunting of the posterior labrum and undersurface cuff abnormalities.

The initial treatment for internal impingement is nonsurgical. Rehabilitation focusing on improved glenohumeral stability through cuff and scapular stabilizer strengthening is the mainstay of treatment. Careful attention to elimination of any posterior capsular contracture is also mandatory.

Surgery for internal impingement refractory to rehabilitation is controversial and is indicated only if there is failure of a minimum of at least 3 to 6 months of appropriate rehabilitation. At the time of arthroscopy the pathognomonic "kissing lesion" of posterior labrum and undersurface of the cuff is noted with the arm abducted and externally rotated. Recommended procedures include débridement of the posterior labrum and undersurface cuff tear, open or arthroscopic capsulolabral stabilization, thermal capsulorrhaphy, and repair of associated SLAP lesions. The key to a successful surgical outcome is recognition and appropriate treatment of associated pathology, including SLAP tears or capsulolabral laxity. If a SLAP tear is present, repair is required. If significant capsulolabral laxity is present, capsular tightening is required. Recently reported data suggest the addition of thermal capsulorrhaphy to SLAP repair in throwing athletes with internal impingment may improve return to play rates.

SLAP Tears

Bennett Lesion

The Bennett lesion was originally described as an extracapsular exostosis at the posterior glenoid rim at the triceps insertion; the lesion has since been localized to the attachment of the posteroinferior capsule to the glenoid and is believed to be a consequence of repetitive traction on the posterior band of the inferior glenohumeral ligament produced by posterior subluxation during cocking, posterior deceleration forces during follow-through, or a combination of both. The diagnosis is made by history and physical examination in conjuction with an axillary lateral radiograph or CT scan showing the lesion. Athletes most often complain of posterior shoulder pain, and tenderness may be present at the posterior inferior glenoid rim, which has a high association with posterior labral tears and undersurface tears of the rotator cuff. Intra-articular pathology is most likely caused by internal impingement, and surgical intervention usually is warranted for the symptomatic thrower with posterior glenoid exostosis.

Little Leaguer's Shoulder

Little leaguer's shoulder is defined as throwing-related pain localized to the proximal humerus in a skeletally immature youth or adolescent baseball player with radiographic findings of widening of the proximal humeral physis. The most common physical finding is pain localized to the proximal lateral humerus. Swelling, weakness, atrophy, and loss of motion are uncommon findings. Bilateral AP internal and external rotation comparison radiographs of the proximal humerus are recommended. Treatment is rest from throwing for at least 3 months.

Elbow Injuries

Elbow injuries in overhead athletes usually result from repetitive stress about the elbow rather than from a single traumatic event. Throwing athletes, in particular baseball pitchers, are most susceptible to elbow injuries (Fig. 1). It appears that learning proper pitching mechanics as early as possible and building strength as the body matures decrease the risk of repetitive stress injuries.

Biomechanics

The phases of pitching, which are similar to the biomechanics of other overhead sport activities, are divided into wind-up, early cocking, late cocking, acceleration, deceleration, and follow-through. During the late cocking and acceleration phases, tremendous valgus forces can be transmitted across the medial aspect of the elbow. Because these forces are greater than the estimated load to failure of the ulnar collateral ligament (UCL), muscle stability is necessary for its protection. Electromyographic studies, however, have shown a limited capacity for dynamic stability across a medially unstable elbow.

Lateral compressive forces across the elbow of up to 1,100 N have been reported during late cocking and acceleration, with shear forces occurring during deceleration. These forces can lead to the development of osteochondral lesions in the radiocapitellar joint, such as osteochondritis dissecans of the capitellum in adults or osteochondrosis of the capitellum in adolescents (Panner's disease). In addition, the combination of

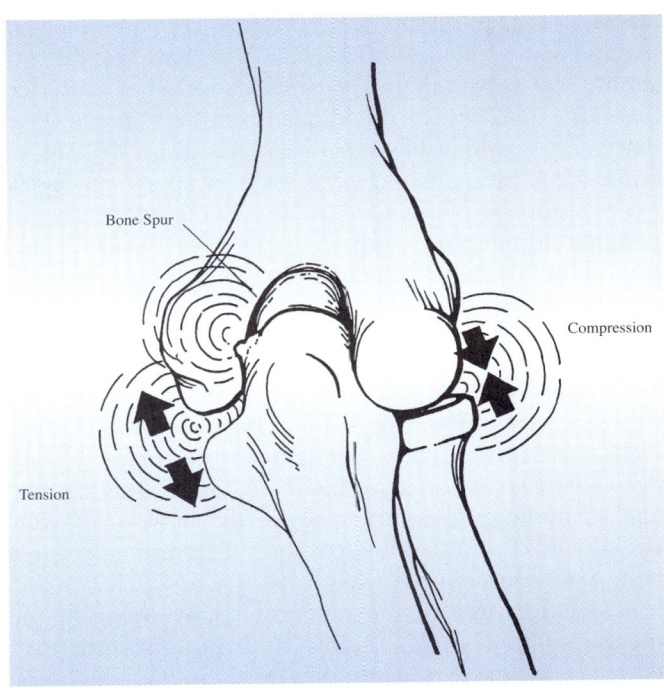

Figure 1 Relationship of the biomechanical forces within the elbow during throwing. *(Adapted with permission from Singer KM, Butters KP: Osteochondroses of the elbow, in DeLee JC, Drez D (eds): Orthopaedic Sports Medicine: Principles and Practice. Philadelphia, PA, WB Saunders, 1994, p 899.)*

compressive and torsional forces may cause impingement of the olecranon by the olecranon fossa, leading to valgus extension overload.

Ulnar Collateral Ligament Injuries

Common complaints include medial elbow pain with overhead activity and decreased velocity, accuracy, and pitch count for pitchers. A positive Tinel's sign has been reported in up to 44% of patients with UCL injuries, whereas clinical laxity with a valgus stress is noted in only 25%. In addition to standard AP, lateral, and axial views, valgus stress views of the elbow are recommended. Increased medial joint laxity can be detected in approximately one half of patients. A recent study of uninjured baseball players, however, demonstrated significant differences between medial joint space opening in the dominant and nondominant elbows with stress radiographs. Contrast MRI is recommended as a routine aspect of the evaluation.

Reconstruction of the ligament is preferred to repair and is most commonly done with a palmaris longus graft passed through bone tunnels. Fixation of the graft with suture anchors has been reported, but there are no long-term clinical studies to support their use. The flexor-pronator mass is elevated anteriorly or through a muscle-splitting approach where a safe zone of 1 cm distal to the sublime tubercle of the ulna can be used. Alternatively, the flexor-pronator mass can be elevated; however, it should not be detached and reflected for exposure. If the ulnar nerve is symptomatic, it should be subcutaneously transposed. The need for excision of a posteromedial osteophyte for valgus extension overload has been reported in up to 25% of patients. A return to previous level of sport activity or better can be expected in approximately 80% of patients, although 1 year of recovery is typically necessary for overhead athletes.

Upper Extremity Stress Fractures

In patients with upper extremity pain associated with overuse, stress fracture should be considered, especially in those who participate in upper limb-dominated sports such as baseball, tennis, racquetball, and swimming. Stress fractures in the upper extremity usually involve the humerus or olecranon and most heal with conservative treatment.

Stress fractures of the olecranon may occur in the olecranon body, tip, or physis. Transverse fractures typically occur in the middle third of the olecranon and are believed to be caused by a traction force from the triceps. Oblique fractures are thought to result from repeated impingement of the intercondylar fossa.

MRI, bone scan, or CT may be indicated for fractures that cannot be readily seen on plain radiographs. In adolescents, recognition of a physeal injury may be difficult. By age 12 the olecranon physis is narrow and usually not wider than 5 mm with congruent borders. With a physeal fracture, the physis may appear widened or fragmented when compared with radiographs of the opposite elbow.

Surgical excision is recommended for olecranon tip fractures because of the risk of nonunion and the formation of loose bodies. Fractures of the body of the olecranon usually can be treated conservatively with 8 to 12 weeks of activity restriction, range of motion and stretching exercises, and an endurance program that does not involve heavy strength training. Light throwing can be allowed in the endurance program, but return to full activity may require 3 to 6 months.

Surgery is indicated when a stress fracture fails to heal, or it can be done in the early clinical presentation if the patient desires as early a return to sport as possible. Surgical techniques include percutaneous placement of a 6.5-mm cannulated screw inserted perpendicularly across the fracture site. Bone grafting usually is not required. For cannulated screw fixation, a screw length of 100 to 110 mm is typically recommended.

Little Leaguer's Elbow

Fractures of the medial epicondylar physis in skeletally immature athletes can be caused by repeated valgus stress or repetitive, violent forearm flexor muscle contractures, as might occur during pitching or a fall. Children with the repetitive form of this injury usually have medial elbow pain with throwing; accuracy and pitch count often are affected. Point tenderness usually is present over the medial condyle, and a flexion contracture may be present in addition to swelling and limited range of motion. On radiographs the epicondylar physis may appear widened or fragmented. A comparison view of the opposite elbow is helpful in identifying abnormalities. The amount of displacement should be critically assessed in a throwing athlete because laxity of the UCL can result.

Treatment depends on the stability of the fragment, which can be evaluated by stress AP radiographs. If the fragment is stable, rest and immobilization are appropriate with a gradual return to throwing. The fracture may heal in as early as 6 to 8 weeks but may take as long as 10 to 12 weeks. If the fragment moves distally and the joint gaps open medially with stressing, the elbow is considered unstable and should be treated with open reduction and internal fixation with a Kirschner wire or cancellous screw through a medial approach. This procedure is most appropriate in treating the dominant arm of a throwing athlete. An interval throwing program is begun after the fracture heals.

Osteochondritis Dissecans

Osteochondritis dissecans of the capitellum occurs in adolescent and young adult athletes who are involved in repetitive activities of the upper extremity, including throwing, weight lifting, and gymnastics. Osteochondritis dissecans manifests as a localized lesion that involves a segment of the articular surface including cartilage and subchondral bone. Although the etiology is uncertain, theories include microtrauma, ischemic events, and genetic factors.

Overuse injuries of the immature elbow are of two types: osteochondrosis of the capitellum (Panner's disease) and osteochondritis dissecans of the capitellum. Panner's disease occurs in children age 4 to 8 years and involves the entire ossific nucleus of the capitellum. The disease often is self-limiting, and conservative treatment usually leads to reossification and resolution of symptoms with time. Osteochondritis dissecans of the capitellum usually occurs in individuals 10 years of age or older and involves a portion of the capitellum. Permanent deformity of the joint surface may result. Some physicians consider the two types to be two separate entities, and others believe that osteochondritis dissecans is a continuum of the process of Panner's disease.

Standard AP and lateral and oblique radiographs of the elbow usually are sufficient in the initial evaluation.

Occasionally, a loose fragment of the central or lateral portion of the capitellum may be noted, as well as loose bodies within the joint. Hypertrophy of the radial head or osteophytes may be noted in more severe and prolonged involvement. MRI and CT are helpful in defining the extent of the lesion. Early changes include low signal intensity on T1-weighted images and no abnormalities on T2-weighted images. Later changes may include intervening fluid on T2-weighted images, indicative of a partially or completely detached fragment.

Treatment of osteochondritis dissecans depends on several factors, including the age of the patient, the radiographic appearance of the lesion, and whether the fragment is attached or loose. Activity modification for 8 to 12 weeks is recommended for treatment of a lesion with intact articular cartilage. A brace can be used and motion is encouraged. Once the pain and swelling have resolved, activities can be resumed, and patients can return to sports, after a period of 3 to 6 months.

Indications for surgery include a partially or completely detached fragment that typically presents as a swollen, painful elbow with mechanical symptoms.

Short- to mid-range follow-up studies report success rates of more than 90% with arthroscopic lesion removal and abrasion chondroplasty. A recent long-term outcome study reported residual elbow symptoms associated with activities of daily living in approximately 50% of patients who had advanced lesions, osteoarthritic changes, and a large osteochondral defect. Successful healing of osteochondritis dissecans lesions after internal fixation has been reported in a small number of patients; however, this technique can be technically demanding.

Valgus Extension Overload

Valgus extension overload, a spectrum of injuries with soft-tissue and bony components, includes posterior medial impingement, UCL injury, flexor pronator injury, and radial capitellar overload. Olecranon impingement occurs as a result of medial elbow stress, cubitus valgus, and a narrowed olecranon fossa from bony hypertrophy. The mechanism of injury is believed to be excessive valgus stress across the elbow during the acceleration phase of pitching, causing a wedging of the olecranon within the olecranon fossa posteriorly. Osteophytes form posterior and posteromedial to the tip of the olecranon and may eventually lead to chondromalacia and loose body formation.

Patients typically report pain during the acceleration phase of pitching. Pitchers report a shortened pitch count as well as problems with accuracy and speed, which are manifested by an early release that causes

them to throw high. Tenderness typically is present along the posterior and posteromedial aspects of the olecranon tip during forced extension. A flexion contracture may be present. Radiographs should include AP, lateral, oblique, and axial views. The elbow should be flexed 110° with the arm lying on the cassette and the beam angled 45° to the ulna. This position gives the best view of the olecranon as it articulates with the trochlea and puts the medial aspect of the olecranon on profile, which may show a posteromedial osteophyte. MRI and CT also may be helpful.

Conservative treatment is recommended initially and should focus on diminishing swelling and pain and restoring elbow motion. Physical therapy should include eccentric exercises to improve strength and control of the elbow flexors to manage the forceful elbow extension that occurs during the deceleration phase of pitching. If conservative treatment fails, arthroscopic or open excision of the osteophytes is indicated. Currently, arthroscopic treatment is favored over open procedures, because it involves less soft-tissue dissection and allows earlier, more aggressive rehabilitation.

Lateral Epicondylitis

Although the term epicondylitis suggests an inflammatory condition, examinations of pathologic specimens generally have found no evidence of acute or chronic inflammation. Patients with lateral epicondylitis usually have pain that is exacerbated by resisted wrist dorsiflexion and forearm supination, and there is pain during a handshake or when grasping objects. Tenderness is present over the lateral epicondyle approximately 5 mm distal and anterior to the midpoint of the condyle. Plain radiographs usually are negative; occasionally calcific tendinitis may be present. MRI demonstrates tendon thickening with increased T1 and T2 signals, but typically is not indicated.

Many nonsurgical modalities have been described for treatment of lateral epicondylitis; however, most are lacking in sound scientific rationale. Initially, conservative treatment, including rest, ice, tennis brace, or injections, is recommended. Physical therapy is centered around modalities such as ultrasound, iontophoresis, electrical stimulation, manipulation, soft-tissue mobilization, friction massage, augmented soft-tissue mobilization, and stretching and strengthening exercises. Augmenting soft-tissue mobilization is becoming more popular since the detection of changes in the soft-tissue texture as patients progress through the rehabilitative process.

In studies of the clinical effectiveness of local corticosteroid injection, standard nonsteroidal anti-inflammatory drugs, and simple analgesics for treatment of lateral epicondylitis, early local corticosteroid injection has been shown to have a high rate of success for lateral epicondylitis. Preliminary data from studies reporting newer treatment methods, such as low-level laser and extracorporeal shockwave therapy and autologous blood injection, are promising, but require further evaluation.

Chronic or resistant symptoms may require surgery. Surgical options for refractory lateral epicondylitis range from percutaneous release of the extensor origin, which can be done in the office with local anesthesia, to arthroscopic release of the extensor carpi radialis brevis to open débridement. An open release is most commonly done. Proponents of arthroscopy report associated elbow pathology in 69% of patients.

Medial Epicondylitis

Medial epicondylitis or "golfer's elbow" is an overuse syndrome of the flexor pronator mass. Although much less common than lateral epicondylitis, medial epicondylitis is also thought to be caused by work- and sports-related repetitive activities. The condition occurs frequently in overhead throwing athletes, racquet sport participants, and golfers. The involved muscles include the flexor carpi radialis, pronator teres, palmaris longus, and infrequently the flexor carpi ulnaris and the flexor digitorum superficialis. Chronic medial epicondylitis is more difficult to treat than lateral epicondylitis.

Physical examination usually reveals medial pain during activities that involve wrist flexion or pronation. Differential diagnoses include injury to the UCL, sprain of the flexor pronator mass, and ulnar nerve injury. The area of maximal tenderness is approximately 5 mm distal and anterior to the midpoint of the medial epicondyle. Resisted wrist flexion and forearm pronation also elicit pain. Loss of range of motion and a flexion contracture may be present. Radiographically, calcification may be seen adjacent to the medial epicondyle, and a traction spur may be present, which may be consistent with a chronic UCL injury.

If conservative treatment fails, surgical treatment may be indicated. Techniques range from a percutaneous release to open débridement with or without release of the flexor pronator origin. A commonly used technique is to release the flexor pronator origin, excise the pathologic tissue, and reattach the flexor pronator origin to bleeding bone. The ulnar nerve should be decompressed and is transposed in patients who have ulnar nerve symptoms preoperatively. Epicondylectomy also can be done, but no more than 20% of the epicondyle should be removed to avoid violation of the UCL. Overall, the results are not as successful as with lateral epicondyle procedures.

Annotated Bibliography

Rotator Cuff Injuries

Barber FA, Morgan CD, Burkhart SS, Jobe CM: Labrum/biceps/cuff dysfunction in the throwing athlete. *Arthroscopy* 1999;15:852-857.

This article presents a point/counterpoint discussion reviewing the ongoing debate regarding the essential lesion of dead arm syndrome in the throwing athlete. The posterior-superior glenoid impingement model of Walch, Jobe, and Sidles in which glenohumeral laxity is the essential lesion is reviewed, as well as the Morgan-Burkhart model of the type II SLAP as the essential lesion.

Bey MJ, Elders GJ, Huston LJ, Kuhn JE, Blasier RB, Soslowsky LJ: The mechanism of creation of superior labrum, anterior, and posterior lesions in a dynamic biomechanical model of the shoulder: The role of inferior subluxation. *J Shoulder Elbow Surg* 1998;7: 397-401.

In this study, a cadaveric model was used to simulate physiologic rotator cuff forces and produce traction on the long head of the biceps. Matched cadaveric pairs (positioned at 20 mm inferior subluxation and at reduced position) were tested to failure using traction forces on the long head of the biceps. The specimens were then assessed for the presence of type II SLAP lesions. Results showed two of eight specimens tested in the reduced position compared with seven of eight tested in the position of inferior subluxation had type II SLAP lesions. The authors concluded that inferior subluxation with biceps traction facilitates generation of type II SLAP lesions.

Burkhart SS, Morgan CD, Kibler WB: Shoulder injuries in overhead athletes: The "dead arm" revisited. *Clin Sports Med* 2000;19:125-158.

This article discusses the authors' philosophical approach to the etiology, pathophysiology, diagnosis, and treatment of dead arm syndrome. A thorough discussion of the Morgan-Burkhart model of the type II SLAP tear as the essential lesion is included.

Cleeman E, Flatow EL: Classification and diagnosis of impingement and rotator cuff lesions in athletes. *Sports Med Arthrosc Rev* 2000;8:141-157.

This review article details rotator cuff lesions, acromion lesions, SLAP lesions, the mechanics of glenohumeral impingement, the classification of impingement including primary, secondary, and internal, the role of the tight posterior capsule, and evaluation and treatment of these conditions in the throwing athlete.

Gartsman GM, Hammerman SM: Superior labrum, anterior and posterior lesions: When and how to treat them. *Clin Sports Med* 2000;19:115-124.

The authors' approach to SLAP lesions, including anatomy, etiology, pathomechanics, classification, evaluation, and treatment is presented in this comprehensive review.

Halbrecht JL, Tirman P, Atkin D: Internal impingement of the shoulder: Comparison of findings between the throwing and nonthrowing shoulders of college baseball players. *Arthroscopy* 1999;15:253-258.

This article reviews a comparison study of gadolinium-enhanced magnetic resonance arthrogram findings in both the throwing and nonthrowing shoulders of 10 asymptomatic college pitchers. The results of the MRI findings correlated with clinical examination findings. Three of 10 throwing shoulders had labral tears with paralabral cysts and 4 of 10 throwing shoulders had an abnormal rotator cuff tendon signal. None of the nonthrowing shoulders had identifiable MRI abnormalities. In all the shoulders, contact was observed between the undersurface of the rotator cuff and the posterior-superior labrum in the abducted/externally rotated position. The authors concluded that MRI findings consistent with internal impingement can be found in the throwing shoulders of asymptomatic throwers.

Mileski RA, Snyder SJ: Superior labral lesions in the shoulder: Pathoanatomy and surgical management. *J Am Acad Orthop Surg* 1998;6:121-131.

This article reviews the pathoanatomy, evaluation, and surgical treatment of SLAP tears.

Musgrave DS, Rodosky MW: SLAP lesions: Current concepts. *Am J Orthop* 2001;30:29-38.

A comprehensive review of SLAP tears including historical perspectives, anatomy, biomechanics/pathophysiology, pathology, clinical history, physical examination, imaging studies, and treatment is presented. This article also includes a discussion of classification subtypes V, VI, and VII and a comprehensive bibliography.

Paley KJ, Jobe FW, Pink MM, Kvitne RS, ElAttrache NS: Arthroscopic findings in the overhand throwing athlete: Evidence for posterior internal impingement of the rotator cuff. *Arthroscopy* 2000;16:35-40.

This article describes the pathologic findings of arthroscopic examination of the symptomatic throwing shoulders of 41 professional overhand throwing athletes. With the arm in the position of the relocation test, contact between the undersurface of the cuff and the posterior-superior labrum was found in 100% of the shoulders. Undersurface cuff fraying was found in 93% of shoulders, fraying of the posterior-superior labrum in 88%, and fraying of the anterior-superior labrum in 36%. The authors concluded that arthroscopic findings supported the concept of internal impingement in the throwing athlete.

Ulnar Collateral Ligament Injuries

Azar FM, Andrews JR, Wilk KE, Groh D: Operative treatment of ulnar collateral ligament injuries of the elbow in athletes, *Am J Sports Med* 2000;28:16-23.

After reconstruction in 78 patients or repair in 13 patients with UCL injuries, 79% returned to previous or higher levels of competition; 9 of 10 patients had complete resolution of ulnar nerve symptoms. Complications occurred in 8 patients. The average time from surgery to initiation of the interval throwing program was 3.4 months. The average time to return to competitive throwing was 9.8 months.

Ellenbecker TS, Mattalino AJ, Elam EA, Caplinger RA: Medial elbow joint laxity in professional baseball pitchers: A bilateral comparison using stress radiography. *Am J Sports Med* 1998;26:420-424.

Both upper extremities in 40 uninjured professional baseball players were tested using a Telos GA-IIE stress radiography device. Joint space width between the trochlea of the humerus and the coronoid process of the ulna was measured on AP radiographs obtained with and without stress. With stress, the dominant elbow opened 1.20 ± 0.97 mm, whereas the nondominant elbow opened 0.88 ± 0.55 mm.

Fleisig GS, Barrentine SW, Zheng N, Escamilla RF, Andrews JR: Kinematic and kinetic comparison of baseball pitching among various levels of development. *J Biomech* 1999;32:1371-1375.

This comparison of kinematic, kinetic, and temporal parameters among 23 youth, 33 high school, 115 college, and 60 professional baseball pitchers found that few of the kinematic positions or temporal parameters differed significantly; however, the kinematic velocity and kinetic parameters showed significant differences. This study supports the philosophy that a child should be taught proper pitching mechanisms for use throughout life, building strength as the body matures.

Kenter K, Behr CT, Warren RF, O'Brien SJ, Barnes R: Acute elbow injuries in the National Football League. *J Shoulder Elbow Surg* 2000;9:1-5.

Review of acute elbow sprains in football players in the National Football League revealed 39 (55.7%) hyperextension injuries, 14 (20%) medial collateral ligament injuries, 2 (2.9%) lateral collateral ligament sprains, and 15 (21.4%) nonspecific strains. The two most common mechanisms of injury for medial collateral ligament injuries were blocking at the line of scrimmage (50%) and the application of a valgus force with the hand planted on the playing surfaces (29%).

Stress Fractures

Brukner P: Stress fractures of the upper limb. *Sports Med* 1998;26:415-424.

Stress fractures of the upper limb are associated with upper limb-dominated sports such as tennis and swimming and with throwing sports. Stress fractures can occur in the clavicle, scapula, humerus, olecranon, ulnar, or radius. Stress fractures should be considered as a possible diagnosis in athletes with upper limb pain.

Osteochondritis Dissecans

Baumgarten TE, Andrews JR, Satterwhite YE: The arthroscopic classification and treatment of osteochondritis dissecans of the capitellum. *Am J Sports Med* 1998;26:520-523.

After arthroscopic treatment of osteochondritis dissecans, the average flexion and extension contractures decreased by 14° and 6°, respectively. Except for three patients, all returned to preoperative levels of activity. Radiographs showed some residual flattening of the capitellum in eight patients. Two patients required reoperation, one for arthrofibrosis and one for a suspected loose body. An arthroscopic classification is proposed.

Kuwahata Y, Inoue G: Osteochondritis dissecans of the elbow managed by Herbert screw fixation. *Orthopedics* 1998;21:449-451.

At an average of 32 months after Herbert screw fixation and cancellous bone grafting, all seven patients (eight elbows) were pain-free and all had returned to previous athletic activities; elbow range of motion was increased an average of 18°.

Peterson RK, Savoie FH III, Field LD: Osteochondritis dissecans of the elbow. *Instr Course Lect* 1999;48:393-398.

This review article discusses the diagnosis, surgical and nonsurgical treatment, and prognosis of osteochondritis dissecans of the elbow. Newer procedures such as osteochondral transplantation, chondrocyte transplantation, and biochemical manipulation of the chondrocyte environment are also discussed.

Takahara M, Ogino T, Fukushima S, Tsuchida H, Kaneda K: Nonoperative treatment of osteochondritis dissecans of the humeral capitellum. *Am J Sports Med* 1999;27:728-732.

Twenty-four patients treated nonsurgically (avoiding heavy use of the elbow for 6 months) were examined at an average follow-up of 5.2 years. Results showed 4 (17%) had no elbow pain, 7 (29%) had pain only with heavy activities, and 13 (54%) had pain with activities of daily living.

Takahara M, Ogino T, Sasaki I, Kato H, Minami A, Kaneda K: Long-term outcome of osteochondritis dissecans of the humeral capitellum. *Clin Orthop* 1999;363:108-115.

In a series of 53 patients with osteochondritis dissecans of the humeral capitellum, 7 of 14 treated conservatively and 18 of 39 treated by surgical removal of a fragment had residual elbow symptoms associated with activities of daily living (poor outcome). On radiographs a poor outcome was seen in 32% of early lesions and in 50% of advanced lesions. A poor outcome was noted in 64% with evidence of osteoarthritis and in 100% of those with large defects after removal of the fragment.

Takahara M, Ogino T, Takagi M, Tsuchida H, Orui H, Nambu T: Natural progression of osteochondritis dissecans of the humeral capitellum: Initial observations. *Radiology* 2000;216:207-212.

In this study 16 patients with conservatively treated osteochondritis dissecans of the capitellum were observed and the earliest characteristic of this condition was subchondral bone flattening over which new bone subsequently forms. The new bone then unites with the underlying bone; however, if subjected to repetitive forces, unstable fragments develop. These fragments, even if not displaced, are unable to unite.

Lateral Epicondylitis

Baker CL Jr, Murphy KP, Gottlob CA, Curd DT: Arthroscopic classification and treatment of lateral epicondylitis: Two-year clinical results. *J Shoulder Elbow Surg* 2000;9:475-482.

Arthroscopic examination identified three types of lesions as intact capsule (type I), linear capsular tear (type II), and complete capsular tear (type III). Of 39 elbows treated with arthroscopic release, clinical results in 37 were rated by patients as "better" or "much better." Patients returned to work in an average of 2.2 weeks. Grip strength of the treated limb averaged 96% of the grip strength of the unaffected limb.

Boyer MI, Hastings H II: Lateral tennis elbow: "Is there any science out there?" *J Shoulder Elbow Surg* 1999;8:481-491.

Despite its frequency, the condition known as tennis elbow as well as the surgical and nonsurgical methods described for its treatment are clouded with a number of fallacies and myths. Objective data on which to base treatment decisions are lacking. This review article examines the myths of tennis elbow.

Hay EM, Paterson SM, Lewis M, Hosie G, Croft P: Pragmatic randomised controlled trial of local corticosteroid injection and naproxen for treatment of lateral epicondylitis of elbow in primary care. *Br Med J* 1999;319:964-968.

One hundred sixty-four patients with a first episode of lateral epicondylitis were randomized to three treatment groups. After 4 weeks, a significantly ($P < 0.01$) greater percentage of patients treated with methylprednisolone injection (92%) were completely improved compared with 57% treated with oral naproxen or 50% with oral placebo ($P < 0.01$). After 12 months, however, outcome was good in all groups ($P > 0.05$) and effective early outcome did not influence this result.

Kuklo TR, Taylor KF, Murphy KP, Islinger RB, Heekin RD, Baker CL Jr: Arthroscopic release for lateral epicondylitis: A cadaveric model. *Arthroscopy* 1999;15:259-264.

Arthroscopic evaluation of the extensor tendon and release of the extensor carpi radialis brevis were done in 10 fresh-frozen cadaveric upper extremities to determine the distance between the cannula and neurovascular structures. The radial nerve was consistently in close proximity to the proximal lateral portal.

Pfahler M, Jessel C, Steinborn M, Refior HJ: Magnetic resonance imaging in lateral epicondylitis of the elbow. *Arch Orthop Trauma Surg* 1998;118:121-125.

Histopathologic analysis of six surgical cases confirmed preoperative MRI findings by showing either focal fibrous degenerative tendon tissue or microruptures of collagenous fibers.

Classic Bibliography

Andrews JR: Bony injuries about the elbow in the throwing athlete. *Instr Course Lect* 1985;34:323-331.

Arroyo JS, Hershon SJ, Bigliani LU: Special considerations in the athletic throwing shoulder. *Orthop Clin North Am* 1997;28:69-78.

Bennett GE: Shoulder and elbow lesions distinctive of baseball players. *Ann Surg* 1947;126:107-110.

Bennett GE: Shoulder and elbow lesions of the professional baseball pitcher. *JAMA* 1941;117:510-514.

Bigliani LU, Codd TP, Connor PM, Levine WN, Littlefield MA, Hershon SJ: Shoulder motion and laxity in the professional baseball player. *Am J Sports Med* 1997;25:609-613.

Bigliani LU, Rodosky MW, Newton PD, O'Boyle MJ, Pollock RG, Flatow EL: Abstract: Arthroscopic coracoacromial ligament resection for impingement in the overhead athletes. *J Shoulder Elbow Surg* 1995; 4(suppl):S54.

Conway JE, Jobe FW, Glousman RE, Pink M: Medial instability of the elbow in throwing athletes: Treatment by repair or reconstruction of the ulnar collateral ligament. *J Bone Joint Surg Am* 1992;74:67-83.

Ferrari JD, Ferrari DA, Coumas J, Pappas AM: Posterior ossification of the shoulder: The Bennett lesion. Etiology, diagnosis, and treatment. *Am J Sports Med* 1994;22:171-175.

Hamilton CD, Glousman RE, Jobe FW, Brault J, Pink M, Perry J: Dynamic stability of the elbow: Electromyographic analysis of the flexor pronator group and the extensor group in pitchers with valgus instability. *J Shoulder Elbow Surg* 1996;5:347-354.

Jobe CM: Posterior Superior glenoid impingement: Expanded spectrum. *Arthroscopy* 1995;11:530-536.

Jobe FW, Stark H, Lombardo SJ: Reconstruction of the ulnar collateral ligament in athletes. *J Bone Joint Surg Am* 1986;68:1158-1163.

King J, Brelsford HJ, Tullos HS: Analysis of the pitching arm of the professional baseball pitcher. *Clin Orthop* 1969;67:116-123.

Kurvers H, Verhaar J: The results of operative treatment of medial epicondylitis. *J Bone Joint Surg Am* 1995;77:1374-1379.

Kvitne RS, Jobe FW, Jobe CM: Shoulder instability in the overhand or throwing athlete. *Clin Sports Med* 1995;14:917-935.

Montgomery WH III, Jobe FW: Functional outcomes in athletes after modified anterior capsulolabral reconstruction. *Am J Sports Med* 1994;22:352-358.

Nirschl RP, Pettrone FA: Tennis elbow: The surgical treatment of lateral epicondylitis. *J Bone Joint Surg Am* 1979;61:832-839.

Ogilvie-Harris DJ, Gordon R, MacKay M: Arthroscopic treatment for posterior impingement in degenerative arthritis of the elbow. *Arthroscopy* 1995;11: 437-443.

Payne LZ, Altchek DW, Craig EV, Warren RF: Arthroscopic treatment of partial rotator cuff tears in young athletes: A preliminary report. *Am J Sports Med* 1997;25:299-305.

Regan W, Wold LE, Coonrad R, Morrey BF: Microscopic histopathology of chronic refractory lateral epicondylitis. *Am J Sports Med* 1992;20:746-749.

Smith GR, Altchek DW, Pagnani MJ, Keeley JR: A muscle-splitting approach to the ulnar collateral ligament of the elbow: Neuroanatomy and operative technique. *Am J Sports Med* 1996;24:575-580.

Snyder SJ, Karzel RP, Del Pizzo W, Ferkel RD, Friedman MJ: SLAP lesions of the shoulder. *Arthroscopy* 1990;6:274-279.

Suzuki K, Minami A, Suenaga N, Kondoh M: Oblique stress fracture of the olecranon in baseball pitchers. *J Shoulder Elbow Surg* 1997;6:491-494.

Tibone JE, Elrod B, Jobe FW, et al: Surgical treatment of tears of the rotator cuff in athletes. *J Bone Joint Surg Am* 1986;68:887-891.

Walch G, Boileau P, Noel E, Donell ST: Impingement of the deep surface of the supraspinatus tendon on the posterosuperior glenoid rim: An arthroscopic study. *J Shoulder Elbow Surg* 1992;1:238-245.

Wilson FD, Andrews JR, Blackburn TA, McCluskey G: Valgus extension overload in the pitching elbow. *Am J Sports Med* 1983;11:83-88.

Chapter 26

Shoulder Trauma: Bone

Douglas R. Dirschl, MD

Proximal Humeral Fractures

Proximal humeral fractures comprise about 4% to 5% of all fractures; approximately 85% of these fractures have minimal displacement. Although nonsurgical management is almost always used for nondisplaced fractures, controversy exists over the most appropriate treatment of the 15% of fractures that are displaced.

Classification and Evaluation

The four-part system of Neer has been used to classify fractures of the proximal humerus. Classification of a fracture requires the identification of anatomic fracture fragments (Fig. 1), as well as determination of the amount of displacement or angulation of each anatomic fragment. A fragment must be displaced more than 1 cm or angulated more than 45°. When the Neer classification system is applied to routine radiographs or CT scans, the result is fair to poor interobserver reliability and intraobserver reproducibility. Although the Neer classification system may be useful for describing fracture types and assessing the severity of injury, caution is urged in using it for comparing outcomes of fractures classified and treated by more than one surgeon.

The shoulder trauma series is the standard for evaluating fractures of the proximal humerus. This series includes scapular AP, scapular/lateral, and axillary radiographs of the glenohumeral joint. The AP and axillary radiographs provide the most useful information. CT scans help to further characterize fractures that involve splitting of the humeral head. MRI is sometimes used to aid in the diagnosis of occult fractures of the greater tuberosity or to assess for the presence of associated rotator cuff injuries. In a recent study of a group of patients with nondisplaced fractures of the greater tuberosity who underwent MRI, no rotator cuff injuries were found. Arthroscopy has also been suggested as a useful tool in fully evaluating the extent of shoulder injury; labral lesions were found in 56% and 31% of patients with fracture-dislocations and displaced two-part fractures of the proximal humerus, respectively.

Treatment

The choice of treatment for a proximal humeral fracture should be based on age and activity level of the patient, the presence and nature of comorbid medical conditions, the general quality of the bone, the presence of other concurrent injuries, and the type of fracture. Humeral head salvage should always be considered in younger patients with good bone quality; in elderly patients with osteoporotic bone or degenerative changes in the rotator cuff or glenohumeral joint, hemiarthroplasty should receive the strongest consideration.

Nonsurgical management with early supervised range of motion is the treatment of choice for nondisplaced or minimally displaced fractures. Initial immobilization in an arm sling or collar and cuff is followed by gentle range of motion exercises as soon as pain allows. Active range of motion is started when the proximal humerus moves as a unit, usually within 4 weeks of injury.

Two-part fractures of the surgical neck are the most common type of displaced proximal humeral fracture. Although closed reduction and immobilization are possible, this treatment is generally reserved for skeletally immature patients. If a closed reduction of the fracture can be obtained, stabilization with terminally threaded percutaneous pins is often advocated. This method of treatment involves little or no soft-tissue disruption, thus possibly reducing the incidence of osteonecrosis and nonunion. Postoperative motion usually is delayed for several weeks until the pins are removed, but excessive stiffness does not appear to be common. Recent studies have reported up to 84% good or excellent results using this technique for selected fractures. However, percutaneous pin stabilization should

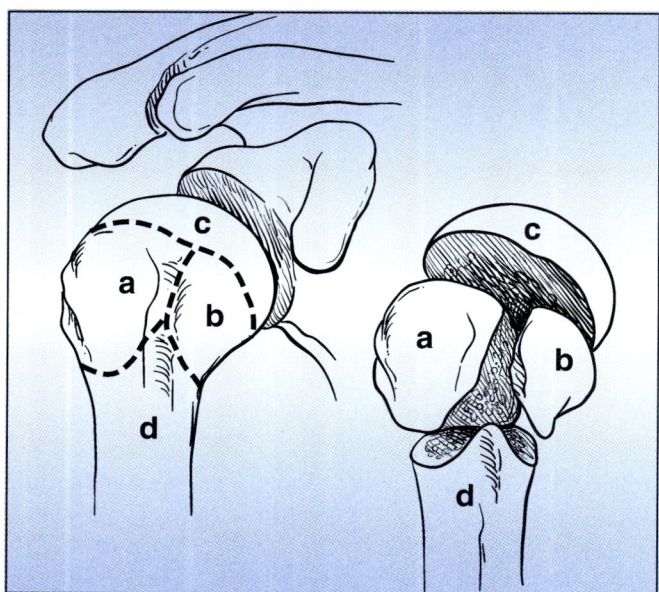

Figure 1 Division of the proximal humerus into four distinct fragments that roughly represent ossification centers during growth and development. **a,** Greater tuberosity; **b,** lesser tuberosity; **c,** humeral head; **d,** humeral shaft.

be used with caution; maintenance of reduction with this technique is much less reliable in patients with poor bone quality.

Open reduction commonly involves use of Ender nails with figure-of-8 tension banding, intraosseous sutures, or plate and screw fixation. However, intramedullary nails and blade plates specifically designed for use in the proximal humerus are being used more frequently.

Two-part fractures of the greater tuberosity often occur in conjuction with a glenohumeral dislocation. After closed reduction of the glenohumeral dislocation, the tuberosity may return to its anatomic position. If superior or posterior displacement greater than 5 mm persists, open reduction and fixation of the tuberosity fragment with repair of the rotator cuff tear should be considered. If left untreated, residual displacement greater than 5 mm can result in impingement of a superiorly displaced tuberosity against the acromion in elevation or abutment of a posteriorly displaced tuberosity against the glenoid in external rotation. Open reduction of greater tuberosity fractures is usually done through a deltoid-splitting approach. Stabilization of the tuberosity can be achieved with intraosseous sutures incorporating the rotator cuff insertion or, if the tuberosity is a single large piece, screw fixation may be used.

Although rare, displaced lesser tuberosity fractures can be associated with posterior shoulder dislocations. Wide displacement of the fragment can lead to loss of active internal rotation, and open reduction with screw

or suture fixation and repair of the rotator interval may be a consideration.

The treatment of three- and four-part fractures of the proximal humerus is controversial. Although results from one recent report show no difference in outcomes between patients treated nonsurgically and with open reduction and internal fixation (ORIF), functional results in anatomically reduced three-part fractures were significantly better than in fractures with residual displacement, according to results from a multicenter study. Although the techniques for reduction and stabilization of these fractures are similar to those for two-part surgical neck fractures, improved results may be achieved with minimal osteosynthesis. Recent reports comparing indirect reduction and plate fixation to classic ORIF have indicated a lower rate of osteonecrosis with the indirect reduction technique.

Four-part fractures usually are treated with humeral head replacement. ORIF usually is reserved for attempts at humeral head salvage in young patients with good bone quality. Results after ORIF of four-part fractures have varied widely, and rates of osteonecrosis from 9% to 11% have been reported. Primary prosthetic replacement for four-part fractures generally has been reported to result in good pain relief but poor range of shoulder motion. Recent reports have indicated that functional outcomes after early hemiarthroplasty are superior to those of late hemiarthroplasty after unsuccessful nonsurgical management.

Fractures of the Clavicle

Although clavicular fractures account for only 4% to 5% of all fractures, they account for 35% of fractures about the shoulder. Eighty-five percent involve the middle third of the clavicle, and nearly all the rest involve the distal third. Associated injuries about the shoulder occur in a very small percentage of patients with clavicular fractures, yet it is these patients for whom surgical treatment is most often beneficial. The most common mechanism of injury in adults is direct trauma, followed by an indirect mechanism of injury (a fall onto the outstretched hand).

Although a single AP radiograph of the shoulder generally is sufficient to establish the diagnosis of and plan treatment for a clavicular fracture, a cephalic tilt radiograph can be obtained to more accurately evaluate AP displacement. CT is rarely indicated for middle third clavicular fractures, but may be helpful in patients with fractures of the medial clavicle to assess the displacement of the medial fragment and the integrity of the sternoclavicular joint.

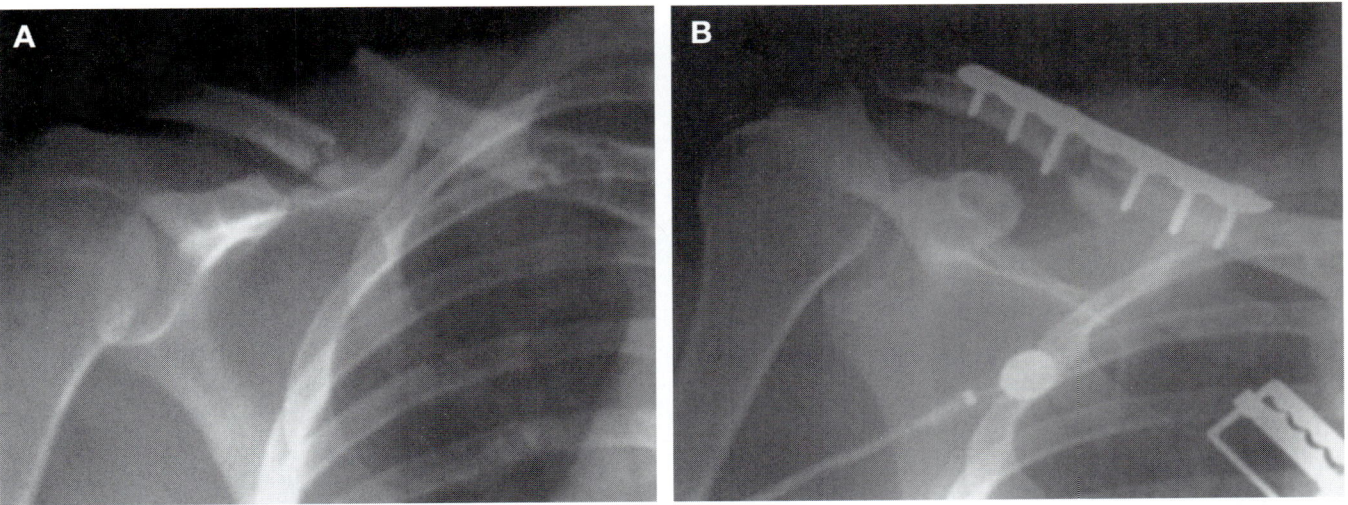

Figure 2 ORIF of a displaced clavicular fracture. **A,** The preoperative radiograph reveals marked displacement of a comminuted fracture of the middle clavicle, with the proximal fragment displaced superiorly. **B,** The postoperative radiograph reveals anatomic alignment and secure stabilization with a pelvic reconstruction plate and screws inserted on the superior surface of the bone.

Treatment

Most middle third fractures are treated with a figure-of-8 bandage or arm sling. The sling or bandage is removed and range of motion exercises started as soon as the patient's comfort allows. Healing will usually be evident on radiographs in about 6 weeks, but return to full function in an adult patient generally takes about 12 weeks. Clavicular shortening and a residual painless deformity, which commonly do not interfere with shoulder function, may result from nonsurgical treatment. Functional outcomes have generally been thought to be good after nonsurgical treatment. Results from a recent study of 17-year follow-up of clavicular fractures treated nonsurgically indicated that 82% of shoulders were asymptomatic and that only 1 of 225 patients had a poor clinical rating.

Open fractures in adults, the presence of neurovascular injury/compromise, and displaced fractures with impending skin compromise are some indications for surgical treatment. ORIF has been suggested as treatment for all widely displaced midclavicular fractures, with the rationale that the shortening generally seen in clavicular fractures treated nonsurgically is likely to result in decreased long-term function and an increase in the rate of nonunion. The evidence supporting this rationale, however, is not consistent. Although one study reported that up to 14 mm of shortening did not impair mobility, strength, or functional rating at 5-year follow-up, another study of completely displaced middle third fractures in adults indicated that shortening of 20 mm or more at the time of injury was a risk factor for the development of nonunion. When ORIF of clavicular fractures is done, plate and screw fixation and intramedullary devices both have been used with

generally good results (Fig. 2). Complications, including infection, nonunion, hardware migration, and an unsightly surgical scar, have been reported. The literature to date does not support the routine surgical treatment of displaced, isolated midclavicular fractures.

Lateral third fractures of the clavicle are grouped according to the location of the fracture relative to the coracoclavicular ligaments. Type I fractures are located between the coracoclavicular and coracoacromial ligaments and are characterized by minimal displacement of the medial fragment. Type I fractures are stable and treated in the same manner as the nonsurgical treatment of middle third clavicular fractures.

Type II fractures are characterized by superior displacement of the medial fragment, because the fracture occurs medial to the coracoclavicular ligaments. The medial clavicular fragment has no bony or ligamentous connection to the remaining shoulder girdle. The weight of the upper extremity pulls the now freed shoulder girdle downward, causing scapular ptosis. The resulting gap between the medial and lateral clavicular fragments can result in nonunion. Nonetheless, there remains disagreement as to the most appropriate treatment for displaced type II fractures. The argument advocating surgical treatment is based on reports of a 30% nonunion rate after nonsurgical treatment. Those advocating nonsurgical treatment, however, point out that the incidence of pain and nonunion after nonsurgical treatment is very low. Plates and screws, intramedullary devices, and methods of reconstructing the coracoclavicular ligaments have been described, with reported success. For very small lateral clavicular fragments, fragment excision, coupled with reconstruction of the coracoclavicular ligaments, has been described.

Type III fractures involve the articular surface of the lateral clavicle at the acromioclavicular joint. An AP view of both shoulders with weights strapped to the wrists may aid in evaluating the integrity of the coracoclavicular ligaments. Type III fractures can be adequately managed nonsurgically, although ORIF or fragment excision may be indicated in the presence of a large fragment with significant articular step-off. If symptomatic degenerative disease of the acromioclavicular joint occurs, distal clavicle resection should be done.

Complications after treatment of clavicular fractures are uncommon, but include nonunion, malunion, neurovascular sequelae, and postoperative degenerative disease of either the acromioclavicular or sternoclavicular joint. The incidence of nonunion is 0.9% to 4.0%; 85% of nonunions occur with middle third clavicular fractures. Inadequate immobilization, significant displacement, increased severity of initial trauma, soft-tissue interposition, refracture, and primary ORIF can predispose patients to nonunion. Asymptomatic nonunion does not require treatment. In the presence of pain, shoulder dysfunction, or neurovascular compromise, compression plating or intramedullary fixation and bone grafting should be considered. Tricortical iliac crest interposition grafting with compression plating has been used with good results in treating atrophic nonunions with large gaps.

Fractures of the Scapula

Because the scapula is protected by the surrounding muscles and chest wall, a large amount of energy is required to cause a scapular fracture. As a result, associated injuries that usually involve the head or shoulder are common in patients with scapular fractures and may be severe and life-threatening. The ipsilateral rib fracture with resulting hemopneumothorax is the most common associated injury, followed by clavicular fracture, closed head injury, injury to the face and skull, and brachial plexus injury. A particularly serious injury combination is fracture of the scapula and first rib because of the risk of pulmonary and neurovascular compromise.

The shoulder trauma series is generally all that is necessary to identify most fractures of the scapula. A chest radiograph is an essential part of the evaluation because of the high incidence of associated injuries involving intrathoracic structures. Because of the complex bony anatomy of the scapula, CT can assist in detecting and defining the extent and/or displacement of intra-articular fractures.

Treatment

Fractures of the scapular body are generally treated nonsurgically and no reduction is attempted, even when the fractures are severely comminuted and displaced. Initial immobilization of the arm in a sling for comfort is followed by progressive range of motion exercises as symptoms allow. Although outcomes after nonsurgical treatment have generally been good, more recent data indicate that surgical treatment of markedly displaced fractures of the scapular body may be warranted.

Fractures of the neck of the scapula are frequently displaced, but usually stable, provided the clavicle and coracoclavicular ligaments are intact. For stable fractures, further displacement is rare and nonsurgical management is the treatment of choice, following the protocol for management of scapular body fractures. Surgery has been suggested if the glenoid fragment is displaced more than 1 cm or angulated greater than 40° because of concerns that shoulder pain and dysfunction will result from nonsurgical treatment. The glenoid fragment is reduced from a posterior approach and stabilized with plates and screws.

Most fractures of the acromion are minimally displaced and can be treated with early range of motion shoulder exercises. Activities involving resisted deltoid function should be avoided until fracture union has been achieved. For depressed acromial fractures that encroach on the subacromial space and interfere with rotator cuff function, ORIF is recommended.

Decision-making regarding the management of scapular fractures is more difficult when a combination of injuries results in instability of the shoulder girdle. The concept of a superior shoulder suspensory complex (SSSC) has been proposed to help describe and understand this group of complex injuries. The SSSC is a bone and soft-tissue ring (the glenoid process, coracoid process, coracoclavicular ligaments, distal clavicle, acromioclavicular joint, and acromial process) at the end of superior (the middle clavicle) and inferior (the lateral scapular body) bony struts. A disruption of the SSSC in a single location will not disrupt the overall integrity of the complex and usually can be treated nonsurgically. Disruptions of the SSSC in two locations may cause instability of the shoulder girdle and make significant displacement more likely to occur. For double disruptions of the SSSC, ORIF is recommended if one or both injury sites have unacceptable displacement. Surgical stabilization at one site is all that is required for satisfactory reduction and stabilization of the entire complex; studies have indicated good results using this treatment. A recent study challenged the recommendation for surgical treatment, reporting 17 excellent and 3 good results in 20 patients with floating shoulders (ipsilateral fracture of the middle third of the clavicle and the scapular neck) treated nonsurgically.

Complications associated with the scapular fracture itself (rather than with associated injuries) are relatively uncommon and generally well tolerated. Malunion of fractures of the scapular body usually causes no symptoms, although painful scapulothoracic crepitus after fracture healing occasionally occurs. Nonunion is extremely rare because the extensive soft-tissue cover of the scapula provides an excellent blood supply for healing. Suprascapular nerve injuries can occur in association with body, neck, or coracoid fractures involving the suprascapular notch; symptoms are often relieved after surgical exploration and decompression.

Humeral Shaft Fractures

Fractures of the humeral shaft comprise approximately 3% of all fractures. Direct blows to the arm, falls, and twisting injuries cause the majority of these fractures. Higher energy mechanisms of injury are more common in young adults, and falls from standing height are the most common mechanism of injury in elderly patients.

Patients with humeral shaft fractures usually complain of arm pain and swelling; deformity may be present but often is not detected, especially in obese patients. A careful examination to assess motor and sensory function of the radial, median, and ulnar nerves should be done; this examination is used as a baseline for subsequent neurologic assessments during treatment of the humeral shaft fracture.

The standard radiographic examination of the humerus includes AP and lateral views that include the entire humerus and the shoulder and elbow joints. These orthogonal radiographs should be obtained by turning the patient's torso, rather than by rotating the injured limb. In fractures that are highly comminuted or severely displaced, traction radiographs may allow better definition of the fragments. Comparison radiographs of the contralateral humerus may assist in determination of normal humeral length before surgical treatment is attempted.

Treatment and Outcomes

Most humeral shaft fractures can be managed nonsurgically, using a coaptation splint, Velpeau dressing, collar and cuff, or a hanging arm cast. Whatever the method of fracture immobilization, the patient is instructed to allow the elbow to hang free, allowing gravity and the weight of the arm to improve fracture alignment. The patient should remain upright as much as possible, either standing or sitting, and not lean on the elbow for support. Within 1 to 2 weeks, as pain allows, the initial immobilization is discontinued and the arm placed in a functional fracture brace. The brace consists of an anterior and a posterior plastic shell, held together with Velcro straps. Fracture stabilization is achieved and fracture alignment improved through compression of the cylinder of soft tissue that comprises the arm. The brace is progressively tightened as swelling decreases. The patient is encouraged to perform range of motion exercises of the shoulder, elbow, wrist, and hand while wearing the brace. Patients with massive soft-tissue or bone loss, the inability to obtain or maintain acceptable fracture alignment, or who are unreliable or uncooperative should not use the functional brace.

Anatomic alignment is not required to achieve satisfactory outcomes after treatment of humeral shaft fractures. Up to 20° of anterior or posterior angulation, 30° of varus or valgus angulation, and 3 cm of shortening may be well tolerated, with varus or valgus angulation better tolerated proximally, near the shoulder joint, than an equal amount of angulation more distally. Similarly, angulation in the plane of elbow joint motion usually does not interfere with function. An obese patient may tolerate more angulation, because the cosmetic deformity is less apparent. Considerable malrotation at the fracture site is well tolerated because of the large amount of rotation at the shoulder joint.

The results of nonsurgical treatment of humeral shaft fractures are generally satisfactory, with a high rate of union. In a recent study, the rate of nonunion was 2% in closed fractures treated with functional bracing. Another study of 158 patients reported good to excellent functional results with nearly full range of shoulder and elbow motion in all patients.

Surgical indications for humeral shaft fractures include open humeral fractures (except those caused by low-velocity gunshot wounds), multiple injuries, spinal cord or brachial plexus injuries, fractures with associated vascular injuries, floating elbow injuries (humeral and forearm fractures), bilateral humeral shaft fractures, fractures extending into the elbow or shoulder joint, impending pathologic fractures, and fractures in which a satisfactory alignment cannot be maintained by nonsurgical means. The floating elbow is best treated by internal fixation of both the humeral and forearm fractures, followed by early range of elbow motion. Surgical stabilization of bilateral humeral fractures is necessary to allow patient self-care. The semisitting position that is necessary for nonsurgical fracture treatment is often unreasonable for the polytrauma patient. Surgical stabilization of the humerus may allow early use of crutches or other aids for ambulation. Neurologic loss after humeral fracture caused by a lacerating injury is an indication for nerve exploration.

Surgical stabilization of humeral shaft fractures using plates and screws offers the advantages of direct fracture reduction, visualization of the radial nerve, and stable fixation of the humeral shaft without violation of the rotator cuff or elbow joint. The use of plates and screws has been considered the gold standard by which all other surgical methods for humeral stabilization should be compared. Plates and screws can be used for almost all humeral shaft fractures requiring surgical treatment, provided the soft-tissue envelope is healthy enough to permit the large surgical exposure required. Plates and screws are also the preferred method for stabilizing nonunions of the humeral shaft. The surgical approach for plating of the humerus depends on the location of the fracture and the need to expose the radial nerve.

Outcomes after plating of acute humeral shaft fractures have in general been good. Recent reports have indicated rates of union of 94% to 100%, times to union of 9 to 20 weeks, and excellent shoulder and elbow function at follow-up. Complications have been infrequent, but have included infection, nonunion, radial nerve palsy, and loss of fixation.

Intramedullary nailing of humeral shaft fractures offers certain biologic and mechanical advantages over plates and screws. Thay can be inserted without direct exposure to the fracture, which minimizes soft-tissue disruption and scarring. An intramedullary device is closer to the mechanical axis of the humerus than a plate; therefore, intramedullary nails are subjected to smaller bending loads than plates. In addition, stress shielding with resultant cortical osteopenia, commonly seen with plates and screws, is minimized. The most frequently cited relative indications for use of intramedullary devices include segmental fractures in which plate and screw stabilization would require considerable soft-tissue dissection, fractures in osteopenic bone, and impending pathologic fractures.

Thin flexible nails and reamed interlocking intramedullary nails are available for use in the humeral shaft. Flexible devices are available in a variety of designs but, because they do not reliably control either fracture shortening or rotation, they are being used with much less frequency than in the past. Reamed, interlocked intramedullary nails prevent fracture shortening and rotation and can be inserted antegrade through the rotator cuff or retrograde proximal to the olecranon fossa.

The potential effects of antegrade humeral nailing on shoulder pain and rotator cuff function currently are being debated. In an increasing number of studies, results have shown a high incidence of shoulder pain after antegrade nail insertion, despite seating of the nail below the rotator cuff. According to the results of a recent study, more than 33% of patients treated with antegrade humeral nailing are reported to have significantly impaired shoulder joint function. The axillary nerve also may be at risk during proximal locking screw insertion. These issues have been examined in anatomic studies and alterations to surgical technique have been recommended in an effort to decrease the incidence of rotator cuff injury and axillary nerve injury with antegrade humeral nailing. Retrograde humeral nailing has been reported as a method for decreasing the incidence of shoulder dysfunction after humeral nailing. Although clinical studies using this retrograde technique are few, anatomic and biomechanical studies have provided recommendations as to entry portal and technique to maximize safety and minimize weakening of the distal humeral shaft. The devastating complication of fractures of the distal humerus around retrograde humeral nails has recently been reported; the possibility of this significant complication should be carefully considered by the surgeon choosing retrograde nailing of the humeral shaft.

Outcomes after interlocked intramedullary nailing of humeral shaft fractures have been mixed. Rates of nonunion in recent series have ranged from 0 to 22%; reported rates of shoulder dysfunction have also varied widely. One recent prospective randomized trial of ORIF with plates and screws versus intramedullary nailing of humeral shaft fractures revealed rates of union of 93% and 87%, respectively, in the ORIF and intramedullary nailing groups; shoulder pain and decreased shoulder range of motion was associated with the intramedullary nailing group, but not with the ORIF group.

Radial nerve injury occurs in up to 18% of patients with humeral shaft fractures. Although the oblique distal third (Holstein-Lewis) fracture is best known for its association with neurologic injury, radial nerve palsy is most commonly observed after middle third humeral fractures. Most nerve injuries are neurapraxias and 90% resolve in 3 to 4 months. Electromyography and nerve conduction studies can help to determine the degree of nerve injury and track the rate of nerve regeneration; ultrasound recently has been reported to be reliable in identifying lacerated or entrapped radial nerves. Radial nerve palsy that develops after manipulation of a closed humeral shaft fracture has historically been an indication for prompt surgical exploration, but observation for return of radial nerve function is currently the recommended course of action. Surgical exploration can be done 3 or 4 months after injury if there is no evidence of neurologic recovery. In a study of 14 patients with open humeral shaft fracture with an associated radial nerve injury, 9 patients (64%) had a radial nerve that was either lacerated or interposed between the fracture fragments.

Nonunion after humeral shaft fracture is rare. Fracture pattern, method of treatment, distraction of the fracture, and overall patient health are factors that may affect the rate of nonunion. Compression plating with bone grafting is the treatment of choice for most established humeral nonunions. Surgical goals include obtaining osseous stability, eliminating the nonunion gap, maintaining or restoring osseous vascularity, and eradicating or avoiding infection. Compression plating combined with cancellous bone grafting to treat humeral nonunions has been effective in two series, with results indicating that 96% and 97% of patients achieved union.

The humeral shaft is commonly involved by metastatic disease, which may result in pathologic fracture. The best way to relieve patient pain, facilitate nursing care, and maximize patient independence is with surgical stabilizaiton of pathologic humeral fractures. The implant of choice for these fractures is the interlocked nail because it provides stable fixation, immediate pain relief, and rapid restoration of upper extremity function. An interlocked nail can be accompanied by adjunctive polymethylmethacrylate in patients with a large tumor defect.

Annotated Bibliography

Proximal Humerus Fractures

Bosch U, Skutek M, Fremerey RW, Tscherne H: Outcome after primary and secondary hemiarthroplasty in elderly patients with fractures of the proximal humerus. *J Shoulder Elbow Surg* 1998;7:479-484.

Thirty-nine patients with three- or four-part fractures of the proximal humerus were treated with hemiarthroplasty. Patients who underwent hemiarthroplasty within 4 weeks of fracture had much better functional outcomes than patients who underwent hemiarthroplasty 4 or more weeks after fracture. The decision to perform hemiarthroplasty should be made as early as possible after fracture.

Chen CY, Chao EK, Tu YK, Ueng SW, Shih CH: Closed management and percutaneous fixation of unstable proximal humerus fractures. *J Trauma* 1998;45: 1039-1045.

Nineteen patients with two- and three-part proximal humeral fractures were treated with closed reduction and percutaneous fixation with cannulated screws. Mean follow-up was 21 months. All but one patient obtained fracture union, and 84% had good or excellent results according to Neer's criteria. No osteonecrosis or collapse was observed.

Hagino H, Yamamoto K, Ohshiro H, Nakamura T, Kishimoto H, Nose T: Changing incidence of hip, distal radius, and proximal humerus fractures in Tottori Prefecture, Japan. *Bone* 1999;24:265-270.

A survey of fracture incidence was done for all patients 35 years of age or older for the years 1986 to 1988 and 1992 to 1994. The incidence per 100,000 population of proximal humeral fractures in women was 42.0 in 1986 and 47.9 in 1992, a statistically significant increase.

Hessmann M, Baumgaertel F, Gehling H, Klingelhoeffer I, Gotzen L: Plate fixation of proximal humeral fractures with indirect reduction: Surgical technique and results utilizing three shoulder scores. *Injury* 1999;30: 453-462.

Ninety-eight patients were evaluated a mean of 34 months after indirect reduction and plating of proximal humeral fractures. Results were good to excellent in 76% of fractures. Osteonecrosis occurred in 4% of cases, and nonunion occurred in one patient.

Lin J, Hou SM, Hang YS: Locked nailing for displaced surgical neck fractures of the humerus. *J Trauma* 1998;45:1051-1057.

Twenty-one consecutive displaced surgical neck fractures of the humerus in patients with a mean age of 66 years were treated with antegrade locked humeral nails. The mean surgical time was 55 minutes. All fractures united at an average time of 14.8 weeks. At 19 months follow-up, excellent or satisfactory results were obtained in 86% of patients.

Mason BJ, Kier R, Bindleglass DF: Occult fractures of the greater tuberosity of the humerus: Radiographic and MR imaging findings. *AJR Am J Roentgenol* 1999;172:469-473.

MRI of patients with nondisplaced greater tuberosity fractures revealed no associated rotator cuff injuries that required surgical treatment. MRI and arthroscopy were unnecessary in the evaluation and treatment of nondisplaced fractures of the greater tuberosity.

Ruch DS, Glisson RR, Marr AW, Russell GB, Nunley JA: Fixation of three-part proximal humeral fractures: A biomechanical evaluation. *J Orthop Trauma* 2000;14: 36-40.

The mechanical stability of fixing three-part fractures of the proximal humerus with tension band wiring with Ender nails, modified clover leaf plating, and intramedullary nailing were compared in fresh frozen cadaveric specimens. In cantilever bending and torsional testing, the plate/screw and intramedullary nail constructs were superior to the tension band technique. There was no difference between the plate/ screw and intramedullary nail constructs in either mode of testing.

Zyto K: Non-operative treatment of comminuted fractures of the proximal humerus in elderly patients. *Injury* 1998;29:349-352.

Seventeen fractures of the proximal humerus in elderly patients treated nonsurgically were evaluated for a minimum of 10 years. The mean Constant score in patients with three- and four-part fractures was 59 and 47, respectively. The mean flexion and abduction were each more than 90°. Only four patients reported mild pain. Although functional scoring was low, the patients' satisfaction with their shoulders was high.

Zyto K, Wallace WA, Frostick SP, Preston BJ: Outcome after hemiarthroplasty for three- and four-part fractures of the proximal humerus. *J Shoulder Elbow Surg* 1998;7:85-89.

Twenty-seven patients who underwent hemiarthroplasty for three- or four-part fractures of the proximal humerus were evaluated at a mean of 39 months. The mean Constant score was 51 and 46 for three- and four-part fractures, respectively. The mean range of abduction and flexion was 70° each. Nine patients had moderate or severe pain, and eight had moderate or severe disability.

Fractures of the Clavicle

Laursen MB, Dossing KV: Clavicular nonunions treated with compression plate fixation and cancellous bone grafting: The functional outcome. *J Shoulder Elbow Surg* 1999;8:410-413.

Fracture healing and outcome were evaluated in 16 patients with clavicular nonunion treated with compression plate fixation and bone grafting. All fractures united uneventfully, but two patients required reoperation for removal of loose screws. Eleven of 12 patients available for clinical assessment had a good or excellent result, and 9 of 12 returned to their preinjury activity level.

Nordqvist A, Petersson CJ, Redlund-Johnell I: Midclavicle fractures in adults: End result study after conservative treatment. *J Orthop Trauma* 1998;12:572-576.

Two hundred twenty-five midclavicular fractures that had been treated nonsurgically were evaluated clinically and radiographically an average of 17 years after injury. At follow-up, 185 shoulders were asymptomatic; 39 were moderately painful, and one was extremely painful. One hundred twenty-five fractures had united in normal position, 53 were malunited with persistent displacement, and 7 were nonunions. Forty malunions and three nonunions were rated clinically as good.

Nowak J, Mallmin H, Larsson S: The aetiology and epidemiology of clavicular fractures: A prospective study during a two-year period in Uppsala, Sweden. *Injury* 2000;31:353-358.

The age- and gender-specific indicence of clavicular fractures were studied during 1989 and 1990. The incidence of clavicular fractures per 100,000 population was 71 in males and 30 in females. Fracture incidence decreased with age in both genders. Seventy-five percent of fractures occurred in the middle third of the clavicle. Ninety-five percent healed uneventfully.

Fractures of the Scapula

Edwards SG, Whittle AP, Wood GW II: Nonoperative treatment of ipsilateral fractures of the scapula and clavicle. *J Bone Joint Surg Am* 2000;82:774-780.

Twenty patients with a floating shoulder were treated either with a sling or a shoulder immobilizer. Eleven clavicular fractures were displaced 10 mm or more, and five scapular fractures were displaced more than 5 mm. Mean follow-up was 28 months. Nineteen of 20 fractures united uneventfully; one clavicular nonunion occurred due to segmental bone loss from a gunshot wound. Eighteen patients had an excellent functional result, one had a good result, and one had a fair result. Eighteen patients had full symmetrical shoulder range of motion. Results were slightly better in those patients with less than 5 mm displacement of the scapular fracture.

Mayo KA, Benirschke SK, Mast JW: Displaced fractures of the glenoid fossa: Results of open reduction and internal fixation. *Clin Orthop* 1998;347:122-130.

Twenty-seven patients with displaced glenoid fractures treated surgically were assessed a mean of 43 months after injury. Anatomic reconstruction was achieved in 89% of patients. Two patients has infraspinatus palsies and one had wound dehiscence following surgery. Functional rating revealed 22% excellent, 60% good, 11% fair, and 7% poor outcomes.

Humeral Shaft Fractures

Chapman JR, Henley MB, Agel J, Benca PJ: Randomized prospective study of humeral shaft fracture fixation: Intramedullary nails versus plates. *J Orthop Trauma* 2000;14:162-166.

A prospective, randomized study of 84 patients treated either with ORIF with plates and screws (PLT) or reamed interlocked intramedullary nailing (IMN) was done. Follow-up averaged 13 months. Healing by 16 weeks occurred in 93% of the PLT group and 87% of the IMN group. Shoulder pain and decreased shoulder function were associated with IMN, but not with PLT. Both methods of treatment provide predictable methods for achieving fracture stabilization and healing.

Crates J, Whittle AP: Antegrade interlocking nailing of acute humeral shaft fractures. *Clin Orthop* 1998;350:40-50.

Seventy-three acute humeral shaft fractures were treated with antegrade humeral nailing. Sixty-nine fractures (94.5%) healed primarily; there were no infections. Two iatrogenic radial nerve palsies occurred, two patients had impingement from proximal locking screws, and one patient had impingement from a prominent nail. Normal elbow function was regained in 96% of patients, and all patients who did not regain normal shoulder and elbow function had concomitant injuries.

Flinkkila T, Hyvonen P, Lakovaara M, Linden T, Ristiniemi J, Hamalainen M: Intramedullary nailing of humeral shaft fractures: A retrospective study of 126 cases. *Acta Orthop Scand* 1999;70:133-136.

Nonunion occurred after primary nailing in 21 of 95 cases followed; nonunion was related to fracture distraction, but not location or implant type. Shoulder function was significantly impaired in 37% of patients. Patients rated results good or satisfactory in 61% of cases at 3 years follow-up.

Lin J, Hou SM, Inoue N, Chao EY, Hang YS: Anatomic considerations of locked humeral nailing. *Clin Orthop* 1999;368:247-254.

The anatomy of the axillary nerve was examined in 20 fresh frozen human cadaveric specimens, which were subsequently nailed with an antegrade technique. The axillary nerve was found an average of 45.6 mm below the greater tuberosity; it was jeopardized by insertion of a proximal interlocking screw in 1 of the 20 specimens. Short humeri, humeri with small heads, and nails inserted too deeply increased the risk of nerve injury.

Ring D, Perey BH, Jupiter JB: The functional outcome of operative treatment of ununited fractures of the humeral diaphysis in older patients. *J Bone Joint Surg Am* 1999;81:177-190.

Twenty-two elderly patients with atrophic humeral nonunions underwent plate and screw fixation and application of autogenous bone graft. In each patient, at least one modification of the standard technique was required because of osteopenia. The fracture united in 91% of patients and the average Constant score improved from 9 to 72 points. It was concluded that surgical treatment can be very successful when techniques are modified to address osteopenia.

Sarmiento A, Zagorski JB, Zych GA, Latta LL, Capps CA: Functional bracing for the treatment of fractures of the humeral diaphysis. *J Bone Joint Surg Am* 2000;82:478-486.

Of 922 patients treated with functional bracing of humeral shaft fractures between 1978 and 1990, 620 were followed at least until fracture union. Six percent of patients with open fractures and 2% of those with closed fractures developed nonunion. Eighty-seven percent of patients healed with less than 16° of varus angulation, and 81% healed with less than 16° anterior angulation. At the time of brace removal, 98% of patients had limitation of shoulder motion of less than 25°.

Strothman D, Templeman DC, Varecka T, Bechtold J: Retrograde nailing of humeral shaft fractures: A biomechanical study of its effects on the strength of the distal humerus. *J Orthop Trauma* 2000;14:101-104.

Nine pairs of fresh frozen human humeri were divided into three groups. Two groups had holes drilled distally at two recommended sites for insertion of retrograde humeral nails; the third group was left intact. Mechanical testing revealed that creation of an entry portal significantly decreased bending strength and ultimate torque of specimens; there was no significant difference between the two distal entry sites.

Classic Bibliography

Balfour GW, Mooney V, Ashby ME: Diaphyseal fractures of the humerus treated with a ready-made fracture brace. *J Bone Joint Surg Am* 1982;64:11-13.

Brumback RJ, Bosse MJ, Poka A, Burgess AR: Intramedullary stabilization of humeral shaft fractures in patients with multiple trauma. *J Bone Joint Surg Am* 1986;68:960-970.

Hill JM, McGuire MH, Crosby LA: Closed treatment of displaced middle-third fractures of the clavicle gives poor results. *J Bone Joint Surg Br* 1997;79:537-539.

Kavanagh BF, Bradway JK, Cofield RH: Open reduction and internal fixation of displaced intra-articular fractures of the glenoid fossa. *J Bone Joint Surg Am* 1993;75:479-484.

Kettelkamp DB, Alexander H: Clinical review of radial nerve injury. *J Trauma* 1967;7:424-432.

Leung KS, Lam TP: Open reduction and internal fixation of ipsilateral fractures of the scapular neck and clavicle. *J Bone Joint Surg Am* 1993;75:1015-1018.

Nordqvist A, Petersson C, Redlund-Johnell I: The natural course of lateral clavicle fracture: 15 (11-21) year follow-up of 110 cases. *Acta Orthop Scand* 1993;64:87-91.

Ogawa K, Yoshida A, Takahashi M, Ui M: Fractures of the coracoid process. *J Bone Joint Surg Br* 1997;79:17-19.

Pollock FH, Drake D, Bovill EG, Day L, Trafton PG: Treatment of radial neuropathy associated with fractures of the humerus. *J Bone Joint Surg Am* 1981;63:239-243.

Rikli D, Regazzoni P, Renner N: The unstable shoulder girdle: Early functional treatment utilizing open reduction and internal fixation. *J Orthop Trauma* 1995;9:93-97.

Rosen H: The treatment of nonunions and pseudarthroses of the humeral shaft. *Orthop Clin North Am* 1990;21:725-742.

Sarmiento A, Horowitch A, Aboulafia A, Vangsness CT Jr: Functional bracing for comminuted extra-articular fractures of the distal third of the humerus. *J Bone Joint Surg Br* 1990;72:283-287.

Chapter 27

Shoulder Instability

R. Sean Churchill, MD

Frederick A. Matsen III, MD

Natural History

Recurrence rates of 60% to 70% have been reported for traumatic anterior instability in patients younger than age 22 years. In this age group, the incidence of recurrent shoulder stability is virtually unaffected by the length of immobilization or maintenance of an organized physical therapy program. These patients often have a detachment of the inferior glenohumeral ligament and labrum, referred to as the Bankart lesion. Patients who are 20 to 30 years of age have somewhat better results with nonsurgical treatment, but the incidence of recurrence remains high at 50% to 64%. Patients older than age 40 years at the time of the initial shoulder dislocation have even lower rates of redislocation. However, 15% of these patients experience a rotator cuff tear at the time of initial dislocation. There is a dramatic increase (to 40%) in the incidence of cuff tears in those patients age 60 years and older. Although recurrent dislocation in patients age 40 years and older is less common than in younger patients, it has been associated with a high incidence of subscapularis and capsular avulsion from the lesser tuberosity.

The extent of soft-tissue injury sustained is not limited to the initial dislocation, but rather has been found to be progressive with each subsequent dislocation. In a recent study, 91 patients (mean age, 31 years) with a history of shoulder instability, ranging from a single dislocation to multiply recurrent dislocations, were evaluated arthroscopically. The soft-tissue injury ranged from an isolated labral detachment with a persistent periosteal hinge to a complete ligament and labrum attachment rupture with degeneration and absence of the labrum. There was a good correlation between the number of shoulder dislocations and the severity of soft-tissue injury, which implies that further damage continues to occur with each subsequent dislocation. The natural history of atraumatic instability is less clear.

Biomechanics

Laxity is the capacity of the humeral head to be translated or rotated from a reference position, and is detected on physical examination. Instability is the inability to maintain the humeral head centered in the glenoid fossa. Instability is determined primarily from the patient's history and is confirmed with the reproduction of symptoms on physical examination.

The principal stabilizers of the shoulder consist of the articular anatomy, capsuloligamentous structures, and the action of the shoulder musculature. The glenoid, a kidney bean-shaped socket, has a nonuniform distribution of articular cartilage (cartilage is thicker at the periphery than in the center, where it is relatively sparse). This in effect enhances the curvature to better match the humeral head. The much larger humeral head has a reciprocal cartilage arrangement where it is thickest at the center and is thinner in the periphery. The flexible labrum further enables the socket to conform to the ball. This combination allows a congruent fit, optimizing stability and contact area. The capsuloligamentous structures consist of the glenoid labrum, superior glenohumeral ligament (SGHL), middle glenohumeral ligament (MGHL), and inferior glenohumeral ligament complex (IGHLC) (Fig. 1). The labrum is a fibrous ring that functions to deepen the glenoid fossa, helping center the humeral head in the glenoid; it also provides the attachment site for the glenohumeral ligaments. Labral attachment in the anterior superior quadrant is variable, but any labral detachment below the glenoid equator is believed to be pathologic and associated with glenohumeral instability.

The SGHL functions primarily as a restraint to inferiorly directed forces while the shoulder is in the adducted position. The MGHL is highly variable and is poorly defined or absent in 40% of the population. This ligament functions as a restraint to translation and rotation in the middle and lower ranges of abduction.

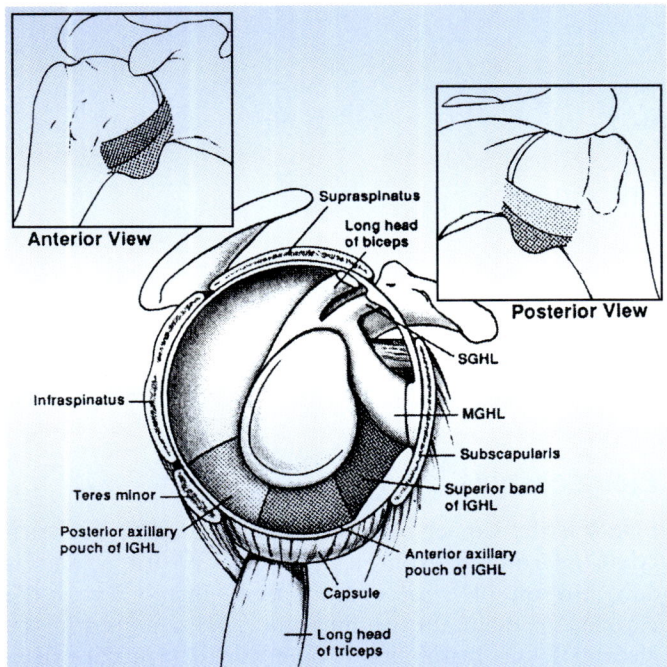

Figure 1 An anatomic drawing of the capsular ligaments. Note the superior band of the inferior glenohumeral ligament, the anterior axillary pouch of the inferior glenohumeral ligament, and the posterior axillary pouch of the inferior glenohumeral ligament collectively form the IGHLC. *(Reproduced with permission from Ticker JB, Bigliani LU, Soslowsky LJ, et al: Inferior glenohumeral ligament: Geometric and strain-rate dependent properties.* J Shoulder Elbow Surg 1996;5:269-279.)

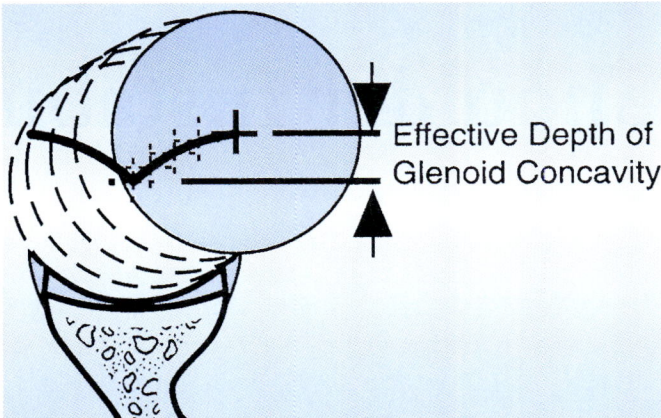

Figure 2 The effective depth of the glenoid concavity. The gull wing-shaped line indicates the path of the center of the head as it is translated from the glenoid center to the top of the lip. The effective depth of the glenoid concavity in a specified direction of translation is equal to the lateral displacement of the humeral head at the top of the lip relative to its starting point centered in the glenoid fossa. *(Reproduced with permission from Matsen FA III, Lippitt SB, Sidles JB, Harryman DT II: Stability, in Matsen FA III (ed):* Practical Evaluation and Management of the Shoulder. Philadelphia, PA, WB Saunders, 1994, pp 59-111.)

The IGHLC consists of a thick anterior band, a thinner, less consistent posterior band, and the thin interposed axillary pouch. This complex acts as a restraint to translation and rotation with the arm abducted 90°; translation is restrained when the arm is abducted, extended, and externally rotated.

The capsule contributes to joint stability, becoming differentially tight in different positions of the upper extremity. The anterior capsule is tight during external rotation, whereas the posterior capsule tightens with internal rotation. These static stabilizers only function when they are under tension at the extremes of joint motion. If they are excessively tight, rotation may cause obligate translation away from the tight capsule. This may be the mechanism of capsulorrhaphy arthropathy following capsular tightening. A recent analysis of the collagen and elastin fibers in the shoulder capsule of patients with anterior instability, multidirectional instability (MDI), failed MDI repair, and those without a history of shoulder instability showed no differences in capsular collagen between the anterior instability group and the MDI group. However, when compared with the failed MDI reconstruction group, the anterior instability group and the MDI group had larger diameter collagen fibrils, increased collagen fibril density, less reducible collagen cross-links, and a

decreased density of elastin. Conversely, the normal capsule tissue had even larger diameter collagen fibrils and no reducible collagen cross-links. These results indicate that those MDI patients in whom surgical reconstruction has failed possibly may represent a subset of patients with a more severe genetic connective tissue abnormality.

Shoulder stability is enhanced by concavity compression, the active compression of the humeral head into the glenoid fossa. For this mechanism to be effective, there must be a competent concavity (similar to the depression in a golf tee) (Fig. 2), and a compressive force passing through the concavity (similar to the force of gravity when a golf tee is vertical). This mechanism can act in all glenohumeral positions. The rotator cuff encircles the humeral head and functions to compress it into the glenoid fossa concavity. Contraction of the rotator cuff allows upper extremity motion while maintaining a concentrically reduced joint. Should injury or fatigue to the rotator cuff muscles occur, or should the concavity be disrupted, this control mechanism will fail and instability will result.

Additionally, shoulder stability is further augmented by the adhesion-cohesion effect of the joint fluid. In the shoulder, the magnitude of the adhesion-cohesion force depends on three separate joint characteristics: the adhesive and cohesive properties of the joint fluid, the "wetability" of the joint surfaces, and the contact area between the joint surfaces. This stabilizing property is most severely affected by traumatic bony and labral injuries, which decrease the contact area available between the humeral head and glenoid.

From a reconstruction standpoint this finely orchestrated system of stability and mobility must be fully understood and appreciated prior to planning treatment. Nonanatomic and nonphysiologic reconstructions may limit motion in an attempt to achieve stability at the risk of early degenerative joint disease. The goal of treatment for glenohumeral instability must be the restoration of the normal stabilizing mechanisms without sacrificing range of motion or articular surface integrity.

Patient Evaluation

History

Patients with anterior instability complain of symptoms during arm abduction and external rotation. Often their initial episode occurred in this position with the application of an external rotation torque. Pitchers with anterior instability have symptoms in the late cocking phase and often beginning in later innings as fatigue ensues. Posterior instability occurs with the arm flexed, adducted, and internally rotated, such as when pushing a heavy cart or pushing open a door. Throwing athletes with posterior instability typically note symptoms of pain and discomfort late in the follow-through phase. Inferior instability may become symptomatic when the patient is carrying heavy objects. Patients with atraumatic instability may have a family history of similar findings and a history of other joint problems such as recurrent atraumatic patellar dislocations.

Physical Examination

The patient should be asked to demonstrate the positions and actions during which the shoulder becomes symptomatic. A thorough neurovascular examination of the entire upper extremity should be included. A screening cervical spine examination with neck range of motion can detect an alternative source of shoulder symptoms. Patients with a history consistent with MDI should be examined for generalized ligamentous laxity (elbow and knee hyperextension, ability to place thumb to forearm, and metacarpophalangeal joint hyperextension).

The three major components of the rotator cuff are tested by isometric examination for strength and comfort, that is, elevation in internal rotation for the supraspinatus, external rotation for the infraspinatus, and internal rotation with the hand on the stomach for the subscapularis.

Provocative examination can be grouped into three basic groups: anterior, posterior, and inferior instability. Results of these tests are compared between the symptomatic and asymptomatic shoulders. Reproduc-

tion of symptoms by provocative tests helps confirm the diagnosis of instability. For anterior instability, the anterior apprehension test is used. The patient is placed supine with the shoulder abducted 90°, elbow flexed 90°, while the extremity is slowly externally rotated until the patient reports symptoms or impending instability.

Posterior instability is evaluated with the jerk test, which involves placing the patient's arm in 90° of elevation and 90° of internal rotation. The arm is then moved from the coronal to the sagittal plane and back while an axial load is applied to the humerus. If posterior instability is present, the humeral head subluxates over the glenoid rim and reproduces the patient's symptoms. Reduction of the humeral head when the arm returns to the coronal plane is often accompanied by a palpable and audible clunk (Fig. 3).

The load and shift test is used to determine the competence of the glenoid concavity. The patient's arm is relaxed in 20° of abduction and 20° of forward flexion and neutral rotation while the humeral head is pressed into the glenoid fossa. Translation of the humeral head anteriorly and posteriorly is attempted while the load is maintained. The resistance to humeral head translation is noted and compared with that of the normal shoulder. Lack of resistance suggests the absence of a functional glenoid cavity (Fig. 4). Laxity tests, such as the AP drawer and the sulcus tests, also are performed.

Imaging

Three views (true AP radiograph, perpendicular to the plane of the scapula, and axillary and apical oblique views) are obtained for characterizing the glenohumeral relationships and bony pathology.

Additional imaging studies may be indicated if necessary to further define suspected pathology. CT can help define humeral and glenoid deficiencies or abnormalities.

Ultrasound or MRI is used to evaluate the rotator cuff in individuals older than age 40 years who have weakness or pain on muscle testing.

Examination Under Anesthesia and Arthroscopy

The physical examination under anesthesia (EUA) can document the translational and rotational laxity of the joint. The awake examination and EUA were compared in a recent study using the load and shift test in patients with traumatic anterior instability. Ninety-two percent of patients had anterior translation at least one grade higher during the EUA as compared with the awake examination. Additionally, the difference between translation on the injured and uninjured side was enhanced on EUA.

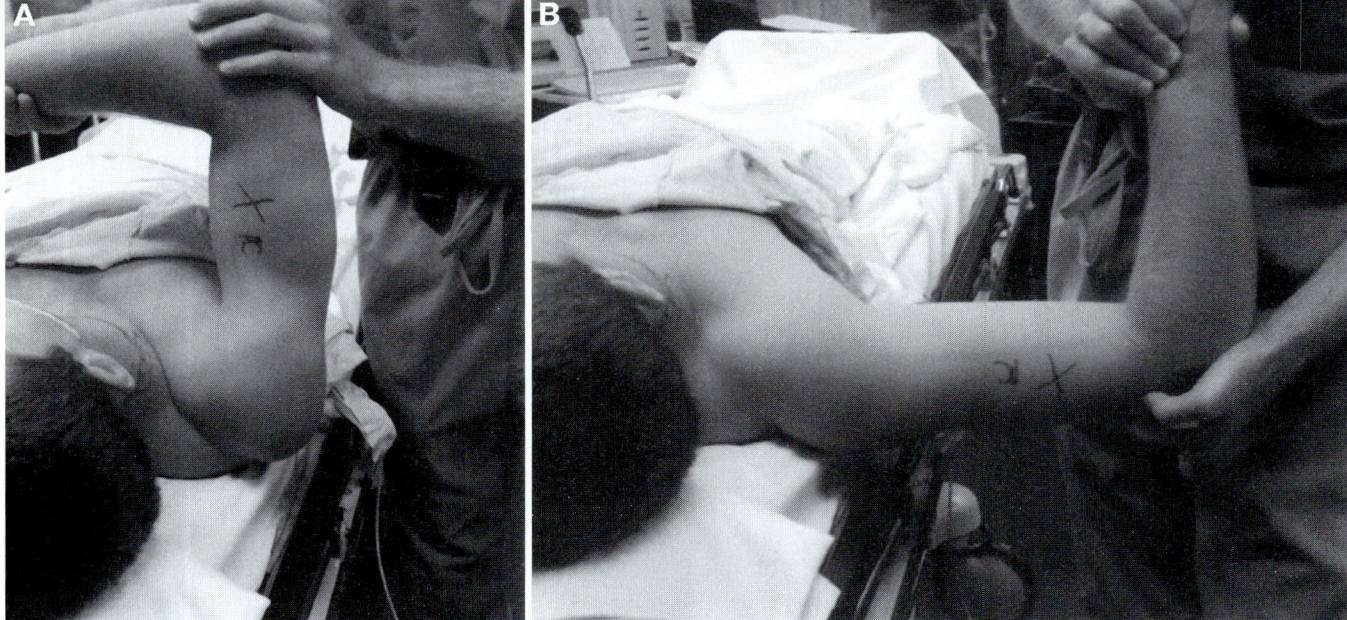

Figure 3 Clinical photographs demonstrating the jerk test. With the patient's arm in 90° of forward elevation and internally rotated, axial pressure is applied to the elbow. **A,** The arm is then brought into abduction. **B,** A positive jerk test occurs when the initial position results in posterior instability, which spontaneously reduces during the abduction positioning.

Additional information regarding pathology associated with shoulder instability may be gained from arthroscopy. A systematic examination of the joint may reveal information regarding labral detachment, articular injury to either the glenoid or humeral head, extent of capsular redundancy, and the status of the rotator cuff.

Treatment

Anterior Instability

Nonsurgical Treatment

Nonsurgical treatment is often used for most first-time shoulder dislocations. After successful reduction and radiographic verification, the arm is placed into a sling and isometric exercises are begun. Because most studies show no benefit to prolonged immobilization, by approximately 3 to 4 weeks patients progress to a strengthening program. The strengthening program should use isometric rotator cuff, deltoid, and scapular stabilizer exercises. Once the injured side has strength and range of motion equal to the contralateral side and after a healing period of 3 months, patients are allowed to return to their preinjury activities while continuing the strengthening program. Recurrent anterior instability after a traumatic dislocation requires limitation of activity, a restrictive brace, more strengthening, or surgical reconstruction. Early surgical stabilization may be considered for those athletes who need to minimize the risks of repeat dislocation.

Arthroscopic Surgery

Arthroscopic treatment of traumatic anterior instability includes the use of staples, transglenoid sutures, cannulated bioabsorbable implants, and suture anchors to reattach or tighten the capsule and labrum. Arthroscopic repairs have a substantially higher rate of failure by recurrence than open repairs. Staple capsulorrhaphy resulted in multiple failures such as staple breakage, loosening, migration, intra-articular penetration, and even painful subscapularis bursitis. For these reasons few surgeons continue to use staple fixation. Transglenoid sutures have the disadvantages of the passage of a drill posteriorly through the glenoid, the tying of sutures posteriorly, and the possibility of suprascapular nerve injury with drilling or suturing. However, a recently published study using multiple transglenoid sutures had good or excellent results in 22 of 24 patients (91.7%) and no serious complications.

An analysis of failed transglenoid suture repair was recently completed. Fifteen of 82 patients treated with arthroscopic transglenoid suturing for traumatic anterior shoulder instability experienced dislocation (13 patients) or subluxation (2 patients) at an average follow-up of 40 months. No bony Bankart lesions (type IV) were included in this study. Factors found to adversely affect the result included the preinjury involvement in contact sports, a ligamentous tear with labral disruption (type III Bankart lesion), an inferior glenohumeral labral complex thickness measuring less than 3 mm, and a repair using five or fewer sutures.

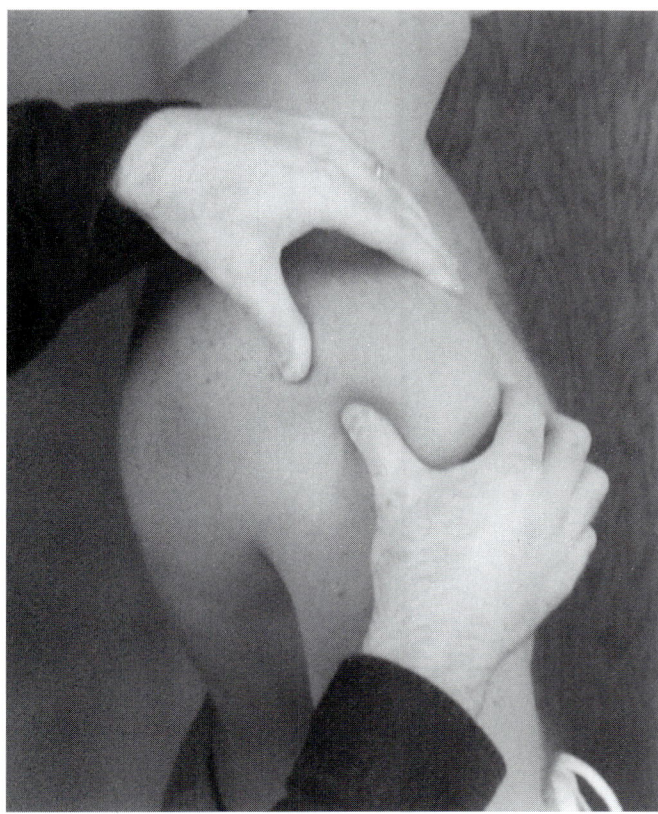

Figure 4 Clinical photograph demonstrating the load and shift test. The examiner stabilizes the scapula and clavicle with one hand, while simultaneously compressing and translating the humeral head with the opposite hand. The magnitude of the translation is assessed in both the anterior and posterior directions.

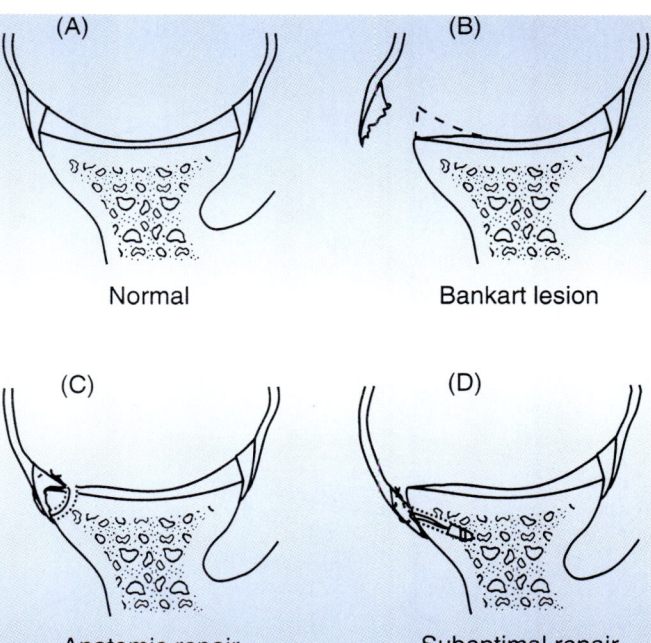

Normal   Bankart lesion

Anatomic repair   Suboptimal repair

Figure 5 Normally, the capsule and labrum deepen the effective glenoid fossa **(A)**. This effect is lost in the presence of a Bankart lesion **(B)**. Anatomic repair of the detached glenoid labrum and glenohumeral ligaments to the glenoid rim helps restore the effective depth of the glenoid concavity **(C)**. In contrast, when the labrum and capsule heal to the neck, concavity is not restored **(D)**. *(Reproduced with permission from Matsen FA III, Lippitt SB, Sidles JB, Harryman DT II: Stability, in Matsen FA III (ed): Practical Evaluation and Management of the Shoulder. Philadelphia, PA, WB Saunders, 1994, pp 59-11.)*

Fixation using cannulated bioabsorbable implants and suture anchors have reports of host foreign body reaction to the bioabsorbable implants and therefore have raised concern regarding their use. A recent arthroscopic and histologic examination in four failed superior labral repairs noted massive synovitis, loose implant fragments throughout the joint cavity, and a hypertrophic synovial membrane with massive infiltration of phagocytic cells.

One of the important aspects of Bankart repair, whether arthroscopic or open, is the accurate and secure reattachment of the glenoid labrum and capsule to the glenoid lip and not the glenoid neck (Fig. 5). Anatomic reconstruction reestablishes the fossa-deepening effect of the labrum.

Open Surgical Procedures

Original techniques involving nonanatomic reconstruction such as the Putti-Platt and Magnuson-Stack showed low rates of redislocation; however, this came at the expense of external rotation and ultimately resulted in dramatically increased rates of early glenohumeral arthritis. As a result, more anatomic reconstruction (Bankart procedure), which preserved rota-

tion and repaired the labrum is advocated. Long-term follow-up with a mean of 12 years has shown 92% good or excellent results with a redislocation rate of less than 5%. The Bankart procedure has become the 'gold standard.' Some modifications have involved capsular tightening by humeral-based, glenoid-based, or central capsular shortening. Each of these methods reduces excessive capsular volume by excising redundant capsular tissue. One modification developed specifically for the throwing athlete involves a subscapularis splitting approach with a glenoid side capsular shift. Theoretically, this approach helps restore stability while preserving motion and allowing a quicker return to competition.

The most important factors in the surgical repair of recurrent traumatic instability appear to be a secure repair of the detached capsule and labrum to the surface of the glenoid from which they were detached, reestablishment of the fossa-deepening effect of the labrum, and avoiding unnecessary capsular tightening, which may predispose the shoulder to capsulorrhaphy arthropathy. Surgical repair is best accomplished through an open Bankart repair, suturing through bone holes. When there is a substantial anterior glenoid lip deficiency, an extracapsular bone graft can restore the competence of the glenoid fossa (Fig. 6).

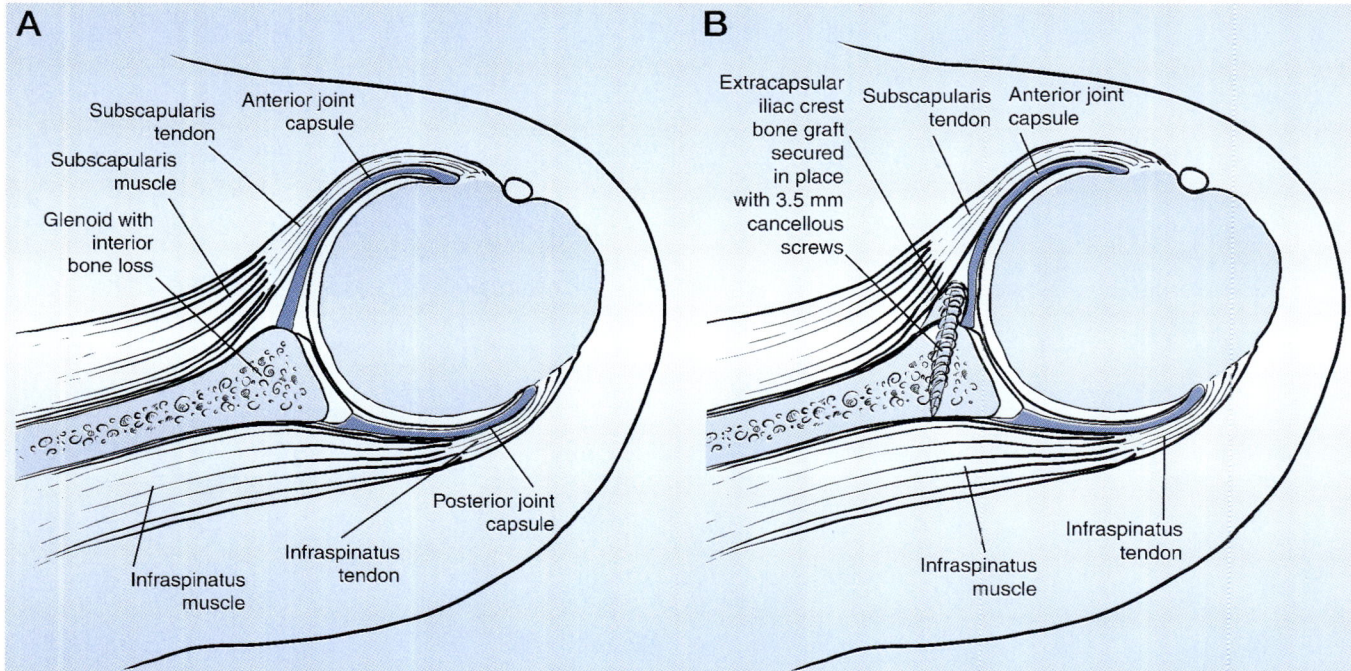

Figure 6 An anteriorly deficient glenoid lacks the depth to allow adequate joint stability through concavity compression **(A)**. By placing an iliac crest bone graft extracapsularly, the glenoid depth is increased, thus improving joint stability **(B)**.

Posterior Instability

Posterior instability occurs less frequently than anterior instability (2% to 12% of all shoulder instability cases). Many cases are atraumatic and best treated with physical rehabilitation. Surgical stabilization is considered for recurrent posterior traumatic instability and for persistent atraumatic posterior instability. The load and shift test may be helpful in determining if the repair needs to augment the posterior glenoid lip; a lack of resistance to posterior translation of the loaded humeral head suggests an insufficient posterior lip.

Arthroscopic techniques for treatment of posterior instability have been described. In a recent study of 14 patients treated with arthroscopic posterior capsular plication, there were 12 excellent and 2 fair results at a minimum 2-year follow-up. The capsular preparation was performed by gentle abrasion of the synovial surface of the posterior capsule with a slotted whisker blade. Then approximately 1 cm of posterior capsule was advanced to the posterior glenoid labrum and sutured in place, using three to eight nonabsorbable sutures to complete the plication. A similar study of 41 patients with posterior instability noted four specific categories of labral lesions: Bankart type detachment (12%), chondral or labral erosion (17%), synovial and capsular stripping (22%), and labral split or flap tear (32%). A similar capsular plication was performed, as described above, resulting in improved stability on physical examination in 86% of patients.

Open surgical stabilization techniques for treating recurrent instability include posterior capsulorrhaphy, posterior bone block, and posterior glenoid osteotomy.

Proximity of neurovascular structures during the posterior approach to the shoulder led to a recent anatomic study of 14 cadaveric shoulders. The surgical approach to the posterior shoulder was through a deltoid split from the posterolateral corner of the acromion followed by an infraspinatous splitting incision. The axillary nerve was isolated and averaged 65 mm from the posterolateral corner of the acromion. This distance decreased by 14 mm (22%) with abduction and 19 mm (29%) with extension. The suprascapular nerve was located 20 mm medial to the glenoid rim and did not change with the position of the upper extremity. This approach is therefore safe to perform an open posterior inferior capsular shift.

When the posterior glenoid lip is deficient, a careful posterior glenoid opening wedge osteoplasty can substantially augment the effective glenoid concavity.

Atraumatic Multidirectional Instability

MDI is usually atraumatic, resulting from some combination of excessive tissue compliance, muscular discoordination, and inadequacy of the glenoid concavity. It often is associated with complaints of pain, which is much less common in traumatic unidirectional instability. For all these reasons atraumatic MDI is more complex to manage. Rehabilitation and education is the standard for most situations. Assessment of these shoulders should include the evaluation of the effectiveness of the glenoid concavity, the directions of true instability (not just laxity), and patient motivation. In patients with voluntary subluxation or dislocation, surgery is not recommended because of poor results from surgical stabilization.

Arthroscopic treatment for MDI includes thermal capsular shrinkage. Thirty patients with symptomatic MDI that had previously undergone 6 months of physical therapy without resolution of their symptoms were treated using a thermal probe for capsular shrinkage of the posterior, inferior, and anterior capsules. To complete the procedure the rotator interval was plicated with interrupted sutures. Gentle, limited range of motion exercises were begun on postoperative day 3, with the initiation of a strengthening program at 3 to 4 weeks. Patients were allowed to return to unrestricted activity when range of motion and strength were equal to that of the contralateral shoulder, usually by 3 to 6 months. At a mean 26-month follow-up, 93% of patients were rated satisfactory and 7% were unsatisfactory.

An all-arthroscopic, glenoid-based capsular shift with transglenoid suture fixation was evaluated in 25 patients. The postoperative protocol consisted of an abduction sling for 6 weeks. During this time limited passive range of motion was allowed beginning at 4 weeks if the motion was nontender. At 6 weeks after surgery, aggressive range of motion and strengthening exercises were begun and continued until range of motion and strength were equal to that of the contralateral side, which typically occurred at 4 to 6 months. Eighty-eight percent of patients at a minimum follow-up of 2 years had a successful outcome.

A common open surgical method for treatment of MDI is the capsular shift. Reports suggest 85% to 90% satisfactory results over the long term. Concern about capsular tightening (arthroscopic or open) for the treatment of MDI lies in the recognition that patients are usually symptomatic when their shoulders are in midrange positions where the glenohumeral ligaments are lax. Because ligaments do not normally stabilize the joint in these positions, tightening ligaments may not be helpful in managing midrange instability.

Acromioclavicular Instability

Acromioclavicular (AC) instability typically occurs as a result of direct trauma to the superolateral aspect of the shoulder. Falls that occur while skiing, cycling, or playing football account for the majority of cases. As the superolateral aspect of the shoulder strikes the ground, the acromion is forcibly inferior with respect to the lateral clavicle. Patients present with their arm held adducted against the body in a 'safe' position and

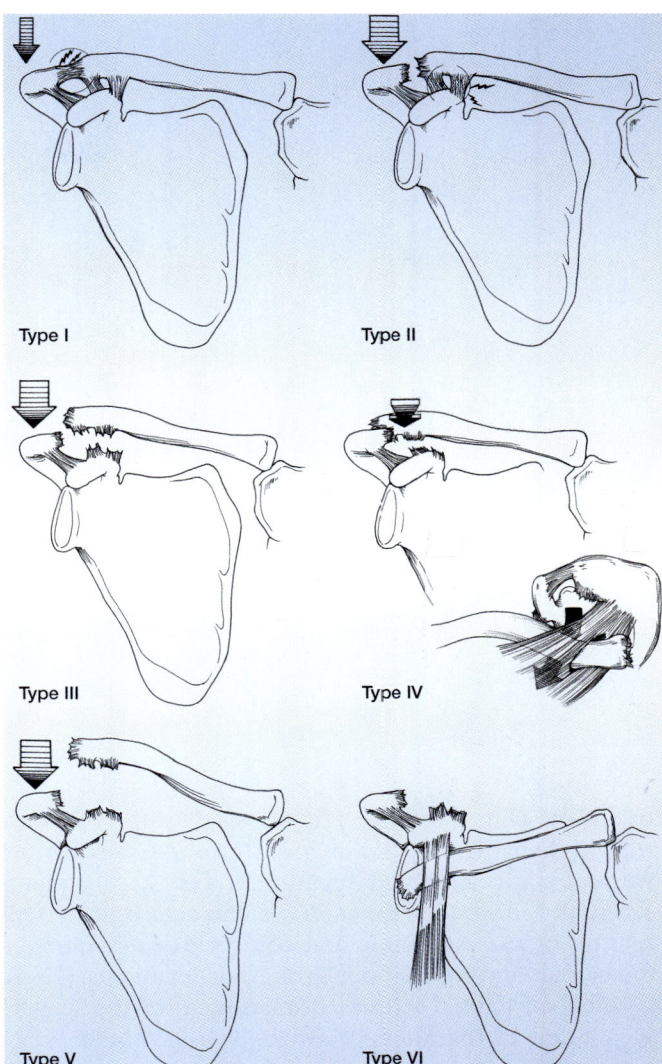

Figure 7 The Rockwood classification of ligamentous injuries to the acromioclavicular joint. *(Reproduced with permission from Rockwood CA, Williams GR, Young DC: Shoulder instability, in Rockwood CA, Green DP, Bucholz RN, Heckman JD (eds): Rockwood and Green's Fractures in Adults. Philadelphia, PA, Lippincott-Raven, 1996, vol 2, p 1354.)*

often have abrasions along the superior aspect of their shoulder. A relatively prominent lateral clavicle may be present in more severe cases, indicating dislocation of the AC joint. Radiographic evaluation consists of an AP radiograph of both AC joints with the arms at the side. (A recent survey of 112 practicing members of the American Shoulder and Elbow Surgeons in the United States and Canada found no value in performing weighted shoulder views.) The injured and normal sides are compared with respect to the separation of the AC joint and the coracoclavicular interval. Increased coracoclavicular separation indicates rupture of the coracoclavicular ligaments.

The AC classification system describes the anatomic basis for the injury as well as directs the appropriate

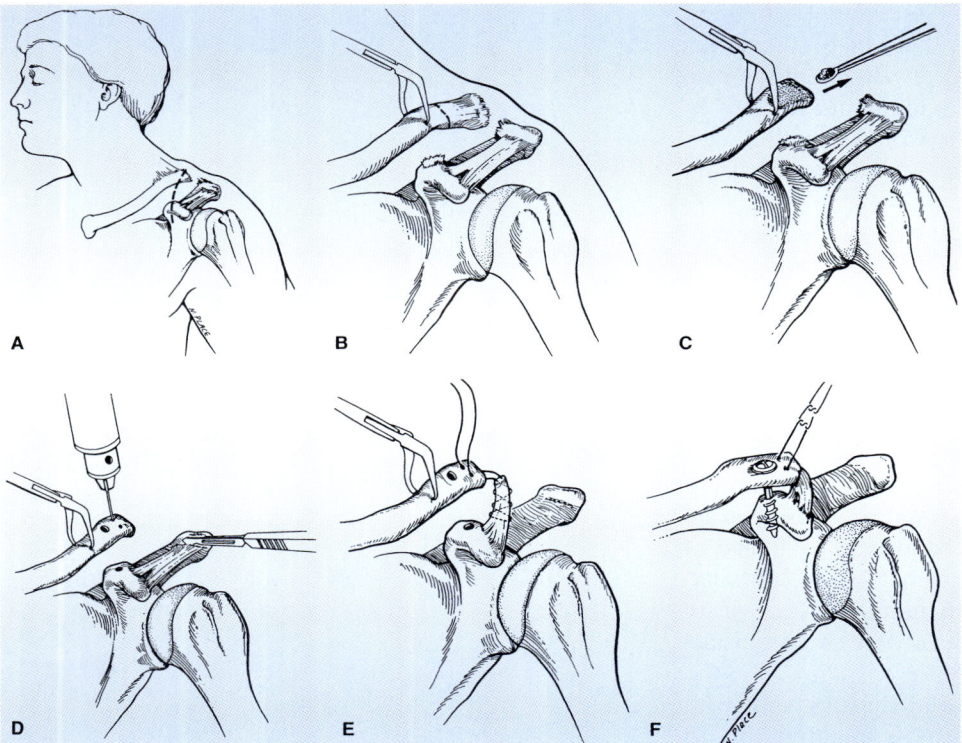

Figure 8 Surgical method of reconstruction for chronic and complete dislocations of the acromioclavicular joint. **A,** Strap-like incision in Langer's lines. **B,** Exposed distal clavicle and site of intended resection. **C,** The medullary canal is curetted to receive the transferred coracoacromial ligament. **D,** The clavicle and coracoid are predrilled with the appropriate size drill bits, and two small drill holes are made through the superior cortex of the clavicle. The acromial attachment of the coracoacromial ligament is released carefully from the acromion. **E,** A heavy nonabsorbable suture is woven through, and the ligament and the suture ends are passed into the medullary canal and out through the two small drill holes in the superior clavicular cortex. **F,** The coracoclavicular lag screw reduces the clavicle to an anatomic position in the relationship to the coracoid. The sutures are used to pull the ligament securely into the medullary canal and are tied over the superior cortex of the distal clavicle. *(Reproduced with permission from Guy DK, Wirth MA, Griffin JL, Rockwood CA Jr: Reconstruction of chronic and complete dislocations of the acromioclavicular joint.* Clin Orthop *1998;347: 138-149.)*

treatment (Fig. 7). Type I injuries have no AC separation. Type II injuries demonstrate AC separation without coracoclavicular separation. The AC ligaments are ruptured. A type III injury is characterized by separation of the AC joints and coracoclavicular interval, indicating rupture of both groups of ligaments. There is often substantial inferior displacement of the scapula in relation to the lateral clavicle. Type IV injuries are a type III injury with posterior displacement of the lateral clavicle into or through the trapezius muscle. A type V AC separation is similar to a type III, but with superior displacement of the lateral clavicle from 100% to 300%. Type VI injuries are very rare and represent complete AC dislocations with the lateral clavicle displaced inferior to the coracoid and the conjoined tendon.

Treatment for type I and II AC joint injuries is nonsurgical. Patients respond well to symptomatic treatment and trapezius rehabilitation, with return to activities as soon as comfort allows. Resection arthroplasty of the AC joint may be necessary in the advent of AC arthritis.

Treatment of type III AC joint injuries remains the topic of debate and investigation. A recent meta-analysis revealed that 88% of surgically treated patients and 87% of nonsurgically treated patients had a satisfactory outcome. Pain, return to activity, range of motion, and strength were all similar between the two groups. Variation occurred in the frequency of complications. Wound or skin breakdown was reported in 6% of surgically treated cases and only 1% of nonsurgically treated cases. Deformity occurred in only 3% of surgically treated patients, whereas 37% in the nonsurgical group experienced deformity. Surgical treatment has been recommended for young laborers, high-demand patients, and athletes. Although the meta-analysis did not specifically address these subsets of the population, it should be noted that the time for both return to work and performance of activities was significantly longer in those treated surgically. There is no literature to support the use of external taping, straps, or bracing for closed reduction and treatment of these injuries. Patients with poor results from the initial closed treatment of a type III injury may respond to surgical intervention.

Because of the severity of injury and extent of displacement, type IV, V, and VI AC joint injuries are treated surgically. Surgical treatment of acute AC separation may consist only of approximation of the coracoid and clavicle using a cerclage suture or a coracoclavicular screw. In chronic dislocations, tissue (either the coracoacromial ligament or a hamstring autograft) usually is added to facilitate healing from the clavicle to the coracoid (Fig. 8). Laboratory testing of the various reconstruction techniques compared with uninjured coracoclavicular ligaments revealed sutures alone provided similar strength but

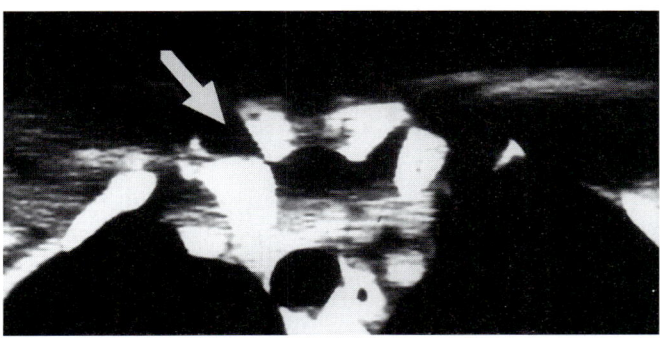

Figure 9 CT scan demonstrating a posterior dislocation of the right sternoclavicular joint. *(Reproduced from Beaty JH (ed): Orthopaedic Knowledge Update 6. Rosemont, IL, American Academy of Orthopaedic Surgeons, 1999, pp 287-297.)*

greater deformation under load. Bicortical screw fixation resulted in comparable stiffness and superior strength whereas the coracoacromial ligament transfers alone were the weakest and least stiff. Soft-tissue procedures should be augmented with a coracoclavicular suture sling or bicortical coracoclavicular screw fixation.

Sternoclavicular Instability

Sternoclavicular instability is classified as anterior or posterior, based on the anatomic location of the medial end of the clavicle in relation to the sternum. Sternoclavicular dislocation often results from direct trauma to the chest or shoulder. Patients with anterior dislocations present with a palpable clavicular head (that becomes more prominent as the arm is abducted and elevated) on their anterior chest wall just lateral to the sternum. Posterior dislocations are characterized by a variety of symptoms, including dyspnea, dysphagia, and upper extremity paresthesias. The physical examination for posterior dislocation shows a relative hollow space lateral to the sternum. Radiographic imaging of the sternoclavicular joint with 40° of cephalic tilt may demonstrate the direction and degree of clavicular displacement. However, a chest CT is the imaging study of choice to accurately determine the extent of the dislocation and evaluate other mediastinal structures for injury (Fig. 9). Treatment of the acute dislocation may include an attempt at reduction by traction on the extended arm. If a stable reduction cannot be achieved, the deformity may be accepted. Posterior dislocations can be managed with an attempt at closed reduction in the operating room. Prior to attempting reduction, the patient can be prepped from the neck to the umbilicus with thoracic surgery personnel on standby to help in the management of potential vascular or airway injuries. After administration of general anesthesia, the reduction maneu-

ver consists of abduction and extension of the involved shoulder. If unsuccessful, grasping the medial clavicle with the fingers or a towel clip and applying an anterior force should complete the reduction. The majority of posterior sternoclavicular dislocations are stable after reduction. If the reduction is unsuccessful or unstable, surgical stabilization may be considered with reconstruction of the sternoclavicular ligaments. The use of hardware for stabilization is not recommended.

Annotated Bibliography

Natural History

Habermeyer P, Gleyze P, Rickert M: Evolution of lesions of the labrum-ligament complex in posttraumatic anterior shoulder instability: A prospective study. *J Shoulder Elbow Surg* 1999;8:66-74.

To evaluate progressive intra-articular damage with recurrent anterior shoulder dislocation, 91 patients were evaluated arthroscopically. Patients ranged from those with a single shoulder dislocation to six or more dislocations. Four 'stages' of lesions were identified of progressively increasing severity. There was good correlation between the frequency of dislocation and extent of injury observed.

Biomechanics

Flatow EL, Warner JJP: Instability of the shoulder: Complex problems and failed repairs: Part I. Relevant biomechanics, multidirectional instability, and severe glenoid loss. *Instr Course Lect* 1998;47:97-112.

A complete review of shoulder biomechanics and factors affecting shoulder stability is presented. Appropriate history, physical examination, and nonsurgical and surgical techniques aimed to produce optimal results in the patient with MDI are addressed. Techniques for managing humeral and glenoid bone loss are briefly discussed.

Rodeo SA, Suzuki K, Yamauchi M, Bhargava M, Warren RF: Analysis of collagen and elastic fibers in shoulder capsule in patients with shoulder instability. *Am J Sports Med* 1998;26:634-643.

Samples of shoulder capsule and skin from 25 patients with anterior instability, MDI, failed MDI surgery, and patients with no history of instability were analyzed for collagen characteristics and elastin density. The anterior instability and MDI groups were not statistically different; however, the failed MDI population had smaller fibrils and decreased density of collagen as well as an increase in elastin density.

Patient Evaluation

Brown GA, Tan JL, Kirkley A: The lax shoulder in females: Issues, answers, but many more questions. *Clin Orthop* 2000;372:110-122.

A complete review of MDI, including epidemiology, voluntary dislocations, patient presentation, and nonsurgical, and surgical management is presented. The commonly held belief that females have increased shoulder laxity is challenged.

Faber KJ, Homa K, Hawkins RJ: Translation of the glenohumeral joint in patients with anterior instability: Awake examination versus examination with the patient under anesthesia. *J Shoulder Elbow Surg* 1999; 8:320-323.

Fifty patients with traumatic anterior shoulder instability were examined using the load and shift test both while awake and under anesthesia. The examination under anesthesia was found to have significantly greater anterior translation and increased side-to-side variation when compared with the awake examination.

Kim SH, Ha KI, Han KY: Biceps load test: A clinical test for superior labrum anterior and posterior lesions in shoulders with recurrent anterior dislocations. *Am J Sports Med* 1999;27:300-303.

A new physical examination test is described to better evaluate the integrity of the superior labrum. In 75 patients with unilateral anterior shoulder dislocations, the test was 90.9% sensitive and 96.9% specific for identifying a superior labrum anterior and posterior lesion.

Wintzell G, Larsson H, Larsson S: Indirect MR arthrography of anterior shoulder instability in the ABER and the apprehension test positions: A prospective comparative study of two different shoulder positions during MRI using intravenous gadodiamide contrast for enhancement of the joint fluid. *Skeletal Radiol* 1998;27: 488-494.

A new radiographic technique is described to better delineate anterior capsulolabral pathology in patients with anterior instability. Patients are placed in the apprehension position and intravenous contrast is used. The initial evaluation in 16 patients found the procedure both accurate and well tolerated.

Treatment

Antoniou J, Harryman DT II: Arthroscopic posterior capsular repair. *Clin Sports Med* 2000;19:101-114.

Forty-one patients with primary posterior inferior instability were treated with arthroscopic capsular repair. At an average follow-up of 28 months, 86% had improved stability on physical examination and the simple shoulder test scores increased from 5.6 to 8.6 after surgery. The surgical technique is described and illustrated.

Bailie DS, Moseley B, Lowe WR: Surgical anatomy of the posterior shoulder: Effects of arm position and anterior-inferior capsular shift. *J Shoulder Elbow Surg* 1999;8:307-313.

The posterior approach to the shoulder was evaluated by dissection of 14 cadaveric shoulders. The axillary nerve and posterior humeral circumflex artery were isolated and found to move by various amounts with arm positioning. The suprascapular nerve was isolated but did not shift with arm position.

Burkart A, Imhoff AB, Roscher E: Foreign-body reaction to the bioabsorbable Suretac device. *Arthroscopy* 2000;16:91-95.

A Case report involving four patients with apparent foreign body reaction to Suretac devices is presented. The patients underwent débridement and restabilization with an alternative device. Each patient had marked synovitis and in three of the four the Suretac was broken. Synovial samples were obtained and the histology reviewed.

Cole BJ, Warner JJ: Arthroscopic versus open Bankart repair for traumatic anterior shoulder instability. *Clin Sports Med* 2000;19:19-48.

This article is a complete review of traumatic anterior shoulder instability that includes proper selection of patients, imaging, and procedure. Multiple arthroscopic repair techniques, implants, and their use are discussed. A treatment algorithm is proposed for patients with traumatic anterior shoulder instability.

Guy DK, Wirth MA, Griffin JL, Rockwood CA Jr: Reconstruction of chronic and complete dislocations of the acromioclavicular joint. *Clin Orthop* 1998;347:138-149.

A new technique using a bicortical clavicular-coracoid lag screw to augment a standard Weaver-Dunn repair is presented. At an average 5.2-year follow-up, 19 of 23 patients experienced good to excellent results. The surgical technique and postoperative protocol are described.

Hamada K, Fukuda H, Nakajima T, Yamada N: The inferior capsular shift operation for instability of the shoulder: Long-term results in 34 shoulders. *J Bone Joint Surg Br* 1999;81:218-225.

Open inferior capsular shift was used on 34 shoulders with a preoperative diagnosis of inferior instability or MDI. At a mean follow-up of 8.3 years, 59% had good or excellent results. Failures included 6 of 12 patients with voluntary subluxation. The authors conclude that voluntary subluxation is a contraindication to surgical treatment.

Harris RI, Wallace AL, Harper GD, Goldberg JA, Sonnabend DH, Walsh WR: Structural properties of the intact and the reconstructed coracoclavicular ligament complex. *Am J Sports Med* 2000;28:103-108.

A cadaver study comparing coracoclavicular ligament properties to various reconstruction techniques using coracoacromial ligament transfer, suture slings, suture anchors, or bicortical clavicular-coracoid screw fixation. The bicortical screw was found to have near-normal stiffness while the coracoacromial ligament transfer had the least stiffness.

Hayashida K, Yoneda M, Nakagawa S, Okamura K, Fukushima S: Arthroscopic Bankart suture repair for traumatic anterior shoulder instability: Analysis of the causes of a recurrence. *Arthroscopy* 1998;14:295-301.

Eighty-two patients treated with transglenoid suture technique for anterior shoulder instability are reviewed. Eighty-four percent good to excellent results are reported at a minimum 2-year follow-up. Analysis of the poor results suggests four predisposing factors that may lead to recurrence if not properly addressed.

Kagaya K, Yoneda M, Hayashida K, et al: Modified Caspari technique for traumatic anterior shoulder instability: Comparison of absorbable sutures versus absorbable plus nonabsorbable sutures. *Arthroscopy* 1999;15:400-407.

Forty-five shoulders underwent stabilization with either all absorbable sutures or a 50:50 combination of absorbable and nonabsorbable sutures. The group with absorbable sutures only had good or excellent results in 74% of cases, compared with 94% for those with a combination of sutures. However, the combination group had a significant decrease in external rotation of 8.4°.

Phillips AM, Smart C, Groom AF: Acromioclavicular dislocation: Conservative or surgical therapy. *Clin Orthop* 1998;353:10-17.

A meta-analysis of 24 articles concerning type III acromioclavicular dislocation treatment is presented. Overall, the results were similar in both the surgical and conservative therapy groups. Range of motion and strength were not significantly different between groups. The outcome analysis detected no significant benefit from surgical intervention for type III AC dislocations.

Savoie FH III, Field LD: Thermal versus suture treatment of symptomatic capsular laxity. *Clin Sports Med* 2000;19:63-75.

A prospective study of 30 patients with MDI treated with thermal capsular shrinkage is presented. At average follow-up of 26 months, 28 of 30 patients rated a satisfactory result. These results compared favorably to an all-arthroscopic capsular shift group as well as a laser-treated capsular shrinkage group.

Treacy SH, Savoie FH III, Field LD: Arthroscopic treatment of multidirectional instability. *J Shoulder Elbow Surg* 1999;8:345-350.

The arthroscopic transglenoid capsular shift technique was performed for treatment of MDI in 25 patients. At average 5-year follow-up, 88% had a satisfactory result. No patient experienced loss of external rotation. Seven of 11 patients returned to sports at their preinjury level of competition.

Wolf EM, Eakin CL: Arthroscopic capsular plication for posterior shoulder instability. *Arthroscopy* 1998;14:153-163.

Fourteen patients with recurrent posterior shoulder instability were treated with arthroscopic posterior capsular plication. At a mean follow-up of 33 months, 86% had good or excellent results. The authors describe a new arthroscopic view, diagnostic of posterior inferior capsular laxity, which was found in all 14 patients.

Yap JJ, Curl LA, Kvitne RS, McFarland EG: The value of weighted views of the acromioclavicular joint: Results of a survey. *Am J Sports Med* 1999;27:806-809.

One hundred twelve members of the American Shoulder and Elbow Surgeons in the United States and Canada were surveyed concerning the clinical relevance of obtaining weighted views of the AC joint for grade II or III AC separations. No correlation was found between the weighted view and the need to perform reconstruction in patients with grade III AC separations.

Yoneda M, Hayashida K, Wakitani S, Nakagawa S, Fukushima S: Bankart procedure augmented by coracoid transfer for contact athletes with traumatic anterior shoulder instability. *Am J Sports Med* 1999;27:21-26.

Eighty-three athletes with traumatic anterior shoulder instability were treated with a Bankart repair and coracoid transfer to the anterior inferior glenoid rim. After 5.8-year follow-up, results were good or excellent in 93%, with 88% of the patients returning to contact sports. Moderate loss of external rotation (7% to 15%) was noted at follow-up.

Classic Bibliography

Bankart ASB: The pathology and treatment of recurrent dislocation of the shoulder-joint. *Br J Surg* 1938;26:23-29.

Burkhead WZ Jr, Rockwood CA Jr: Treatment of instability of the shoulder with an exercise program. *J Bone Joint Surg Am* 1992;74:890-896.

Hovelius L, Augustini BG, Fredin H, Johansson O, Norlin R, Thorling J: Primary anterior dislocation of the shoulder in young patients: A ten-year prospective study. *J Bone Joint Surg Am* 1996;78:1677-1684.

Lippitt S, Matsen F: Mechanisms of glenohumeral joint instability. *Clin Orthop* 1993;291:20-28.

Morgan CD, Bodenstab AB: Arthroscopic Bankart suture repair: Technique and early results. *Arthroscopy* 1987;3:111-122.

Neer CS II, Foster CR: Inferior capsular shift for involuntary inferior and multidirectional instability of the shoulder: A preliminary report. *J Bone Joint Surg Am* 1980;62:897-908.

Rockwood CA Jr: Part II: Subluxations and dislocations about the shoulder: Injuries to the acromioclavicular joint, in Rockwood CA Jr, Green DP (eds): *Fractures in Adults,* ed 2. Philadelphia, PA, JB Lippincott, 1984, pp 860-910.

Rowe CR: Prognosis in dislocations of the shoulder. *J Bone Joint Surg Am* 1956;38:957-977.

Thomas SC, Matsen FA III: An approach to the repair of avulsion of the glenohumeral ligaments in the management of traumatic anterior glenohumeral instability. *J Bone Joint Surg Am* 1989;71:506-513.

Tossy JD, Mead NC, Sigmond HM: Acromioclavicular separations: Useful and practical classification for treatment. *Clin Orthop* 1963;28:111-119.

Weaver JK, Dunn HK: Treatment of acromioclavicular injuries, especially complete acromioclavicular separation. *J Bone Joint Surg Am* 1972;54:1187-1194.

Zuckerman JD, Matsen FA III: Complications about the glenohumeral joint related to the use of screws and staples. *J Bone Joint Surg Am* 1984;66:175-180.

Chapter 28

Shoulder Reconstruction

Frances Cuomo, MD

Joel A. Shapiro, MD

Rotator Cuff Disease

Anatomy and Function

The advent of MRI in the understanding of rotator cuff pathology has had a dual effect. On one hand, it has proved highly sensitive and specific for cuff pathology, to the degree that arthrography is now rarely used for this purpose. On the other hand, studies have documented the presence of partial- or full-thickness tears in a large percentage of asymptomatic patients.

Histologic studies of the rotator cuff have revealed a complex microanatomic structure consisting of five layers. It is suggested that this architecture not only contributes to normal function, but also plays a role in both tendon failure and repair. The vascular anatomy of the rotator cuff also has been investigated; although classically described as an avascular "critical zone," several studies have confirmed that the vascular supply reaches the tendinous insertions of the rotator cuff. The primary vascular supply to the cuff includes branches of the anterior and posterior humeral circumflex arteries, along with contributions from the suprascapular, subscapular, and suprahumeral arteries.

The rotator cuff has two principal functions: maintenance of humeral head position on the glenoid, and rotational power at the shoulder. The rotator cuff compresses the humeral head into the glenoid fossa, stabilizing the humeral head against superior migration and providing a stable fulcrum against which rotational forces may be applied. The rotator cuff resists the upward force of the deltoid, allowing rotation instead of translation. A recent radiographic investigation compared glenohumeral kinematics in three groups: those with asymptomatic cuff tears, symptomatic tears, and intact cuffs. The authors found a significant difference in superior humeral translation between the group with intact cuffs and each of the groups with torn cuffs. There was no significant difference between the groups with torn cuffs.

The concept of force couples has refined the understanding of rotator cuff function. Cadaveric studies have demonstrated that the anterior and posterior cuffs must work in concert to achieve normal function. Loss of one or the other creates translational movement and reduces the effect of compression. Although the primary function of the supraspinatus is to initiate abduction of the shoulder, several studies have shown that loss of supraspinatus function alone does not prevent elevation of the arm and does not create superior migration of the humeral head. These results have led to the suggestion that the supraspinatus acts principally to provide compression of the glenohumeral joint, thereby augmenting stability.

The role of the long head of the biceps tendon continues to be investigated. Studies have reported conflicting data regarding this structure as it relates to rotator cuff function. One electromyographic study found little activity in the biceps muscle during isolated shoulder motion. A cadaveric study, however, demonstrated decreased anterior to posterior translation of the glenohumeral joint with loading of the biceps tendon. Some authors continue to assert that the biceps is an active depressor of the humeral head. Others believe its significance lies in a potentially unrecognized source of pain, distinct from the rotator cuff. The current trend seems to be to view the long head of the biceps as a component of the rotator cuff, and to view its pathology as fitting within the spectrum of rotator cuff disease. Its exact role and optimum treatment remain to be determined.

Pathoanatomy

The structures implicated in rotator cuff pathology include the cuff itself and the coracoacromial arch, consisting of the acromion, coracoacromial ligament, and acromioclavicular (AC) joint. Although histologic studies of torn rotator cuff tissue have shown degenerative changes, there is little evidence of inflammation.

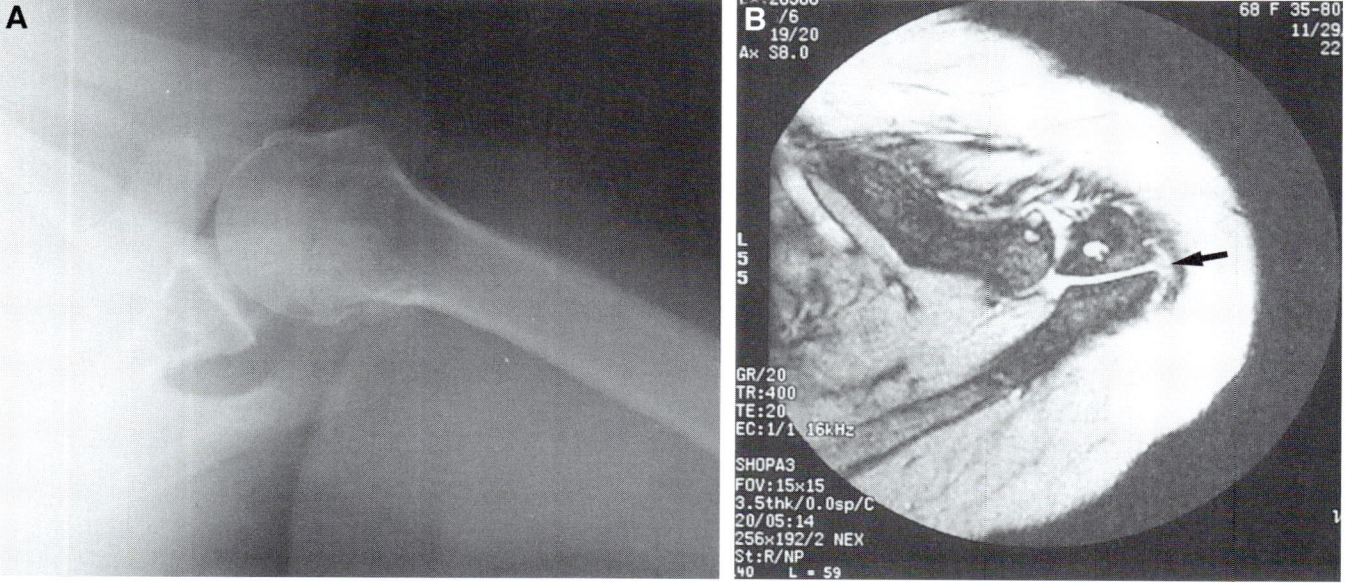

Figure 1 **A,** Axillary view demonstrating an os acromiale (mesoacromion type) located at the posterior aspect of the acromioclavicular joint. **B,** Axial MRI of an os acromiale (*arrow*).

The acromion is often implicated in cuff pathology. The shape of the acromion does not change with age; in contrast, anterior acromial spurs are age-dependent, found in 7% of patients 50 years old or younger versus 30% of patients older than 50 years according to a recent study. Studies of contact forces demonstrate increased pressure on the rotator cuff in association with increasing curvature of the acromion. The thickness, length, and elasticity of the coracoacromial ligament have been shown to be associated with rotator cuff tears. The incidence of an unfused os acromiale has been reported to be 8% in a cadaveric study; at least 33% of these are bilateral. A mobile os acromiale has been implicated as a cause of mechanical impingement (Fig. 1). Another potential cause of impingement is a degenerative AC joint. A recent cadaveric study found a significant association between degenerative AC joint spurs larger than 2 mm and full-thickness rotator cuff tears.

Extrinsic and intrinsic mechanisms have been implicated in rotator cuff pathology. The anatomy of the acromial arch is believed to be related to rotator cuff pathology. Clear associations have been documented between acromial morphology and rotator cuff tears. Similarly, altered microanatomy and biomechanical properties of the rotator cuff and surrounding tissues are associated with rotator cuff tears. A causal relationship, however, has yet to be demonstrated. It seems likely that these mechanisms are not independent, but rather represent interrelated processes that contribute to the deterioration and eventual failure of the rotator cuff.

Imaging

Conventional radiography remains the initial modality of choice. A complete series includes AP views of the scapula in neutral, internal, and external rotation, along with outlet and axillary lateral views. The outlet view allows assessment of the acromial morphology and confirms the presence of an anterior spur. Studies have associated an increased curvature of and/or presence of a spur in the acromion with an increased incidence of rotator cuff tear. MRI is the modality of choice for imaging the soft tissues about the shoulder, and is highly sensitive and specific for the detection of rotator cuff pathology (Fig. 2). Although ultrasound has been demonstrated to be sensitive and specific, before and after surgery, in the diagnosis of rotator cuff pathology, its use currently is limited to a small number of centers with expertise in this area. Arthrography has been largely supplanted by MRI; it remains useful for patients for whom MRI is not an option. CT has limited use in the workup of rotator cuff disease.

Impingement

Neer's classic description of impingement included three stages that represent points along a spectrum from irritation and inflammation of the subacromial bursa to failure of the rotator cuff tendons. Although knowledge of this condition has expanded, these stages remain a framework for diagnosis and treatment.

The inciting cause of impingement may be a combination of mechanical abrasion and pathologic changes within the rotator cuff tissue itself. The focus of treat-

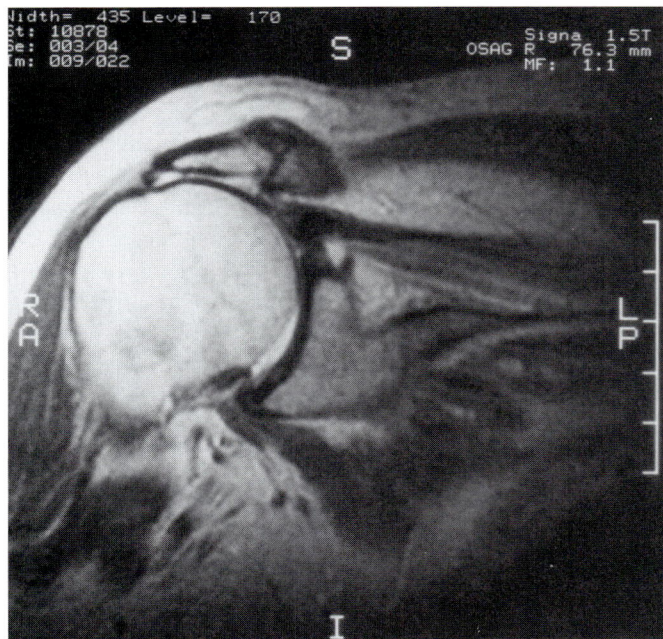

Figure 2 MRI study of massive rotator cuff tear with retraction, atrophy, and fatty degeneration of supraspinatus.

ment on mechanical causes may be partly because of the inability to alter intrinsic tendon pathology.

The initial diagnosis of rotator cuff impingement is clinical. Patients usually present with shoulder pain accentuated by overhead activities. The pain often radiates down the arm and precludes sleeping on the affected side. A study of the clinical tests for impingement found the Hawkins sign to have 92% and 88% sensitivity for bursitis and cuff tear, respectively. Neer's sign had 75% and 85% sensitivity, respectively. Both examinations were found to have low specificity, however. MRI is of questionable value in the diagnosis and initial treatment of impingement syndrome. A recent prospective, blinded, controlled study documented supraspinatus pathology on MRI in similar proportions of age-matched symptomatic and asymptomatic patients.

Nonsurgical management remains the foundation for treatment of impingement. Reported success rates are as high as 90%. One large retrospective study reported 67% good results using nonsteroidal anti-inflammatory medication combined with physical therapy. Poor results correlated with older age and increased acromial curvature. Other studies have documented the efficacy of subacromial lidocaine/steroid injections in relieving pain and improving range of shoulder motion.

When nonsurgical treatment fails, surgical decompression (both open and arthroscopic) has yielded consistently good results. A recent prospective study comparing nonsurgical care with arthroscopic subacromial decompression revealed a greater success rate with sur-

gery, with a 50% failure rate of nonsurgical care over 2.5 years. In a recent meta-analysis, subjectively good outcomes were found in 90% of open and 89.3% of arthroscopic subacromial decompressions for Neer stage II impingement. The question of what period of time constitutes an adequate trial of conservative care is controversial, with recommendations ranging from 3 to 18 months.

A 9-year follow-up study of 96 shoulders treated with open decompression for impingement (no tears initially) revealed a rotator cuff tear in 17 on ultrasound despite an initial excellent result. The majority of the patients with tears began to have pain an average of 5 years after the index procedure. The authors suggest that decompression does not preclude progression of rotator cuff pathology.

Rotator Cuff Tears

Rotator cuff tears may occur as the final event in a long-standing degenerative process or as a result of a single traumatic episode. The latter scenario occurs primarily in younger patients and there is little controversy as to treatment; most authors advocate prompt surgical repair. The majority of clinically significant tears, however, occur in patients older than age 40 years who likely have trauma to the tendon superimposed on an underlying tendinopathy. Decision making as to the most appropriate treatment is more controversial in this patient population. Treatment recommendations have included nonsurgical management (with or without steroid injections), decompression, débridement, and decompression with tendon repair.

Partial-Thickness Tears

Prior to the advent of MRI, definitive identification of the majority of partial-thickness tears could only be made at surgery (Fig. 3). The presentation of partial-thickness tears is similar to that of impingement. A study of the natural history of partial-thickness tears documented progression in 80% ultrasonographically. Most reports recommend débridement of tears judged to comprise less than 50% of the thickness of the tendon. Excision and repair are advocated for more significant tears. A study comparing these treatment modalities (in tears greater than 50% thickness) found no recurrence in the group undergoing excision and repair, but 3 of 32 patients undergoing débridement (combined with decompression) later progressed to complete tears.

An important distinction must be made between the typical patient older than age 40 years who presents with classic impingement syndrome and the younger overhead athlete who may have impingement second-

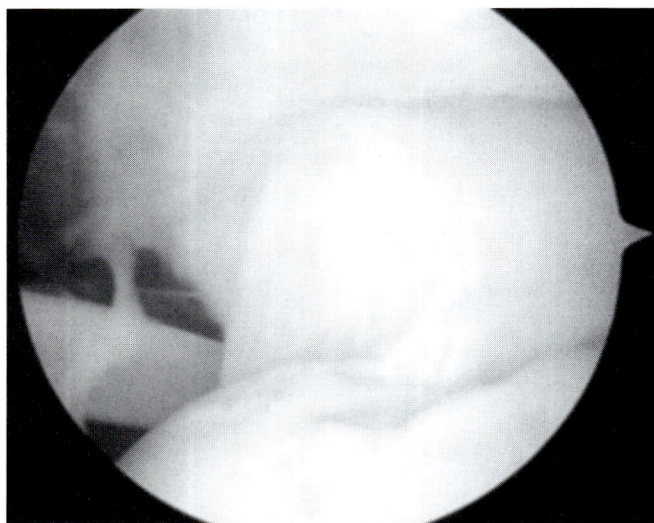

Figure 3 Partial-thickness undersurface rotator cuff tear found posterior to the biceps tendon during arthroscopic examination.

ary to glenohumeral instability, a process termed internal impingement. The hallmark of internal impingement is partial-thickness tearing of the articular side of the posterosuperior cuff along with fraying of the posterosuperior labrum. It is postulated that anteroinferior instability allows the greater tuberosity to abut the posterosuperior aspect of the glenoid during abduction and external rotation. Treatment of the impingement alone in this condition is not likely to prove effective.

Full-Thickness Tears

The treatment of full-thickness tears depends on several factors. The ideal setting for repair is an acute tear in a younger, healthy patient with good quality tissue. In a prospective outcome study, significant improvement was noted after rotator cuff repair at 2-year follow-up based on the SF-36 and limb-specific questionnaires. Another retrospective study with 54-month average follow-up demonstrated 96% good and excellent results following rotator cuff repair. The authors noted worse results correlated with a tear size greater than 5 cm and with female patients with associated biceps tendon rupture. Other authors have described worse results to be correlated with tear size and delay in treatment.

A massive rotator cuff tear is defined as one extending more than 5 cm or including two or more tendons. A recent prospective study documented the long-term durability of repairs of massive tears in 30 patients. At 65-month average follow-up, all patients retained significant improvements in pain, function, and range of motion over preoperative values, and all remained satisfied with the results. Another prospective study reported on 27 patients with massive tears followed up

for a minimum of 2 years. Seventeen patients had intact rotator cuffs at follow-up and had an excellent result. Despite a documented repeat tear in 10 patients, the authors reported that these patients were significantly improved from their preoperative state in terms of pain and function. A report on massive tears in patients older than age 70 years found a 78% satisfactory outcome at a mean follow-up of 3 years.

Some authors have suggested that repair of all cuff tears may be unnecessary. The results of arthroscopic subacromial decompression and rotator cuff débridement in 210 patients with a mean age of 61 years and a mean follow-up of 26.6 months was reported. Seventy-three percent of patients were considered to have satisfactory results by objective criteria. Poor prognostic indicators were identified as preoperative stiffness, workers' compensation, younger age, delay in presentation longer than 4 years, and postoperative pain "crises". Another report from the same group revealed 92% good and excellent results from decompression and débridement in 283 patients at a minimum 3-year follow-up. Fewer good results were noted in older patients.

Despite these results, enthusiasm for débridement of rotator cuff tears remains limited. In multiple previous studies, débridement has consistently yielded results that, while satisfactory, did not match those of rotator cuff repair. Other concerns include the inability to predict which patient will do well with more limited treatment, and the documented worse results associated with late attempts at repair. The current trend is to attempt to repair any full-thickness tear that causes persistent pain or loss of function.

The current focus has been on various less-invasive techniques for repair and on the problem of irreparable tears. The mini-open technique differs from the traditional open technique in that it minimizes detachment of the deltoid from the acromion. A study examining the long-term results of 60 rotator cuff tears of varying sizes repaired using a mini-open technique found no deterioration of good results (80% satisfactory) at an average 62-month follow-up.

Arthroscopic rotator cuff repair appears to be gaining popularity. Proponents of this technique emphasize the need for adherence to established repair principles, including appropriate mobilization and secure tendon-to-bone or tendon-to-tendon fixation. Several recent studies have reported medium-term follow-up. One study, with 53 patients, reported 49 good and excellent results at a minimum 2-year follow-up.

Irreparable tears of the rotator cuff have remained a difficult problem. Although no exact definition of irreparable exists, there is a population of patients who fit this category. Treatment of the truly irreparable tear can include nonsurgical management, débridement, tendon grafts or substitutes, and local or regional tendon transfers. Nonsurgical care is unlikely to be of benefit, although physical therapy may play a role in maintaining range of shoulder motion while awaiting further treatment. Substitutes for the cuff tendons, including autograft, allograft, and prosthetic substitutes usually perform poorly. Débridement combined with a modest subacromial decompression yielded good results in one study, with 26 of 33 patients experiencing significant improvement in pain and motion at short-term follow-up. This appears to be a viable treatment alternative in the low-demand patient.

Concern for the fate of the glenohumeral joint in the younger patient with an irreparable tear has prompted efforts at tendon transfer to maintain humeral head depression and improve function. Transfer of the superior portion of the subscapularis has been recommended to assist with abduction, supported by a recent biomechanical study, although this method has not been shown clinically to be effective. In addition, the pectoralis major, trapezius, and portions of the deltoid have been suggested as transfer candidates, although these structures are rarely used in this manner.

Transfer of the latissimus dorsi has attracted attention because of its biomechanical potential to act as an active humeral head depressor and humeral elevator. In a study of 16 shoulders treated with transfer of the latissimus dorsi, all demonstrated significant improvement at 33-month average follow-up. The average function was 73% of normal and 80% in patients with a functional subscapularis. In a more recent study, 14 of 17 patients were satisfied, demonstrating significant improvement in pain and function.

Long Head of the Biceps Tendon

The long head of the biceps tendon (LHB) continues to generate interest and controversy. Although the LHB is a known source of pain, its exact function and in particular its role as a humeral head depressor has been debated. Results from cadaver and electromyographic studies do not agree; several retrospective clinical studies have reported success with tenodesis or tenolysis, whereas others recommend preservation of the tendon in order to reinforce a rotator cuff repair.

The LHB is subject to a number of problems that may be divided into two broad groups: those associated with rotator cuff disease and those isolated to the area of the tendon origin. Several authors have noted degeneration and tearing of the LHB in association with rotator cuff disease. Treatment recommendations focus on appropriate management of the rotator cuff.

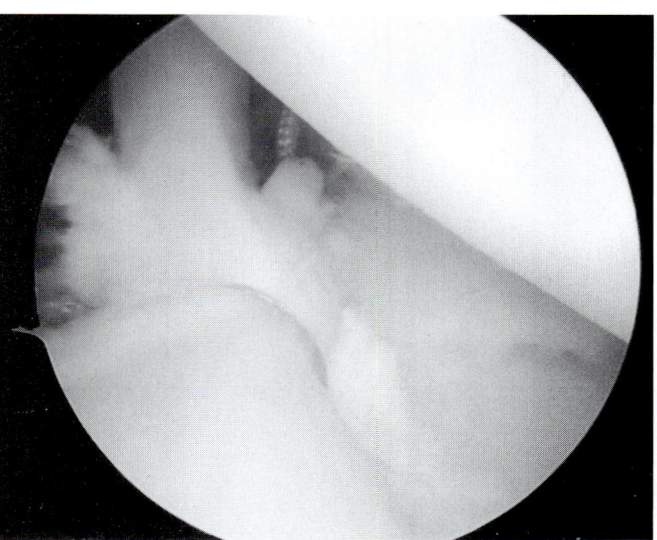

Figure 4 Arthroscopic repair of type II SLAP lesion. Anchors are placed posterior and anterior to the biceps origin to secure repair.

The LHB may be repaired or débrided as required. Tenodesis has been recommended when the tendon is noted to subluxate into the joint, as is commonly seen with tears involving the subscapularis.

Disorders about the origin of this tendon have been termed superior labrum anterior and posterior (SLAP) lesions. The etiology of this disorder includes acute trauma and overuse phenomenon that is more common in overhead athletes. A recent cadaver study found that SLAP lesions were more likely to occur in the presence of anterior subluxation. Another study reported a 6% incidence of SLAP lesions in patients undergoing shoulder arthroscopy for any reason. A recent radiologic study using magnetic resonance arthrography demonstrated a sensitivity of 89% and specificity of 91% and found that magnetic resonance classification correlated with arthroscopic findings 76% of the time.

Classification of the SLAP lesion addresses tears of the labrum and integrity of the biceps origin. Treatment protocols have been proposed based on the classification. Those lesions involving detachment of the biceps origin appear to require repair. Several authors have reported good short-term results with arthroscopic techniques (Fig. 4).

Failure of treatment of rotator cuff pathology can often be traced to failure of the repair, inadequate decompression, AC joint pathology, deltoid dehiscence, or postoperative infection. Successful treatment requires identification of the cause of failure. Even with this knowledge, one study documented only 60% satisfactory results after repeat surgery for failed rotator cuff repair.

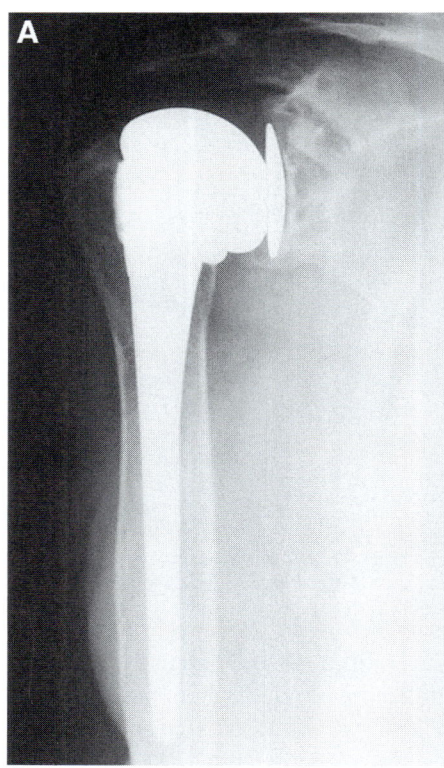
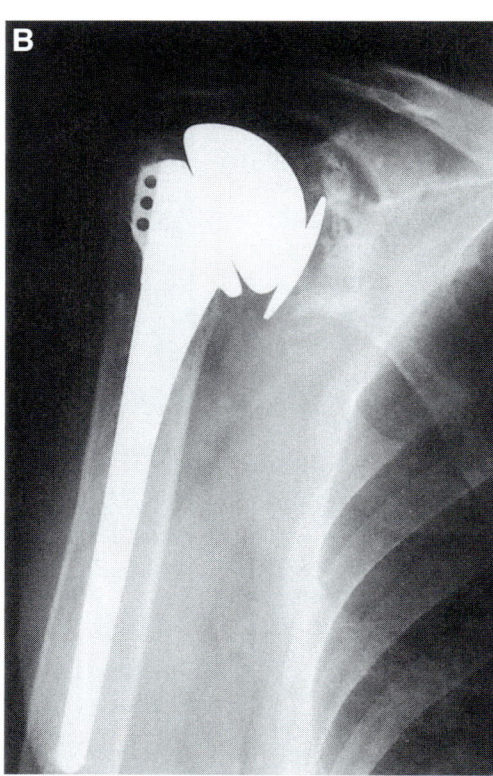

Figure 5 **A,** Radiolucent line noted at the bone-prosthesis interface of the glenoid. **B,** Eighteen months later, gross glenoid component loosening is noted by a shift in the glenoid implant.

Acromioclavicular Joint

Degeneration of the AC joint is a well-known cause of pain and is closely associated with other shoulder pathology. A recent arthroscopic study found that 213 of 218 patients with a painful AC joint had a concomitant pathologic lesion in the shoulder. Failure to address AC pathology is a cause of failure of reconstructive surgery about the shoulder. However, several studies have documented evidence of AC joint degeneration in a large proportion of asymptomatic individuals. This dilemma can be addressed through careful correlation of clinical findings, such as pain on palpation of the joint, with radiographic evidence of pathology. The response to selective lidocaine injections can aid in deciding on the appropriate treatment.

Prosthetic Arthroplasty

Prosthetic arthroplasty of the shoulder continues to be a valuable solution to end-stage degeneration of various etiologies. Since its introduction by Neer for treatment of severe proximal humerus fractures, the indications have widened. Research currently is directed toward improving prosthetic design and on evaluating surgical outcomes.

Basic Science

The majority of prosthetic designs in current use have a metallic, stemmed humeral endoprosthesis with a metal-bearing surface. The glenoid designs favor an all-polyethylene component with either a keel or pegs. Conformity of the prosthetic joint varies among systems, but typically involves a slight degree of mismatch.

Fixation was originally described using cement for both humeral and glenoid components. The trend is toward press-fitting the humeral component (except in fracture cases). Results from several studies have shown no increase in rates of aseptic loosening with press-fitting, although there was shifting of 50% of press-fit components after 15 years in one study. The glenoid is routinely cemented, but problems persist and bone ingrowth glenoids have been studied. A recent study comparing cemented versus noncemented glenoid components revealed similar rates of aseptic loosening. None had required revision at 4- to 7-year followup and functional results were not significantly different. Two of 26 glenoids required revision for component dissociation with the authors reporting focal osteolysis under the metal trays, suggesting that this situation may result in loosening.

Aseptic loosening of the glenoid component remains a complication associated with total shoulder arthroplasty. A rate of revision for loosening of cemented components of up to 11% has been reported at 3- to 5-year follow-up. Radiolucent lines have been reported, although their significance is disputed (Fig. 5). Efforts continue to be directed toward understanding the causes and identifying solutions to this problem. The focus has been on biomechanical issues of component design and limited fixation available in the glenoid. A recent study examining glenoid component biomechanics showed improved stress transfer with all-polyethylene components. Another model demonstrated improved glenoid edge loading characteristics with less constrained designs and roughened fixation surfaces. The recent development of sophisticated mathematical models of glenohumeral joint motion may aid in future designs. Several cases of osteolysis in the presence of polyethylene debris resulting in aseptic loosening and revision (at average 12 years) have been documented. Histologic analysis shows a process similar to that in the hip, although the particles from the shoulder were noted to be larger and more fibrillar.

The current trend is toward increased modularity. The stability of a shoulder arthroplasty is entirely dependent on proper soft-tissue balance. Improved reproduction of normal anatomy may provide better stability and motion. One study of humeral head sizing found that motion in a cadaver model was better with sizing matched to humeral head volume rather than diameter. Components that allow intraoperative adjustments such as neck-shaft angle and humeral offset are available with short-term follow-up only. Increased modularity allows for more intraoperative choices, but carries with it the potential for intracomponent wear and failure.

Bipolar prostheses have been developed for the shoulder. One hundred eight patients treated for various diagnoses with an average 2.9-year follow-up had results and revision rates on par with hemiarthroplasty. Other authors report improved results in the subset of rheumatoid patients with irreparable rotator cuff tears. The role of this design requires further study.

Indications

The main indication for shoulder arthroplasty is unremitting pain, caused by a degenerative glenohumeral joint, that is refractory to nonsurgical measures. The diagnoses commonly associated with end-stage disease include osteoarthritis (OA), rheumatoid arthritis, osteonecrosis, posttraumatic arthrosis, rotator cuff tear arthropathy, arthritis of dislocations, and chronic dislocation. Each disorder has unique considerations with regard to prosthetic arthroplasty.

Contraindications to total shoulder arthroplasty include active infection, intractable instability, paralysis of both deltoid and rotator cuff musculature, and neuropathic arthropathy. Relative contraindications to glenoid replacement in particular include a young patient, inadequate bone stock, and irreparable rotator cuff tears.

Disease-Specific Recommendations

OA is the most common indication for shoulder arthroplasty. The typical presentation is in an older patient with an insidious onset of progressive shoulder pain that worsens with activity. Classic radiographic findings of OA include joint space narrowing, osteophytes, subchondral sclerosis, and cysts. A predilection for posterior glenoid wear often is noted on the axillary view and clinical studies show that patients often lack full external rotation.

Prosthetic replacement has yielded consistently good results in most reports. Various authors have reported good results with routine use of either total arthroplasty or hemiarthroplasty. A recent prospective, randomized trial demonstrated slightly superior results in the group that included glenoid resurfacing. Specifically, there was better pain relief, internal rotation, and overall subjective satisfaction with total shoulder replacement. At an average follow-up of 35 months, 12% of the hemiarthroplasty group required revision for pain. None of the total shoulder arthroplasty patients had required revision within the same time. The authors noted, however, that evaluation with University of California at Los Angeles and American Shoulder and Elbow Surgeons scoring systems revealed no significant difference in outcomes between the two groups.

Rheumatoid arthritis frequently affects the shoulder. Early diagnosis and aggressive medical management are the mainstays of treatment. Failure to respond to medical management is best treated by early surgical intervention, which reliably provides pain relief. Functional improvement is less predictable and related to the status of the rotator cuff and the patient's overall condition. End-stage disease with corresponding severe bone and soft-tissue deficits leads to a worse outcome. Therefore, many authors have recommended early reconstruction in hopes of improving outcomes.

Most reports have shown better pain relief and range of motion with resurfacing of the glenoid in patients with intact rotator cuffs. This parallels the experience with knee arthroplasty regarding the patella, and probably reflects the global joint involvement with rheumatoid arthritis. Because of severe central wear, inadequate bone stock may preclude glenoid fixation. Several authors have emphasized the importance of rotator cuff function to outcome and every effort should be made to repair tears found at surgery. Good results may be achieved when an acceptable repair is obtained. An irreparable rotator cuff tear is a relative contraindication to glenoid resurfacing. A preoperative MRI study may assist surgical planning and patient counseling.

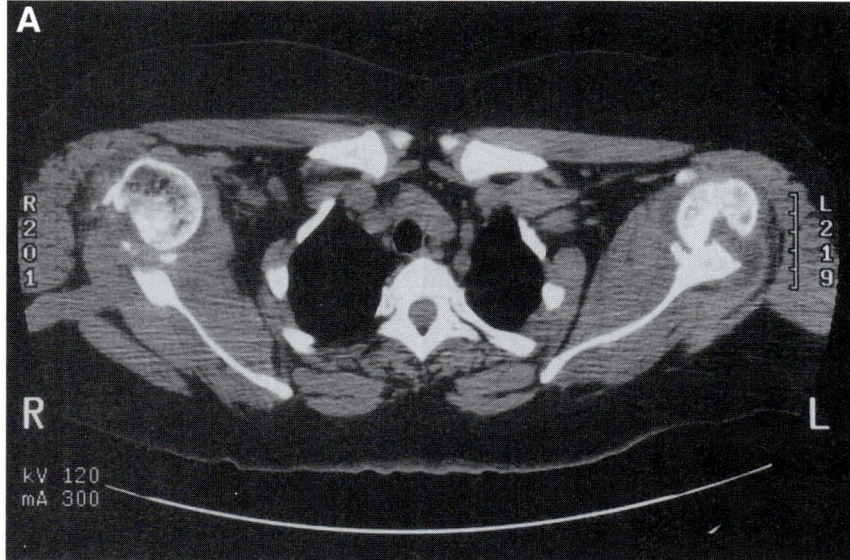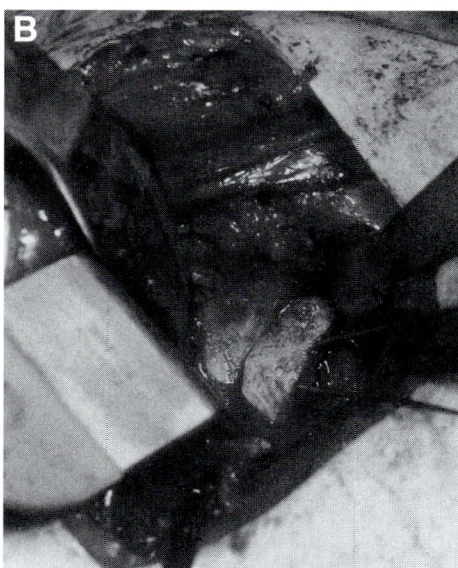

Figure 6 **A,** CT scan of chronic locked bilateral anterior dislocations of 6 months' duration. The left shoulder demonstrates a 40% articular surface defect on the humeral head and destruction of the anterior 30% of the glenoid. **B,** Intraoperative photograph of anterior glenoid bone graft during replacement surgery. The remainder of the osteotomized humeral head was used as glenoid graft and held with cannulated headless screws.

Rotator cuff tear arthropathy is a well-recognized entity with a reported incidence of 4% to 7%. Symptomatic patients may be treated effectively with arthroplasty. Glenoid resurfacing is controversial, but because of increased loosening rates is generally not recommended. Loosening is believed to be a result of shearing forces generated with loss of rotator cuff function. This phenomenon has been termed "rocking-horse glenoid" and describes the repeated edge loading leading to early loosening. Hemiarthroplasty with a humeral head that matches the "acetabularized" glenoid-coracoacromial arch anatomy seems to provide predictable pain relief, albeit with limited function. Preservation of the coracoacromial arch is critical for preventing superior instability. Bipolar components have not demonstrated improved results over monopolar prostheses. Semiconstrained prostheses have shown unacceptable early loosening. Reverse ball-and-socket prostheses are available but have had unacceptable rates of failure.

When osteonecrosis is diagnosed early, prior to secondary glenoid degeneration, the results of hemiarthroplasty have been consistently good. Later treatment in the presence of glenoid destruction may benefit from total shoulder replacement. A recent long-term questionnaire follow-up study found 79.5% satisfaction at an average 8.9-year follow-up. The study did not report a difference in results between total shoulder arthroplasty and hemiarthroplasty.

Although recurrent instability is believed to have a relatively low rate of secondary arthrosis, the results of overtightening the glenohumeral joint after instability procedures are well reported. Any technique that lim-

its glenohumeral motion (ie, Putti-Platt) has the potential for late arthropathy. Shoulder arthroplasty is recommended as the treatment of choice for secondary arthrosis. The results may be jeopardized by the young age of most patients with this diagnosis. Soft-tissue resurfacing of the glenoid has been suggested as an alternative to prosthetic replacement (in conjunction with humeral head replacement) as a means of avoiding the issue of loosening. Good short-term results have been reported with this technique.

Prosthetic replacement for fracture treatment was described by Neer and spurred the subsequent development of shoulder arthroplasty. This treatment has since been applied primarily to four-part fractures and fracture-dislocations of the proximal humerus in the elderly. Additional indications include three-part fractures when stable internal fixation cannot be obtained. Earlier studies reported over 80% good and excellent results. Several recent reports, however, have not been able to duplicate these results. One long-term follow-up study of arthroplasty for fracture found a significant number of patients with continued pain and loss of function, leading the authors to caution against viewing this procedure as a panacea. Significantly better objective and subjective outcomes have been noted when hemiarthroplasty was performed within 4 weeks of injury.

Chronic glenohumeral dislocation is considered an indication for arthroplasty in an appropriately functional patient (Fig. 6). Most authors use 6 months of dislocation as criteria for replacement. Although this number is somewhat arbitrary, it is believed that prior to this time the joint may be salvageable. An additional indication for replacement is an articular impression defect greater than 40% to 45% of the articular surface, causing instability. The complexity of arthroplasty in this population has been noted because of the presence of bony and soft-tissue deformities.

Glenohumeral Arthrodesis

As the indications for shoulder replacement have widened, the indications for glenohumeral fusion have narrowed. This procedure was once advocated for many end-stage shoulder disorders, including massive rotator cuff tears. It is now reserved primarily for those cases in which a shoulder arthroplasty is contraindicated. Current indications include septic arthritis, combined deltoid and rotator cuff paralysis (such as brachial plexus injury and postpolio syndrome), failed arthroplasty, recurrent dislocation, tumor reconstruction, and for the young, heavy laborer with severe arthropathy.

Several recent studies have shown reliably good function, within limited parameters, with shoulder fusion. Children in particular are able to compensate extremely well for the lack of glenohumeral motion. Various authors have made recommendations as to position for fusion. A classic functional study noted that rotation was the key parameter and recommended internal rotation between 25° and 30°, abduction 25° to 40°, and flexion 20° to 30°. Other studies have recommended position on the lower end of these ranges, in particular abduction, noting pain associated with a more abducted position.

Technically, numerous techniques are available to achieve fusion. One important functional criteria is that the hand be able to reach the mouth and the midline of the body; technique descriptions emphasize the importance of draping such that the location of the patient's mouth may be identified intraoperatively.

Frozen Shoulder Syndrome

Frozen shoulder syndrome is a common disorder that remains poorly understood. Despite the common finding of inflamed synovium on arthroscopy, several recent studies have demonstrated that the predominant cells found in the abnormal capsule are fibroblasts and myofibroblasts. Inflammatory cells are not present in significantly increased numbers. It has been suggested that the disease process is similar to Dupuytren's contracture. Cytokines, growth factors, and metalloproteinases have been found to be increased over normal capsular control samples. These increases were similar, but not identical to samples from cases of Dupuytren's contracture. This avenue of research may hold promise for developing molecular biological treatments for this condition.

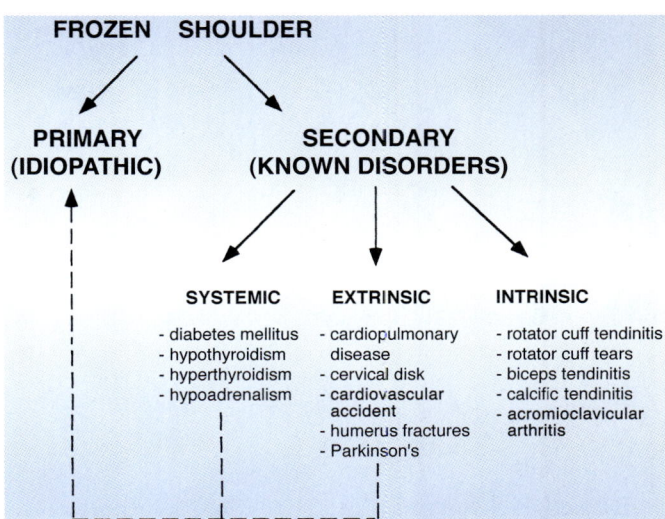

Figure 7 Classification system proposed for frozen shoulder syndrome with primary and secondary etiologies suggested. *(Reproduced with permission from Zuckerman JD, Cuomo F, Rokito AS: Abstract: Definition and classification of frozen shoulder: A consensus approach. J Shoulder Elbow Surg 1994;3:S72.)*

The diagnosis of frozen shoulder is primarily a clinical one; the hallmark is limitation of both passive and active range of shoulder motion. The etiology may be primary (idiopathic) or secondary to a variety of medical conditions or traumatic events. An arthrogram demonstrating reduced capsular volume is the classic study. Insidious onset of severe pain on shoulder motion marks the early phase of the disease, followed by resolution of pain accompanied by loss of shoulder motion. Previous reports have asserted that the disease resolves spontaneously within 2 years. More recent studies, using strict criteria, have found that as many as 50% of patients experience some degree of chronic pain and stiffness. A classification system has been proposed, dividing the etiology as primary or secondary, with secondary causes subdivided as intrinsic, extrinsic, or systemic (Fig. 7). This stratification may facilitate a logical treatment plan.

Treatment options include anti-inflammatory medication, physical therapy, intra-articular steroid injection, manipulation under anesthesia, and capsular release, either open or arthroscopic (Fig. 8). Studies documenting the effectiveness of each of these treatments have been published. In one study, arthroscopic release was evaluated in 73 patients, with restoration of full range of motion and relief of pain in most patients at 8.9 weeks postoperatively. These results were maintained in 89% of patients at 12-month follow-up. Despite these somewhat optimistic results, the mainstay of treatment continues to be diligent nonsurgical management, consisting of daily range of motion exercises.

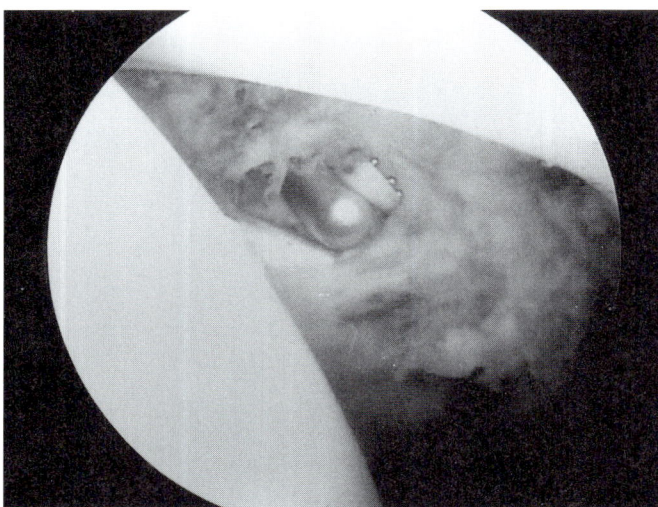

Figure 8 Arthroscopic capsular release with electrothermal wand releasing a scarred, contracted rotator interval just superior to the subscapularis.

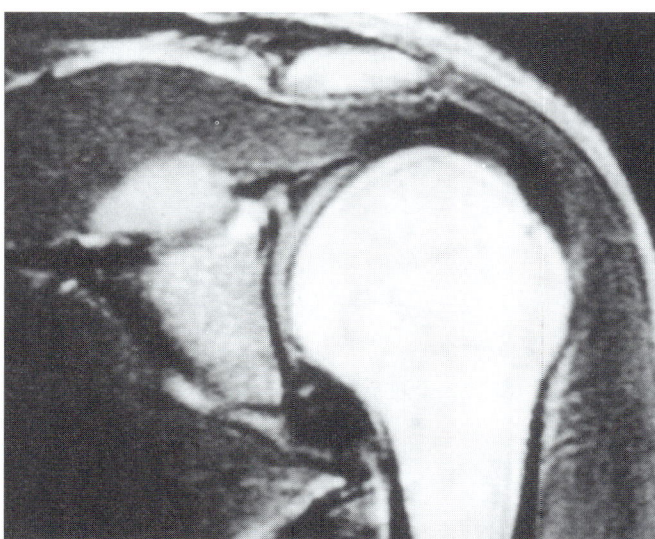

Figure 9 A ganglion cyst at the suprascapular notch associated with superior labral tear identified on coronal cut of MRI study.

Miscellaneous Problems

Nerve Compression About the Shoulder

Nerve compression syndromes about the shoulder are uncommon. The two most often reported involve the long thoracic and suprascapular nerves.

The long thoracic nerve supplies the serratus anterior musculature and interruption of its function leads to the clinical finding of scapular winging. The cause is often a traumatic neurapraxia, but may be idiopathic. Most patients recover function, although the recovery period is lengthy, taking up to 2 years. Many treatments have been proposed, including bracing, scapulothoracic fusion, and a variety of tendon transfers. Several recent studies have reported consistent success with transfer of the sternal head of the pectoralis major to the inferior angle of the scapula.

There are many reports of suprascapular nerve compression in the literature. The sites of compression are the suprascapular and spinoglenoid notches. The etiology of the compression may be a ganglion cyst (secondary to labral pathology) or a thickened traversing ligament (Fig. 9). Fracture callus has also been reported as a cause. The typical clinical scenario involves an overhead athlete (baseball, swimming, or volleyball) with vague posterior shoulder pain and mild external rotation weakness. In long-standing cases, atrophy may be noted in the supraspinatus and/or infraspinatus fossa, depending on the site of nerve compression. Electromyographic studies may be helpful in confirming the diagnosis and localizing the site of compression. A recent report noted improvement of pain in all patients after decompression of the suprascapular notch. There was minimal improvement in

atrophy when present. Early decompression is recommended for symptomatic patients.

Brachial Plexus Palsy

Brachial plexus palsy in children is most frequently the result of birth injury and is addressed elsewhere in this book. In adults, trauma is the most frequent cause, usually characterized by high-energy injuries and is often accompanied by other potentially life-threatening problems. Other reported etiologies include viral (Parsonage-Turner syndrome), tumor, radiation, and iatrogenic.

Several classification schemes exist for these injuries. Brachial plexus injury may be classified as neurapraxia, axonotmesis, or neurotmesis. The location of the injury may be described as preganglionic or postganglionic. Injuries that occur between the spinal cord and the dorsal root ganglion (preganglionic) often represent avulsion of the nerve root, which is not amenable to direct repair and has no potential for spontaneous recovery. The prognosis of postganglionic lesions is dependent on the specific type of neuronal damage.

Another system divides the injury pattern into two groups: supraclavicular or infraclavicular. This anatomic division reflects two common patterns of closed injury; the supraclavicular type commonly involves higher energy and affects the root, trunk, or division level of the plexus. (These may represent preganglionic or postganglionic injuries.) Infraclavicular injuries are associated with lower energy, fracture, or dislocation mechanisms and typically localize to the cords or peripheral nerve branches (postganglionic). Overall, infraclavicular injuries carry a better prognosis, and reportedly show functional improvement over a 3-year period, with 95% of patients recovering proximal musculature, and median nerve and ulnar nerve recovery occurring in 80% and 60%, respectively.

History and detailed physical examination are important tools in patient evaluation. Often, localization of the injury can be made on careful physical examination. Physical examination signs of a preganglionic lesion include a Horner sign, lack of a Tinel sign (tapping over plexus fails to produce tingling distally) and paralysis of the rhomboid and serratus anterior musculature.

Additional testing can aid in diagnosis and decision making. Electromyography and nerve conduction velocity examinations at 3 weeks after injury can confirm diagnosis and delineate preganglionic from postganglionic lesions. Serial electrical examinations can objectively assess recovery or lack thereof. MRI can provide anatomic information that may assist with surgical planning. Traditional myelographic studies can demonstrate meningoceles in the presence of a root avulsion, although MRI has largely supplanted this technique.

Treatment of these injuries is often complex. Options include nonsurgical care, surgical repair of the plexus, neurologic reconstruction (grafting or neurotization), orthopaedic reconstruction (tendon transfers, fusion), and palliation. Guiding principles include the need for a functional, sensate hand followed by the ability to position the hand in space. The varied nature of the injury along with its relative infrequence make controlled studies difficult. Studies of treatments report widely varied results and often lack control groups, randomization, and long-term follow-up.

Early experience with aggressive plexus reconstruction was poor. The treatment regimen that evolved in the wake of these failures included early conservative care followed by tendon transfers as needed. However, functional results in these patients have been disappointing. Improved microsurgical techniques and more success in pediatric cases have led to renewed enthusiasm for surgical nerve reconstruction of these injuries in adults. With increasing experience, it has been recognized that these injuries are often postganglionic, and therefore potentially repairable. Several recent studies have reported improved results of nerve repair and nerve grafting. The results appear to be best for reconstruction of the lateral cord. Surgery within 6 months of injury correlated with improved results. Preganglionic injuries are not amenable to anatomic repair, but neurotization has shown promising results, in particular for the lateral cord.

A recently proposed treatment algorithm includes early exploration for open injuries (with potential for direct repair) and for documented preganglionic lesions (with concurrent neurotization). For postganglionic lesions, 3 months of observation are recommended. If no improvement or electromyographic evidence of recovery is seen, surgery is performed within 6 months of injury with nerve grafting or neurotization.

Annotated Bibliography

Bentolila V, Nizard R, Bizot P, Sedel L: Complete traumatic brachial plexus palsy: Treatment and outcome after repair. *J Bone Joint Surg Am* 1999;81:20-28.

A retrospective review of treatment of complete closed brachial plexus palsy, with a minimum 3-year follow-up, is presented. A mix of pathoanatomic lesions were included. The treatment regimen included neurolysis, nerve repair or grafting when possible, and nerve transfer in the remainder. A good result was defined as at least 3+/5 motor power. Good results were found in 63% of patients for biceps function, 35% for triceps function, and less than 20% for wrist or finger flexor function. Significantly better results were found with respect to the biceps when surgery was performed within 6 months of the injury.

Bunker TD, Reilly J, Baird KS, Hamblen DL: Expression of growth factors, cytokines and matrix metalloproteinases in frozen shoulder. *J Bone Joint Surg Br* 2000;82:768-773.

Using reverse transcription and polymerase chain reaction techniques, expression of cytokines, growth factors, and matrix metalloproteinases (MMP) were assessed in tissue from patients with frozen shoulder, Dupuytren's contracture, and in control subjects. The levels of proinflammatory cytokines (IL-beta, TNF-alpha and TNF-beta) were near control levels in the frozen shoulders, and lower than that of the Dupuytren's tissue. The most notable difference in the frozen shoulder samples was the absence of MMP-14, which is an activator of other proteinases.

Dodenhoff RM, Levy O, Wilson A, Copeland SA: Manipulation under anesthesia for primary frozen shoulder: Effect on early recovery and return to activity. *J Shoulder Elbow Surg* 2000;9:23-26.

In this prospective study, there was significant early improvement after shoulder manipulation. Of 39 shoulders, 59% had no or mild disability at 3 months, 28.2% had moderate disability, and 12.8% had severe disability. Ninety-four percent of patients were satisfied, and improvements in the Constant-Murley scores were maintained at average 11-month follow-up. Interestingly, there was no correlation between the initial Constant-Murley score or range of motion and the final outcome.

Gartsman GM, Roddey TS, Hammerman SM: Shoulder arthroplasty with or without resurfacing of the glenoid in patients who have osteoarthritis. *J Bone Joint Surg Am* 2000;82:26-34.

Results from a prospective, randomized study of 51 shoulder replacements comparing hemiarthroplasty to total shoulder replacement are presented. At a mean follow-up of 35 months, there was significantly better pain relief and internal rotation in the total shoulder group. The authors also noted trends toward better function, strength, and satisfaction with glenoid resurfacing, although these were not statistically significant. The glenoid resurfacing added $1,177, 30 minutes of operating room time, and a 150-mL blood loss to the procedure. No total shoulders had been revised at the most recent follow-up. Three of the 25 hemiarthroplasties (12%) required revision to total shoulder arthroplasty for pain at a mean cost of $15,998.

Hattrup SJ, Cofield RH: Osteonecrosis of the humeral head: Results of replacement. *J Shoulder Elbow Surg* 2000;9:177-182.

In this retrospective review of 127 shoulder arthroplasties for osteonecrosis, hemiarthroplaties were performed in 71 and total shoulder replacements in 56. At average follow-up of 8.9 years, 79.5% reported subjective improvement and 77.3% noted either no or only occasional moderate pain. Better results were noted in steroid-induced osteonecrosis, while worse results were noted with a posttraumatic etiology. Minimal difference was found in outcomes between hemiarthroplasty and total shoulder replacement. Postoperative rotator cuff tears were found in 18.1% of patients, and this complication was more common in shoulders that had undergone prior surgery.

Kido T, Itoi E, Konno N, Sano A, Urayama M, Sato K: The depressor function of biceps on the head of the humerus in shoulders with tears of the rotator cuff. *J Bone Joint Surg Br* 2000;82:416-419.

Radiographic evidence of a depressor function of the long head of the biceps tendon was demonstrated during active forward elevation in patients with an MRI-documented rotator cuff tear. Less humeral head proximal migration was found with biceps contraction at elevations of 0°, 45° and 90°.

Rokito AS, Cuomo F, Gallagher MA, Zuckerman JD: Long-term functional outcome of repair of large and massive chronic tears of the rotator cuff. *J Bone Joint Surg Am* 1999;81:991-997.

Thirty patients with large or massive cuff tears underwent strength testing preoperatively and postoperatively at 12 months and 65 months (average). Findings included significant increases in strength, range of motion, and function at 1 year. Gains continued past 1 year. Strength was approximately 80% of unaffected side at final follow-up. The mean University of California at Los Angeles shoulder score increased from 12.3 to 31.0 at most recent follow-up. All patients reported satisfaction with the outcome.

Sojbjerg JO, Frich LH, Johannsen HV, Sneppen O: Late results of total shoulder replacement in patients with rheumatoid arthritis. *Clin Orthop* 1999;366:39-45.

In this retrospective outcome study of more than 500 total shoulder replacements for rheumatoid arthritis with 2- to 15-year follow-up, most patients had satisfactory outcomes, with nearly all having good pain relief. Functional results as measured by active range of motion were less predictable, but correlated with extent of disease progression. The authors found deterioration in results over time, which appeared to correlate with progressive rotator cuff failure, proximal migration of the humeral head, and resultant increased rates of late glenoid loosening.

Stone KD, Grabowski JJ, Cofield RH, Morrey BF, An KN: Stress analyses of glenoid components in total shoulder arthroplasty. *J Shoulder Elbow Surg* 1999;8: 151-158.

A comparison was made as to stress patterns in cemented all-polyethylene versus uncemented metal-backed polyethylene glenoid components. The all-polyethylene components had a stress pattern more closely approximating the native glenoid. Metal-backed prostheses were found to have regions of high stress at the plastic/metal interface. It was concluded that metal-backed glenoids had a higher potential for stress shielding and polyethylene wear.

Yamaguchi K, Sher JS, Andersen WK, et al: Glenohumeral motion in patients with rotator cuff tears: A comparison of asymptomatic and symptomatic shoulders. *J Shoulder Elbow Surg* 2000;9:6-11.

In radiographic comparison of normal shoulders, asymptomatic cuff tears and symptomatic cuff tears, the symptomatic and asymptomatic cuff tear groups demonstrated significantly more superior migration than the group without tears. There was no significant difference in migration between the symptomatic and asymptomatic tear groups. The authors conclude that although rotator cuff tears result in abnormal kinematics, this alteration does not account for symptoms.

Classic Bibliography

Blair B, Rokito AS, Cuomo F, Jarolem K, Zuckerman JD: Efficacy of injections of corticosteroids for subacromial impingement syndrome. *J Bone Joint Surg Am* 1996;78:1685-1689.

Codman EA, Akerson IB: The pathology associated with rupture of the supraspinatus tendon. *Ann Surg* 1931;93:348-359.

Gartsman GM: Arthroscopic acromioplasty for lesions of the rotator cuff. *J Bone Joint Surg Am* 1990;72: 169-180.

Groh GI, Williams GR, Jarman RN, Rockwood CA Jr: Treatment of complications of shoulder arthrodesis. *J Bone Joint Surg Am* 1997;79:881-887.

Harryman DT II, Mack LA, Wang KY, Jackins SE, Richardson ML, Matsen FA III: Repairs of the rotator cuff: Correlation of functional results with integrity of the cuff. *J Bone Joint Surg Am* 1991;73:982-989.

Hawkins RJ, Neer CS II: A functional analysis of shoulder fusions. *Clin Orthop* 1987;223:65-76.

Leffert RD, Seddon H: Infraclavicular brachial plexus injuries. *J Bone Joint Surg Br* 1965;47:9-22.

McCoy SR, Warren RF, Bade HA III, Ranawat CS, Inglis AE: Total shoulder arthroplasty in rheumatoid arthritis. *J Arthroplasty* 1989;4:105-113.

McLaughlin HL: Lesions of the musculotendinous cuff of the shoulder: I. The exposure and treatment of tears with retraction. *J Bone Joint Surg Am* 1944;26:31-51.

Neer CS II: Anterior acromioplasty for the chronic impingement syndrome in the shoulder: A preliminary report. *J Bone Joint Surg Am* 1972;54:41-50.

Neer CS II: Replacement arthroplasty for glenohumeral osteoarthritis. *J Bone Joint Surg Am* 1974;56: 1-13.

Neer CS II, Watson KC, Stanton FJ: Recent experience in total shoulder replacement. *J Bone Joint Surg Am* 1982;64:319-337.

Neer CS II: Impingement lesions. *Clin Orthop* 1983; 173:70-77.

Neviaser JS: Adhesive capsulitis of the shoulder: A study of the pathological findings in periarthritis of the shoulder. *J Bone Joint Surg* 1945;27:211-222.

Sher JS, Uribe JW, Posada A, Murphy BJ, Zlatkin MB: Abnormal findings on magnetic resonance images of asymptomatic shoulders. *J Bone Joint Surg Am* 1995;77:10-15.

Snyder SJ, Karzel RP, Del Pizzo W, Ferkel RD, Friedman MJ: SLAP lesions of the shoulder. *Arthroscopy* 1990;6:274-279.

Zuckerman JD, Cuomo F, Rokito S: Abstract: Definition and classification of frozen shoulder: A consensus approach. *J Shoulder Elbow Surg* 1994;3:S72.

Chapter 29

Elbow: Pediatric Aspects

Michael G. Vitale, MD, MPH

David L. Skaggs, MD

Pediatric Elbow Fractures

As one of the most frequent causes of medical liability claims, elbow injuries deserve careful consideration. A recent retrospective cohort study of 6,493 pediatric fractures documented a marked increase in percutaneous fixation of these common injuries. For example, rates of pinning of supracondylar elbow fractures increased from 4% to 40% over the 10-year period of the study. This shift toward fixation of these fractures presumably reflects an increased awareness of the range of potential complications that may occur in the closed management of some of these fractures.

Radiographic Anatomy

The secondary centers of ossification of the bones about the elbow appear in a relatively predictable order, with girls reaching skeletal maturity approximately 2 years before boys. The capitellum appears first, usually by 1 year of age. The epiphysis of the radial head and the medial epicondylar epiphysis appear at about age 5 years, followed by the trochlea and olecranon epiphysis at age 8 or 9 years. The lateral condyle usually appears last, ossifying at about age 10 years (Fig. 1).

There has been substantial disagreement in the interpretation of radiographs of trauma about the pediatric elbow. A systematic assessment of the known anatomic relationships can help to identify and better define the fracture lines that pass through the often unossified, radiolucent cartilage of the pediatric elbow. The following anatomic relationships should be assessed in all radiographs of children's elbows as part of a trauma evaluation: (1) The proximal radius should point to the capitellum in all views (Fig. 2, A). Malalignment here suggests a lateral condyle fracture (Fig. 2, B), a radial neck fracture, a Monteggia fracture or equivalent, or an elbow dislocation (Fig. 2, C). (2) The long axis of the ulna should line up with or be slightly medial to the long axis of the humerus on a true AP view (Fig. 2, A). If not, a transphyseal injury (Fig. 2, D) should be suspected if the radial head and capitellum remain in correct alignment, or more commonly, an elbow dislocation if they do not. (3) The anterior humeral line bisects the capitellum on the lateral view (Fig. 3). Malalignment here suggests a supracondylar, lateral condyle, or transphyseal fracture. When examining this relationship, it is important to be certain that the radiograph is a true lateral view of the distal humerus because any rotation will make the capitellum appear more posterior relative to the anterior humeral line. (4) The humeral-capitellar (Baumann's) angle should be within the range of 9° to 26° of valgus (Fig. 3). Despite this rather wide range of normal values, it is a sensitive indicator of varus angulation of the distal humerus, and is useful in assessing the adequacy of reduction in supracondylar and transphyseal fractures.

Occult fractures can sometimes only be inferred from the fat pad on the lateral radiograph, which represents subperiosteal bleeding. Although a normal elbow flexed at 90° may show an anterior fat pad, the posterior fat pad is not normally visible. When a posterior fat pad is visible, a recent study found that a fracture about the elbow is present 76% of the time. Supracondylar fractures (53%), proximal ulna fractures (26%), and lateral condyle fractures (9%) account for the majority of these occult injuries. Routine comparison radiographs of the uninjured elbow have not proved to be useful in making the correct diagnosis.

Supracondylar Fractures

Supracondylar fractures account for about 10% of all pediatric fractures, and are commonly seen in both the community and referral setting. Extension type injuries account for approximately 98% of pediatric supracondylar fractures. Flexion type injuries are rare and are characterized by anterior displacement of the condyles

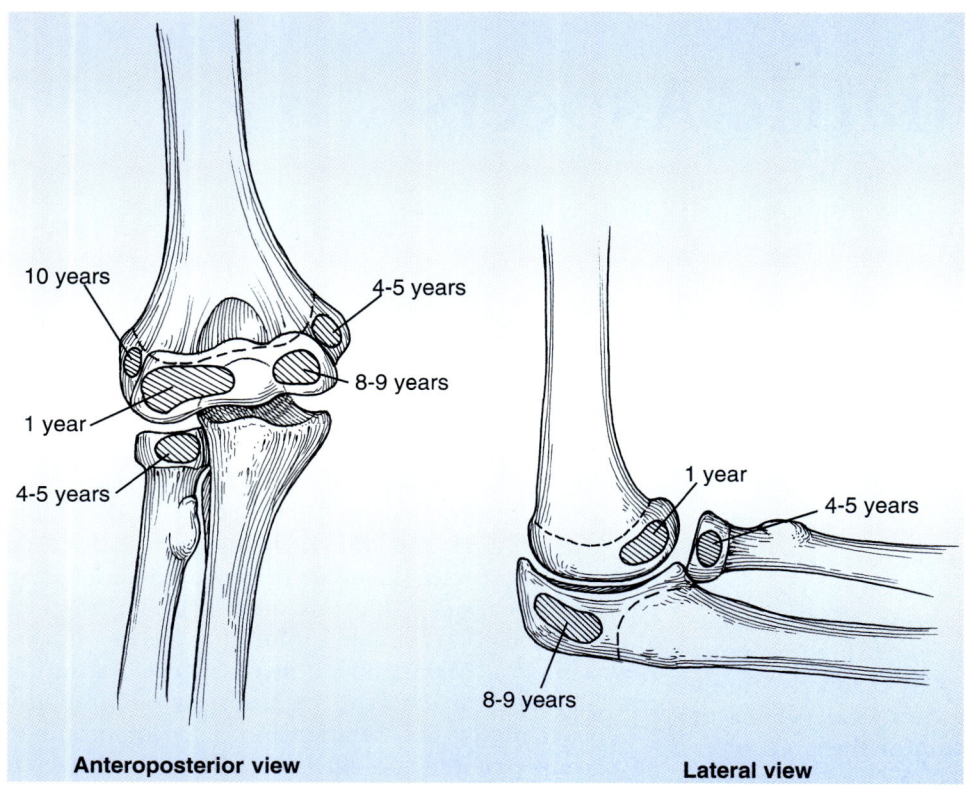

10 years

4-5 years

8-9 years

1 year

4-5 years

Anteroposterior view

1 year

4-5 years

8-9 years

Lateral view

Figure 1 Secondary ossification centers of the elbow with range of ages of appearance. *(Reproduced with permission from Skaggs DL: Elbow fractures in children: Diagnosis and management. J Am Acad Orthop Surg 1997;5: 303-312.)*

as a result of a fall on a flexed elbow. It is reported that flexion type supracondylar fractures are more likely than extension type to require open reduction.

Classification

The most commonly used classification system of extension type supracondylar fractures is a modification of Gartland's, based on fracture displacement. Type I fractures are nondisplaced, whereas type II fractures exhibit anterior gapping, limited rotational malalignment, and an intact posterior hinge. Type III fractures have no cortex in continuity.

Treatment

Restoration of sagittal alignment is verified on the lateral radiograph by the passage of the anterior humeral line through the capitellum. Coronal plane displacement is restored when Baumann's angle is restored. A limited degree of rotational malalignment (less than 20°) is well compensated by shoulder motion and often results in few clinical problems. In contrast, varus malalignment does not significantly remodel. Baumann's angle less than 9° or a difference of greater than 10° compared with the contralateral side usually should not be accepted. The carrying angle of the arm relative to the other arm may also serve as a guide.

Nonsurgical Treatment
Stable fractures without significant soft-tissue injury may be treated nonsurgically. Athough type I fractures are universally treated in a long arm cast, there is some controversy as to which, if any, type II fractures can be treated nonsurgically. In order to maintain reduction, it is often necessary to immobilize the elbow in a position of extreme flexion, which is associated with neurovascular compromise and compartment syndrome. These concerns, as well as the possibility of malunion, have led many pediatric orthopaedists to choose percutaneous pinning of most type II fractures as the more "conservative" approach. If a reduction is needed, closed reduction and casting of displaced supracondylar fractures is associated with higher rates of both early and late complications than those fractures treated with closed reduction and pinning.

Surgical Treatment
After closed reduction, smooth Kirschner wires are used to maintain fixation. In the past, cross pins were used most commonly, but reports highlighting iatrogenic ulnar nerve injuries have prompted the increased use of multiple pins placed from the lateral side alone. Biomechanical studies suggest that cross pins are more rigid than two lateral pins. However, a retrospective review of 345 surgically treated supracondylar fractures found that the use of lateral pins alone provided clin-

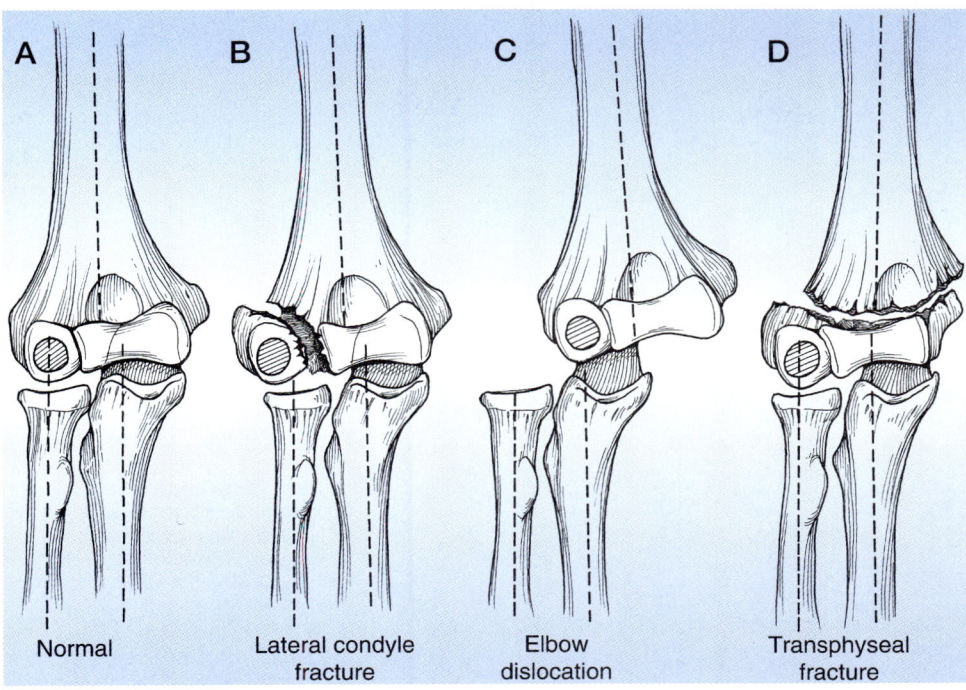

Figure 2 Schematic representation to compare injuries about the elbow on AP radiographs. Note the relationship between the radius and the capitellum, as well as the midshaft ulna and midshaft humerus. **A,** Normal elbow. **B,** Displaced lateral condyle fracture. **C,** Elbow dislocation. **D,** Transphyseal (Salter I) fracture. *(Reproduced with permission from Skaggs DL: Elbow fractures in children: Diagnosis and management. J Am Acad Orthop Surg 1997;5:303-312.)*

ically equivalent fixation to cross pins in both type II and type III supracondylar fractures, while avoiding iatrogenic injury to the ulnar nerve. It was found that if a medial pin was placed when the elbow was hyperflexed, there was a 17% incidence of iatrogenic ulnar nerve injury. This incidence is presumably a result of ulnar nerve subluxation during hyperflexion, which has been shown to occur in 61% of children age 6 years or younger. In contrast, this series reported no iatrogenic ulnar neurapraxia in patients treated with lateral pins alone, but a 4% incidence of ulnar neurapraxia in patients treated with cross pins when the medial pin was inserted without elbow hyperflexion. The authors concluded that the use of lateral pins alone is an equally effective, but safer way to treat type II and III fractures and strongly advised against the placement of a medial pin while the elbow is hyperflexed. Collectively these results suggest that the use of a medial pin is not necessary, and certainly should not be placed with the elbow flexed more than 90°.

One series identified interposition of the brachialis muscle at the fracture site as the cause of initial irreducibility of 18 of 20 fractures. By "milking" the brachialis off the proximal spike of the humerus, 85% of "irreducible" fractures were reduced. A comparison of immediate versus delayed (at least more than 8 hours after fracture) reduction and pinning of type III fractures has shown no difference in rates of failed closed reduction or outcome between groups, leading the authors to conclude that treatment of these fractures can be safely delayed.

Various approaches have been described for open reduction. Generally, reduction is facilitated by an approach from the side opposite the direction of displacement of the distal fragment to preserve the remaining periosteum. However, the anterior approach is preferable if the surgeon is concerned about interposition of the neurovascular structures.

There is some controversy regarding the approach to the patient who has a pulseless, but well-perfused, warm hand after reduction of the fracture. Several recent studies have documented excellent outcomes without an attempt at exploration and reanastomosis as long as the extremity remains viable and perfused. Furthermore, it has been shown that arterial repair often does not result in long-term patency. However, arterial exploration and repair are clearly indicated if the hand is not well perfused. Obviously, careful observation with frequent neurovascular checks and attention to the early signs of loss of circulation or compartment syndrome is warranted in this setting.

Neurologic Injuries

Recent literature suggests a 10% to 20% incidence of neurologic injuries in displaced extension type supracondylar fractures, with the anterior interosseous nerve cited as the most common neurologic injury. These nerve injuries typically spontaneously recover within 12 weeks, though recovery may take as long as 6 months. It has been suggested that upon acute recognition of iatrogenic ulnar nerve injury, the medial pin may be

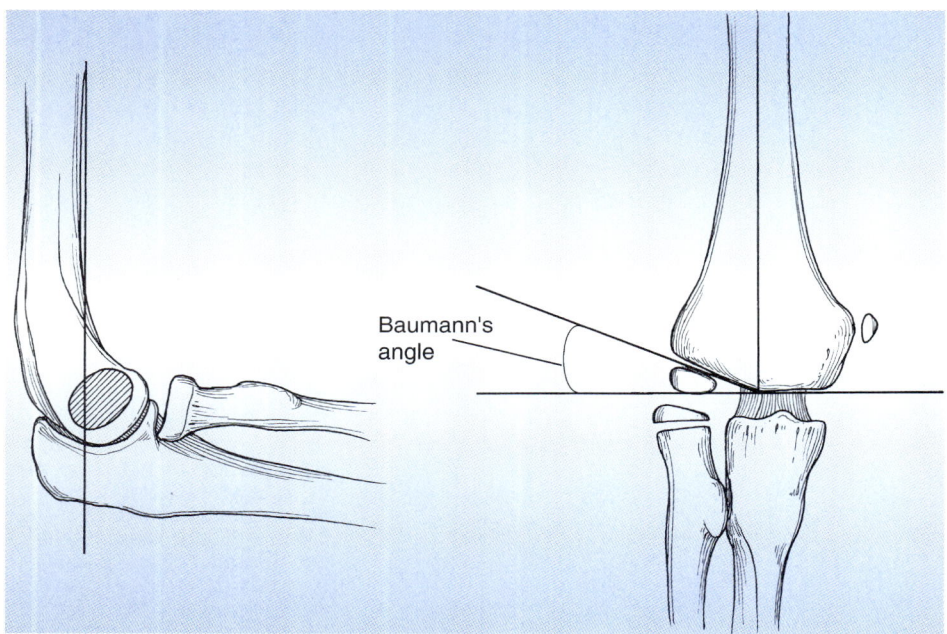

Figure 3 Lateral view of the elbow. Note a line drawn along the anterior humeral cortex bisects the capitellum. Baumann's angle is formed by the intersection of the capitellar physis and the perpendicular to the humeral axis. *(Reproduced with permission from Skaggs DL: Elbow fractures in children: Diagnosis and management. J Am Acad Orthop Surg 1997;5:303-312.)*

left in place, with recovery expected. Although the majority of iatrogenic ulnar nerve injuries resolve over time, permanent palsies have been reported. If there is no clinical or electromyographic evidence of recovery in 5 months, exploration and neurolysis lead to good results for nerves in continuity.

Malunion

It is generally accepted that cubitus varus occurs secondary to malreduction, and not growth disturbance. Cubitus varus may occasionally impact function, and the cosmetic appearance is often disturbing to the patient and family. Persistent posterior angulation can lead to hyperextension and some loss of flexion. Although malunion rarely affects function and often remodels, some children are bothered by the cosmetic appearance or loss of motion. Many osteotomies and fixation techniques have been described to correct deformity following malunion of the supracondylar fracture. Although high complication rates have been documented in previous studies, more recent series have shown good results with late osteotomies to correct cubitus varus.

Lateral Condyle Fractures

Fracture of the lateral condyle is second to supracondylar fracture as the most common pediatric elbow fracture. Recognition of the high rate of complications in this seemingly benign fracture should guide decision making.

Although several classification systems describe this fracture, grading by the amount of displacement seems to be most useful. The Milch classification, which describes these fractures based on the location of the fracture at the articular surface, has been shown to inaccurately describe these fractures more than half of the time. Oblique views are particularly helpful in the assessment of displacement. MRI has been reported to be a useful adjunct in assessing fracture stability, with potentially unstable fractures showing the fracture line passing though the physis and exiting at the joint.

Treatment

In fractures with less than 2 mm of displacement, treatment with cast immobilization is generally successful. One must be certain that the fracture is minimally displaced, with AP, lateral, and oblique radiographs showing no more than 2 mm of displacement. All lateral condyle fractures being treated nonsurgically should be reassessed with AP, lateral, and oblique views out of plaster 5 to 7 days after injury to check for displacement, which is not uncommon and which requires surgical treatment. Fractures with greater than 2 mm of displacement are most commonly treated surgically. An intraoperative arthrogram can be used to assess the integrity of the articular surface before and after reduction. In a recent report on 12 children with lateral condylar fractures displaced more than 2 mm and intact articular surfaces on arthrogram, results were uniformly excellent with closed reduction and percutaneous pinning. However, with greater degrees of fracture displacement or extension of the fracture into the articular surface, open reduction is warranted. Although a posterolateral approach to this fracture has been advocated, the possibility of injury to the posterior vascular supply of the lateral condyle raises obvious concerns regarding this approach. A direct lateral approach is recommended.

In the past, surgical treatment more than 3 weeks after injury was avoided secondary to concerns about the development of osteonecrosis and decreased range of motion associated with late open reduction. However, it is currently believed that delayed open reduction of lateral condyle fractures can result in good outcomes if posterior dissection is avoided and early range of motion is instituted.

Complications

Delayed union and nonunion are not uncommon. Fortunately, many children with nonunions are asymptomatic, and thus require no treatment. Tarda ulnar nerve palsy may develop years after a lateral condyle fracture complicated by progressive cubitus valgus resulting from a growth disturbance or nonunion. Treatment includes nerve transposition accompanied by supracondylar closing wedge osteotomy. Cubitus varus deformity is thought to result from either overgrowth of the lateral column or osteonecrosis of the lateral trochlea. Delayed union or nonunion are not necessarily symptomatic and motion is not necessarily always significantly impaired. Osteotomy is reserved for patients who have pain, are dissatisfied with their cosmetic appearance, or for patients who develop late ulnar nerve symptoms.

Medial Epicondyle Fractures

Up to 50% of these fractures may be associated with an elbow dislocation. Nonsurgical treatment is appropriate for most medial epicondyle fractures, even those that are widely displaced. Immobilization should be limited to less than 3 weeks, and it is often possible to remove the long arm cast at 7 to 10 days and begin active range of motion.

A 35-year follow-up of 56 unreduced, displaced (mean, 6 mm) fractures of the medial epicondyle treated by immobilization alone reported very good function and range of motion despite the fact that pseudarthrosis occurs commonly. In a study that compared nonsurgically and surgically treated children, the surgically treated group demonstrated higher rates of radiographic union, but more minor symptoms than those treated conservatively. Historically, the amount of displacement has been a key factor guiding the decision toward surgical treatment. However, recent literature has deemphasized the importance of displacement and has leaned toward a conservative approach to these injuries.

Irreducible incarceration of the medial epicondyle within the joint and the rare open fracture comprise the only two absolute indications for surgical treatment in these fractures. One additional possible indication for treatment of the medial epicondyle fracture involves the child who is expected to make excessive demands of valgus stress on the elbow, such as a pitcher or gymnast.

Olecranon Fractures

These rare fractures occur in combination with other fractures about the elbow in about 20% of cases. Metaphyseal displacement of 5 mm or articular step-off of 2 mm or more comprise commonly agreed-upon indications for surgical intervention, though intra-articular displacement may be underappreciated on plain radiographs. In fractures treated nonsurgically, immobilization should be in about 20° of flexion to relax the triceps. Surgical options include the use of tension band fixation with suture or wires, cancellous screws, or plate fixation depending on the geometry and stability of the fracture pattern.

Proximal Radius Fractures

Proximal radius fractures are commonly seen in children between the ages of 8 and 12 years. In contrast to the adult fracture pattern, radial neck fractures are more common than fractures of the radial head.

Angulation of the radial neck of less than 30° is best treated closed and excellent results can be expected, but attention should be given to limiting the period of immobilization to 3 weeks and to restoration of motion. Closed reduction under general anesthesia is usually successful when less than 60° of angulation exists. The Israeli technique is often successful for closed reduction. The surgeon's thumb is used to place direct pressure on the radial head with the elbow flexed to 90°, while rotating the forearm from full supination to pronation.

If either passive pronation or supination are less than 60° after attempted closed reduction, if there is greater than 60° of initial angulation, or if there is greater than 1 cm of translation, percutaneous reduction may be attempted. Using the image intensifier, a stout Kirschner wire is used to gently push the radial head into a reduced position. Favorable results at reduction have also been reported with the use of an intramedullary pin, which can catch the proximal fragment when inserted in a retrograde manner.

Open reduction is indicated in the minority of fractures where less invasive means have failed to provide a stable reduction, allowing 50° to 60° each of pronation and supination. An aversion to open treatment of radial neck fractures is a result of an appreciation of the less favorable prognosis associated with open treatment, specifically loss of supination and pronation of the forearm. A recent review of 116 children with a fracture of the proximal radius included 23 fractures of the radial head. These fractures were found to be more common when the proximal radial physis was closed, and results were generally worse in those children with open physes (Salter-Harris III and IV). In contrast to fractures of the radial neck, these fractures demand anatomic reduction, usually by open means. Excision of the radial head should be avoided in the immature skeleton, as synostosis, cubitus valgus, and radial deviation of the wrist may develop.

Monteggia Fracture

In contrast to the adult Monteggia fracture, these fractures in children are more commonly the result of low-energy trauma, can have a broader, more atypical presentation, and are more often successfully treated through closed means. When an apparently isolated radial head dislocation is encountered in children, plastic deformation of the ulna is often present. Reduction of the ulna is a prerequisite for stable reduction of these fractures, and plating and intramedullary fixation have been used with good results.

Dislocation of the radial head can result from either trauma or congenital causes. Acute dislocation is usually associated with a fracture of the proximal ulna (Monteggia) and closed reduction can be performed for up to 3 weeks after this injury with the focus on anatomic reduction of the ulna by whatever means necessary. Between 3 weeks and 3 months, open reduction is supported by most studies. The Bell-Tawse reconstruction with a slip of triceps fascia has been advocated as one treatment option for the chronic radial head dislocation. Recently, a new procedure for the treatment of these injuries, which involves reconstruction of the annular ligament using a strip of triceps fascia passed through drill holes in the proximal ulna, showed excellent results even after prolonged dislocation as long as the radial head retained a normal shape and contour.

Transphyseal Fractures of the Distal Humerus

Although transphyseal fractures are rare, they merit special attention for a number of reasons. These fractures can occur as sequelae of birth trauma in the newborn or as a result of child abuse; the diagnosis can be challenging (Fig. 2, *D*). Prior to the ossification of the capitellum, the appearance on plain radiograph is indistinguishable from that of an elbow dislocation, although elbow dislocation in this age group is rare. In

contrast to elbow dislocations (Fig. 2, *C*), the normal alignment of the radius and the capitellum is preserved in transphyseal fractures. Ultrasonography or arthrogram can be helpful in identifying the transphyseal fracture in the very young child with a completely unossified elbow. Treatment principles are similar to those for supracondylar fractures, with an attempt made to minimize trauma to the physis during reduction.

Annotated Bibliography

Pediatric Elbow Fractures

Cheng JC, Ng BK, Ying SY, Lam PK: A 10-year study of the changes in the pattern and treatment of 6,493 fractures. *J Pediatr Orthop* 1999;19:344-350.

A retrospective review of a large cohort of pediatric fractures in Hong Kong showed that the pattern of injury has not changed significantly over the 10 years of this study. However, there was a tenfold increase in the rate of closed reduction and percutaneous pinning of supracondylar elbow fractures in children during this period.

Skaggs DL, Mirzayan R: The posterior fat pad sign in association with occult fracture of the elbow in children. *J Bone Joint Surg Am* 1999;81:1429-1433.

Thirty-four (76%) of forty-five patients with no initial radiographic evidence of a fracture other than an elevated posterior fat pad were found to have a fracture at radiographic reevaluation 3 weeks after injury. Supracondylar fractures accounted for 53% of these fractures, with proximal ulna (26%) and lateral condyle fractures (9%), accounting for other significant occult fracture patterns.

Supracondylar Fractures

Amillo S, Mora G: Surgical management of neural injuries associated with elbow fractures in children. *J Pediatr Orthop* 1999;19:573-577.

The authors document 25 cases of nerve injury associated with pediatric elbow fracture, 17 of which involved a constrictive lesion and 8 of which involved discontinuity at surgical exploration at a later date. In the subgroup of cases where the nerve was found to be compressed, results were generally excellent with surgical neurolysis. Results of nerve grafting deteriorated when the procedure was attempted more than 1 year after the original injury.

Iyengar SR, Hoffinger SA, Townsend DR: Early versus delayed reduction and pinning of type III displaced supracondylar fractures of the humerus in children: A comparative study. *J Orthop Trauma* 1999;13:51-55.

In this uncontrolled, retrospective study of children with type III supracondylar fractures, radiographic and clinical outcomes between a group of patients who were treated early (less than 8 hours after fracture) were compared with patients treated with delayed (more than 8 hours) reduction and pinning. No differences in the rate of open reduction, carrying angle, nonunion or grip strength were noted between groups, leading to the authors' conclusion that supracondylar fractures of the humerus can be safely treated in a delayed manner.

Lyons JP, Ashley E, Hoffer MM: Ulnar nerve palsies after percutaneous cross-pinning of supracondylar fractures in children's elbows. *J Pediatr Orthop* 1998;18: 43-45.

Nineteen of 375 supracondylar fractures treated with percutaneous pin fixation were found to have postoperative ulnar nerve palsies. The majority of patients were treated with removal of the medial pin. All patients available for follow-up had complete spontaneous return of function, though sometimes complete return of function took up to 4 months.

Rasool MN: Ulnar nerve injury after K-wire fixation of supracondylar humerus fractures in children. *J Pediatr Orthop* 1998;18:686-690.

This is a series describing six cases of ulnar nerve injury after crossed Kirschner wire fixation of displaced supracondylar humeral fractures in children. All cases were immediately explored. In two of these, the nerve was found to be directly penetrated by the pin, in three it was constricted by the retinaculum of the cubital tunnel, and in the sixth it was found to be displaced anterior to the epicondyle. Three children had complete recovery, two had partial recovery, and one had no recovery at follow-up. Early exploration, repositioning of the pin under direct vision, and decompression of the nerve rather than simple pin removal is advocated.

Skaggs DL, Hale JM, Bassett J, Kaminsky C, Kay RM, Tolo VT: Operative treatment of supracondylar fractures in children: The consequences of pin placement. *J Bone Joint Surg Am* 2001;83:735-740.

A retrospective review of 345 operatively treated supracondylar fractures found that the use of only lateral pins provided clinically equivalent fixation to cross pins in both type 2 and type 3 supracondylar fractures, while avoiding iatrogenic injury to the ulnar nerve. It was found that if a medial pin was placed when the elbow was hyperflexed, there was a 17% incidence of iatrogenic ulnar nerve injury, presumably because of ulnar nerve subluxation during hyperflexion.

Lateral Condyle Fractures

Bast SC, Hoffer MM, Aval S: Nonoperative treatment for minimally and nondisplaced lateral humeral condyle fractures in children. *J Pediatr Orthop* 1998;18:448-450.

Ninety-eight percent of lateral condyle fractures showing displacement of less than 2 mm in three planes were amenable to treatment in a long arm cast.

Kamegaya M, Shinohara Y, Kurokawa M, Ogata S: Assessment of stability in children's minimally displaced lateral humeral condyle fracture by magnetic resonance imaging. *J Pediatr Orthop* 1999;19:570-572.

The authors used MRI to aid in the determination of fracture stability in 12 children with minimally displaced lateral condyle fractures. The fractures were thought to be unstable if MRI revealed that the fracture line passed through the growth plate into the joint space. Percutaneous pin fixation is recommended for this subgroup.

Radial Head and Neck Fractures

Evans MC, Graham HK: Radial neck fractures in children: A management algorithm. *J Pediatr Orthop Br* 1999;8:93-99.

A management algorithm is presented that suggests the appropriate role of closed reduction, percutaneous and intramedullary fixation, and open reduction of these injuries.

Leung AG, Peterson HA: Fractures of the proximal radial head and neck in children with emphasis on those that involve the articular cartilage. *J Pediatr Orthop* 2000;20:7-14.

Although intra-articular fractures of the radial head are much more common if the proximal radial physis is closed, this review demonstrates that the outcome of these fractures in children with open physis is much more guarded. The authors suggest that this may be related to the difficulty appreciating the true degree of displacement in the unossified elbow. Treating physicians should maintain a high index of suspicion and should opt for anatomic reduction and fixation if necessary to restore congruity.

Mohan N, Hunter JB, Colton CL: The posterolateral approach to the distal humerus for open reduction and internal fixation of fractures of the lateral condyle in children. *J Bone Joint Surg Br* 2000;82:643-645.

This is a study of 20 patients who have undergone a posterolateral approach to the distal humerus for open reduction and internal fixation of displaced fractures of the lateral condyle. At a mean follow-up of 12 months, no cases of clinical or radiographic malunion or nonunion were noted.

Seel MJ, Peterson HA: Management of chronic posttraumatic radial head dislocation in children. *J Pediatr Orthop* 1999;19:306-312.

A new procedure for the management of chronic posttraumatic radial head dislocation is described which reconstructs the annular ligament using two drill holes in the proximal ulna. In contrast to the Bell-Tawse procedure, which has been associated with constriction or "notching" of the radial neck limiting growth, this procedure is reported to result in fixation which more closely mimics the normal biomechanics of the radioulnar joint. In seven children treated in this manner, results were good at an average of 30 months after their original injury. It was concluded that this procedure can be successfully applied even to late dislocations if the shape of the radial head is not deformed.

Transphyseal Fractures of the Distal Humerus

Oh CW, Park BC, Ihn JC, Kyung HS: Fracture separation of the distal humeral epiphysis in children younger than three years old. *J Pediatr Orthop* 2000;20: 173-176.

At a mean follow-up of almost 2 years, 7 of 12 children who had sustained a fracture separation of distal humeral epiphysis were found to have a cubitus varus deformity. Cubitus varus did not seem to be associated with surgical or nonsurgical treatment but was related to osteonecrosis of the medial condyle in almost all cases.

Classic Bibliography

Archibeck MJ, Scott SM, Peters CL: Brachialis muscle entrapment in displaced supracondylar humerus fractures: A technique of closed reduction and report of initial results. *J Pediatr Orthop* 1997;17:298-302.

Cramer KE, Green NE, Devito DP: Incidence of anterior interosseous nerve palsy in supracondylar humerus fractures in children. *J Pediatr Orthop* 1993;13:502-505.

Dormans JP, Squillante R, Sharf H: Acute neurovascular complications with supracondylar humerus fractures in children. *J Hand Surg Am* 1995;20:1-4.

Foster DE, Sullivan JA, Gross RH: Lateral humeral condylar fractures in children. *J Pediatr Orthop* 1985;5:16-22.

France J, Strong M: Deformity and function in supracondylar fractures of the humerus in children variously treated by closed reduction and splinting, traction, and percutaneous pinning. *J Pediatr Orthop* 1992;12:494-498.

Gaddy BC, Strecker WB, Schoenecker PL: Surgical treatment of displaced olecranon fractures in children. *J Pediatr Orthop* 1997;17:321-324.

Garbuz DS, Leitch K, Wright JG: The treatment of supracondylar fractures in children with an absent radial pulse. *J Pediatr Orthop* 1996;16:594-596.

Kissoon N, Galpin R, Gayle M, Chacon D, Brown T: Evaluation of the role of comparison radiographs in the diagnosis of traumatic elbow injuries. *J Pediatr Orthop* 1995;15:449-453.

Lincoln TL, Mubarak SJ: Isolated traumatic radial-head dislocation. *J Pediatr Orthop* 1994;14:454-457.

Pirone AM, Graham HK, Krajbich JI: Management of displaced extension-type supracondylar fractures of the humerus in children. *J Bone Joint Surg Am* 1988;70:641-650.

Roye DP Jr, Bini SA, Infosino A: Late surgical treatment of lateral condylar fractures in children. *J Pediatr Orthop* 1991;11:195-199.

Sabharwal S, Tredwell SJ, Beauchamp RD, et al: Management of pulseless pink hand in pediatric supracondylar fractures of humerus. *J Pediatr Orthop* 1997;17:303-310.

Williamson DM, Coates CJ, Miller RK, Cole WG: Normal characteristics of the Baumann (humerocapitellar) angle: An aid in assessment of supracondylar fractures. *J Pediatr Orthop* 1992;12:636-639.

Zionts LE, McKellop HA, Hathaway R: Torsional strength of pin configurations used to fix supracondylar fractures of the humerus in children. *J Bone Joint Surg Am* 1994;76:253-256.

Chapter 30

Elbow and Forearm: Adult Trauma

Gregory J. Schmeling, MD

Distal Humeral Fractures

Distal humeral fractures have a bimodal age and energy distribution. In elderly patients, low energy fractures usually are the result of a fall. In younger patients, high energy fractures usually result from a motor vehicle accident or a fall from a height.

Initial evaluation should include a careful neurovascular examination. The AP and lateral radiographs are rarely adequate because the limb is shortened and fragments overlap, creating a very confusing picture. Traction AP and lateral radiographs are used for preoperative planning.

Treatment of displaced distal humeral fractures begins with anatomic articular and mechanical axis reduction with rigid internal fixation that allows early motion for optimal outcome. Although injury dictates the maximal possible outcome, reconstruction and rehabilitation determine how close to that maximal outcome the patient gets.

Several techniques are used for exposure of the distal humerus, including olecranon osteotomies (transverse intra-articular, chevron intra-articular, extra-articular), triceps splitting, and triceps sparing approaches.

The distal humerus can be thought of as two columns connecting the epiphyseal segment to the shaft. In elderly patients, these columns are composed of dense cortical bone; the epiphyseal segment is dense cancellous bone in young patients, making excellent purchase possible in the columns and the epiphyseal segment. In the elderly patient, the quality of fixation in the epiphyseal segment is often less than ideal, but secure fixation can be expected along the columns of the distal humerus.

Internal fixation usually consists of lag screw and neutralization plate fixation in two planes. One plate is placed posteriorly on the radial column and the other is placed medial on the ulnar column. This 90° to 90° construct is preferred but the fracture pattern dictates the reconstruction construct and 90° to 90° positioning is not always possible. One study demonstrated that the strongest construct was a radial dynamic compression plate combined with an ulnar pelvic reconstruction plate. An alternative to this combination is a pelvic reconstruction plate on the radial column and a one-third tubular plate on the ulnar column. Column screws placed from distal to proximal up the columns improves the stability of the reconstruction.

The extent of the soft-tissue injury is more important in determining outcome than the fracture pattern. High-energy injuries are characterized by greater soft-tissue injury and as a group are associated with poorer outcomes when compared with low-energy injuries. Pain with exertion has been reported in 25% of patients studied.

The perception that age affects outcome resulted in many elderly patients treated with a short period of immobilization followed with motion, the so-called "bag of bones" technique, an approach that may lead to a painful malaligned nonunion. Recent evidence suggests that outcome is not affected by age and that anatomic reduction and stable fixation may lead to a good outcome in an elderly patient if stable fixation can be achieved.

In the elderly patient with a comminuted distal humeral fracture, open reduction and internal fixation is difficult; a primary total elbow arthroplasty is an alternative. A recent study evaluated the results of primary total elbow arthroplasty in 20 patients age 48 to 92 years. Using the medial triceps reflecting exposure, all patients had excellent or good results.

Complications reported in conjunction with treatment of distal humeral fractures include failure of fixation, malunion, nonunion, olecranon osteotomy nonunion, infection, prominent painful hardware, and ulnar nerve neuritis. Most fixation failures are a result of improper fixation. Malunion and nonunion are uncommon but are associated with high-energy injuries and inadequate fixation. Most nonunions will heal with revision fixation and bone grafting. Olecranon osteotomy nonunion has been reported as high as 30% in some studies. Lower rates of olecranon osteotomy nonunion are reported with a chevron osteotomy or when an intramedullary screw is used for fixation. The implants that stabilize the olecranon osteotomy are most likely to become painful and are easily removed. The incidence of infection ranges from 0 to 6% and is more frequent in high-grade open fractures. The incidence of ulnar nerve damage is reportedly 15% and can occur at injury or during surgery, and can be caused by the implants and as a result of postoperative scarring. An incidence of 15% has been reported. Transposition of the nerve should be considered if hardware is placed distally on the medial column.

Capitellum Fractures

Fractures of the capitellum are rare injuries that result from a shear force generated by an axial load applied through the radius to the radial head. Twenty percent of these injuries are accompanied by radial head fractures. Concomitant injury to the interosseous ligament and membrane, medial collateral ligament (MCL) of the elbow, and the distal radioulnar joint may also occur.

Capitellar fractures have a presentation similar to that of radial head fractures. Pain, swelling, and crepitus with motion are common complaints. Routine radiographs will demonstrate the fracture, although the radial head capitellum view may be needed. A CT scan with AP and lateral reconstructions is very important to further define the injury and assist with preoperative planning with displaced fractures. The incidence of associated injuries mandates complete evaluation of the wrist, forearm, and elbow.

Three types of capitellar fractures were initially described. The type I fracture is a complete fracture of the capitellum with a large bone fragment (Hahn-Steinthal I injury). The type II fracture is a thin osteochrondral wafer of the capitellum (Kocher-Lorenz injury). The type III fracture is a comminuted capitellar fracture. Added to the classification was a fourth type, in which the fracture line extends into the trochlea past the lateral trochlear ridge (Hahn-Steinthal II).

Nondisplaced fractures of the capitellum can be treated with immobilization followed by controlled motion. Closed reduction of a displaced fragment is difficult because little or no soft tissue is attached to the fragment and open reduction and internal fixation via lateral approach is usually required. A fascial-periosteal sleeve is developed to elevate the common extensor origin. The fragment can be stabilized using lag screws (minifragment or Herbert) or Kirschner wires. Study results indicated better function and earlier mobilization with screw fixation when compared with Kirschner wires. On occasion, an antiglide plate is added to support a large fragment or significant comminution.

Every effort should be made to reconstruct the capitellum if there is an associated injury to the interosseous ligament or membrane, the MCL of the elbow, or the radial head. Late instability of the elbow as a result of capitellar resection is difficult to treat. Should the fracture of the capitellum lead to posttraumatic radiocapitellar arthritis, late radial head or capitellar resection in a stable elbow is a salvage option for pain relief.

Loss of some elbow motion may result after a capitellar fracture, and usually is greater with acute excision than open reduction and internal fixation (ORIF). Diffuse elbow weakness and pain with exertion are also expected although most symptoms are usually mild and not disabling. Osteonecrosis of the capitellum is rare and usually without clinical consequences. Malunion is usually a result of closed treatment or delayed recognition of the nature of the injury. Excision of the fragments and an elbow release usually provide pain relief.

Radial Head Fractures

Radial head fractures are common injuries comprising 20% to 30% of fractures about the elbow. They can be isolated injuries or occur in combination with other injuries including carpal fractures, elbow dislocation, capitellar fractures, olecranon and ulnar shaft fractures (Monteggia equivalent), distal humerus fractures, and disruption of the distal radioulnar joint and the interosseous membrane (Essex-Lopresti lesion).

Physical findings commonly consist of pain at the lateral elbow, swelling, joint effusion, and pain with elbow motion. Careful examination for tenderness and stability of the MCL of the elbow, the distal radioulnar joint, and interosseous membrane (ligament) is critical. Associated injury to any of these structures has significant impact on treatment planning. The radial head is a secondary stabilizer to valgus load at the elbow and also resists proximal migration of the radius when there is associated injury to the distal radioulnar joint and interosseous membrane. Resection of the radial head as primary treatment when these associated injuries are present will result in instability at the elbow or wrist, pain, and poor function.

Radiographic evidence of fracture may be very subtle. Oblique views of the elbow and the radiocapitellar view compliment standard AP and lateral views because nondisplaced fractures are often difficult to diagnose radiographically. With the appropriate history and physical examination, a positive posterior fat pad sign is sufficient for the diagnosis. When radiographs

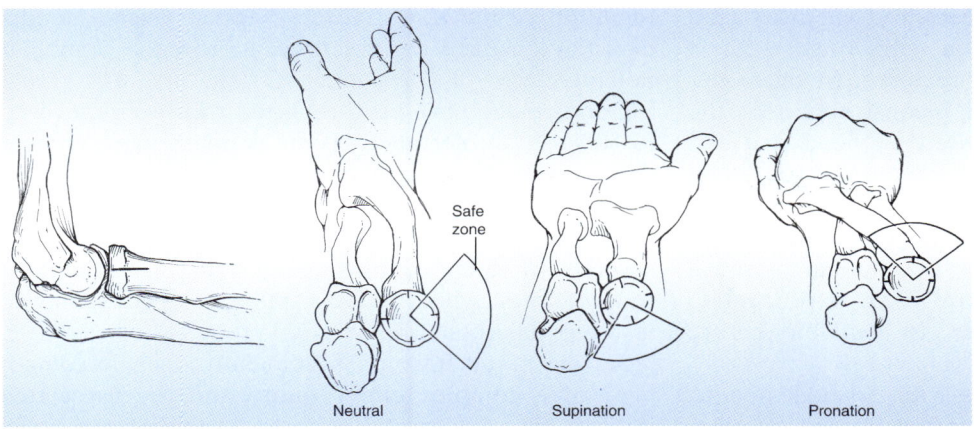

Figure 1 The safe zone for hardware placement can be found by bisecting the midline of the radial neck in neutral forearm rotation. *(Reproduced from Hotchkiss RN: Displaced fractures of the radial head: Internal fixation or excision? J Am Acad Orthop Surg 1997;5:1-10.)*

Neutral   Supination   Pronation

are negative, a radial head fracture should not be ruled out and a high index of suspicion is required.

When an isolated radial head fracture is present or suspected, initial evaluation should include an assessment of elbow range of motion. A mechanical block to motion may be the result of osteochondral fragments and is an indication for surgical treatment.

Although multiple classification systems exist for radial head fractures, they fail to incorporate the often associated injuries. The Mason classification with Johnson's modification is the most common; only Johnson's modification associated the radial head fracture with an elbow dislocation.

Treatment of radial head fractures may consist of early motion, ORIF, prosthetic replacement, or excision. A treatment plan can be formulated with an understanding of the fracture pattern, whether a mechanical block is present, or whether an associated injury exists.

Nondisplaced fractures or those displaced less than 2 mm without a mechanical block or associated injury are treated with early motion and functional rehabilitation. These patients regain motion slowly but progressively as their pain subsides. Nondisplaced fractures with an associated injury do not require internal fixation unless the potential for future instability exists. If the fragment is greater than one third of the radial head articular surface, the potential for instability exists. Nondisplaced fractures with a mechanical block on physical examination may benefit from an examination under anesthesia.

Displaced fractures with more than 2 mm of articular step-off, more than 20% to 30% of depression, or a bony block to motion require surgical treatment. Surgical options include excision (complete or partial), ORIF, or hemiarthroplasty. The presence or absence of an associated injury is also important in the treatment decision, when an associated injury is present, excision is contraindicated.

Two-part fractures may be treated with minifragment lag screws or variable pitch screws. Multifragment or comminuted fractures are reconstructed with lag screws and plate fixation. Kirschner wires (threaded or smooth) are not recommended unless the fragments are so small that lag screws cannot be placed.

Care must be taken to place hardware in the nonarticular safe zone of the radial head to prevent impingement on the ulnar sigmoid fossa and forearm rotation. The safe zone is a 100° arc that bisects the midline of the lateral radial neck with the forearm in neutral position (Fig. 1). Inspection will show a bare spot along the lateral radial neck that is nonarticular. If placement of hardware outside of the safe zone or in the radiocapitellar articular surface is required, subchondral countersinking of screws or use of a diamond-tipped burr to recess Kirschner wires is needed.

The reconstruction of comminuted fractures or fractures with disassociation of the head from the radial neck can involve either removal of the free fragments, reconstruction on the back table, and reimplantation or prosthetic replacement. It is unclear whether one option or the other offers a better outcome.

Incomplete or complete excision of the radial head, may be necessary in severely comminuted fractures that cannot be reconstructed. When an interosseous ligament injury (Essex-Lopresti lesion) is present, the radial head helps to maintain radial length and prevents proximal migration. Even in the face of severe comminution or incongruity, late excision of the head is superior to primary excision. The radial head also is a secondary stabilizer to valgus stress and may become the primary stabilizer with MCL injury. If more than half of the radial head remains intact, partial excision is acceptable. When neither the interosseous ligaments or MCL are injured and the radial head is irreparable, primary excision followed by early motion is an acceptable alternative.

Hemiarthroplasty may be necessary when an axial forearm (Essex-Lopresti lesion) or valgus elbow (elbow dislocation) stabilizer is required. Metal modular prostheses allow improved reconstruction of the patient's preinjury anatomy based on head size and degree of neck involvement. Silicone or Silastic hemiarthroplasty have been largely abandoned because of prosthesis failure, synovitis, and joint destruction. Radiographs may underestimate the amount of radial head comminution present; therefore, it is prudent to ensure that a metal prosthesis is available before surgery.

Outcome is variable. Patients with isolated, nondisplaced fractures may have near-normal motion, whereas patients with associated injuries experience much greater loss of motion, weakness, and more pain. The patient with a nondisplaced radial head fracture may have a greater loss of motion than would be expected. Occult injuries, such as osteochondral fractures of the distal humerus, may explain this result.

Complications after excision of the radial head include muscle weakness, wrist pain, valgus elbow instability, heterotopic bone, and arthritis. These complications can be prevented by recognizing associated injuries and avoiding early excision as a treatment option.

Olecranon Fractures

Olecranon fractures occur as a result of a tension-bending moment, producing a transverse or oblique fracture. The other common mechanism is direct load applied to the olecranon often resulting in comminuted fractures with depressed articular segments. Tension-bending fractures are low energy whereas direct load injuries are high energy.

The initial evaluation should include a careful neurologic examination. In most cases, an AP and lateral radiograph are adequate for evaluation and preoperative planning. When depressed intra-articular fragments are identified, a CT scan with AP and lateral reconstruction views may be helpful.

Nondisplaced fractures (less than 2 mm) with an intact extensor mechanism can be treated with nonsurgical methods, including a long arm cast for 4 to 6 weeks or splinting for a few days followed by early motion in a brace. Significant stiffness will result after wearing the long arm cast. There is only a small risk of fracture displacement with early motion.

Displaced fractures without an intact extensor mechanism require surgical treatment. These methods include ORIF with either a tension band or a lag screw and neutralization plate, or fragment excision with extensor mechanism reconstruction. Plates and screws are more commonly used when there is extensive comminution of the dorsal cortex because overtightening of a tension band construct will narrow the semilunar notch.

Good results have been reported with excision of up to 50% of the olecranon. There is no clear recommendation as to how much or little of the olecranon can safely be removed. Excision and extensor mechanism repair should be considered in older patients with severely comminuted fracture patterns that cannot be reduced or in whom stable fixation has been achieved in osteopenic bone.

An olecranon fracture is frequently a single component of a complex elbow injury and the associated injuries must be treated as well. A multiplanar single axis of rotation elbow external fixator may be used if the elbow remains unstable after reconstruction.

Patients typically experience a 10° loss of extension and a 5° loss of flexion. Supination and pronation loss are usually equal (5°). Strength is decreased when compared with the contralateral side. Union rates of 76% to 98% have been reported. Revision reduction and fixation for nonunions should only be considered if they are painful.

Excellent or good results were noted in 85% to 88% of patients with olecranon fractures. Outcome was influenced by patient age, malreduction, comminution, and timing of surgery. Complications associated with the treatment of olecranon fractures include painful hardware in 22% to 80% of patients, but hardware is removed in only 33% to 66%. Hardware failure and infection are uncommon (0 to 6%). Ulnar nerve neuritis and heterotopic ossification are more common (2% to 13%).

Elbow Dislocation

Nearly 50% of the stability of the elbow is provided by the skeletal anatomy of the trochlea and the olecranon. The MCL or ulnar collateral ligament, the lateral (radial) collateral ligament, and the annular ligament provide soft-tissue stability. The MCL is composed of three bands: anterior, posterior, and oblique. The anterior band is responsible for stability of the elbow. Most studies document complete disruption of the MCL in an elbow dislocation as well as injury to the lateral collateral ligament. Other soft-tissue structures typically injured include the anterior elbow capsule, the brachialis muscle insertion, articular cartilage, and the flexor-pronator origin. There is a 20% incidence of ulnar or median nerve neurapraxia. Arterial injuries occur, but are rare.

The elbow is swollen, deformed, and painful. The mechanism of injury is thought to be either forced hyperextension with the elbow extended or axial loading with the elbow slightly flexed. The evaluation should include a neurovascular examination and radiographs.

Elbow dislocations are classified as either simple (no associated fracture) or complex (associated fracture). Simple elbow dislocations have been classified by the position of the distal segment on the radiographs. The majority of simple dislocations are posterolateral.

The goal of treatment is a stable joint that tolerates early motion. Treatment of the simple elbow dislocation is closed reduction. Conscious sedation followed by axial traction of the arm with gentle manipulation of the olecranon is usually all that is needed to obtain a reduction. Rarely, general anesthesia and paralysis may be required. After reduction, the stability of the elbow should be assessed. If postreduction radiographs suggest a chondral or osteochondral injury, MRI, CT, or CT arthrogram may define the extent of the injury. A short period of immobilization to calm the acute soft-tissue inflammation is followed by early range of motion. The initial range of motion allowed is the stable arc found on the postreduction examination. Studies have demonstrated a better outcome when simple elbow dislocations are treated nonsurgically rather than with surgical repair.

Simple elbow dislocations usually have an excellent outcome (return of functional range of motion with normal strength). A loss of terminal extension is the most common sequelae. Recurrent dislocation is rare. Most nerve injuries (approximately 90%) recover. Persistent pain and muscle weakness are correlated with the period of immobilization rather than the injury. Most good and excellent results occur when the elbow is immobilized for less than 2 weeks. The incidence of heterotopic ossification is 5%, but increases dramatically with associated injuries about the elbow and head injuries.

Complex elbow dislocations often are high-energy injuries. Fractures of the radial head or neck or coronoid fracture or dislocation are the most commonly associated injury. The elbow will remain unstable unless the associated fractures are treated with ORIF or hemiarthroplasty (comminuted radial head fracture). Unfortunately, the elbow may remain unstable even after anatomic reduction and stable internal fixation of the associated fractures. Repair of the MCL may restore stability. If the elbow remains unstable after soft-tissue and ligament repair, a hinged external fixator may allow early motion while maintaining reduction of the elbow. Some authors have advocated temporary ulnohumeral screw fixation for gross persistent instability at the elbow. A constrained or semi-constrained total elbow arthroplasty is an alternative for older patients with a severely comminuted complex elbow dislocation.

The outcomes after a complex elbow dislocation are worse than those after simple dislocation. The final range of motion is variable but is usually less than that seen with simple dislocations. In addition, the incidence of recurrent instability, heterotopic ossification, posttraumatic arthritis, persistent pain, and muscle weakness all are much higher.

Coronoid Fractures

Fracture of the coronoid usually is caused by hyperextension of the humerus and is associated with an elbow dislocation 10% to 33% of the time. The coronoid is the anterior portion of the greater sigmoid notch of the olecranon and plays an important role in elbow stability. A congruent articulation of the greater sigmoid notch and the trochlea provides up to 50% of elbow stability. In addition, the anterior elbow capsule, the anterior band of the MCL, and a portion of the brachialis insert on the coronoid.

There are three types of coronoid fractures. Type I is a fracture of the intra-articular tip of the coronoid. This injury usually represents a hyperextension injury of the elbow, a near-dislocation, or "perched" subluxation. It is not likely to result in long-term instability. Because the tip of the coronoid is intra-articular without any soft-tissue attachments, the type I fracture is treated in the same manner as a simple elbow dislocation with early mobilization unless symptoms of a loose body develop.

A type II fracture involves less than 50% of the coronoid. This injury may have an effect on stability of the ulnohumeral joint. If the ulnohumeral joint is stable, the fracture is treated in the same manner as a type I injury. ORIF is indicated when the joint is unstable or the fragment blocks full elbow motion. A portion of the triceps reflecting anconeus pedicle approach may be used for exposure. A posterior incision is used. The deep dissection consists of a modified Kocher dissection of the lateral side between the extensor carpi ulnaris and the anconeus with care to preserve the lateral collateral ligament complex, capsule, and annular ligament to expose the lateral side of the coronoid. A part of the medial triceps reflecting exposure is opened to reveal the medial side of the coronoid. A suture or wire is passed through drill holes in the ulna posterior to anterior, through or around the fragment, and then back through the ulna. The suture or wire is then tied on the dorsal ulnar surface.

A type III fracture involves more than 50% of the coronoid and often is associated with posterior elbow instability. Treatment should consist of ORIF. An anterior approach or the triceps reflecting anconeus pedicle approach as previously described can be used. Severely comminuted fractures may require an articulated external fixator; however, excision of the fragments should be avoided.

The two basic tenets for treatment of all types of coronoid fractures are joint stabilization and early mobilization. If joint stability is maintained, early motion is initiated. If stability is compromised, the coronoid and associated injuries are repaired, and early controlled motion initiated. In cases of comminution or poor stability despite repair, motion is initiated with the aid of a distraction external hinged fixator. The patient should expect an outcome similar to that of a simple elbow dislocation with a type I fracture. The patient with a type II fracture does less well than a patient with a type I injury and the majority of patients with a type III injury have a poor outcome.

Forearm Axis Injuries

The term forearm axis refers to the wrist, forearm, and elbow as a functional unit used to place the hand in space. A forearm injury may involve one or all components of the axis. All components of the forearm axis should be assessed when dealing with forearm, elbow, and wrist injuries.

Simple Axis Injuries

Isolated diaphyseal ulna fractures have an excellent record of healing with functional bracing or splinting, which allows elbow and wrist motion. Nondisplaced (less than 50% translation) fractures can be treated with immobilization whereas displaced fractures are treated with ORIF.

Nonsurgical treatment of completely nondisplaced isolated radial shaft fractures is with a long arm cast for 4 to 6 weeks. Significant wrist and elbow stiffness may result, along with loss of motion and forearm axis dysfunction if residual angulation and translation are present. ORIF is advantageous because it leads to anatomic reduction, immediate motion, and a high rate of union, and is recommended for displaced fractures.

Both-bone forearm fractures in adults are treated with ORIF to restore the anatomy of the bones and the interosseous ligament. Immediate motion of the forearm axis is well tolerated and a union rate of 95% to 99% is expected.

The addition of bone graft to forearm fractures, associated with a loss of more than 30° of the diameter of the bone, is recommended. However, two recent studies investigating the use of immediate bone graft for forearm fractures found that comminuted forearm fractures have the same union rate whether acute bone graft is used or not.

Complicated Axis Injuries
Galeazzi Fracture

A Galeazzi fracture is a diaphyseal radius fracture near the junction of the middle and distal thirds of the radius and an injury through the distal interosseous ligament and the distal radioulnar joint. Careful assessment of radiographs of the wrist and a physical examination of the distal radioulnar joint are required when an isolated radius fracture is found in the distal one half of the forearm. Radiographic evidence that suggests a Galeazzi fracture includes radial shortening compared with the contralateral wrist, an ulnar styloid fracture, and incongruity or subluxation of the distal radioulnar joint. Clinical findings consist of wrist pain and increased AP motion of the radius on the ulna. These physical findings often are difficult to assess in the acute setting without an anesthetic.

The Galeazzi fracture is treated with ORIF after anatomic stabilization of the radius fracture. If radiographic reduction and clinical stability are apparent, early range of motion is indicated. If the joint is stable only in supination (rarely in pronation), the forearm can be immobilized for up to 6 weeks in a long arm cast. In the event the joint does not become stable in supination or pronation, the joint is stabilized by fixation of the ulnar styloid avulsion (if present) or pinning of the distal radius and ulna with reduction of the distal radioulnar joint reduced to allow healing of the injured soft tissues.

Monteggia Lesion

The Monteggia lesion is an ulna fracture associated with an injury to the proximal radioulnar joint. The most common presentation is a proximal ulna fracture and radial head dislocation. Treatment is with ORIF of the ulna fracture. Anatomic reduction of the ulna restores forearm length. Restoration of forearm length usually reduces the radial head. After reduction of the ulna, the radial head is evaluated for stability in elbow flexion/extension and supination/pronation. Immobilization of the forearm and elbow for approximately 6 weeks is necessary to allow healing of the proximal radioulnar joint. Because the Monteggia lesion may include injury to the interosseous ligament, radial head resection for treatment of a comminuted radial head fracture should be considered carefully.

Essex-Lopresti Fracture-Dislocation

The Essex-Lopresti fracture-dislocation involves injury to all three components of the forearm axis. This diagnosis is frequently missed and outcome is worse when treatment is delayed.

The most common presentation is a radial head fracture after a fall onto the outstretched hand. Clinical findings include wrist and forearm pain, increased anteroposterior translation of the distal radius on the ulna, and pain with compression of the radius and ulna (squeeze test of the forearm). Subtle radiographic findings may include radial shortening, separation or incongruity of the distal radioulnar joint, or ulnar styloid fracture. Clenched-fist radiographs may be necessary to reproduce and see the radial shortening secondary to interosseous ligament injury.

The treatment of this combination injury involves restoration of radial length, treatment of the radial head fracture with fixation or replacement, and reduction with or without fixation of the distal radioulnar joint. Primary radial head resection without replacement is contraindicated. Treatment of the distal radioulnar joint is as described for Galeazzi fractures.

Late reconstruction and salvage of an unrecognized Essex-Lopresti injury is unrewarding. Options include attempted reconstruction of the interosseous ligament (which, to date, has been largely unsuccessful), late metallic radial head replacement, Suave-Kapandji procedure, and creation of a one-bone forearm. The key to treatment of this lesion is immediate diagnosis and treatment of the underlying pathology.

Heterotopic Ossification

Heterotopic ossification, myositis ossificans (heterotopic bone formed in inflammatory muscle), and periarticular calcification all describe extraosseous bone formation. Heterotopic ossification can have significant impact on outcome after trauma to the elbow and forearm. The development of heterotopic ossification is most clearly associated with a fracture-dislocation of the elbow, with concomitant head or spinal cord injury, or burns. The association of heterotopic ossification with postoperative passive range of motion exercises is less well defined.

The treatment of heterotopic ossification about the elbow and forearm has focused on prevention. Anticipating injuries with a predisposition for the formation of heterotopic ossification and treatment with postoperative radiation therapy, nonsteroidal anti-inflammatory drugs (NSAIDs), or diphosphonates has been recommended. Avoiding passive extension of the elbow in the immediate postoperative period and early surgical treatment (less than 72 hours after injury) for complex elbow injuries also has been recommended as a preventive measure.

Traditionally, heterotopic ossification resection has been delayed until the bone has matured. Postoperative radiation and/or NSAIDs are used to prevent recurrence. Bony maturation is not well defined, but negative bone scan, normal serum alkaline phosphatase, stable pattern on serial radiographs, or a time period of 12 to 18 months after injury are indicative factors. However, a high rate of recurrence and significant loss of motion are still seen after 18 months. Delay of treatment has recently been challenged because of the risk of progressive contracture, cartilage loss, and prolonged disability.

In a small series of eight patients, significant improvement in range of motion with little recurrence of symptoms was found when the heterotopic ossification was resected 3 to 10 months after injury coupled with the administration of five 200-cGy doses of radiation postoperatively. In other studies, radiation administered in a single dose of 700 to 800 cGy produced similar results.

In another study, "simple" release of contractures about the elbow associated with heterotopic ossification was defined as resection of the heterotopic ossification and restricting soft tissues. Fifteen elbows in 14 patients were treated less than 32 weeks after injury. Indomethacin was administered for 5 days postoperatively. The mean improvement in the flexion-extension arc of motion was 80° and there was no recurrence of heterotopic ossification. Patients with burns or significant persistent neurologic injury were excluded. Postoperative prophylaxis for heterotopic ossification may not be required in select patients.

Exactly how the time to surgical treatment plays a role in the development of heterotopic ossification remains unclear. One retrospective study identified 17 patients with significant elbow injuries surgically treated less than 48 hours after injury and 24 patients treated more than 48 hours after injury. None of the patients treated less than 48 hours after injury developed significant heterotopic ossification, whereas 33% of those treated more than 48 hours after injury developed heterotopic ossification. While certainly not definitive, this study suggests that timing may play a role in preventing the development of heterotopic ossification.

Prevention of heterotopic ossification remains the mainstay of treatment, and prophylaxis should be considered for patients with risk factors (delay in surgical treatment, head or spinal cord injury, burns, injury severity). Early resection (4 to 6 months after injury) of significantly disabling heterotopic ossification with postoperative prophylaxis can result in significant functional improvement with a low risk of recurrence.

Annotated Bibliography

Distal Humeral Fractures

Kuntz DG Jr, Baratz ME: Fractures of the elbow. *Orthop Clin North Am* 1999;30:37-61.

A comprehensive review on the treatment of distal humeral fractures, radial head fractures, coronoid fractures, and olecranon fractures is presented.

McKee MD, Kim J, Kebaish K, Stephen DJ, Kreder HJ, Schemitsch EH: Functional outcome after open supracondylar fractures of the humerus: The effect of the surgical approach. *J Bone Joint Surg Br* 2000;82:646-651.

In a retrospective review, 13 patients underwent ORIF by triceps splitting and 13 by olecranon osteotomy. The patients with a triceps splitting approach had a better outcome as measured by the Mayo elbow score, Disabilities of the Arm, Shoulder, and Hand score (DASH) optional module score, and SF-36 role-physical and bodily pain scores.

McKee MD, Wilson TL, Winston L, Schemitsch EH, Richards RR: Functional outcome following surgical treatment of intra-articular distal humeral fractures through a posterior approach. *J Bone Joint Surg Am* 2000;82:1701-1707.

Twenty-five patients with distal humeral fracture treated with posterior approach at 18 to 75 months after injury were studied. Outcomes were measured using DASH, SF-36, and manual muscle testing. Patients had decreased range of motion and strength. The DASH score and SF-36 results demonstrated mild residual physical impairment.

Mehdian H, McKee MD: Fractures of the capitellum and trochlea. *Orthop Clin North Am* 2000;31:115-127.

Diagnosis and treatment are discussed.

Morrey BF: Fractures of the distal humerus: Role of elbow replacement. *Orthop Clin North Am* 2000;31:145-154.

A comprehensive analysis of indications, methods, and results of arthroplasty for the treatment of distal humeral fractures is presented.

O'Driscoll SW: The triceps-reflecting anconeus pedicle (TRAP) approach for distal humeral fractures and nonunions. *Orthop Clin North Am* 2000;31:91-101.

An extensile exposure of the distal humerus is described.

Ring D, Jupiter JB: Fracture-dislocation of the elbow. *J Bone Joint Surg Am* 1998;80:566-580.

This comprehensive analysis of fracture-dislocations of the elbow, includes a discussion of treatment options and associated complications.

Radial Head, Capitellum, Trochlea, Olecranon, and Coronoid Fractures

Closkey RF, Goode JR, Kirschenbaum D, Cody RP: The role of the coronoid process in elbow stability: A biomechanical analysis of axial loading. *J Bone Joint Surg Am* 2000;82:1749-1753.

The authors demonstrated that the elbow was more stable when less than 50% of the coronoid was fractured than it was when more than 50% was fractured.

Frankle MA, Koval KJ, Sanders RW, Zuckerman JD: Radial head fractures associated with elbow dislocations treated by immediate stabilization and early motion. *J Shoulder Elbow Surg* 1999;8:355-360.

The authors describe the treatment of unstable elbow associated with a radial head fracture in 21 patients. Nondisplaced radial head fractures were treated with benign neglect while displaced fractures were treated with ORIF or arthroplasty. Six elbows required primary repair of the MCL, and three of these six required a hinged elbow external fixation. Initial radial head displacement predicted outcome.

Furry KL, Clinkscales CM: Comminuted fractures of the radial head: Arthroplasty versus internal fixation. *Clin Orthop* 1998;353:40-52.

This article reviews the current literature.

Hak DJ, Golladay GJ: Olecranon fractures: Treatment options. *J Am Acad Orthop Surg* 2000;8:266-275.

This article presents a comprehensive review of treatment options.

Ikeda M, Oka Y: Function after early radial head resection for fracture: A retrospective evaluation of 15 patients followed for 3-18 years. *Acta Orthop Scand* 2000;71:191-194.

All 15 patients studied lost elbow power and two thirds had pain.

Janssen RP, Vegter J: Resection of the radial head after Mason type-III fractures of the elbow: Follow-up at 16 to 30 years. *J Bone Joint Surg Br* 1998;80:231-233.

Twenty-one patients age 16 to 30 years were studied after radial head resection. There were 20 excellent/good and one fair result. Radial head resection viable option unless there is valgus instability of the elbow.

Elbow Dislocation

Cohn MS, Hastings H II: Acute elbow dislocation: Evaluation and management. *J Am Acad Orthop Surg* 1998;6:15-23.

A comprehensive review of the treatment of acute elbow dislocations is presented.

Hildebrand KA, Patterson SD, King GJ: Acute elbow dislocations: Simple and complex. *Orthop Clin North Am* 1999;30:63-79.

Simple and complex elbow dislocations are discussed.

McKee MD, Bowden SH, King GJ, et al: Management of recurrent, complex instability of the elbow with a hinged external fixator. *J Bone Joint Surg Br* 1998;80: 1031-1036.

The authors report the use of a hinged external fixator for recurrent elbow instability in 16 patients. Follow-up ranged from 14 to 40 months. The Morrey score cataloged the results as excellent in 2 patients, good in 10, fair in 3, and poor in 1.

Morrey BF: Complex instability of the elbow. *Instr Course Lect* 1998;47:157-164.

A comprehensive review of complex elbow instability, including treatment protocols for the injuries associated with elbow dislocations, is presented.

O'Driscoll SW: Classification and evaluation of recurrent instability of the elbow. *Clin Orthop* 2000;370: 34-43.

The author outlines a classification of elbow instability including posterolateral rotatory instability. Diagnosis and mechanism of recurrent instability are emphasized.

Ring D, Jupiter JB: Reconstruction of posttraumatic elbow instability. *Clin Orthop* 2000;370:44-56.

A comprehensive review of the principles required to reconstruct complex elbow instability is presented.

Ross G, McDevitt ER, Chronister R, Ove PN: Treatment of simple elbow dislocation using an immediate motion protocol. *Am J Sports Med* 1999;27:308-311.

The authors report the results for 20 consecutive patients with simple elbow dislocations treated with early motion without immobilization. Redislocation was noted in one patient. Range of motion was within 5° of the opposite side.

Viola RW, Hanel DP: Early "simple" release of posttraumatic elbow contracture associated with heterotopic ossification. *J Hand Surg Am* 1999;24:370-380.

The authors report excision of heterotopic ossification about the elbow followed by a 5-day course of indomethacin within 32 weeks of injury in 15 elbows. The motion obtained at surgery was maintained at follow-up 2 years later.

Forearm Axis Injuries

Graham TJ, Fischer TJ, Hotchkiss RN, Kleinman WB: Disorders of the forearm axis. *Hand Clin* 1998;14:305-316.

A comprehensive review of complicated forearm lesions is presented.

Sarmiento A, Latta LL, Zych G, McKeever P, Zagorski JP: Isolated ulnar shaft fractures treated with functional braces. *J Orthop Trauma* 1998;12:420-424.

In a retrospective review of 287 isolated ulnar fractures treated by functional bracing, union occurred in 99%. Radial angulation ranged from 0° to 18° and dorsal angulation ranged from 0° to 20°. Loss of pronation ranges from 5° to 12°.

Wei SY, Born Ct, Abene A, Ong A, Hayda R, DeLong WG Jr: Diaphyseal forearm fractures treated with and without bone graft. *J Trauma* 1999;46:1045-1048.

In a study of 56 fractures, all of the grafted and nongrafted comminuted fractures healed. The addition of bone graft did not alter the rates nor time to union in comminuted forearm fractures.

Heterotopic Ossification

Beingessner DM, Patterson SD, King GJ: Early excision of heterotopic bone in the forearm. *J Hand Surg Am* 2000;25:483-488.

The authors report the successful excision of heterotopic ossification from the forearm 4 months after injury in conjunction with the administration of 500 to 1000 cGy of radiation and indomethacin postoperatively. Patients maintained an average arc of motion of 136° at 3-year follow-up.

Ilahi OA, Strausser DW, Gabel GT: Post-traumatic heterotopic ossification about the elbow. *Orthopedics* 1998;21:265-268.

The authors evaluated the incidence of heterotopic ossification after elbow trauma in 41 patients. None of the 17 patients who had surgical treatment less than 48 hours after injury developed grade II, III, or IV heterotopic ossification compared with 8 of 24 patients who had surgical treatment more than 48 hours after injury.

Ippolito E, Formisano R, Caterini R, Farsetti P, Penta F: Resection of elbow ossification and continuous passive motion in postcomatose patients. *J Hand Surg Am* 1999;24:546-553.

The authors report the results of excision of heterotopic ossification in 16 elbows in brain-injured patients at the end of coma 4 to 67 months after injury. No prophylaxis to prevent recurrence was used. A continuous passive motion machine was used after excision and believed to be the reason motion was maintained at 12 to 60 months.

Viola RW, Hastings H II: Treatment of ectopic ossification about the elbow. *Clin Orthop* 2000;370:65-86.

This article presents a review of the current treatment of heterotopic ossification about the elbow. The authors discuss pathophysiology, indications for treatment, and treatment methods.

Classic Bibliography

An KN, Morrey BF, Chao EY: The effect of partial removal of proximal ulna on elbow constraint. *Clin Orthop* 1986;209:270-279.

Broberg MA, Morrey BF: Results of delayed excision of the radial head after fracture. *J Bone Joint Surg Am* 1986;68:669-674.

Cage DJ, Abrams RA, Callahan JJ, Botte MJ: Soft tissue attachment of the ulnar coronoid process: An anatomic study with radiographic correlation. *Clin Orthop* 1995;320:154-158.

Cobb TK, Morrey BF: Total elbow arthroplasty as primary treatment for distal humeral fractures in elderly patients. *J Bone Joint Surg Am* 1997;79:826-832.

Edwards GS Jr, Jupiter JB: Radial head fractures with acute distal radioulnar dislocation: Essex-Lopresti revisited. *Clin Orthop* 1988;234:61-69.

Hastings H II, Engles DR: Fixation of complex elbow fractures: Part I. General overview and distal humerus fractures. *Hand Clin* 1997;13:703-719.

Hotchkiss RN, An KN, Sowa DT, Basta S, Weiland AJ: An anatomic and mechanical study of the interosseous membrane of the forearm: Pathomechanics of proximal migration of the radius. *J Hand Surg Am* 1989;14:256-261.

Hotchkiss RN: Displaced fractures of the radial head: Internal fixation or excision? *J Am Acad Orthop Surg* 1997;5:1-10.

Josefsson PO, Gentz CF, Johnell O, Wendeberg B: Surgical versus non-surgical treatment of ligamentous injuries following dislocation of the elbow joint: A prospective randomized study. *J Bone Joint Surg Am* 1987;69:605-608.

McAuliffe JA, Wolfson AH: Early excision of heterotopic ossification about the elbow followed by radiation therapy. *J Bone Joint Surg Am* 1997;79:749-755.

McKee MD, Jupiter JB, Bamberger HB: Coronal shear fractures of the distal end of the humerus. *J Bone Joint Surg Am* 1996;78:49-54.

Morrey BF: Acute and chronic instability of the elbow. *J Am Acad Orthop Surg* 1996;4:117-128.

Morrey BF: Current concepts in the treatment of fractures of the radial head, the olecranon, and the coronoid. *J Bone Joint Surg Am* 1995;77:316-327.

Pereles TR, Koval KJ, Gallagher M, Rosen H: Open reduction and internal fixation of the distal humerus: Functional outcome in the elderly. *J Trauma* 1997;43:578-584.

Smith GR, Hotchkiss RN: Radial head and neck fractures: Anatomic guidelines for proper placement of internal fixation. *J Shoulder Elbow Surg* 1996;5:113-117.

Tornetta P III, Hochwald N, Bono C, Grossman M: Anatomy of the posterior interosseous nerve in relation to fixation of the radial head. *Clin Orthop* 1997;345:215-218.

Wallenbock E, Potsch F: Resection of the radial head: An alternative to use of a prosthesis? *J Trauma* 1997;43:959-961.

Wright RR, Schmeling GJ, Schwab JP: The necessity of acute bone grafting in diaphyseal forearm fractures: A retrospective review. *J Orthop Trauma* 1997;11:288-294.

Chapter 31

Elbow Reconstruction

Robert N. Hotchkiss, MD

Ken Yamaguchi, MD

Imaging

Proper radiographs and well-aligned CT scans continue to be invaluable techniques for the diagnosis and treatment of most conditions of the elbow. In most cases, plain radiographs are sufficient; however CT scans can be useful in the localization of heterotopic bone about the elbow. In cases of medial or posterolateral instability, stress radiographs and fluoroscopic spot films can assist in determining the diagnosis. Medial collateral ligament (MCL) insufficiency has been demonstrated on stress radiographs using a standardized valgus force, with side-to-side differences as little a 0.5 mm reported to be significant (Fig. 1). Posterolateral rotatory instability has been demonstrated on fluoroscopic films, where posterior dislocation of the radial head as well as ulnar-humeral joint space widening can be demonstrated on a pivot shift maneuver during fluroscopic examination. Both of these radiographic modalities can be important adjuncts to making the diagnosis of ligament insufficiency. MRI has been used to view the medial and lateral collateral ligaments and can confirm or deny the presence of injury. However, there is no substitute for a careful history and physical examination in pursuit of diagnosis and proper treatment.

Surgical Exposures

Well-defined exposures for contracture release, osteophyte débridement, ligament reconstruction, and total elbow arthroplasty provide a wide range of treatment options. Several extensile approaches have been described, such as a posterior incision with either a medial or lateral triceps takedown, the Bryan-Morrey approach, consisting of a medial to lateral triceps release in continuity with the distal forearm fascia, and the Kocher approach, consisting of a lateral to medial takedown. Direct lateral or medial exposures can be useful for specific surgical indications, particularly for contracture release or ligament reconstruction. The direct lateral and medial exposures can protect the important anterior bundle of the MCL and the lateral ulnar collateral ligament (LUCL).

Elbow Biomechanics and Kinematics

Much of the recent research on elbow biomechanics and kinematics has focused on elbow joint stability and the anatomy and biomechanics of the medial and lateral collateral ligament complexes.

Historically, the anterior bundle of the MCL has been considered the primary stabilizer of the elbow, with all other structures having secondary roles. However, studies on primary LUCL injuries and overhead throwing athletes, and biomechanical testing indicate that other structures may play a greater role in elbow stability. Structures responsible for elbow stability recently have been divided into primary and secondary constraints. The primary constraints consist of the anterior bundle of the MCL, the LUCL, and the ulnohumeral articulation. Secondary constraints are the radiocapitellar articulation, anterior and posterior capsule, and dynamic muscular forces. Dynamic constraints are not completely understood but are certainly more important than previously realized. Simple elbow dislocations, in which all ligamentous and capsular structures have been torn, can be rendered stable after reduction if normal muscular contraction is present. In addition, biomechanical analysis of valgus forces encountered by the MCL during high performance overhead throwing have shown the ligament to approach load to failure with each repetitive activity. It is clear that muscular dynamic forces must help share these loads.

One reason for an oversimplified understanding of instability has been the lack of studies on rotational forces on stability. The present understanding of posterolateral rotatory instability has highlighted the importance of supination in the development of instability. Recently, a study found rotatory forces to be

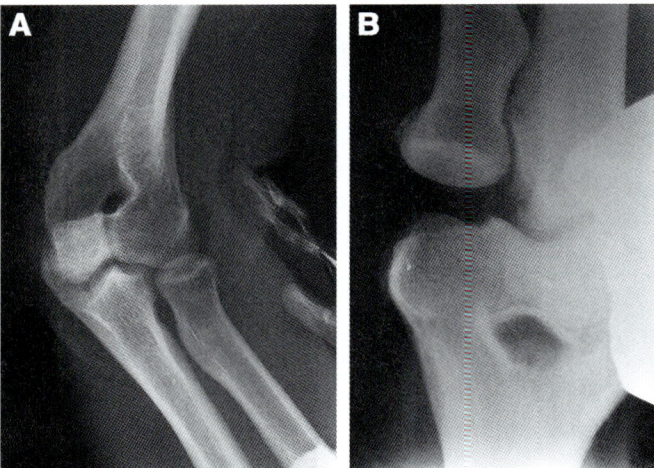

Figure 1 **A,** Medial collateral ligament deficiency demonstrated with valgus stress. **B,** Lateral collateral ligament insufficiency demonstrated with varus stress. *(Reproduced from Morrey BF: Acute and chronic instability of the elbow. J Am Acad Orthop Surg 1996:117-128.)*

important in MCL-deficient elbows. After transection of the MCL, there was a significant increase in internal-external rotation of the elbow during passive flexion. Forearm supination significantly reduced this instability. These results were analogous to previous studies that showed pronation was important in reducing instability following LUCL injuries.

Recent anatomic and biomechanical studies have verified the original concepts of posterolateral rotatory instability proposed by O'Driscoll and Morrey. The lateral collateral ligament complex as a sheet of tissue on the lateral side extending to the ulna is unequivocally important in rotatory instability. Reconstruction of the LUCL with autogenous grafting has reliably restored stability.

On the medial side, the anterior bundle of the MCL, which was previously thought to be posterior to the isometric axis of flexion, has been shown to be isometric throughout the flexion extension arc. This structure was believed to be the major ligament that resisted valgus and internal rotatory stress. However, partial transection of the anterior bundle does not result in significant instability.

Arthroscopy

Arthroscopy of the elbow is developing into a safe and helpful tool to care for loose body extraction, the release of elbow contractures, and synovectomy in inflammatory arthritis. Recent studies have documented its relative safety in the hands of experienced surgeons. However, concerns for nerve injury, especially the radial nerve with the lateral portal, are still warranted.

Arthroscopic synovectomy is especially helpful in younger patients with rheumatoid arthritis who have

disease limited to the elbow, or who have poor elbow motion despite newer anti-inflammatory agents. Access to the entire joint is especially crucial and the use of scopes (both 30° and 70°) permits greater visual flexibility. After synovectomy, the elbow may drain for an extended period. In cases of hemophilia, synovectomy may be beneficial to reduce the incidence of bleeding and proliferative synovitis in the elbow. If arthroscopic synovectomy is undertaken in this patient population, care must be taken to keep the factor VIII levels at a therapeutic level for at least 2 weeks. Otherwise, bleeding may occur during the rehabilitation program.

Débridement of posterior and anterior osteophytes in primary osteoarthritis can also be facilitated with the use of the arthroscope. Excellent visualization of the coronoid osteophyte permits burring of the bony projection. In the posterior fossae, the posterior medial osteophytes can also be removed, but care must be taken to ensure that the ulnar nerve is safe and protected. It may be advisable to make a small incision over the cubital tunnel, decompressing the ulnar nerve, before proceeding with débridement.

Elbow Instability

Ligamentous Insufficiency: Lateral Versus Medial

It is helpful to distinguish MCL insufficiency, which usually is seen in the throwing athlete, from LUCL instability, which often is discovered late, following a dislocation. These conditions are not mirror images of one another, and share only a reference to ligamentous insufficiency. They should be thought of as having distinct presentations, methods of assessment, and treatment options (Table 1).

Lateral Ulnar Collateral Ligament Insufficiency

Recurrent instability resulting in joint subluxation or recurrent dislocation is usually the result of a lesion in the posterolateral ligament complex. The cause of recurrent dislocation or subluxation is usually a traumatic event such as a fall on the outstretched hand, but can also occur iatrogenically when the posterolateral ligament complex is compromised during surgery on the radial head or to correct tennis elbow. Although there is debate about the exact anatomy of the lateral ligamentous complex, there is little controversy as to the essential role of the LUCL. A tear noted at the time of surgery is usually a separation off the humeral origin of the ligament. In acute cases, retraction of the ligament is minimal and the complex can be reattached through drill holes, placed at the axis of rotation. In many cases, the chronic attenuation of the complex has occurred, requiring tendon graft reconstruction (Fig. 2).

TABLE 1 | Medial Versus Lateral Ligamentous Insufficiency

	MCL Insufficiency	LUCL Insufficiency
Symptoms	Medial elbow pain with throwing History of a "pop" Locking if loose bodies present Possible ulnar nerve neuritis	Giving way Painful episode (subluxation) with pushup or lifting with outstretched hand
History	Repetitive throwing or racquet sports	Traumatic fall Often history of dislocation Previous lateral elbow surgery
Pathoanatomy	Midsubstance failure (usually)	Avulsion of humeral origin of ligament
Physical examination	Medial elbow pain along the ligament Possible ulnar nerve sensitivity	Apprehension to supination, load, and extension
Other diagnostic measures	X-ray for loose bodies or calcifications in MCL MRI	Stress views to look for posterolateral subluxation MRI
Surgical treatment decision	Failed rehabilitation Return to high-level sports	Often disabling in daily activities Activity and position modification or surgery

Postoperative care and rehabilitation must be carefully monitored and adjusted to each patient. Excessive stress on the reconstruction may result in failure, whereas prolonged immobilization may result in stiffness. The protection and rehabilitation period is 3 to 5 months depending on the ultimate demands of the patient. Successful stabilization often results in a slight (less than 20°) flexion contracture. In most published series, over 80% of patients achieve a stable elbow and return to activity with minimal loss of motion.

Valgus Instability

Medial instability results from repeated and excessive overload in valgus and extension. Tennis strokes and overhead throwing motion can maximally load the medial ligament and lateral joint in the late cocking and early acceleration phases. The rate of strain at angular velocities, estimated to be at 2,000°/s to 3,000°/s, can gradually attenuate the anterior portion of the MCL and begin to load the lateral joint in with injurious compression forces. As the ligament gradually attenuates, the posterior medial corner of the ulnohumeral joint can be impacted in late deceleration as the joint moves into full extension. This continued impaction may result in the formation of painful posteromedial osteophytes, diminishing the player's throwing capacity (Fig. 3).

The primary complaint of MCL insufficiency is pain, as opposed to giving way or instability as seen in LUCL insufficiency. Medial elbow pain typically is felt only during the throwing motion and at the larger extremes of effort. Patients usually do not complain of pain with activities of daily living, nor do they have any symptoms such as popping or clicking that may indicate instability; rather, the pain is seen as 80% to 100% of effort is approached during overhead motions. These patients no longer can achieve the same velocity, either with a thrown ball or with a racket. In contrast to LUCL injuries that do affect activities of daily living, loss of the MCL appears to affect only overhead throwing activities. Although a tendon weave through both ulnar and humeral bone tunnels is the standard of care for ligament reconstructions, a "docking" procedure has recently become popular as an alternative way to obtain accurate tensioning of the palmaris tendon graft without the use of a humeral tendon weave. This procedure may help decrease the risk of iatrogenic fractures of the medial humeral condyle.

The treatment of the MCL-insufficient elbow in the patient who participates in throwing or racquet sports is dependent on the level of competition. In the elite baseball pitcher, rehabilitation is seldom effective and MCL reconstruction is usually needed for an effective return to high-level competition. For the more recreational athlete, a trial of nonsurgical treatment with modalities such as phonophoresis, electrical stimulation, and iontophoresis should be instituted in an attempt to decrease swelling. Strengthening exercises should focus on the medial sided flexor/pronator muscle mass as well as the shoulder musculature. The ulnar nerve may also be aggravated and require a

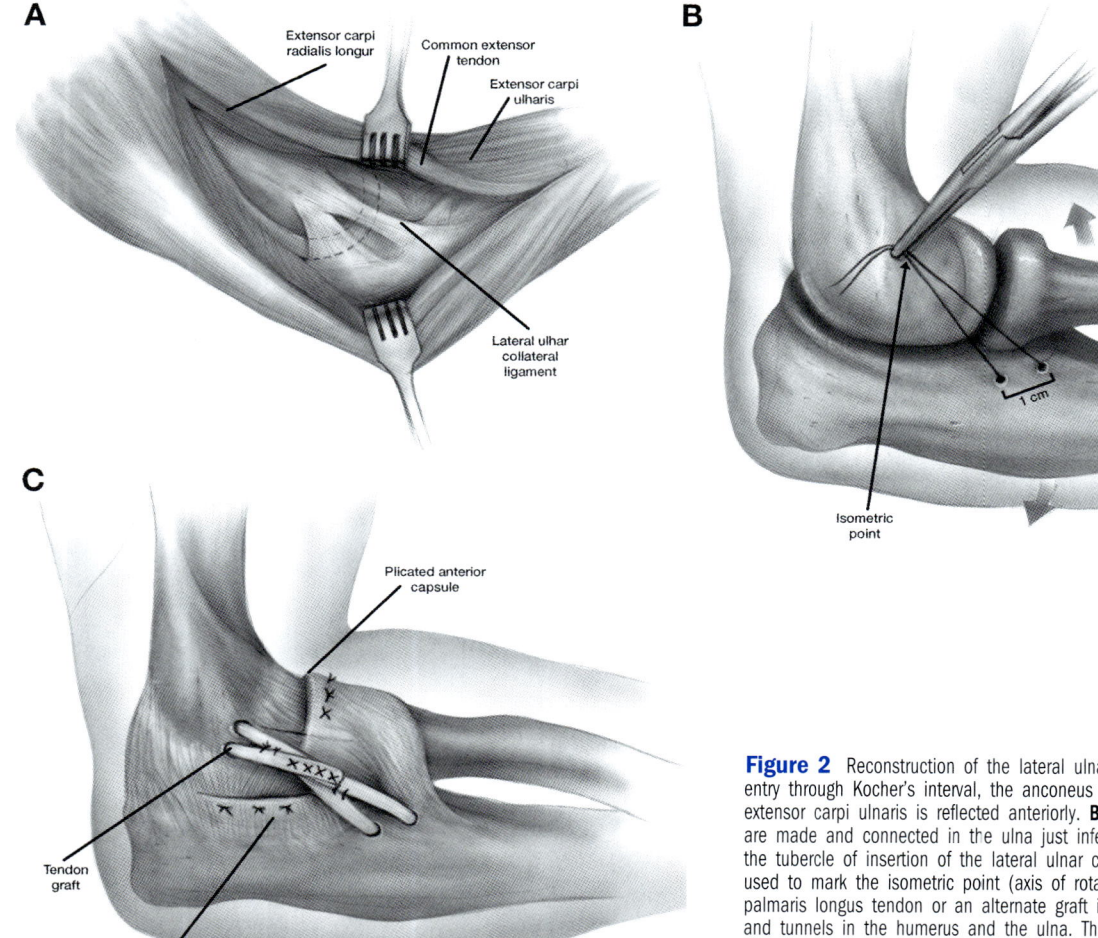

Figure 2 Reconstruction of the lateral ulnar collateral ligament. **A,** After entry through Kocher's interval, the anconeus is reflected posteriorly, and the extensor carpi ulnaris is reflected anteriorly. **B,** Two holes (3-mm diameter) are made and connected in the ulna just inferior to the crista supinatoris at the tubercle of insertion of the lateral ulnar collateral ligament. A suture is used to mark the isometric point (axis of rotation) on the humerus. **C,** The palmaris longus tendon or an alternate graft is woven through these holes and tunnels in the humerus and the ulna. Three-ply fixation is considered ideal. *(Reproduced from Morrey BF: Acute and chronic instability of the elbow. J Am Acad Orthop Surg 1996;4:117-128.)*

short period of splinting to reduce the associated neuritis.

Surgical treatment of the MCL-insufficient elbow is dictated by the demands of the athlete. The primary indication for MCL reconstruction is the need for the elite athlete to return to competition. Although rehabilitation efforts may improve symptoms in the lower-demand patient, a return to previous velocity and control is often impossible without surgical reconstruction. The ulnar nerve may require transposition if symptoms warrant. A muscle-splitting approach is preferred to avoid exposure and risk to the ulnar nerve during reconstruction. Rehabilitation requires a coordinated effort between the coach, therapist, and athlete over a 9- to 12-month period. Most reports of the procedure document a 70% to 80% rate of success, defined as the player returning to their previous level of performance.

The Stiff Elbow

A stiff elbow limits the ability of the patient to position the hand in space. Loss of flexion is more disabling than loss of extension because there is less opportunity for accommodation. A flexion/extension arc of a minimum of 100° is required to perform activities of daily living. In general, more that 120° of elbow flexion and extension to at least 30° is required. With loss of flexion, actions such as buttoning a collar, washing hair, or eating with the affected hand become difficult. The neck can only bend so far and flexion of the wrist adds little to the effective reach of the digits. Alternatively, loss of extension (beyond 30°) can be accommodated by moving the trunk closer to the intended object.

In general, contractures of the elbow can be divided into those with primarily extrinsic or intrinsic pathologies. With extrinsic contractures, the articular surfaces and bony anatomy are relatively well preserved and the primary source of stiffness is contracture of the surrounding soft tissues including instances of significant heterotopic ossification. With intrinsic contractures, there is disruption of the articular surfaces and bony anatomy, usually secondary to severe arthrosis or in posttraumatic situations.

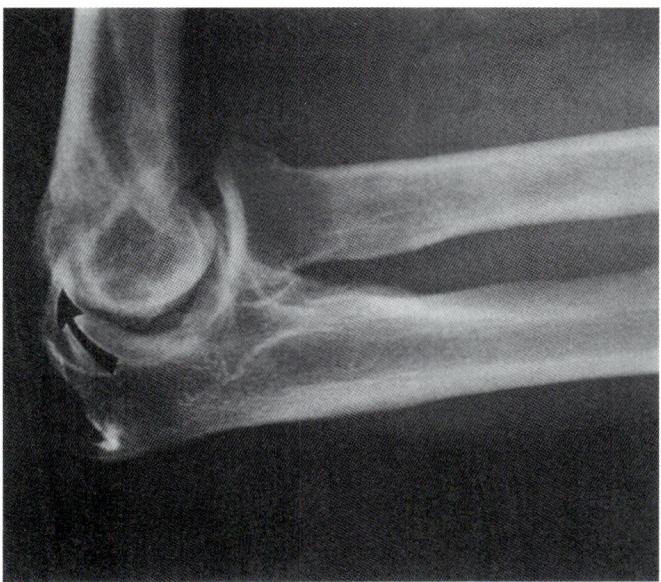

Figure 3 Lateral radiograph demonstrates osteophytes on the olecranon (arrow). *(Reproduced from O'Driscoll SW: Loose bodies of the elbow, in Norris TR (ed): Orthopaedic Knowledge Update Shoulder and Elbow. Rosemont, IL, American Academy of Orthopaedic Surgeons, 1997, pp 355–362.)*

Most uncomplicated posttraumatic contractures are not very painful. There may be discomfort at the end range, but the zone of limited motion is generally comfortable. If significant pain is present, intrinsic or posttraumatic arthrosis or joint inconcruity should be suspected. Patients who have had excessively forceful manipulations or passive mobilization in a misguided attempt to restore motion at a later date may have reactive pain and swelling. However, as scar maturation and tissue equilibrium occur, this inflammatory response usually abates.

Posttraumatic Contractures

The surgical treatment of the posttraumatic stiff elbow has become more routine and predictable. The main reasons for progress in this area have been improved surgical exposures and a better understanding of the factors that result in stiffness. The primary indications for surgical contracture release are an elbow range of motion less than 30° to 120° and failure to improve with a properly supervised physical therapy program using static splinting. Most authors report that 90% of patients can achieve substantial improvement with surgical intervention. Failures are now less common and when they occur are usually the result of inadequate exposure and release, a poor or deteriorating joint surface, or related to a small group of patients who seem to form a rapid fibrosis or who are unable to participate in the postoperative rehabilitation regimens.

Posttraumatic contractures can be caused by a loss of cartilage, joint incongruity, malalignment, or intrinsic contractures. Extrinsic to the joint surface itself, the thickened capsule usually tethers the joint, both on the posterior and anterior surface. Heterotopic bone formation may also block flexion and/or extension, depending on location. If the joint surface is judged to be inadequate for congruous motion because of loss of cartilage or incongruity, resurfacing must be considered. In the elderly patient, total elbow replacement may be the best alternative. In the younger patient, distraction interposition arthroplasty should be considered.

In those patients in whom the ulnohumeral joint is preserved, the capsule can be excised via either a medial and/or lateral approach depending on what is needed to safely excise the blocking/tethering tissue while preserving the stabilizing ligaments and protecting the ulnar and radial nerves, which are vulnerable.

Imaging Studies

The quality of the joint and relative health of the cartilage, location of hardware and whether it is impeding motion, the location of heterotopic ossification, and whether or not fractures have united are important radiologic features that need to be assessed before surgery is considered.

The quality of the articular surfaces in the stiff posttraumatic elbow is another important factor. The ulnohumeral joint is probably more important than the radiocapitellar joint, though having both structures intact and functional is optimal. Assessment of this joint and the quality of the cartilage is best done using plain radiographs. If this method is insufficient, CT scans with thin slices in the sagittal and coronal plains may be needed.

Surgical Approaches and Strategy

A variety of surgical approaches and techniques can be considered for contracture release as categorized in Table 2. For simple contractures (with minimal heterotopic bone and no ulnar nerve involvement), arthroscopic capsular release has proved to be quite effective. The surgeon must be experienced in arthroscopic techniques and be conscious of the proximity of major neurovascular structures.

The radial nerve is at particular risk during the anterior portion of the capsular release and the ulnar nerve is vulnerable to injury at the posterior and medial aspect of the joint. The median nerve and brachial artery are relatively safe because they are protected by the interposed brachialis muscle belly.

Open capsular release (from the medial or lateral exposure) is the most common and effective procedure. Both of these surgical exposures can be achieved

TABLE 2	Surgical Approaches for Contracture Release

Arthroscopic release

Open capsular release

   Medial column approach

   Lateral column approach

   Combined approach

Adjuvant devices/implants for instability or resurfacing

   Hinged external fixation

   Distraction interposition arthroplasty

   Total elbow replacement

   Allograft replacement

through a posterior skin incision. If the ulnar nerve is involved, the medial approach is preferred so that the ulnar nerve may be protected. Using a split in the flexor-pronator muscle, the anterior portion of the MCL can be protected while safely excising the capsule from the anterior and posterior joint surfaces. The lateral joint may be preferred, especially if the radial head was injured or requiring excision. Using the lateral exposure, care is taken to protect the LUCL, while excising anterior and posterior capsule and heterotopic bone.

There are instances where massive amounts of heterotopic bone or severe contracture require excision or incision of the stabilizing ligaments, and where the elbow may be both dislocated and stiff. Hinged external fixation is needed to maintain joint reduction and permit immediate postoperative mobilization. However, as more has been learned about elbow stability, the need for hinged external fixation in this circumstance has declined.

The Ulnar Nerve and Contracture Release

The ulnar nerve is quite vulnerable to injury, scarring, and dysfunction after any major trauma to the distal humerus or elbow region. Because of this vulnerability, a careful preoperative assessment is mandatory. Sometimes it is not possible to ascertain whether the nerve has been transposed. Even if the previous operative note states that a transposition was performed, the nerve may have slipped back into a more posterior position.

If the ulnar nerve is entrapped or shows signs of significant dysfunction, neurolysis at the time of contrac-

ture release can be quite helpful and restore sensibility and strength in the proximal muscles innervated by the ulnar nerve. The more distal, intrinsic muscles of the hand are less likely to recover, although dramatic improvement may be seen in younger patients.

Rehabilitation After Contracture Release

The judicious application of regional blocks, continuous passive motion, and static progressive splints has improved results of surgical release. Each patient requires an individualized approach; some require a few days of intermittent continuous passive motion (CPM) along with resting positional splints and others may require turnbuckle type splints early in the rehabilitation period. Most patients require some form of splinting and therapy for at least 3 months after treatment.

Adjuvant Therapy for Heterotopic Ossification Prevention

The efficacy of nonsteroidal medication or radiation for the prevention of heterotopic ossification has never been established after contracture release of the elbow. Although many authors have reported the use of indomethacin for 6 to 8 weeks after surgical release, to date there has not been a controlled trial of its use in combination with contemporary methods of postoperative mobilization. The use of gentle CPM, passive turnbuckle splinting, or dynamic external hinged fixation has probably diminished the incidence of heterotopic ossification, irrespective of adjuvant therapy. Most surgeons who treat the stiff elbow on a regular basis use either low-dose radiation immediately after surgery or a 3- to 6-week course of indomethacin, 25 mg three times daily, or 75 mg (slow-release) once a day.

The Arthritic Elbow
Primary Osteoarthritis

Primary osteoarthritis of the elbow is seen in men age 40 to 60 years and is characterized by osteophytic projections off the coronoid, olecranon tip, and occasionally the radial neck. This condition may be exacerbated by weight lifting or racquet sports. The ulnar nerve may also be under tension-compression, as the cubital tunnel fills with bone along the posteromedial joint line of the olecranon, leading to an insidious ulnar neuropathy. Pain is usually present at the end range of flexion and extension, as the osteophytes impact against bone. In most instances, the majority of the distal humeral surface and articulating ulna are covered with healthy cartilage, unlike other joints afflicted by primary osteoarthritis. The symptom usually noted first is loss of extension and/or flexion without much pain. If pain is prominent at mid range, there should be greater concern for a more aggressive form of the condition and the beginning of total loss of cartilage.

Studies have shown that surgical removal of the osteophytes generally results in substantial pain relief and improved mobility. Several techniques have been reported that either remove the osteophytes directly, using a medial approach, or create a transhumeral decompression from a posterior approach (the Outerbridge-Kashiwagi procedure). There have been reports of distal humeral fracture if the transhumeral bone trephination inadvertently weakens one of the columns of the distal humerus. Arthroscopic débridement has also been successfully used, but is technically challenging.

For more aggressive forms of primary arthritis, there is usually a patient history of heavy repetitive loading (such as weight lifting, throwing, or heavy labor, for example using a jackhammer), suggesting that there is a component of microtrauma accelerating the breakdown of the cartilage. As a result, the entire surface of the joint requires resurfacing. Total elbow replacement for these patients is quite problematic using linked designs. These patients are generally quite active and are not anxious to abide by a 10-lb weight limit. The optimal design for resurfacing prostheses of the elbow remains elusive. Continued work in this area may lead to a more enhanced performance design than is currently available.

Posttraumatic Arthritis

The location and extent of posttraumatic arthritis dictates the options for treatment. For arthritis localized to the radial head and radiocapitellar joint, radial head resection is often quite effective for pain relief and improvement of motion. Even with relief of pain, however, patients often experience arm weakness. The use of metallic implants for radial head replacement following fracture is now becoming commonplace, especially for instability. If the radial head excision appears to create excessive varus-valgus instability, or proximal migration of the radius (tear of the interosseous ligament), a metallic prosthesis should be considered. The size of the radial head replacement should be considered carefully, balancing the need to share load with the ulna, but not create excessive loading by overstuffing the lateral compartment.

If the ulnohumeral joint has no cartilage, the options are less attractive. Although distraction interposition arthroplasty using hinged fixation has been described and practiced for many years, the results are unpredictable and are seldom overwhelmingly gratifying. Nonetheless, for the painful posttraumatic elbow compli-

cated by dislocation and loss of articular congruity, the use of fascial resurfacing with hinged distraction is often the only possible treatment for improved function. Unless there is rampant infection, elbow fusion should be considered infrequently.

Distal Nonunion of the Humerus in the Elderly

In elderly patients with painful, stiff, or unstable elbows caused by humeral nonunion, there is often little chance that open reduction, internal fixation, and bone grafting of the nonunion would be of benefit. Instead, total elbow replacement in this group of patients using a semiconstrained, linked design has been beneficial. Surgical treatment of this patient population is technically challenging, demanding, and requires careful exposure and protection of the ulnar nerve, maintenance of triceps function, and precautions to minimize the opportunity for infection. Antibiotic-impregnated cement should be considered in all patients. Postoperatively, recovery is slow. Many patients have splints or casts in a fixed position of flexion for an extended period of time prior to joint replacement.

Rheumatoid Arthritis

Rheumatoid arthritis varies greatly in its presentation and degree of joint involvement. Newer agents being used to treat this condition have reduced the number and intensity of synovial flares, but it is not clear that the destructive component of the condition has been changed. The patient with rheumatoid arthritis who could benefit from elbow surgery generally is described according to four types of conditions as shown in Table 3.

The clinical course of rheumatoid arthritis is changing dramatically as newer disease-modifying agents become available. Implant design for joint replacement of the elbow needs to evolve to permit wider application to patients with increased physical demands and longevity.

Total Elbow Arthroplasty

The primary indication for total elbow arthroplasty is pain relief in an arthritic or injured joint. The cause of joint destruction can vary from inflammatory arthritis to trauma. Because the implants currently available have a shortened life span with vigorous use, the more likely the replacement will be of sustained benefit for a low-demand, elderly patient. The prospect of implant failure or infection must be considered for each patient.

The ideal indications for total elbow arthroplasty are inflammatory arthrosis in a patient with multijoint disease of the upper limb (low demand), and nonunion or acute

TABLE 3 | Patient Conditions Present in Rheumatoid Arthritis of the Elbow

Type	Description	Treatment	Special Considerations
Proliferative synovitis	No cartilage destruction; single or pauciarticular pattern; minimal stiffness; elbow not responsive to remittive agents	Arthroscopic synovectomy Open synovectomy	Open synovectomy may result in more stiffness; the radial head should be maintained if possible and excised only if identifiable pain and arthrosis are present
Stiff elbow with joint space narrowing	Bony architecture is preserved often in pauciarticular pattern; pain	Total elbow arthroplasty Distraction interposition arthroplasty	Goal is to rely on intact ligaments and minimize bone resection; optimal implant or procedure not yet developed
Painful elbow joint	Complete loss of joint space; bony architecture preserved; multiple joint involvement	Total elbow arthroplasty (linked semiconstrained design)	None
Grossly unstable elbow	Destructive bone loss of the elbow; inability to abduct shoulder or control elbow; weakness and pain	Total elbow arthroplasty (linked semiconstrained design)	Ulnar canal may be small; architecture of remaining bone stock may present a challenge

fracture of the distal articular surface in the elderly patient. Other indications to be considered include inflammatory arthrosis with more limited disease but disabling pain; primary osteoarthritis with complete loss of cartilage in the low-demand patient; and failed interposition arthroplasty in the low-demand patient.

Implant Selection

Total elbow designs can be divided into several broad categories: unconstrained and unlinked; semiconstrained and unlinked; semiconstrained and linked; and semiconstrained with the option of being linked or unlinked.

Currently the most reliable implant is the linked semiconstrained design. Although there are promising designs of semiconstrained unlinked implants, the problem of postoperative instability and dislocation still warrant concern. More experience and published results are necessary to provide more information concerning the other options for implants.

Clinical Results

The survivorship analyses published on the linked semiconstrained design are encouraging in the low-demand elbow. The 5-year survival rate at one institution was 94% (78 patients) and 92% at 10 years. Substantial pain relief and restoration of function was reported in over 90% of patients. The majority of these patients had rheumatoid arthritis.

In patients with primary osteoarthritis, implant failure and loosening required revision surgery in nearly 50% of the patients after 3 years. Presumably, these patients subject the implant to greater loads on a repetitive basis, leading to mechanical failure, including bushing wear and aseptic loosening.

Complications of Total Elbow Arthroplasty

The most devastating complication after total elbow replacement is complete removal of the implant without the possibility for revision. The resulting flail arm has limited strength in flexion, absent extension power, and virtually no control of the forearm with shoulder abduction.

Management of infection following total elbow arthroplasty depends on the causative organism and fixation of the implants. Implant removal, aggressive débridement, and intravenous antibiotics should be used for all loose implants. The timing of staged reimplantation depends on the causative organism and demonstrated eradication of the infection. Removal of well-fixed implants can result in destruction of bone stock, making reimplantation difficult or impossible. In one large report on infections of total elbow replacements, either revision replacement or irrigation and débridement and component retention were unsuccessful if the affected organism was *Staphylococcus epidermidis*. Reasonably good revision rates were obtained with other organisms.

Triceps weakness and insufficiency can be quite symptomatic in some patients after total elbow replacement. It is difficult to know the incidence of this complication because a direct measurement is required. Nonetheless, many patients will report a loss of extension control in a recumbent or supine position. Those who require a crutch or cane also may complain of a lack of control. If triceps function noticeably and abruptly declines, surgical reattachment of the insertion should be strongly considered. It is sometimes necessary to perform a turndown type of reconstruction if there has been a gradual separation for the proximal ulna, leading to a permanent shortening of the triceps.

Ulnar nerve neuritis and palsy is reported in 10% to 25% of patients. Care must be taken to expose and protect the nerve. The medial exposure (Bryan-Morrey) for total elbow replacement may be more advantageous because the nerve is first seen as a part of the surgical exposure. If a lateral approach or triceps-splitting approach is used, the ulnar nerve can be safely exposed and protected to minimize this complication.

Mechanical failure, either in the form of implant breakage, bushing wear/disassembly, or aseptic loosening can occur based on the level of use and duration of implantation. Problems with the axel/bushing assembly have been noted in all sloppy hinge designs, prompting modifications designed to improve stability and durability. If revision of the axel assembly is required, this is generally a relatively simple procedure. When mechanical failure results in aseptic loosening with bone loss around the stems, revision surgery becomes much more challenging. Revision of the ulnar component is especially problematic because of the narrow canal of the ulna. In most cases of revision surgery, a sloppy hinge design is needed as a result of loss of bone stock and attached ligaments.

Annotated Bibliography

Surgical Exposures

Cohen MS, Hastings H II: Operative release for elbow contracture: The lateral collateral ligament sparing technique. *Orthop Clin North Am* 1999;30:133-139.

This article describes the technique of elbow release and débridement using a lateral approach designed to spare the lateral collateral ligament complex and extensor tendon origins of the elbow. This exposure allows for complete exposure of the anterior and posterior ulnohumeral and radiocapitellar joints through a single incision.

Elbow Biomechanics and Kinematics

Armstrong AD, Dunning CE, Faber KJ, Duck TR, Johnson JA, King GJ: Rehabilitation of the medial collateral ligament-deficient elbow: An in vitro biomechanical study. *J Hand Surg Am* 2000;25:1051-1057.

The effect of forearm position on stability of the MCL-deficient elbow was evaluated in a cadaver model. Following MCL transection, the elbow was more stable with the forearm in supination than in pronation. This effect was decreased during active flexion as opposed to passive flexion. The authors concluded that active mobilization of the elbow during rehabilitation of an MCL-deficient elbow is safe in either the fully supinated or pronated position. However, splinting and passive mobilization of the MCL-deficient elbow should be done in supination.

Eygendaal D, Olsen BS, Jensen SL, Seki A, Söjbjerg JO: Kinematics of partial and total ruptures of the medial collateral ligament of the elbow. *J Shoulder Elbow Surg* 1999;8:612-616.

The authors showed that increase in joint opening was significant only after complete transection of the anterior part of the MCL and that joint opening was detected during valgus and internal rotatory stress only. No significant opening could be detected in the presence of partial ruptures.

Arthroscopy

Kelly EW, Morrey BF, O'Driscoll SW: Complications of elbow arthroscopy. *J Bone Joint Surg Am* 2001;83:25-34.

Four hundred seventy-three consecutive elbow arthroscopies were performed at a single institution. Procedures performed included 184 synovectomies, 180 joint surface débridements, 164 excision of osteophytes, 144 loose body removals, 154 diagnostic arthroscopies, and 73 capsular procedures including capsular releases. There were four joint space infections (0.8%) and 50 (11%) minor complications such as prolonged drainage or minor temporary contractures. There were also 12 transient nerve palsies included in the minor complication category.

Savoie FH III, Nunley PD, Field LD: Arthroscopic management of the arthritic elbow: Indications, technique, and results. *J Shoulder Elbow Surg* 1999;8:214-219.

Twenty-four patients with painful restricted motion of the elbow joint because of an arthritic process were treated with an arthroscopic modification of the open Outerbridge-Kashiwagi procedure. Arthroscopic ulnohumeral arthroplasty provided satisfactory results in terms of pain control and improved motion. Careful attention to technique and preoperative evaluation of the ulnar nerve is crucial for success.

Elbow Instability

Azar FM, Andrews JR, Wilk KE, Groh D: Operative treatment of ulnar collateral ligament injuries of the elbow in athletes. *Am J Sports Med* 2000;28:16-23.

Over a 6-year period, 91 ulnar collateral ligament reconstructions and repairs were performed with approximately 80% of patients able to return to a competitive throwing sport. All patients were male and between the ages of 15 and 39 years (average age of 21.6 years). Thirty-seven patients (41%) were professional baseball players, 41 (45%) were collegiate baseball players, and 7 (7.7%) were high school or recreational players. Subcutaneous ulnar nerve transposition with stabilization of the nerve with fascial slings of the flexor pronator mass was performed in all patients and additional procedures were performed in 27 patients (29.7%), including 22 excisions of posteromedial olecranon osteophytes. Ten patients had preoperative ulnar nerve symptoms, nine of whom had complete resolution of symptoms after surgery. The average time from surgery to initiation of the interval throwing program was 3.4 months, and the average time to return to competitive throwing was 9.8 months.

O'Driscoll SW, Jupiter JB, King GJW, Hotchkiss RN, Morrey BF: The unstable elbow. *J Bone Joint Surg Am* 2000;82:724-738.

This is a comprehensive review of acute and chronic elbow instability that addresses posterolateral instability and an algorithm of treatment.

The Stiff Elbow

Cheng SL, Morrey BF: Treatment of the mobile, painful arthritic elbow by distraction interposition arthroplasty. *J Bone Joint Surg Br* 2000;82:233-238.

Thirteen patients with mobile painful arthritic elbows were treated by distraction interposition arthroplasty using fascia lata. An elbow distractor/fixator was applied for 3 to 4 weeks to separate the articular surfaces and to protect the fascial graft. Nine of the 13 patients (69%) had satisfactory relief from pain; eight (62%) had an excellent or good result by the objective criteria of the Mayo Elbow Performance score. Four have required revision to total elbow arthroplasty at a mean of 30 months with good results to date. Instability of the elbow, both before and after surgery, was found to be associated with unsatisfactory results.

Fox RJ, Varitimidis SE, Plakseychuk A, Vardakas DG, Tomaino MM, Sotereanos DG: The Compass Elbow Hinge: Indications and initial results. *J Hand Surg Br* 2000;25:568-572.

The Compass Elbow Hinge uses Ilizarov's methods of fixation to externally hold the elbow reduction and allow both passive and active motion. Eleven patients with degenerative disease, contracture or instability, were treated with the Compass Elbow Hinge and were retrospectively evaluated at an average follow-up of 29 months (range, 18 to 62 months). Patients with degenerative changes underwent fascia lata interposition while those treated for contractures underwent anterior and posterior capsular release with or without fascia lata interposition. Those with elbow instability underwent ligament reconstruction. The device was removed after 6 weeks and 7 of the 11 patients were satisfied with the outcome of the operation. Stability could not be achieved in two patients with coronoid fractures that were not reconstructed.

Mansat P, Morrey BF: The column procedure: A limited lateral approach for extrinsic contracture of the elbow. *J Bone Joint Surg Am* 1998;80:1603-1615.

Thirty-eight elbows (37 patients) with an extrinsic contracture were treated surgically with a limited lateral approach to the anterior and posterior aspects of the capsule. The mean total gain in the arc of flexion-extension was 45°; 34 elbows (89%) had an improved range of motion. Understanding both the medial and lateral approaches is important for care of these patients.

Ring D, Jupiter JB: Reconstruction of posttraumatic elbow instability. *Clin Orthop* 2000;370:44-56.

Successful reconstruction of posttraumatic elbow instability is dependent on restoration of the radial head and coronoid and lateral collateral ligament complex. This structure can be reattached to its origin from the lateral epicondyle. Patients with long-standing subluxation or dislocation may require temporary hinged external fixation or reconstruction of the collateral ligaments with tendon grafts.

Gill DR, Morrey BF: The Coonrad-Morrey total elbow arthroplasty in patients who have rheumatoid arthritis: A ten to fifteen-year follow-up study. *J Bone Joint Surg Am* 1998;80:1327-1335.

Sixty-nine patients (78 elbows) who had rheumatoid arthritis underwent total elbow replacement and were followed for 10 to 15 years. Seventy-six of the 78 elbows had long-term radiographic evaluation; the two remaining elbows were excluded because a resection arthroplasty had been performed. Five bushings (7%) were completely worn, and six (8%) were partially worn. Serious complications occurred in eleven elbows (14%) necessitating reoperation in ten (13%). Delayed complications included three avulsions of the triceps, two deep infections, two ulnar fractures, and one fracture of an ulnar component. In addition, two elbows were revised because of aseptic loosening. Forty-three of the 78 elbows had an excellent result; 26, a good result; 7, a fair result; and 2, a poor result. The rate of survival of the prosthesis was 92.4%.

Total Elbow Arthroplasty

Hildebrand KA, Patterson SD, Regan WD, MacDermid JC, King GJ: Functional outcome of semiconstrained total elbow arthroplasty. *J Bone Joint Surg Am* 2000;82:1379-1386.

Thirty-six of 47 consecutive patients who underwent total elbow arthroplasty in a single institution were followed-up at an average of 50 months. Eighteen patients (21 elbows) had inflammatory arthritis and 18 patients (18 elbows) had either an acute fracture or posttraumatic condition. Results showed that significant improvements in function and patient satisfaction can be achieved with the total of both inflammatory and posttraumatic conditions. However, patients who underwent arthroplasty for inflammatory arthritis had significantly higher functional outcomes. Of concern, 11 of 34 elbows had changes in the bone cement interface consistent with loosening.

Kudo H, Iwano K, Nishino J: Total elbow arthroplasty with use of a nonconstrained humeral component inserted without cement in patients who have rheumatoid arthritis. *J Bone Joint Surg Am* 1999;81:1268-1280.

A modification of the Kudo design total elbow was used in 43 elbows with rheumatoid arthritis. This modification did not require cement for fixation. The elbows were followed for an average of 3 years and 10 months. The overall result was excellent for 6 elbows, good for 31, and fair for 6. There was almost complete relief of pain in 29 elbows and mild or occasional pain in the remaining 14 elbows. Flexion increased but extension worsened. Surprisingly, no loosening was reported and only one dislocation was noted.

Schneeberger AG, Hertel R, Gerber C: Total elbow replacement with the GSB III prosthesis. *J Shoulder Elbow Surg* 2000;9:135-139.

Total elbow replacement with the GSB III implant was used to treat 14 consecutive elbows with either rheumatoid arthritis (9 elbows) or posttraumatic osteoarthritis (5 elbows). Ten of 14 elbows had a functioning GSB III implant at follow-up (average follow-up was 6 years); 7 of them were rated satisfactory and 3 unsatisfactory with the Mayo elbow performance score. Aseptic loosening requiring revision occurred in 4 (29%) elbows. This study reflects the difficulty of total elbow replacement.

Yanni ON, Fearn CB, Gallannaugh SC, Joshi R: The Roper-Tuke total elbow arthroplasty: 4- to 10-year results of an unconstrained prosthesis. *J Bone Joint Surg Br* 2000;82:705-710.

This article reports the results of 59 unconstrained total arthroplasties of the elbow after a mean follow-up of 6.5 years (4 to 10). All the patients had rheumatoid arthritis and the indication for surgery was pain in all but one patient. Two patients developed instability, but neither required further surgery. There was a mean increase of 21° in flexion and of 7° in extension. The overall rate of complications was 33.9% (deep infection in two patients).

Classic Bibliography

Bryan RS, Morrey BF: Extensive posterior exposure of the elbow: A triceps-sparing approach. *Clin Orthop* 1982;166:188-192.

Indelicato PA, Jobe FW, Kerlan RK, Carter VS, Shields CL, Lombardo SJ: Correctable elbow lesions in professional baseball players: A review of 25 cases. *Am J Sports Med* 1979;7:72-75.

Kasparyan NG, Hotchkiss RN: Dynamic skeletal fixation in the upper extremity. *Hand Clin* 1997;13:643-663.

Lee BP, Morrey BF: Arthroscopic synovectomy of the elbow for rheumatoid arthritis: A prospective study. *J Bone Joint Surg Br* 1997;79:770-772.

O'Driscoll SW, Bell DF, Morrey BF: Posterolateral rotatory instability of the elbow. *J Bone Joint Surg Am* 1991;73:440-446.

Potter HG, Weiland AJ, Schatz JA, Paletta GA, Hotchkiss RN: Posterolateral rotatory instability of the elbow: Usefulness of MR imaging in diagnosis. *Radiology* 1997;204:185-189.

Chapter 32

Forearm, Wrist, and Hand: Pediatric Aspects

Michelle A. James, MD

Richard A.K. Reynolds, MD, FRCSC

Congenital Upper Extremity Malformations

Introduction

Recent developments in the care of children with upper extremity malformations include the use of distraction lengthening and free vascularized tissue transfer. However, few surgical operations have been conclusively proved to improve function in a malformed hand. Often the biggest challenge to the family is the psychological adjustment to the appearance of the child's hand.

In large population studies, the reported incidence of congenital anomalies of the upper extremity varies between 3.4 and 16 cases per 10,000 live births. Most congenital malformations are more common in boys and are caused by genetic and/or environmental factors.

In the human embryo, upper limb buds appear 26 to 28 days after fertilization. During the next 25 days, the upper limb is completely differentiated; the same mutagenic insult occurring at the various stages of differentiation will cause different malformations.

Consultation with a geneticist is a very important component in the care of children with congenital hand malformations. The geneticist helps diagnose anomalies outside the musculoskeletal system (which are associated with more than 80% of heritable limb deficiencies) and provides genetic counseling. Although many hand anomalies are visible on prenatal ultrasound, they are frequently overlooked.

General Principles

The surgeon must be familiar with normal developmental milestones to assess the functional abilities of a child with a malformed upper extremity. Most children younger than age 3 years do not notice their hand difference, and early motor development is unaffected by most upper extremity malformations. Children between 4 and 8 years of age with transverse and longitudinal deficiencies may have difficulty performing advanced dressing and hygiene activities, and benefit from goal-directed occupational therapy.

Complex malformations are most effectively treated using a team approach. The hand surgeon directs the child's care, with the assistance and support of the nursing and social services staff, who help educate the family and coordinate care. Other team members include the occupational therapist, the orthotist and prosthetist, child life and therapeutic recreation specialists, a geneticist, a pediatric anesthesiologist, and a medical librarian.

Classification and Terminology

The most commonly used classification system for congenital upper limb malformations is descriptive, and based on morphology. It was originally proposed in 1968 and was adopted in a modified form by the American Society for Surgery of the Hand and the International Federation of Societies for Surgery of the Hand (ASSH/IFSSH) in 1983 (Table 1). Only a few large studies of congenital hand anomalies have used this scheme. This classification system has several disadvantages: it is too complex; several well-described conditions include anomalies that fit into more than one category; some anomalies defy classification; and it provides only very broad guidelines for prognosis and treatment.

Synostosis of Proximal Radius and Ulna

The proximal radius and ulna fail to separate in this rare condition, resulting in a forearm fixed in varying degrees of pronation. Sixty percent of cases are bilateral, with an equal incidence in males and females.

Congenital radioulnar synostosis is caused by a longitudinal arrest of segmentation, with several underlying causes. In children with bilateral congenital radioulnar synostosis, surgeons traditionally recommended repositioning one forearm into supination. This position is no longer recommended, however, because

TABLE 1	ASSH/IFSSH Classification of Congenital Upper Limb Malformations

Failure of formation of parts (arrest of development)

    Transverse arrest

    Longitudinal arrest

Failure of differentiation (separation) of parts

Congenital tumorous conditions

Duplication

Overgrowth

Undergrowth

Congenital constriction ring syndrome

Generalized skeletal abnormalities

(Adapted with permission from Swanson AB: A classification for congenital limb malformation. J Hand Surg 1976;1:8–22.)

bilateral pronation is necessary for computer keyboarding. Most children with congenital radioulnar synostosis require no surgical intervention, because of the ability of the shoulder to adapt by abduction.

Transverse Forearm Deficiency

Transverse failure of formation occurs when the upper limb fails to form below a certain level. Finger nubbins usually form at the distal end of the limb, regardless of level; their presence helps differentiate this condition from congenital constriction ring syndrome, in which nubbins do not form. Transverse failure of formation is not inheritable. The most common level of transverse failure of formation is proximal forearm (below elbow), followed by transcarpal, distal forearm, and through humerus (above elbow). This condition is almost always unilateral, and the left side is more commonly affected. Children with unilateral congenital below-elbow deficiency have remarkably few functional deficits, and surgery has not been proved to improve function. A prosthesis enhances prehension, and possibly appearance, but blocks sensory feedback. Goal-directed occupational therapy may help the school-aged child learn to perform activities of daily living with and without a prosthesis.

The child with unilateral congenital below-elbow deficiency should be assessed by a prosthetic team (which includes a physician, prosthetist, and occupational therapist, and may include a recreation therapist and social worker) at around age 6 months, and fitted with a prosthesis with a passive hand or mitt when he or she is able to sit independently. Parents are encouraged to gradually increase wearing time until the child tolerates the prosthesis for the majority of waking hours. Children with more proximal or distal failure of formation usually are not fitted with a prosthesis in infancy. If the deficiency is at shoulder level, the prosthesis is too heavy for comfortable wear; if the deficiency is at the distal forearm or through the carpus, the child functions better without a prosthesis. At age 2 to 3 years, the child with unilateral congenital below-elbow deficiency is evaluated for readiness for an active terminal device. If the child readily bears weight on the passive prosthesis when crawling and uses it for pulling up, balance, and two-handed activities such as throwing and catching, an active terminal device probably can be introduced.

Longitudinal Deficiency of the Ulna

Children with this rare anomaly (approximately 1 in 100,000 live births) have hypoplasia of the entire upper extremity. The elbow is malformed or absent (humeroradial synostosis) in the majority of cases. Deficiency of the ulna may be partial or complete, and a cartilaginous ulna anlage often is present. All children with this deficiency have hand and carpal anomalies; about 90% of hands are missing digits, 30% have syndactyly, and 70% have thumb abnormalities. Unilateral involvement is twice as common as bilateral. This condition is often associated with other musculoskeletal anomalies, most commonly proximal femoral focal deficiency, fibula deficiency, phocomelia, and scoliosis, but is rarely associated with anomalies of other organ systems. Despite their upper extremity malformation, children with ulna deficiency usually function well. Thumb reconstruction, release of syndactyly, and external rotation osteotomy of the humerus are well-accepted treatments for malformations associated with ulna deficiency. Lengthening may improve the appearance of a short forearm, but is indicated only in the presence of a stable elbow with active flexion.

Longitudinal Deficiency of the Radius

Radius deficiency is a rare condition, occurring in approximately 1 in 30,000 live births. Although thumb deficiency is not always associated with radius deficiency, radius deficiency is nearly always associated with thumb and carpal deficiencies, and frequently associated with other upper extremity anomalies, anomalies of other organ systems, and syndromes. The newborn with radius deficiency should be carefully examined for thrombocytopenia-absent radius syndrome (autosomal dominant or recessive inheritance of completely absent radius with a near-normal thumb and thrombocytopenia) in addition to the syndromes associated with isolated thumb deficiency. Radius defi-

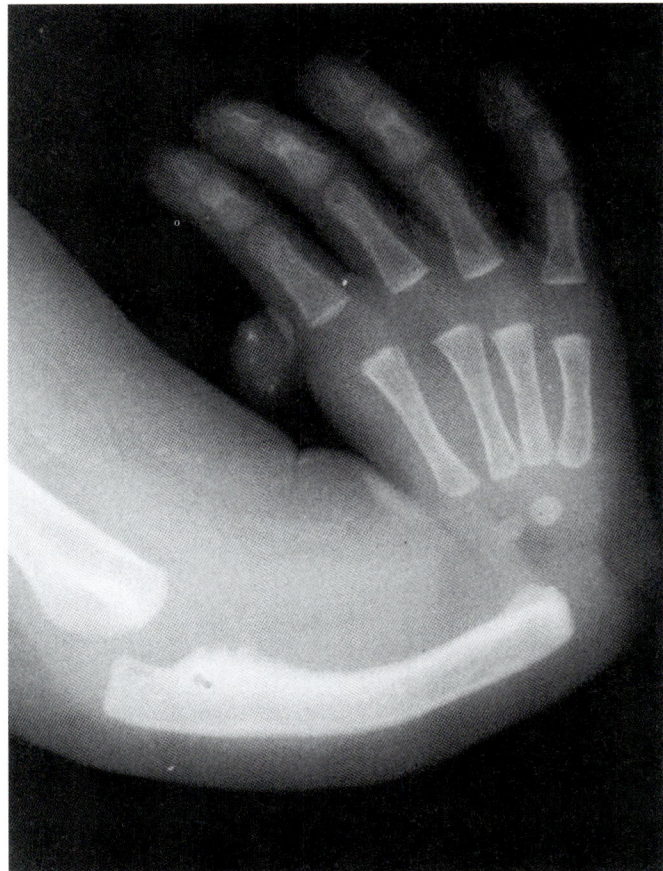

Figure 1 Type 4 radial deficiency with complete absence of the radius.

ciency is usually bilateral, although the two sides are frequently asymmetric; when unilateral, it is more common on the right side.

The wrist instability and radial deviation associated with types 3 and 4 deformity (near-complete and complete absence of the radius, respectively) are treated with centralization of the carpus on the end of the ulna (Fig. 1). The best results are obtained if aberrant radial wrist extensors are transferred to help maintain the new position, before 1 year of age. Most wrists require stretching of the tight radial soft tissue and joint capsule prior to centralization. Traditionally serial casting has served this purpose, but more recently, distraction of the radial structures with an external fixator has been done. Stabilization of the wrist enhances the appearance and possibly the function of the hand, but is difficult to maintain throughout growth. Radial deviation tends to recur unless the wrist is quite stiff.

Thumb Deficiency and Absence

Thumb deficiency and absence are part of longitudinal radial deficiency, which may involve the thumb alone, or the entire radial hand, wrist, and forearm. This condition is rare, occurring in 1 in 30,000 to 1 in 100,000 live births, frequently bilateral, and often associated with congenital anomalies of the lower extremities, spine, and other organ systems. Several syndromes are characterized by hypoplastic or absent thumbs, usually combined with radius deficiency, including the VACTERL association (*V*ertebral, *A*nal, *C*ardiac, *T*racheo-*E*sophageal, *R*enal, *L*ung) and Holt-Oram syndrome.

The deficient thumb must be examined carefully for the presence or absence of thenar intrinsic muscles, metacarpophalangeal joint-ulnar collateral ligament stability, extrinsic muscles (flexor and extensor pollicis longus), and carpometacarpal joint stability, because the presence of these components determines whether the thumb is surgically reconstructible, or whether the child's hand would function better if the thumb were ablated and the index finger pollicized.

Madelung Deformity

Madelung deformity is caused by a growth disturbance of the ulnar and palmar aspects of the distal radial epiphysis (Fig. 2). This condition may be caused by a combination of a bony lesion in the ulnar portion of the distal radius physis and an abnormal palmar ligament tethering the lunate to the radius proximal to the physis. It is the final common pathway for many different disorders, including dysplasia, trauma, chromosomal abnormalities, infection, and tumors (Table 2). Madelung deformity is most commonly caused by dysplasia associated with Leri-Weill syndrome (dyschondrosteosis), which is inherited in an autosomal dominant fashion with 50% penetrance. Repetitive loading of the wrist in the growing child may cause Madelung-like deformity in gymnasts (gymnast wrist). Madelung deformity may be classified into typical and atypical types.

The normal distal radial epiphysis appears at age 2 years and begins to flatten at age 6 years, but in typical Madelung deformity the ulnar third of the epiphysis does not ossify. The characteristic wedge-shaped distal epiphysis persists, and can be quite severely angulated, with the distal articular surface tilted as much as 80° palmar and 90° ulnar. The entire carpus is shifted toward the ulna, and may be interposed into the space between the ulna and radius. Wrist deformity is the most common presenting complaint, becoming noticeable between 8 and 12 years of age. Pain is uncommon but weakness resulting from subluxation of the wrist into the radioulnar space and limited rotation are common complaints.

With atypical or reverse Madelung deformity, the distal radius is tilted dorsally, and the distal ulna is displaced palmarward. Dorsiflexion is excessive, but palmar flexion

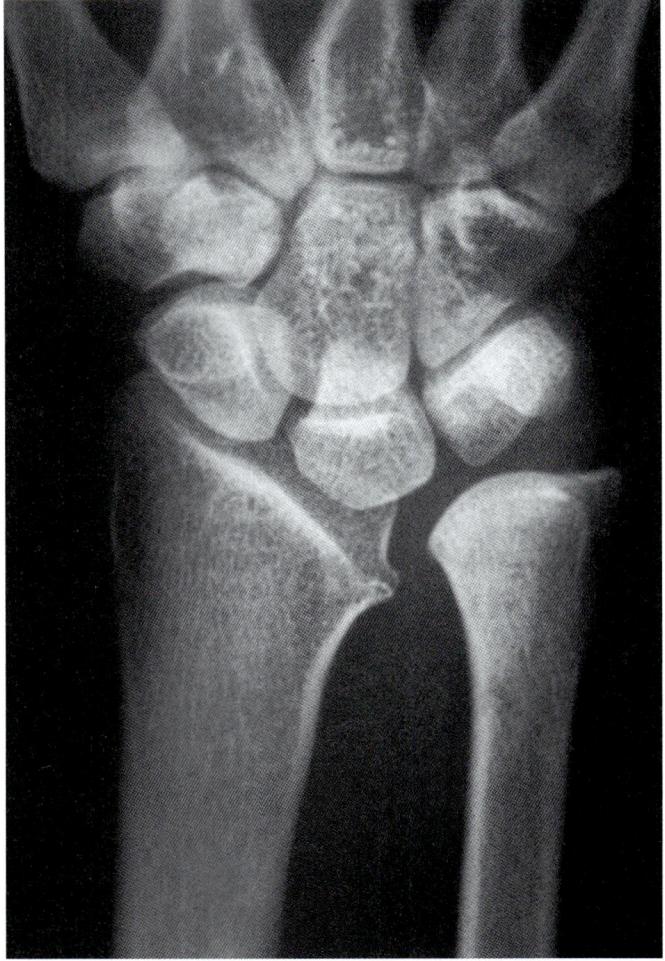

Figure 2 Madelung deformity is a congenital deformity caused by a growth abnormality of the ulnar-volar aspect of the distal radial epiphysis.

TABLE 2	Differential Diagnosis of Madelung Deformity of the Distal Radius and Ulna

Trauma	Metabolic	Inflammatory
Dislocation of the distal radioulnar joint	Rickets	Rheumatoid arthritis
Infection	**Osteochondrodysplasias**	**Neoplasm**
Distal radius infection	Leri-Weill syndrome Ollier's disease	Osteochondromas

and pronation are limited. Weakness may be caused by radiocarpal or distal radioulnar instability.

If the deformity is not painful, no treatment is necessary, although untreated Madelung deformity has been associated with spontaneous extensor tendon rupture, probably because of the ulna-plus deformity and disruption of the distal radioulnar joint. If the deformity is painful and the patient has not achieved skeletal maturity, physiolysis (resection of the section of arrested growth plate to allow correction of the growth plate alignment through growth) may reduce pain and, with additional growth, improve the deformity. In the skeletally mature patient with wrist pain associated with Madelung deformity, correction of the deformity with radial and dorsal closing wedge osteotomy and ulnar shortening may be helpful.

Symbrachydactyly

Symbrachydactyly is characterized by fingers that have failed to form normally; this condition differs from constriction ring syndrome, in which fingers have prenatal deformation. Transverse failure of formation, or terminal deficiency, occurs in about 1.5 in 10,000 births and 98% of cases are unilateral. One characteristic is incomplete separation of short digits. Parents and children frequently request lengthening of short fingers, and several methods to augment length have been devised. However, no single procedure is superior, normal appearance is usually unattainable, and lengthening the digits of a child with a normal contralateral hand does not improve function. Surgical reconstruction is not recommended for digits that have failed to develop metacarpals, with the exception of the thumb.

Web deepening may enhance pinch and grasp. Distraction lengthening of the phalanges usually is not indicated because stiff fingers should be short, or they will interfere with the function of more flexible fingers. Distraction lengthening of short metacarpals may enhance function and appearance. Nonvascularized toe phalanx transfers are possible when a soft-tissue tube large enough to hold bone graft has developed distal to the metacarpal. The indications for toe-to-hand free transfer for transverse defects and symbrachydactyly are controversial, and the arterial supply, venous drainage, nerves, and muscles in a malformed hand are always abnormal, and sometimes nonexistent.

Syndactyly

Syndactyly is the most common congenital hand malformation, occurring in 1 in 2,500 births. It may occur as an isolated anomaly or as part of a syndrome. Up to 40% of cases are inherited in an autosomal dominant pattern. Syndromes commonly associated with syndactyly include Poland's syndrome (sporadic occurrence of symbrachydactyly associated with variable deficiency of the pectoralis major muscle) and Apert's syndrome (acrocephalosyndactyly). If radiographs reveal a partial duplication hidden in the syndactyly, it is likely to be inheritable.

Release of complete syndactyly requires full-thickness skin grafts. Timing of surgery is determined by the digits involved, and the degree and complexity of the syndactyly. Syndactyly of border digits (especially thumb-index) is released early, usually by 6 months of age, because length discrepancy may cause the longer digit to develop flexion and angulatory deformities with growth. Although there is no urgency to release long-ring or index-long syndactyly, parents may prefer early surgery. The etiology of web creep, or partial recurrence of syndactyly, is unclear, but it probably is not related to the patient's age at the original operation.

Polydactyly

Polydactyly is the second most common congenital hand malformation in the United States, and the thumb is the most common duplicated, or split, digit. Thumb polydactyly is most often sporadic; when it is associated with syndactyly, or when one or both of the bifid thumbs is triphalangeal, it is more likely to be caused by a genetic mutation. Finger polydactyly is slightly less common, and more commonly associated with a syndrome than thumb polydactyly. The small finger is the most commonly duplicated finger. Duplication of the index, long, or ring finger is rare, and is usually associated with other limb or nonlimb defects or syndromes.

Split thumbs are thinner and shorter than normal, and have stiff joints, hypoplastic tendons with anomalous interconnections, and abnormal vascular anatomy. Usually neither thumb has completely normal function. The ulnar thumb is usually larger and more functional than the radial thumb, but when the two "halves" are equal in size, or when both are triphalangeal, both are likely to be severely hypoplastic.

Thumb polydactyly has been classified by level of duplication. Thumbs duplicated at the level of the distal phalanx may be treated with a combination (Bilhaut) procedure, in which a central wedge of tissue (including bone, joint, physis, and nailbed and skin) is removed, and the two remaining parts are joined together. For other types of thumb polydactyly, simple ablation of one split thumb is inadequate. Elements of the excised thumb, including collateral ligament, skin, and/or tendons, are used to augment the preserved thumb to reduce the risk of angulation and joint instability. Even the carefully reconstructed thumb may angulate or develop joint instability with growth; the child should be evaluated until skeletal maturity has been achieved.

Infantile Trigger Digit

Trigger thumb is a relatively common condition, with an incidence estimated to be less than 3 in 1,000 live births. Trigger thumb in children is probably acquired, not congenital.

The infant's affected thumb rarely triggers, or snaps, but instead usually presents as a fixed flexion contracture at the interphalangeal joint. A palpable nodule in the flexor pollicis longus at the metacarpophalangeal joint flexion crease of the thumb is almost always present and is probably caused by bunching up and swelling of the flexor pollicis longus after chronic pressure from the proximal pulley. Secondary metacarpophalangeal joint hyperextensibility frequently results. Surgical release of the A1 pulley is successful, but up to 49% of trigger thumbs will spontaneously resolve, so initial observation is warranted.

Trigger fingers may also occur in older children, but they are much rarer than trigger thumbs and more likely to resolve spontaneously. They reportedly are associated with mucopolysaccharide storage disorders, juvenile arthritis, and diabetes mellitus. Triggering may occur at the A2 pulley, and treatment may require excision of one slip of the flexor digitorum superficialis.

Camptodactyly

Camptodactyly is a nontraumatic flexion contracture of the proximal interphalangeal joint, usually of the small finger. The incidence of camptodactyly is unknown. Malformations of several different anatomic structures have been cited as the underlying cause of this deformity, including the lumbrical, flexor digitorum superficialis, and extensor mechanism.

Camptodactyly is classified by the age of the patient at presentation, and whether it is associated with a syndrome. Type I, which is most common, is an isolated anomaly affecting the small finger that presents in infancy and almost always improves with splinting and stretching. Type II is similar to type I, except that the patient with type II camptodactyly first presents in adolescence. Type II also improves with splinting, and even if the deformity is severe, it rarely interferes with function. In type III camptodactyly, multiple digits are involved, the contractures are more severe than types I and II, and the child has an associated syndrome. Type III also improves with splinting, but is the most likely of the three types to require surgery. Failure of the patient to use a splint is not an indication for surgery, because postoperative management requires therapy and splinting. Surgery should be considered only when the contracture worsens despite splinting and interferes with function. The results of surgical release are often poor (less than 50% of fingers with increased range of motion postoperatively) and tend to deteriorate with follow-up.

Clinodactyly and Longitudinal Epiphyseal Bracket (Delta Phalanx)

Clinodactyly is the deviation of a finger in the radio-ulnar plane. The condition usually is caused by malformation of the distal end of the middle phalanx, but also may be caused by a longitudinal epiphyseal bracket (or delta phalanx) or soft-tissue contracture. A longitudinal epiphyseal bracket is an abnormal epiphysis that occurs in bones with a proximal epiphysis, and extends longitudinally along the diaphysis, and transversely across the opposite end of the affected bone, forming a "C" shape. Although it can occur in any finger, it is most common in the small finger. In the United States, radial deviation of the small finger at the distal interphalangeal joint may occur in up to 1% of normal children and 10% of children with other congenital anomalies. Familial clinodactyly is autosomal dominant with reduced penetrance, and usually is not associated with other anomalies. Clinodactyly usually does not interfere with function. Splinting does not affect the deformity. Surgical treatment is indicated for worsening clinodactyly caused by a longitudinal epiphyseal bracket, or when crossing of the flexed fingers is bothersome. Clinodactyly caused by longitudinal epiphyseal bracket is likely to progress, and simple division of the abnormal longitudinal epipheseal bracket is not reliably successful. If the patient has not reached skeletal maturity, a portion of the mid zone, or isthmus, of the continuous epiphysis may be removed and replaced with fat graft (physiolysis). For clinodactyly of any etiology, regardless of skeletal maturity, an ulnar closing wedge osteotomy will correct the angulation. If modest lengthening is desired in addition to straightening, in the larger hand a reversed wedge osteotomy can be performed by removing a wedge of bone from the convex (usually ulnar) side, reversing it and inserting it on the concave (usually radial) side.

Constriction Ring Syndrome

The incidence of this syndrome has been estimated at 1 in 15,000 live births. The etiology of constriction ring syndrome is unclear; however, it is not genetic. This condition frequently affects both arms or all four limbs, and is associated with clubfoot and craniofacial clefts. Anomalies similar to those seen in this syndrome reportedly are associated with maternal cocaine use and chorionic villus sampling. Digits may be amputated, constricted by a partial or complete ring (a tight band of tissue) and/or webbed. Surgical treatment includes z-plasty of constriction rings and release of acrosyndactyly, usually when the child is older than 1 year of age. Deep circumferential rings may need to be released earlier if lymphedema is severe, if the vascular supply of the digit or extremity is compromised, or if the ring is causing a peripheral nerve palsy. Release of a circumferential ring can be performed at one operation. Free vascularized toe transfers may be indicated; unlike finger hypoplasia, proximal neurovascular and musculotendinous structures are probably normal.

Central Deficiency (Cleft Hand)

Cleft hand is rare, with an incidence between 1 in 90,000 and 1 in 150,000 live births. It is frequently inherited in an autosomal dominant pattern. The deficiency varies from absent long finger phalanges to absent index, long, and ring finger rays, to monodactyly or even absence of all digits.

Cleft hand usually is associated with syndactyly (especially thumb-index) and cleft feet, and frequently associated with other musculoskeletal anomalies including central polydactyly, camptodactyly, longitudinal epiphyseal bracket, and absence of the tibia, and anomalies of other organ systems including cleft lip and palate. Cleft hand also is frequently associated with various syndromes. Surgical treatment is not always indicated, and surgical planning is complex, because various operations (including syndactyly release, cleft closure, and excision of a transverse phalanx) may be needed.

Trauma
Distal Radius Fractures

Distal radius fractures are the most common long bone fractures in children and are classified by location, amount of displacement, angular alignment, rotational alignment, and completeness of the fracture. Closed reduction and cast immobilization are usually the only treatments required. Complete bayonet apposition is acceptable for children with at least 2 years of growth remaining, as long as angulation after reduction does not exceed 20°. Surgery is done when the fracture is open or when acceptable alignment cannot be achieved or maintained.

Forearm Fractures

Most pediatric forearm fractures are treated with closed reduction. In one series of 730 forearm fractures, 300 required reduction and only 22 had to be remanipulated because of loss of reduction; 12 required pinning. Reductions with up to 15° of angulation and 45° of malrotation can be accepted in children younger than age 9 years. In children 9 years of age or older, 30° of malrotation and up to 10° of angulation for proximal fractures and 15° for more distal fractures are acceptable. Nonunion is extremely rare.

Intramedullary (IM) rods for the treatment of forearm fractures in children are increasingly popular.

Advantages of IM rodding over open reduction include preservation of soft tissue and indirect reduction. Complications of IM rodding include infection, loss of reduction and extensor pollicis longus rupture. Plate fixation has many drawbacks, including more prominent surgical scars, high refracture rates with plate removal, and nerve injuries, especially with more proximal fractures.

Hand Injuries
Burns

Pediatric hand burns are common injuries. Although the hand represents less than 5% of the total body surface area, hand burns are considered major injuries by the American Burn Association because of the importance of hand function, and usually should be treated by an experienced burn team. Aggressive range of motion exercises and splinting, and for full-thickness burns, prompt autograft coverage and long-term hand therapy and follow-up including reconstructive surgery are the mainstays of treatment. Dorsal burns and thumb web burns have a poorer prognosis.

Flexor Tendon Lacerations

Past reports of flexor tendon repair in children have indicated that most results are satisfactory. Associated digital nerve lacerations do not affect the results. Children younger than age 5 years should be immobilized in a long arm cast. Although early mobilization is not necessary, immobilization should not be continued beyond 4 weeks postrepair.

Triangular Fibrocartilage Injuries

These injuries are more common in children than previously believed. Arthroscopic examination is necessary for diagnosis in many cases. The most common type of tear is Palmer 1B (ulnar peripheral). Common associated injuries included distal radius fracture and ulnar styloid fracture nonunion. A high rate of success has been reported with surgical repair of the triangular fibrocartilage complex lesions, provided that associated injuries are also appropriately treated.

Fingertip Injuries

Fingertip injuries are most common in children younger than age 5 years. Definitive treatment can result in good functional and cosmetic results after a delay of up to 2 weeks, but these injuries should be treated urgently. Indications for surgical exploration include a displaced distal phalanx fracture, disruption of the nail or nailfold, or leverage of the proximal nail out of the nailfold. In the absence of these findings,

size of subungual hematoma was not associated with outcome; thus, formal nailbed exploration and reconstruction is no longer recommended for hematomas larger than 25% of the nailbed surface area as long as the nail and nail margin are intact.

Carpal Fractures

Carpal fractures are uncommon in children. The scaphoid is fractured most frequently, with a low-energy fall the most common mechanism. Most pediatric scaphoid fractures occur in the 11- to 13-year age group, and most are nondisplaced distal pole fractures. The majority of fractures heal in a thumb spica cast in 8 weeks or less. Nonunions occasionally occur, most often in scaphoid waist fractures; excellent results can be achieved with open reduction, internal fixation with a small Herbert screw, and bone grafting.

Physeal Fractures

The most common epiphyseal fracture in the hand is Salter-Harris type II (through the physis and metaphysis). Salter-Harris type III (through physis and epiphysis, an intra-articular injury) fractures are rare, but typically occur at the base of the proximal phalanx. The proximal phalanx is especially susceptible to physeal injury because of collateral ligament anatomy; although the collateral ligaments of the interphalangeal joints span the epiphyseal plate, the same ligaments of the metacarpophalangeal joints insert on the epiphysis of the proximal phalanx. An avulsion force at this joint causes type III fractures, especially in adolescents, and most commonly during athletics. Unless these fractures are nondisplaced, which is uncommon, open reduction and internal fixation of the avulsed and rotated epiphyseal fragment is required.

Digital Replantation

Long-term follow-up of children with replanted digits indicates excellent recovery of sensibility, good grip and pinch strength, and 93% of normal bone growth, according to a study of mostly sharp amputations (as opposed to crush or avulsion injuries, which have a worse prognosis). Amputation of digits in children is a strong indication for replantation, regardless of level of amputation or number of digits involved.

Infection

The most common infection in the toddler and preschooler's hand is herpetic whitlow, a viral infection caused by herpes simplex virus. Painful vesicles appear over the distal phalanx of a single digit, without systemic signs of infection. Herpetic whitlow is self-limited and surgical treatment is not indicated. Children are also susceptible to hand infections as a result of bite wounds. The treatment for bite wounds in children (débridement and prophylactic antibiotics) is the same as for adults.

Cerebral Palsy

Several different patterns of cerebral palsy may be manifested in the upper extremity, resulting in impairment of hand function. The most common pattern affecting the upper extremity is spastic hemiplegia, which is most likely to have a prepartum etiology. In spastic hemiplegia, the affected upper extremity is typically spastic, and deformities include shoulder internal rotation, elbow flexion, forearm pronation, wrist flexion, and thumb-in-palm. The affected arm is always smaller, but the amount of the discrepancy is unpredictable.

A recent review of a large number of procedures in children with cerebral palsy showed a significant improvement in functional level following surgery, provided that surgical planning was tailored to the needs of the individual child, and that surgery was based on the following principles: soft-tissue releases of deforming spastic muscles, tendon transfers to augment antagonistic activity, and joint stabilization. In this study, patients with fair and good voluntary control had significantly greater improvement in functional use scores than those with poor voluntary control.

Selective injection of botulinum toxin (Botox) temporarily weakens or paralyzes a muscle by preventing the release of acetylcholine at the neuromuscular junction for 3 to 6 months, until nerve terminal sprouting occurs. The associated decrease in spasticity may allow stretching of the contractures to improve function, and may help in predicting the effect of muscle-tendon lengthening.

Annotated Bibliography

Cardon LJ, Ezaki M, Carter PR: Trigger finger in children. *J Hand Surg Am* 1999;24:1156-1161.

The authors review a large population of children with trigger digits. The thumb is the most commonly involved digit. Trigger fingers are uncommon, and may not respond to A-1 pulley release, requiring exploration of the flexor mechanism and resection of one slip of the flexor digitorum superficialis.

Dunsmuir RA, Sherlock DA: The outcome of treatment of trigger thumb in children. *J Bone Joint Surg Br* 2000;82:736-738.

The authors note 49% spontaneous recovery, leading to the recommendation of initial observation. Surgical outcomes were satisfactory.

Fitoussi F, Lebellec Y, Frajman JM, Pennecot GF: Flexor tendon injuries in children: Factors influencing prognosis. *J Pediatr Orthop* 1999;19:818-821.

The authors report that the results of flexor tendon repair in children are usually excellent. Short arm postoperative immobilization in younger children is associated with a higher rupture rate, and early mobilization and digital nerve injury do not affect the outcome. The authors recommend 4 weeks of immobilization.

James MA, McCarroll HR, Manske PR: The spectrum of radial longitudinal deficiency: A modified classification. *J Hand Surg Am* 1999;24:1145-1155.

The authors propose amending the Bayne classification of radius deficiency to include the carpal anomalies and thumb deficiency commonly seen with radius deficiency, based on review of radiographs of a large number of children with these conditions.

Jones K, Weiner DS: The management of forearm fractures in children: A plea for conservatism. *J Pediatr Orthop* 1999;19:811-815.

This articles presents the position that the incidence of complications with conservative treatment is very low and remains the gold standard for routine fracture treatment.

Kanaya F, Ibaraki K: Mobilization of a congenital proximal radioulnar synostosis with use of a free vascularized fascio-fat graft. *J Bone Joint Surg Am* 1998;80:1186-1192.

This article describes a new mobilization technique that has produced excellent results.

Kay S, McGuiness C: Microsurgical reconstruction in abnormalities of children's hands. *Hand Clin* 1999;4:563-583.

This is a comprehensive review of the application of microsurgical techniques to children's hand problems. The authors have a lower threshold than most surgeons for using these techniques in children.

Luhmann SJ, Gordon JE, Scoenecker PL: Intramedullary fixation of unstable both-bone forearm fractures in children. *J Pediatr Orthop* 1998;18:451-456.

Fracture management of skeletally immature patients who underwent only intramedullary fixation showed 84% of patients had excellent results and 16% had good results, using a grading scheme developed by Price.

McLaurin TM, Bukrey CD, Lovett RJ, Mochel DM: Management of thrombocytopenia-absent radius (TAR) syndrome. *J Pediatr Orthop* 1999;19:289-296.

This article discusses upper and lower extremity management. Lower extremity surgery is usually rejected.

Noonan KJ, Price CT: Forearm and distal radius fractures in children. *J Am Acad Orthop Surg* 1998;6:146-156.

Acceptable limits of deformity are defined and indications for surgical intervention are discussed in this article.

Pugh DM, Galpin RD, Carey TP: Intramedullary Steinman pin fixation of forearm fractures in children: Long-term results. *Clin Orthop* 2000;376:39-48.

Results of this study showed that time to union averaged 6 weeks; longer times were noted in patients older that 10 years of age.

Roser SE, Gellman H: Comparison of nail bed repair versus nail trephenation for subungual hematomas in children. *J Hand Surg Am* 1999;24:1166-1170.

Based on a prospective sequential study, the authors report that the size of a subungual hematoma is not predictive of the need for nailbed exploration and repair. If the nail is in place and the nail margin intact, then exploration and repair of the nail bed probably is not necessary.

Ruedi TP, Sommer C, Leutenegger A: New techniques in indirect reduction of long bone fractures. *Clin Orthop* 1998;347:27-34.

This article presents a discussion of indirect techniques of reduction and emphasizes preservation of blood supply to the bone.

Sheridan RL, Baryza MJ, Pessina MA, et al: Acute hand burns in children: Management and long-term outcome based on a 10-year experience with 698 injured hands. *Ann Surg* 1999;229:558-564.

Treatment recommendations for hand burns are provided.

Terry CL, Waters PM: Triangular fibrocartilage injuries in pediatric and adolescent patients. *J Hand Surg Am* 1998;23:626-634.

A series of children with triangular fibrocartilage complex tears are reviewed. This injury is more common than previously recognized, and diagnosis is often delayed. In children and adolescents, triangular fibrocartilage complex tears are usually repairable and the results of repair are good, but concomitant wrist injuries must also be appropriately treated.

Vilkki SK: Distraction and microvascular epiphysis transfer for radial club hand. *J Hand Surg Br* 1998;23:445-452.

The author describes free microvascular transfer of the second metatarsophalangeal joint to the distal ulna following correction of radial deviation by distraction, in a small number of children with Bayne type 4 radius deficiency (absent radius). Preliminary results are promising, but the technique is demanding and not yet widely applicable.

Wulff RN, Schmidt TL: Carpal fractures in children. *J Pediatr Orthop* 1998;18:462-465.

The authors report that the scaphoid is the carpal bone most commonly fractured in adolescents. The mechanism of injury is usually a low-energy fall, the fracture usually occurs in the distal pole, and cast immobilization usually results in successful union.

Classic Bibliography

Bayne LG, Klug MS: Long-term review of the surgical treatment of radial deficiencies. *J Hand Surg Am* 1987;12:169-179.

Benson LS, Waters PM, Kamil NI, Simmons BP, Upton J III: Camptodactyly: Classification and results of nonoperative treatment. *J Pediatr Orthop* 1994;14:814-819.

Buck-Gramcko D: Pollicization of the index finger: Method and results in aplasia and hypoplasia of the thumb. *J Bone Joint Surg Am* 1971;53:1605-1617.

Cheng JC, Shen WY: Limb fracture pattern in different pediatric age groups: A study of 3,350 children. *J Orthop Trauma* 1993;7:15-22.

Cole RJ, Manske PR: Classification of ulnar deficiency according to the thumb and first web. *J Hand Surg Am* 1997;22:479-488.

De Billy B, Gastaud F, Repetto M, Chataigner H, Clavert JM, Aubert D: Treatment of Madelung's deformity by lengthening and reaxation of the distal extremity of the radius by Ilizarov's technique. *Eur J Pediatr Surg* 1997;7:296-298.

Hahn MP, Richter D, Muhr G, Ostermann PA: Pediatric forearm fractures: Diagnosis, therapy and possible complications. *Unfallchirug* 1997;100:760-769.

Horii E, Nakamura R, Sakuma M, Miura T: Duplicated thumb bifurcation at the metacarpophalangeal joint level: Factors affecting surgical outcome. *J Hand Surg Am* 1997;22:671-679.

James MA, McCarroll HR Jr, Manske PR: Characteristics of patients with hypoplastic thumbs. *J Hand Surg Am* 1996;21:104-113.

Manske PR, Rotman MB, Dailey LA: Long-term functional results after pollicization for the congenitally deficient thumb. *J Hand Surg Am* 1992;17:1064-1072.

Manske PR, Halikis MN: Surgical classification of central deficiency according to the thumb web. *J Hand Surg Am* 1995;20:687-697.

Murphy MS, Linscheid RL, Dobyns JH, Peterson HA: Radial opening wedge osteotomy in Madelung's deformity. *J Hand Surg Am* 1996;21:1035-1044.

Ogino T, Kato H: Clinical and experimental studies on teratogenic mechanisms of congenital absence of digits in longitudinal deficiencies. *Cong Anom* 1993;33:187-196.

Slakey JB, Hennrikus WL: Acquired thumb flexion contracture in children: Congenital trigger thumb. *J Bone Joint Surg Br* 1996;78:481-483.

Chapter 33

Wrist and Hand: Trauma

Keith A. Glowacki, MD

Michael Hausman, MD

Julie A. Katarincic, MD

Kavi Sachar, MD

John Gray Seiler III, MD

Patrick Casey, MD

Distal Radius Fractures

Distal radius fractures are the most common fracture seen in orthopaedics and are characterized by a bimodal age distribution. Accurate reduction, whether it be through closed or open techniques, is correlated with prognosis.

The fracture pattern, degree of displacement, and stability of the fracture are factors that determine whether surgical treatment is necessary. Radial inclination, volar tilt, radial height, and amount of comminution all are standard methods to measure and determine existing or potential instability (Figs. 1 and 2).

Imaging techniques available to assess distal radius fractures include CT, arthrography, plain radiographs, fluoroscopy, and MRI. With the advent of arthroscopy and its use in reducing intra-articular distal radius fractures, associated carpal injuries are now being diagnosed more frequently. A CT scan can be used to determine the degree of intra-articular displacement and fracture fragment delineation. Approximately 50% of radial fractures are accompanied by soft-tissue injuries including those to the lunotriquetral ligament, scapholunate ligament, and triangular fibrocartilage complex (TFCC) which may be seen with MRI (Fig. 3).

Biomechanical testing in several studies has produced data that support the use of external fixation to augment surgical management of distal radius fractures. External fixation enhances stability with the addition of percutaneous Kirschner wires and bone grafting. Excessive traction on the capsuloligamentous structures of the wrist should be avoided. Pin tract infections and stiffness (complications of external fixation alone) should occur less often when external fixation is used to augment surgical treatment. In a study of augmented external fixation in a biomechanical analysis, augmentation with a single Kirschner wire in a cadaver model was significant. This model may be used to study other patterns and types of augmentation. Calcium-phosphate bone cement, compared with

Kirschner wires, produced results comparable to fixation with Kirschner wires in preventing settling of a comminuted distal radius fracture. Augmentation with both Kirschner wires and cement may allow for even less shortening. In a cadaver model, the tension placed across the wrist with application of an external fixator was studied. Most surgeons measure fluoroscopic carpal height during surgery and the ability to fully flex the fingers to determine appropriate tension. These techniques may not allow the surgeon to detect when excess traction is applied. This is an important factor in the prevention of stiffness and associated complex regional pain syndrome.

Nonsurgical treatment with cast immobilization is commonly used for extra-articular distal radius fractures. In one study in which the length of cast application was randomized, no significant difference between 1 and 3 weeks of plaster treatment on minimally displaced distal radius fractures was found, therefore supporting early mobilization for restoration of full function in this fracture type. Supportive splints were used in this study. Classification systems of distal radius fractures are numerous and there are great interobserver and intraobserver differences. The classification of extra-articular and intra-articular type fractures with increasing degree of instability and severity is the most common system used to determine treatment (Table 1). The options for surgical treatment include open reduction and internal fixation, percutaneous pinning, external fixation, augmentation with Kirschner wires or cannulated screws, and bone grafting (autogenous or allograft with or without bone substitutes).

Arthroscopically-assisted reduction was compared with open reduction and internal fixation. Thirty-four fractures were treated arthroscopically and 48 were treated with conventional open reduction and internal fixation. After an average follow-up of 31 months, accurate reduction with minimal capsular and soft-

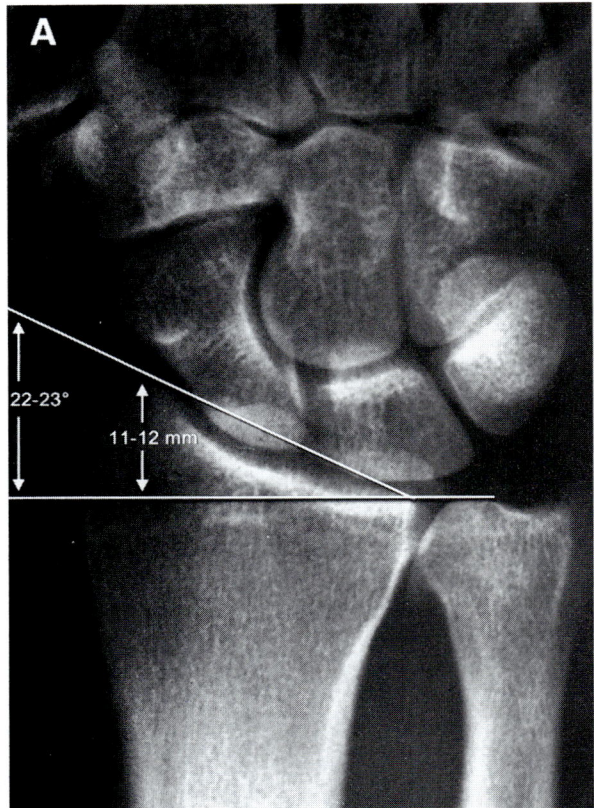

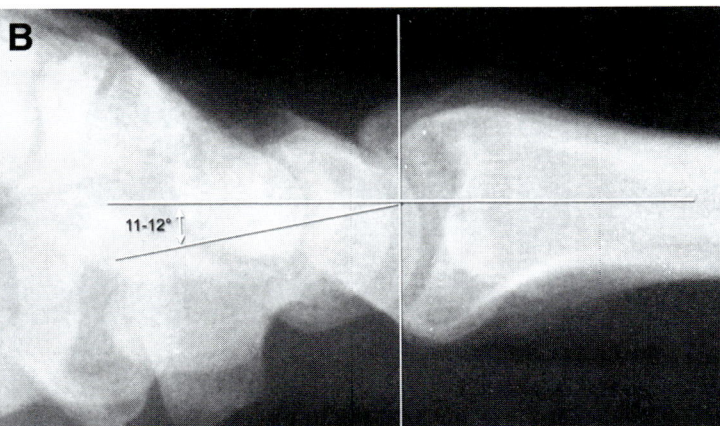

Figure 1 **A,** AP and **B,** lateral radiographs of the wrist showing normal angles, inclination 22° to 23°, tilt 11° to 12°, and length 11 to 12 mm.

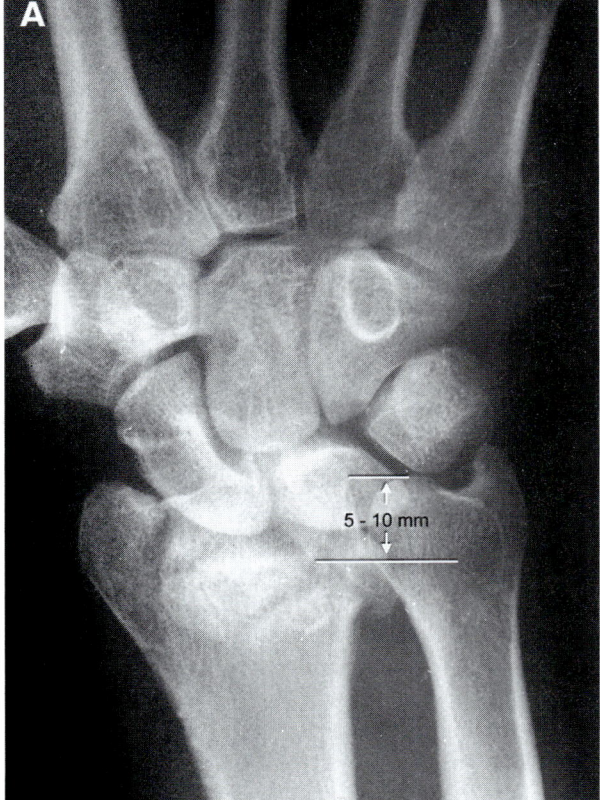

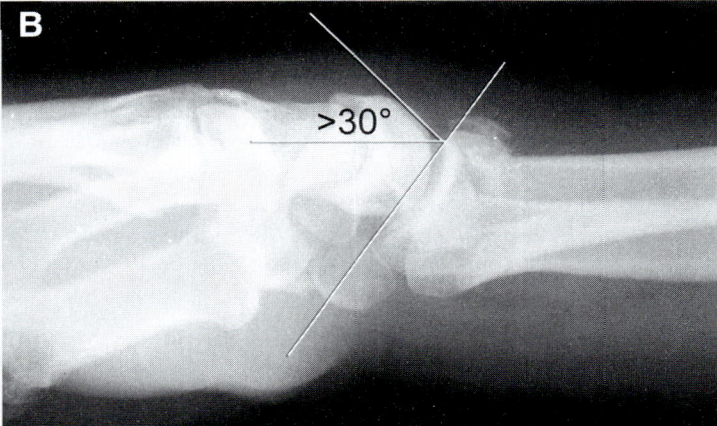

Figure 2 **A,** AP and **B,** lateral radiographs of the wrist showing instability, 5- to 10-mm shortening, > 25° dorsal tilt, and 2-mm articular step-off.

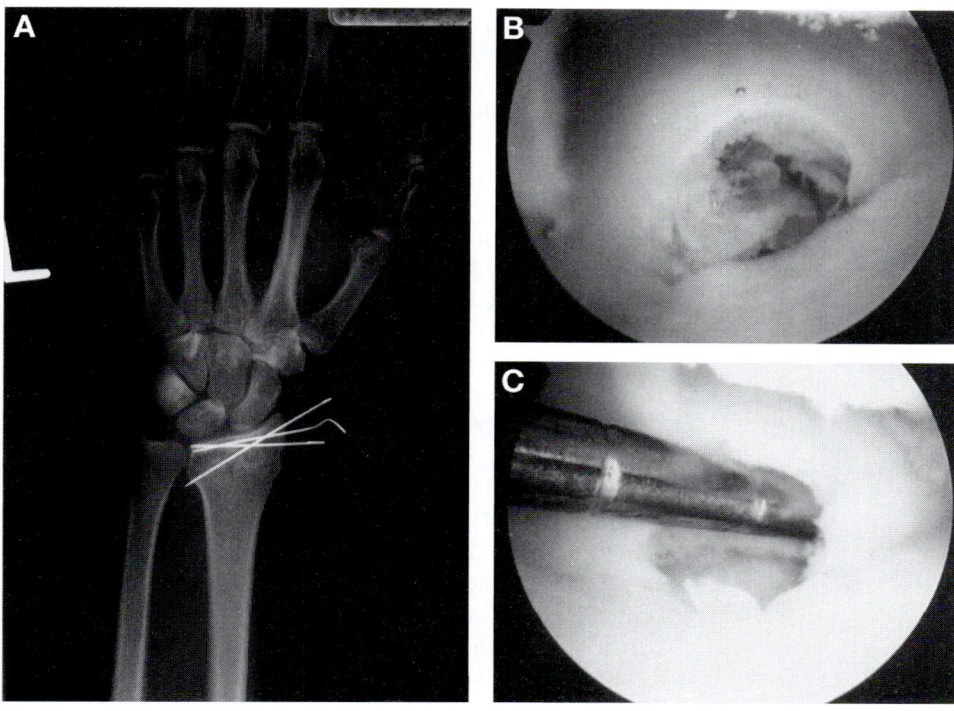

Figure 3 **A,** Plain radiograph, and **B** and **C,** arthroscopic view of intra-articular distal radius fracture and radial-sided TFCC tear in a young adult.

tissue scarring with arthroscopic assistance was noted, improving the overall results. With the high incidence of associated ligament injuries in high-energy distal radius fractures, arthroscopy is becoming more important in diagnosis and treatment.

Injuries About the Distal Ulna

Acute instability of the distal radioulnar joint (DRUJ) can occur with distal radius fractures, with distal ulnar articular and shaft fractures, and with forearm fractures such as the Galeazzi and Essex-Lopresti injuries. Radiographs of the wrist should always be obtained with complex elbow fractures/dislocations to avoid the pitfalls and delayed diagnosis of DRUJ instability. Simple reduction and pinning can be done acutely as opposed to a complex reconstruction of a chronically dislocated distal ulna. Distal radius fractures that include the sigmoid notch and basilar ulnar styloid fractures need to be examined for instability.

The imaging studies most often used, other than standard radiographs, include CT scans in various positions of pronation, neutral, and supination compared with the opposite uninvolved side. These studies can detect instability and/or subluxation at the DRUJ.

The primary factor predicting instability is the degree of dorsal dislocation and shortening in a distal radius fracture. When greater than 25° of dorsal angulation and 5 mm of shortening are found, there is a high incidence of TFCC injuries. Basilar ulnar styloid fractures, articular ulnar dome fractures, and sigmoid

notch injuries are also likely to involve the TFCC. Significant complications can occur after wrist fractures as a result of continued ulnar-sided wrist pain.

Acute instability with dislocation or subluxation can be in both a dorsal and volar direction. The DRUJ will dislocate when there is volar translation of the radiocarpal unit and dorsal displacement of the ulna known as a dorsal DRUJ dislocation. Dorsal subluxation of the radiocarpal unit with volar dislocation of the ulna would be termed a volar dislocation. Treatment includes closed reduction and, if stable on examination and by radiographic evaluation, casting for 6 weeks with a long arm cast in either supination for a dorsal dislocation or pronation for a volar dislocation. Should instability persist, surgical reduction and removal of interposed soft tissue with pinning of the DRUJ just proximal to the sigmoid notch and immobilization for 6 weeks are recommended. Widening of the DRUJ and displacement of the distal ulna on lateral radiographs also are signs of instability at the DRUJ.

Carpal Instability

Carpal instability is classified into two major instability patterns associated with scapholunate and lunotriquetral ligament injury: dorsal intercalary segment instability (DISI) and volar (or palmar) intercalary segment instability (VISI or PISI). This classification describes common instability patterns caused by rupture of the scapholunate and lunotriquetral ligaments, respectively. Perilunate instability is caused by forceful loading of

TABLE 1	Treatment Recommendations for Distal Radius Fractures

Extra-articular

Nondisplaced	Cast immobilization (early splint fabrication with range of motion exercises)
Displaced	
Reducible	Cast without comminution
Stable	Pinning/bone graft with comminution
Unstable	Closed reduction/percutaneous pinning
	+/− Ex-Fix
	+/− Bone graft
	Intrafocal pinning

Intra-articular

Nondisplaced	Pin fixation/cannulated screws
Displaced	
Simple (two parts)	AAR-P arthroscopy
	Cannulated screws
	+/− Bone graft/Ex-Fix
Complex (more than two-part)	
Volar fracture/dislocation	Volar plate
	+/− Bone graft
	+/− Ex-Fix
Die-punch	AAR; bone graft
	+/− Ex-Fix
Severe comminution	ORIF
	+/− Ex-Fix
	+/− Bone graft

Ex-fix = external fixation; AAR-P = arthroscopically-assisted reduction and pin fixation; AAR = arthroscopically-assisted reduction; ORIF = open reduction and internal fixation

the wrist in dorsiflexion. Injury progresses in a predictable, clockwise manner from the scaphoid or scapholunate ligament across the midcarpal joint and lunatotriquetral joint, with the end result being a transscaphoid perilunate fracture dislocation, or its purely ligamentous variant, perilunate dislocation.

Scapholunate Instability

Scapholunate instability is caused by injury to the scapholunate interosseous ligament, comprising three distinct sections. The dorsal part of the ligament, with transversely oriented collagen fibers, is the strongest segment, effectively hinging the two bones together while permitting limited rotation about the dorsal lig-

ament and separation of the palmar surfaces. Continued loading beyond the yield point of the ligament will cause permanent deformation or rupture that propagates in a palmar to dorsal direction. The degree of injury to the scapholunate ligament, as well as to the secondary restraints such as the radioscaphocapitate ligament, determines whether a static deformity with a scapholunate diastasis (Terry-Thomas sign), called carpal instability-dissociative will occur or whether the instability will be of a more subtle, dynamic form, carpal instability-nondissociative (CIND) which becomes apparent only when the wrist is loaded (Fig. 4).

Radiographic hallmarks of scapholunate instability include an increased scapholunate angle (normally 30° to 57°) and diastasis between the scaphoid and lunate bones, which may be apparent only in grip stress radiographs (Fig. 4). A fixed, static deformity assumes the characteristic DISI pattern, with an increased scapholunate angle and dorsally tilted lunate. Over time, a characteristic degenerative pattern will occur with arthrosis at the radial styloid-scaphoid interval, followed by capitolunate arthrosis. This pattern is known as scapholunate advanced collapse (SLAC) and the changes are attributed to incongruity between the boat-shaped scaphoid and the scaphoid fossa of the radius (Fig. 5). The minimum injury conditions necessary to cause progressive collapse are unknown and isolated scapholunate injury may not progress to SLAC without concomitant injury to the radioscaphocapitate or radiolunate ligaments.

Patients with scapholunate instability complain of radial-sided and dorsoradial wrist pain that is aggravated by forceful use and gripping. There may be subtle swelling due to chronic synovitis over the scapholunate joint. The scaphoid shift test is done by pressing over the distal pole of the scaphoid as the wrist is moved from ulnar to radial deviation. If scapholunate instability is present, flexion of the scaphoid will be blocked and cause dorsal subluxation of the proximal pole that spontaneously reduces with a clunking sound when pressure is removed from the distal pole. Triple injection arthrography can demonstrate scapholunate lunotriquetral ligament tears with an accuracy and specificity of 60% and 83%, respectively, compared to arthroscopy.

Lunotriquetral Instability

Rupture of the lunotriquetral ligament, also thought to occur from forceful dorsiflexion or a sudden twisting injury, is associated with volar instability and tilting of the lunate (VISI). Isolated lunotriquetral ligament rupture alone will not result in a VISI deformity without collateral damage to the ulnar arcuate ligament complex or dorsal radiotriquetral and scaphotriquetral lig-

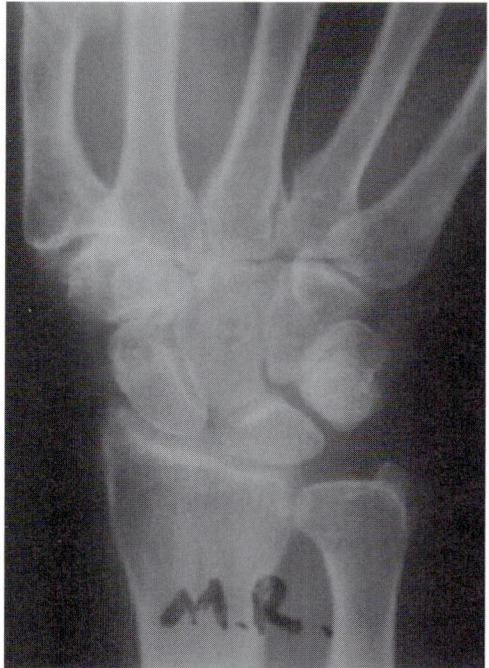
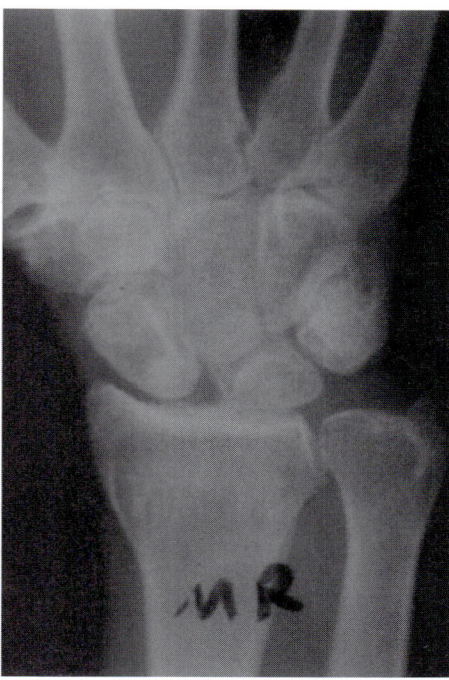

Figure 4 Dynamic scapholunate instability. The foreshortening of the scaphoid and Terry-Thomas sign are apparent in the grip-stress view on the right.

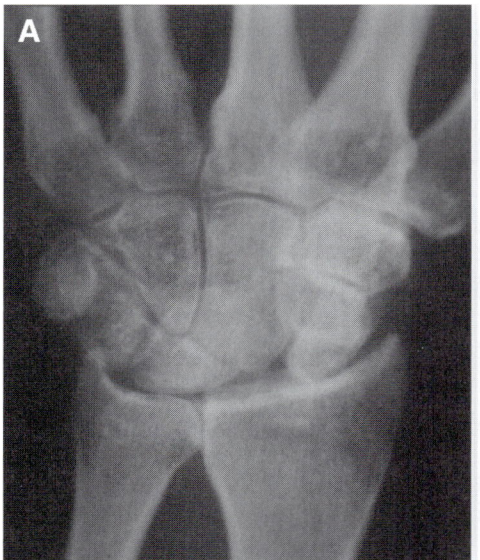
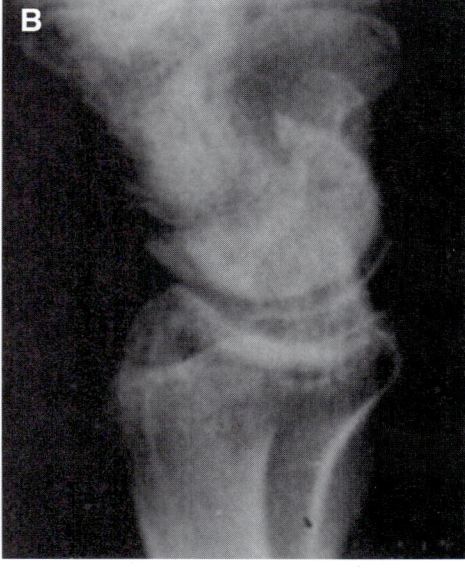

Figure 5 SLAC wrist. Note the characteristic radioscaphoid and capitolunate arthrosis, loss of carpal height and DISI instability pattern **(A)**. These conditions are easily seen on the lateral view **(B)**, but the quadrangular lunate, and triquetrum in the "high" or distal position on the hamate indicate that the lunate is dorsiflexed.

aments. Injury to the luntotriquetral ligament also has resulted from palmar flexion.

An established VISI deformity will be apparent on plain radiographs as a palmar tilted lunate. The scapholunate angle may be decreased and the longitudinal axis drawn through the third metacarpal and capitate will pass palmar to the longitudinal axis of the radius. Posteroanterior and lateral radiographs in radial and ulnar deviation frequently demonstrate asynchronous motion of the proximal carpal row and a break in Shenton's line of the wrist. Lunotriquetral lig-

ament rupture is best observed with triple-injection arthrography or MRI (Fig. 6).

Midcarpal Instability

Patients with midcarpal instability complain of ulnar-sided wrist pain and grip weakness, especially while twisting against resistance. The injury is caused by forced dorsiflexion or twisting. On physical examination, a dorsal-palmar shear force across the midcarpal joint may also produce a pronounced clunking sound

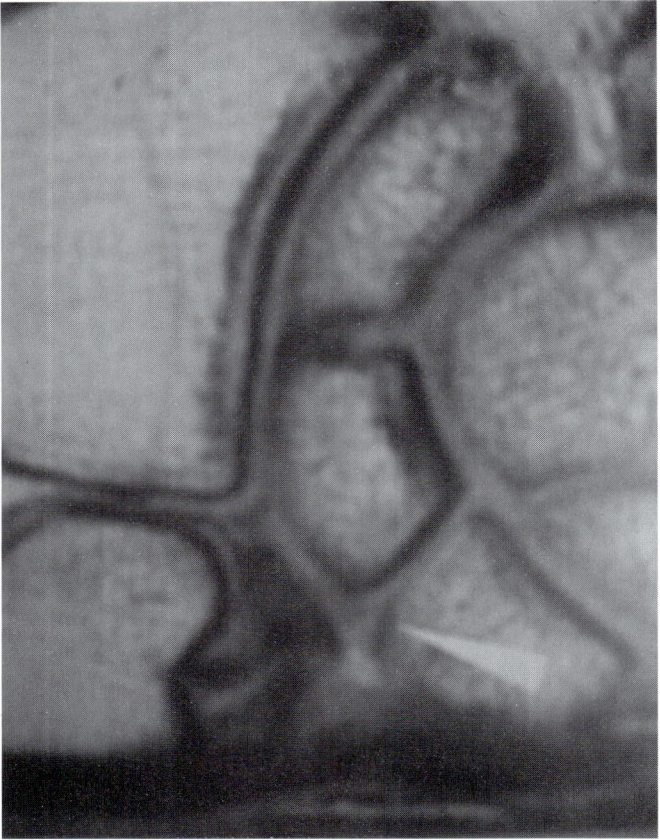

Figure 6 Gradient-echo MRI technique demonstrates low signal intensity in the intact scapholunate ligament, but rupture of the lunotriquetral ligament (*arrow*).

indicative of instability. Moving the wrist from radial to ulnar deviation also can result in instability.

Cineradiography in the lateral projection is the best imaging study to assess midcarpal instability. As the wrist is moved from radial to ulnar deviation, a sudden shift of the midcarpal joint is seen with the hamate and capitate perched on the dorsum of their respective articular surfaces with the triquetrum and lunate. MRI and arthroscopy may show synovitis and capsuloligamentous degeneration in the dorsum of the midcarpal joint. Midcarpal instability also has been reported after malunion of distal radial fractures with dorsal angulation. However, it is not known if bony malalignment alone will cause midcarpal instability without a concomitant ligament injury. Midcarpal instability has been classified into dorsal (original capitolunate instability pattern), palmar, nondissociative, and extrinsic variants with different pathologic findings and treatments (Table 2).

Treatment

Open reduction and anatomic repair are advocated for acute scapholunate, lunatotriquetral, or perilunate instabilities, but the results are variable and recurrence of the deformity is frequently seen. For the correction of chronic or static deformities, various intercarpal arthrodeses, including scaphocapitate, scapholunate, and scaphotrapezial-trapezoid have been attempted; good results have been reported in more than 90% of cases. All intercarpal arthrodeses compromise motion to some degree, with motion after scaphotrapezial-trapezoid fusion reported in 65% to 80% of the uninjured wrist.

The results of ligament reconstruction using tendon grafts show variable relief of symptoms but frequent radiographic failure, reflecting the challenge of reproducing the function of the intact scapholunate ligament complex. Bone-ligament-bone graft complexes from the dorsum of the hand or the foot are currently under investigation. Scapholunate arthrodesis has a nonunion rate as high as 60%. However, the observation that even nonunions may remain stable and asymptomatic led to proposal of the reduction and association of the scaphoid and lunate procedure, which intentionally recreates a fibrous pseudarthrosis between the scaphoid and lunate using a Herbert screw. A small amount of rotation of the scapholunate joint is preserved, which may account for the good results reported, although long-term review is lacking.

There seems to be consensus on the treatment of dynamic instability. Dorsal capsulodesis or some variation of the procedure seems to confer symptomatic relief in more than 90% of cases, even in the presence of persistent or recurrent scapholunate diastasis, although some series report less success.

Treatment of lunotriquetral instability is also controversial. Primary ligament repair or reconstruction with a distally based slip of the extensor carpi ulnaris tendon in chronic cases with degenerated ligaments has been advocated. Lunotriquetral arthrodesis has a nonunion and failure rate of up to 50%. Other problems that may complicate treatment include ulnar impaction, which may require concomitant ulnar shortening and TFCC repair, or symptomatic lunatohamate arthrosis.

Ligament Injuries of the Hand

The classification system for ligamentous injuries of the digits is based on whether or not the ligament tear is incomplete or complete and whether or not the accessory stabilizing structures are injured. Grade I injuries represent intrasubstance or partial ligament tears. Grade II injuries represent a complete proper collateral ligament tear but with integrity of the volar plate attachment and accessory collateral ligament. Grade III injuries represent a complete ligament tear with instability secondary to rupture of the volar plate and accessory collateral ligament.

TABLE 2 | Classification of Midcarpal Instability

Suggested Terminology	Original Terminology and Reference	Proposed Etiology	Direction of Subluxation	Suggested Surgical Treatment
Palmar midcarpal instability	Ulnar midcarpal instability	Laxity of: Ulnar arm arcuate ligament Dorsal radiolunotriquetral ligament	Palmar	Limited carpal arthrodesis
Dorsal midcarpal instability	Capitolunate instability pattern Chronic capitolunate instability	Laxity of palmar radioscaphocapitate ligament	Dorsal	Palmar capsular reefing (radioscaphocapitate to radiolunotriquetral)
Midcarpal CIND	CIND	Either of above or ulnar minus variant	Palmar and/or dorsal	Depending on etiology (arthrodesis, ligament repair, or ulnar lengthening)
Extrinsic midcarpal instability	Midcarpal instability secondary to radial malunion	Dorsal displacement and angulation of distal radius; adaptive Z deformity of carpus	Dorsal	Corrective radial osteotomy

CIND is a more inclusive category of carpal instabilities, including palmar and dorsal midcarpal instability and radiocarpal instabilities, but excluding proximal row dissociative lesions
(Reproduced with permission from Lichtman DM, Bruckner JD: Palmar midcarpal instability: Results of surgical reconstruction. J Hand Surg Am 1993;18:307–315.)

Proximal Interphalangeal Joint Dislocations and Ligament Injuries

Isolated collateral ligament injuries of the distal interphalangeal (DIP) and proximal interphalangeal (PIP) joints may result in prolonged discomfort and stiffness. Gross instability in a border digit may require surgical repair.

Most PIP joint ligament injuries occur during PIP joint dislocations. Dorsal dislocations result in distal rupture of the volar plate with or without a bony fragment. In pure dorsal dislocations, the collateral ligaments remain intact. Posterolateral PIP dislocations result in a tear of the volar plate, accessory collateral ligament, and proper collateral ligament. An inability to obtain a concentric closed reduction in dorsal dislocations implies soft-tissue interposition by the volar plate, lateral band, or collateral ligament. This situation may require open reduction. Treatment of stable dorsal and posterolateral PIP joint dislocations that have been reduced closed should focus on early controlled motion, edema control, and avoidance of a flexion contracture.

In contrast to dorsal dislocations, palmar dislocations may injure the central slip. Treatment requires immobilization of the PIP joint with either an extension splint or Kirschner wire for 4 weeks, allowing DIP motion.

Metacarpophalangeal Joint Collateral Ligament Injuries

Metacarpophalangeal (MCP) joint collateral ligament injuries most commonly involve the radial collateral ligament (RCL) of the index or small finger accompanied by a malrotated or deviated digit. Sagittal band ruptures may coexist. The digit is examined in full flexion to place the collateral ligament under maximum tension. Grade I and II injures can be treated with buddy taping and early motion. If there is any evidence of malrotation or uncorrectable lateral deviation, surgical repair is necessary. The ligament can be repaired directly, with a pull-out button or suture anchor. Early active motion should be started to avoid a flexion contracture and extensor lag. Small finger RCL injuries have a greater likelihood to remain unstable because of the pull of the abductor digit minimi.

Chronic collateral ligament instability of the MCP joint can be successfully treated with a tendon graft. Long-term results show excellent return of function, pain relief, and absence of degenerative changes.

Thumb Metacarpophalangeal Joint Collateral Ligament Injuries

Ulnar collateral ligament injuries of the thumb occur as a result of forceful radially deviated stress across the partially flexed thumb MCP joint. If the ulnar collateral ligament is displaced superficial to the adductor aponeurosis (Stener's lesion), surgical repair is necessary to reapproximate the ligament ends. The MCP joint is tested in 30° of flexion to isolate the proper collateral ligament and full extension to test the accessory collateral ligament and palmar plate. Clinically unstable MCP joints are treated with surgical repair.

Surgical techniques include direct repair, repair over a pull-out button, arthroscopic reduction of the Stener's lesion, and repair using suture anchors. In a series of 36 patients in whom a suture anchor technique was used, loss of MCP motion averaged 10° and collateral ligament stability was restored in all patients. No complications were encountered with use of the suture anchor.

Ulnar collateral ligament injuries can be associated with fractures of the base of the proximal phalanx. A Stener's lesion should be suspected with a widely displaced avulsion fragment. Clinical examination continues to be important because nondisplaced fractures can be associated with grade III injuries.

Surgery is necessary to stabilize clinically unstable complete tears of the RCL. These injuries can involve associated injuries to the dorsal capsule and abductor pollicis brevis as evidenced by radiographic palmar subluxation. Persistent painful instability may require repair or arthrodesis.

Thumb Carpometacarpal Dislocations

Thumb carpometacarpal (CMC) dislocations result in injuries to the volar beak ligament and dorsal RCL. Closed reduction is often easy to achieve. Treatment options consist of cast immobilization, closed pinning of the CMC joint, or early ligament reconstruction. According to one study, closed pinning alone resulted in CMC instability or arthritis in 50% of patients; immediate ligament reconstruction with a flexor carpi radialis weave resulted in preservation of motion, grip strength, and absence of pain.

Metacarpal and Phalangeal Fractures

Most fractures of the digits and hand can be treated nonsurgically with short-term cast immobilization followed by early protected motion. Indications for surgical intervention include significant malrotation or angulation, displaced articular fractures, open fractures, fractures combined with tendon injuries, and multiple fractures.

Fractures involving the distal phalanx are often the result of crush injuries and involve nailbed lacerations. Comminuted tuft fractures are treated by repair of the nail bed, which aligns the comminuted fragments. Solid bony union is rare, but fibrous union will result in stability and pain relief. Transverse fractures at the base

of the distal phalanx are unstable secondary to the pull of the profundus tendon on the distal fragment and usually involve avulsion of the germinal matrix. Fracture fixation is achieved with a Kirschner wire that crosses the DIP joint.

Stable shaft fractures of the proximal and middle phalanx can be treated with cast immobilization followed by early protected motion. Angulation or shortening of unstable fractures may result in an extensor lag. When internal fixation is necessary, Kirschner wires minimize soft-tissue trauma, thereby reducing tendon adhesions. When plate fixation is used, immediate motion must be instituted to prevent dorsal extensor tendon adhesions.

In fifth metacarpal neck fractures, up to 50° of angulation can be tolerated. Lesser degrees are acceptable in the more radial metacarpals. No malrotation is acceptable. For stable fractures, intermittent splint immobilization or functional bracing are as effective as cast immobilization. The complications from plate fixation are lower in the fifth metacarpal neck than in the phalanges, yet extensor tendon adhesions are still problematic.

Articular fractures of the MCP and interphalangeal joints require anatomic alignment. Condylar fractures of the PIP joint have characteristic fracture patterns. Fixation usually requires open reduction to correct malrotation that is often present.

Thumb Metacarpal Base Fracture Dislocations

Fractures at the base of the thumb metacarpal include nondisplaced intra-articular fractures, fracture-dislocations involving separation between the ulnar beak ligament fragment and the dislocation of the remaining metacarpal (Bennett's fracture), and Y-shaped intra-articular fractures (Rolando's fracture). Treatment of the entire injury spectrum focuses on anatomic reduction of the articular component and reduction of the dislocation.

Nondisplaced Bennett's fractures can be treated with a well-molded cast. Frequent radiographs are necessary to evaluate articular displacement and joint subluxation. Displaced Bennett's fractures are often easy to reduce but are inherently unstable because the main stabilizing ligament, the beak ligament, is attached to the ulnar fragment. Closed reduction and pinning is achieved with traction, pronation, and downward pressure over the dorsal radial base of the extended, palmarly abducted thumb. Anatomic reduction is important to minimize the risk of CMC arthritis. Kirschner wire fixation should cross the CMC joint and pin the thumb to the second metacarpal. It is not necessary to pin the Bennett's fragment as long as an anatomic, stable reduction is obtained. Screw fixation can be used in large fragments and allows for early CMC motion.

Proximal Interphalageal Joint Fracture Dislocations

PIP fracture dislocations remain one of the most difficult injuries to treat in the hand. The mechanism of injury involves an axial load applied to a hyperextended PIP joint. Treatment centers around adequate contour of the joint surfaces and maintaining stability of the PIP joint while encouraging motion.

With volar lip fragments consisting of less than 30% of the articular surface, dislocation can usually be prevented with extension block splinting that is gradually diminished over 3 to 4 weeks. The congruency of the volar fragment is less important than regaining a full arc of flexion.

Larger fragments often result in gross instability of the PIP joint. Treatment options consist of open reduction and internal fixation, dynamic traction, dynamic external fixation, and volar plate arthroplasty. Joint reduction, whether closed or open, is the best treatment. Open reduction may be carried out through a midlateral or Brunner approach. The joint reduction can then be maintained with small Kirschner wires. Bone grafting may be necessary to elevate the volar fragment. Fixation should allow for early motion and a dynamic external fixator should be applied if necessary. According to one series in which this technique was used, the average PIP range of motion was 12° to 84°. Complications included redislocation, septic arthritis, pin tract infections, and breakage of the compass hinge.

When comminution is high or a pilon type injury exists, exposure can be obtained through a volar gunstock approach, allowing complete dislocation of the joint and bone repair with a cerclage wiring technique with or without bone grafting.

For comminuted fragments that cannot be fixed, volar plate arthroplasty is an alternative. Either a pullout suture or minianchor can be used to reattach the volar plate. Long-term results revealed a high incidence of posttraumatic arthritis in one series. Despite poor motion and radiographic arthritis, there were few functional deficits.

Flexor Tendon Repair

Transection of the flexor tendons in zone 2 continues to be one of the more challenging problems in hand surgery. By using recent advances in the basic science of tendon repair, surgical methods of repair, and rehabilitation, satisfactory outcomes can be obtained in 80% of patients with zone 2 flexor tendon injuries. Despite precise surgical technique and strict adherence

to a rehabilitation program, additional problems such as adhesions and rupture still occur.

Basic Science

Investigations reporting on the biology of flexor tendon repair have been focused in three general areas: biologic substances that modulate tendon repair, ways to prevent peritendinous adhesion formation, and suture methods. Several experimental studies have demonstrated substantial roles for endothelial growth factor (EGF), basic fibroblast growth factor (bFGF), and transforming growth factor (TGF) in modulating tendon cells and the repair environment (Table 3).

Prevention of adhesions after flexor tendon surgery continues to be a significant focus for basic science research. Peritendinous flexor tendon adhesions formed after injury are associated with fibroblast upregulation in the synovial sheath that is caused by increased production of cytokines (TGF-β1). Treatment with TGF-β1 Ab increases range of motion. 5-fluorouracil also appears to decrease peritendinous adhesions without affecting the structural integrity of the healing tendon.

The use of externally applied devices has also been investigated to control adhesion formation. Expanded polytetrafluoroethylene has been used to reconstruct the synovial sheath in the zone of the repair and demonstrate decreased adhesion formation.

Recent biomechanical studies have concluded that the application of load to the tendon influences the composition of the extracellular matrix. Unloaded tendons demonstrated progressive matrix degradation and decreased proteoglycan and collagen content.

Repair site gliding is another important biomechanical stimulus to tendon healing. In a recent study that examined partially lacerated flexor tendons of chickens, tendons exposed to both motion and tension showed the greatest amount of repair site strength, collagen deposition and cell proliferation at the repair site.

Surgical Principles

The suture material, suture size, number of suture strands crossing the repair site, and geometry of the repair all affect the initial tensile strength of the repair site. The location of the core suture in the tendon is important. Several studies have reported that placement of the core stitch in the dorsal portion of the tendon increases repair site strength. The number of strands crossing a tendon repair site correlates with improved initial tensile strength in flexor tendon repairs. Two-strand suture methods were associated with significantly greater gap formation than four or

TABLE 3	Stages of Repair for Intrasynovial Flexor Tendons

Inflammatory phase (0 to 14 days)

Fibrin clot forms at the repair site

Macrophage migration and leukocyte migration to the repair site

Fibronectin production peaks (chemotaxis)

bFGF production peaks

Cells from the epitenon proliferate and migrate to the repair site

Gliding surface is restored

Immediately following repair the strength of the repair is related to the strength of the suture and the suture method

Reparative phase (2 to 6 weeks)

Intense collagen production, mostly type I

Fibers of collagen are laid down randomly and gradually orient themselves along the axis of tensile forces

Neovascularization of the repair site occurs

TGF production peaks

At 2 weeks following repair the repair site strength may decrease but it increases during this period as collagen deposition occurs at the repair site

Remodeling phase (6 weeks or longer)

Collagen remodelling

Decreased rates of cell division

Increase in repair site strength

Nerve entubulation: advantages

Minimizes trauma to nerve ends

Allows resection of up to 3 cm of total nerve tissue

Isolates the zone of repair

Allows accumulation of trophic factors

Fibrin matrix that forms orients itself in a longitudinal direction

Gap offers options for advancing axons

Nerve entubulation: disadvantages

May result in compression of the nerve ends

May require a second procedure for removal of the tube

six strands. Although gap formation of less than 3 mm did not promote adhesion formation or impair range of motion, it may be associated with an increased rate of rupture.

Six- and eight-strand suture methods reportedly are associated with significantly improved early repair strength compared with two-strand repair methods. A running epitendinous suture significantly adds to the strength of the repair. Neither time from repair nor suture method significantly affected interphalangeal

(distal and proximal) joint rotation or linear tendon excursion. The effect of suture strength is most significant during the first 3 weeks after repair.

The treatment of partial flexor tendon lacerations is controversial. Although results from animal studies show successful management of partial lacerations of up to 70% of the tendon with protected motion, repair of lacerations of more than 50% of the tendon is recommended to prevent entrapment or triggering.

Pediatric flexor tendon injuries have poorer outcomes in patients younger than 5 years, when the injury is in zone 2, when both tendons are lacerated, or when a below-elbow splint is used. The overall repair site rupture rate is 9%. Based on this finding, use of a postoperative above-elbow cast for 4 weeks is recommended.

Postoperative Rehabilitation

Most programs use dorsal splint protection with passive or early active motion protocols. According to a prospective, randomized multicenter trial with 1-year follow-up, multistrand, multigrasp repair methods and controlled active digital mobilization are associated with improved postoperative range of motion, less joint contracture, and an improved outcome with similar rupture rates compared with passive mobilization.

Delayed Flexor Tendon Reconstruction Using Tendon Grafting

Occasionally, primary tendon repair is unsuccessful or not possible, and delayed tendon reconstruction may be necessary. In the use of silicone rods for flexor tendon reconstruction, stage I rod implantation had a complication rate of 16.5%, whereas stage II rod implantation for graft exchange had a complication rate of 10%. Several authors have reported that intrasynovial donor tendons can be repaired by intrinsic mechanisms, are associated with less peritendinous adhesion formation when compared with extrasynovial tendon grafts, and have superior functional and mechanical characteristics.

Extensor Tendon Repair

Experimental studies have shown that the strength of extensor and flexor tendon repairs after load application is similar. The beneficial effects of controlled motion after extensor tendon repair have been reported. The feasibility of two-stage extensor tendon reconstruction achieving acceptable proximal interphalangeal joint flexion with minimal extensor lag also has been reported.

Nerve Repair

Basic Science

The beneficial effects of various growth factors improve nerve regeneration in animal models. Recent basic science and clinical studies have suggested that peripheral nerve entubulation can be a reasonable alternative to peripheral nerve repair. This method, which secures cut nerve ends within a hollow tube, can be used for peripheral nerve repair and for the reconstruction of peripheral nerves, which would traditionally require a short nerve graft.

Vein grafts and hollow synthetic tubes have been used successfully in experimental nerve reconstruction with defects less than 4 cm. In a prospective, randomized clinical trial that compared conventional nerve repair with nerve entubulation using a silicone tube for patients who had sustained median or ulnar nerve injuries at the wrist, touch perception was improved with entubulation at 3 months; no other differences were found.

Methods of Nerve Repair

Epineural suture repair is currently the most common method of peripheral nerve repair. Short-term immobilization (3 weeks) after nerve repair is often instituted. A cadaver study of human digital nerve defects found that the repair site could withstand full digital range of motion if less than 2.5 mm of nerve was resected at the time of repair.

Clinical Results of Nerve Repair

The best results of nerve repair occur in young patients with clean, sharp nerve transactions. The digital nerve is the most commonly injured in the upper extremity. Injuries to major mixed peripheral nerves are less common and are associated with a poorer outcome. Results from a study of 15 patients with combined median nerve, ulnar nerve, and flexor tendon injuries showed that the majority only achieved protective sensation with modest motor recovery. Motor recovery showed continued improvement for at least 4 years after repair.

Results of median and ulnar nerve repair in children are superior to those of adults. Eighteen children (average age, 6.1 years) with median nerve injury underwent epineural repair and were evaluated 1 year after repair. Five mm, two-point sensation was reported 1 year after median nerve repair. Similar results were reported after ulnar nerve repair. Good motor recovery was observed.

Fingertip Injuries

Treatment for fingertip injuries should be individualized to each patient, considering such factors as age, general health, occupation, and the patient's wishes. The goals of treatment should be the return of near-normal sensibility, early bone healing, good digital motion, and satisfactory appearance that will allow for the early return to activity. The most simple and efficacious classification system involves classifying the injury as either soft tissue only or soft-tissue and bony involvement.

Conservative treatment that allows healing by secondary intention continues to be effective. In fingertip injuries involving isolated skin and pulp loss, healing by primary closure and secondary intention (letting the wound granulate) remains the preferred method of treatment, with 90% good or excellent results. This treatment regimen is typically used for clean wounds of less than 1 cm² in area. Healing takes approximately 1 month. A number of occlusive dressings that protect the fingertip during the healing process are available. The use of split-thickness skin grafting has been reported to lead to poor results when compared with closed or open treatment because of loss of sensibility at the tip and possible complications that could be avoided by conservative management.

In soft-tissue and bony involvement, the primary goals are to reduce pain, prevent infection, and allow for reasonable long-term function. If there is only a minimal amount of exposed bone, healing by secondary intention may be successful, especially in children. The other common option is the use of local flaps including volar V-Y advancement flap, double V-Y flap, thenar flap, cross finger flaps, and a homodigital island flap. In addition, some bone shortening followed by primary closure or healing by open techniques have provided good results.

Infections

Elevation, immobilization, and antibiotic therapy combined with surgical débridement, if necessary, have been the mainstay of treatment for hand infections. The most common organism present in upper extremity soft-tissue infections is *Staphylococcus aureus.* There have been increasing reports of methicillin-resistant *S aureus,* atypical mycobacterium, and group A streptococcus (sometimes associated with necrotizing fasciitis).

An additional and continuing problem is mycobacterial upper extremity infections. Approximately one third of the world's population has tuberculosis; 40% to 50% of these individuals have extrapulmonary involvement. According to the literature, *Mycobacte-*

rium marinum is the most common pathogen in superficial infections, followed by *Mycobacterium avium-intracellulare* as the pathogen for deep infections. One complicating factor in the treatment of these infections is delay in diagnosis; the symptoms are often treated as a synovitis. Identification requires a prolonged incubation time of up to 8 to 10 weeks for mycobacteria with special cultures incubated at 30°C to 32°C on Lowenstein-Jensen agar. "Red snappers" (groups of acid-fast bacilli) may also be seen on a Ziehl-Neelson stain. If these particular organisms are not tested for in the initial culture, results are often negative.

The majority of patients who develop atypical mycobacterial infections require surgical débridement and antimicrobial therapy. An additional atypical organism is *Mycobacterium septicum,* which carries an association to patients at risk for colon cancer.

Infections remain a challenge in the patient with diabetes. Multiple studies have shown that increased rates of amputations are associated with deep infections, renal failure, and infections with gram-negative anaerobes or polymicrobes. In addition, it is not atypical for multiple surgeries to be required before the infection can be completely treated. Patients with human immunodeficiency virus are at risk for upper extremity infections from skin flora and *Pseudomonas.*

The incidence of group A streptococcus infections has been increasing in recent years. These patients may or may not develop necrotizing fasciitis and typically have severe infections that are rapidly progressive, with or without minor preceding trauma. These patients usually are older with chronic diseases, are on prolonged steroids, or are immunosuppressed for other reasons. Necrotizing fasciitis can be seen without soft-tissue air on the radiographs. If present, rapid surgical débridement with amputation, if necessary, is required to prevent a limb-threatening disease from becoming life-threatening.

Burns

Approximately 100,000 patients per year are admitted to the hospital with burns; the mortality rate is 5%. In children, scalding is the most frequent mechanism of burn injury, and males between 17 and 30 years old are most frequently seriously burned by flammable liquids. Structural fires account for 45% of burn-associated deaths. The American Burn Association's criteria for referral to a specialized burn center are listed in Table 4.

Pathophysiology

Burn severity relates to the depth of tissue destruction, with thermal energy a function of temperature

TABLE 4	American Burn Association's Criteria for Referral to a Specialized Burn Center

> 10% TBSA burned if younger than 10 years or older than age 50 years

> 20% TBSA burned in other ages

> 5% TBSA full-thickness burns

Burns of privileged areas (hands, feet, face, genitalia, perineum)

Electrical/lightning burns

Inhalational injuries

Patients with significant underlying medical problems

and time. The zones of coagulation, stasis, and hyperemia describe the depth of burning. Coagulated areas are irreversibly damaged, whereas the hyperemic zone will survive. In the static zone, timely intervention may limit burn damage. Histamine and bradykinin that is released upon activation of the complement and coagulation systems increase capillary permeability, producing edema that further decreases perfusion.

Capillary leakage with major burns (> 30% total body surface area [TBSA]) causes generalized edema due to "third-spacing" or extracellular accumulation of fluid. Paradoxical hypovolemia further decreases tissue perfusion and may cause multiple organ failure. Other effects include tumor necrosis factor-β depression of myocardial contractility, impaired pulmonary function, and generalized immunosuppression that results in fatal infections.

Initial Treatment

First Degree

The epidermis remains intact (no dermal injury) and is dry, red, and sensate. No therapy beyond analgesia is required.

Second Degree

Burns destroying the epidermis and penetrating the dermis are sensate, red, moist and edematous. Superficial partial-thickness burns will heal in 7 to 10 days with minimal risk of scarring. Deep, partial-thickness burns take up to 21 days or more to heal. The risk of hypertrophic scarring increases with time to healing. Necrotic debris and ruptured blisters should be removed and the wound washed with mild soap and water. Small, clean, superficial partial-thickness burns less than 24 hours old can be managed with any of the semipermeable membrane dressings available until healed. Wounds that are too large, deep, old, or otherwise unsuitable for occlusive dressings require daily dressings along with a topical antimicrobial agent. Silver sulfadiazine has a broad spectrum of activity and is the agent of choice. Mafenide has better eschar penetration, but can cause metabolic acidosis. Mobile surfaces such as the hands or elbows are splinted until epithelial coverage is reestablished and motion is begun. Protracted splinting and the use of silicone sheeting or elastomer pressure molds may be necessary for scar remodeling to prevent contracture.

Third Degree

Third degree (full-thickness) burns appear dry, white or brown, contracted, and are insensate. Major burns require fluid resuscitation. The Parkland formula (intravenous Ringer's lactate solution, 4 mL/kg body weight/% burn) is the accepted standard in fluid requirement calculation for the first 24 hours. Half of the solution is administered over the first 8 hours from the time of burn, with the remainder administered over the next 16 hours. Low-dose dopamine infusions (3 to 5 mg/kg/min) help to restore renal and splanchnic blood flow. At 24 hours after the time of the burn, the endothelium is less leaky and colloids are administered (5% albumin in Ringer's lactate at 0.5 mL/kg/% burn) to maintain intravascular volume. Urinary output of 30 to 50 mL per hour (1 mL/kg/h in children) indicates adequate resuscitation. The serial hematocrit is not used because hemoconcentration is expected. When patients fail to respond, a serious underlying medical condition or a significant inhalation injury is indicated and invasive monitoring is necessary. Carbon monoxide intoxication requires 100% oxygen and respiratory support for chemical pneumonitis.

Escharotomies

Inextensable eschar, combined with generalized edema, jeopardizes circulation to the extremities and must be decompressed. Escharotomies should be done in the midlateral lines of limbs and digits to prevent joint exposure. With massive edema, fasciotomies may also be required, particularly if multiple trauma has occurred.

Nutritional Support

Nasogastric (or preferably nasojejunal) feeding is begun as soon as possible and is critical to maintain mucosal integrity and prevent bacterial translocation from the gut, causing systemic sepsis. Initial caloric requirements are based on the Curreri formula (25 kcal/kg + 40 kcal/% TBSA). A kcal to nitrogen ratio of 100:1 and at least 2 g of protein/kg/day are supplied. Prealbumin levels are used to monitor nutritional support.

Wound Management

Surgical intervention is indicated for full-thickness burns and in those unlikely to heal in less than 3 weeks (to decrease the likelihood of unacceptable scarring). Tangential excision down to viable tissue is the treatment of choice. Tourniquets, topical thrombin, phenylephrine hydrochloride, or 1:1,000,000 epinephrine infiltration will minimize bleeding. Deep and large burns can be débrided at the fascial level to limit bleeding at the expense of late contour deformities and decreased mobility. Autologous split-thickness skin grafts (8/1,000 to 12/1,000 of an inch) remain the gold standard for wounds that cannot be directly closed. Thin grafts have better rates of healing but cause more late contracture. In cosmetically sensitive areas and small to moderate wounds, sheet grafting should be considered. Otherwise, meshed grafts are used to increase graft healing, coverage, and decrease graft loss if the wound becomes infected.

Skin Substitutes

Various products and combinations of products are available or are undergoing active investigation. Temporary skin substitutes decrease water loss, prevent wound desiccation, promote faster reepithelialization, and decrease mechanical trauma and pain. Porcine xenografts adhere to clean superficial wounds via fibrin bonding during reepithelization. Porcine xenografts do not vascularize and are held in place under dry dressings. Various proprietary single-layer synthetic membranes are available that function similarly. Biobrane is a bilayer of nylon fabric partially embedded in a silicone film. Blood and sera clot in the fabric, attaching the dressing to the wound. The dressing is trimmed during reepithelialization and the dressing separates. All of these products are effective occlusive dressings and are subject to submembrane purulence if used to cover devitalized tissue. Several temporary allogeneic substitutes incorporating live human fibroblasts currently are being investigated.

Electrical Injury

Electrical injury is associated with multiple trauma in 15% of affected patients. The apparent cutaneous injury does not necessarily reflect the degree of tissue involvement. Cardiac monitoring is indicated if the patient has a history of arrest, arrhythmia, or abnormal electrocardiogram. Myocardial damage can be ruled out by serial creatinine kinase (MB) fractions. Muscle damage, most commonly occurs around the electrical current entry and exit points. Technetium Tc 99m muscle scanning can be used to diagnose the extent of muscle damage. Resuscitation requirements are based on the apparent cutaneous injury. Additional fluid is given when underlying muscle damage is present. If the urine is pigmented, a single treatment of 2 ampules of sodium bicarbonate and 2 ampules of mannitol are given in intravenous Ringer's lactate. Urine output should be maintained between 100 to 125 mL/h until pigmentation disappears. Close observation of the extremities is warranted because compartment syndrome is a distinct possibility. Mafenide is used topically because of its tissue penetration and gram-negative bacterial action.

Chemical Burns

The extent of chemical burns is often underestimated on initial examination. The immediate treatment of chemical injuries consists of copious tap water irrigation. Some chemicals will continue to burn until specific additional measures to neutralize the burning process are applied. Burns caused by hydrofluoric acid require topical or subcutaneous administration of calcium carbonate gel. Phosphorus-induced burns must be kept wet until emergent surgical débridement. Polyethylene glycol or vegetable oil should be applied to phenol burns. Appropriate texts should be consulted for all chemical burns.

High-Pressure Injection Injuries

High-pressure injection injuries can cause vascular compression, compartment syndrome, and severe necrosis in addition to the direct toxic effect of the injected substance. These injuries are severe and the amputation rate may approach 48%.

Clinical Presentation

The patient may notice only a small puncture wound, which belies the severity of the injury, and results in a delay of treatment until pain, swelling, dysesthesias or dysvascular changes become apparent. Injected material frequently contains solvents and petroleum distillates, which have a direct cytotoxic effect in addition to provoking an inflammatory reaction. Vascular thrombosis is common. The severity of the injury correlates with the amount of material injected, which can be substantial with fluid nozzle speeds approaching 600 ft/s and operating pressures of up to 12,000/psi. The injected substance travels along paths of least resistance, including fascial planes and tendon sheaths, and the toxin may thus spread over a considerable distance from the site of injury (Fig. 7). Radiographs may show the extent of infiltration of radiopaque substances. Palmar injection sites have a better prognosis than digital entry points.

Treatment

Tetanus toxoid is administered, if indicated by the patient's immunization history, and immediate and aggressive surgical débridement of foreign material and necrotic tissue is done along with copious irrigation. Wide exposure is critical to adequately decompress affected compartments and to remove toxic material.

Mircrosurgery and Replantation

Microsurgery has become more commonplace as a part of orthopaedic practice. Historically, its primary use

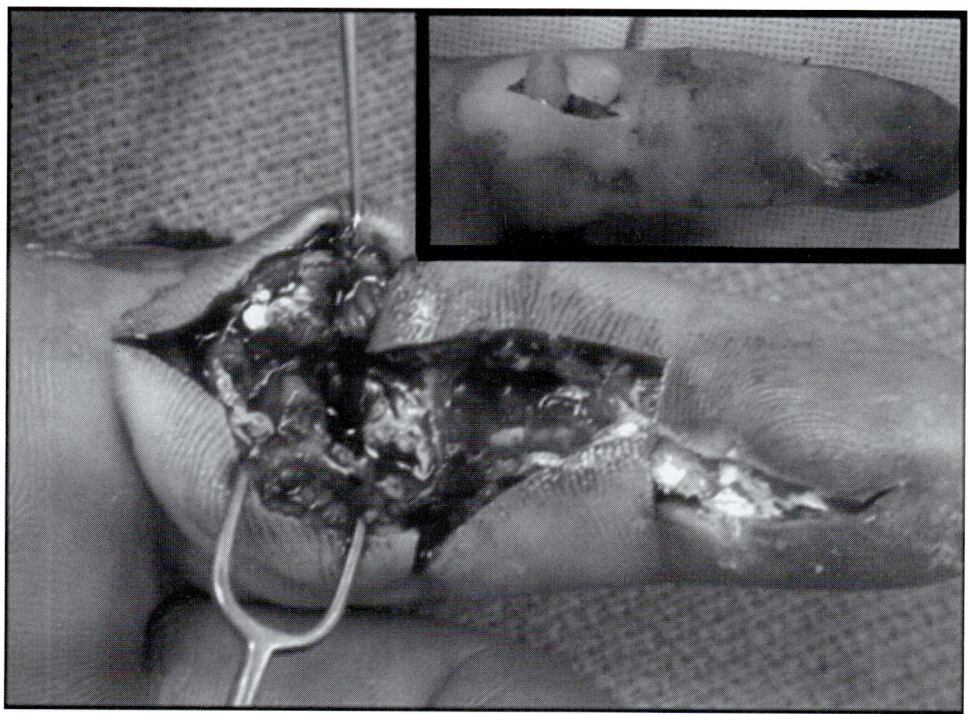

Figure 7 Inset, left index finger at presentation 3 days after high-pressure paint gun injury. Entry at the fingertip and abscess draining paint/pus at proximal phalanx. Main photo shows paint at the time of initial débridement.

has been in reconstruction of digits in trauma and tumor patients and extremity replantation and revascularization. Recently, the use of neurotized free muscle transfers for the reconstruction of paralyzed limbs, primarily in patients with brachial plexus injuries, has become more prevalent. The survival rate for elective free flaps continues to be about 95%. This rate is somewhat lower in the trauma situation and the success rate is even lower with replants or revascularizations.

It is important when using free flaps in the trauma situation that adequate débridement of all potentially nonviable tissues is performed before soft-tissue coverage. In addition, it is critical to ensure that the anastomoses is performed out of the zone of injury to minimize the chances of failure. Monitoring flap survival by inspection is still vital. Recent reports have discussed the use of implantable Doppler probes placed on the venous anastomoses in the first 48 hours after surgery, allowing for 100% detection of a thrombus and salvage of all compromised flaps. Experimental rat studies demonstrate no difference in patency between the end-to-side and end-to-end anastomoses.

The latissimus dorsi is the main muscle used in free tissue transfers. It is a large muscle for transfer and may be potentially neurotized with minimal morbidity related to the harvest site. Shoulder function remains excellent with minimal scarring. Seroma formation is the most common complication.

With more stringent safety precautions in the workplace, replantation has decreased over the past decade. Typically, indications for replantation are a single digit amputated distal to the superficialis insertion, multiple digits, any thumb injury, or any replanted digit in children.

An amputated part should be wrapped in a saline-soaked gauze in a sturdy plastic bag placed on ice. Patient age, any associated medical conditions, smoking status, type of injury, and duration of ischemia are factors to consider before replantation is done. Warm ischemia time should typically be less than 6 hours. Because of the minimal muscle present in fingertips, they remain potentially viable up to 12 hours. Ischemia time can be prolonged to 24 hours by cooling the digits. Poor long-term function may also preclude replantation. Amputation requiring arthrodesis may be unsatisfactory for patients with occupations that require grip. Patients in cooler climates or with jobs requiring prolonged cold exposure may find the pain associated with a replanted digit to be so debilitating that they request an elective amputation.

In children, the success rate tends to be slightly lower than that of adults for several reasons. The mechanism of injury is typically an avulsion, which has poorer success rates compared with clean lacerations.

The vessels are much smaller and more prone to vasospasm. If the revascularized vessels did not look viable immediately after repair, the chances of survival of the replanted digit are quite low. Forty-one percent of children require a transfusion, so diligent overall medical care is necessary. Long-term bone growth was reported to be 88% of the normal digit if the joint was involved and 93% if the joints were not involved.

A recent study compared patients treated with replantation in a matched set to those treated with amputation for injuries at or proximal to the wrist level. In evaluating these patients and considering total function, replantation produced better functional results than amputation and prosthesis. This study noted that prehension should be the goal of primary treatment. It is doubtful that a similar study examining digital replantation versus amputation would show similar results secondary to increased problems of stiffness at this level.

Annotated Bibliography

Distal Radius Fractures

Doi K, Hattori Y, Otsuka K, Abe Y, Yamamoto H: Intra-articular fractures of the distal aspect of the radius: Arthroscopically assisted reduction compared with open reduction and internal fixation. *J Bone Joint Surg Am* 1999;81:1093-1110.

Thirty-four fractures were treated arthroscopically and 48 with conventional open reduction and internal fixation. The average follow-up was 31 months. Outcome scores were assessed by various systems. Functional and radiographic results showed that patients who had an arthroscopically assisted procedure had better reduction of volar tilt, ulnar variance, and articular displacement. The arthroscopically-assisted group also showed significantly better range of motion in flexion, extension, and radial deviation of the wrist.

Dunning CE, Lindsay CS, Bicknell RT, Patterson SD, Johnson JA, King GJ: Supplemental pinning improves the stability of external fixation in distal radius fractures during simulated finger and forearm motion. *J Hand Surg Am* 1999;24:992-1000.

This study created an unstable fracture model in cadavers. Fracture motion was measured when postoperative finger and forearm motions were simulated. The addition of radial styloid pins to a construct of an external fixator significantly improved fragment stability approaching that of a dorsal plate. Regardless of technique, fragment motion occurred with finger and forearm motion.

Herrera M, Chapman CB, Roh M, Strauch RJ, Rosenwasser MP: Treatment of unstable distal radius fractures with cancellous allograft and external fixation. *J Hand Surg Am* 1999;24:1269-1278.

Seventeen patients had freeze-dried or irradiated cancellous bone allograft used to treat unstable distal radius fractures with metaphyseal comminution. The outcome using the modified Mayo Wrist Score demonstrated three excellent, eight good, six fair, and no poor results. The average follow-up was 23 months.

Kawaguchi S, Sawada K, Nabeta Y, Hayakawa M, Aoki M: Recurrent dorsal angulation of the distal radius fracture during dynamic external fixation. *J Hand Surg Am* 1998;23:920-925.

Thirty-three fractures of the distal radius were treated with dynamic external fixation, allowing motion between 2 and 4 weeks after surgery. Attention was paid to the loss of fracture reduction, specifically dorsal angulation. Fractures with preoperative dorsal angulation greater than 20° had significantly larger loss of reduction than those fractures with less severe dorsal angulation or those with an intact DRUJ. Preoperative shortening greater than 2 mm and involvement of the radiocarpal joint did not significantly increase the loss of dorsal angulation with dynamic fixation.

Ladd AL, Pliam NB: Use of bone-graft substitutes in distal radius fractures. *J Am Acad Orthop Surg* 1999;7:279-290.

This study reviews the present bone graft substitutes available for distal radius fractures and describes their composition and use.

Spence LD, Savenor A, Nwachuku I, Tilsley J, Eustace S: MRI of fractures of the distal radius: Comparison with conventional radiographs. *Skeletal Radiol* 1998;27:244-249.

In 21 patients with distal radius fractures, conventional radiographs and MRI scans were compared. Forty-eight percent of these patients had associated soft-tissue injuries (six scapholunate ligament ruptures, two TFCC disruptions, and one tear of a dorsal radiocarpal ligament). The study found that MRI evaluated not only the osseous injury but the accompanying soft tissue injuries.

Trumble TE, Wagner W, Hanel DP, Vedder NB, Gilbert M: Intrafocal (Kapandji) pinning of distal radius fractures with and without external fixation. *J Hand Surg Am* 1998;23:381-394.

Sixty-one patients with dorsally displaced extra-articular distal radius fractures were treated with either intrafocal pinning alone or in combination with external fixation. Older patients had significantly improved results when external fixation was used even when only one cortex of the radius was comminuted. Younger patients showed good results with interfocal pinning alone when only one surface was comminuted. When more than two sides were comminuted, the younger patients had better results with external fixation. This study also found that restoration of radial length had the most significant effect on range of motion and grip strength.

Wolfe SW, Lorenze MD, Austin G, Swigart CR, Panjabi MM: Load-displacement behavior in a distal radial fracture model The effect of simulated healing on motion. *J Bone Joint Surg Am* 1999;81:53-59.

This biomechanical study observed the load-displacement behavior of a distal radial fracture model in which they simulated partial healing with caulk to mimic the effect of early removal of an external fixator in a partially healed fracture model. Various constructs were augmented with Kirschner wire fixation. All augmented constructs were significantly more stable than nonaugmented constructs. Results of this study support early removal of external fixation when augmentation is performed with either bone graft or Kirschner wires in a partially healed fracture.

Injuries About the Distal Ulna

Faierman E, Jupiter JB: The management of acute fractures involving the distal radio-ulnar joint and distal ulna. *Hand Clin* 1998;14:213-229.

Fracture pattern recognition is discussed, which will help to determine treatment based on a stable or unstable injury.

Carpal Instability

Berger RA: Arthroscopic anatomy of the wrist and distal radioulnar joint. *Hand Clin* 1999;15:393-413.

This article provides a review of normal arthroscopic anatomy and pathologic findings in patients with TFCC and intercarpal ligament injuries.

Ligament Injuries of the Hand

Deitch MA, Kiefhaber TR, Comisar BR, Stern PJ: Dorsal fracture dislocations of the proximal interphalangeal joint: Surgical complications and long-term results. *J Hand Surg Am* 1999;240:914-923.

Short-term results and long-term complications were evaluated in patients treated with either volar plate arthroplasty or open reduction and internal fixation for dorsal PIP fracture-dislocations. The postoperative complication rate was 18%; redislocation was the most frequent complication. Over the long term, 96% of patients had degenerative changes but few had functional deficits.

Hansen PB, Hansen TB: The treatment of fractures of the ring and little metacarpal necks: A prospective randomized study of three different types of treatment. *J Hand Surg Br* 1998;23:245-247.

Three different treatment methods were evaluated in ring and small metacarpal neck fractures: ulnar gutter splint, functional wrist brace, and elastic bandage. There was no difference in patient satisfaction. Functional bracing led to faster mobilization and less pain, making it the authors' treatment of choice.

Kuz JE, Husband JB, Tokar N, McPherson SA: Outcome of avulsion fractures of the ulnar base of the proximal phalanx of the thumb treated nonsurgically. *J Hand Surg Am* 1999;24:275-282.

Avulsion fractures of the base of the ulnar collateral ligament were treated nonsurgically. The nonunion rate was 25% and instability rate 10%. Patients with nonunions tended to have larger fragments with greater initial rotation. Despite the nonunion and instability rates, all patients were satisfied with their treatment.

McDermott TP, Levin LS: Suture anchor repair of chronic radial ligament injuries of the metacarpophalangeal joint of the thumb. *J Hand Surg Br* 1998;23: 271-274.

Five cases of chronic instability of the thumb radial collateral ligament are discussed. Repair consisted of use of a Mitek anchor to reattach the avulsed ligament. A stable thumb MCP joint was achieved in each case.

Page SM, Stern PJ: Complications and range of motion following plate fixation of metacarpal and phalangeal fractures. *J Hand Surg Am* 1998;23:827-832.

In this retrospective study of modern plate fixation techniques in the hand, major complications including stiffness, nonunion, plate prominence, infection, and tendon rupture were encountered in 36% of fractures. Complications were highest in open phalangeal fractures.

Riederer S, Nagy L, Buchler U: Chronic post-traumatic radial instability of the metacarpophalangeal joint of the finger: Long-term results of ligament reconstruction. *J Hand Surg Br* 1998;23:503-506.

The authors discuss results from 24 patients who underwent radial collateral ligament reconstruction of the index MCP joint using a free tendon graft. Eighty percent of patients had excellent or good results, with relief of pain, return of stability, a near normal range of motion, and absence of degenerative changes.

Rosenstadt BE, Glickel SZ, Lane LB, Kaplan SJ: Palmar fracture dislocation of the proximal interphalangeal joint. *J Hand Surg Am* 1998;23:811-820.

Thirteen patients were followed for an average of 55 months. PIP motion averaged 91° for acute injuries and 70° for chronic injuries. Complications included loss of reduction, swan neck deformity, and DIP extensor lag.

Vahey JW, Wegner DA, Hastings H III: Effect of proximal phalangeal fracture deformity on extensor tendon function. *J Hand Surg Am* 1998;23:673-681.

The effects of proximal phalangeal fracture angulation on extensor function was evaluated in a cadaver study. A linear relationship between extensor tendon lengthening and resulting PIP lag was observed. Similarly, a linear relationship between proximal phalangeal shortening and the lag was observed.

Flexor Tendon Repair

Bidder M, Towler DA, Gelberman RH, Boyer MI: Expression of mRNA for vascular endothelial growth factor at the repair site of healing canine flexor tendon. *J Orthop Res* 2000;18:247-252.

Canine flexor tendons that were repaired were analyzed for mRNA of vascular EGF. The highest concentration of vascular EGF was seen at the repair site, while a smaller concentration was seen in the uninjured area of tendon.

Boardman ND, Morifusa S, Saw SS, McCarthy DM, Sotereanos DG, Woo SL: Effects of tenorraphy on the gliding function and tensile properties of partially lacerated canine digital flexor tendons. *J Hand Surg Am* 1999;24:302-309.

Tendon repair was not beneficial if up to 70% of the tendon was lacerated. These flexor tendons could be treated without primary repair.

Chang J, Thunder R, Most D, Longaker MT, Lineaweaver WC: Studies in flexor tendon wound healing: Neutralizing antibody to TGF-beta 1 increases postoperative range of motion. *Plast Reconstr Surg* 2000;105: 148-155.

Flexor tendons in rabbits were transected and repaired and given either phosphate buffer solution (control), TGF-β1 antibodies, or TGF-β1 and TGF-β2 antibodies. TGF-β1 may reduce adhesion formation following flexor tendon repair.

Gelberman RH, Boyer MI, Brodt MD, Winters SC, Silva MJ: The effect of gap formation at the repair site on the strength and excursion of intrasynovial flexor tendons: An experimental study on the early stages of tendon healing in dogs. *J Bone Joint Surg Am* 1999;81: 975-982.

Sixty-four canine flexor tendons were lacerated, repaired, and examined for gap formation at the repair site at 10, 21, and 42 days. Tendon repairs that had a gap formation of 3 mm or more were noted to have decreased tensile strength and stiffness 42 days after repair compared with tendons with less gap formation. Gap formation of 3 mm or more was not associated with an increase in adhesions or impaired range of motion. Gap formation of 3 mm or more at the repair site may be associated with an increased risk for rupture.

Moran SL, Ryan CK, Orlando GS, Pratt CE, Michalko KB: Effects of 5-fluorouracil on flexor tendon repair. *J Hand Surg Am* 2000;25:242-251.

Flexor tendons of chickens were lacerated, repaired, and a topical dose of 0, 5, 25, or 50 mg/mL of 5-fluorouracil was given. The tendons were immobilized for 3 weeks after repair. The 25 mg/mL dose appeared to be the most effective at reducing the work of flexion and preventing postoperative adhesions. Histologic specimens of the tendons that had 5-fluorouracil application demonstrated satisfactory tendon repair.

Strickland JW: Development of flexor tendon surgery: Twenty-five years of progress. *J Hand Surg Am* 2000;25: 214-235.

An excellent review of flexor tendon basic science, repair techniques, and postoperative rehabilitation is presented.

Extensor Tendon Repair

Crosby CA, Wehbe MA: Early protected motion after extensor tendon repair. *J Hand Surg Am* 1999;24: 1061-1070.

Thirty hands with 50 extensor tendon injuries in zones 3 to 7 were treated with early passive motion and dynamic splinting. Forty-five of the 50 tendon injuries regained full range of motion, and five patients had extensor lags of less than 10°. All patients returned to full activity, and 93% of patients regained full strength.

Nerve Repair

Bolitho DG, Boustred M, Hudson DA, Hodgetts K: Primary epineural repair of the ulnar nerve in children. *J Hand Surg Am* 1999;24:16-20.

Nineteen children who were 13 years of age or younger with ulnar nerve injuries underwent epineural repair. The average muscle grade for the first dorsal interosseous and abductor digiti minimi were 4.0 and 3.9 respectively (scale 0-5). The average two-point sensation was 6 mm. Proximal ulnar nerve injuries carried a worse prognosis.

Polatkan S, Orhun E, Polatkan O, Nuzumlali E, Bayri O: Evaluation of the improvement of sensibility after primary median nerve repair at the wrist. *Microsurgery* 1998;18:192-196.

Twenty-eight patients with sharp median nerve lacerations at the wrist underwent epiperineural repair and were evaluated an average of 25 months after repair. Excellent results were seen in 35.7%, good results in 28.5%, fair results in 14.2%, and poor results in 21.4%. Younger age correlated with better outcome.

Rosen B, Dahlin LB, Lundborg G: Assessment of functional outcome after nerve repair in a longitudinal cohort. *Scand J Plast Reconstr Surg Hand Surg* 2000;34: 71-78.

Nineteen patients with either median or ulnar nerve injuries were followed up periodically from the time of injury to 4 years postoperatively.

Fingertip Injuries

Adani R, Busa R, Scagni R, Mingione A: The heterodigital reversed flow neurovascular island flap for fingertip injuries. *J Hand Surg Br* 1999;24:431-436.

This type of flap is an option for patients who have limited reconstructive options short of free tissue transfer.

Martin C, Gonzalez del Pino J: Controversies in the treatment of fingertip amputations: Conservative versus surgical reconstruction. *Clin Orthop* 1998;353:63-73.

This article presents a summary of the treatment options for patients with fingertip amputations.

Infections

Gonzalez MH, Bochar S, Novotny J, Brown A, Weinzweig N, Prieto J: Upper extremity infections in patients with diabetes mellitus. *J Hand Surg Am* 1999;24: 682-686.

A review of 45 diabetic patients with 46 infections is presented. Twenty-three required more than one operation with the presence of polymicrobial infection, renal failure, and deep infections being associated with an increased rate of amputation.

Hoyen HA, Lacey SH, Graham TJ: Atypical hand infections. *Hand Clin* 1998;14:613-634.

A summary of atypical infections including mycobacteria, fungus, and other opportunistic infections that may be seen in the upper extremity is presented.

Karanas YL, Bogdan MA, Chang J: Community acquired methicillin-resistant Staphylococcus aureus hand infections: Case reports and clinical implications. *J Hand Surg Am* 2000;25:760-763.

Four cases of community acquired methicillin-resistant *S aureus* in patients without preceding risk factors are reviewed.

Burns

Kao CC, Garner WL: Acute burns. *Plast Reconstr Surg* 2000;105:2482-2493.

A comprehensive summary of diagnosis, evaluation, resuscitation, and treatment of thermal burns is presented.

Purna SK, Babu M: Collagen based dressings: A review. *Burns* 2000;26:54-62.

An exhaustive review of dressing products and their classification with particular emphasis on collagen products is presented.

Sheridan RL, Tompkins RG: Skin substitutes in burns. *Burns* 1999;25:97-103.

This article presents a thorough review of currently available skin substitutes and ongoing efforts to create a permanent skin substitute.

High-Pressure Injection Injuries

Schnall SB, Mirzayan R: High-pressure injection injuries to the hand. *Hand Clin* 1999;15:245-248.

A historical review of high-pressure injection injuries including emergency, surgical, and antibiotic management is presented.

Microsurgery and Replantation

Boulas HJ: Amputations of the fingers and hand: Indications for replantation. *J Am Acad Orthop Surg* 1998;6:100-105.

Replantation including care of parts, variables affecting outcome, risks, indications, and contraindications as well as results are discussed.

Cheng GL, Pan DD, Zhang NP, Fang GR: Digital replantation in children: A long-term follow-up study. *J Hand Surg Am* 1998;23:635-646.

This article presents long-term results of replantation in children showing 88% to 93% of longitudinal growth.

Doi K, Muramatsu K, Hattori Y, et al: Restoration of prehension with the double free muscle technique following complete avulsion of the brachial plexus: Indications and long-term results. *J Bone Joint Surg Am* 2000;82:652-666.

Thirty-two patients had a staged double free latissimus transfer for restoration of elbow flexion, finger extension, and finger flexion; 96% regained satisfactory elbow flexion and 65% satisfactory prehension.

Dotson RJ, Bishop AT, Wood MB, Schroeder A: End-to-end versus end-to-side arterial anastomosis patency in microvascular surgery. *Microsurgery* 1998;18:125-128.

The patency of microsurgical end-to-end and end-to-side anastomoses in the rat carotid artery were both found to be 100%. The decision of the anastomoses type should, therefore, be based on the situation presented by each particular surgical case.

Graham B, Adkins P, Tsai T-M, Firrell J, Breidenbach WC: Major replantation versus revision amputation and prosthetic fitting in the upper extremity: A late functional outcomes study. *J Hand Surg Am* 1998;23:783-791.

A group of 22 patients undergoing successful upper extremity replantations were compared with 22 amputees. On a functional level, replantation produced superior results. Young patients with more distal levels of injury regained better function.

Kind GM, Buntic RF, Buncke GM, Cooper TM, Siko PP, Buncke HJ Jr: The effect of an implantable Doppler probe on the salvage of microvascular tissue transplants. *Plast Reconstr Surg* 1998;101:1268-1273.

A miniature Doppler ultrasonic probe was used to monitor the venous anastomoses in the first 48 hours postoperatively. In the 147 flaps monitored, 20 cases of thrombus were identified and all 20 flaps were able to be salvaged.

Classic Bibliography

Adams BD: Staged extensor tendon reconstruction in the finger. *J Hand Surg Am* 1997;22:833-837.

Berger RA: The gross and histologic anatomy of the scapholunate interosseous ligament. *J Hand Surg Am* 1996;21:170-178.

Blatt G: Capsulodesis in reconstructive hand surgery: Dorsal capsulodesis for the unstable scaphoid and volar capsulodesis following excision of the distal ulna. *Hand Clin* 1987;3:81-102.

Bowers WH: Instability of the distal radioulnar articulation. *Hand Clin* 1991;7:311-327.

Flotre M: High-pressure injection injuries of the hand. *Am Fam Physician* 1992;45:2230-2234.

Fortin PT, Louis DS: Long-term follow-up of scaphoid-trapezium-trapezoid arthrodesis. *J Hand Surg Am* 1993;18:675-681.

Gelberman RH, Posch JL, Jurist JM: High-pressure injection injuries of the hand. *J Bone Joint Surg Am* 1975;57:935-937.

Hudson DA, Bolitho DG, Hodgetts K: Primary epineural repair of the median nerve in children. *J Hand Surg Br* 1997;22:54-56.

Jackson D: The diagnosis of the depth of burning. *Br J Surg* 1953;40:588-596.

Janzekovic Z: A new concept in the early excision and immediate grafting of burns. *J Trauma* 1970;10:1103-1108.

Kleinman WB: Long-term study of chronic scapho-lunate instability treated by scapho-trapezio-trapezoid arthrodesis. *J Hand Surg Am* 1989;14:429-445.

Kozin SH, Bishop AT: Atypical Mycobacterium infections of the upper extremity. *J Hand Surg Am* 1994;19:480-487.

Lichtman DM, Bruckner JD, Culp RW, Alexander CE: Palmar midcarpal instability: Results of surgical reconstruction. *J Hand Surg Am* 1993;18:307-315.

Lichtman DM, Schneider JR, Swafford AR, Mack GR: Ulnar midcarpal instability: Clinical and laboratory analysis. *J Hand Surg Am* 1981;6:515-523.

Linscheid RL, Dobyns JH, Beabout JW, Bryan RS: Traumatic instability of the wrist: Diagnosis, classification, and pathomechanics. *J Bone Joint Surg Am* 1972;54:1612-1632.

Lundborg G, Rosen B, Dahlin L, Danielsen N, Holmberg J: Tubular versus conventional repair of median and ulnar nerves in the human forearm: Early results from a prospective, randomized, clinical study. *J Hand Surg Am* 1997;22:99-106.

Mayfield JK: Mechanism of carpal injuries. *Clin Orthop* 1980;149:45-54.

Reagan DS, Linscheid RL, Dobyns JH: Lunotriquetral sprains. *J Hand Surg Am* 1984;9:502-514.

Seiler JG, Chu CR, Amiel D, Woo SL, Gelberman RH: Autogenous flexor tendon grafts: Biologic mechanisms for incorportation. *Clin Orthop* 1997;345:239-247.

Simonian PT, Trumble TE: Traumatic dislocation of the thumb carpometacarpal joint: Early ligamentous reconstruction versus closed reduction and pinning. *J Hand Surg Am* 1996;21:802-806.

Sotereanos DG, Mitsionis GJ, Giannakopoulos PN, Tomaino MM, Herndon JH: Perilunate dislocation and fracture dislocation: A critical analysis of the volar-dorsal approach. *J Hand Surg Am* 1997;22:49-56.

Soucacos PN, Beris AE, Malizos KN, Xenakis T, Touliatos A, Soucaços PK: Two-stage treatment of flexor tendon ruptures: Silicone rod complications analyzed in 109 digits. *Acta Orthop Scand Suppl* 1997;275:48-51.

Watson HK, Ballet FL: The SLAC wrist: Scapholunate advanced collapse pattern of degenerative arthritis. *J Hand Surg Am* 1984;9:358-365.

Watson HK, Ryu J, Akelman E: Limited triscaphoid intercarpal arthrodesis for rotatory subluxation of the scaphoid. *J Bone Joint Surg Am* 1986;68:345-349.

Weiland AJ, Berner SH, Hotchkiss RN, McCormack RR Jr, Gerwin M: Repair of acute ulnar collateral ligament injuries of the thumb metacarpophalangeal joint with an intraosseous suture anchor. *J Hand Surg Am* 1997;22:585-591.

Zawacki BE: Immersion time to produce full thickness burns, in Boswick JA Jr (ed): *The Art and Science of Burn Care.* Rockville, MD, Aspen Publishers, 1987, pp 25-36.

Chapter 34

Wrist and Hand Reconstruction

Brian D. Adams, MD

Mark E. Baratz, MD

Scott H. Kozin, MD

John A. McAuliffe, MD

Kevin D. Plancher, MD

Christopher C. Schmidt, MD

Nerve Compression Syndromes

Upper extremity compression neuropathies are related to trauma, medical conditions, and occupational factors. In a series of women having carpal tunnel release, however, work practices did not influence the incidence of tenosynovial thickening or fibrosis on histologic examination. In another study, histologic abnormalities in either the retinaculum or tenosynovium were rare. Based on epidemiologic studies, carpal tunnel syndrome is believed to be more closely correlated with health status and factors such as obesity and use of tobacco and caffeine than to occupational factors. Documented intrinsic risk factors for compressive neuropathies are female gender, pregnancy, diabetes, hypothyroidism, and rheumatoid arthritis. The importance of risk factors is indicated by the high prevalence of bilateral occurrence or multiple nerve involvement even when only one extremity is predominantly involved in an activity. Aging lowers the threshold for the manifestation of a compressive neuropathy.

Compression at specific anatomic sites can tether a nerve and prevent its normal movement, resulting in nerve traction during joint motion. Nerve mobility can generate a friction-neuritis, typically found at joints where acute changes in nerve direction occur. The double crush phenomenon occurs when a compressive lesion at one site lowers the threshold for tolerance of compression at a more distal site. The most commonly cited pattern is coexistent cervical radiculopathy and carpal tunnel syndrome. Recent reports suggest that the concept of the double crush phenomenon is not supported by good experimental evidence and the diagnosis is offered clinically too often.

An ischemic pathway of compression is indicated by exacerbation of symptoms with provocative clinical maneuvers and rapid clinical resolution often seen after surgery. Patients in the early stage of compression with intermittent symptoms should be treated with conservative management such as steroid injection, activity modification, and splinting. Patients in the intermediate stage of compression, which is characterized by impaired intraneural circulation and constant paresthesias and numbness, are best treated with decompression. Patients with extended or advanced compression develop intraneural fibrosis, which explains the slow or incomplete recovery after surgery. The goal of surgery in such cases is to halt progression of symptoms. Although internal neurolysis was once advocated for severe compressive neuropathy, recent studies indicate there is no benefit.

The clinical presentation is typically either exertional or insidious. Acute, unresolving compression results from trauma or a dramatic spontaneous event such as internal bleeding or infection; these situations require urgent management. A number of clinical tests are available to confirm the diagnosis of a compressive neuropathy (Table 1).

Unless the patient has a history of trauma or physical examination reveals skeletal deformity or limited joint motion, radiographs of the upper extremity have a low yield for demonstrating causative factors for neuropathies. In a patient with a history of smoking, shoulder pain, and ulnar nerve symptoms, radiographs of the chest are indicated to rule out a Pancoast's tumor. Radiographs of the neck are useful to evaluate cervical spondylosis. Similarly, CT and MRI can be used to evaluate complex cases such as nerve compression caused by tumors or skeletal deformities.

Electrophysiologic testing, with both nerve conduction velocity and electromyography (EMG) assessment, is indicated if there is difficulty confirming a diagnosis, more than one compression site is suspected, or a polyneuropathy coexists. Conduction velocities and latencies are related to nerve myelination; values can be compared to established population norms, the contralateral nerve, other nerves in the same extremity, or previous tests. Decreased electrical amplitude indicates axonal damage. Normal variations are associated with

TABLE 1 | Clinical Tests for Compressive Neuropathy

Test	Mechanism
Tinel's percussion test	Elicit paresthesias
Phalen's test	Indirect creation of nerve compression or traction
Static two-point discrimination test	Evaluate innervation density of slowly adapting nerve fibers
Moving two-point discrimination test	Evaluate rapidly adapting nerve fibers
Vibrometry	Evaluate rapidly adapting nerve fibers
Semmes-Weinstein monofilaments	Evaluate slowly adapting nerve fibers

age and limb temperature. In early stages of entrapment, electrical testing may be normal even when symptoms are present.

Carpal Tunnel Syndrome

The mean age at diagnosis of carpal tunnel syndrome is 51 years, with women accounting for 79% of cases. The incidence of bilateral clinical carpal tunnel syndrome was 87% in one study population. Raynaud's phenomenon has been found to be coexistent in more than half of patients with carpal tunnel syndrome. Nocturnal pain is the most sensitive predictor of carpal tunnel syndrome; it is the most reliably relieved symptom after decompression and therefore is the best indication for surgery. The carpal tunnel compression test is a more sensitive predictor than the traditional Tinel's sign and Phalen's test. The most specific tests are the hand diagram and Tinel's sign. Two-point discrimination has low sensitivity.

Conservative therapy includes activity modification, splinting, and steroid injection. Steroid injection provides transient relief to 80% of patients; however, only 22% of them will be symptom free after 12 months. Steroid injection is most effective when symptoms have been present less than 1 year, numbness is diffuse and intermittent, two-point discrimination is normal, there is no weakness, thenar atrophy, or denervation potentials on EMG examination, and there is less than 2 ms of prolongation of distal motor and sensory latencies. Forty percent of patients meeting these criteria will remain symptom free longer than 12 months. Pyridoxine (vitamin B_6) does not appear to alter the natural history of the disease.

Carpal tunnel release has been successful in relieving symptoms. Studies suggest that earlier surgical intervention leads to better results. Patients who had surgery more than 3 years after initial diagnosis were less

than half as likely to have resolution of symptoms than patients who had surgery within 3 years of diagnosis. Patients with intermittent preoperative numbness and paresthesias had much better sensory recovery than patients with constant numbness. Improvements in electrical measurements were shown to be dependent on the degree of preoperative impairment, with complete recovery observed only in patients with mild carpal tunnel syndrome. Prospective randomized studies have indicated no additional benefit from epineurotomy. An hourglass deformity of the nerve did not correlate with chronicity of symptoms or electrical studies, nor was it a negative prognostic indicator of response to surgery.

Endoscopic techniques for carpal tunnel release have not been shown to reduce pillar pain or eliminate palmar tenderness. Reports vary regarding the accelerated recovery of grip and pinch strength with endoscopic versus open release; however, it is clear the outcome is equivalent by 6 months after surgery. Endoscopic surgery has led to the use of smaller incisions and the development of instrumentation to better facilitate the procedure; endoscopic surgery is as effective as open procedures that use larger incisions. In a prospective, randomized study of patients treated surgically for idiopathic carpal tunnel syndrome, no benefit was obtained from postoperative splinting. Bowstringing of tendons and delayed wound healing were not observed in either the splinted or unsplinted wrists. Patients with splinted wrists experienced a longer delay in return to activities of daily living, return to light and full occupational duty, and in recovery of grip and pinch strength. Patients with splinted wrists also had more pain and scar tenderness in the first month after surgery. Otherwise, there were no differences in outcome between the two groups.

Incomplete division of the transverse carpal ligament, unrecognized proximal nerve entrapment, severe or persistent compression, advanced age, and workers' compensation are factors that reduce relief of symptoms. MRI studies have shown a 20% to 30% increase in carpal tunnel volume after surgery. The results of reoperation are worse than those of the primary surgery, with only about half of patients achieving good results. Preoperative factors that correlate with a better result after reoperation are incomplete primary release of the transverse carpal ligament and abnormal electrophysiologic studies.

Pronator Syndrome

Potential sites of median nerve compression in the proximal forearm are between the ligament of Struthers and supracondylar process, beneath the bicipital aponeurosis, within the pronator teres, and under the flexor digitorum superficialis arch. Pronator syndrome is more common in women and in the fifth decade of life. Patients have vague pain in the anterior proximal forearm but hand numbness or nocturnal paresthesias, along with objective findings of numbness or weakness, are rare. Specific provocative maneuvers help localize the site of entrapment. Nerve conduction velocity in the forearm can be misleading because it may be reduced in up to 32% of patients with carpal tunnel syndrome. All four sites of potential entrapment should be considered in surgical treatment. Electrodiagnostic studies are a poor predictor of outcome from surgery.

Anterior Interosseous Nerve Compression Syndrome

The anterior interosseous nerve is a pure motor branch of the median nerve. Anterior interosseous nerve compression syndrome is characterized by variable weakness or paralysis of the flexor pollicis longus, flexor digitorum profundus to the index finger and, to a lesser extent, the middle finger, and the pronator quadratus. Only one digit may be involved, leading to misdiagnosis as a tendon rupture. The distal joints of the thumb and index finger collapse into extension during tip-to-tip pinch, creating pulp-to-pulp contact (inability to make "OK" sign). The differential diagnosis includes Parsonage-Turner syndrome (brachial neuritis), which often is heralded by intense pain. Surgical decompression in the proximal forearm is indicated if clinical or electrical recovery are not achieved within 12 weeks, unless a neuritis is suspected.

Cubital Tunnel Syndrome

Ulnar neuropathy at the elbow is second to carpal tunnel syndrome as the most common type of peripheral nerve entrapment and is generally considered a compression or entrapment neuropathy. A variety of anatomic and physiologic factors may contribute to the development of ulnar neuropathy, therefore, the term cubital tunnel syndrome is frequently used when a specific cause is not identified. Recurrent subluxation or dislocation of the ulnar nerve over the medial epicondyle, a known cause of neuritis, especially in the throwing athlete, is a common and frequently asymptomatic finding, occurring in 16% of the general population. Work-related activities involving repetitive elbow flexion and extension may aggravate cubital tunnel syndrome but there are no scientific data to support work-related activities as a true cause. A severe flexion contracture of the elbow may produce a delayed neuropathy. Posttraumatic conditions can involve the nerve through incarceration in callous, heterotopic bone or scar. Synovitis or osteophytes from

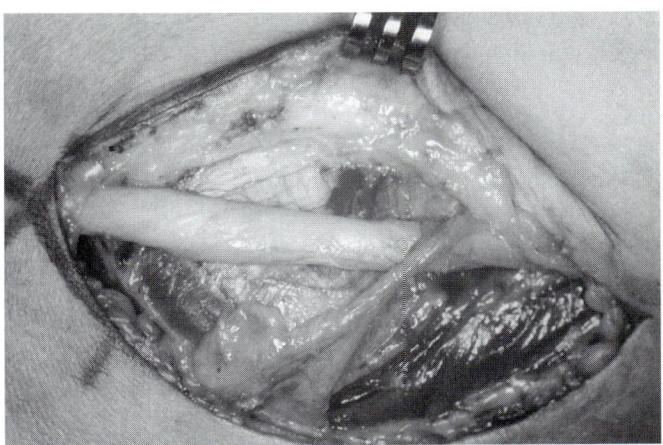

Figure 1 The ulnar nerve passes beneath a stout band (Osborne's ligament) connecting the heads of the flexor carpi ulnaris muscle, a source of compression.

arthritis can encroach on the nerve at the epicondylar groove. Similarly, ganglions and other space-occupying lesions can cause compression. Although polyneuropathy often affects the ulnar nerve, the potential for coexisting entrapment at the elbow should be considered.

There are several potential sites for entrapment. The nerve enters the elbow region by passing through the medial intermuscular septum. Although the septum is rarely associated with entrapment, it marks the proximal extent of the arcade of Struthers, which has been implicated in ulnar nerve compression. After exiting the arcade of Struthers, the nerve continues anteriorly to the medial head of the triceps. The muscle may be prominent or hypertrophic, and with elbow flexion it can compress the nerve. The muscle can also snap over the medial epicondyle, causing local inflammation that involves the nerve. The nerve then passes through the epicondylar groove where there are a variety of mechanical and structural causes for neuropathy. Accessory muscles in this area, in particular the anconeus epitrochlearis, are a source of constriction. The nerve passes between the humeral and ulnar heads of the flexor carpi ulnaris muscle. The humeral and ulnar heads are connected superficially by a stout fibrous band known as Osborne's ligament (Fig. 1). This passageway, the true cubital tunnel, is often implicated as a site of compression. Approximately 5 cm into the flexor capri ulnaris, the nerve courses under the deep flexor-pronator muscle fascia, presenting the most distal site for compression near the elbow.

Any one or a combination of these sites may produce nerve entrapment; however, the pathogenesis of entrapment neuropathy at sites of normal anatomic narrowing is poorly understood. Nerve compression, nerve traction, and conditions intrinsic to the nerve probably are involved in the process.

Symptoms vary, including mild numbness or paresthesias in the ring and small fingers to severe medial elbow pain. Muscle weakness generally develops after the onset of numbness and it is typically a late complaint, affecting intrinsic function long before any deterioration in the flexor digitorum profundus. Nocturnal paresthesias that routinely awaken the patient are less common than in carpal tunnel syndrome. In the elderly, pain and paresthesias occur less often than numbness and weakness, which may partially explain why neuropathy is more advanced in this age group.

Physical examination should begin at the neck and proceed distally, looking for evidence of cervical disease, brachial plexopathy, and thoracic outlet syndrome. A Tinel's sign is sought over the course of the nerve; however, approximately one fourth of asymptomatic patients will have a positive test. The elbow flexion test is best performed with the elbow at maximum flexion, the forearm in supination, and the wrist in comfortable extension. This test is falsely positive in up to 24% of the normal population. Applying gentle compression to the nerve at the epicondylar groove with the index and long fingers increases the sensitivity of the elbow flexion test but may increase the false-positive rate. Abnormal two-point discrimination testing indicates a more established neuropathy. Vibratory perception and light touch with Semmes-Weinstein monofilament are more sensitive tests during the early stage of neuropathy. Atrophy or significant weaknesses of pinch or grip are usually late findings. However, an abducted small finger (Wartenberg's sign) may occur early and indicates intrinsic muscle weakness. Weakness may be masked by a Martin-Gruber anastomosis through which the ulnar intrinsic muscles receive partial innervation from the median nerve. Intrinsic muscle atrophy is a normal process of aging; thus comparison with the opposite side and the thenar eminence is important. Clawing of the small and ring fingers and increased flexion of the thumb interphalangeal joint during pinch (Froment's sign) are indications of chronic neuropathy. MRI has no proven role in the diagnosis of cubital tunnel syndrome.

In patients with classic symptoms but without clinically measurable sensibility or motor deficits, the false-negative rate for electrodiagnosis is more than 50%. Slowing of motor conduction is indicated when the velocity across the flexed elbow is less than 50 m/s or the across-elbow segment is 10 m/s slower than the adjacent forearm segment. A reduction in amplitude of compound muscle action potentials often accompanies slowed motor conduction. A Martin-Gruber anastomosis can be expected in approximately 7% of patients. A reduction in sensory nerve action potential is a sensitive indicator of early neuropathy.

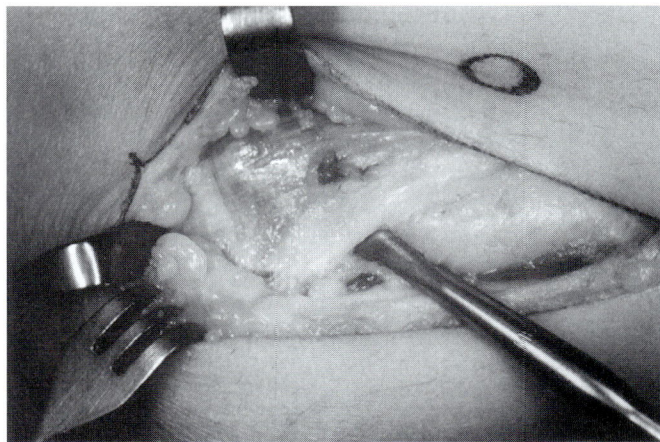

Figure 2 The medial antebrachial cutaneous nerve often lies within the surgical exposure; its branches should be identified and protected.

Patients with mild to moderate symptoms are best treated nonsurgically, which includes splinting the elbow at 45°, padding the nerve, and avoiding irritating elbow positions. For chronic neuropathy associated with muscle weakness, nonsurgical treatment generally is not warranted. In patients treated with surgery, all sites of compression must be eliminated and the nerve must be tension free and allowed to glide. Results of one study showed improved clinical and electrical results when the extrinsic vascular supply was mostly preserved.

Complications are minimal when the most simple effective procedure is chosen and performed correctly. Failed surgery is most often attributed to incomplete decompression or perineural scarring. Injury to the medial antebrachial cutaneous nerve may result in hyperesthesia, a painful scar, or hyperalgesia (Fig. 2). The medial collateral ligament of the elbow is easily injured in a submuscular transposition. Subluxation of the nerve may occur with simple decompression and subcutaneous transposition. Submuscular and intramuscular transpositions may result in recurrent entrapment from perineural scarring.

In most patients with neuropathy, improvement after surgery occurs when any of the accepted procedures is used. In one prospective randomized comparison of in situ release, subcutaneous transposition, and submuscular transposition for the treatment of cubital tunnel syndrome, no one procedure had a statistically significant advantage; however, the results were slightly better in patients having transpositions. In situ decompression is appropriate only for patients with mild symptoms and a nonsubluxating nerve. Patients with objective weakness and decreased sensibility achieve intermediate results with surgery whereas those with atrophy have the worst prognosis. Pain and dysesthesias are most reliably improved, followed by sensibility.

Duration of symptoms affects outcome only if the neuropathy is severe. Some symptomatic improvement can be expected in a chronic neuropathy associated with atrophy, but the objectives of surgery are more palliative than curative. Improvement in atrophy occurs in only 17% to 43% of patients. Although revision surgery provides some benefit, the results are unpredictable, with residual symptoms present in 75% of patients. Submuscular transposition has been the recommended revision technique; however, a recent study found subcutaneous transposition to be effective in 15 of 20 patients.

Ulnar Tunnel Syndrome

Ulnar nerve entrapment at the wrist is rare. Guyon's tunnel extends from the palmar carpal ligament to the fibrous arch of the hypothenar muscles. The nerve divides into motor and sensory branches within the tunnel. The ulnar artery and sensory branch may pass over or radial to the hook of the hamate, increasing risk of injury to this structure. The more commonly reported causes of neuropathy include chronic repetitive trauma, ganglia, ulnar artery aneurysms, and fracture of the hook of the hamate. Ulnar artery thrombosis (ulnar hammer syndrome) may cause a neuritis. Patients may have pure motor, pure sensory, or mixed symptoms, depending on the site of involvement. Allen's, Phalen's, and nerve compression tests are used in the physical examination. Carpal tunnel radiographs and CT for hamate fractures and Doppler studies for ulnar artery conditions are useful in diagnosis. Surgical decompression should follow the nerve through the entire tunnel. Ulnar artery aneurysm or thrombosis is treated by resection or vein grafting, depending on palmar arch competency.

Posterior Interosseous Nerve Compression Syndrome

The potential sites of compression of the posterior interosseous nerve near the elbow are the radial recurrent vessels (leash of Henry), fibrous edge of extensor carpi radialis brevis, arcade of Frohse, and distal edge of the supinator. The compression is usually idiopathic but may be caused by a lipoma, ganglia, or elbow synovitis. The extensor carpi radialis longus and usually the extensor carpi radialis brevis and supinator are innervated proximal to the arcade of Frohse and thus not involved. The typical history is an insidious onset of finger extension weakness and radial wrist deviation without pain. The syndrome may be incomplete, with only loss of small and ring finger extension. In patients with rheumatoid arthritis, the differential diagnosis is tendon rupture at the wrist and elbow synovitis causing

posterior interosseous nerve compression. Electrical studies will confirm the diagnosis. The sensory action potential should be normal. MRI is useful to confirm the presence of suspected elbow tumors or synovitis. If there is no improvement after 1 to 3 months, surgical release of all potential sites of compression is indicated. Recovery may continue for 18 months.

Radial Tunnel Syndrome

The main differential diagnosis in radial tunnel syndrome is lateral epicondylitis, which may be difficult to differentiate because the symptoms are similar and provocative tests for both conditions are unreliable. In radial tunnel syndrome, tenderness should be distal to the epicondyle and over the course of the nerve. Provocative tests are painful resisted supination and resisted middle finger extension. Although electrical studies are typically normal, one study found that differential latency testing, in which latencies are compared in different forearm positions, increased the test's sensitivity. Diagnosis is best made by injection of anesthetic into the radial tunnel, which should produce a posterior interosseous nerve palsy and relieve pain. Nonsurgical treatment is appropriate for most patients because the diagnostic criteria for the condition are unreliable and the outcome of surgical treatment is unpredictable. In one study, only 39% of patients achieved good or excellent results by objective assessments; however 64% reported good or excellent results by questionnaire.

Scaphoid Nonunion
Natural History

The proximal and distal fracture fragments of the scaphoid are both inherently unstable and prone to displacement or angulation. The proximal pole tends to rotate into extension via the influence of the triquetro-hamate articulation. In contrast, the distal pole is pulled into flexion by means of the scaphotrapeziotrapezoid articulation. These reverse manipulations create intrascaphoid angulation. The scaphoid is almost completely covered by cartilage and possesses an odd, undulating shape, which creates a small margin of error to maintain bony coaptation. Fracture displacement or intrascaphoid angulation further diminishes the contact area for healing. The scaphoid is intracapsular and primary union is required for fracture healing. Fracture displacement further diminishes the scaphoid's limited blood supply and jeopardizes the vascularity of the proximal pole. Approximately one third of waist fractures and virtually all proximal fifth fractures develop osteonecrosis. All of these factors counteract healing after fracture.

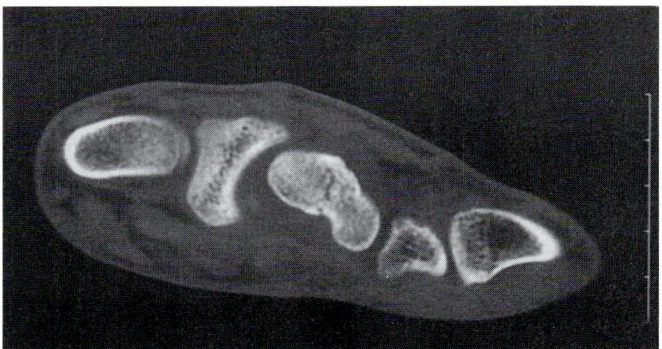

Figure 3 CT scan performed along the longitudinal axis of the scaphoid fracture to assess position and union of fracture fragments. *(Reproduced with permission from Kozin SH: Internal fixation of scaphoid fractures. Hand Clin 1997;13:573-586.)*

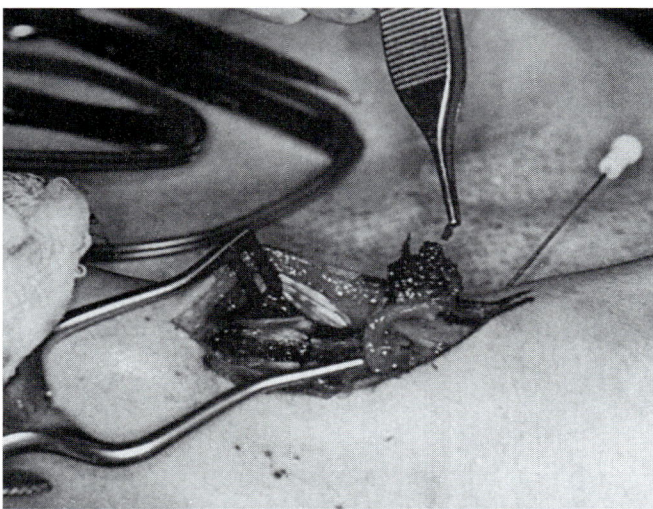

Figure 4 Vascularized bone graft harvested from distal radius for avascular scaphoid nonunion. *(Reproduced with permission from Kozin SH: Internal fixation of scaphoid fractures. Hand Clin 1997;13:573-586.)*

Most nondisplaced scaphoid fractures heal with strict immobilization. Displaced fractures have a propensity for nonunion. A small amount of displacement (1 mm) or angulation (15°) has a deleterious effect on healing. Therefore, open reduction is recommended to achieve anatomic alignment to promote healing and prevent nonunion. Union rates after open reduction and internal fixation of acutely displaced fractures are more than 90%.

Diagnosis

Advances in imaging modalities have been integrated with treatment selection and outcome. CT provides excellent detail of the fracture fragments and is useful to assess union (Fig. 3). The sagittal scan must be performed parallel to the longitudinal axis of the scaphoid using 1-mm intervals. Additional coronal images are recommended to assess biplanar deformity. CT is a more precise method to evaluate union when compared with plain radiographs.

MRI has been used to predict healing after acute scaphoid fractures by evaluating the initial pattern of vascularity after fracture and monitoring the subsequent bony response using sequential studies. In fractures with ischemic changes, failure of the revascularization front to extend from the fracture into the avascular fragment line by 8 weeks is associated with nonunion. MRI is also used to assess the vascular status of the proximal fragment. Gadolinium-enhanced MRI improves the overall accuracy to approximately 83%.

Treatment

The duration of nonunion influences the probability of surgical success. Nonunion present for 5 years or longer is associated with a decreased union rate, compared with nonunion present for less than 5 years. The choice of an internal fixation device is less important

than the surgical technique. Proper resection of all fibrous material, removal of sclerotic bone, and adequate bone grafting appears paramount to obtain union. Correct positioning of the internal fixation device is necessary to obtain adequate fixation and bony union.

Vascularized bone grafts are being used with increased frequency, especially in proximal third or avascular nonunions. The bone can be harvested from a distance as a free graft or rotated on a regional pedicle (Fig. 4). The vascular anatomy of the wrist has been further defined to offer potential sources for pedicled bone grafts. A canine model has been developed that simulates a scaphoid fracture nonunion with osteonecrosis. Using this model, a conventional (nonvascularized) technique was compared with a vascularized method using a local reverse-flow arteriovenous pedicle. Union was achieved in 73% of the limbs treated with vascularized bone grafting; union was not achieved after conventional bone grafting.

Free vascularized bone grafting from a distant source also has been developed for the treatment of scaphoid nonunion associated with an avascular fragment. Potential donor sites include the supracondylar region of the femur and iliac crest. Microsurgical anastomosis is done on the radial artery and its venae comitans. Union can be achieved in the majority of cases, with good to excellent results in approximately 80%.

Wrist Imaging

Various imaging modalities are available to a surgeon when evaluating the wrist. Interpretation of results can be technique-, equipment-, and reader-dependent. The presence of an abnormality on imaging is not necessarily equated with clinically relevant lesions.

CT has proved useful in the assessment of scaphoid healing, hamate fractures, and complex carpal injuries. Wrist arthrography should be performed using a triple injection technique and a postexercise phase for optimal interpretation. Despite precision methods, sensitivity and specificity, when compared with that of arthroscopy, is fair to good.

MRI may be useful in detecting osteonecrosis, soft-tissue injuries, triangular fibrocartilage complex tears, and ulnar collateral ligament injuries.

Wrist Arthroscopy

Wrist arthroscopy is a useful technique for evaluating intra-articular injuries and has proved beneficial in the diagnosis and treatment of chronic wrist pain. Arthroscopy allows excellent visualization of radiocarpal and midcarpal joint anatomy.

Arthroscopic débridement with or without repair of an ulnar-sided triangular fibrocartilage complex perforation has shown good to excellent results. Arthroscopically-assisted repairs of radial-sided lesions are now being reported with favorable initial results. Arthroscopic débridement of the arthritic wrist is being done. Removal of loose bodies and radial styloidectomy for focal arthritis are fairly well established procedures.

Arthroscopic excision of dorsal wrist ganglions has had encouraging early results. The recurrence rate is equal to that with open techniques.

Wrist arthroscopy may be useful in the treatment of intra-articular distal radius fractures by facilitating fragment reduction and in the evaluation and potential treatment of associated soft-tissue injuries (scapholunate ligament tears, triangular fibrocartilage complex tears, osteochondral lesions, and lunotriquetral tears).

Complications associated with wrist arthroscopy are uncommon and can be minimized with the establishment of correctly placed skin portals. Adequate padding and special attention to patient positioning is important to avoid traction injuries to the peripheral nerves of the wrist and forearm.

Kienböck's Disease

Kienböck's disease, originally termed lunatomalacia, is an incompletely understood process characterized by osteonecrosis and fragmentation of the lunate, ultimately leading to carpal collapse and generalized wrist arthrosis. The precise etiology of Kienböck's disease is uncertain, although predispositions are known. Notable among these are the effects of increased mechanical stress on the lunate associated with negative ulnar vari-

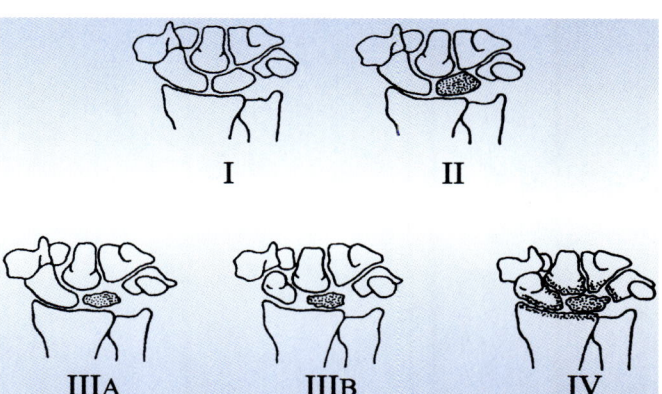

Figure 5 Radiographic classification of Kienböck's disease according to Lichtman and associates. Stage I: The lunate appears normal on conventional radiographs or there may be a nondisplaced fracture; MRI demonstrates loss of signal consistent with osteonecrosis. Stage II: Increased lunate radiodensity without loss of contour. Stage IIIA: Increased lunate radiodensity and fragmentation without loss of carpal height. Stage IIIB: Lunate fragmentation with proximal migration of the capitate and rotation of the scaphoid. Stage IV: Lunate fragmentation, carpal collapse, and degenerative changes at joints surrounding the lunate. *(Reproduced with permission from Weiss AP, Weiland AJ, Moore JR, Wilgis EF: Radial shortening for Kienböck's disease. J Bone Joint Surg Am 1991;73:384-391.)*

ance and high radial inclination angles, and precarious patterns of interosseous vascularity. Repetitive microtrauma is also thought to play a role; however, it remains unclear whether lunate fracture is the cause or result of osteonecrosis.

The natural history of Kienböck's disease also is poorly understood. Although good results after simple immobilization of wrists in early stages of the disease have been described, it is possible that such treatment only resolves inflammatory symptoms, allowing lunate fragmentation and carpal collapse to continue unchecked. Unfortunately, the ability of any of the available surgical treatments to predictably halt the progression of Kienböck's disease is far from certain. In the rare case of Kienböck's disease in the preadolescent wrist, early immobilization has been shown to arrest the process and preserve normal anatomy. The radiographic classification of Kienböck's disease is shown in Figure 5.

In early Kienböck's disease, prior to fragmentation of the lunate (stages I and II), the goal of treatment is to preserve normal wrist architecture if possible. Surgical procedures designed to unload the lunate are the mainstays of this treatment. In the ulnar negative wrist, radial shortening is usually preferred to ulnar lengthening, because bone grafting is not required and nonunion is less likely. In the unusual circumstance of ulnar neutral or positive variance, options include radial wedge osteotomy or limited intercarpal arthrodesis (most commonly scaphoid-trapezium-trapezoid). These alternatives have been shown to produce acceptable symptom relief, although the lunate is not always

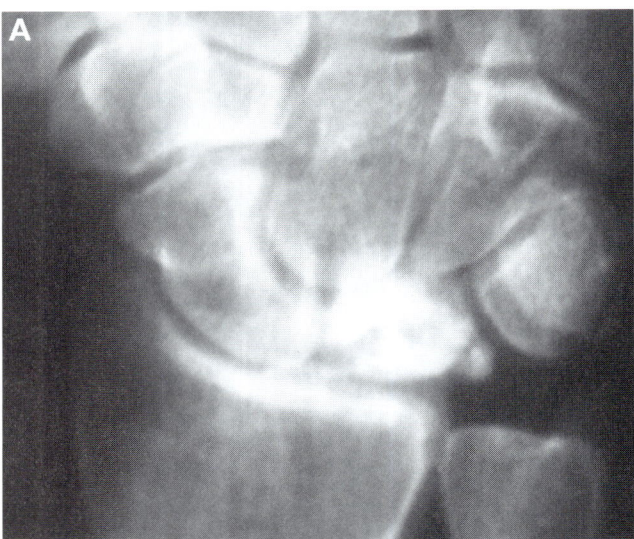
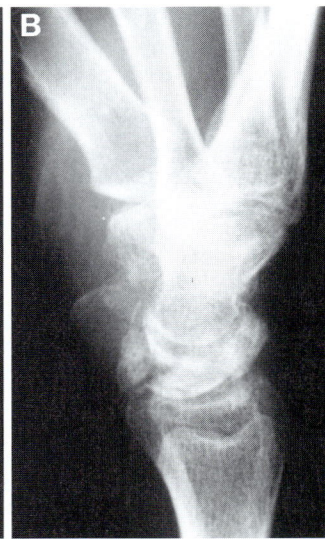

Figure 6 **A,** AP, and **B,** lateral radiographs of the wrist of a patient with stage IIIB Kienböck's disease. Note the increased radiodensity and fragmentation of the lunate, and flexion of the scaphoid on the lateral view.

restored to its normal architecture and some measure of fragmentation may still occur.

Promising results of bone grafting and revascularization prior to lunate collapse have been reported, although there is not sufficient experience with these techniques to recommend them without reservation. The recent description of pedicled dorsal distal radius bone grafts has renewed interest in the role of restoring blood supply in an effort to maintain normal lunate architecture.

The lunate unloading procedures described have also provided symptom relief even in the face of lunate fragmentation (stage IIIA). Lunate excision has fallen out of favor, as has Silastic arthroplasty, because of high complication rates. Once proximal migration of the capitate and scaphoid rotation have occurred (stage IIIB), lunate unloading procedures are sometimes helpful but less predictable (Fig. 6). At this stage, and almost certainly in the presence of degenerative changes at the intercarpal or radiocarpal joints surrounding the lunate (stage IV), salvage surgery in the form of proximal row carpectomy or wrist arthrodesis may be necessary.

Wrist Arthritis

The surgical treatment of wrist arthritis includes wrist denervation, arthroplasty, and limited and complete wrist fusion. The choice of procedure depends, in part, on the stage of wrist arthritis. In stage I arthritis, which is caused by scapholunate advanced collapse (SLAC), and is more typically seen in scaphoid nonunion advanced collapse, the worn radial half of the scaphoid fossa can be resected via radial styloidectomy. Stage II arthritis, involving the entire scaphoid fossa, can be surgically treated with either proximal row carpectomy

or scaphoid excision and capitolunate-triquetrohamate fusion. Proximal row carpectomy was found to be superior to scaphoid excision and capitolunate-triquetrohamate fusion in terms of pain relief, wrist motion, grip strength, and the need for subsequent surgery.

When the arthritis caused by SLAC extends to the midcarpal joint (stage III), the conventional approach has been to perform scaphoid excision with capitolunate-triquetrohamate fusion (Fig. 7). A technique for combining proximal row carpectomy with resection of the head of the capitate and interposition of dorsal capsule between the distal carpal row and the articular surface of the radius has been described. This procedure provided pain relief and preserved wrist motion to a greater degree than scaphoid excision and capitolunate-triquetrohamate fusion.

Partial wrist denervation via excision of the posterior and anterior interosseous nerves seems to provide at least partial relief from wrist pain caused by arthritis. Access to the anterior and posterior interosseous nerves is possible through a small incision centered 2 cm proximal to the wrist joint. The procedure is simple to perform and can be completed under regional anesthesia, which is an attractive option for the older patient with medical problems that preclude a major reconstructive procedure.

Wrist arthrodesis is an option for individuals who have pancarpal arthritis or radiocarpal arthritis that develops after proximal row carpectomy or scaphoid excision and capitolunate-triquetrohamate fusion. Because wrist fusion is a time-tested procedure, many techniques are available. Wrist arthrodesis with plate fixation has resulted in high union rates with minimal morbidity from immobilization. A 100% rate of union

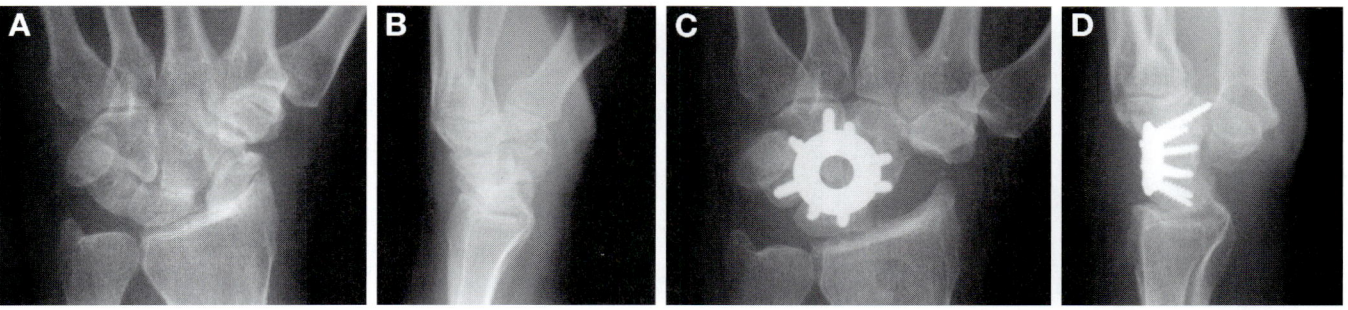

Figure 7 **A** through **D**, Preoperative and postoperative views of a wrist with stage III arthritis caused by SLAC. Scaphoid excision and capitolunate-triquetrohamate fusion was done.

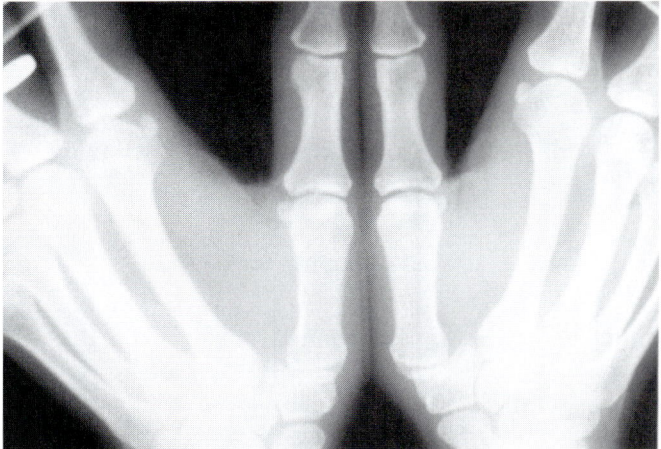

Figure 8 Stress radiograph of the CMC joints of both thumbs showing radial subluxation of the metacarpal bases. Minimal arthritic changes are seen. This patient would be an excellent candidate for ligament reconstruction.

was achieved using plate fixation and local bone graft. In a companion study, hand function after wrist fusion approximated that of a normal wrist with the exception of perineal care and manipulating the hand in tight spaces.

Degenerative Arthritis of the Small Joints

Thumb Carpometacarpal Joint

The importance of instability in the production of the classic pattern of joint degeneration seen in the thumb carpometacarpal (CMC) joint has been clearly described. Postmortem and biomechanical studies have shown that attenuation of the critical volar beak ligament allows dorsoradial subluxation of the metacarpal base and initiates a pattern of articular cartilage degeneration that begins volarly and progresses dorsally. Long-term follow-up of patients with symptomatic joint instability in the absence of degenerative changes (Fig. 8) who are treated with ligament reconstruction indicates that the appearance of clinically symptomatic arthritis can be delayed.

Silastic arthroplasty of the thumb CMC joint has fallen out of favor; tendon interposition, often combined with some form of ligament reconstruction, has become the common method of treatment after trapezial excision. Compressive and shear forces on Silastic implants at this level create wear debris and a resultant inflammatory reaction that is capable of producing synovitis and osteolysis.

Thumb CMC arthrodesis is the generally favored treatment for younger patients who require strength and durability. Thumb metacarpal extension osteotomy is a viable alternative for selected patients with early degenerative changes confined to the volar aspect of the joint.

Proximal Interphalangeal Joints

Arthrodesis of the proximal interphalangeal (PIP) joint provides a stable, pain-free digit, and is preferred for younger, high-demand patients, and in the presence of lateral joint instability. Even in the absence of these indications, the index PIP joint may be best treated with arthrodesis because of the significant stress placed on this articulation by key pinch activities.

When soft-tissue stability is present, Silastic arthroplasty of the PIP joints can provide excellent pain relief and fair range of motion. Resurfacing joint arthroplasty remains an elusive goal, although recently developed devices seem to hold some promise.

Distal Interphalangeal Joints

Nonsurgical treatment of the swollen, painful distal interphalangeal joint will often yield a joint that is stiff but asymptomatic. Indications for surgical reconstruction include unrelieved pain, instability, and angular deformity, and these symptoms are most predictably relieved by joint arthrodesis. The use of intramedullary compression screws provides excellent initial stability and predictable fusion rates. Silastic arthroplasty can be considered in the rare instance that joint mobility is a vocational necessity.

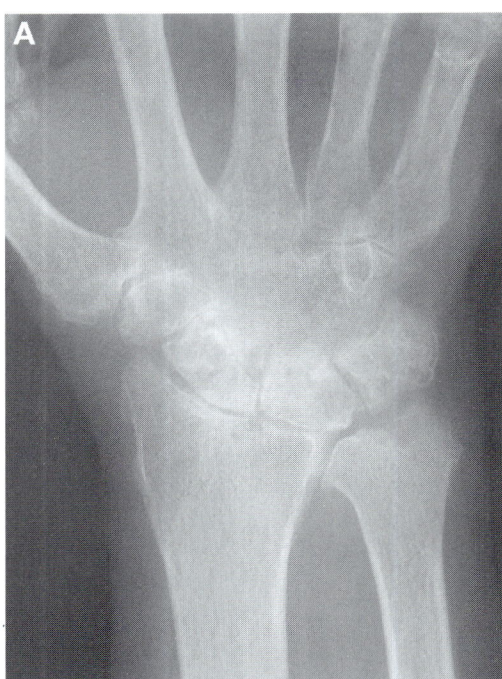
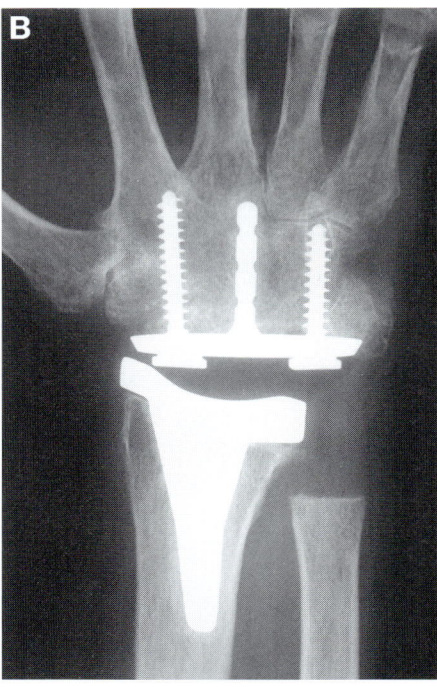

Figure 9 **A** and **B,** Preoperative and postoperative radiographs of a rheumatoid patient treated with a newer generation total wrist replacement in which the carpal component is fixed with osteointegrative screws, resulting in reliable long-term fixation.

Rheumatoid Reconstruction

The goals of surgical reconstruction of the rheumatoid wrist and hand are pain relief, improvement of function, prevention of deformities, and improvement of appearance. Early surgical intervention should be considered to slow or prevent the progression of deformities. However, the presence of a deformity is not itself always an indication for surgery. The shoulder and elbow generally should be operated on before the hand and wrist.

A classification of wrist arthritis (ankylosis, osteoarthritis, or disintegration types) is based on disease progression. The type is determined from radiographic changes over time, including carpal height ratio, ulnar translocation, and scapholunate dissociation. The disintegration type should be stabilized early.

Distal radioulnar joint arthritis is associated with dorsal subluxation of the ulnar head, and supination and ulnar translation of the carpus. An irregular, prominent ulnar head can cause attrition rupture of the finger extensor tendons (Vaughn-Jackson syndrome). Controversy exists over whether ulnar head resection increases the risk of ulnar translation of the carpus and whether the Sauvé-Kapandji procedure provides protection against its occurrence. Partial wrist arthrodesis (radiolunate or radioscapholunate) should be considered in conjunction with distal ulnar resection procedures. However, results from a 1- to 15-year review indicated that although radiolunate fusion improves radial deviation deformity of the wrist, restrains ulnar translation, and prevents wrist dislocation, the procedure has limited influence on the progression of radiologic changes in the carpus. Radiolunate arthrodesis is indicated in the intermediate stages of arthritis, especially in the osteoarthritis type, but this procedure has a restricted role in the disintegration type.

In contrast to open wrist synovectomy, arthroscopic synovectomy does not cause joint stiffness. Arthroscopic synovectomy reduced pain and improved range of motion in 24 wrists (19 patients) with a follow-up of 2 to 6 years. Progressive radiographic changes of arthritis were less common in patients with no or very early changes at the time of surgery.

Wrist arthrodesis is a reliable procedure that corrects deformity and leads to satisfactory function. In a recent study of wrist fusion in patients with rheumatoid arthritis, fused wrists received high satisfaction scores and fusion did not create additional functional loss, compared with nonfused wrists. Other studies have found that wrist arthroplasty is preferred over wrist arthrodesis because of the improved dexterity in both wrists. The ellipsoidal articulation present in newer prosthetic designs has reduced the wrist imbalance problems associated with older designs. The range of motion typically achieved with this type of articulation is approximately 35° of flexion and 35° of extension. One newer prosthetic design has not had the carpal component loosening problems common with other designs (Fig. 9). The distal component is supported by the entire width of the carpus and it is fixed into the carpus, primarily with deep threaded screws, rather

TABLE 2 | Tetraplegia Classification and Treatment Recommendations

ICSHT	ASIA	Key Muscle	Tendon Transfer for Hand Function
0	C5	None	None
1	C5	Brachioradialis	Active wrist extension, passive pinch
2	C6	Brachioradialis + extensor carpi radialis longus	Active pinch
3	C6	Above + extensor carpi radialis brevis	Active pinch, active grasp
4	C6	Above + pronator teres	Active pinch, active grasp, active release
5	C6	Above + flexor carpi radialis	Active pinch, active grasp, active release
6	C7	Above + extensor digitorum comminus	Active pinch, active grasp, possible intrinsic transfer
7	C7	Above + extensor pollicis longus	Active pinch, active grasp, possible intrinsic transfer
8	C8	Above + finger flexors	Active pinch, possible intrinsic transfer
9	C8-T1	Lacking only intrinsics	Intrinsic transfer

Cutaneous (Cu) and ocular (O) modifiers are added to the group to indicate intact sensibility (two-point discrimination < 10 mm in thumb and index) and/or visual feedback (eg, O(Cu): 2 indicates ocular and cutaneous input and presence of brachioradialis and extensor carpi radialis longus)

than cemented into the metacarpal canals. An intercarpal fusion is performed to provide solid bony support. In a series of 57 implants with a 4- to 10-year follow-up, there was no evidence of carpal component loosening. Salvage of a failed total wrist arthroplasty by arthrodesis requires internal fixation; extensive bone grafting is often required to fill the defect. One group achieved a high union rate using femoral head allograft and an intramedullary Steinmann pin, which reduced the surgical morbidity.

Tendon ruptures may be caused by erosion of bony prominences, synovial infiltration, or ischemia. A frequent site for an extensor tendon rupture is at the distal end of the retinaculum. One report concluded that dorsal subluxation of the ulna, erosive change at the distal radioulnar joint (scallop sign), and tenosynovitis persisting for at least 6 months were associated with ruptures. Fifty percent of patients undergoing prophylactic extensor tenosynovectomy have synovial invasion of the tendons. The incidences of tendon rupture and recurrent tenosynovitis following tenosynovectomy are 5%.

New implants for digital arthroplasty have been designed in an attempt to improve stability, durability, and function. Short-term studies have demonstrated improved arc of motion, however, there are no long-term follow-up studies to demonstrate improved outcome. In a randomized trial of standard dynamic splinting versus continuous passive motion for postoperative rehabilitation following silicone arthroplasty, use of the continuous passive motion machine did not produce greater motion. In a recent review of the literature, complications after silicone arthroplasty were few. The most frequent complication is osteolysis at the bone-implant interface (4%). Implant fracture ranges from 0 to 38%. Infection (usually caused by *Staphylococcus aureus*) is rare (< 1%). Early results of PIP joint replacement are encouraging in fingers without severe injury or static deformity; loosening has not been a problem. However, ultimate joint motion was unpredictable and recurrent deformity was common in severely afflicted joints.

Tetraplegia

Restoration of upper extremity function remains a high priority for people with tetraplegia. The treatment algorithm depends on the level of injury and availability of muscles for transfer. The International Classification of Surgery of the Hand in Tetraplegia (ICSHT) continues to increase in popularity and is more detailed than the American Spinal Injury Association (ASIA) classification (Table 2). The ICSHT defines 10 groups of tetraplegia based on segmental key muscle return (grade four or better), beginning with the brachioradialis muscle.

Restoration of elbow extension is independent of hand reconstruction and an integral part of upper extremity surgical reconstruction in persons with tetraplegia. The ability to control the elbow will increase the available work space for functional activities, improve the ability to perform pressure relief maneuvers, allow better manual wheelchair propulsion, and facilitate independent transfer. Posterior deltoid-to-triceps transfer has been the preferred technique to regain active elbow extension. However, prolonged immobilization time, inadequate elbow extension strength, and attenuation of the transfer are potential problems. The biceps-to-triceps transfer has been rediscovered as an alternative method to restore elbow extension. Previously, the biceps tendon was routed laterally around the humerus to the triceps tendon and olecranon. However, there were reports of radial nerve injury resulting in loss of available forearm muscle (brachioradialis and wrist extensors) function. Technical modifications and medial routing of the biceps tendon over the nonfunctioning ulnar nerve has led to its resurgence. However, intact supinator and brachialis muscles are prerequisites to biceps transfer to compensate for the approximately 50% decrease in forearm supination and elbow flexion strength.

Functional electrical stimulation is an option to restore functional grasp (palmar and lateral grasp patterns) and release in high-level tetraplegia without available donor muscles (ICSHT 0 or 1). Functional electrical stimulation uses intact lower motor neuron pathways below the level of injury to electrically excite viable muscles. Denervated muscles within the zone of injury cannot be stimulated. Indwelling electrodes are placed intramuscularly or on the muscles (epymysial) to be stimulated. The standard muscles implanted include the primary flexors and extensors of the fingers and thumb (flexor digitorum profundus and superficialis, flexor pollicis longus, adductor pollicis, flexor pollicis brevis, abductor pollicis brevis, extensor digitorum communis, and extensor pollicis longus). Electrode leads are tunneled proximally up the arm and attached to an implant stimulator unit placed in the infraclavicular subcutaneous tissue. The sequence for grasp and release is programmed and contraction of each muscle regulated by the intensity (amplitude), pulse duration, and frequency of their respective signal. A radiofrequency inductive link provides the communication and power to the implant stimulator via external components. Contralateral shoulder motion is used to control grasp and release by variations in shoulder elevation-depression and protraction-retraction.

Brachial Plexus Injuries

The decision to proceed with surgical intervention is not always straightforward in brachial plexus traction injuries. The accuracy of CT scan and MRI can be improved with the use of contrast. In addition, indirect MRI findings of nerve root avulsion (spinal cord edema, syrinx, hemorrhage, absent roots, meningoceles, erector spinae denervation) can be used to increase its accuracy.

Early surgical exploration affords the opportunity to repair (graft) nerve ruptures and perform nerve transfers to circumvent nerve root avulsions. Nerve transfers can use a variety of axonal sources, such as the spinal accessory nerve, intercostal nerves, a portion of the ulnar nerve, medial pectoral nerve, phrenic nerve, and contralateral C7 nerve root, depending on the level of injury.

The use of local nerve transfers (ulnar nerve fascicle, medial pectoral nerve) has certain advantages over traditional transfers (spinal accessory nerve, intercostal nerves). Local nerves are closer to the motor end plates, are dispensable, and are pure motor nerves. Transfer of an ulnar nerve fascicle to the musculocutaneous nerve is an effective treatment for upper root avulsions (C5, C6). Clinical recovery of elbow flexion tends to occur relatively early (between 2 and 5 months) secondary to proximity of transfer to the motor end plates. Transient ulnar nerve parasthesias can occur, but no permanent loss of sensibility is apparent. Local nerve transfer also spares the spinal accessory nerve for reconstruction about the shoulder joint.

Contralateral C7 nerve transfer has been used in total root avulsions because of the considerable deficiency in viable axons. C7 nerve transfer does not result in permanent donor deficit and possesses a large number of nerve fibers for reinnervation. This technique is usually combined with other nerve transfers (such as the spinal accessory nerve to musculocutaneous nerve) to enhance likelihood of muscle recovery. The clinical results of C7 root transfer to the median nerve have been encouraging with reference to return of sensibility but disappointing with regard to forearm and hand motor recovery. This difference in results between motor sensory recovery relates to the distance and time required for axonal regeneration, which results in irreversible changes in the neuromuscular junction and motor end plates.

Free muscle transfer is another option to restore hand function after severe brachial plexus injuries. The double free muscle technique consists of staged muscle transfers to restore prehensile function. This sophisticated approach requires considerable expertise, prolonged rehabilitation, and a motivated patient. The usual muscle donors are the gracilis, contralateral latissimus dorsi, or rectus femoris muscles. Double free muscle can result in ample elbow motion, modest finger movement, and limited sensibility. This amount of motion can provide voluntary movement and stability of the shoulder and elbow, basic grasping, and improved function.

Tumors

Dorsal ganglions of the wrist can be treated with arthroscopic resection. Benefits include less scarring, limited immobilization, and decreased stiffness. The ganglion stalk can be visualized in approximately two thirds of the cases. Open ganglionectomy is necessary if doubt exists about whether resection is complete. Recurrence rates of arthroscopic resection for primary ganglions appear comparable, or even somewhat less, than open surgery rates.

Lymphatic mapping is changing the standard of care of many malignant disorders including melanoma, squamous cell carcinoma, breast cancer, colon cancer, parathyroid tumors, and bone lesions. Malignant melanomas tend to metastasize to regional lymph nodes in an orderly progression beginning with the sentinel lymph node. The role of elective lymph node dissection is controversial because of associated morbidities (risk of infection, seroma formation, and chronic lymphedema). Preoperative lymphoscintigraphy and intraoperative lymphatic plotting allow identification of the first node in the chain (sentinel) receiving afferent lymph flow. Selective lymphadenectomy of the sentinel lymph node allows delineation of any metastatic disease and permits staging of the disease. However, the sentinel lymph node must be examined closely using immunohistochemical stains to identify micrometastases and avoid false-negative interpretations. Lymphatic mapping is minimally invasive, identifies the lymphatic drainage pattern, has a low morbidity, and avoids unnecessary radical lymph node dissection in patients with a biopsy-proven negative sentinel lymph node.

Soft-tissue sarcomas of the upper extremity are rare, but errant biopsy must be avoided. Inadequate local treatment and local recurrence is more likely when a surgeon inexperienced in tumor management performs the procedure. Malignant fibrous histiocytoma is the most common histotype and grade IV (four-grade scale) is the most common malignancy grade. Tumor size larger than 5 cm and vascular invasion significantly increase the likelihood of metastasis (the lungs are the most common localization of first metastasis).

Cerebral Palsy

Cerebral palsy is characterized by spasticity secondary to loss of upper motor neuron regulatory control. Options for treatment include neuropharmacologic agents (oral, injectable, intrathecal), surgery (selective neurectomy, tenotomy, tendon lengthening, tendon transfer), or physical therapy modalities (stretching, strengthening, electrical stimulation). Because oral agents are often poorly tolerated, other options to control spasticity have been explored. Intrathecal baclofen infusion has been effective in reducing upper and lower extremity spasticity in a randomized, double-blinded study. Adverse effects (such as hypotonia, somnolence, and vomiting) were common, but manageable.

Neuromuscular electrical stimulation can be combined with dynamic bracing to treat upper extremity spastic hemiplegia. Neuromuscular electrical stimulation stimulates the antagonist wrist and finger extensors to address the overpull of the flexion force, whereas dynamic traction stretches the tight spastic flexors. This treatment regimen reduces spasticity and enhances upper extremity function. However, the duration of effectiveness is unclear and a maintenance program is recommended.

The needs, goals, and expectations of each child and family must be considered before surgery. Soft-tissue releases of deforming spastic muscles, tendon transfers to augment deficient activity, and joint stabilization procedures are the mainstays of treatment. In properly selected patients, surgery improves limb control and enhances function.

Vascular Disorders

The natural history and management of radial artery thrombosis has received limited attention in contrast to that of ulnar artery thrombosis. Symptomatic occlusion (pain, cold sensitivity, weakness, and tissue loss) may occur in the absence of sufficient collateral flow from the ulnar artery or a persistent median artery. When nonsurgical management is unsuccessful, radial artery reconstruction (interpositional vein graft) to the deep arch can be done. This treatment regimen results in significant recovery of digital microvascular perfusion, along with symptomatic and functional improvement.

Digital artery sympathectomy remains a useful, although not always predictable, treatment for severe Raynaud's phenomenon refractory to medical management. A positive response to a preoperative sympathetic nerve blockade is not an essential prerequisite as secondary extrinsic vascular compression may negate any effect from the block. Digital sympathectomy addresses both the sympathetic overtone and any extrinsic compression from the fibrotic adventitia. Vascular bypass grafting of occlusive areas of disease may also be required to salvage the digits.

Annotated Bibliography

Nerve Compression Syndromes

Arons JA, Collins N, Arons MS: Results of treatment of carpal tunnel syndrome with associated hourglass deformity of the median nerve. *J Hand Surg Am* 1999;24:1192-1195.

The implications of an hourglass deformity of the median nerve at surgery did not correlate with chronicity of symptoms or electrophysiologic severity. Patients with the deformity responded well to surgery, indicating that deformity is not a negative prognostic indicator.

Aulisa L, Tamburrelli F, Padua R, Romanini E, Lo Monaco M, Padua L: Carpal tunnel syndrome: Indication for surgical treatment based on electrophysiologic study. *J Hand Surg Am* 1998;23:687-691.

In patients treated surgically for idiopathic carpal tunnel syndrome, all showed electrophysiologic improvement but the amount of improvement was dependent on the degree of preoperative impairment. Complete restoration of clinical and electrophysiologic function only occurred in mild cases.

Caputo AE, Watson HK: Subcutaneous anterior transposition of the ulnar nerve for failed decompression of cubital tunnel syndrome. *J Hand Surg Am* 2000;25: 544-551.

Fifteen patients had a good or excellent outcome and five had a fair or poor outcome after anterior subcutaneous transposition for previous failed surgery. Subcutaneous transposition is effective for recurrent cubital tunnel syndrome regardless of the type of initial failed procedure.

Kupfer DM, Bronson J, Lee GW, Beck J, Gillet J: Differential latency testing: A more sensitive test for radial tunnel syndrome. *J Hand Surg Am* 1998;23: 859-864.

Radial nerve latencies were measured with the forearm in neutral, supination, and pronation in asymptomatic volunteers, and preoperative and postoperative symptomatic patients. Radial nerves that were compressed demonstrated a significantly greater latency versus controls; latency normalized after decompressive surgery.

Padua L, Padua R, Nazzaro M, Tonali P: Incidence of bilateral symptoms in carpal tunnel syndrome. *J Hand Surg Br* 1998;23:603-606.

In 133 patients with unilateral carpal tunnel syndrome complaints, 87% presented with clinical and electrophysiologic evidence of carpal tunnel syndrome on the opposite side at follow-up. Bilateral involvement had been underestimated.

Sotereanos DG, Varitimidis SE, Giannakopoulos PN, Westkaemper JG: Results of surgical treatment for radial tunnel syndrome. *J Hand Surg Am* 1999;24: 566-570.

Only 11 of 28 patients (39%) had a good or excellent result as measured by objective assessments; however, 64% were satisfied after surgical treatment for radial tunnel syndrome. A high rate of morbidity is associated with both the disease and its treatment.

Szabo RM, Slater RR Jr, Farver TB, Stanton DB, Sharman WK: The value of diagnostic testing in carpal tunnel syndrome. *J Hand Surg Am* 1999;24:704-714.

The typical signs and tests for carpal tunnel syndrome were subjected to a critical analysis. The tests with the highest sensitivity were the compression test, Semmes-Weinstein monofilament test, and hand diagram scores. Night pain was a highly sensitive predictor. The most specific tests were the hand diagram and Tinel's sign.

Scaphoid Nonunion

Cerezal L, Abascal F, Canga A, Garcia-Valtuille R, Bustamante M, del Pinal F: Usefulness of gadolinium-enhanced MR imaging in the evaluation of the vascularity of scaphoid nonunions. *AJR Am J Roentgenol* 2000;174:141-149.

Thirty consecutive patients with scaphoid nonunions were examined by unenhanced and enhanced MRI. Images were correlated with surgical findings. Unenhanced imaging demonstrated little correlation with surgical findings. Gadolinium sequences improved sensitivity, specificity, and accuracy to 66%, 88%, and 83%, respectively.

Doi K, Oda T, Soo-Heong T, Nanda V: Free vascularized bone graft for nonunion of the scaphoid. *J Hand Surg Am* 2000;25:507-519.

Ten patients with scaphoid nonunion and osteonecrosis were treated with free vascularized bone graft from the supracondylar region of the femur based on a branch of the geniculate artery and vein. Union was achieved in all patients and good to excellent results in 80%.

Gabl M, Reinhart C, Lutz M, et al: Vascularized bone graft from the iliac crest for the treatment of nonunion of the proximal part of the scaphoid with an avascular fragment. *J Bone Joint Surg Am* 1999;81:1414-1428.

Fifteen patients underwent free vascularized bone grafting from the iliac crest for scaphoid nonunion with avascularity. Union was achieved in 12 patients (80%) with improved subjective outcome. Bone grafting failed in three patients and resulted in progressive arthritis and carpal collapse.

Gunal I, Oz elik A, Gokturk E, Ada S, Demirtas M: Correlation of magnetic resonance imaging and intraoperative punctate bleeding to assess the vascularity of scaphoid nonunion. *Arch Orthop Trauma Surg* 1999; 119:285-287.

Preoperative MRI studies were correlated with intraoperative observations in 32 patients. Consistent findings were present in 19 patients, although 13 patients had no correlation.

Kulkarni RW, Wollstein R, Tayar R, Citron N: Patterns of healing of scaphoid fractures: The importance of vascularity. *J Bone Joint Surg Br* 1999;81:85-90.

Acute scaphoid fractures were evaluated with serial MRI. Different MRI patterns were noted and correlated to the vascular status. In fractures with ischemic changes, failure of the revascularization front to extend into avascular fragment by 8 weeks was associated with nonunion.

Rajagopalan BM, Squire DS, Samuels LO: Results of Herbert-screw fixation with bone-grafting for the treatment of nonunion of the scaphoid. *J Bone Joint Surg Am* 1999;81:48-52.

A cohort of 21 patients with scaphoid nonunion were treated with Herbert screw fixation and bone grafting. Union was achieved in 18 (86%) with good or excellent results. Nonunion persisted in three patients (14%).

Schuind F, Haentjens P, Van Innis F, Vander Maren C, Garcia-Elias M, Sennwald G: Prognostic factors in the treatment of carpal scaphoid nonunions. *J Hand Surg Am* 1999;24:761-776.

A multicenter study of 138 patients was done to assess prognostic factors for scaphoid nonunion. Delay between initial trauma and treatment was most predictive. If the nonunion was present for 5 years or longer, the success of surgery was diminished.

Sunagawa T, Bishop AT, Muramatsu K: Role of conventional and vascularized bone grafts in scaphoid nonunion with avascular necrosis: A canine experimental study. *J Hand Surg Am* 2000;25:849-859.

A canine experimental model was developed to simulate scaphoid fracture nonunion with osteonecrosis. Subsequently, nonvascularized or vascularized pedicled bone grafting was performed bilaterally in 12 dogs. Seventy-three percent of the vascularized bone grafting procedures united compared to none with the conventional graft.

Wrist Imaging

Freedman DM, Dowdle J, Glickel SZ, Singson R, Okezie T: Tomography versus computed tomography for assessing step off in intraarticular distal radial fractures. *Clin Orthop* 1999;361:199-204.

Trispiral tomography is more accurate and cost effective than CT and should be the modality of choice when evaluating a fracture of the intra-articular distal radius.

Grechenig W, Peicha G, Fellinger M, Seibert FJ, Preidler KW: Wrist arthrography after acute trauma to the distal radius: Diagnostic accuracy, technique, and sources of diagnostic errors. *Invest Radiol* 1998;33:273-278.

Arthrography is used to identify interosseous carpal ligaments and triangular fibrocartilage complex tears in the posttraumatic wrist.

Plancher KD, Ho CP, Cofield SS, Viola R, Hawkins RJ: Role of MR imaging in the management of "skier's thumb" injuries. *Magn Reson Imaging Clin N Am* 1999; 7:73-84.

This article presents a current concepts review of ulnar collateral ligament rupture, including a study of 34 ulnar collateral ligament injuries in which MRI was used as the main diagnostic tool.

Wrist Arthroscopy

Culp RW: Wrist and hand arthroscopy. *Hand Clin* 1999;15:393-535.

All aspects of wrist arthroscopy for the novice and advanced surgeon are discussed. The latest technique of laser-assisted as well as metacarpophalangeal arthroscopy are covered.

Doi K, Hattori Y, Otsuka K, Abe Y, Yamamoto H: Intra-articular fractures of the distal aspect of the radius: Arthroscopically assisted reduction compared with open reduction and internal fixation. *J Bone Joint Surg Am* 1999;81:1093-1110.

Accurate reduction of intra-articular fractures of the distal radius is discussed. Overall functional results are improved because of decreased soft-tissue scarring and minimal capsular contracture.

Grechenig W, Peicha G, Fellinger M, Seibert FJ, Weiglein AH: Anatomical and safety considerations in establishing portals used for wrist arthroscopy. *Clin Anat* 1999;12:179-185.

Eight safe portals are made with the use of external landmarks.

Haugstvedt JR, Husby T: Results of repair of peripheral tears in the triangular fibrocartilage complex using an arthroscopic suture technique. *Scand J Plast Reconstr Surg Hand Surg* 1999;33:439-447.

Arthroscopic suture technique to repair peripheral triangular fibrocartilage complex lesions had good objective results.

Luchetti R, Badia A, Alfarano M, Orbay J, Indriago I, Mustapha B: Arthroscopic resection of dorsal wrist ganglia and treatment of recurrences: *J Hand Surg Br* 2000;25:38-40.

This article presents a review of 30 patients with dorsal wrist ganglia treated with arthroscopic resection. There were two recurrences. Mean follow-up was limited to 16 months with no complications reported.

Mehta JA, Bain GI, Heptinstall RJ: Anatomical reduction of intra-articular fractures of the distal radius: An arthroscopically-assisted approach. *J Bone and Joint Surg Br* 2000;82:79-86.

The wrist arthroscope was used in diagnosis and treatment of a compilation of injuries. Arthroscopic débridement of necrotic scaphoids, lunotriquetral, scapholunate, and triangular fibrocartilage complex tears and 31 intra-articular fractures of the distal radius with percutaneous Kirschner wire fixation are discussed. Outcomes are reviewed with recommendations.

Kienböck's Disease

Jafarnia K, Collins ED, Kohl HW, Bennett JB, Ilahi OA: Reliability of the Lichtman classification of Kienbock's disease. *J Hand Surg Am* 2000:25:529-534.

In a study of 64 sets of radiographs of patients with Kienböck's disease and 10 normal controls, the results indicated substantial reliability and reproducibility of the classification.

Lamas C, Mir X, Llusa M, Navarro A: Dorsolateral biplane closing radial osteotomy in zero variant cases of Kienbock's disease. *J Hand Surg Am* 2000;25:700-709.

Twenty-six patients with stage II and III Kienböck's disease underwent biplane radial closing wedge osteotomy to reduce radial inclination and volar tilt. Clinical follow-up, radiographs, and MRI showed promising results, roughly equivalent to conventional radial shortening osteotomy in ulnar negative patients.

Shin AY, Bishop AT: Treatment of Kienbock's disease with distal radius pedicled vascularized bone graft. *Atlas Hand Clin* 1999;4:91-118.

This preliminary report describes surgical technique and briefly discusses the results of surgery in nine patients. MRI showed progressive signs of revascularization over time, and radiographic measures showed no deterioration in modified carpal height, lunate index, or scapholunate angle during 32 months average follow-up.

Wrist Arthritis

Berger RA: Partial denervation of the wrist: A new approach. *Tech Hand Upper Extrem Surg* 1998;2:25-35.

The method of partial wrist denervation via resection of the anterior and posterior interosseous nerves is described.

Berger RA, Imeada T, Berglund L, An K-N: Constraint and material properties of the subregions of the scapholunate interosseous ligament. *J Hand Surg Am* 1999;24:953-962.

This study measured the biomechanical properties of the three anatomic regions of the scapholunate ligament. The measurements were made using a servohydraulic testing machine incorporating a rotatory actuator. The dorsal region offered the greatest constraint to differential translation, but both the dorsal and palmer regions showed statistically significant combined constraints to differential rotation between the scaphoid and lunate. The dorsal region showed the greatest yield strength.

Schmidt CC, Kleinman WB: Lunatotriquetral fusion. *Atlas Hand Clin* 1998;3:115-127.

This article presents an overview of the diagnosis and treatment of lunatotriquetral injuries.

Weiss A-P: Scapholunate ligament reconstruction using a bone-retinaculum-bone autograft. *J Hand Surg Am* 1998;23:205-215.

The use of a bone retinaculum-bone autograft for patients with partial or complete tears of the scapholunate ligament with normal radiographs, resulted in improvement of pain in all patients, a slight decline in wrist range of motion, and a 46% increase in grip strength. Results were less favorable in patients with a static scapholunate deformity on plain radiographs.

Wyrick JD, Youse BD, Kiefhaber TR: Scapholunate ligament repair and capsulodesis for the treatment of static scapholunate dissociation. *J Hand Surg Br* 1998; 23:776-780.

With an average interval between injury and surgery of 3 months, results of the study showed that no patients were pain free. The average wrist motion was 60% and grip strength 70% of the opposite side. The radiographic correction obtained at surgery was not maintained over time.

Degenerative Arthritis of the Small Joints

Foucher G, Long Pretz P: Proximal interphalangeal joint denervation. La Main 1998;3:55-60.

PIP joint denervation was performed on 34 PIP joints of 26 patients who exhibited a functional range of motion with intractable pain. Eighty-five percent of operated joints showed a mean improvement in pain of 88% as measured on a visual analog scale.

Freedman DM, Eaton RG, Glickel SZ: Long-term results of volar ligament reconstruction for symptomatic basal joint laxity. *J Hand Surg Am* 2000;25:297-304.

Twenty-four thumb CMC joints in 19 patients were followed up for an average of 15 years after volar ligament reconstruction. Only 8% of thumbs advanced to radiographic stage III or IV basal joint arthritis, which compares favorably with the 17% to 33% reported incidence of arthritis of this degree in the general population.

Hobby JL, Lyall HA, Meggitt BF: First metacarpal osteotomy for trapeziometacarpal osteoarthritis. *J Bone Joint Surg Br* 1998;80:508-512.

Results from a study of 41 thumbs in 33 patients with a mean follow-up of 7 years showed that 93% of patients reported improved hand function, and grip and pinch strength were normal in 82% of cases. First metacarpal osteotomy is a simple procedure that is useful in patients with early or moderate trapeziometacarpal osteoarthritis.

Moller K, Sollerman C, Geijer M, Branemark PI: Early results with osseointegrated proximal interphalangeal joint prostheses. *J Hand Surg Am* 1999;24:267-274.

Excellent osseointegration was achieved with a titanium screw fixation device in phalangeal bone. The flexible silicone spacer that allows joint motion has, however, shown disappointing rates of fracture and deformation and is presently being redesigned.

Schmidt CC, McCarthy DM, Arnoczky SP, Herndon JH: Basal joint arthroplasty using an allograft tendon interposition versus no interposition: A radiographic, vascular, and histologic study. *J Hand Surg Am* 2000;25: 447-457.

In this primate study, all joints had the anterior oblique ligament reconstructed after trapezial excision. Those animals treated without tendon interposition allograft showed a significantly greater decline in trapezial height. Filling the trapezial void with an interposition tendon spacer may aid in maintaining normal wrist anatomy.

Uchiyama S, Cooney WP, Linscheid RL, Niebur G, An KN: Kinematics of the proximal interphalangeal joint of the finger after surface replacement. *J Hand Surg Am* 2000;25:305-312.

The kinematics of the PIP joint after resurfacing metal-polyethylene prosthetic replacement were found to be similar to those of the normal joint when nine cadaver specimens were evaluated. The center of rotation was nearly identical to that of the normal joint, and normal motion was restored.

Wachtl SW, Guggenheim PR, Sennwald GR: Cemented and non-cemented replacements of the trapeziometacarpal joint. *J Bone Joint Surg Br* 1998;80:121-125.

In this study of 43 de la Caffiniere cemented implants and 45 noncemented Ledoux implants, substantial rates of dislocation and loosening were seen. The survival rate for the Ledoux implant was 59% at 16 months and 66% for the de la Caffiniere implant at 68 months. Ball and socket joints are not suitable for trapeziometacarpal joint replacement.

Yang SS, Weiland AJ: First metacarpal subsidence during pinch after ligament reconstruction and tendon interposition basal joint arthroplasty of the thumb. *J Hand Surg Am* 1998;23:879-883.

Fifteen arthroplasties were evaluated radiographically at rest and with maximal effort key pinch stress at a mean follow-up of 32 months. With axial compressive loading of the arthroplasty, minor increases (10.5%) in proximal migration of the first metacarpal were seen, but these increases did not correlate with functional outcome. Key and tip pinch measurements were both improved 17% from preoperative values.

Rheumatoid Reconstruction

Adams BD: Total wrist arthroplasty. *Semin Arthroplasty* 2000;11:72-81.

A newer total wrist prothesis studied in this article demonstrates reliable long-term fixation. In the 57 previously reported cases with 4- to 10-year follow-up and in 18 additional cases, there were no distal component loosenings. Flexion averaged 46° and extension 35°.

Barbier O, Saels P, Rombouts JJ, Thonnard JL: Long-term functional results of wrist arthrodesis in rheumatoid arthritis. *J Hand Surg Br* 1999;24:27-31.

After wrist arthrodesis in a series of rheumatoid patients, no difference in sensory or motor impairment ratings were found between the fused and unoperated wrists. The results indicate that fusion does not create additional impairment when compared with an arthritic wrist, nor does it necessarily produce a significant improvement in function.

Flury MP, Herren DB, Simmen BR: Rheumatoid arthritis of the wrist: Classification related to the natural course. *Clin Orthop* 1999;366:72-77.

Rheumatoid wrist disease was classified into three types based on the progression of several radiographic parameters. The more stable osteoarthritic and ankylosis types progress slower whereas the disintegration type leads to more rapid instability and is indicated for earlier surgical intervention.

Tetraplegia

Friden J, Ejeskar A, Dahlgren A, Lieber RL: Protection of the deltoid to triceps tendon transfer repair sites. *J Hand Surg Am* 2000;25:144-149.

Stainless steel sutures were placed into the posterior deltoid, graft, and triceps insertion at surgery in 11 patients. Distances between the markers were measured and significant tendon elongation was observed, primarily in the proximal connection site.

Kuz JE, Van Heest AE, House JH: Biceps-to-triceps transfer in tetraplegic patients: Report of the medial routing technique and follow-up of three cases. *J Hand Surg Am* 1999;24:161-172.

Technique of biceps-to-triceps transfer using a medial route and results in three patients (four elbows) are described. All patients had a marked increase in activities that require elbow extension and all transfers were at least a grade 4.

Revol M, Briand E, Servant JM: Biceps-to-triceps transfer in tetraplegia: The medial route. *J Hand Surg Br* 1999;24:235-237.

Eight tetraplegic patients (13 elbows) were treated with biceps-to-triceps transfer via a medial route. There were no complications, but a 47% reduction in elbow flexion power was noted.

Brachial Plexus Injuries

Doi K, Muramatsu K, Hattori Y, et al: Restoration of prehension with the double free muscle technique following complete avulsion of the brachial plexus: Indications and long-term results. *J Bone Joint Surg Am* 2000;82:652-666.

Twenty-six patients who underwent double free muscle transfer to restore prehension were followed for at least 2 years. Satisfactory elbow flexion was restored in 96% and modest prehension in 65%.

Hems TE, Birch R, Carlstedt T: The role of magnetic resonance imaging in the management of traction injuries to the adult brachial plexus. *J Hand Surg Br* 1999;24:550-555.

MRI of the cervical spine and brachial plexus was compared with intraoperative neurophysiology, surgical findings, and clinical progress in 26 patients. MRI had no false-positive interpretations, but the number of individual root avulsions (sensitivity, 81%) was underestimated.

Leechavengvongs S, Witoonchart K, Uerpairojkit C, Thuvasethakul P, Ketmalasiri W: Nerve transfer to biceps muscle using a part of the ulnar nerve in brachial plexus injury (upper arm type): A report of 32 cases. *J Hand Surg Am* 1998;23:711-716.

Transfer of one or two ulnar nerve fascicles was done in 32 patients. Thirty patients (93%) regained grade 4 elbow flexion. No permanent impairment in ulnar nerve function was noted.

Waikakul S, Orapin S, Vanadurongwan V: Clinical results of contralateral C7 root neurotization to the median nerve in brachial plexus injuries with total root avulsions. *J Hand Surg Br* 1999;24:556-560.

This article presents a prospective study of contralateral C7 nerve root transfer to the median nerve in 96 patients with total root avulsions. The return of sensibility was encouraging, but forearm and hand motor function was poor.

Waikakul S, Wongtragul S, Vanadurongwan V: Restoration of elbow flexion in brachial plexus avulsion injury: Comparing spinal accessory nerve transfer with intercostal nerve transfer. *J Hand Surg Am* 1999;24: 571-577.

This article presents a prospective randomized series (205 patients) comparing spinal accessory nerve transfer with intercostal nerve transfer. Spinal accessory nerve advantages included less surgical time, fewer blood transfusions, and better motor function. Intercostal nerves produced earlier reinnervation, protective sensation, and pain reduction.

Tumors

Gustafson P, Arner M: Soft tissue sarcoma of the upper extremity: Descriptive data and outcome in a population-based series of 108 adult patients. *J Hand Surg Am* 1999;24:668-674.

A referral center reviewed population-based database for soft-tissue sarcomas. The 5-year metastasis-free survival rate was 72%. Tumor size greater than 5 cm and vascular invasion were independent prognostic factors for metastasis. Referral to an experienced tumor or cancer center was recommended for deep-seated tumors or masses larger than 5 cm prior to biopsy.

Joseph E, Brobeil A, Cruse CW, Wells K, Costello D, Reintgen DS: Lymphatic mapping for melanomas of the upper extremity. *J Hand Surg Am* 1999;24:675-681.

This article details the approach to upper extremity melanomas using preoperative lymphoscintigraphy and intraoperative lymphatic mapping to identify the sentinel node, which is removed for biopsy. Immunohistochemical stains are used to identify micrometastases, which parallels the status of the regional lymph node basin.

Luchetti R, Badia A, Alfarano M, Orbay J, Indriago I, Mustapha B: Arthroscopic resection of dorsal wrist ganglia and treatment of recurrences. *J Hand Surg Br* 2000;25:38-40.

Arthroscopic resection was attempted on 43 patients. Nine patients required conversion to open ganglionectomy. The ganglion stalk was seen in 79% of the cases. There were two recurrences after arthroscopic resection.

Cerebral Palsy

Gilmartin R, Bruce D, Storrs BB, et al: Intrathecal baclofen for management of spastic cerebral palsy: Multicenter trial. *J Child Neurol* 2000;15:71-77.

This article presents a randomized, double-blinded study of intrathecal baclofen for spasticity in cerebral palsy. There was decreased upper and lower extremity spasticity with manageable side effects, including vomiting, hypotonia, and somnolence.

Scheker LR, Chesher SP, Ramirez S: Neuromuscular electrical stimulation and dynamic bracing as a treatment for upper-extremity spasticity in children with cerebral palsy. *J Hand Surg Br* 1999;24:226-232.

Neuromuscular electrical stimulation was combined with dynamic bracing to treat a series of 19 patients with spastic hemiplegia. A reduction in spasticity of the wrist and fingers was obtained, along with an improvement in upper extremity function.

Van Heest AE, House JH, Cariello C: Upper extremity surgical treatment of cerebral palsy. *J Hand Surg Am* 1999;24:323-330.

Surgical treatment of cerebral palsy was done in 134 patients. Outcome was measured by upper extremity functional use scale. Individuals with fair and good voluntary control had significantly greater improvement than patients with poor control.

Vascular Disorders

McCall TE, Petersen DP, Wong LB: The use of digital artery sympathectomy as a salvage procedure for severe ischemia of Raynaud's disease and phenomenon. *J Hand Surg Am* 1999;24:173-177.

Digital artery sympathectomy was performed as a last resort to prevent amputation in seven patients with severe digital ischemia. Salvage was successful in six of the seven patients.

Ruch DS, Aldridge M, Holden M, Smith TL, Koman LA, Smith BP: Arterial reconstruction for radial artery occlusion. *J Hand Surg Am* 2000;25:282-290.

The history, subjective complaints, and objective findings were reviewed in 13 patients with symptomatic radial artery occlusion. Arterial reconstruction provided a substantial decrease in symptoms and improvement in function. Graft patency was 100% at follow-up (average of 22 months).

Yee AM, Hotchkiss RN, Paget SA: Adventitial stripping: A digit saving procedure in refractory Raynaud's phenomenon. *J Rheumatol* 1998;25:269-276.

Advential stripping provided long-term improvement (mean follow-up 28 months) in 13 ischemic digits (nine patients). There was no clinical response to preoperative sympathetic nerve blockade in 10 digits.

Classic Bibliography

Adolfsson L, Frisen M: Arthroscopic synovectomy of the rheumatoid wrist: A 3.8 year follow-up. *J Hand Surg Br* 1997;22:711-713.

Burgess RC: The effect of rotatory subluxation of the scaphoid on the radio-scaphoid contact. *J Hand Surg Am* 1987;12:771-774.

Chung KC, Zimmerman NB, Travis MT: Wrist arthrography versus arthroscopy: A comparative study of 150 cases. *J Hand Surg Am* 1996;21:591-594.

Johnson RP, Carrera GF: Chronic capitolunate instability. *J Bone Joint Surg Am* 1986;68:1164-1176.

Kilgore KL, Peckham PH, Keith MW, et al: An implanted upper-extremity neuroprosthesis: Follow-up of five patients. *J Bone Joint Surg Am* 1997;79:533-541.

Kirschenbaum D, Sieler S, Solonick D, Loeb DM, Cody RP: Arthrography of the wrist: Assessment of the integrity of the ligaments in young asymptomatic adults. *J Bone Joint Surg Am* 1995;77:1207-1209.

Kleinman WB, Carroll C IV: Scapho-trapezio-trapezoid arthrodesis for treatment of chronic static and dynamic scapho-lunate instability: A 10-year perspective on pitfalls and complications. *J Hand Surg Am* 1990;15:408-414.

Larsen CF, Jacoby RA, McCabe SJ: Nonunion rates of limited carpal arthrodesis: A meta-analysis of the literature. *J Hand Surg Am* 1997;22:66-73.

Lichtman DM, Bruckner JD, Culp RW, Alexander CE: Palmar midcarpal instability: Results of surgical reconstruction. *J Hand Surg Am* 1993;18:307-315.

Mulcahey MJ, Betz RR, Smith BT, Weiss AA, Davis SE: Implanted functional electrical stimulation hand system in adolescents with spinal injuries: An evaluation. *Arch Phys Med Rehabil* 1997;78:597-607.

Nakamura T, Yabe Y, Horiuchi Y, Takayama S: Magnetic resonance myelography in brachial plexus injury. *J Bone Joint Surg Br* 1997;79:764-769.

Rosenwasser MP, Miyasaka KC, Strauch RJ: The RASL procedure: Reduction and association of the scaphoid and lunate using the Herbert Screw. *Tech Hand Upper Extrem Surg* 1997;1:263-272.

Salomon GD, Eaton RG: Proximal row carpectomy with partial capitate resection. *J Hand Surg Am* 1996; 21:2-8.

Weiss A-P, Akelman E, Lambiase R: Comparison of the findings of triple-injection cinearthrography of the wrist with those of arthroscopy. *J Bone Joint Surg Am* 1996;78:348-356.

Weiss A-P, Hastings H II: Wrist arthrodesis for traumatic conditions: A study of plate and local bone graft application. *J Hand Surg Am* 1995;20:50-56.

Weiss A-P, Sachar K, Glowacki KA: Arthroscopic debridement alone for intercarpal ligament tears. *J Hand Surg Am* 1997;22:344-349.

Weiss APC, Wiedeman G Jr, Quenzer D, Hanington KR, Hastings H II, Strickland JW: Upper extremity function after wrist arthrodesis. *J Hand Surg Am* 1995; 20:813-817.

Wyrick JD, Stern PJ, Kiefhaber TR: Motion-preserving procedures in the treatment of scapholunate advanced collapse wrist: Proximal row carpectomy versus four-corner arthrodesis. *J Hand Surg Am* 1995;20:965-970.

Section 4

Lower Extremity

Section Editors:
Jay R. Lieberman, MD
Paul Tornetta III, MD
Elly Trepman, MD
James G. Wright, MD

Chapter 35

Evaluation of Lower Extremity Deformity

David S. Feldman, MD

Introduction

Although the clinical implication of long-term mechanical malalignment of the lower extremity as a cause of osteoarthritis and pain is not completely understood, understanding of lower extremity alignment has improved over the past 2 decades. It is increasingly important to be able to understand and quantify lower extremity long bone and joint malalignment to achieve safe and effective correction of deformity.

History and Physical Examination

The evaluation of the deformity begins with the medical history of the patient, including factors such as whether or not the patient has a history of diabetes, peripheral vascular disease, or previous surgeries. The nature of the injury or congenital problem and the extent of disability and pain associated with the deformity should be determined.

The physical examination should assess for overall appearance of limb alignment (varus, valgus, procurvatum, recurvatum). The vascularity of the limb/bone and scarring as well as compromised skin play critical roles in deformity assessment and correction. Passive and active range of motion as well as the presence of pain with motion and apparent joint contractures are recorded. Ligamentous instability of the knee and ankle is important. The patient's gait and single limb stance should be observed for ligamentous instability, that is, a lateral or medial thrust of the knee. The patient's muscle strength as well as neurologic status (including sensation, proprioception, and peroneal nerve dysfunction) should be examined.

Radiographic Evaluation

The first radiograph obtained in the coronal plane is a standing full lower extremity film from the pelvic rim to the floor. The patellae should be facing forward, a factor that is particularly important if concomitant internal tibial torsion or femoral anteversion is present. For cases in which the patella forward view cannot be used, the axis of the knee should be perpendicular to the plate.

A 3-ft film is sufficient in children, and a 51-in plate may be required in adults. If a limb-length discrepancy is present, a lift should be used under the short leg in order to level the pelvis. Limb-length inequality may be measured with a full-length film, standard radiographic scanogram, or a CT scanogram. The CT scanogram exposes the patient to the least amount of radiation and is the most accurate method.

In a patient with a limb-length discrepancy, foot height should be considered. A lateral foot radiograph is obtained and measurement from the plafond of the ankle to the base of the heel is obtained. A full-length lower limb hyperextension lateral radiograph is also obtained, which is particularly important to determine if a flexion deformity or recurvatum is a soft-tissue or bony type.

The overall alignment and knee joint orientation can be determined from the standing view; however, joint alignment of the hip and ankle should be determined from separate orthogonal views of the tibia and the femur to avoid parallax. If a patient has ligamentous laxity, then a single limb stance view should be obtained in order to determine the contribution of the laxity to the mechanical axis deviation. When measuring joint alignment the beam should be centered over the joint being considered.

The relationship of the calcaneus (hindfoot) to the tibia is best assessed through a PA view that is obtained with the foot flat on the plate and the beam canted 45° off the horizontal. Alternatively, the beam is canted 20° from the horizontal and the plate is canted 20° off the vertical. This method reduces setup distortion and is a more anatomic way of measuring the calcaneal-tibial relationship.

Mechanical Malalignment

The mechanical axis of the limb is defined as a line drawn from the center of the femoral head to the center of the ankle joint. Normally this line falls just medial to the medial tibial spine of the knee. Any deviation of this line means that in the limb there is an axis deviation; that is, if the line falls through the medial compartment of the knee then there is overall varus of the limb and if the line falls lateral this represents valgus. The location of the deformity cannot be determined from this test. It simply means that the sum of all deformities is either normal, varus, or valgus. The magnitude of mechanical axis deviation can be determined by measuring the distance between the center of the knee and the mechanical axis line. The mechanical axis deviation determines the extent of overall malalignment and effect on the knee joint. Deformity arising about the knee causes the greatest deviation of the mechanical axis, whereas deformities about the ankle or hip may cause joint malorientation but do not contribute greatly to mechanical axis deviation such as in coxa vara or ankle valgus. Similarly, there can be a normal mechanical axis when drawn from the center of the hip to the center of the ankle but the joints themselves are not parallel to each other or the floor. These deformities are periarticular or intra-articular and are important to recognize.

A deformity may arise in the tibia, femur, hip joint, knee joint, ankle joint, subtalar joint, or from ligamentous laxity. The deformity can be defined in six planes: frontal angulation, sagittal angulation, transverse angulation (rotation), transverse translation (length), frontal translation (medial/lateral), and sagittal translation (anterior/posterior).

In order to evaluate abnormal alignment, the relationship between the weight-bearing axis of the lower extremity in the coronal, sagittal, and transverse planes as well as the position of the joints (joint alignment) must be understood. Dynamic single leg weight bearing as well as the way the patient walks may alter the effect on the joint and change the mechanical axis of that limb.

Each limb deformity has an apex of deformity that is the intersection of normal mechanical or anatomic axes coming from proximal and distal directions. A bone may have more then one apex of deformity, called a multiapical deformity (Fig. 1).

Joint Alignment

In order to assess limb deformity, the orientation of the joints with respect to the femur and tibia and the joint's relationship to the ground must be understood. The proximal femur, distal femur, proximal tibia, distal tibia, and talar dome should be addressed. Nomencla-

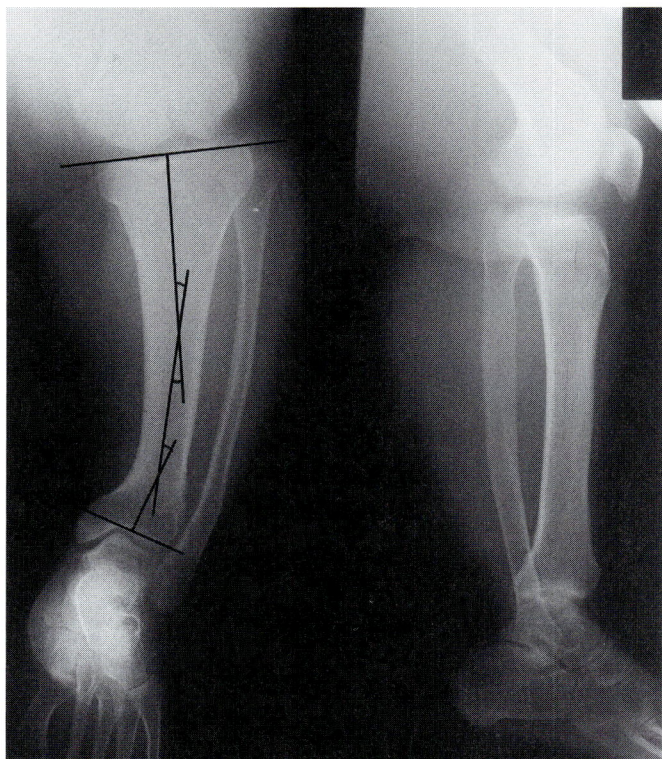

Figure 1 Multiapical deformity of the tibia with two apices outlined.

ture for the angles is provided in Fig. 2. In an adult in whom the greater trochanter is ossified, there is a line drawn from the tip of the trochanter to the center of the femoral head, which indicates an approximate 90° angle with the mechanical axis. Anatomically the mid-diaphyseal line of the femur and a line drawn from the tip of the trochanter and the center of the femoral head meets at the piriformis fossa at a medial angle of an average of 84°. In children, in whom the greater trochanter is not ossified, the neck shaft angle must be used or intraoperative evaluation must be done with a wire from the tip of the nonossified trochanter to the center of the femoral head. The distal femur creates an approximate 88° angle on the lateral side of the mechanical axis and an 81° anatomic axis. The proximal tibia has an 88° angle on its medial side. The distal tibia and plafond should create a 90° angle with the anatomic plane in the coronal plane.

In the sagittal plane the relationship between the joint and the diaphyseal line is equally important. A line drawn from the anterior intersection of the lateral femoral condyle to the anterior cortex to the top of the posterior condyles (the flattened part of the posterior condyles) intersects the mid-diaphyseal line approximately one third back on the femur. In children, this line can be drawn by connecting the anterior and posterior physis with the mid-diaphyseal line; this normally portends an angle of 83° posteriorly.

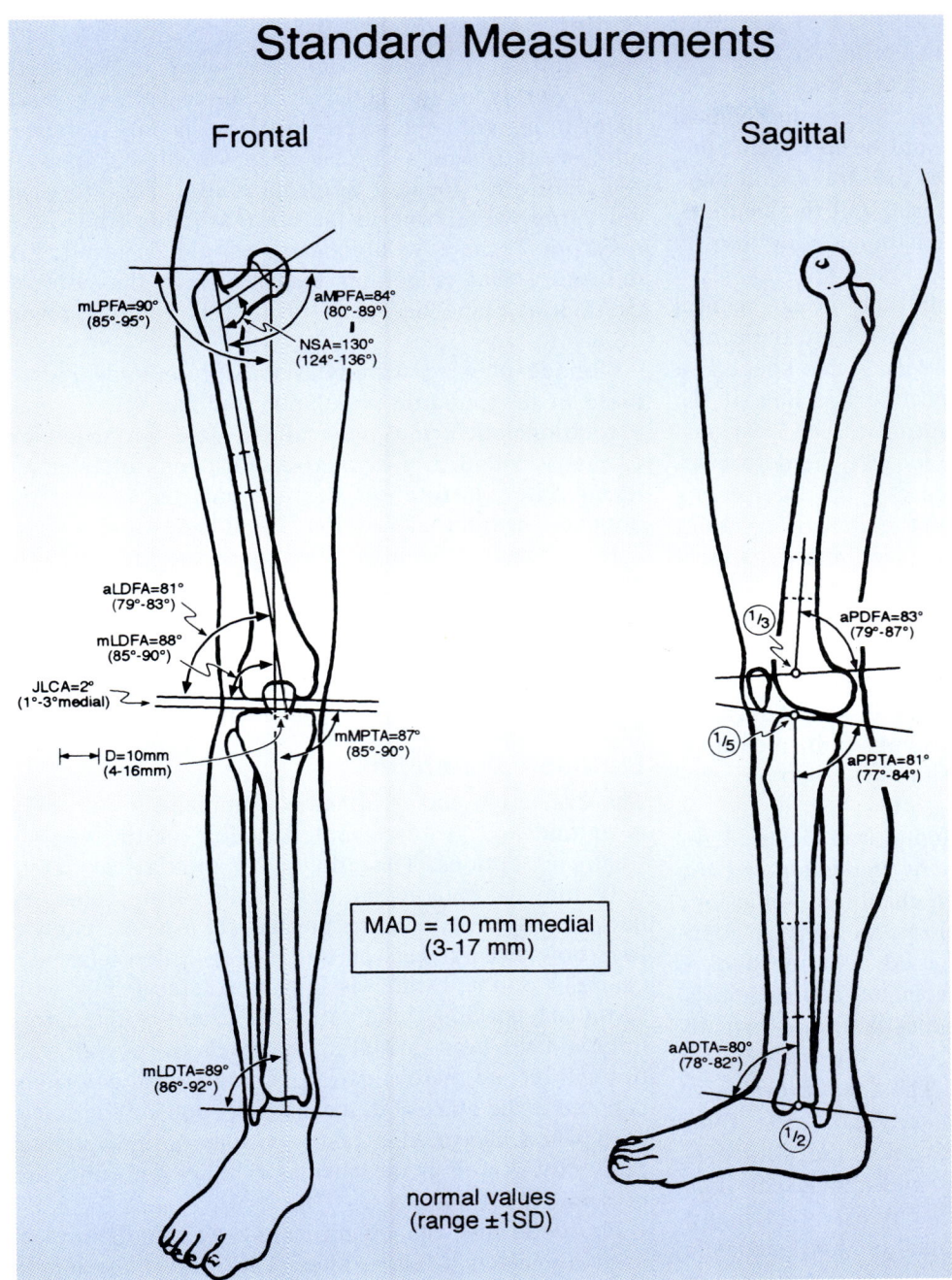

Figure 2 Standard measurements of mechanical axis and joint alignment. See text for details. mLPFA = mechanical lateral proximal femoral angle; aMPFA = anatomic medial proximal femoral angle; NSA = neck shaft angle; aLDFA = anatomic lateral distal femoral angle; mLDFA = mechanical lateral distal femoral angle; JLCA = joint line congruence angle; mMPTA = mechanical medial proximal tibial angle; mLDTA = mechanical lateral distal tibial angle; aPDFA = anatomic posterior distal femoral angle; aPPTA = anatomic posterior proximal tibial angle; aADTA = anatomic anterior distal tibial angle; MAD = mechanical axis deviation; SD = standard deviation. (© Maryland Limb Length Institute.)

The mid-diaphyseal line on the sagittal plane of the tibia intersects with the tibial plafond one fifth back. This creates an average posterior angle of 81°. The distal tibia angle off the anatomic axis on the sagittal plane has an angle of 80° anteriorly. This angle allows dorsiflexion of the ankle without impingement. These angles are population averages and have variability of a few degrees.

When evaluation of a patient reveals that the contralateral side is normal, then the joint measurements should be determined and used when assessing the deformity on the affected side. These lines and angles may not be as accurate in young children who have less ossification of the epiphyses and if correction of a deformity is to be undertaken, intraoperative arthrograms may be helpful.

Malalignment Test

The malalignment test systematically resolves the deformity into its component parts. A standing leg length film is obtained to determine overall alignment and axes about the knee as previously described.

Plain radiographs of the affected bone(s) are taken 90° to each other. A line is drawn from the center of the femoral head to the center of the ankle to determine mechanical axis deviation. If there is mechanical axis deviation, the deformity should be localized using a systematic approach. Joint lines are drawn and measured with respect to the mechanical and the anatomic axes, which will determine which bone(s) or joint(s) are involved in creating the deformity.

The femur can be assessed from both the mechanical and the anatomic axis. A line is drawn from the center of the femoral head to the center of the knee. The joint line is measured with respect to this line. If the angle is abnormal then the deformity is at least partially arising from the femur. To localize the deformity, mid-diaphyseal lines can be used and the intersecting point(s) will be the location of the deformity. Joint lines need to be measured from these mid-diaphyseal lines to rule out metaphyseal or intra-articular deformity as well. A metaphyseal deformity can be quantified by drawing a joint line and its corresponding "normal" diaphyseal line. This line will intersect with the mid-diaphyseal line at the location of the deformity. The joint axes of the distal femur are measured mechanically from the center of the knee and anatomically from 1 cm medial to the center.

The mechanical axis of the femur can be used for deformity measurement as well by understanding the relationship between the mechanical and anatomic axes. If the patient has bilateral disease, then a population average for joint axis is used. The mechanical axis is on average 7° of varus from the anatomic axis.

The tibia anatomic and mechanical axes are virtually the same (the anatomic axis is a few millimeters medial to the mechanical axis). The tibia is evaluated by drawing intersecting mid-diaphyseal lines. Even with an obvious diaphyseal deformity, the joint axes must be measured off of the mid-diaphyseal lines drawn. If there is an obvious diaphyseal or metaphyseal deformity, an intra-articular or juxta-articular deformity must be ruled out. This is done in the same fashion as in the femur, by drawing joint lines and the normal line down from the proximal tibia and up from the distal tibia.

In the sagittal plane the measurements are made in a similar fashion. The unique requirement in the sagittal view is to define the center of knee rotation, which is defined as the intersection point of a line drawn parallel and on the posterior cortex of the femur with the midpoint of the condyles if viewed as a circle. The condyles should overlap on the lateral knee radiograph, and this usually requires a few degrees of external rotation.

Oblique Plane Deformity

Few deformities other than iatrogenic deformities occur purely in the coronal or sagittal plane; most deformities are somewhere in between. For instance, adolescent Blount's disease occurs with the apex of the deformity located anterolaterally. Therefore, if correction were done in the coronal plane (the varus deformity), there would be a residual deformity. A deformity that is neither exclusively in the coronal or sagittal plane has been termed an oblique plane deformity.

Oblique plane deformity is most commonly recognized in the pediatric population and can often mimic a rotational deformity clinically. Adolescent Blount's disease is found in the anterolateral plane, often mimicking internal rotation of the limb. A radiograph obtained in internal rotation will demonstrate a view with maximal deformity. This radiograph can also be analyzed and understood in conjunction with orthogonal AP and lateral radiographs of the tibia. The magnitude and direction of the deformity can be assessed via a simple graph (Fig. 3). Understanding of all components of the deformity in all planes is essential.

Multiapical Deformity

The evaluation and treatment of multiapical deformity is unique and requires understanding of the various treatment options. The etiology of multiapical deformity may be a congenital anomaly with secondary deformity that restores the mechanical axis, or simply a long bow as in rickets or osteogenesis imperfecta. An example of the former is an anterolateral bow with secondary proximal tibia vara. The extent of the deformity and the bow as well as the levels of the deformities will dictate the evaluation. A multiapical deformity is noted if the apex of deformity falls outside the bone, or if when measured a juxta-articular or metaphyseal deformity as well as the obvious primary deformity are present.

The deformity can be measured via mid-diaphyseal lines connected to each other. The greater the length of the bow, the greater the number of lines that can be drawn and apices defined. The deformity can also be defined by a single angle drawn with normal joint orientation lines from above and below (Fig. 4, A). The number of apices does not define the number of osteotomies that need to be performed; this number is determined by the magnitude and direction of the curve as well as the clinical situation. Therefore, at times a multiapical deformity may be treated by restoring the mechanical axis via a single osteotomy (Fig. 4, B) that resolves all deformities or by two osteotomies, one proximal and one distal to the resolution angle of the deformity.

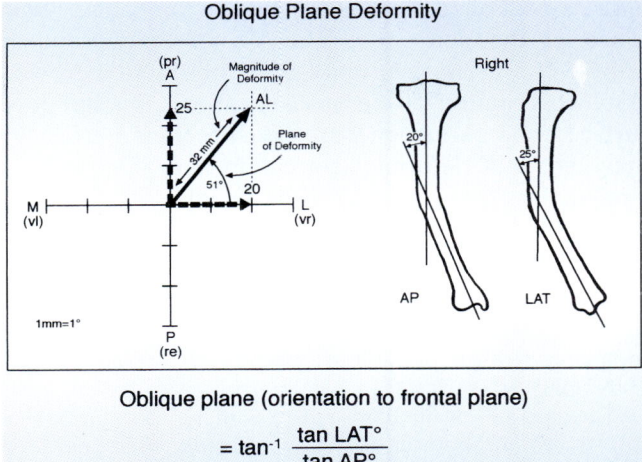

Figure 3 Oblique plane measurement and graph. (© Maryland Limb Length Institute.)

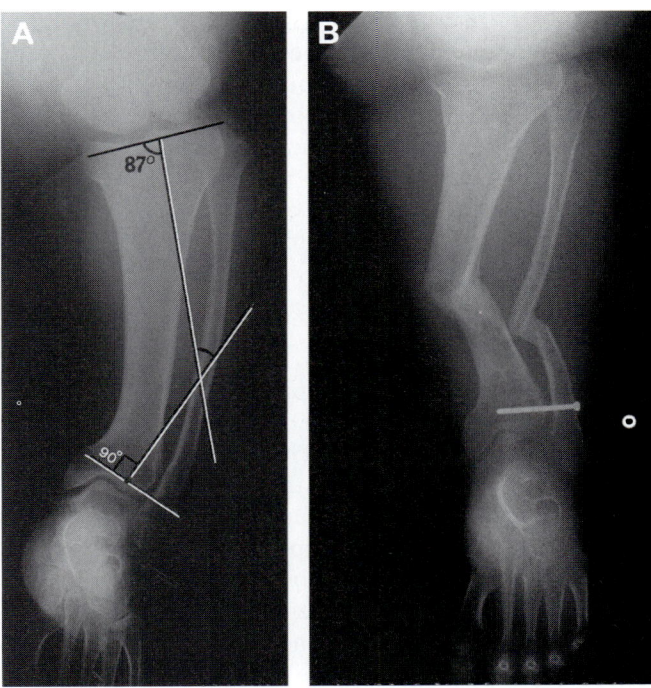

Figure 4 **A,** Resultant deformity of multiapical deformity noting the apex lateral to the tibia. **B,** Correction of the deformity with a single osteotomy.

Joint Laxity/Contracture Deformity

Joint laxity secondary to ligamentous laxity about the knee is quite common in various deformities. It is essential to determine the contribution of mechanical axis deviation from bony deformity versus ligamentous laxity or contracture. Varus deformities about the knee can have both medial collateral ligament laxity and/or lateral collateral ligament laxity. Single leg stance will help determine the contribution of ligament laxity to overall deformity. Treatment of joint laxity may be by correction of the deformity, primarily tightening ligaments or indirectly tightening ligaments (such as via fibula transport to tighten the lateral collateral ligament). Correction of the laxity by overcorrection of the bony malalignment should be done with caution because an oblique joint line will result, which may create shear within the joint.

Deformity of the joint may arise from an intra-articular depression such as in a tibial plateau fracture or untreated severe Blount disease. The evaluation of this contributing factor must be taken into account when assessing overall limb alignment. An intra-articular correction as opposed to an osteotomy below the deformity may be required.

The evaluation of a knee flexion contracture requires a lateral radiograph that includes the knee and proximal tibia and distal femur. A hyperextension lateral radiograph of the lower extremity may be beneficial. With a maximum extension lateral radiograph of the knee a line is drawn along the anterior border of the distal femur and an anterior line is drawn along the proximal tibia. These lines intersect and define the degree of lateral deformity. Sagittal plane measurements are then taken of the distal femur and proximal

tibia. A simple way to look at this deformity is that the apparent flexion or extension contracture may be bony or soft tissue or a combination of the two. Total joint deformity equals soft-tissue contracture plus bony angulation. This is especially important for a knee flexion contracture in determining the contribution from hamstring and capsular tightness versus bony malalignment.

Assessment of ankle valgus also requires differentiation of ankle joint valgus, joint line malorientation, subtalar deformity, and distal tibia bony deformity. Ankle valgus can be assessed with a standing radiograph of the distal tibia that includes the ankle. The standing leg length film is inaccurate in assessing ankle deformity because of parallax.

Translational Deformity

If intersecting anatomic lines do not cross at the obvious site of deformity, then there is either a second deformity, which is not as obvious, or translation is involved in the deformity. Isolated translational deformity is the most difficult to recognize and often requires innovative techniques for treatment.

A parallelization of the mechanical axes with normal joint lines defines a pure translational deformity. Therefore, there is a normal joint line angulation with continued mechanical axis deviation. This scenario would occur, for example, from a proximal varus derotational osteotomy of the hip without medialization of the distal fragment. There would be a varus moment at the knee even though the knee joint angulation would be normal. Correction using either a translational osteotomy or a double osteotomy would be required. The first osteotomy of the double osteotomy creates a deformity and then the correction of the deformity at a different site could correct both the new deformity as well as the pre-existing translation.

Rotational Deformity

The assessment of either a pure rotational deformity or a deformity that has a rotational component is most often performed clinically. The extent of rotation of the femur is best tested with the patient prone and the examiner rotating the hip internally and externally with a hand on the patient's ipsilateral greater trochanter. When the trochanter becomes parallel to the ground, this represents hip version. The CT scan accurately assesses for femoral and acetabular version for preoperative planning.

Tibial rotation is best assessed clinically using the bimalleolar axis and the foot progression angle. The examiner must not be fooled by an oblique plane deformity appearing as rotation in the tibia.

Correction of Limb Deformity

The correction of limb deformity is less difficult if the surgeon is able to correct a single-level deformity at the level of the deformity. This may not always be possible because of poor skin and soft-tissue quality or because the deformity is juxta-articular or at the level of the physis. Therefore, correction away from the site of deformity is often clinically ideal. If the mechanical axis is to be restored with an osteotomy away from the apex of the deformity, then translation of the bone onto the mechanical axis is essential. Osteotomies, such as a dome osteotomy, use this principle to allow the osteotomy to match the arc of translation and angulation required. If the mechanical axis were restored with an osteotomy away from the site of deformity without translation, then the angulation will by necessity cause an oblique joint line. This situation should be avoided. For example, in infantile Blount disease, the center of the deformity is often at the level of the physis and therefore a valgus osteotomy away from the deformity is required. The correction of the angulation should be of the angle measured at the deformity and the translation should occur laterally back onto the mechanical axis. Parallel joint lines and restoration of the mechanical axis will be achieved.

When performing angular correction in children, future potential growth must be considered. The pres-ence of continued asymmetric growth will cause recurrence of the deformity. The use of epiphyseodesis often will prevent recurrence of deformity in a growing child. Restoration of the mechanical axis, parallel joint surfaces, and permanence of the correction are the primary goals of deformity correction and, if possible, a straight long bone is a secondary goal.

Annotated Bibliography

Heijens E, Gladbach B, Pfeil J: Definition, quantification, and correction of translation deformities using long leg, frontal plane radiography. *J Pediatr Orthop* 1999;8:285-291.

The unique evaluation and treatment of translational deformities of the lower extremity is clearly described.

Classic Bibliography

Chao EY, Neluheni EV, Hsu RW, Paley D: Biomechanics of malalignment. *Orthop Clin North Am* 1994;25:379-386.

Cooke TD, Li J, Scudamore RA: Radiographic assessment of bony contributions to knee deformity. *Orthop Clin North Am* 1994;25:387-393.

Green SA, Green HD: The influence of radiographic projection on the appearance of deformities. *Orthop Clin North Am* 1994;25:467-475.

Henderson RC, Kemp GJ: Assessment of the mechanical axis in adolescent tibia vara. *Orthopedics* 1991;14:313-316.

Hollister AM, Jatana S, Singh AK, Sullivan WW, Lupichuk AG: The axes of rotation of the knee. *Clin Orthop* 1993;290:259-268.

Moreland JR, Bassett LW, Hanker GJ: Radiographic analysis of the axial alignment of the lower extremity. *J Bone Joint Surg Am* 1987;69:745-749.

Paley D, Herzenberg JE, Tetsworth K, McKie J, Bhave A: Deformity planning for frontal and sagittal plane corrective osteotomies. *Orthop Clin North Am* 1994;25:425-465.

Paley D, Bhatnagar J, Herzenberg JE, Bhave A: New procedures for tightening knee collateral ligaments in conjunction with knee realignment osteotomy. *Orthop Clin North Am* 1994;25:533-555.

Puno RM, Vaughan JJ, Stetten ML, Johnson JR: Long-term effects of tibial angular malunion on the knee and ankle joints. *J Orthop Trauma* 1991;5:247-254.

Saltzman CL, el-Khoury G: The hindfoot alignment view. *Foot Ankle Int* 1995;16:572-576.

Wright JG, Treble N, Feinstein AR: Measurement of lower limb alignment using long radiographs. *J Bone Joint Surg Br* 1991;73:721-723.

Chapter 36

Hip, Pelvis, and Femur: Pediatric Aspects

Michael B. Millis, MD

Mininder S. Kocher, MD

Introduction

Disorders of the hip in childhood and adolescence are relatively common. The three most frequently encountered developmental hip disorders, dysplasia, Legg-Calvé-Perthes disease (LCPD), and slipped capital femoral epiphysis (SCFE), are important not because of the dysfunction they can cause prior to skeletal maturity, but also because they are associated with a majority of cases of osteoarthritis of the adult hip.

Developmental Dysplasia of the Hip

Developmental dysplasia of the hip (DDH) comprises a spectrum, ranging from mild ultrasound or radiographic abnormality in a clinically normal infant to frank dislocation that is clinically evident. Risk factors include family history, female gender, constrained intrauterine environment (breech position), primiparity, increased birth weight, or oligohydramnios.

Diagnosis

Physical examination is the classic method for detecting neonatal and infant hip instability, although ultrasound is a more sensitive method. The Ortolani and Barlow tests are useful in the diagnosis of frankly unstable infant hips. Signs of instability (ie, the Barlow and Ortolani signs) become less clear and less frequent as the patient gets older, whereas the classic finding of limitation of abduction becomes more prominent. The greatest diagnostic dilemma lies in identifying the anatomically dysplastic but clinically stable hip that may not become symptomatic until adolescence or early adulthood.

Ultrasound is an excellent method of screening for DDH in the infant up to 6 months of age. Operator skill is, however, quite important in assessing the reliability of the study. In addition, in infants up to about 2 months of age, mild ultrasonographic dysplasia may be difficult to distinguish from physiologic immaturity.

In some parts of Europe, hip ultrasound is used for universal infant hip screening, even of clinically normal hips. Its role for universal screening in this country is controversial.

Ultrasound is useful in following the progress of treatment in dislocated and dysplastic hips in the infant up to 6 months of age. The appearance of the capital femoral ossification center after age 6 months reduces the resolution of the ultrasound, so plain radiography becomes the standard diagnostic modality in children 6 months of age or older.

A complete ultrasound examination has static and dynamic components. Important static measurements include the alpha angle (analogous to acetabular angle in an AP radiograph) and the percentage of femoral head coverage. The dynamic assessment of stability, done with a gentle on-line Barlow type maneuver, which attempts to detect pathologic instability of the femoral head, is much more subjective but can be useful. The presence of dysplasia noted on ultrasound, in the absence of clinically detectable instability, may not require immediate treatment, but does require careful follow-up clinically and with imaging.

Treatment

The Pavlik harness is commonly used for the initial treatment of the dislocated, unstable, or dysplastic hip from birth to about 6 months of age. Although reduction will be achieved in most dislocated infant hips treated with the Pavlik harness, careful clinical and ultrasound monitoring is mandatory. The anterior straps of the harness are adjusted tightly enough to flex the hips approximately 90° and the posterior straps adjusted tightly enough to prevent the hips from abducting to neutral. The side-lying position tends to adduct the hips and must be avoided. Moreover, keeping the treated infant supine tends to gently abduct the hips, mechanically encouraging reduction.

Ultrasound is recommended 2 to 3 weeks after placement of the Pavlik harness to confirm hip reduction. Splinting is continued usually for at least 3 months, until imaging studies are normal. Clinical testing of residual instability by the Barlow maneuver is not advisable during early treatment because of the risk of iatrogenic stretching of the capsule, with possible recurrent instability. If the Pavlik harness has affected reduction of a dislocated hip, but the hip remains positionally unstable, then the use of a fixed abduction device (either a brace or a cast) is the treatment of choice.

If reduction of a dislocated hip has not been achieved after about 3 weeks of treatment with the Pavlik harness, based on careful clinical and ultrasonographic monitoring, then the harness should be removed to prevent iatrogenic erosion of the posterior acetabular wall, which can make stability extremely difficult to achieve once the reduction is ultimately accomplished. Treatment choices at this point include closed or open reduction.

Closed Reduction

Closed reduction of an infant hip dislocation is done using the Ortolani maneuver with the patient under general anesthesia. With any form of reduction of a dislocated hip, attempts should be made to position the hip in the so-called "safe zone", which is a position where the hip is not only located and stable, but the femoral head and proximal femoral growth centers have an adequate vascular supply. Closed reduction carries a risk of vascular disturbance (noted in long-term follow-up studies) that is somewhat higher than that of either open reduction or reduction with the Pavlik harness, although exact comparisons are difficult. Whether closed or open reduction of a dislocated hip should be delayed until appearance of the proximal femoral ossification center is controversial because the presence of the ossification center is believed to exert a protective effect against ischemic necrosis. Recent studies suggest that reduction of a dislocated hip with an absent proximal femoral ossification center should not be delayed until the ossification center appears.

The use of preliminary traction, at home or in the hospital, before closed reduction is also controversial. Percutaneous adductor longus tenotomy is advocated as a minimal risk factor that results in increased abduction and a larger safe zone. Positioning the hip in a stable and vascularly safe position is critical for success of closed reduction. The usual "best" position, the so-called "human position", tends to approximate more than 90° of hip flexion, 60° or so of abduction, and approximately neutral rotation. Extreme positioning, particularly extremes of abduction, which are associated with an increased risk of osteonecrosis, is contra-

indicated. Positioning the hips midway in abduction between maximum passive abduction and the point in abduction where the hip dislocates is reasonable. A carefully fitted spica cast is crucial in maintaining reduction. Reduction can be confirmed using CT scans or, more recently, MRI. Intraoperative arthrography is occasionally useful. The first spica cast is usually changed 3 to 6 weeks after reduction, with subsequent cast changes every 6 to 8 weeks, with the patient under a general anesthetic, until the joint is stable.

Open Reduction

Certain dislocated hips are resistant to closed reduction or treatment with a Pavlik harness and may be reducible only with unacceptable force or extreme positioning. Anatomic obstacles including an hourglass constriction in the capsule, a tight psoas tendon, interposed labrum, hypertrophic ligamentum teres, tight transverse acetabular ligament, and hypertrophic pulvinar fat within the joint may preclude closed reduction. Acetabular dysplasia, coxa valga, and pathologic femoral anteversion may also render stable reduction difficult. Open reduction can be performed through an anterolateral, medial, or anteromedial approach. The anterolateral approach has the advantage of avoiding the medial circumflex vessels, as well as allowing a capsule repair or a pelvic osteotomy through the same incision. It is the approach of choice if there has been a previous failure of open reduction because it allows the most extensile approach to the acetabulum. The more medial approaches can be useful in a very young child in whom reduction may require division of the psoas tendon and the medial capsule.

An absolute requirement of any open reduction is the achievement of concentric reduction of the femoral head within the acetabulum. No stabilizing osteotomies should be carried out until complete concentric reduction has been achieved. Femoral shortening may be necessary to relax contracted soft tissues before a perfect reduction is possible in the older child (older than 2 years of age) or in a previously treated hip.

An inverted acetabular labrum may represent an obstacle to deep concentric reduction. However, an inverted or deformed labrum should not be excised but should be everted manually, making radial cuts in the labrum. Excision of the labrum may frequently lead to long-term growth disturbance in the anterolateral acetabular growth centers and acetabular dysplasia in late childhood and adolescence.

Open Reduction in Older Children

After a certain age, even the most skillful reduction of a dislocated hip is unlikely to produce a mobile, pain-free hip over the long term. Conversely, many high dislocations may remain mobile and pain free for decades, despite an inefficient gait. Bilateral pain-free dislocations discovered after age 6 or 7 years probably should not be reduced. Unilateral dislocations usually create additional difficulties with limb-length discrepancy and spinal malalignment. Unilateral dislocation therefore should be strongly considered for reduction when discovered at any age up to adolescence. After skeletal maturity, arthroplastic reconstruction is usually the primary treatment of choice for the symptomatic dislocation.

Osteotomies for Hip Dysplasia

In the child younger than 15 to 18 months of age, the predominant structural abnormality is often capsular laxity rather than bony deformity. Once a concentric reduction has been achieved, whether by closed or open means, spica immobilization with or without capsule repair is often enough to achieve stability.

In the dislocated hip that is reduced at age 15 months or older, usually there is enough associated bony deformity, either femoral, acetabular, or both, to require stabilizing osteotomy to maintain the concentric reduction. In general, up to about age 3 years, the more deformed element, either femoral or acetabular, should be corrected. An acetabular redirection often is more convenient because it can be done through the anterior incision used for the anterolateral approach.

If a child of walking age has a mechanically stable hip that is reduced but dysplastic, it is important to determine whether the dysplasia is improving, stable, or worsening. Serial radiographs, therefore, are ideal in determining the status of the developing hip. If there is no spontaneous improvement, then surgical correction of the dysplasia is indicated. If acetabular dysplasia is more severe radiographically than the proximal femoral deformity, then a pelvic osteotomy would be more appropriate than intertrochanteric osteotomy. If the femoral deformity seems more severe than the acetabular deformity, then intertrochanteric osteotomy would be more appropriate.

Before osteotomy of the pelvis or proximal femur to correct the residually dysplastic hip can be done, the hip must be evaluated in three dimensions, paying particular attention to the sagittal plane. Posterior instability or subluxation is difficult to detect in plain films, and CT analysis often is helpful in analyzing the problematic dysplastic hip. If a femoral osteotomy is done, care should be taken to prevent retroversion and excessive varus, along with excessive medialization of the distal femoral fragment, to avoid impingement by the lateral femoral neck or greater trochanter on the acetabular rim.

The Salter innominate osteotomy involves pure redirection of the acetabulum without change in the acetabular size or shape, and it requires internal fixation

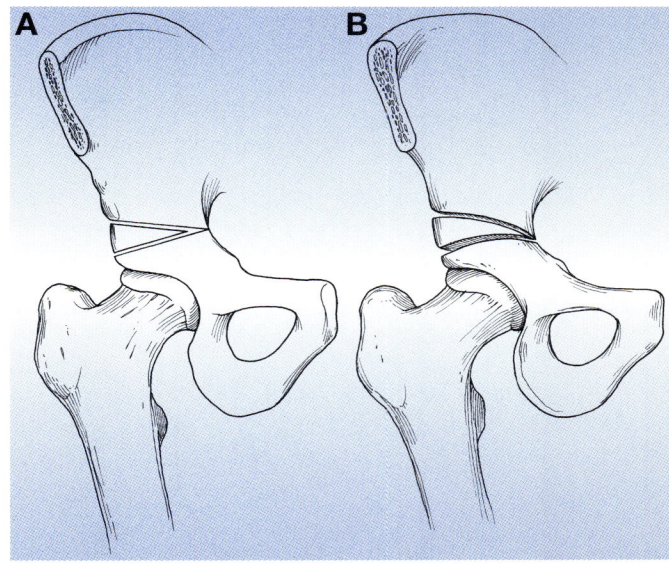

Figure 1 **A,** Salter single innominate osteotomy allows simple uniplanar redirection through a complete pelvic osteotomy. **B,** The Pemberton osteotomy achieves redirection and reduction in size of the dysplastic acetabulum through an incomplete osteotomy. *(Reproduced with permission from Gillingham BL, Sanchez AA, Wenger D: Pelvic osteotomies for the treatment of hip dysplasia in children and young adults.* J Am Acad Orthop Surg *1999;7:325-337.)*

to hold the wedge-shaped interposition bone graft into the supra-acetabular osteotomy site (Fig. 1). Its classic indication is stabilization of a well reduced femoral head that is congruous with an anteriorly maldirected acetabulum in which the acetabular radius is the same as that of the femoral head.

The Pemberton and Dega osteotomies are similar in concept and indication, representing supra-acetabular opening wedge osteotomies that both redirect and reshape the dysplastic acetabulum (Fig. 1). In these osteotomies, both iliac cortices are divided anteriorly, the medial cortex is left intact more posteriorly, and the lateral iliac portion of the osteotomy continues more posteriorly than the medial portion. The osteotomy should extend to but not through the posterior limb of the triradiate cartilage. Because these osteotomies not only tend to redirect the anterior and lateral portions of the acetabulum into a more horizontal position but also tend to reduce its size and radius of curvature, their best indication is a hip in which the femoral head easily reduces into the depths of the acetabulum for which the radius of curvature is slightly larger than that of the femoral head. These incomplete osteotomies tend to exert more of a lengthening effect than does the Salter innominate osteotomy. Osteotomies done in the presence of a slightly short femur or in conjunction with an intertrochanteric osteotomy that allows some degree of simultaneous shortening are preferable because the placement of too much pressure on the femoral head is prevented.

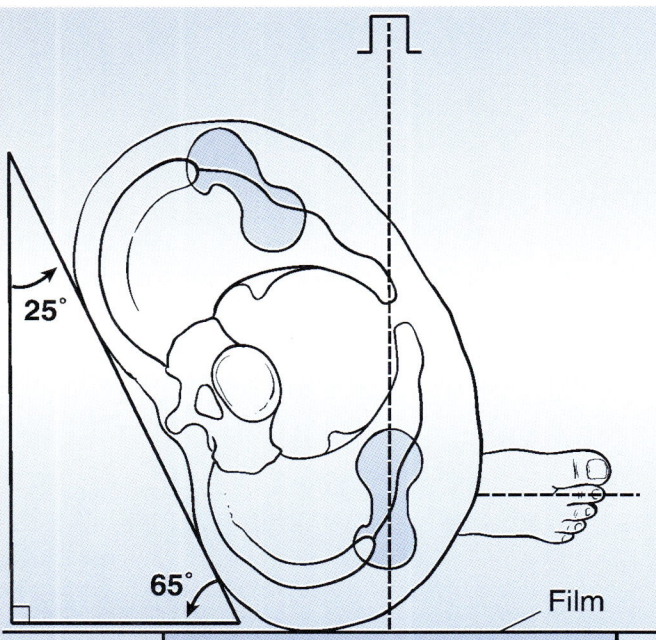

Figure 2 Diagram of the faux profil view originally described by DeSeze and associates in 1962. A standing lateral view of the acetabulum is taken with the hip to be examined placed against the x-ray plate, with the pelvis rotated 25° toward the x-ray beam. An anterior center edge angle can be measured from the resulting image. *(Reproduced with permission from Tonnis D: Congenital Dysplasia and Dislocation of the Hip in Children and Adults. New York, NY, Springer-Verlag, 1987.)*

In the child with a dysplastic hip, it is important to consider changes in the hip over time, rather than basing treatment decisions on one isolated radiographic and clinical examination. Clinical and radiographic follow-up to skeletal maturity is mandatory in all treated cases, because growth arrest of either the proximal femur or acetabular rim may become clear at any point until the end of growth.

The goal of treatment of hip dysplasia is to obtain a both clinically and radiographically normal hip at skeletal maturity. Long-term follow-up studies suggest that any subluxation or dysplasia with a lateral center edge angle of less than 20° will lead to osteoarthritis before or during middle age. As the growth centers of the proximal femur and acetabular rim close in late adolescence, predictions about the long-term prognosis of most hips can be made. Clinical examination of the hip should be supplemented with at least two radiographic views: a standing AP view (demonstrating lateral coverage) and a faux profil view (demonstrating anterior acetabular coverage) (Fig. 2). If the lateral center edge angle is less than 20°, the obliquity of the weight-bearing zone of the acetabulum in the AP view is more than 10°, the anterior center edge angle on the faux profil view is less than 10°, or if there is any subluxation at skeletal maturity, redirectional osteotomy should be considered.

Osteotomies of the Hip in Adolescence and Early Adulthood

The Salter innominate osteotomy and the incomplete hinge periacetabular osteotomies of Dega and Pemberton are useful in the child with open triradiate cartilage, but the relative stiffness of the pelvis in the adolescent and adult makes these osteotomies much less useful for the child older than 10 years of age. All redirectional osteotomies require either maintenance or establishment of congruity to achieve good long-term results. In the adolescent and young adult dysplastic hip, incongruity is much more common and problematic than in the young child with the potential for remodeling.

Radiographic acetabular dysplasia is treated in symptomatic individuals with acetabular obliquity, low center edge angle, or subluxation. In asymptomatic individuals, surgical treatment may be indicated. The treatment of asymptomatic dysplasia in adolescents is controversial; close radiographic and clinical follow-up is mandatory because most of these patients will ultimately develop symptoms. Prophylactic treatment may be justified on an individual basis.

Acetabular reorienting osteotomies are indicated to correct symptomatic congruous acetabular dysplasia in the nearly mature or mature hip with closed triradiate cartilage. Though the Salter innominate and Steel osteotomies are done in the adolescent and young adult, more reliable major multiplanar corrections can be achieved by spherical osteotomy, the Tonnis triple pelvic osteotomy, and the Bernese periacetabular osteotomy (Fig. 3). The closer to the acetabulum the osteotomy cuts are located, there is more freedom of acetabular redirection.

The Tonnis triple pelvic osteotomy, like the Steel osteotomy, requires both an anterior and buttock incision, and requires some abductor dissection. The Bernese periacetabular osteotomy can be done through one anterior incision, and without abductor dissection. The spherical osteotomy allows excellent correction, but the osteotomy is located very close to the acetabulum and requires major abductor dissection. All of these osteotomies allow excellent multiplanar corrections, stable fixation, and early function without external mobilization. The triple pelvic and Bernese periacetabular osteotomies allow an anterior arthrotomy if labral tears or anterior acetabular rim problems are suspected. There may be some capsular blood supply that is important to the acetabular fragment in the spherical osteotomies, and therefore it is not clear whether anterior simultaneous arthrotomy should be done in conjunction with spherical osteotomies.

Although acetabular dysplasia is more common in adolescence and early adulthood than femoral dyspla-

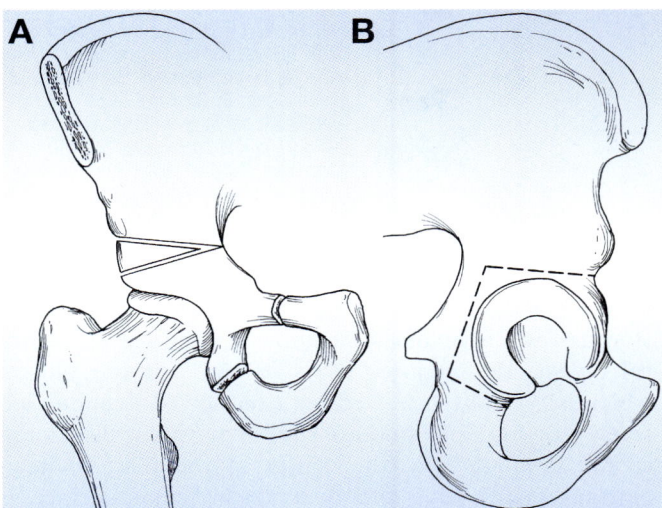

Figure 3 **A,** The triple pelvic osteotomy uses three separate osteotomy cuts. The first is very similar to the classic Salter-innominate osteotomy; the second and third cuts involve osteotomies through the superior pubic ramus and ischium proximal to the tuberosity. **B,** The Bernese periacetabular osteotomy uses a sequence of cuts that leave the posterior column intact. The anterior osteotomy begins just below the anterior superior iliac spine and lies higher than the classic innominate osteotomy line. A satellite osteotomy is made of the superior pubic ramus just medial to the tear drop, similar to that used in the triple pelvic osteotomy. *(Reproduced with permission from Gillingham BL, Sanchez AA, Wenger D: Pelvic osteotomies for the treatment of hip dysplasia in children and young adults. J Am Acad Orthop Surg 1999;7:325-337.)*

sia, femoral deformities do occur, both as a part of the spectrum of primary dysplasia and occasionally as a result of early growth disturbance associated with treatment. Overcorrection of coxa valga does not compensate for residual acetabular dysplasia.

Legg-Calvé-Perthes Disease

LCPD is a poorly understood hip disorder of unknown etiology that is associated with disturbance of the blood supply to the capital femoral epiphysis. The condition is five times more common in boys age 3 to 8 years old.

Diagnosis

LCPD involves a characteristic sequence of radiographic stages that include epiphyseal growth retardation, sclerosis, fragmentation, and reossification, with variable coxa magna and deformation. There is no absolute diagnostic test. Although LCPD occurs bilaterally in as many as 20% of cases, it is rarely at the same stage in both hips. When LCPD is symmetrical, other diagnoses, including variants of epiphyseal dysplasia and hypothyroidism, should be considered.

Evolution and Prognosis

The blood supply to the epiphysis is usually reestablished, and reossification of the epiphysis usually

occurs, although it is rare that a patient is left with a central femoral head lesion resembling osteochondritis dissecans. A variable amount of residual deformity occurs as a sequela of LCPD. The more spheroid the femoral head, the better the prognosis. As many as 50% of hips affected by LCPD will develop osteoarthritis in adulthood. In these cases, the osteoarthritis is associated with impingement by the aspherical femoral head on the anterolateral acetabular rim and labrum.

A major indication for treatment of LCPD is a poor prognosis. The younger the child at the onset of the disease, the smaller the portion of the femoral head involved, and the better the range of motion, the less likely are residual head deformity and osteoarthritis in adulthood.

The lateral pillar classification is quite useful during the active stage of the disease in determining final outcome, and it may be more useful than the percentage of the femoral head involved. This classification follows from the observation that fragmentation of the head in LCPD usually occurs in distinct anatomic portions of the femoral head, leading to a classification based on the AP radiograph. The AP projection of the femoral head is divided into three parts (pillars). The lateral pillar occupies the lateral 25% of the femoral head; the central pillar occupies approximately 50% of the central portion of the femoral head; and the medial pillar occupies the remaining medial portion of the femoral head. The classification focuses on the amount of the involvement of the lateral pillar, dividing patients with LCPD into three groups, A, B, and C. In group A, there is no involvement of the lateral pillar; group B, more than 50% of the lateral pillar height is maintained; group C, less than 50% maintenance of lateral pillar height (Fig. 4).

Treatment

Maintaining a physiologic range of motion, particularly abduction, and physical contact are the mainstays of treatment. Activity limitation, physiotherapy, and abduction splinting or casting can be useful in reestablishing a physiologic range of motion. Containment bracing has not been proved effective in altering the natural history of LCPD, but the Scottish Rite brace has been used. Physical containment, either by innominate osteotomy, shelf arthroplasty, or intertrochanteric varus osteotomy or combinations, may be effective in improving prognosis in hips at risk.

Limited abduction, internal rotation, and flexion are quite common in severe cases of LCPD when the femoral head has overgrown anteriorly and laterally. In such hips, the limitation of movement is secondary to impingement of the overgrown portions of the femoral head with the anterior and anterolateral acetabular

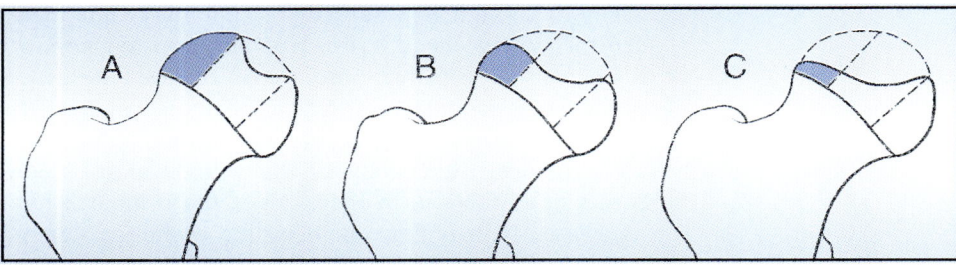

Figure 4 Lateral pillar classification of LCPD. The femoral head is divided into three pillars. **A,** Normal height of the lateral pillar is maintained. **B,** Greater than 50% of the lateral pillar height is maintained. **C,** Less than 50% of the lateral pillar height is maintained. (*Adapted with permission from Herring JA, Neustadt JB, Williams JJ, Early JS, Brown RH: The lateral pillar classification of Legg-Calve-Perthes disease. J Pediatr Orthop 1992;12:143-150.*)

rim. Mechanical disturbance in the growth centers of the acetabular rim and subsequent secondary acetabular dysplasia can occur. Valgus flexion intertrochanteric osteotomy can eliminate the impingement in such hips, with excellent short-term results reported, although long-term results are still lacking.

In the older adolescent and young adult, the impingement from deformed femoral heads can lead to acetabular labral tears, which are associated with intermittent sharp groin pain, locking, and clicking. Labral tears may be diagnosed with contrast MRI. If labral tears are present, débridement of the acetabular rim and labrum by either arthrotomy or arthroscopy may lead to functional improvement, though osteotomy or osteoplasty may also be needed to prevent recurrent impingement.

Slipped Capital Femoral Epiphysis

This mechanical disorder of the capital femoral physis usually occurs in an adolescent who has increased femoral retroversion and is often obese. Initial symptoms are vague, involving some aching in the groin, thigh, and knee. An asymmetric out-toeing gait and variable limp are almost universal. AP and frog lateral radiographs of both hips are the initial imaging studies of choice. The direction of displacement of the capital femoral epiphysis is posterior, with variable degrees of external rotation of the femoral neck from under the epiphysis. The appearance on the AP radiograph is often an apparent varus deformity. CT scans are useful in determining the exact direction and degree of displacement.

SCFE is classified into mechanically stable and unstable groups, with different prognoses in the two groups. A patient with a stable SCFE is able to bear weight; the patient with an unstable SCFE is unable to bear any weight on the affected extremity. Associated osteonecrosis of the femoral head is extremely rare in the stable group and relatively common in the unstable group. A stable SCFE can become unstable at any time until it is stabilized either by fixation or by spontaneous healing.

The long-term results of SCFE correlate with the avoidance of complications and anterior impingement.

Because SCFE involves instability of the capital femoral physis, the major goal is to stabilize the physis, which is typically achieved with one or two cannulated screws, or multiple smooth Kirschner wires. Placement of the implants into the center of the femoral head without penetrating the neck or articular surface is essential. Screws or pins in the anterosuperior quadrant of the femoral head should be avoided because this area does not provide mechanical stability, and because implants placed in this region tend to jeopardize the blood supply to the epiphysis.

Reduction or Realignment in Slipped Capital Femoral Epiphysis

Unstable SCFE is characterized by the inability to bear weight that often is associated with gross mechanical instability of the physis. With the patient under anesthesia, reduction of any posterior tilt of the femoral head to the position present before the unstable slip, or even beyond, may be quite easy, though not necessarily safe. Though placement of the patient on a fracture table or internal rotation of the hip in the patient under anesthesia may lead to partial or complete reduction, such reduction is controversial and may increase the risk of osteonecrosis. If a traumatic episode has occurred in association with the unstable slip, then aspiration of a possible hematoma should be considered at the time of stabilization. Leaving some degree of residual posterior tilt of the femoral head is somewhat controversial, but may be safer than achievement of complete reduction. The use of two screws rather than one may be considered. Placing three screws into the adolescent epiphysis is probably excessive, because satisfactory stability is almost always achievable with two screws, and the third screw often jeopardizes the blood supply to the epiphysis.

Residual deformity of the proximal femur may require surgery at a later time. Acute realignment at the level of the physis should be done before any surgical stabilization is achieved. Unstable slips can be treated with no reduction, closed reduction to a stable position, or open reduction with or without simultaneous osteotomy. Although the so-called cuneiform osteotomy allows the most anatomic reduction of severe SCFE, occurring at the site of the deformity, it is a technically demanding procedure with some risk to the blood supply to the femoral head. If done correctly, the procedure must achieve enough shortening of the femoral neck and/or resection of any posterior callus to allow a reduction of the epiphysis onto the femoral neck without tension or disruption of the lateral retinacular vessels to the femoral head. Virtually any degree of deformity may be corrected with this procedure, although with the aforementioned risk to the blood supply. A less aggressive approach to major realignment involves the use of flexion intertrochanteric osteotomy. With cuneiform osteotomy, two screws should be lagged into the femoral head to achieve some compression and good stability. If intertrochanteric osteotomy is done while the physis is still open, then one or two screws must be used for physeal stabilization, in addition to a different implant used to stabilize the intertrochanteric osteotomy itself.

A major principle in realignment of the severe SCFE is that the deformity is largely or entirely in the sagittal plane and involves an extension deformity of the femoral epiphysis. Realignment is used to prevent anterior impingement of the femoral neck or head/neck junction on the anterior acetabulum and rim. Because the direction of correction is flexion, a pure flexion intertrochanteric osteotomy is the best treatment, with varying degrees of internal rotation of the distal femoral fragment; with simultaneous valgus correction is almost never indicated. A 90° intertrochanteric blade plate is the most useful implant. Anterior capsular release is also useful to avoid postoperative flexion deformity. No wedge should be removed from the proximal fragment. Placement of the blade and the proximal screw into the proximal fragment is necessary for optimal stability. Anterior translocation of the distal fragment on the proximal fragment is important for mechanical axis considerations and supplemental bone graft should be curetted from the medullary canal of the distal fragment to place around the osteotomy site to optimize healing. Internal rotation of the distal fragment should be carried out to a degree to allow reestablishment of at least some internal rotation.

In patients who have developed osteonecrosis of the anterolateral portion of the femoral head associated with SCFE, excellent preservation of the sphericity of the posterior and posteromedial femoral head is almost universal. In these patients, flexion valgus intertrochanteric osteotomy can be useful in eliminating pain and restoring a functional range of motion if the procedure is carried out before impingement has destroyed the joint. Basilar neck osteotomy is an alternative realigning procedure in SCFE with or without osteonecrosis, but it is too limited in degree of correction to be useful for major corrections, and more dangerous than intertrochanteric osteotomy because of its proximity to the cervical vessels in the trochanteric sulcus.

Annotated Bibliography

Developmental Dysplasia of the Hip

Jaramillo D, Villegas-Medina O, Laor T, Shapiro F, Millis MB: Gadolinium-enhanced MR imaging of pediatric patients after reduction of dysplastic hips: Assessment of femoral head position, factors impeding reduction, and femoral head ischemia. *AJR Am J Roentgenol* 1998;170:1633-1637.

Documentation of the usefulness of MRI in the immediate postoperative period was done to assess both adequacy of reduction and femoral blood flow after both open and close reductions. Accuracy of determination of femoral head position compared well with previously used CT scans. Determination of femoral head vascularity allowed monitoring unavailable with other techniques.

Luhmann SJ, Schoenecker PL, Anderson AM, Bassett GS: The prognostic importance of the ossific nucleus in the treatment of congenital dysplasia of the hip. *J Bone Joint Surg Am* 1998;80:1719-1727.

A careful multicenter analysis of 153 dislocated hips treated by open or closed reduction was done to determine whether the presence of the ossific nucleus of the femoral head at the time of reduction was associated with a lowered rate of ischemic necrosis. No difference in the rate of osteonecrosis could be detected between the group of 90 hips in which the ossific nucleus was present at reduction and the 63 hips in which the ossific nucleus was absent. It was suggested that surgical reduction of a congenitally dislocated hip should be done when a child can be safely placed under anesthesia and without regard to the presence or absence of the ossific nucleus.

Siebenrock KA, Scholl E, Lottenbach M, Ganz R: Bernese periacetabular osteotomy. *Clin Orthop* 1999;363:9-20.

Long-term follow-up (mean, 11.3 years) of 75 symptomatic dysplastic hips treated with Bernese periacetabular osteotomy confirmed positive results. Unfavorable outcome correlated with moderate or severe preoperative osteoarthritis, labral lesions, and incomplete corrections. Major complications occurred only in the first 18 patients and included two intra-articulate osteotomies, three postoperative femoral head subluxations, and three losses of correction. This study confirms the importance of correction of residual dysplasia before the onset of osteoarthritis and labral tear.

Tonnis D, Heinecke A: Acetabular and femoral anteversion: Relationship with osteoarthritis of the hip. *J Bone Joint Surg Am* 1999;81:1747-1770.

Versional abnormalities of the proximal femur and acetabulum in pathogenesis of osteoarthritis of the hip are documented. Diagnostic and therapeutic approaches are clearly outlined.

Wood MK, Conboy V, Benson MK: Does early treatment by abduction splintage improve the development of dysplastic but stable neonatal hips? *J Pediatr Orthop* 2000;20:302-305.

Most hips in a series of mechanically stable but radiographically and ultrasonographically dysplastic infant hips normalize spontaneously with or without abduction splinting. A few hips in each group had persisting dysplasia, documenting that careful imaging follow-up is indicated in any hip that is documented to be dysplastic, although active treatment can be withheld initially in any hip documented to be mechanically stable.

Legg-Calvé-Perthes Disease

Bankes MJ, Catterall A, Hashemi-Nejad A: Valgus extension osteotomy for "hinge abduction" in Perthes' disease: Results at maturity and factors influencing the radiological outcome. *J Bone Joint Surg Br* 2000;82:548-554.

A study of painful hips with residual limitation of abduction caused by asphericity confirms the usefulness of valgus extension intertrochanteric osteotomy to both restore abduction and reduce pain. Best results occurred in patients with open triradiate cartilage at the time of osteotomy. The authors believed that osteotomy should not be done during the stage of fragmentation nor carried out simultaneously with shelf acetabuloplasty.

Slipped Capital Femoral Epiphysis

Leunig M, Casillas MM, Hamlet M, et al: Slipped capital femoral epiphysis: Early mechanical damage to the acetabular cartilage by a prominent femoral metaphysis. *Acta Orthop Scand* 2000;71:370-375.

Abrasive damage to the anterior acetabular cartilage by a prominent femoral metaphysis was noted in a consecutive series of patients with mild and moderate SCFE in whom anterior arthrotomy and surgical subluxation was carried out during the course of their surgical stabilization. The abrasive damage is suggested as an etiology of chondrolysis and osteoarthritis in some patients with SCFE.

Rab GT: The geometry of slipped capital femoral epiphysis: Implications for movement, impingement, and corrective osteotomy. *J Pediatr Orthop* 1999;19:419-424.

Metaphyseal impingement is implicated as a source of impingement in high-grade SCFE in this three-dimensional computer modeling study of the relationship between the metaphyseal prominent and the acetabular rim during computer simulation of ambulation and sitting. Simulated angular corrections by osteotomy using sagittal flexion, combined valgus and distal fragment internal rotation, or combined flexion valgus and internal rotation achieved elimination of impingement. This study confirms an accumulating clinical experience documenting impingement as etiology of osteoarthritis of some patients with SCFE.

Classic Bibliography

Aronsson DD, Loder RT: Treatment of the unstable (acute) slipped capital femoral epiphysis. *Clin Orthop* 1996;322:99-110.

Bradley J, Wetherill M, Benson MK: Splintage for congenital dislocation of the hip: Is it safe and reliable? *J Bone Joint Surg Br* 1987;69:257-263.

Ganz R, Klaue K, Vinh TS, Mast JW: A new periacetabular osteotomy for the treatment of hip dysplasias: Technique and preliminary results. *Clin Orthop* 1988;232:26-36.

Graf R: Fundamentals of sonographic diagnosis of infant hip dysplasia. *J Pediatr Orthop* 1984;4:735-740.

Harcke HT, Kumar SJ: The role of ultrasound in the diagnosis and management of congenital dislocation and dysplasia of the hip. *J Bone Joint Surg Am* 1991;73:622-628.

Herring JA: The treatment of Legg-Calve-Perthes disease: A critical review of the literature. *J Bone Joint Surg Am* 1994;76:448-458.

Herring JA, Neustadt JB, Williams JJ, Early JS, Browne RH: The lateral pillar classification of Legg-Calve-Perthes disease. *J Pediatr Orthop* 1992;12:143-150.

Malvitz TA, Weinstein SL: Closed reduction for congenital dysplasia of the hip: Functional and radiographic results after an average of thirty years. *J Bone Joint Surg Am* 1994;76:1777-1792.

Millis MB, Murphy SB, Poss R: Osteotomies about the hip for the prevention and treatment of osteoarthrosis. *J Bone Joint Surg Am* 1995;77:626-647.

Murphy SB, Ganz R, Muller ME: The prognosis in untreated dysplasia of the hip: A study of radiographic factors that predict the outcome. *J Bone Joint Surg Am* 1995;77:985-989.

Ninomiya S: Rotational acetabular osteotomy for the severely dysplastic hip in the adolescent and adult. *Clin Orthop* 1989;247:127-137.

O'Hara JN: Congenital dislocation of the hip: Acetabular deficiency in adolescence (absence of the lateral acetabular epiphysis) after limbectomy in infancy. *J Pediatr Orthop* 1989;9:640-648.

Schai PA, Exner GU, Hansch O: Prevention of secondary coxarthrosis in slipped capital femoral epiphysis: A long-term follow-up study after corrective intertrochanteric osteotomy. *J Pediatr Orthop Br* 1996;5:135-143.

Tonnis D: Treatment of residual dysplasia after developmental dysplasia of the hip as a prevention of early coxa arthrosis. *J Pediatr Orthop Br* 1993;2:133-144.

Chapter 37

Pelvis and Acetabulum: Trauma

Paul Tornetta III, MD

David Templeman, MD

Pelvic Fractures

Evaluation

The orthopaedic surgeon should become involved in the management of patients with pelvic injury as early as possible, preferably in the emergency department. The evaluation begins with a history of the accident and determination of the patient's hemodynamic status. The goal of the initial physical examination is to identify associated injuries.

Concomitant urologic injury occurs in approximately 15% of pelvic fractures, and is more common in men than women. The lower urinary tract is usually affected. The most common physical findings of urethral disruption are blood at the meatus and a high prostate. Hematuria also is indicative of injury, most commonly to the bladder. Results from one study indicated no bladder rupture in patients with less than 25 red blood cells per high-power field. In hemodynamically stable male patients, a retrograde urethrogram is performed before Foley catheter placement. In hemodynamically unstable male patients, a single attempt to pass a catheter is made. Because the urethra is very short in females, catheter placement may be attempted without a urethrogram.

The AP radiograph of the pelvis may indicate complete pelvic instability, eliminating the need for manual examination. Physical examination of the pelvic ring should be done to assess stability of the pelvis. Gross instability may be apparent with manual examination; subtle instability may be detected with stress radiographs. Because repeated manipulation of an unstable injury may displace clots, lead to greater blood loss, or cause neurologic injury, physical and manual examination should be done only once.

Radiographic evaluation begins with an AP view of the pelvis. The need for inclusion of a standard AP pelvic radiograph in trauma patients has been confirmed in a recent study. Pelvic injuries can be further evaluated with inlet, outlet, and Judet views (45° obliques), and CT scans. Pelvic CT scans, usually obtained in conjunction with the trauma abdominal CT scan, should include 5-mm cuts through the sacrum and sacroiliac (SI) joints, if possible. In addition to identifying the location of pelvic hematomas, the bony windows of the scan clarify the bony injuries and displacements. Sacral fractures, posterior iliac fractures, avulsions, and the degree of posterior displacement are best seen on the CT. The lower lumbar spine also can be viewed and coincident injuries recognized.

Classification

Pelvic ring injuries are classified according to anatomic location, stability, or mechanism of injury (Fig. 1). Because each classification has advantages and disadvantages, they should be used together. The anatomic system identifies the bony and ligamentous structures injured. Assessment of the rotational and vertical stability of the pelvic ring assists in determination of immediate and definitive treatment. The mechanism of injury system is most helpful in the acute phase of injury, with injury pattern recognition and prediction of blood loss.

Initial Treatment

Resuscitation/Hemorrhage

Patients in shock (systolic blood pressure less than 90 mm Hg) have mortality rates up to 10 times those of normotensive patients. Therefore, the response to the initial resuscitation also may be predictive of mortality. The time that it takes for a hemodynamically unstable patient's blood pressure to rise correlates with mortality.

Hemorrhage occurs in the thoracic, abdominal, and retroperitoneal (including pelvis) cavities as well as external sites. The abdominal cavity can be evaluated using a miniopen supraumbilical tap and lavage, a CT scan, or ultrasound. According to one study, the false negative rate for the Focused Assessment for the

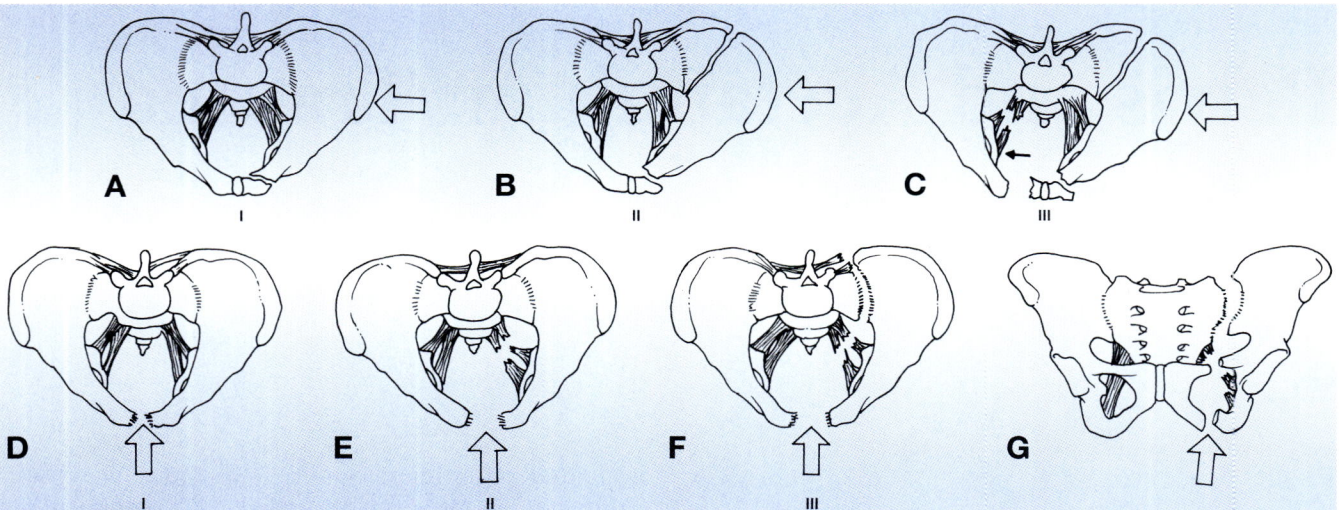

Figure 1 The Young and Burgess classification of pelvic injuries. The arrows indicate the direction of the force causing the injury. **A** through **C** represent lateral compression injuries. Type I is a stable injury that includes rami fractures. Further displacement results in a type II injury with hemipelvic instability usually from a fracture-dislocation posteriorly. If the force continues across the body, a type III injury with an opening of the contralateral pelvis occurs. **D** through **F** depict the increasing injury to the ligaments of the pelvis with anteroposterior compression injuries. A type I injury is stable with only the symphysis disrupted. As the force and displacement increases, the sacrospinous and sacrotuberous ligaments rupture and allow rotational instability, a type II injury. Last, the posterior sacroiliac ligaments fail, creating a completely unstable hemipelvis, a type III injury. **G** shows a vertical shear injury, which ruptures the pelvis anteriorly and posteriorly. *(Reproduced from Beaty JH (ed): Orthopaedic Knowledge Update 6. Rosemont, IL, American Academy of Orthopaedic Surgeons, 1998, pp 427-439.)*

Sonographic examination of the Trauma patient (FAST) examination was 18% (13 of 70 patients). With the exclusion of other areas of potential hemorrhage, further blood loss is likely to be from the pelvic injury.

Head and thorax injuries are the most common direct causes of mortality in patients with pelvic fractures. In up to 65% of patients with pelvic fractures, hemorrhage from pelvic injuries is considered to be a significant contributing factor to mortality. Most pelvic bleeding is venous and can be controlled by avoiding coagulopathy and providing a tamponade. Arterial bleeding may require angiographic control.

External Treatment
External immobilization is indicated only if the pelvic ring is skeletally unstable. Initial external treatment, which may consist of sandbags and straps, beanbags, or military antishock trousers (MAST), may be applied in the field. Although MAST stabilize the pelvis, they have been associated with decreased ventilatory ability, significant delay in transport time, and compartment syndromes of the lower extremities. Deflation of MAST must be gradual to avoid a sudden increase in the intravascular space, which can cause shock or cardiac arrest.

External stabilization in the emergency department may consist of a sheet tied around the iliac crest for open book injuries or an external fixator or pelvic clamp with traction for more unstable injuries. The goal is to provide as much skeletal stabilization as early as possible. External stabilization decreases blood loss by providing a tamponade, opposing bleeding fracture edges, and limiting motion of the soft tissues so as not to break up the initial pelvic clot. External stabilization should be considered part of the resuscitation effort, and external fixation has been demonstrated to decrease injury severity score-dependent mortality and transfusion requirements.

Angiography
Candidates for angiography with selective embolization include patients with stable pelvic fractures or unstable pelvic fractures that have been stabilized with external fixation and in whom other sources of bleeding (for example, in the chest, abdomen, and retroperitoneum) have been ruled out.

Patients without unstable pelvic injury may also have arterial bleeding. Up to 18% of patients with stable pelvic injuries needing more than six units of blood in the first 24 hours required angiographic embolization.

Definitive Treatment
In patients with stable pelvic injuries (Tile type A), nonsurgical treatment is indicated. Because most pelvic fractures are caused by a lateral compression mechanism causing pubic ramus fractures and stable sacral impaction, this group comprises the majority of pelvic fractures. In stable impacted sacral fractures with less than 1 cm of displacement, observation is indicated if there is no neurologic deficit. If nonsurgical management is chosen, immediate mobilization with progressive ambulation should be implemented. Repeat AP

and inlet radiographs of the pelvis are obtained within the first week to rule out further displacement.

External Fixation

In patients with rotationally unstable injuries (Tile type B), external fixation is effective. However, in obese patients, failures have been reported, resulting from difficulty in application and loss of reduction. External fixation is not effective for unstable posterior ring injuries (Tile type C). Union of bony posterior injuries generally will occur in an external fixator, but in a displaced position, and may lead to an increase in long-term disabilities. External fixation sometimes may be used to control the anterior ring in conjunction with internal fixation of the posterior ring.

Internal Fixation

Internal fixation of the pelvic ring is the most stable form of stabilization, with the main emphasis on an accurate reduction. Internal fixation of the pelvis poses several risks, including neurologic injury, vascular injury, infection, wound complications, nonunion, malunion, and loss of reduction.

Injury to the anterior pelvic ring can occur as symphyseal disruptions, ramus fractures, or a combination of both. Complete symphyseal disruptions with or without unstable posterior pelvic ring injury should be stabilized. Open reduction and internal fixation (ORIF) using single, double, and right angle plates has been successful, with the use of a single superiorly placed plate via a rectus splitting approach being the simplest approach. Fixation of ramus fractures rarely is indicated. If a ramus fracture occurs medial to the pubic tubercle, then separation of the fracture may occur because Poupart's and Cooper's ligaments do not cross the fracture site. If the fracture is lateral to the pubic tubercle, then the soft-tissue attachments generally provide sufficient stability. However, if after posterior internal fixation is performed a significant gap remains at the site of a ramus fracture, fixation of the ramus is recommended. The most common method is to use a plate, but intramedullary screws provide equivalent stability. External fixation is another option.

Surgical approach and type of fixation used is determined by the anatomic location of the injury. The type of unstable posterior pelvic ring fracture (sacral, sacroiliac dislocation, sacroiliac fracture-dislocation, iliac) and its particular anatomy will dictate the treatment options.

The use of closed reduction and percutaneous fixation in the management of pelvic fractures is controversial. The reported soft-tissue complication rate is 4% because a large incision and stripping are not used. However, the technique is applicable only if the fracture is addressed early, because a delay in its use may prohibit acceptable closed reduction, and only if the injury can be treated with iliosacral screw fixation. Percutaneous screw fixation is associated with significant risks and usually is used only if the posterior injury is unstable (Tile type C). Closed reduction and percutaneous fixation is most effective for posterior ring disruptions with concomitant soft-tissue injury that are addressed within the first few days after injury. ORIF of posterior pelvic ring injuries results in accurate reductions, but the risk of wound complications is higher than with closed methods. Infection rates for ORIF of the posterior pelvic ring reportedly are less than 3%. Significant soft-tissue injury should be considered a relative contraindication to open reduction. Reduction of unstable posterior injuries also presents a risk of neurologic injury. Intraoperative neurologic monitoring for early identification of noxious stimuli has been recommended in an attempt to avoid iatrogenic neurologic injury.

Iliac Wing Fractures

Iliac wing fractures usually are minimally displaced stable injuries that can be treated nonsurgically; ORIF is indicated only for iliac fractures with significant displacement. These fractures are reduced and fixed through the lateral window of the ilioinguinal approach separating the abdominal from the abductor musculature. Plates and/or lag screws can be used for fixation.

Sacroiliac Joint Dislocations

It is difficult in many cases to determine whether the displacement of the SI joint is complete based on the initial AP radiograph. Significant displacement of the anterior ring (usually the symphysis) and the anterior SI joint may occur in the presence of intact posterior soft tissues. These injuries are rotationally unstable, with the posterior SI ligaments intact and disruption of the anterior ligaments (Tile type B). ORIF of the symphysis is all that is required because the intact posterior SI ligaments will support the posterior pelvis after anterior reduction and fixation. Tile type C injuries have no remaining ligamentous support. The SI joint may be approached and fixed anteriorly, posteriorly, or via percutaneous techniques. With the anterior approach, direct observation of the superior portion of the joint is permitted, but excessive traction may place the L5 nerve root at risk. Plates with screws in the ilium and the lateral sacrum are used for fixation. This technique cannot be used to treat fractures of the sacral ala. The posterior approach allows for visualization of the posterior SI joint and palpation of the anterior SI joint. Fixation is achieved with iliosacral lag screws placed under fluoroscopic control or with transiliac bars or plates.

Of the types of posterior injury, SI dislocation is the best indication for closed reduction and internal fixation. The reduction must be carefully evaluated with all three views of the pelvis. The earlier the procedure is done, the more likely the reduction can be obtained closed. If the reduction can be obtained, then fixation is with iliosacral screw(s) placed through small stab incisions. If the anterior ring injury is a symphyseal separation, then anterior fixation is generally done first to aid in the posterior alignment.

Fracture-Dislocations

Fracture-dislocations of the SI joint are a combination of an iliac fracture and a partial SI joint injury. The smaller the intact iliac fragment, the more the injury resembles a pure dislocation. The larger the intact iliac fragment, the closer it is to an iliac fracture. If the fragment is large enough to maintain the integrity of the posterior SI ligaments, then fixation of the ilium is all that is required. This injury is called a crescent fracture. If there is a question about the integrity of the posterior SI ligaments or the size of the intact fragment is small, then the fixation should include at least one iliosacral screw in conjunction with iliac fixation, or the anterior ring should be reduced and fixed.

Sacral Fractures

Sacral fractures are the most common posterior pelvic injury. Most of these fractures are stable and occur as a result of a lateral compression mechanism. These injuries can be managed nonsurgically. Open reduction is recommended for displaced and unstable (Tile type C) fractures, but closed reduction and percutaneous fixation also have been advocated. Open reduction facilitates débridement of the fracture site and decompression of the neural foramina before fixation. Iatrogenic neurologic injury may occur if bony fragments remain in the foramen during compression of the fracture. If an open anatomic reduction in conjunction with decompression is done, then fracture fixation is done with lag screws without the risk of overcompression. A percutaneous technique has the risk of neural injury if the fracture is overcompressed. The use of percutaneous fixation for sacral fractures has been criticized in one report because many of the fractures in the series were not unstable. Intrasacral plate fixation also has been described, but with limited use in the United States. A unique technique in which standard sacral fixation with iliosacral screws, intrasacral plates, or transiliac plates was combined with an internal vertical verte-

bropelvic distractor made from a pedicle screw system has been used in 23 patients.

Iliosacral Screw Fixation

Iliosacral screws may be indicated in pure SI dislocations, sacral fractures, and in fracture-dislocations with very small crescent fractures. The goal is an anatomic reduction of the posterior ring. Whether the reduction is performed closed or open, iliosacral lag screw placement is technically demanding. Common bony abnormalities such as lumbarization of S1, sacralization of L5, and hypoplastic sacral deformities must be recognized. One study showed that the average distance from iliosacral lag screws to the S1 neural foramen was only 3 mm, highlighting the need for precise placement.

The angle of the sacral pedicle has been studied extensively. The S1 foramen has more available space for screws than the S2 foramen. Screws placed perpendicular to the body in the horizontal plane are the least safe. The safest screw placement is from inferior on the outlet view and posterior on the inlet view to be as close as possible to the center of the narrow portion of the sacrum.

In 177 patients studied, malposition as a result of surgeon error was reported in 2% of the screws. The radiologic landmarks were difficult to assess in 18%. Open plate fixation was required in half of these patients because it was deemed unsafe to insert the screws. The noncritical malreduction rate (more than 1 cm displacement) was 11% (19 of 177 patients). Late displacement occurred in patients with head injuries and in those who were noncompliant.

In a series of vertically unstable fractures, 13% (5 of 38) of iliosacral screws were misplaced. Three of these were anterior to the sacrum and two were in the S1 foramen. An additional 12% had a malreduction of greater than 1 cm. At the end of treatment, 44% of fractures were malunited. The use of iliosacral screws has been well established, but is not without significant risks.

Open Pelvic Fractures

Studies have found an association between pelvic skeletal instability and sepsis. When possible, external fixation should be used for the anterior injury if fecal contamination of the pelvis has occurred. In a large multicenter study, mortality was 75% if the diverting colostomy was delayed beyond 48 hours and 20% if done within 48 hours. It is reasonable to consider that not all open wounds in association with pelvic fractures require diversion. In particular, anterior wounds in the proximal thigh and those associated with iliac wing injuries do not require fecal diversion.

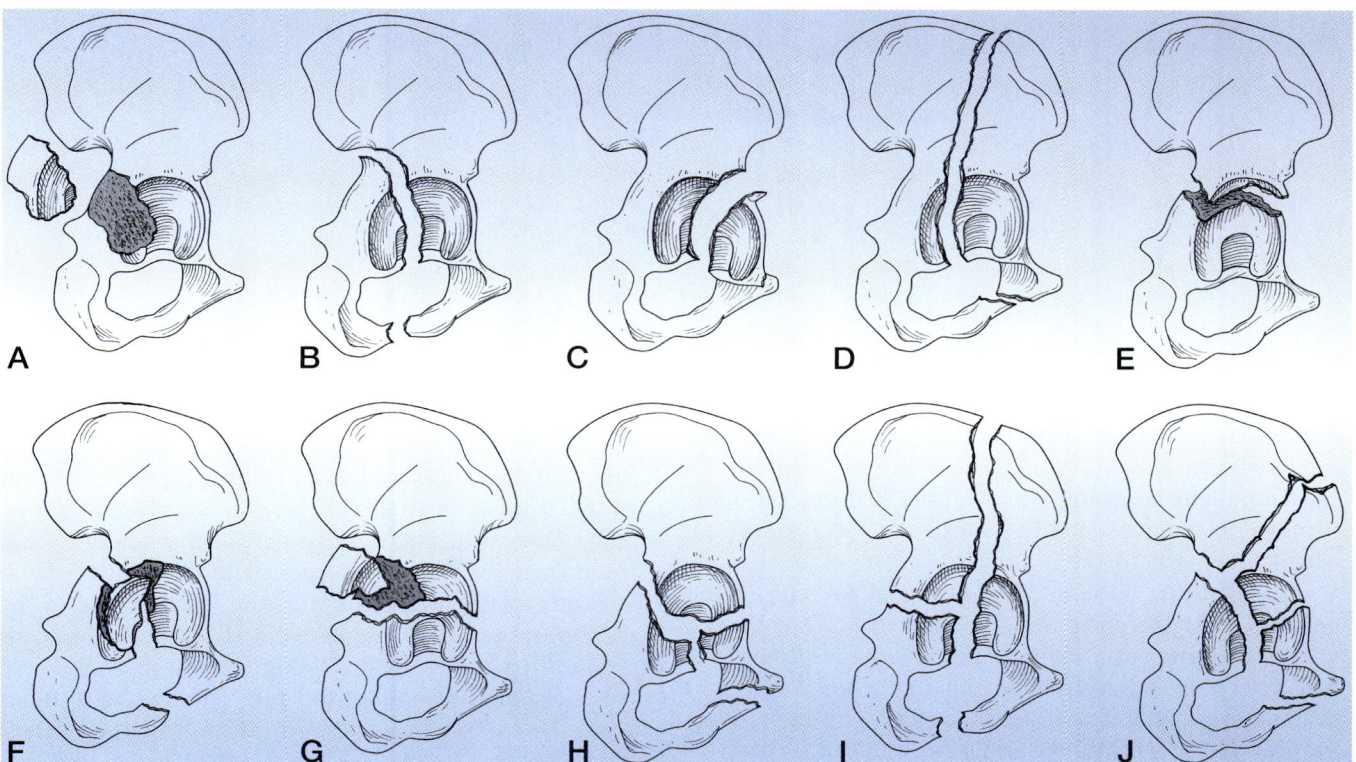

Figure 2 Letournel and Judet classification of acetabular fractures. **A,** Posterior wall. **B,** Posterior column. **C,** Anterior wall. **D,** Anterior column. **E,** Transverse. **F,** Posterior column and posterior wall. **G,** Transverse and posterior wall. **H,** T-shaped. **I,** Anterior and posterior hemitransverse. **J,** Complete both-column. *(Reproduced with permission from Matta J: Surgical treatment of acetabulum fractures, in Browner B, Jupiter J, Levine A, Trafton P (eds): Skeletal Trauma. Philadelphia, PA, WB Saunders, 1992, pp 899-922.)*

Outcome

Studies indicate that the overall outcome for patients depends more on the associated injuries than on the pelvic fracture. In a study of Dutch patients, those with a pelvic injury were statistically different from the normal control population in six of the eight categories of the SF-36 outcome instrument. Only 40% of patients could sit without pain. In another study, low scores were seen in the areas of pain, general health, and physical functioning scales at 4 years.

Clinical results appear to decline with increasing instability of the initial injury, with good or excellent results after fixation of rotationally unstable type B injuries ranging from 80% to 96%. Acceptable results occur in only 27% to 66% of patients with type C injuries. Pelvic pain has been associated with residual displacement, but this finding is not confirmed unless the displacement is more than 1 cm. However, pelvic pain is rarely the reason for the fair and poor results.

Associated neurologic, urologic, and lower extremity injuries are the most common causes of disability, pain, and loss of function. Neurologic injury may affect gait as well as sexual function and cause pain. After 3 years, symptoms resolve in approximately 50% of neu-rologic injuries; however, the L5 nerve root is least likely to regain normal function.

Significant sexual dysfunction has been noted in women who have had pelvic fracture, with dyspareunia in 43% of those with more than 5 mm of residual displacement. Up to 40% of patients with unstable pelvic injuries may complain of a change in sexual function. In men, genitourinary complications after urethral tear include urethral strictures in as many as 60% of patients. Early realignment procedures may help to minimize this problem, but impotence may occur in up to 36%.

In males with pelvic injury, impotence has been reported in as many as 11% of patients. Disruption of the cavernosal nerves has been implicated as the cause of impotence. Concomitant lower extremity fractures, particularly of the foot and ankle, are a significant source of disability.

Acetabular Fractures

Most fractures of the acetabulum are caused by high-energy injuries. Motor vehicle accidents account for 50% to 70% of these injuries. Associated injuries are frequent and approximately half of the patients with

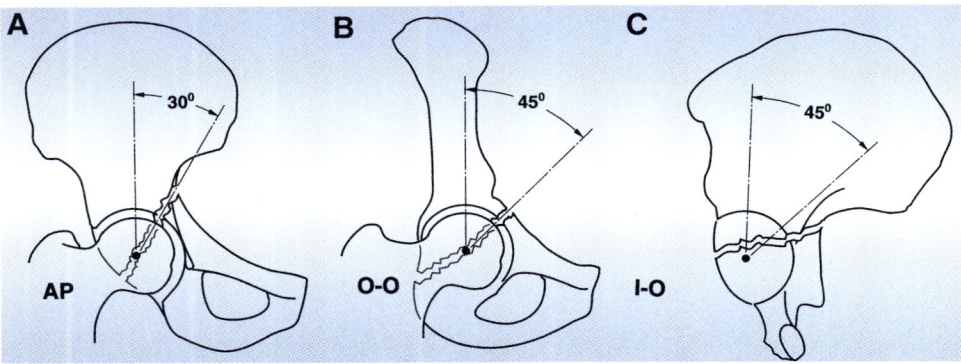

Figure 3 Roof arcs as initially described by Matta. **A,** Medial roof arc 30°. **B,** Anterior roof arc 45°. Obturator oblique AP view. **C,** Posterior roof arc 45°. Iliac oblique view.

acetabular fractures will have an injury to another organ system.

A complete neurologic evaluation is necessary, particularly in the presence of a posterior hip dislocation, because damage to the sciatic nerve occurs in as many as 20% of these patients. The peroneal division of the nerve is most often injured. Fracture displacement into the sciatic notch can cause injury to the superior gluteal artery; in this setting unexplained blood loss can be diagnosed and treated with angiography and embolization. Hip dislocations should be reduced as soon as possible in order to reduce the risk of osteonecrosis. Skeletal traction is used to maintain reduction in unstable hips, or for distraction of the femoral head when it is abutting a fracture edge or incarcerated fragment.

Morel-Lavallé lesions are closed degloving injuries of the skin and subcutaneous tissue off the underlying fascia. Although these injuries are not easily recognized at the time of presentation, they become evident as a fluctuant and ecchymotic area over the greater trochanter or surrounding area. The liquefied collection of hematoma and tissue necrosis in these injuries is culture positive for bacteria in 46% of cases; this is a risk factor for infection with surgical treatment. If incisions are necessary through these wounds, recommended treatment should include surgical evacuation of the hematoma and débridement. ORIF should be delayed until the skin appears viable, usually after 1 week.

Diagnosis and Classification

The diagnosis and classification of acetabular fractures require the accurate interpretation of plain radiographs and CT scans. Plain radiographs include AP and Judet views of the pelvis and 45° iliac oblique and obturator oblique projections. The use of three-dimensional CT reconstructions to display the relative position of the fracture fragments is on the rise. The Letournel and Judet classification is used, comprising five elemental and five associated fracture types (Fig 2).

Nonsurgical Treatment

Using AP and Judet radiographs of the pelvis, a series of roof arcs is constructed to define the weight-bearing dome. A vertical line is drawn from the center of the acetabulum and then a second line is drawn from the center of the acetabulum to the fracture line in the subchondral bone; the angle formed by the two lines is measured to the nearest 5° (Fig 3). These angles, the roof arcs, are measured for the AP and two Judet views. CT scans of the superior 10 mm of the acetabulum display a series of subchondral rings that are equivalent to the area of the roof defined by 45° roof arcs. Fracture displacement within this area of the dome should be less than 2 mm for nonsurgical treatment to be effective. When the injury pattern includes a posterior wall fracture, a minimum of 50% of the posterior wall, as defined by CT, must be intact. Clinical studies indicate that these criteria define the minimum articular surface area required for a good clinical result. The addition of dynamic stress views to the above criteria may further define an additional subset of patients with unstable hips that will require surgical treatment. These stress examinations are performed under general anesthesia with fluoroscopic imaging because subtle instability may not be palpable.

Additional criteria to be considered for possible nonsurgical management of a fracture include the patient's age and health. Because the option of a total hip replacement is available for the older patient population, nonsurgical treatment with a total hip replacement planned if symptomatic arthritis occurs is reasonable.

Open Reduction and Internal Fixation

Open reduction is indicated if a patient does not meet the criteria for nonsurgical management (Fig 4). The goal of surgery is to obtain an anatomic reduction with stable fixation, while avoiding associated complications. Comparison of published results indicates that reductions with less than 1 mm of displacement are obtained in 55% to 75% of patients. Based on findings indicat-

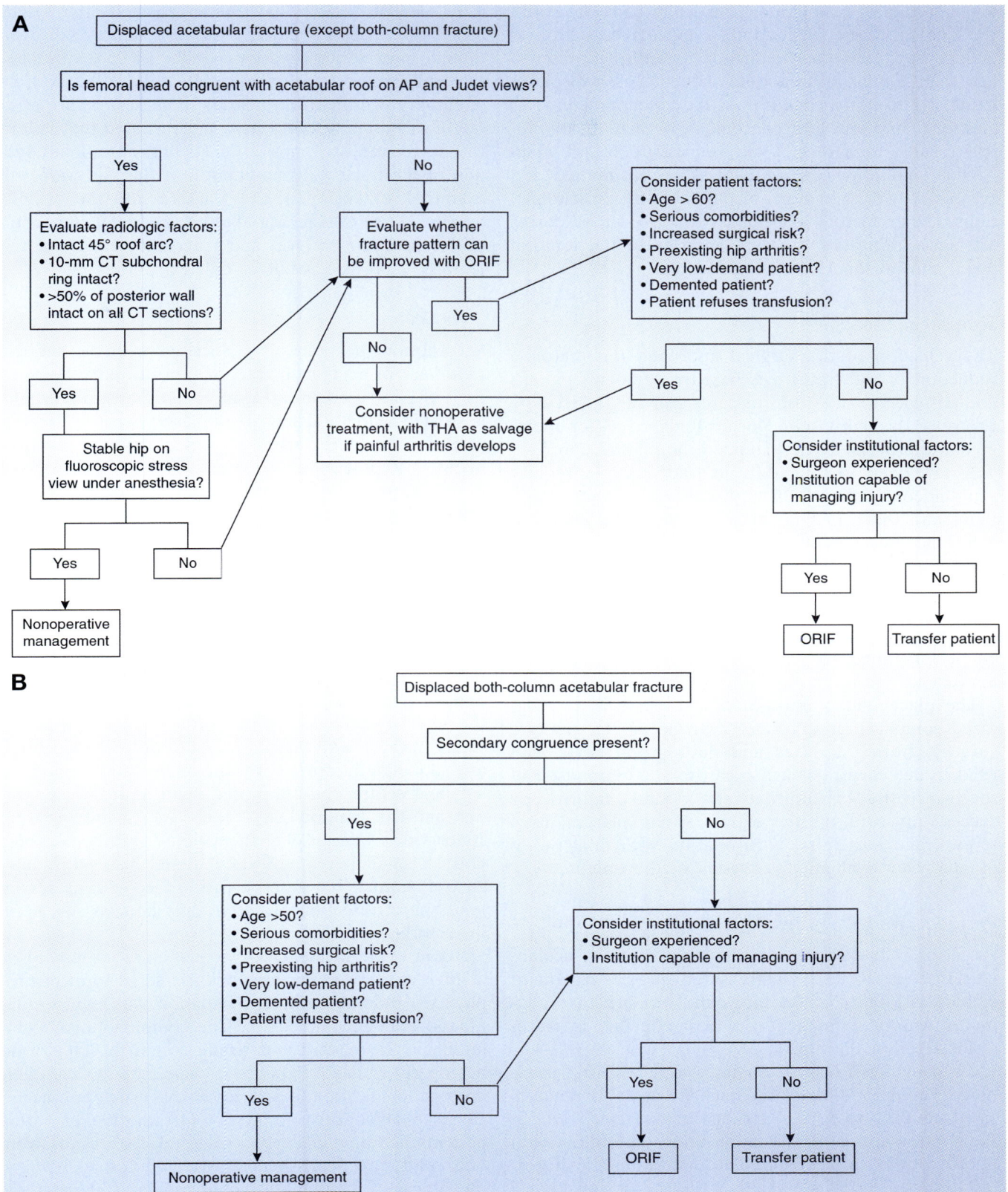

Figure 4 **A,** Algorithm for treatment of displaced acetabular fractures (except both-column fractures). **B,** Algorithm for treatment of displaced both-column acetabular fractures. THA = total hip arthroplasty. *(Reproduced from Tornetta P: Displaced acetabular fractures: Indications for operative and nonoperative management. J Am Acad Orthop Surg 2001;9:18-28.)*

ing that clinical results are statistically correlated with the quality of the reduction, a perfect reduction is defined as an anatomic reduction or a displacement of less than 1 mm; an imperfect reduction is a displacement of 2 to 3 mm; and a poor reduction is defined as greater than 3 mm of displacement. In analyses of clinical results, the greatest differences are found when perfect and imperfect reductions are combined and compared with the results of patients with poor reductions. Other factors associated with poorer outcomes are age older than 40 years, injuries to the femoral head, and postoperative complications.

Surgical Approaches

The selection of the surgical approach for anatomic reduction of the fracture is based on fracture pattern and displacement. Most fractures can be reduced by exposure through either Kocher-Langenbeck or ilioinguinal approaches. The extended iliofemoral approach was developed to treat difficult fractures that require simultaneous exposure of both columns of the acetabulum and the articular surface of the hip. Theoretically, the presence of a traumatic injury or preoperative embolization of the superior gluteal artery could result in necrosis of the abductor muscles when the extended iliofemoral approach is done. Studies do not support obtaining routine preoperative arteriograms when planning to use the extended iliofemoral approach.

The placement of intra-articular screws is a recognized complication associated with acetabular fracture surgery. Both CT scans and fluoroscopy have been used to detect intra-articular hardware. Comparison of the two methods found that intraoperative fluoroscopy successfully confirms the extra-articular placement of screws, and has a 100% correlation with final radiographs when evaluating reduction of the fracture.

Posterior Wall Fractures

Posterior wall fractures are the most common acetabular fractures. The indications for surgical treatment include instability of the hip joint, intra-articular fragments, marginal impaction, and irreducible fracture-dislocations of the hip.

CT scans have correlated defect size with hip instability. The defects that sometimes are unstable range in size from 20% to 50% of the articular surface width of the posterior wall. Examination under anesthesia with fluoroscopy often is required to define hip stability or instability to determine whether surgical or nonsurgical treatment should be used.

Fractures of the posterior wall represent a large proportion of fractures that have poor results. Failure rates of 18% to 32% have been reported after ORIF in a large series of patients. These fractures fail even though most series report that 80% to 96% of posterior wall fractures are anatomically reduced at the time of surgery. Results from a study of clinical failure after ORIF of posterior wall fractures concluded that failure was associated with intra-articular hardware, malreduction of the fracture, comminution of the posterior wall fragment, extension of the fracture into the weight-bearing dome of the acetabulum, marginal impaction of the articular surface, and early subluxation of the femoral head as a result of failed fixation.

Complications

Several complications are associated with the surgical treatment of acetabular fractures; posttraumatic arthritis is the most common. Symptomatic arthritis usually is treated with total hip arthroplasty; because of poor patient acceptance, arthrodesis is performed less frequently. Radiographic evidence of arthritis is present in 15% to 45% of acetabular fractures that are observed for 5 years or longer. Arthritis is more common after an unacceptable reduction than after an anatomic reduction. With an excellent reduction, arthritis usually occurs more than 10 years after injury; in contrast, arthritis develops within 10 years after an imperfect reduction.

The development of heterotopic ossification is thought to be related to dissection and stripping of the abductor muscles because extensile approaches have the highest incidence of heterotopic bone formation. Other factors associated with heterotopic ossification are associated injuries to the chest and abdomen, T-type fracture pattern, closed head injury, male gender, and trochanteric osteotomies. AP radiographs and Judet views best display the volume of ectopic bone. Only a small percentage of patients lose more than 20% of normal hip motion. In the face of a preserved joint space, resection of heterotopic bone is successful in restoring motion.

Because the incidence of heterotopic ossificiation is as high as 80%, many surgeons use some form of prophylaxis. Indomethacin or irradiation alone or in combination are recommended. The combination of indomethacin 25 mg/day and irradiation with 700 Gy on postoperative day 1 eliminated clinically significant heterotopic ossification in a series of extensile approaches. Because of concerns related to irradiation in young patients, indomethacin alone is used, but results from one randomized prospective study failed to confirm the efficacy of indomethacin in reducing hetrerotopic ossification.

Deep vein thrombosis is reported in a high incidence of patients with a pelvic or acetabular fracture. The incidence of pulmonary embolism is reported to be as high as 10% and that of fatal pulmonary embolism as high as 2%. The use of duplex ultrasound has led to additional study of these patients. However, duplex ultrasound is limited in evaluating proximal pelvic thrombi. Preliminary studies with magnetic resonance venography suggest that this may be a more sensitive screening tool, especially for the detection of pelvic thrombi. With magnetic resonance venography, as many as 34% of patients with acetabular fractures were found to have thrombi within their pelvic veins.

When a venous thrombosis is diagnosed prior to surgery, the placement of an inferior vena caval filter before surgery is recommended. Complication rates associated with vena caval filters are reported to be 1% or 2%. The long-term efficacy of filters placed for patients with trauma was 93% according to one study.

Both mechanical and pharmacologic methods are used before and after surgery to reduce the incidence of deep vein thrombosis in patients with pelvic trauma. Currently there is wide variability in how these different treatments are used. There is no consensus regarding the standard of care for the prevention of venous thrombosis in patients with pelvic or acetabular fractures. However, these patients should receive some form of prophylaxis.

Annotated Bibliography

Pelvic Fractures

Asci R, Sarikaya S, Buyukalpelli R, Saylik A, Yilmaz AF, Yildiz S: Voiding and sexual dysfunctions after pelvic fracture urethral injuries treated with either initial cystostomy and delayed urethroplasty or immediate primary urethral realignment. *Scand J Urol Nephrol* 1999;33:228-233.

Type 3 (membranous) urethral injuries accounted for 73% of all injuries. Treatment by suprapubic cystostomy and delayed reconstruction was compared with primary realignment. Strictures and the need for open uroplasty were more common after cystostomy and delayed repair than after primary realignment. Eighty-nine percent and 90% eventually achieved normal urination and approximately 20% in both groups developed impotence.

Ballard RB, Rozycki GS, Newman PG, et al: An algorithm to reduce the incidence of false-negative FAST examinations in patients at high risk for occult injury: Focused Assessment for the Sonographic examination of the Trauma patient. *J Am Coll Surg* 1999;189:145-151.

Thirteen of 70 patients (30%) with pelvic fractures had false-negative FAST examinations. CT scanning was more sensitive in detecting occult injuries in the face of pelvic fractures and is recommended to supplement negative FAST examinations. Of the 13 false-negative FAST examinations, four patients required surgery based on CT findings.

Dujardin FH, Hossenbaccus M, Duparc F, Biga N, Thomine JM: Long-term functional prognosis of posterior injuries in high-energy pelvic disruption. *J Orthop Trauma* 1998;12:145-151.

This article presents a review of 88 patients with unstable pelvic injuries treated nonsurgically with traction and external fixation. Outcome after bony injuries such as fracture-dislocations and iliac wing fractures was better than ligamentous disruptions of the SI joint. The quality of reduction in SI joint injuries correlated with results.

Hamill J, Holden A, Paice R, Civil I: Pelvic fracture pattern predicts pelvic arterial haemorrhage. *Aust NZJ Surg* 2000;70:338-343.

Angiographic embolization was used in 76 of 364 patients (21%) with pelvic fractures. These patients required greater than 6 units of packed red cells over the first 24 hours. The patients in the embolization group were older (42 years versus 29 years) and had a higher abbreviated injury score for pelvic injury (three versus two). Forty-four percent of patients with major ligamentous disruption underwent embolization versus 18% of those with less severe injuries.

Hupel TM, McKee MD, Waddell JP, Schemitsch EH: Primary external fixation of rotationally unstable pelvic fractures in obese patients. *J Trauma* 1998;45:111-115.

Uniplanar external fixation is unable to maintain a reduction of open book rotationally unstable pelvic injuries in the obese patient.

Kaneriya PP, Schweitzer ME, Spettell C, Cohen MJ, Karasick D: The cost-effectiveness of routine pelvic radiography in the evaluation of blunt trauma patients. *Skeletal Radiol* 1999;28:271-273.

A carefully performed analysis confirming the need for a standard AP pelvic radiograph in trauma patients is presented. Pelvic fractures were suspected on clinical grounds in 47% of patients.

Keating JF, Werier J, Blachut P, Broekhuyse H, Meek RN, O'Brien PJ: Early fixation of the vertically unstable pelvis: The role of iliosacral screw fixation of the posterior lesion. *J Orthop Trauma* 1999;13:107-113.

Thirty-eight vertically unstable fractures were treated with posterior iliosacral fixation. All but four had anterior stabilization with either internal or external fixation. Screw misplacement occurred in five patients (13%). Fifteen patients (44%) had a malunion; most developed postoperatively. Malunion was slightly less common if internal fixation was used anteriorly. At follow-up, 85% of patients had pain and only 46% returned to their preinjury occupation.

Moed BR, Anders MJ, Ahmad BK, Craig JG, Jacobson GP: Intraoperative stimulus-evoked electromyographic monitoring for placement of iliosacral implants: An animal model. *J Orthop Trauma* 1998;12:85-89.

A follow-up report to a clinical series previously reported is presented. The authors demonstrate that stimulus-evoked electromyogram threshold closely correlates with the proximity of implants to the nerve roots.

Morgan DE, Nallamala LK, Kenney PJ, Mayo MS, Rue LW III: CT cystography: Radiographic and clinical predictors of bladder rupture. *AJR Am J Roentgenol* 2000;174:89-95.

In hemodynamically stable patients with hematuria, no bladder ruptures were seen if there were less than 25 red blood cells per high-powered field. All patients with rupture demonstrated pelvic fluid on contrast-enhanced CT.

Noojin FK, Malkani AL, Haikal L, Lundquist C, Voor MJ: Cross-sectional geometry of the sacral ala for safe insertion of iliosacral lag screws: A computed tomography model. *J Orthop Trauma* 2000;14:31-35.

Analysis of 13 pelvic CT scans demonstrated that the inclination angle for iliosacral screw placement averaged 45° and ranged from 25° to 65°. The dimensions of the narrowest portion of the safe placement area was 28-mm high by 28-mm wide.

Pell M, Flynn WJ Jr, Seibel RW: Is colostomy always necessary in the treatment of open pelvic fractures? *J Trauma* 1998;45:371-373.

Nine patients with open pelvic fractures and nonperineal wounds were treated without fecal diversion and none developed infectious complications.

Schildhauer TA, Josten C, Muhr G: Triangular osteosynthesis of vertically unstable sacrum fractures: A new concept allowing early weight-bearing. *J Orthop Trauma* 1998;12:307-314.

The authors describe a novel construct including vertebropelvic distraction via pedicle screws in combination with standard sacral fixation to maintain vertical stability and allow for early weight bearing. Nineteen patients were studied, with a loosening rate of 9%.

Schmidt AH, Templeman DC, Kyle RF: Blood conservation in hip trauma. *Clin Orthop* 1998;357:68-73.

An excellent review of the current methods of blood conservation in the trauma patient undergoing pelvic or acetabular fixation is presented. The use of hypotension and Cell Saver yielded a transfusion rate of only 54%. The theoretical advantages of iron and erythropoietin are discussed.

Spain DA, Bergamini TM, Hoffmann JF, Carrillo EH, Richardson JD: Comparison of sequential compression devices and foot pumps for prophylaxis of deep venous thrombosis in high-risk trauma patients. *Am Surg* 1998;64:522-526.

Foot pumps were found to result in similar rates of deep vein thrombosis to standard sequential compression devices in a very small series of 118 patients. Foot pumps were most helpful in patients with lower extremity injuries.

Van den Bosch EW, Van der Kleyn R, Hogervorst M, Van Vugt AB: Functional outcome of internal fixation for pelvic ring fractures. *J Trauma* 1999;47:365-371.

Thirty-seven patients with 16 type B and 21 type C pelvic injuries were evaluated at an average of 36 months. Twelve (40%) reported changes in sexual intercourse and 24 (60%) had complaints related to sitting. The combination of anterior and posterior internal fixation had better results than anterior internal and posterior external fixation on general health scores. Overall, 68% of patients returned to their original job.

Velmahos GC, Kern J, Chan LS, Oder D, Murray JA, Shekelle P: Prevention of venous thromboembolism after injury: An evidence-based report. Part II: Analysis of risk factors and evaluation of the role of vena caval filters. *J Trauma* 2000;49:140-144.

A review of the observational studies of the use of vena caval filters in trauma patients is presented, demonstrating a diminution of pulmonary embolism in patients treated with filters (0.2% versus 1.5%).

Woods RK, O'Keefe G, Rhee P, Routt ML Jr, Maier RV: Open pelvic fracture and fecal diversion. *Arch Surg* 1998;133:281-286.

Pelvic instability was found to correlate with infectious complications in open pelvic fractures when analyzed using regression analysis.

Wong YC, Wang LJ, Ng CJ, Tseng IC, See LC: Mortality after successful transcatheter arterial embolization in patients with unstable pelvic fractures: Rate of blood tranfusion as a predictive factor. *J Trauma* 2000;49:71-75.

Of 507 patients, 17 (3%) underwent angiographic embolization with a 100% success rate in controlling arterial bleeding. The mortality rate was 18% in this group. Mortality was predicted by increased transfusion requirements prior to embolization (11 units versus 3 units in nonsurvivors and survivors, respectively).

Acetabular Fractures

Moed BR, Carr SE, Watson JT: Open reduction and internal fixation of posterior wall fractures of the acetabulum. *Clin Orthop* 2000;377:57-67.

This report documents the results of treatment of a large series of posterior wall fractures. The presence of comminuted unreconstructable fragments resulted in residual defects (greater than 3 mm) in 41% of the 92 fractures reviewed. Additional findings included injury to the femoral head in 13%; marginal impaction in 47%; and comminution of the posterior wall in 47%.

Reilly MC, Olson SA, Tornetta P III, Matta JM: Superior gluteal artery in the extended iliofemoral approach. *J Orthop Trauma* 2000;14:259-263.

Intraoperative Doppler study revealed pulsatile flow of the superior gluteal artery during the extended iliofemoral approach in 40 of 41 patients. There were no instances of abductor necrosis. The authors concluded that preoperative angiography is not routinely required.

Saterbak AM, Marsh JL, Nepola JV, Brandser EA, Turbett T: Clinical failure after posterior wall acetabular fractures: The influence of initial fracture patterns. *J Orthop Trauma* 2000;14:230-237.

This retrospective review emphasizes the potential complications and adverse outcomes associated with posterior wall acetabular fractures. Comminuted posterior wall fractures and fractures extending into the acetabular roof had a high risk of failure.

Tornetta P III: Non-operative management of acetabular fractures: The use of dynamic stress views. *J Bone Joint Surg Br* 1999;81:67-70.

Examination during anesthesia using dynamic fluoroscopy to detect hip instability was used as additional criteria for the nonsurgical treatment of acetabular fractures. Nonsurgical treatment consisted of early mobilization and 91% of patients had a good or excellent result at a mean follow-up of 2.7 years.

Classic Bibliography

Agolini SF, Shah K, Jaffe J, Newcomb J, Rhodes M, Reed JF III: Arterial embolization is a rapid and effective technique for controlling pelvic fracture hemorrhage. *J Trauma* 1997;43:395-399.

Brenneman FD, Katyal D, Boulanger BR, Tile M, Redelmeier DA: Long-term outcomes in open pelvic fractures. *J Trauma* 1997;42:773-777.

Draijer F, Egbers HJ, Havemann D: Quality of life after pelvic ring injuries: Follow-up results of a prospective study. *Arch Orthop Trauma Surg* 1997;116:22-26.

Eastridge BJ, Burgess AR: Pedestrian pelvic fractures: 5-year experience of a major urban trauma center. *J Trauma* 1997;42:695-700.

Jones AL, Powell JN, Kellam JF, McCormack RG, Dust W, Wimmer P: Open pelvic fractures: A multicenter retrospective analysis. *Orthop Clin North Am* 1997;28:345-350.

Montgomery KD, Potter HG, Helfet DL: The detection and management of proximal deep venous thrombosis in patients with acute acetabular fractures: A follow-up report. *J Orthop Trauma* 1997;11:330-336.

Rogers FB, Shackford SR, Ricci MA, Huber BM, Atkins T: Prophylactic vena cava filter insertion in selected high-risk orthopaedic trauma patients. *J Orthop Trauma* 1997;11:267-272.

Routt ML Jr, Simonian PT, Mills WJ: Iliosacral screw fixation: Early complications of the percutaneous technique. *J Orthop Trauma* 1997;11:584-589.

Taffet R: Management of pelvic fractures with concomitant urologic injuries. *Orthop Clin North Am* 1997;28:389-396.

Whitbeck MG Jr, Zwally HJ II, Burgess AR: Innominosacral dissociation: Mechanism of injury as a predictor of resuscitation requirements, morbidity, and mortality. *J Orthop Trauma* 1997;11:82-88.

Chapter 38

Hip: Trauma

Kenneth A. Egol, MD

Kenneth J. Koval, MD

Hip Dislocations

A significant force is required to cause a hip disloca-tion. Severe associated injuries commonly occur. Radiographic evaluation of the pelvis and entire femur identifies the most commonly associated musculoske-tal injuries, which are fractures of the ipsilateral fem-oral head, neck and shaft, pelvis, and acetabulum. Outcome depends on several variables, including time to reduction, presence of associated fracture, and postinjury management.

The incidence of osteonecrosis associated with hip dislocation is reported to be 2% to 40%; osteonecrosis can occur up to 5 years after injury. The risk of osteo-necrosis decreases to 2% to 10% if reduction of the dislocated hip is performed within 6 hours of injury. The role of MRI in determining the risk of osteone-crosis after hip dislocation is controversial.

Anterior Dislocations

Anterior dislocations account for 10% to 18% of all hip dislocations and can be classified as either superior or inferior. Treatment is with closed reduction by trac-tion in line with the femur, followed by hip extension and internal rotation. Associated fractures of the fem-oral head occur in 22% to 77% of cases and are clas-sified as either transchondral or indentation fractures. For displaced transchondral fractures that result in a nonconcentric reduction, treatment is with open reduc-tion and either excision or internal fixation, depending on size and location of the fragment. There is no spe-cific treatment for indentation fractures. Larger frag-ments involving the articular surface have a poorer prognosis.

The incidence of osteonecrosis in patients with ante-rior dislocations is reportedly 10%. Delayed reduction and repeated attempts at reduction are risk factors for osteonecrosis. Transchondral fracture, indentation frac-ture with a depth greater than 4 mm, and osteonecrosis

are some of the risk factors for posttraumatic degen-erative arthritis.

Posterior Dislocations

Posterior dislocations account for up to 90% of all hip dislocations and are classified based on the presence or absence of an associated acetabular and/or femoral head fracture. Treatment is with closed reduction by traction on the adducted and flexed hip. Radiographs obtained after reduction should be assessed to ensure a concentric reduction, and to check for intra-articular fragments and associated fractures. Closed reduction under general anesthesia with muscle paralysis should be done when the initial reduction is unsuccessful. The proximal femur can be manipulated with a percutane-ous Schanz pin at the subtrochanteric level. Open reduction, preceded by a CT scan, is done when closed reduction is unsuccessful or nonconcentric.

After closed or open reduction is done, the stability of the hip must be assessed. Dislocations without frac-tures are inherently stable. CT can be used to assess stability after reduction of posterior wall fracture-dislocations. Stability is inversely related to the size of the posterior wall fragment; cadaveric CT studies have indicated that fragments involving less than 20% to 25% of the acetabular wall do not affect hip stability. Fragments that involve more than 40% to 50% of the acetabular wall result in instability. The condition of the posterior capsule may determine stability for frag-ments of intermediate size. If a posterior wall fracture exists, stress views under fluoroscopy may be consid-ered because posterior wall fragments involving as lit-tle as 15% of the acetabular wall have been associated with instability.

Posterior Dislocations Associated With a Femoral Head Fracture

Approximately 7% of posterior dislocations have asso-ciated fractures of the femoral head or neck that result

TABLE 1	Pipkin Classification of Femoral Head Fractures	
Category	**Description**	**Initial Treatment**
Type I	Fracture of the femoral head caudad to fovea	Closed reduction
Type II	Fracture of the femoral head cephalad to fovea	Closed reduction
Type III	Type I or II associated with a femoral neck fracture	Open reduction
Type IV	Type I, II, or III associated with a fracture of the acetabulum	Closed reduction

from an axial force applied to the flexed knee with the hip adducted and flexed less than 50°. The Pipkin classification system groups these fractures into four types as outlined in Table 1.

Open reduction is required when closed reduction (including under general anesthesia) is unsuccessful or nonconcentric. Type I fractures require either excision or fixation (Fig 1). Type II fractures generally require open reduction from an anterior approach and internal fixation using well recessed cancellous or headless screws. Type III fractures in young (age 50 years or younger), active patients require open reduction and internal fixation of the femoral neck fracture, followed by internal fixation of the femoral head fracture. In the elderly or low functional demand patient, prosthetic replacement is indicated. With type IV fractures, treatment depends on the acetabular fracture pattern and stability and concentricity of the reduction. In the presence of an unstable hip or nonconcentric reduction, open reduction with fixation of the femoral head and posterior acetabular fracture is indicated.

Posterior hip dislocations with an associated femoral head fracture are at high risk for the development of osteonecrosis and posttraumatic degenerative arthritis. Type I and II fractures reportedly have the same prognosis as a simple dislocation. Type IV fractures have about the same prognosis as acetabular fractures without a femoral head fracture. Type III fractures have a 50% rate of posttraumatic osteonecrosis; prognosis is poor.

Hip Fractures

Risk Factors

Most hip fractures occur in the elderly population and are the result of low-energy trauma. Hip fractures in patients younger than age 50 years are rare and usually caused by high-energy trauma. The incidence of hip fracture increases with age, doubling for each decade beyond age 50 years. Women are two to three times more likely to be affected than men. The incidence in white women is two to three times higher than that reported for black and Hispanic women. Additional risk factors are outlined in Table 2. In general, osteoporosis should not be considered a cause of hip frac-

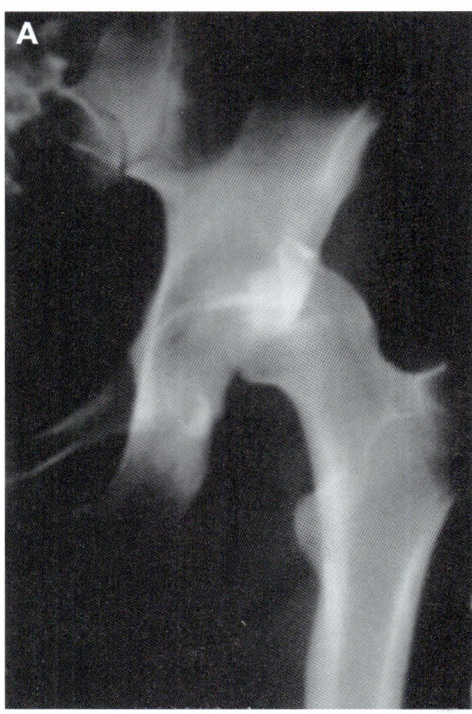
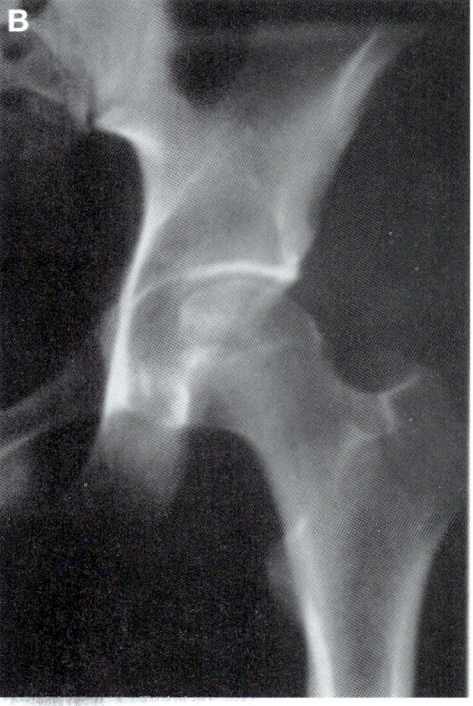

Figure 1 A, AP radiograph of the hip showing a posterior hip dislocation. **B,** Post-reduction films clearly show an associated infrafoveal femoral head fracture (type I Pipkin fracture).

TABLE 2 | Risk Factors for Hip Fracture

Age 50 years or older

Caucasian female

Urban dwelling

Smoking

Excessive alcohol or caffeine intake

Physical inactivity

Previous hip fracture

Significant weight loss in midlife

Use of psychotropic medication

Senile dementia

Postmenarche

Institutionalization

Osteoporosis

Inadequate dietary intake of calcium

tures in the elderly, but rather a potential contributing factor. Osteomalacia has not been shown to be a risk factor for hip fracture. Arthritis of the ipsilateral hip is rarely associated with an intracapsular femoral neck fracture, whereas intertrochanteric fractures are associated with the presence of degenerative changes.

Age-related changes in neuromuscular function may increase the likelihood that a fall will result in a hip fracture. Fall characteristics (factors that increase or lessen the force of impact) and body habitus have been implicated as factors that influence the risk of hip fracture after a fall. Results from a recent study indicate that the use of external hip protectors may decrease the risk of hip fracture in the elderly, particularly in the nursing home population.

In addition, the demographic profile for patients with a femoral neck fracture differs from those with an intertrochanteric hip fracture. According to one study, patients with an intertrochanteric fracture were more likely to be older, in poorer health, and have four or more comorbid conditions.

Mortality

The overall 1-year mortality rate after hip fracture in the elderly ranges from 14% to 36%, which is greater than that for age-matched controls. The risk of mortality is highest within the first 4 to 6 months after fracture. After 1 year, the mortality rate approaches that for age- and sex-matched controls. The lowest mortality rates have been reported in elderly patients who are community dwellers with intact cognitive skills. In one study, a 1-year mortality rate of 12.6% was

reported in this patient population. Factors associated with increased mortality include advanced age, poorly controlled systemic disease, male sex, institutionalized living, and psychiatric illness. Although the effect on mortality of delayed surgery after hip fracture remains controversial, it appears that this delay is appropriate only to permit stabilization of existing medical problems. According to one study, a surgical delay of 3 calendar days approximately doubled the risk of death before the end of the first postoperative year. Nutritional status has been shown to impact on 1-year mortality.

Treatment Principles

Return of the patient to prefracture level of function usually can best be accomplished with surgery. Nonsurgical management has resulted in an excessive rate of medical morbidity and mortality, malunion, and nonunion, and is appropriate only in selected nonambulators with minimal discomfort from their injury. However, the complications associated with prolonged recumbency (decubiti, thrombophlebitis, atelectasis, urinary tract infection) can be avoided with early patient mobilization.

All comorbid medical conditions must be evaluated and corrected prior to surgery in the elderly patient with a fractured hip. The goal of postoperative management is early patient mobilization. The ability to walk within 2 weeks after surgery is associated with living at home 1 year after surgery. Elderly patients with hip fractures should be allowed to bear weight as tolerated because it is difficult for these patients to limit weight bearing. Negative effects of full weight bearing after either internal fixation or prosthetic replacement have not been reported.

Thromboembolic Disease

The reported incidence of lower extremity deep vein thrombosis and fatal pulmonary embolism ranges from 40% to 83%, and 4% to 38%, respectively, in hip fracture patients who do not receive thromboprophylaxis. In 133 hip fracture patients who underwent venography at the time of hospital admission, 13 (10%) had evidence of a deep vein thrombosis; in patients with a delay of more than 2 days from injury to hospital presentation, the risk for deep vein thrombosis was increased significantly: 55% versus 6%.

Warfarin sodium is one agent used for thromboprophylaxis; 10 mg usually are administered orally the night prior to surgery and then an appropriate dose given to maintain an International Normalizing Ratio (INR) between 2 and 3. Low molecular weight heparins (LMWH), another thromboprophylactic agent, is an injectable derivative of heparin and require no monitoring of prothrombin or partial thromboplastin time, or INR. LMWHs can be self-administered upon discharge from the hospital. Subcutaneous injection of LMWH has been an effective prophylaxis in patients undergoing total joint and hip fracture surgery. Low dose subcutaneous heparin has not been shown to be effective. Aspirin has not been recommended for thromboprophylaxis after hip fracture in the past; however, more recent literature may support its use. Intermittent external pneumatic compression also is effective, but the cost of specialized equipment and the need for recumbency may limit its usefulness. Thromboprophylactic medication usually is continued until hospital discharge.

Imaging Studies

Most hip fractures can be identified on standard radiographs. However, occult hip fractures require additional imaging studies. A combination of T1- and T2-weighted images that optimize anatomic detail and depict bone marrow edema is essential. MRI is very sensitive in the diagnosis of musculoskeletal pathology and is more accurate and cost-effective than bone scanning in the identification of occult fractures of the hip. Another advantage is that MRI can be performed within 24 hours of injury. In one study, 67% of emergency room patients with posttraumatic hip pain and negative plain films had MRI findings that were positive for occult hip fracture. However, MRI within 48 hours of fracture does not appear useful for assessing femoral head viability or vascularity, or for predicting the development of osteonecrosis or healing complications.

Functional Recovery

Forty percent to 60% of elderly patients with hip fracture are able to return home immediately after hospitalization and this same percentage will regain their prefracture ambulatory status within 1 year after fracture. Factors predictive of a hospital to home discharge are younger age, independent ambulation before and immediately after fracture, ability to perform activities of daily living (ADLs), and the presence of another person at home. Younger age, male sex, and the absence of preexisting dementia are some factors associated with regaining prefracture ambulatory status. Patients younger than age 85 years who have an American Society of Anesthesiologists rating of operative risk I or II, or those who had intertrochanteric fracture are likely to regain prefracture ambulatory status at 1 year after fracture. A recent study indicated that the following factors were associated with regaining prefracture ambulatory status at 1 year: age younger than 80 years, ambulation restricted to indoors, independence with dressing, ability to perform ADLs within 2 weeks of injury, absence of dementia, and no history of contralateral fracture.

Functional independence is defined as being able to perform ADLs. Of those patients who can independently perform ADL before fracture, only 20% to 35% will regain this status. Younger age, absence of dementia or delirium in nondemented patients, and greater contact with a social network are factors predictive of recovery of ADL.

Stress Fractures

Femoral neck stress fractures are rare in patients younger than age 50 years and more common in elderly women. Treatment depends on the type of fracture present. Tension stress fractures occur along the superior aspect of the femoral neck and are at risk for displacement, whereas compression fractures occur along the inferomedial neck and are thought to be stable.

Although tension femoral neck stress fractures can be treated nonsurgically with no weight bearing and frequent observation until the patient is pain free and there are radiographic signs of healing, the potential complications of displacement (osteonecrosis, malunion, and nonunion) outweigh the risk of surgical intervention. A tension femoral neck stress fracture should be internally stabilized. The area of the stress fracture can be curetted or reamed under radiologic control to induce a biologic reaction.

Compression stress fractures are considered stable and may be treated nonsurgically. Nonsurgical management includes serial radiographs to detect any displacement, and several days of rest, followed by protected weight bearing. If serial radiographs show evidence of fracture widening or displacement, internal fixation should be performed.

Femoral Neck Fractures

Femoral neck fractures occur in two distinct patient populations: the patient younger than age 50 years who experiences high-energy trauma, and the elderly patient who experiences low-energy trauma. A femoral neck fracture in a young person is an orthopaedic emergency that requires prompt evaluation and definitive management. Nondisplaced fractures should be stabilized with multiple lag screws placed parallel. Nonunion and osteonecrosis are uncommon after nondisplaced fractures, except in cases where the fracture was not identified initially. An intracapsular hematoma may be the pathophysiologic mechanism; therefore, capsulotomy or joint aspiration should be considered. Successful treatment of displaced fractures is related to achieving an anatomic reduction and stable internal fixation as soon as possible after the injury. A gentle, closed reduction should be attempted. If closed reduction is not effective, an open reduction, followed by multiple lag screw fixation, should be done.

The Garden classification of femoral neck fractures is the one most commonly used for elderly patients in the literature. However, there is difficulty in differentiating the four types of fractures as shown by studies of interobserver reliability. Therefore, it may be more accurate to classify femoral neck fractures as impacted or nondisplaced (Garden types I and II) or displaced (Garden types III and IV).

Treatment of impacted and nondisplaced femoral neck fractures (Garden types I and II) is with internal stabilization using multiple lag screws placed in parallel. Successful use of three or four screws for both nondisplaced and displaced fractures has been reported in some studies. Nonunion and osteonecrosis are uncommon complications following nondisplaced fractures, with nonunion occurring in less than 5% of cases, and osteonecrosis in less than 10%.

Treatment of displaced femoral neck fractures remains controversial. Closed/open reduction and internal fixation in younger active patients, and primary prosthetic replacement in older, less active patients has been advocated, but there is general agreement that when internal fixation is chosen, achieving anatomic reduction is the most important factor in avoiding healing complications. An acceptable reduction may have up to 15° of valgus angulation and less than 10° of anterior or posterior angulation. Open reduction via an anterolateral or anterior approach is required when closed reduction is not acceptable. Urgent reduction with capsulotomy has consistently been shown to be beneficial in optimizing femoral head blood flow in laboratory models. Benefit of these principles, however, has not been conclusively demonstrated in clinical studies of adequate design and statistical power. Nonunion and osteonecrosis continue to be problematic after fracture displacement. The incidence of nonunion ranges from 10% to 30% and for osteonecrosis, 15% to 33%. The need for reoperation after internal fixation of displaced fractures has been variable. Approximately 33% of patients with osteonecrosis will require additional surgery; approximately 75% of patients with nonunion or early fixation failure will require reoperation.

Prosthetic Replacement

Prosthetic replacement should be used to treat displaced femoral neck fractures in older and less active patients. Results with methylmethacrylate generally are superior to those with noncemented prosthetic replacement. In some series of unipolar hemiarthroplasties, progressive acetabular erosion has been problematic. The factors that have best correlated with the severity of acetabular erosion are patient activity level and duration of follow-up.

The bipolar prosthesis (an endoprosthesis with an inner bearing) was designed to decrease the incidence of acetabular erosion. Early results have been satisfactory, demonstrating that the bipolar design is at least as good as a unipolar design. Although dislocation rates of the unipolar and bipolar designs are similar, the bipolar design makes closed reduction much more difficult. Several studies have questioned whether or not bipolar motion actually occurs after insertion. In a prospective, randomized trial comparing unipolar and bipolar endoprostheses in patients older than 80 years, no differences in outcome could be found with regard to pain, satisfaction, complication rate, and functional ability. Because of the high cost of the bipolar prosthesis, a cemented modular unipolar endoprosthesis has been advocated.

The results of primary cemented total hip replacement after femoral neck hip fracture have been less than optimal. At an average follow-up of 56 months, 18 of 37 patients (49%) younger than 70 years who had a primary total hip replacement after fracture had undergone or were awaiting revision surgery in one uncontrolled series. A prospective study comparing range of hip motion after total hip replacement for arthritis and fracture reported significantly greater motion in the fracture group, a possible predisposing factor for early loosening and dislocation. Primary total hip arthroplasty is indicated for treatment of acute femoral neck fractures in patients with preexisting acetabular disease (rheumatoid arthritis, osteoarthritis, and Paget's disease).

Special Problems

Neurologically impaired patients include those with Parkinson's disease, previous stroke, severe dementia, and Paget's disease. The choice of treatment for patients with Parkinson's disease should be based on patient age, fracture type, and disease severity. Patients who have had a stroke are at increased risk for hip fracture, primarily because of residual problems with balance and gait and osteoporosis of the paretic limb. When the fracture occurs within 1 week of the stroke, poor functional recovery can be anticipated. If prosthetic replacement is chosen to treat patients with Parkinson's disease or a history of strokes, tenotomy should be used to correct hip contractures. An anterior approach may be preferred to decrease the risk of dislocation.

In institutionalized patients with severe dementia, in-hospital mortality reportedly has been as high as 50%. Treatment of nondisplaced fractures is with internal fixation. For treatment of displaced fractures, prosthetic replacement should be done through an anterior approach to decrease the risk of dislocation and infection from wound contamination in incontinent patients. Nonambulatory patients with severe dementia who do not experience significant discomfort from the injury should be treated with nonsurgical management. Nondisplaced and displaced femoral neck fractures in patients with chronic renal disease or hyperparathyroidism are at increased risk for complications of internal fixation because of the associated metabolic bone disease. In these patients, cemented primary prosthetic replacement or total hip arthroplasty is recommended.

Femoral neck fractures in patients with Paget's disease should be carefully evaluated because of the potential for preexisting acetabular degeneration and deformity of the proximal femur. Nondisplaced fractures can be treated with internal fixation, and prosthetic replacement is preferred for displaced fractures. If prefracture symptoms of hip pain occur in the presence of acetabular degeneration, total hip arthroplasty is indicated; if acetabular deformity or degeneration is not present, cemented hemiarthroplasty should be performed.

Basicervical Fractures

Basicervical (base of the neck) fractures are extracapsular and less likely to result in the complications associated with femoral neck fractures. Biomechanically, these fractures behave as intertrochanteric hip fractures and thus are treated with sliding and intramedullary hip screws. If a screw and side plate are used, the technique should be modified. Because there is less cancellous bone in this region in comparison with the intertrochanteric region, there is the tendency for the head to spin with screw placement. The use of an antirotation screw or guide wire is recommended.

Intertrochanteric Fractures

Intertrochanteric fractures occur with approximately the same frequency as femoral neck fractures in patients with similar demographic characteristics. Determination of stability is the most important aspect of intertrochanteric fracture classification. Stability is provided by an intact or a reconstructible posteromedial cortical buttress. Loss of the posteromedial buttress, subtrochanteric extension, and reverse obliquity

fractures are factors that indicate unstable fracture patterns.

Sliding Hip Screw and Medoff Plate

The sliding hip screw is the implant of choice for the treatment of stable and unstable intertrochanteric fractures, except for the reverse obliquity subtrochanteric fracture. Sliding hip screw side plate angles are available in 5° increments from 130° to 150°, with the 135° plate being the one used most often because it is easier to insert in the desired central position of the femoral head and neck. The insertion point in metaphyseal bone produces less of a stress riser than the diaphyseal insertion point required for the 150° plate. Clinical studies have not shown a significant difference in the amount of sliding and impaction between these two plate angles.

The question of side plate length has recently been addressed. Previous biomechanical studies have shown no advantage of four screws over three. According to recent reports, both laboratory biomechanical and a prospective consecutive series support the use of two-hole side plates whether stable or unstable fracture patterns are present.

Secure placement of the sliding hip screw within the proximal fragment (insertion of the screw to within 1 cm of the subchondral bone) is paramount. A central position within the femoral head and neck is most commonly recommended. Because shortening and trochanteric displacement can affect gait and mobility, techniques to preserve proximal femoral anatomy while obtaining firm fixation are being investigated. In one study, a synthetic calcium sulfate bone cement tested favorably to methylmethacrylate in preventing screw cutout in the laboratory. A pilot study using the calcium sulfate cement showed a decrease in fracture collapse compared with controls.

There is no need to perform a medial displacement osteotomy when a sliding hip screw is used. The sliding hip screw allows controlled fracture collapse; therefore, unstable fractures anatomically reduced can be expected to impact into a stable pattern that often is medially displaced, resulting in less shortening of the extremity than with a formal medial displacement osteotomy. Clinical studies indicate no advantage of medial displacement over anatomic reduction for unstable fractures.

Use of the sliding hip screw is associated with a small incidence (4% to 12%) of loss of fixation, usually with unstable fractures. Technical problems such as poor fracture reduction and screw placement are usually the reason for failure. The tip-apex distance, which is the sum of the distance from the tip of the lag screw to the apex of the femoral head on the AP

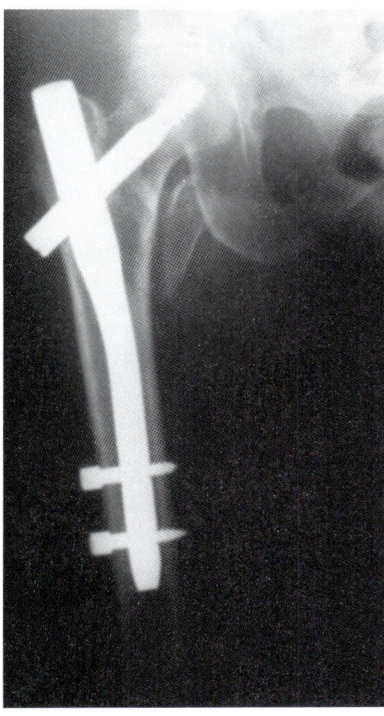

Figure 2 AP radiograph of the right hip that shows an intramedullary hip screw device.

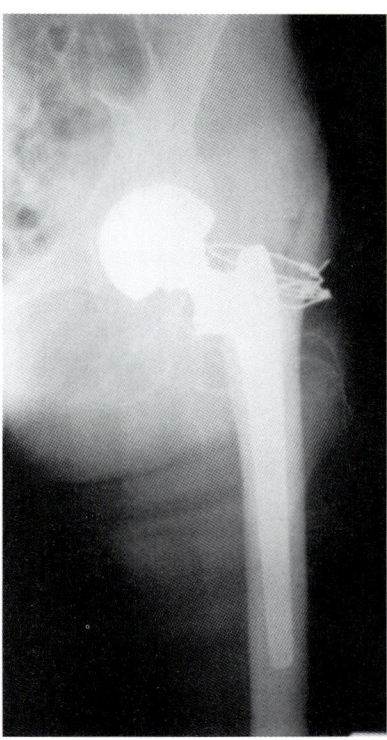

Figure 3 Comminuted intertrochanteric hip fracture in an 80-year-old woman who underwent primary prosthetic replacement with a calcar-replacing unipolar hemiarthroplasty.

and lateral views, corrected for magnification, is predictive of screw cutout after intertrochanteric fracture. If the tip-apex distance is 25 mm or less, screw cutout and resultant loss of fixation will be minimized.

An impacted reduction should be obtained at the time of surgery to avoid excessive postoperative collapse that may exceed the sliding capacity of the device. The minimum amount of available screw/barrel slide, which is necessary to reduce the risk of fixation failure with use of a compression hip screw, is about 10 mm. In one study, intertrochanteric fractures stabilized using a compression hip screw with less than 10 mm of available slide had three times the risk of fixation failure than those stabilized with more than 10 mm of slide.

The Medoff plate, a modification of the compression hip screw, uses the same lag screw as the compression hip screw to allow compression along the axis of the femoral neck. However, the side plate of the compression hip screw has been replaced with a sliding component that enables the fracture to impact parallel to the longitudinal axis of the femur. A randomized, prospective trial comparing the Medoff plate to a standard sliding hip screw was performed on 160 intertrochanteric hip fractures. Results showed a statistically lower failure rate in unstable fractures stabilized with the Medoff plate. There was no difference in stable fracture patterns.

Intramedullary Devices

The advantages of using intramedullary hip screws (intramedullary nail/sliding hip screw devices) for the treatment of intertrochanteric hip fractures (Fig 2), compared with the sliding hip screw, are both technical and mechanical. Most studies comparing these two devices have found no differences in surgical time, duration of hospital stay, infection rate or wound complications, implant failure, transfusion requirements, screw cutout, or screw sliding. However, the intramedullary hip screw does increase the risk of thigh pain and for femoral shaft fracture at the nail tip and the insertion sites of the distal locking bolts. Treatment of comminuted intertrochanteric fractures with subtrochanteric extension, reverse obliquity fractures, and high subtrochanteric fractures may be the best use for the intramedullary hip screw. In a randomized, prospective study in 100 patients with intertrochanteric hip fractures in which intramedullary hip screws were compared with sliding hip screws, there was no difference with regard to outcome or complications. The intramedullary hip screw group had less limb deformity (shortening) when unstable fracture patterns were identified.

Prosthetic Replacement

Primary prosthetic replacement for comminuted, unstable fractures has been used successfully in a limited number of patients (Fig 3). The disadvantages include a larger and more extensive surgical procedure and the potential for dislocation. Prosthetic replacement for intertrochanteric fractures is an attractive option when open reduction and internal fixation fails. The generally good to excellent results afforded by traditional modes of fracture fixation has minimized the use of this treatment option. The use of a calcar replacing prosthesis may be precluded by newer, stronger prosthetic designs and superalloys.

Annotated Bibliography

Hip Dislocations

Konrath GA, Hamel AJ, Guerin J, Olson SA, Bay B, Sharkey NA: Biomechanical evaluation of impaction fractures of the femoral head. *J Orthop Trauma* 1999;13:407-413.

Contact pressures in intact hips were compared with those in hips with varying degrees of simulated impaction fractures created in the femoral head. The hips were loaded in conditions that simulated single limb stance. Statistically significant increases in mean maximum pressures were seen in the superior dome of the acetabulum with an impaction deficit of more than 1 mm². The peripheral load distribution is unchanged regardless of the size of the defect.

Pape HC, Rice J, Wolfram K, Gansslen A, Pohlemann T, Krettek C: Hip dislocation in patients with multiple injuries: A follow-up investigation. *Clin Orthop* 2000; 377:99-105.

In this study of 29 multiple trauma patients with 31 traumatic hip dislocations, all of the patients had injury severity scores of 18 or greater. Initial closed reductions were satisfactorily achieved in 23 patients. Follow-up data were obtained for 13 patients for a mean 8 years after injury. Clinical results were good although seven patients had evidence of osteonecrosis.

Stannard JP, Harris HW, Volgas DA, Alonso JE: Functional outcome of patients with femoral head fractures associated with hip dislocations. *Clin Orthop* 2000;377:44-56.

A series of 26 femoral head fractures were reviewed using standard functional outcome measures. Patients who underwent stabilization with 3.0 mm cannulated screws with washers had poor results. Those who had a Kocher-Langenbach approach were more likely to develop osteonecrosis than if a Smith-Peterson approach were used.

Hip Fractures

Cameron ID, Stafford B, Cumming RG, et al: Hip protectors improve falls self-efficacy. *Age Ageing* 2000; 29:57-62.

External hip protectors were randomized for use in 131 elderly women.

Fox KM, Magaziner J, Hebel JR, Kenzora JE, Kashner TM: Intertrochanteric versus femoral neck hip fractures: Differential characteristics, treatment, and sequelae. *J Gerontol A Biol Sci Med Sci* 1999;54: M635-M640.

According to this prospective study of 923 elderly hip fracture patients, demographic evaluation revealed patients who sustained intertrochanteric hip fractures were more likely to be older and have four or more comorbid conditions. In addition, intertrochanteric hip fracture patients were more likely to have experienced a fall leading to fracture, have longer hospital stays, be discharged to a nursing home, and not recover their prefracture level of function at 2 months after injury.

Gilbert TB, Hawkes WG, Hebel JR, et al: Spinal anesthesia versus general anesthesia for hip fracture repair: A longitudinal observation of 741 elderly patients during 2-year follow-up. *Am J Orthop* 2000;29: 25-35.

In a retrospective, multicenter observational study, 741 patients underwent hip fracture repair; 430 received spinal anesthesia and 311 received general anesthesia. Regression models were created to compare functional outcomes and complications between the two groups. No differences between the two groups were found.

Kannus P, Parkkari J, Niemi S, et al: Prevention of hip fracture in elderly people with use of a hip protector. *N Engl J Med* 2000;343:1506-1513.

The authors randomly assigned 1,801 frail, elderly patients to an anatomically designed hip protector group or a control group. They found that use of the hip protector reduced the risk of hip fracture from 46 per 1,000 person-years to 21.3 per 1,000 person-years. The risk of pelvic fracture was less as well but not significant. In addition, 9 of the 13 patients in the hip protector group fractured their hip while the protectors were off.

Kitamura S, Hasegawa Y, Suzuki S, et al: Functional outcome after hip fracture in Japan. *Clin Orthop* 1998;348:29-36.

This observational study involved 1,669 elderly hip fracture patients in Japan. Mortality rates at 1 and 2 years after surgery were 6% and 11%, respectively. At 1 year, ambulatory status was restored to preinjury levels in two thirds of patients. Ability to regain preinjury functional status correlated with ability to walk at 2 weeks after surgery.

Koval KJ, Aharonoff GB, Su ET, Zuckerman JD: Effect of acute inpatient rehabilitation on outcome after fracture of the femoral neck or intertrochanteric fracture. *J Bone Joint Surg Am* 1998;80:357-364.

The cost effectiveness of acute inpatient rehabilitation was studied in this report. The authors compared functional outcomes in patients who had undergone a structured inpatient rehabilitation program versus a historic control group that had not. The results showed no differences in discharge status, ambulatory ability, need for home assistance and the regaining of ADL.

Koval KJ, Maurer SG, Su ET, Aharonoff GB, Zuckerman JD: The effects of nutritional status on outcome after hip fracture. *J Orthop Trauma* 1999;13:164-169.

The authors performed a retrospective review of prospectively collected data to determine the effect of nutrition on patient outcome after hip fracture. Patients with an abnormal albumin level and total lymphocyte count were 2.9 times more likely to have a length of hospital stay that was longer than 2 weeks, 3.9 times more likely to die within 1 year after surgery, and 4.6 times less likely to recover prefracture level of independence in basic activities of daily living.

Koval KJ, Sala DA, Kummer FJ, Zuckerman JD: Postoperative weight-bearing after a fracture of the femoral neck or intertrochanteric fracture. *J Bone Joint Surg Am* 1998;80:352-356.

The authors performed a prospective study to quantify weight bearing and other gait parameters during the early postoperative period in 60 patients with hip fractures who were allowed to bear weight as tolerated, and to determine if weight bearing was related to fracture type and treatment. Computerized gait testing was done at 1, 2, 3, 6, and 12 weeks after surgery. By 6 weeks, there were no significant differences in weight bearing or other measured gait parameters between the groups studied.

Lavernia CJ: Hemiarthroplasty in hip fracture care: Effects of surgical volume on short-term outcome. *J Arthroplasty* 1998;13:774-778.

The results of 5,604 hip fractures were examined in order to assess the effect that volume of hip fracture surgery has on short-term outcome. Physicians were divided into three groups: low, medium, and high volume based on the number of hemiarthroplasty surgeries performed. Surgeons in the low volume group had a statistically significant longer length of stay and in hospital charges than the other two groups.

Pandey R, McNally E, Ali A, Bulstrode C: The role of MRI in the diagnosis of occult hip fractures. *Injury* 1998;29:61-63.

Thirty-three patients with posttraumatic hip pain and negative plain films were assessed in a prospective study. MRI was done within 48 hours of admission to the hospital. Fractures about the hip were detected in 67% of patients. A tumor was detected in one patient. Fractures of the neck of the femur were detected in 40% of patients and fracture in the intertrochanteric region in 15%.

Parker MJ, Pryor GA, Myles J: 11-year results in 2,846 patients of the Peterborough Hip Fracture Project: Reduced morbidity, mortality and hospital stay. *Acta Orthop Scand* 2000;71:34-38.

This prospective study of 3,025 consecutive hip fracture patients admitted to a dedicated hip fracture service showed a decrease in the length of hospital stay from 51 to 21 days, reduction in 30-day mortality from 22% to 7%, and no significant readmission rate or significant proportion of patients requiring institutional care. The authors recommend development of designated multidisciplinary hip fracture care programs to reduce costs and morbidity.

Prevention of pulmonary embolism and deep vein thrombosis with low dose aspirin: Pulmonary Embolism Prevention (PEP) trial. *Lancet* 2000;355:1295-1302.

This randomized, placebo-controlled trial conducted in multiple countries between 1992 and 1998 looked at the effect of low-dose aspirin on hip fracture patients and hip and knee arthroplasty patients. One hundred forty-eight hospitals randomized over 13,000 hip fracture patients. Aspirin was effective in reducing the rate of fatal pulmonary embolus and deep vein thrombosis when compared with placebo and was as effective as other deep vein thrombosis prophylaxis protocols.

Intertrochanteric Fractures

Bolhofner BR, Russo PR, Carmen B: Results of intertrochanteric femur fractures treated with a 135-degree sliding screw with a two-hole side plate. *J Orthop Trauma* 1999;13:5-8.

Seventy of 103 patients with intertrochanteric hip fractures treated with a sliding hip screw and two-hole side plate were assessed in a prospective, nonrandomized study. Stable and unstable fractures were treated with the two-hole plate. The device failed in three fractures secondary to screw cutout, but no failures occurred secondary to plate pulloff. The authors concluded that use of the device was advantageous because of less potential blood loss and shorter surgical time.

Goodman SB, Bauer TW, Carter D, et al: Norian SRS cement augmentation in hip fracture treatment: Laboratory and initial clinical results. *Clin Orthop* 1998;348: 42-50.

A pilot study was done on 52 patients (mean age, 79 years) with displaced femoral neck fractures and 39 patients with intertrochanteric hip fractures. These patients were injected with adjuvant Norian SRS cement during the course of fracture fixation. Nine patients in the femoral neck group underwent revision surgery for healing compliations. All fractures in the intertrochanteric group healed without loss of fixation. The amount of screw sliding was decreased in patients treated after technique of delivery was improved. Laboratory studies have shown enhanced fracture stability with this nonexothermic, carbonic apatite cement.

Hardy DC, Descamps PY, Krallis P, et al: Use of an intramedullary hip-screw compared with a compression hip-screw with a plate for intertrochanteric femoral fractures: A prospective, randomized study of one hundred patients. *J Bone Joint Surg Am* 1998;80: 618-630.

This prospective, randomized study comparing use of an intramedullary hip screw with a sliding hip screw for the treatment of intertrochanteric hip fractures evaluated outcomes at 1, 3, 6, and 12 months postoperatively. There was less hip screw sliding in unstable patterns and thus, less deformity with the intramedullary hip screw. No differences were found with regard to mortality, complications, functional outcome, and ambulatory ability at 1 year. The intramedullary hip screw group did have better mean mobility scores in the early postoperative period.

Watson JT, Moed BR, Cramer KE, Karges DE: Comparison of the compression hip screw with the Medoff sliding plate for intertrochanteric fractures. *Clin Orthop* 1998;348:79-86.

The authors performed a randomized, prospective study on 160 consecutive patients with intertrochanteric hip fractures. Ninety-one patients received a dynamic hip screw and 69 were treated with a Medoff sliding plate. Stable fracture patterns united without problem in both groups. Unstable fracture patterns had an overall failure rate of 9.6%. Fourteen percent of the dynamic hip screws failed while only 3% of the Medoff plates failed. There was an associated increase in surgical time and blood loss with the Medoff plate.

Classic Bibliography

Aharonoff GB, Koval KJ, Skovron ML, Zuckerman JD: Hip fractures in the elderly: Predictors of one-year mortality. *J Orthop Trauma* 1997;11:162-165.

Aune AK, Ekeland A, Odegaard B, Grogaard B, Alho A: Gamma nail vs compression screw for trochanteric femoral fractures: 15 reoperations in a prospective, randomized study of 378 patients. *Acta Orthop Scand* 1994;65:127-130.

Baumgaertner MR, Curtin SL, Lindskog DM, Keggi JM: The value of the tip-apex distance in predicting failure of fixation of peritrochanteric fractures of the hip. *J Bone Joint Surg Am* 1995;77:1058-1064.

Baumgaertner MR, Solberg BD: Awareness of tip-apex distance reduces failure of fixation of trochanteric fractures of the hip. *J Bone Joint Surg Br* 1997;79:969-971.

Blair B, Koval KJ, Kummer F, Zuckerman JD: Basicervical fractures of the proximal femur: A biomechanical study of 3 internal fixation techniques. *Clin Orthop* 1994;306:256-263.

Broeng L, Bergholdt Hansen L, Sperling K, Kanstrup IL: Postoperative Tc-scintimetry in femoral neck fracture: A prospective study of 46 cases. *Acta Orthop Scand* 1994;65:171-174.

Brumback RJ, Holt ES, McBride MS, Poka A, Bathon GH, Burgess AR: Acetabular depression fracture accompanying posterior fracture dislocation of the hip. *J Orthop Trauma* 1990;4:42-48.

Calder SJ, Anderson GH, Jagger C, Harper WM, Gregg PJ: Unipolar or bipolar prosthesis for displaced intracapsular hip fracture in octogenarians: A randomised prospective study. *J Bone Joint Surg Br* 1996;78:391-394.

Delamarter R, Moreland JR: Treatment of acute femoral neck fractures with total hip arthroplasty. *Clin Orthop* 1987;218:68-74.

Desjardins AL, Roy A, Paiement G, et al: Unstable intertrochanteric fracture of the femur: A prospective randomised study comparing anatomical reduction and medial displacement osteotomy. *J Bone Joint Surg Br* 1993;75:445-447.

Dreinhofer KE, Schwarzkopf SR, Haas NP, Tscherne H: Isolated traumatic dislocation of the hip: Long-term results in 50 patients. *J Bone Joint Surg Br* 1994;76:6-12.

Gebhard JS, Amstutz HC, Zinar DM, Dorey FJ: A comparison of total hip arthroplasty and hemiarthroplasty for treatment of acute fracture of the femoral neck. *Clin Orthop* 1992;282:123-131.

Gerhart TN, Yett HS, Robertson LK, Lee MA, Smith M, Salzman EW: Low-molecular-weight heparinoid compared with warfarin for prophylaxis of deep-vein thrombosis in patients who are operated on for fracture of the hip: A prospective, randomized trial. *J Bone Joint Surg Am* 1991;73:494-502.

Leung KS, So WS, Shen WY, Hui PW: Gamma nails and dynamic hip screws for peritrochanteric fracture: A randomised prospective study in elderly patients. *J Bone Joint Surg Br* 1992;74:345-351.

Lu-Yao GL, Keller RB, Littenberg B, Wennberg JE: Outcomes after displaced fractures of the femoral neck: A meta-analysis of one hundred and six published reports. *J Bone Joint Surg Am* 1994;76:15-25.

Marchetti ME, Steinberg GG, Coumas JM: Intermediate-term experience of Pipkin fracture-dislocations of the hip. *J Orthop Trauma* 1996;10: 455-461.

Moore DC, Frankenberg EP, Goulet JA, Goldstein SA: Hip screw augmentation with an in-situ setting calcium phosphate cement: An in vitro biomechanical analysis. *J Orthop Trauma* 1997;11:577-583.

Rizzo PF, Gould ES, and Lyden JP, Asnis SE: Diagnosis of occult fractures about the hip: Magnetic resonance imaging compared with bone-scanning. *J Bone Joint Surg Am* 1993;75:395-401.

Swiontkowski MF, Thorpe M, Seiler JG, Hansen ST: Operative management of displaced femoral head fractures: Case-matched comparison of anterior versus posterior approaches for Pipkin I and Pipkin II fractures. *J Orthop Trauma* 1992;6:437-442.

Upadhyay SS, Moulton A, Srikrishnamurthy K: An analysis of the late effects of posterior dislocation of the hip without fractures. *J Bone Joint Surg Br* 1983;65:150-152.

Chapter 39

Hip and Pelvis Reconstruction

Robert Barrack, MD

Corey Burak, MD

Gracia Etienne, MD

William Maloney, MD

Robert T. Trousdale, MD

Daniel Berry, MD

John J. Callaghan, MD

Paul Khanuja, MD

Michael A. Mont, MD

Alternatives to Total Hip Arthroplasty

Structural hip disorders, including dysplasia and abnormal acetabular and femoral torsion problems, often lead to the development of degenerative joint disease. Although total hip arthroplasty (THA) has proved to be successful in the older, more sedentary patient population, the results of this procedure have been much less satisfying in younger, more active patients. It is premature to state that "enhanced" polyethylenes or alternative bearing surfaces will improve the results in these patients. If possible, younger patients, especially those with structural changes around the hip, should rely on alternative procedures to THA.

Clinical Assessment

A thorough evaluation of the hip should initially include an evaluation for other conditions that may mimic hip pathology. These conditions include lumbosacral spine disease, sacroiliac joint pathology, nerve pathology, vascular ischemic conditions, and abdominal or pelvic pathology. Once the potential causes of referred pain have been excluded, focus should be directed at whether the patient's pain is intra-articular or extra-articular. Extra-articular discomfort may originate from bursitis, tendinitis, or muscular or bony pathology. Intra-articular discomfort can originate from osteoarthritis, osteonecrosis, synovial disease, labral or articular pathology, and structural abnormalities such as dysplasia, slipped capital femoral epiphyses, or impingement problems secondary to abnormal femoral or acetabular version. Most hip pathology can be diagnosed by a thorough history, physical examination, and appropriate plain films. The history should check for factors known to lead to hip pathology. Systemic metabolic, myelogenous, and rheumatic conditions, a history of steroids, alcohol abuse, trauma, and a family history of dysplasia are all important conditions to consider in the etiology of hip pathology.

Patients with hip pathology may complain of pain, most typically in the groin or buttock area. The pain may localize or radiate to the anteromedial thigh or knee. Other symptoms include limping, hip stiffness associated with difficulties in arising from a chair, entering or exiting a car, tying shoes, or putting on socks. Pain with weight bearing and activity is typical for arthritis, fracture, or subluxation pain from dysplasia. Pain at rest is common with synovitis, tumor-related problems, or bursitis. Catching or locking can often be noted with chondral injuries or labral pathology.

Physical examination should include assessment of gait, leg length, range of motion, palpation about the hip, and neural and vascular examination of the extremity. Patients with significant hip pathology will lean to the affected side while in the stance phase (Duchenne sign) in order to unload the hip joint. Certain maneuvers may be indicative of hip pathology. Groin pain with forcing the hip into the figure-of-4 position (Patrick's test), resisted straight leg raise (Stinchfield test), or pain with flexion and internal rotation of the hip all are indicative of hip pathology. Patients with hip arthritis typically will lose internal rotation initially and pain will be produced with internal rotation and flexion of the hip joint. Pain from labral pathology or abnormal retroversion of the acetabulum or femur may be elicited with flexion, adduction, and internal rotation of the hip as the femoral neck impinges on the anterior acetabulum. Pain caused by tendinitis or bursitis may be increased by stretching the muscle in question or by direct palpation of the bursa. Severe pain in patients who have minimal radiographic changes is a cause for suspicion. Hip reconstruction in these patients will often be unsuccessful because these patients' pain is likely referred from a distant source or they have soft-tissue pain that will not be amenable to surgical reconstruction.

Radiographic Assessment

Initial radiographic evaluation should include an AP view of the pelvis, and AP and lateral views of the hip and proximal femur, checking for the presence of trauma, abnormal joint space, and structural changes about the hip. Most patients with osteoarthritis have a structural abnormality in the hip joint. Dysplasia, slipped capital femoral epiphysis, osteonecrosis, and a dysmorphic hip all can be causes of hip arthritis. Dysplasia typically will be characterized by a lateralized hip center of rotation, a poorly covered femoral head laterally and anteriorly (as noted on the false profile radiograph), superior inclination of the weight-bearing surface, increased femoral anteversion, and coxa valga. Abnormalities in acetabular and/or femoral version may be a potential source of anterior impingement and play a role in the development of secondary degenerative changes. Assessment of acetabular version is easily done on a true AP radiograph (Fig. 1). Functional views with the hip abducted or adducted are helpful in determining what the joint space will look like after a reorientation osteotomy. Osteonecrosis may first be noted on a frog-leg lateral view of the hip joint. CT, MRI, and bone scan should be obtained only if plain films are unable to document the pathology and guide appropriate treatment. Bone scans are useful in identifying occult fractures, tumors, or early degenerative disease not visible on plain films. CT scans are useful in assessing complex pelvic trauma or mapping out the size of a necrotic femoral head lesion. MRI is the test of choice in the diagnosis of early osteonecrosis, femoral neck stress fractures, bony contusions, and transient osteoporosis. MRI with intra-articular contrast is the best test to assess labral integrity. Dynamic interventional MRI has been described to assess hip stability, which may be helpful in the planning of osteotomies. Intra-articular injections of the hip with an anesthetic is an invaluable diagnostic test to determine whether a patient's pain originates from an intra-articular source.

Arthroscopy

The role of arthroscopy in the treatment of hip disorders continues to evolve. Arthroscopy is most useful in the diagnosis and treatment of labral pathology (in the absence of marked dysplasia or structural abnormalities), loose bodies, synovial disease, and potentially for limited chondral lesions of the acetabulum or femoral head. Recently arthroscopy has been shown to be helpful in the evaluation and treatment of the adult with hip pain of uncertain etiology. In one recent study, the results of 328 hip arthroscopies were reviewed. Unrecognized pathology was revealed in 75 patients: osteochondral defects (34), torn labra (23), synovitis (11),

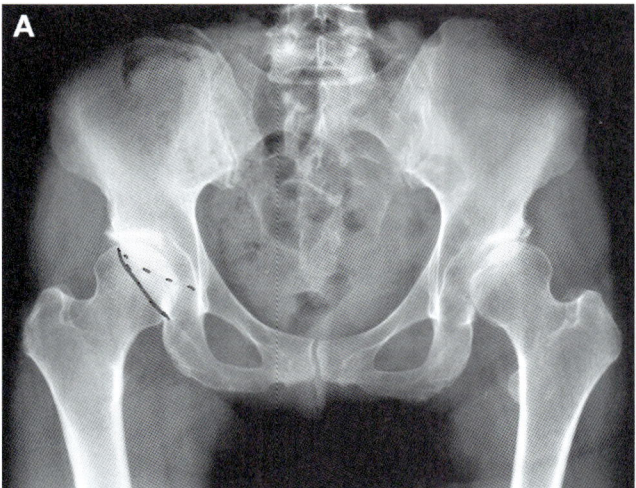

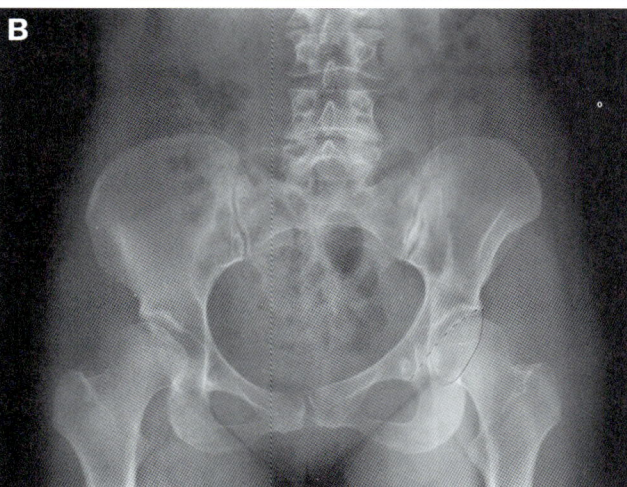

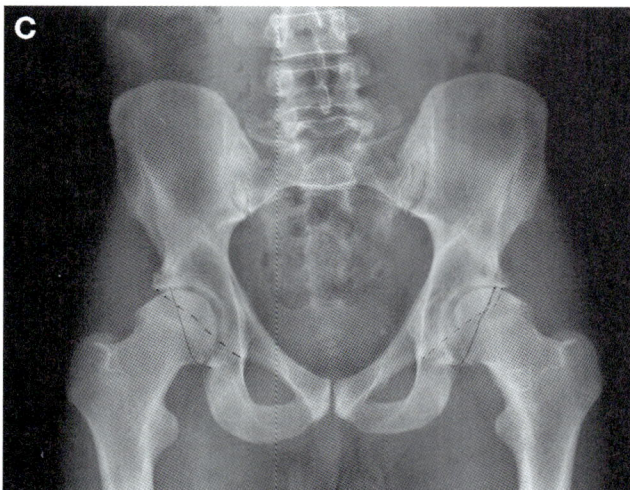

Figure 1 Acetabular version is seen on a true AP pelvic radiograph. **A,** AP radiograph of a normally anteverted right acetabulum. The anterior and posterior acetabular margins are approximately 1.5 cm apart with the anterior rim covering less of the femoral head than the posterior rim. **B,** AP radiograph of an excessively anteverted left acetabulum. Acetabular margins are further apart than normal suggesting increased acetabular anteversion. **C,** AP radiograph showing bilateral retroverted acetabulae. The posterior acetabular margin is more medial than the anterior margin at the superior lateral aspect of the acetabular rim indicating a retroverted acetabulum. In this pelvic radiograph of a 41-year-old man, degenerative changes secondary to impingement are seen.

and loose bodies (9). In the treatment of labral pathology, which is most commonly located anteriorly, it is imperative to rule out poor anterior femoral head coverage or retroversion problems of the acetabulum and femur. Hips that have poor anterior coverage as noted on the AP and false profile radiographs as well as those that have impingement secondary to a retroverted acetabulum or femoral neck are probably more prone to the development of anterior articular cartilage and labral problems. These patients are better treated with a reorientation osteotomy and open treatment of labral pathology. In the absence of these structural problems, arthroscopy offers a less invasive treatment option. Hip arthroscopy is somewhat more challenging than arthroscopy of most other joints secondary to the geometry of the hip joint and its relatively far location from the skin. Furthermore, the long-term outcome of arthroscopy for various conditions has not been well established. Complications from hip arthroscopy may include nerve injuries, patient positioning problems, and inadvertent chondral damage to the acetabulum and/or femoral head.

Resection Arthroplasty

Resection arthroplasty is rarely used in the treatment of hip problems, but remains useful for the nonambulatory patient with severe spasticity. Resection arthroplasty provides pain relief, more optimal positioning of the hip, and improved peroneal care. It is also commonly used for the control of infection in a minimally ambulatory patient. The drawbacks of resection arthroplasty include instability, limb shortening, weakness, slightly unpredictable pain relief, a high dependence on ambulatory aids, and increased oxygen consumption with ambulation.

Hip Arthrodesis

The primary indication for a hip arthrodesis is isolated unilateral hip disease in a young, active patient. Although it provides a durable alternative to THA, it often is not accepted by patients. Contraindications include ipsilateral knee pathology, contralateral hip involvement, or spinal pathology. Multiple techniques to obtain an arthrodesis have been described. Most surgeons believe it is imperative to preserve the abductor mechanism and avoid distortion of the proximal femoral anatomy should conversion to a THA be considered in the future. Fixation can be obtained with a compression hip screw with ancillary fixation, a lateral Cobra plate placed via trochanteric osteotomy with secondary trochanteric attachment, or a ventral plate placed through an anterior approach, allowing preservation of the abductor mechanism. Most agree that

placing the hip in approximately 30° of flexion, neutral abduction-adduction, and slight external rotation is ideal. Conversion of a hip fusion to a total joint arthroplasty is technically challenging and may be fraught with complications.

Osteotomy

Osteotomies about the hip continue to play a critical role in the treatment of patients with structural hip abnormalities such as dysplasia, torsion problems, osteonecrosis, and femoral neck nonunions, as well as sequelae of childhood diseases including Legg-Calvé-Perthes disease and slipped capital femoral epiphysis.

Pelvic Osteotomy

Pelvic osteotomies have historically been divided into two subgroups. Reconstructive osteotomies have the goal of redirecting the acetabulum, thereby obtaining a weight-bearing area of hyaline cartilage. A hip in which congruency can be obtained with a reorientation procedure is a prerequisite for reconstructive osteotomy. Some viable articular cartilage must be available to bring into the weight-bearing surface of the hip. A salvage osteotomy is done in the patient with established arthritis in whom congruency is not possible. The goal of the salvage osteotomy is to add functional years of life to the hip until a definitive procedure, either arthroplasty or arthrodesis, is required. Historically, patients with developmental dysplasia who experienced degenerative changes have been considered candidates for salvage osteotomy (Chiari or shelf), THA, or arthrodesis. Recent work has shown that when acetabular insufficiency is the primary cause of joint incongruity, pelvic osteotomy offers a biologic solution that may prevent or delay the progression of arthritis.

A Chiari salvage osteotomy medializes the hip center of rotation, which decreases the joint contact forces and provides some lateral femoral head coverage with the hip joint capsule. Unlike reconstructive osteotomy, the Chiari osteotomy does not cover the femoral head with articular cartilage; therefore the Chiari osteotomy should be considered only in patients who have unsatisfactory acetabular anatomy (marked out of round acetabulum and/or femoral head), superior hip subluxation, or when articular cartilage for reconstructive osteotomy is not available for coverage of the femoral head.

The most physiologic solution for a young adult who has a dysplastic hip seems to be redirection of the acetabulum into a more normal position that will allow coverage of the femoral head by hyaline articular cartilage. Previously described reconstructive procedures have included single, double, and triple innominate

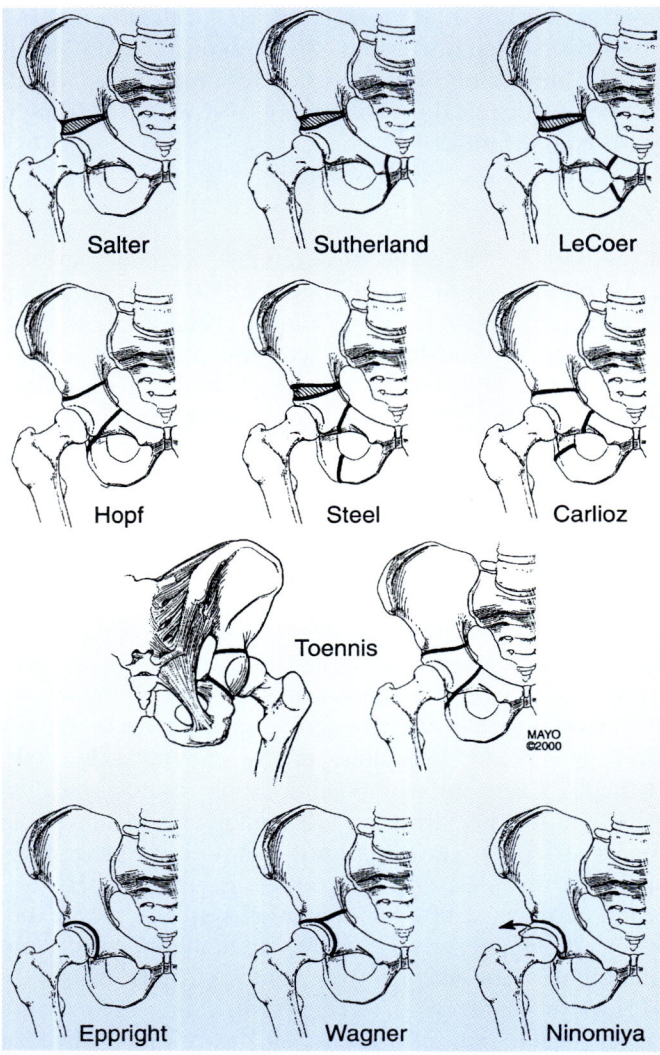

Figure 2 Schematic representation of some of the previously described reorientation pelvic procedures. *(Reproduced with permission from The Mayo Foundation, Rochester, MN.)*

osteotomies, and various types of periacetabular osteotomies (Fig. 2). A single innominate osteotomy is beneficial for children but often is insufficient for adolescents and adults. It also can lateralize the hip joint, an undesirable effect in the dysplastic hip.

Double and triple osteotomies have the disadvantage of necessitating bone cuts at a distance from the acetabulum. The large acetabular fragment allows limited rotational correction and when rotated creates some pelvic deformity. Spherical osteotomies about the hip are technically difficult and minimize the amount of medialization that can be obtained.

The Bernese periacetabular osteotomy, developed in 1983, has many advantages compared with previously described osteotomies. The ideal patient is a relatively young individual with symptomatic dysplasia with little or no arthritis. There should be a relatively round ace-

tabulum and femoral head in which congruency is possible. The series of straight reproducible cuts can be performed through one incision, leaving the abductor mechanism completely unviolated to facilitate healing and rehabilitation. The posterior column of the hemipelvis remains intact, allowing for immediate mobilization of the patient without the need for a cast or brace postoperatively. A considerable degree of correction can be obtained laterally and anteriorly with medialization of the hip joint. The shape of the true pelvis is not altered to a major degree. The vascularity of the acetabular fragment is preserved, allowing intra-articular inspection of the labrum without risk of further devitalization of the osteotomized fragment. This pelvic osteotomy is technically challenging and may be best reserved for centers and surgeons with specific interest and expertise. Reported complications include neurovascular injuries, intra-articular osteotomies, delayed union, especially of the pubic bone, and heterotopic ossification. The most common complication is poor correction. Retroversion and excessive anterior correction of the acetabular segment should be avoided. Accurate assessment of femoral head coverage, including normalizing the angle of the weight-bearing surface and checking the amount of medialization and acetabular anteversion, is critical. Midterm results recently have been reported and are extremely favorable with acceptable complication rates.

Femoral Osteotomy

Intertrochanteric osteotomies are named according to the direction of rotation through the osteotomy site. For example, a varus intertrochanteric osteotomy rotates the proximal femur to a varus position, and an extension osteotomy directs the femoral head posteriorly. A prerequisite for intertrochanteric osteotomy is that adequate hip motion be present in the planned plane of correction to allow the hip to return to a functional position after osteotomy. Proximal femoral osteotomies usually combine correction in several planes with displacement to allow a more precise corrective procedure as well as to maintain proper mechanical axis of the limb. When performing a varus-producing osteotomy, it is important to medialize the femoral shaft and in valgus osteotomies to lateralize the femoral shaft in order to keep the mechanical axis of the leg going through the middle of the knee (Fig. 3). The role of femoral osteotomy for dysplasia has diminished as more sophisticated pelvic procedures have become available and because most of the bony deformity seen in dysplasia is on the acetabular side of the joint. A pelvic procedure allows correction at the primary location of the deformity.

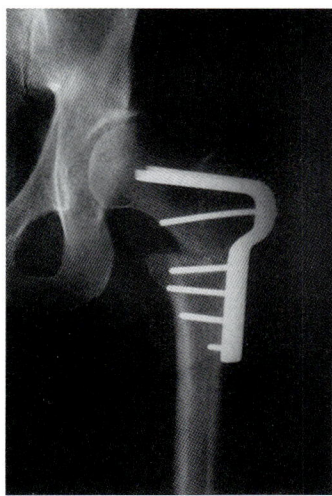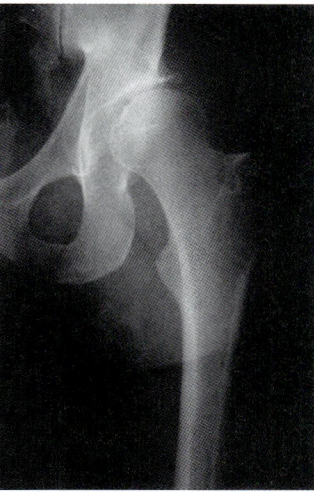

Figure 3 AP radiograph of the left hip before and after varus intertrochanteric osteotomy. The preoperative radiograph shows that the patient has a marked coxa valga deformity, minimal acetabular involvement, and minimal degenerative changes.

General contraindications to femoral osteotomy include poor motion, inflammatory joint conditions, significant metabolic disease, and severe degenerative joint disease. The patient should be relatively pain-free after osteotomy (if a varus osteotomy is planned the patient should be comfortable in abduction). Functional radiographs in abduction and adduction should show improvement of joint congruity.

Dysplasia

Varus intertrochanteric osteotomy is still indicated in the rare patient with symptomatic dysplasia with coxa valga with minimal acetabular involvement. It is more commonly used in combination with a pelvic procedure when maximal acetabular correction has been obtained and the femoral head is still subluxated. The recovery after a varus osteotomy is much more prolonged than after a reconstructive pelvic procedure, especially those pelvic procedures that maintain the integrity of the abductor muscles. Varus osteotomy will shorten the limb and techniques that do not remove a large wedge of bone of the femur are preferred. A prolonged abductor limp can be present after a varus osteotomy, especially if an excessive amount of correction has been obtained. Valgus intertrochanteric osteotomy is reserved for the rare patient with femoral head deformities that become more congruent with the hip in an adducted position, and for the young patient with a mushroom-shaped femoral head in which the large osteophyte can be placed into the weight-bearing surface. Valgus osteotomy may also be appropriate for the young patient with primary acetabular protrusio. It is also the procedure of choice for young patients with femoral neck nonunions with a slightly vertical orientated fracture line.

Osteonecrosis

The role of proximal femoral osteotomy in the treatment of osteonecrosis of the femoral head remains limited. Varus, valgus, flexion, and various rotational osteotomies have been developed, all with the idea of moving the necrotic segment away from the weight-bearing surface of the femoral head and/or obtaining increased coverage of the necrotic segment. Only those patients who have relatively small lesions are amenable to a femoral osteotomy. The size of the lesion can be measured on both AP and lateral radiographs. If the necrotic arc of the lesion on a combined AP and lateral view is more than 200°, a successful osteotomy is unlikely. The use of tomography and CT scan may allow for better mapping of the lesion and assist in proper patient selection. Recent studies have reported satisfactory results in 70% to 84% of patients with osteonecrosis treated with intertrochanteric osteotomy and results are slightly improved with smaller involvement of the femoral head and the earlier the stage of the disease.

Osteonecrosis

Osteonecrosis, also known as avascular necrosis, is a disease process characterized by a poorly understood derangement of the osseous circulation. Approximately 400,000 to 600,000 patients in the United States are afflicted. Although osteonecrosis is not life-threatening, it is extremely debilitating because of its onset in 30- to 40-year-old patients and the relatively high historic failure rate of THA in this patient population.

Etiology, Associated Factors, and Pathogenesis

Although the exact mechanism for osteonecrosis is not well understood, there are multiple associated risk factors and these are listed in Table 1. A small percentage (less than 10%) of individuals with these risk factors will develop osteonecrosis. Most authors believe that osteonecrosis has a multifactorial etiology.

The pathology of the disease leads to death of the cells in the marrow and osteocytes. There is eventual collapse of the necrotic segment, leading to loss of congruence and subsequent degenerative arthritis.

Diagnosis

Prompt diagnosis is important in the management of osteonecrosis because early treatment results in better outcomes. A high index of suspicion is essential and risk factors should be sought during the initial evaluation. The most common presenting complaint is a deep throbbing pain in the groin associated with an antalgic gait. During the physical examination, pain on hip

TABLE 1	Risk Factors of Osteonecrosis

Exposure to radiation

Space-occupying myeloproliferative disorders such as leukemia and Gaucher's disease

Caisson's disease

Sickle cell disease

Use of corticosteroids

Use of alcohol

Use of nicotine

Hypofibrinolysis

Thrombophilia

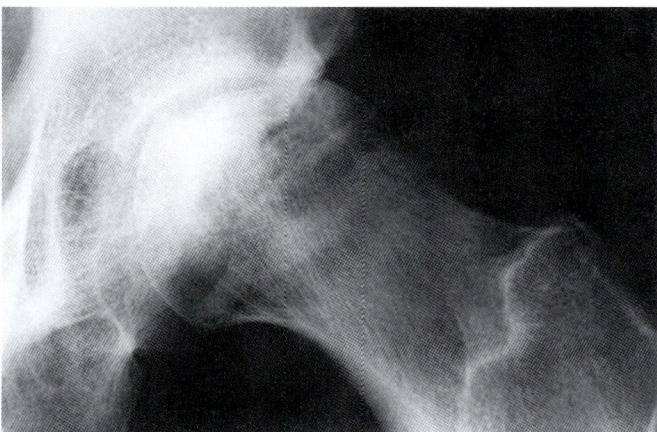

Figure 4 Crescent sign. Radiograph of a 45-year-old man with a history of corticosteroid use. Note the significant subchondral collapse with minimal head depression.

internal rotation as well as a decreased range of motion may be elicited.

Plain radiographs are the first step in the diagnostic evaluation. Adequate AP and frog-leg lateral radiographs are essential. Changes in the femoral head usually occur many months after the onset of the disease and radiographs may show cysts, mottled sclerosis, or a crescent sign (Fig. 4). The crescent sign results from subchondral collapse of the necrotic segment.

MRI is the best diagnostic method for the detection of osteonecrosis, with greater than 98% sensitivity and specificity. A single-density line on the T1-weighted image demarcates the normal-ischemic bone interface. On the T2-weighted image, a double-density line represents the hypervascular granulation tissue.

Staging and Classification

Multiple classification systems are based on radiographic and/or MRI findings (Table 2). No classification system has been uniformly accepted, because each has its limitations.

The Ficat and Arlet classification system has been the most widely used, predating MRI. In stage I no changes are noted on plain radiographs. In stage II disease, sclerotic or cystic lesions are present without subchondral collapse. Stage III femoral heads have a crescent sign, which is indicative of early subchondral collapse. There may or may not be changes in the contour of the femoral head. In hips with stage IV disease, there is narrowing of the joint space with secondary degenerative changes in the acetabulum. This classification system is limited because it does not take into account the size or location of the lesion, both of which have been shown to play a role in prognosis.

The University of Pennsylvania System expands on that of Ficat and Arlet. The two major contributions of this system are the addition of information regarding the size of the lesion, and its characterization of Ficat

stage III lesions into those without femoral head depression (stage III) and those with head depression (stage IV).

The Association Research Circulation Osseous has adopted a classification system that incorporates the University of Pennsylvania system and adds the location of the lesion and other radiographic parameters. The Marcus classification is similar to the Ficat and Arlet classification, except that stage III is divided into two stages: crescent sign only, and crescent sign with step-off. The Japanese classification emphasizes the location of the lesions with the larger, more lateral lesions carrying the worst prognosis.

Treatment

The best treatment methods are not agreed on except for the most advanced stages of the disease. It is difficult to compare the results of the various methods for several reasons: (1) the inconsistency as well as the lack of reproducibility of the classification systems; (2) the patient population from any one center is relatively small; (3) technical differences in how procedures are performed at various institutions; and (4) incomplete understanding of the disease process and its natural history.

The goal of surgery is to relieve pain and maintain congruity of the hip joint. Because of the young age of patients with osteonecrosis, the general practice should be to avoid THA. Less destructive methods or procedures should be used so that joint replacement is delayed.

Most authors agree that there are four radiographic characteristics important to predict prognosis and to formulate a treatment plan. First, it is necessary to classify lesions into precollapse and postcollapse disease. A crescent sign with or without a change in con-

TABLE 2 | Radiographic Classification of Osteonecrosis of the Femoral Head

Stage	Description
	Ficat and Arlet
I	Normal
II	Sclerotic or cystic lesions, without subchondral fracture
III	Crescent sign (subchondral collapse) and/or step-off in contour of subchondral bone
IV	Osteoarthrosis with decreased articular cartilage, osteophytes
	Marcus and Associates (modified)
	The modification is that symptoms are not included in the radiographic staging because they have been found to be variable within stages in any system. Same as Ficat and Arlet except that stage III is divided into:
III	Crescent sign only
IV	Step-off in contour of subchondral bone
V	Stage IV of Ficat and Arlet
	University of Pennsylvania Staging System
	Same as Marcus and associates except:
V	Divided into early and late arthritis (V and VI)
	Each lesion is divided into A, B, and C depending on size of lesion (small, moderate, large)
	Association Research Circulation Osseous (ARCO)
	Three distinct systems published from 1990 to 1992, most recently as follows:
	Same as University of Pennsylvania except each lesion is also classified as a, b, or c depending on location (medial, central, or lateral)
	Quantification of various factors:
a	Amount of head depression
b	Length of crescent arc
c	Size of lesion
	Japanese Investigation Committee on Osteonecrosis Characterized by Location of Lesion
A	Medial one third or less of weight-bearing head
B	Medial two thirds or less of weight-bearing head
C	Greater than two thirds of weight-bearing head

(Reproduced from Mont MA, Jones LC, Sotereanos DG, Amstutz HC, Hungerford DS: Understanding and treating osteonecrosis of the femoral head. Instr Course Lect 2000;49:169–185.)

tour of the femoral head is indicative of postcollapse disease. Second, the size of the necrotic segment is important because small and medium-sized lesions have a better prognosis. A necrotic segment involving less than 15% of the femoral head is considered small. A medium-sized lesion measures between 15% and 30% of the femoral head; large lesions involve more than 30% of the femoral head. The Kerboul angle is often used to quantify the size of the lesion. Small lesions have a Kerboul angle smaller than 150°. Lesions with a Kerboul angle larger than 200° are considered large. A third important feature is the amount of change in head contour, with more than 2 mm of head depression conferring worse prognosis. Finally, disease with acetabular involvement implies advanced arthritic changes, and the only viable treatment option is total hip replacement.

Nonsurgical Treatment

Protected Weight Bearing

Protected or non-weight bearing plays a limited role in the treatment of this disease. In a large review of 21 studies, unsatisfactory results were obtained by limiting weight bearing. Of 819 hips, only 182 (22%) had successful results at a mean follow-up of 34 months (range, 20 months to 10 years).

Pharmacologic Treatment

Current approaches to medical management are based on what the possible etiology might be. For example, if a thrombophilic disorder is present, treatment with an anticoagulant such as warfarin might be beneficial. Results with these modalities are presently experimental or at best anecdotal.

Early Surgical Treatment

Core Decompression

The proposed mechanism of this procedure is based on the reduction of intraosseous pressure to prevent further ischemia and resultant infarction. Core decompression can be done alone or with bone grafting. This method is best suited for precollapse radiographic disease. Patients experience a consistent decrease in hip pain immediately after this procedure. The long-term effects of this modality are not entirely known. Most recent reports conclude that core decompression can be useful in small and medium sized precollapse disease.

Nonvascularized Grafting Procedures

The goal of these procedures is to maintain articular congruity, prevent collapse, and provide a scaffold for the repair and remodeling of subchondral bone. This is done by removing the necrotic area and replacing it with bone graft. Structural cortical bone grafts most commonly come from the fibula and iliac crest. These grafts can be placed through the track of the core decompression. In one study, the results of 20 hips were reported in which structural tibial autografts and a combination of fibular autogenous and fibular allografts were used. A 90% success rate was reported in 20 hips with Ficat stage I or II disease at an average of 8 years follow-up (range, 2 to 19 years).

Vascularized Grafting Procedures

Vascularized grafts theoretically allow for decompression of an osteonecrotic lesion, structural support, and enrichment of the vascular supply to enhance healing. In one report on 88 hips, clinical success was found in 61 hips at a mean of 5.5 years. The survival rate for subgroups was 100% for stages IC and IIA, 94% for stage IIB, 50% for stage IIC, 80% for stage IIIB, 58% for stage IIIC, 72% for stage IVA, and 58% for stage IVB. In another study, 103 hips were followed at least 5.5 years. Average Harris Salter hip scores improved at all stages and there was a high patient satisfaction rate of 81%. Vascularized fibular grafting is a technically demanding procedures that is time-consuming and can lead to donor site morbidity. Nevertheless, at experienced centers the results can be quite satisfactory in hips that do not have significant head depression.

Osteotomies

The rationale for the use of proximal femoral osteotomies is to move the necrotic segment of the femoral head from the weight-bearing area to a less loaded region. Several methods have been described in the literature. The two main types are varus/valgus and transtrochanteric osteotomies. The best results have been found in small or medium sized lesions (less than 30% of the femoral head, combined necrotic angle on AP and lateral views of less than 200°) in the earlier stages (Ficat I, II, and early III).

The transtrochanteric osteotomy as described by Sugioka is difficult to perform. In Japan the success rate is reported to be greater than 80% at long-term follow-up. In the United States, multiple centers have reported greater than 80% failure rates at approximately 5 years mean follow-up.

Osteotomies are difficult to perform, and have a high potential for morbidity, including nonunion. If the procedure fails, good results can be obtained with THA. However, these procedures are technically more demanding than primary replacements.

Late Surgical Treatment

With larger lesions and when significant collapse is present, the previously mentioned procedures do not have high success rates; therefore, prosthetic replacement is recommended. Unfortunately, in this patient population the limited survival of these implants needs to be recognized because patients may have a life expectancy of 35 to 40 years or more. Options for treatment include limited femoral resurfacing arthroplasty and THA.

Limited Femoral Resurfacing Arthroplasty

A recent review of 33 femoral head resurfacings for Ficat stage III and early stage IV lesions showed good or excellent results for 61% of the hips overall at a mean of 10.5 years postoperatively. The mean interval between limited femoral resurfacing and THA was 60 months. The authors concluded that femoral head resurfacing is a useful interim procedure for Ficat and Arlet stage III and early stage IV lesions that would otherwise only be treated with THA (Fig 5). Good or excellent results were reported in 22 of 25 hips (88%) that had been followed for a mean of 37 months (range, 25 to 60 months). Results from yet another study showed good or excellent results in 28 of 30 hips at a mean of 5 years (range, 2 to 6 years).

Hip Fusion and Endoprostheses

Hip fusion is difficult because of the necrotic bone, and results are poor. Its use is limited in this disease in which close to 80% of patients have bilateral disease. The results with monopolar and bipolar femoral endo-

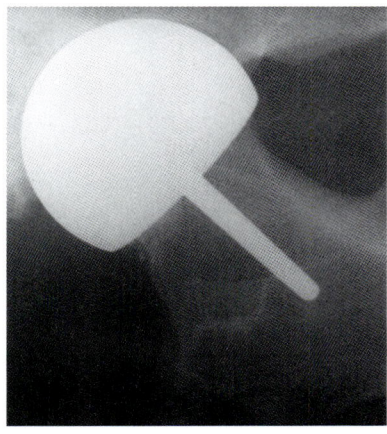

Figure 5 Radiograph of a femoral head resurfacing. There is minimal involvement of the acetabulum.

prostheses historically have been poor. In a review of the results of 19 Austin Moore prostheses, 12 hips (63%) had proximal migration at 5-year follow-up. Bipolar arthroplasties also have poor results; in one study of 31 hips treated with bipolar endoprostheses, only 15 (48%) had good and excellent results at a mean follow-up of 4.6 years.

Total Hip Arthroplasty

Although THA is the most definitive treatment for the arthritic stage of osteonecrosis, results have not been as successful as for age-matched controls with other diseases. Most studies found 30% to 50% failure rates at less than 7 years mean follow-up. The outcome of THA in patients with osteonecrosis may be influenced by the etiology of the disease. For example, transplant patients may perform differently with THA than those patients with posttraumatic osteonecrosis. Recently, better results have been found with modern prosthetic designs and techniques. Although the results in these studies are only midterm, they still show inferior success rates when compared with studies of other patient populations.

Despite these less than optimal results, THA is the most reliable treatment option for advanced osteonecrosis with degenerative changes.

Primary Total Hip Arthroplasty

Measuring Outcome

A number of recent studies have evaluated factors that affect the patient's level of satisfaction with the results of THA. One prospective study showed that approximately 50% of patients were frustrated for a 3-month period postoperatively despite clinical improvement as measured by standard ratings. Results steadily improved during the course of the first year, but it was at a year after surgery that most patients achieved the expected subjective benefits.

Another study assessed 100 patients after primary THA using a disease-specific score (The Harris Hip Score) and compared it to a health-related quality of life score (Nottingham Health Profile) at 1, 3, and 5 years after primary THA. Results from both scoring systems correlated highly and were heavily influenced by the functional classification of Charnley (A, B, or C rating). After 5 years both scores reflected the function of the implant and the general state of the patient, but a higher degree of sensitivity was necessary to distinguish between the performance of different implants. These authors concluded that despite the number of available hip scores and quality of life scoring systems, the ideal system of clinical assessment has yet to be developed.

Cost

THA is one of the most common and costly procedures covered by Medicare and therefore it has been the target of constant economic scrutiny and the subject of numerous cuts in reimbursement to both the hospital and the surgeon over the past decade. Previous studies on the clinical outcome or cost effectiveness of THA have objectively rated it among the most efficacious and cost-effective medical interventions. In one recent study, cost utility ratios were used to judge the efficacy of THA. This methodology basically judges the value to the patient of having their symptoms alleviated and divides this by the expenditure necessary to achieve this result. The test administered was the quality of well-being index, which is used to calculate the cost of a quality well year (QWY). The average cost of a QWY for THA at 2 years was approximately $7,000. Hip procedures were economically superior to knee procedures and both primary and revision hip arthroplasty rated extremely well compared with other medical interventions using this cost utility ratio.

Strategies found to be economically effective without apparent decline in clinical results include clinical pathways, implant standardization, and the use of a single price/case price purchasing program. Certain tests, including the routine pathologic examination of tissue, routine autologous blood donation for primary THA, and the use of routine postoperative radiographs and the radiologist's interpretation of these radiographs, have been evaluated and were determined not to be necessary on a routine basis. The necessity of routine office follow-up after THA has also been questioned. Submitting a combination of routine radiographs and self-administered outcomes questionnaires was found to be effective and preferred by a high percentage of patients.

Acetabular Components

Cemented Acetabular Components

Cemented acetabular components currently comprise a very small percentage of acetabular components implanted in the United States but continue to be popular in many parts of Europe. Long-term data on cemented total hips continue to show that acetabular component loosening is generally more of a problem than femoral stem loosening beyond 10 years. In one recent study of patients in whom 62 Charnley total hips were still in place more than 25 years postoperatively, the prevalence of acetabular revision was 15% compared with 7% for femoral stems. Another study examined the results of metal-backed cemented acetabular components and reported a 9.2% incidence of revision at 9 years among 86 primary total hips in 74 patients. An additional 24 components (31.6%) had evidence of radiographic loosening for a total failure rate of 40.8%. There is generally a higher rate of loosening reported for metal-backed cups compared to analogous reports of cemented all-polyethylene components.

The consensus has developed in recent years that when a cemented acetabular component is used, there is no advantage to metal backing, which may, in fact, be counterproductive. The metal backing decreases the polyethylene thickness and introduces another interface for the potential generation of wear debris. Apparently the interface between the metal-backed component and cement is no better and may be worse than the interface between an all-polyethylene component. Most surgeons prefer to use an all-polyethylene component, therefore, when a cemented acetabular component is selected in primary THA. Cemented all-polyethylene components seem to function best over the long term in older, less active patients. One recent study examined 112 patients (132 hips) who were 75 years or older at the time of THA. Clinical follow-up (on average 14.6 years for the patients who were still living) showed that no acetabular component had required revision for aseptic loosening. For younger, more active patients, there is evidence that a cemented component may not perform as well as press-fit, porous-coated, cementless components. Recent matched-pair studies comparing cemented acetabular components to cementless porous-coated components have shown a lower revision rate and lower incidence of radiographic loosening for porous-coated components compared with cemented components.

Cementless Acetabular Components

The clinical results of the use of porous-coated cementless acetabular components in a 5- to 10-year time frame has been reported from a number of centers. Reliable fixation is generally obtained in 95% to 99% of cases. These results apply to the general population of patients but the results may not be as good in younger, more active patients. This is particularly true when the incidence of osteolytic lesions is reported. The component that has been studied most extensively is the Harris-Galante I (Zimmer, Inc, Warsaw, IN). This component comprises a titanium metal shell with a titanium fiber mesh coating that was usually implanted with line-to-line reaming and screw fixation. Most of the reports in the 5- to 10-year time frame in recent literature used this technique.

Similar results have been reported with other acetabular cementless designs. In a study of the Acetabular Reconstruction Component (ARC, Howmedica, Rutherford, NJ) in 72 hips (67 patients) at average 12-year follow-up, the incidence of both aseptic loosening and acetabular lysis was only 4%, compared with a much higher incidence of lysis and revision with the PCA component (Howmedica, Rutherford, NJ) also fabricated of cobalt-chrome with a similar sintered bead coating. These results emphasize the importance of design differences in the clinical performance of cementless porous coated acetabular components. Another study of a large group of cementless Omnifit components (Osteonics Corporation, Allendale, NJ) reported results from a group of 350 cementless total hips. The use of a 32-mm head and thin polyethylene correlated with a high wear rate. The authors questioned the acetabular component design which they believed contributed to the high incidence of osteolysis observed. The same component was used in a multicenter study of 316 hips in 282 patients. Only three porous-coated cups (2.7%) were revised while 25 (11.9%) hydroxyapatite-coated non-porous cups were revised at 7.9 years.

The effect of the backside surface finish and the metal type on the wear performance of cementless modular acetabular liners was evaluated in a laboratory study. The results of the study showed no difference in wear rate between cobalt-chrome and titanium acetabular metal shells and in addition found no appreciable effect of polishing of the components in reducing backside wear. There are advantages and disadvantages to using screws as adjunctive fixation with cementless acetabular components. There is no clear consensus at this point and either approach is acceptable. Recently there has been emphasis on improving the locking mechanism and the liner conformity, ensuring adequate polyethylene thickness and avoidance of 32-mm heads.

Acetabular Components With Alternative Bearing Surfaces

The clinical performance of cementless porous-coated acetabular components over 10 years indicates that problems with component fixation are rare. The resulting osteolysis associated with polyethylene wear has continued to be a concern and has led to heightened interest in alternative bearing surfaces to substitute for polyethylene as the articulation with the femoral head. These alternatives include metal-on-metal and ceramic bearing surfaces, and cross-linked polyethylene.

In a clinical study of metal-on-metal hip replacements, 70 hips were evaluated at an average of 5.2 years. There was one revision for acetabular loosening, two acetabular component revisions for dislocation, and no femoral component loosening. There was no measurable wear on radiographs and there was no evidence of acetabular osteolysis. It should be noted that these were cemented acetabular components. Although the absence of radiographic wear or osteolysis was promising, a number of previously quoted series of conventional metal on polyethylene articulations have also noted the absence of component revision or lysis in the same time frame. A much larger study at longer term follow-up will be necessary to demonstrate any advantage over metal on polyethylene. These results certainly do demonstrate an improvement over early metal-on-metal designs, however.

The other potential hard-on-hard bearing surface is ceramic. The two primary materials are aluminum oxide and zirconium oxide. Both materials have been used as femoral head bearing surfaces against polyethylene but alumina has also been used in a ceramic-on-ceramic configuration. Polyethylene wear against ceramic heads has been reported to be 5 to 10 times lower than that against metal heads in wear simulator studies; however, in clinical radiographic wear measurements the results have been extremely variable. There is conflicting data regarding ceramic bearing surfaces. Some studies have shown significantly lower radiographic wear rates of the ceramic head against the polyethylene, while an equal number of studies have not shown any significant difference in wear rate. Two major issues associated with the use of ceramic heads are cost and breakage. There have been a number of case reports of fracture of ceramic heads; however, with current specifications fractures should be a rare occurrence. When ceramic heads were initially released on the American market, the cost was approximately three times that of a comparable metal head. While the costs are declining, the ceramic heads continue to be markedly more expensive than metal heads. Ceramic-on-ceramic wear rates have been reported to be 10 times less than the lowest polyethylene wear rates. Other drawbacks of ceramic-on-ceramic include limited head and neck sizes. Because of the extremely low wear rates reported, it is possible that larger heads can be used with metal-on-metal and ceramic-on-ceramic articulations. The use of such hard-on-hard articulations does not necessarily eliminate the problem of wear debris and osteolysis. A high incidence of lysis and wear has been documented for at least one alumina-on-alumina hip of early design.

The most popular approach to enhance the wear characteristics of standard ultra-high molecular weight polyethylene has been to use various methods of cross-linking of polyethylene. A number of highly cross-linked polyethylenes have recently been approved by the Food and Drug Administration and are currently available on the American market. Cross-linked polyethylene has been used overseas for many years. One recent study reported on the results of 14 cross-linked polyethylene cemented acetabular components combined with alumina ceramic femoral heads. After an initial period of 2 years there was a remarkably low rate of head penetration, only 0.02 mm per year. This finding did not represent any change from the wear rate previously reported at 6 years to the present study at 10 to 11 years. Numerous studies are expected in the coming years that will better delineate the expected rate of wear and osteolysis using the alternative bearing surfaces of metal-on-metal, ceramic-on-ceramic, ceramic-on-polyethylene, metal-on-cross-linked polyethylene, and ceramic-on-cross-linked polyethylene.

Femoral Components
Cemented Stems
The cement technique is recognized as an important factor in increasing the longevity of cemented stem fixation. In the late 1970s, the so-called "second-generation" cement technique was introduced and included the use of an intramedullary plug, pulsatile lavage of the medullary canal, the use of a cement gun, retrograde filling of the femoral canal with doughy cement, pressurization of the cement, and use of a forged cobalt-chrome stem with rounded corners. Long-term studies at 10 to 15 years and beyond document excellent results with cemented stems implanted with this technique. In one study, 131 hips were examined and followed for 10 to 15 years (mean 12 years) in patients (average age, 67 years) with the Harris Design II femoral stem (HD2, Howmedica, Rutherford, NJ). Only 2% of femoral components were loose while 9% of acetabular components were loose. One hundred forty patients (161 hips) using second-generation cement were examined in another study. Eighty-four hips in 72 patients were followed for an average of 18 years (range, 17 to 20 years). Only 7% of stems were revised for loosening compared with 27% of acetabular components. Similar results have been reported in younger patients (age 50 years or younger).

Despite the excellent long-term results of second-generation cementing, a number of changes in stem design and cement technique occurred in an attempt to further improve fixation of cemented stems. Laboratory evidence indicated that debonding of cement from the stem was potentially the initiating factor in failure of many cemented stems. This provided the rationale for increasing the strength of the bond between stem and cement, which was achieved in some stem designs by increasing the surface roughness of the stem, usually over the proximal portion, and/or the addition of a thin layer of polymethylmethacrylate (precoating). Porosity reduction also was introduced in an attempt to increase the fatigue strength of the cement. The major methods of achieving this were with either centrifugation or vacuum mixing. An enhanced stem surface and porosity reduction were components of what was termed "third-generation" cement technique. Although no clinical series have, as yet, demonstrated improvement in results of cemented stems using third-generation cement compared with second-generation cement, some studies have at least demonstrated equivalent results in the 5- to 10-year time frame. In one study of 100 hips in 86 patients followed for an average of 120 months (range, 84 to 153 months), centrifugation of the cement and a precoated femoral stem was used. Only one stem had been revised for loosening and an additional three stems were loose radiographically but were asymptomatic. In another study of precoated femoral components, 82 patients (98 hips) with an average age of 67 years and average follow-up of 6.5 years (range, 5 to 9 years) were examined. Definite failures occurred in 2% (2 of 98) in this group of femoral components. Other studies have reported a higher rate of loosening of osteolysis with precoated stems attributed to thin cement mantles leading to cement fracture, fragmentation, and subsequent osteolysis or progressive circumferential bone interface osteolysis with relative preservation of the cement-metal interface. As a result, awareness of the importance of stem surface finish as a potential factor in the success or failure of cemented stems has increased.

Surface Finish

A number of clinical series have indicated that at least some stem designs are associated with a higher failure rate with a roughened surface compared with a smooth surface. The Exeter, Iowa, and T-28 stems have had a higher incidence of loosening and osteolysis reported with a rough stem surface finish than with a smooth stem. However, some stems with roughened surfaces have performed well in the 5- to 10-year time frame. One stem with a grit blast surface in the proximal third has had a reported 10-year survival rate of 99%

according to the Swedish Joint Registry. A grit blast surface, in itself, is therefore not necessarily associated with a high incidence of lysis or loosening. Apparently there is an interaction of surface finish with other factors such as stem geometry and length that is important in achieving long-term stability of cemented stems. If a roughened or grit blast surface is applied to a cemented stem it is apparently important that the stem be rotationally stable so that debonding does not occur. Once debonding does occur, a rough stem is more likely to generate wear debris leading to aggressive osteolysis.

Charnley Cemented Stem

The most extensively documented results in the literature are with the use of the Charnley cemented stem. A number of studies have appeared in recent years documenting the long-term results of the Charnley cemented stems used in young patients. In one 10-year follow-up study of 258 matte finish Charnley cemented stems (58.5% flanged, 41.5% nonflanged) in 221 patients with an average age of 41 years, a 99% survival at 10 years, a 94% survival at 15 years, and a revision rate of 3.5% at an average of 13.4 years were reported. These stems were implanted using an intramedullary bone block. In another study of polished flatback Charnley cemented stems, 69 patients (93 hips) younger than 50 years old were followed for 20 to 25 years. Only 5% of stems had been revised whereas an additional 8% were radiographically loose. The cemented acetabular components did not fare as well, with 19% revised for loosening and an additional 15% radiographically loose. Even the Charnley cemented stem has been less successful in extremely young patients (age 30 years or younger). In one series of 83 Charnley cemented stems in 55 patients with an average age 24.9 years, at 20-year average follow-up, 23% of stems had been revised, with an 18% incidence of lysis.

Although the Charnley cemented stem has been frequently referred to as the "gold standard," higher stem survival rates have been reported with other cemented stems. In one prospective randomized study of 206 flanged matte finish Charnley cemented stems and 204 Spectron (Smith & Nephew, Memphis, TN) stems, radiographic follow-up at 10 years revealed 10 loose Charnley stems and only one loose Spectron stem. The difficulty in positioning the Charnley stem with an adequate cement mantle in the absence of a trochanteric osteotomy was suggested as a possible explanation for its inferior stem longevity.

In one recent study, the results of the Charnley cemented stem were evaluated across an entire health region rather than from a single dedicated total joint center. The results were dramatically different than previous reports, with a known rate of aseptic loosening of 2.3% at 5 years, infection rate of 1.4%, dislocation rate of 5%, revision rate of 3.2%, and a radiographic gross failure rate of 5.2%. These results represented an overall failure rate of approximately 10% within 5 years, which may be more representative of the norm rather than the typical reports in the literature that originate from dedicated total joint centers.

Cementless Stems

The use of cementless fixation for primary THA continues to be a popular approach. Most early failures of cementless components have occurred on the acetabular side and have been associated with accelerated polyethylene wear and osteolysis. There have been relatively fewer major problems with porous-coated cementless femoral stems; these stems have been quite successful in achieving fixation consistently. The major problems observed with cementless stems are thigh pain and stress shielding. A number of different uncemented stem designs have been in widespread clinical use for which midterm clinical results of 5 to 10 years have recently become available.

Extensively Coated Stems

Uncemented stems that have a porous coating extending over most or all of the surface previously have been fabricated of cobalt-chrome because of the difficulty in obtaining adequate stem strength with an extensively coated titanium stem. Long-term results beyond 10 years with a fully coated cobalt-chrome stem are documented in the literature. Previous reports on the Anatomic Medullary Locking stem (AML, DePuy, Warsaw, IN) have reported a 97% stem survival at 12 years. Recent follow-up studies on the use of this stem in patients 65 years of age or older document a similar excellent success rate with 196 hips followed for more than 5 years (mean, 8.5, range, 5 to 14 years). Only one stem was revised for loosening and one additional stem was radiographically loose. Stress shielding was seen radiographically in 26% of the 174 hips followed for at least 2 years. Nine percent of patients had pain that limited activity but this pain was localized to the thigh in only 3%. In another recent study that specifically examined the issue of thigh pain in extensively coated stems, a proximally coated stem was found to have twice the incidence of thigh pain as a fully coated stem. The incidence of thigh pain with a fully coated stem was equivalent to that of a cemented stem. A number of studies have suggested that cylindrical cobalt-chrome stems seem to have the best clinical results in terms of thigh pain when they are fully coated rather than proximally coated.

Proximally Coated Stems

Certain proximally coated stems have been associated with a higher incidence of osteolysis, loosening, and revision. One design feature that has been associated with a higher incidence of distal osteolysis is the presence of noncircumferential proximal porous coating. The Harris-Galante uncemented femoral stem (Zimmer, Inc, Warsaw, IN) had pads of coating in the proximal portion anteriorly, medially, and posteriorly. A study of 77 such hips in 72 patients at an average of 126 months revealed a 60% incidence of lysis with a 19% stem revision rate. Better results have been documented for proximally coated titanium hips with a circumferential coating. In one series of 100 anatomic proximally coated titanium hips in 88 patients followed for an average of 7.1 years, there was only one revision for loosening, a 5% incidence of thigh pain, and no incidence of femoral osteolysis. Proximally circumferentially coated cobalt-chrome stems also have been successful. One of the earliest designs was the Porous Coated Anatomic hip (PCA, Howmedica, Rutherford, NJ). A 10-year follow-up study of this implant in 71 patients (77 hips) revealed there were two femoral revisions for loosening, and three additional loosenings for proximal osteolysis. There was also a 12% incidence of thigh pain. Another proximally coated implant system with recently documented long-term results is the Omnifit cementless total hip (Osteonics Corporation, Allendale, NJ). In one series of 76 hips in 67 patients with an average age of 45 years at surgery who were followed for an average of 10 years, two stems and one cup were revised for aseptic loosening for an incidence of 2.6% on the femoral side and 1.3% on the acetabular side. Thigh pain was present in only three patients. There was, however, a 17% reoperation rate primarily for bone grafting of the proximal osteolytic lesions. Again, the major problem with this particular component was similar to that of the PCA in that accelerated wear of the modular cementless acetabular component frequently used with this stem was the apparent cause of the femoral osteolytic lesions. Because osteolysis and thigh pain have been encountered with some early generation cementless components, second-generation components have emerged. Changes have occurred in sizing and geometry of the femoral stems. On the acetabular side the focus has been on improving the locking mechanism and the liner conformity, ensuring adequate polyethylene thickness and avoidance of 32-mm heads. Such a second-generation cementless system has been described with intermediate term clinical results. The PCA E (Howmedica, Rutherford, NJ) stem is modified by widening of the proximal flare and modification of the curve of the tip to reduce the incidence of stem tip abutment. A

5- to 7-year follow-up study of 109 hips in 102 patients (average age, 56 years) demonstrated one femoral stem loosening and one radiographically loose stem with this system. No osteolytic lesions were observed in this time frame.

Tapered Stems

Another approach to cementless stem fixation has been the use of a stem with a tapered geometry to achieve mechanical stability in the proximal portion of the femur by wedging the component into place rather than using a cylindrical reamer. This design has been a popular concept in Europe for many years. Tapered stems have been used with traditional porous-coated surfaces and roughened titanium surfaces, with or without hydroxyapatite coating. Intermediate-term results are now available for a number of tapered stems with proximal porous coating. Both titanium and cobalt-chrome tapered proximally porous-coated stems have been used with a high degree of success.

In one series of 100 hips (average age of patient, 37 years) followed for a mean of 10.2 years, results showed no femoral loosening. Femoral cortical lysis occurred in seven patients but was considered to be a major event in one. The component used in this study was a plasma spray proximally coated titanium hip (Taperloc, Biomet, Warsaw, IN). Similar results have been reported with a proximally coated tapered cobalt-chrome hip (Trilock, DePuy, Inc, Warsaw, IN). Results of a review of 66 hips followed for an average of 10 years (range, 8.3 to 11.6; average patient age 62 years) showed only one stem revised for loosening and no cases of distal lysis. One study compared the clinical results of a cobalt-chrome versus a titaniumtapered stem. The same type of acetabular component and polyethylene were implanted in all hips. Although clinical results were equivalent between the two stems, the calculated average linear wear rate was significantly higher for titanium stems with a plasma spray porous surface compared with the cobalt-chrome stems with a sintered bead surface. The average wear rate was 0.22 mm per year for the titanium stems versus 0.07 mm per year for the cobalt-chrome stems. The prevalence of periprosthetic osteolysis was 16% for the titanium stems compared to none for the cobalt-chrome stems. A potential cause of the higher wear rate and higher incidence of osteolysis is accelerated polyethylene wear secondary to third body particulates from either the modular head/neck interface or the plasma spray porous coating.

Hydroxyapatite

The use of hydroxyapatite to help achieve fixation of uncemented femoral stems is a subject of interest. Hydroxyapatite has been used on a textured or "nor-malized" surface as well as on a traditional porous-coated surface. The possibility that hydroxyapatite could increase polyethylene wear and increase the incidence of osteolysis is cause for concern, as well as the possibility that the hydroxyapatite coating may resorb over time and thus fail to maintain long-term fixation. A multicenter study of 316 hips in 282 patients in which a hydroxyapatite coated stem was used assessed patients for an average 8.1 years (range, 5.6 to 9.9 years). The average patient age was 50 years. Only one stem (0.3%) was revised for aseptic loosening and there were no instances of intramedullary femoral osteolysis. The results of the use of hydroxyapatite with this particular stem did not support concerns over increased wear or osteolysis with a hydroxyapatite stem. Questions were raised, however, regarding the use of hydroxyapatite-coated acetabular components when used without porous coating. Several studies have compared porous-coated femoral stem fixation with and without the addition of hydroxyapatite to the porous coating. None of the studies to date have demonstrated a clinical advantage in terms of hip score, thigh pain, or revision rate.

Total Hip Arthroplasty in Special Cases

Rheumatoid Arthritis

Recent studies indicate that results of primary THA in patients with rheumatoid arthritis are roughly equivalent to those of patients with osteoarthritis in terms of revision rate. Although the patients tend to be younger and their bone quality often is not as good, this factor is offset by the fact that they are usually of smaller stature and less active, with a higher proportion of female patients than in the population with osteoarthritis. In one study of 103 cemented total hips in patients with adult-onset rheumatoid arthritis followed for a minimum of 10 years, only one femoral stem and one acetabular component had been revised for loosening. Radiographic loosening was present, however, in 8% of acetabular components compared with 2% of femoral stems. In another study of over 1,500 Charnley cemented stems placed in patients with rheumatoid arthritis, the survival rate of the femoral stem at 10 and 15 years was 93.2% and 89.9%, respectively, compared with 93.6% and 87.1% for the acetabular component.

Acetabular Dysplasia

The presence of a shallow dysplastic acetabulum predisposes to the development of osteoarthritis at a relatively early age. The presence of anatomic variations requires modification of the standard technique for primary THA to be successful. On the femoral side there is often an exaggerated degree of anteversion. This situation can be addressed in a number of ways, including subtrochanteric osteotomy and femoral shortening if necessary. If this approach is used, the proximal femur can be derotated to a more anatomic degree of version at the time of implantation of the stem. Other options for adjusting the anteversion include using a modular stem, a cemented stem, or an anteverted neck designed for the contralateral hip. The latter technique allows for adjustment for moderate degrees of excessive anteversion. The use of a 10° anteverted right femoral stem in a left hip, for instance, would effectively decrease the amount of femoral anteversion by 20°, which may be adequate for mild to moderate degrees of excessive anteversion.

The other major challenge is the shallow acetabulum. Results from previous studies using femoral head autograft have demonstrated a high rate of loosening after 10 to 15 years. Results from recent studies report a higher degree of success with the use of a femoral head autograft and a cemented acetabular component. In one study of 45 Charnley cemented components in 41 patients (mean age, 41 years), no revisions were reported after 11-year follow-up. The autograft of the femoral head covered only 26% of the acetabular component (range, 16% to 35%). In patients in whom less than 40% of the acetabular component is covered by autograft, a higher success rate can be expected. Similar results were reported from a group in Japan. In a large study of 112 patients with 103 dysplastic hips, after a mean follow-up of 12.3 years (range, 8 to 24 years) 15-year survivorship of the acetabular component was 90%.

Other approaches to the dysplastic acetabulum include the use of an uncemented acetabular component with screw fixation, a medial protrusio technique with a hemispherical uncemented component, and the use of a reenforcement ring. In one series of 24 hips in 21 patients, an uncemented hemispherical component with screw fixation was used and up to 30% uncoverage of the component was accepted. At an average follow-up of 83 months (range, 64 to 102 months) there were no cases of revision, loosening, or pelvic osteolysis. An alternative approach is to ream through the medial wall of the acetabulum using a so-called "medial protrusio" technique. The use of such a technique was reported in 24 hips in 19 patients followed for a minimum of 5 years. The amount of the surface of the cup beyond Köhler's line averaged over 40%. At follow-up averaging 7 years (range, 5 to 13 years) there were no revisions. This technique is faster and simpler but does sacrifice bone stock for future revisions. The final technique that has been described is the use of a metal roof-reenforcement ring with or without autograft of the femoral head in combination with a cemented all-polyethylene component. Such a technique was used in 123 consecutive hips followed for an average of 9.4 years (range, 5 to 15 years). There was only one revision for acetabular component loosening but two other hips had radiographic evidence of loosening. The literature supports a number of viable options available in dealing with the anatomic variations present in patients with dysplastic acetabulum that require THA.

Complications After Total Hip Arthroplasty

Although THA has been successful, some complications associated with the procedure cannot be completely eliminated. The patient should be made aware of these complications as well as postoperative expectations. One of the goals of the orthopaedic surgeon must be to minimize these complications as much as possible. The major complications associated with THA that can compromise the end result and diminish patient satisfaction include death, dislocation, severe heterotopic ossification, infection, nerve palsy, and leg length inequality.

Death

Accurate diagnosis of mortality rates after surgical procedures, including THA, has become a topic of interest. Evaluations have been categorized in various studies to include in-hospital mortality, 30-day postoperative mortality, and 90-day postoperative mortality. In-hospital mortality rates after primary THA have been reported in the range of 0.1% to 0.8%, 30-day rates between 0.15% and 1.42%, and 90-day rates between 0.2% and 0.74%. (The study with 1.42% 30-day mortality rates did not report 90-day results.) Ninety-day mortality rates after revision hip surgery range from 0.6% to 0.9%. Patients at increased risk for death after the procedure include elderly patients (older than age 70 years according to one study), patients with a history of malignancy, and patients with hip fractures. Cause of death has most commonly been attributed to cardiac problems and thromboembolic disease (see chapter 6). Further investigation is needed to adequately evaluate the relationships between comorbidities, diagnoses at surgery, surgical volume, age at surgery, type of fixation, cause of death, and the mortality rates reported after THA in the studies where this subject is investigated.

Dislocation

Dislocation after THA is stressful to the patient and surgeon. The reported occurrences in various series ranges from zero to 10% in primary surgery and rates of up to 20% have been reported in revision surgery. Patient risk factors, including alcohol use and cerebral dysfunction,

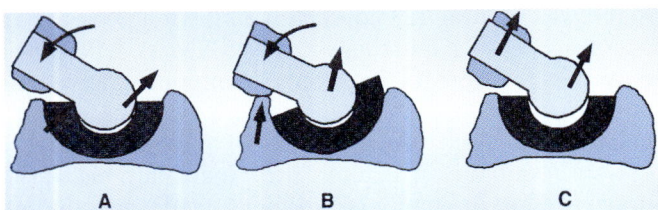

Figure 6 Three mechanisms of hip dislocation. **A,** Impingement of the prosthetic femoral neck on the cup liner. **B,** Impingement of the osseous femur on the osseous pelvis. **C,** Spontaneous dislocation. *(Reproduced with permission from Bartz RL, Noble PC, Kadakia NR, Tullos HS: The effect of femoral component head size on posterior dislocation of the artificial hip joint. J Bone Joint Surg Am 2000;82: 1303.)*

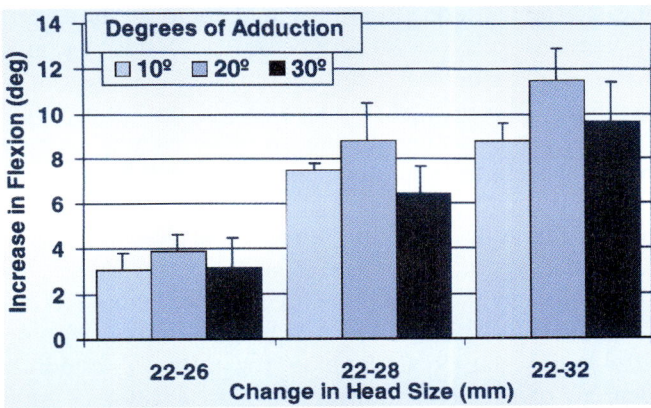

Figure 7 Bar graph depicting the increase in hip flexion at dislocation with changes in the head diameter of the femoral component. *(Reproduced with permission from Bartz RL, Noble PC, Kadakia NR, Tullos HS: The effect of femoral component head size on posterior dislocation of the artificial hip joint. J Bone Joint Surg Am 2000;82:1303.)*

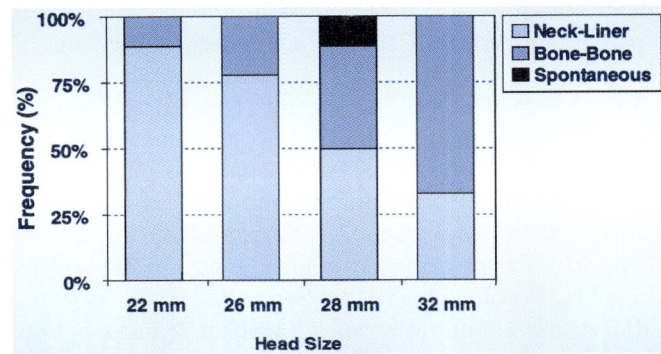

Figure 8 Bar graph depicting the effect of the head diameter of the femoral component on the mechanism of dislocation. *(Reproduced with permission from Bartz RL, Noble PC, Kadakia NR, Tullos HS: The effect of femoral component head size on posterior dislocation of the artificial hip joint. J Bone Joint Surg Am 2000; 82:1303.)*

have been well established recently. Results from most series have demonstrated higher dislocation rates when a posterior approach rather than an anterior-lateral or lateral approach was used; however, with the recent techniques described to repair the posterior capsule and external rotators to the hip, dislocation rates of less than 0.5% have been reported with the posterior approach. There are no definitive data available to date that document an increased incidence of dislocation since modularity has been introduced as a factor in THA. However, laboratory data suggest a decrease in motion before neck-liner impingement occurs when modular head-neck connections are used because they require a lower head-neck ratio (a wider neck) than monolithic components because of neck strength issues. The use of skirted heads is associated with significant decreases in motion prior to impingement. Extended lip liners have been shown in the laboratory to allow more motion in one direction before neck-liner impingement; however, they limit the motion before impingement in the opposite direction. In one large series of patients who had undergone THA, those with extended liners had a lower rate of dislocation than did those without extended liners (2.2% versus 3.85%). The use of trial components to determine the need for such components as well as to help in the optimal positioning of the extended liner currently are available. Use of trial components and femoral components with greater offset should help reduce dislocation rates; however, clinical data to support this statement are not yet available.

Recent laboratory data on head size and the propensity for dislocation have demonstrated a greater chance for bony impingement with larger head sizes (28 and 32 mm) versus a greater chance for cup liner impingement with smaller sizes (22 mm) (Figs. 6 through 8). In a clinical study of modular hip components, patients with larger outer cup diameters had a higher dislocation rate than those with smaller cup diameters and patients with 22-mm heads had a higher rate than did those with 28-mm heads.

Constrained liners are being used more often to treat recurrent dislocation after THA. Use of a tripolar type of constrained device was associated with only a 4%

failure rate in one series; in other studies where other operations were performed to treat recurrent dislocations, the rate of success in preventing further dislocation was 61%. However, not all types of constrained liners have been as successful. Dissociation of the capturing mechanism as well as accelerated wear and loosening are possible. Bipolar and unipolar replacements also have been used with success rates of 81% reported in one relatively large case series. Case reports of capsular augmentation with allograft tendon also have been reported in the treatment of recurrent dislocation.

Heterotopic Ossification

Three percent to 10% of THA patients experience functional impairment in the form of diminished range of motion or pain related to the inflammatory reaction that accompanies the process of heterotopic ossification. Several prophylactic methods aimed at inhibiting heterotopic ossification, including pharmacologic measures and radiation therapy, have been investigated.

Indomethacin remains the most studied nonsteroidal anti-inflammatory drug (NSAID) but others have demonstrated effectiveness in limiting heterotopic ossification. Aspirin was demonstrated to be beneficial in one study but a recent, large, randomized trial demonstrated no effect. A 10-day short course of indomethacin in high-risk patients demonstrated no grade III or IV heterotopic ossification in a recent study.

Although the initial dose of irradiation recommended to prevent heterotopic ossification after THA was 2000 cGy, one 800- or 700-cGy dose has now been shown to be efficacious. Lower doses (550 cGy) have not been efficacious. Recent basic and clinical studies have demonstrated the efficacy of preoperative irradiation; cementless components should be shielded as well as any trochanteric osteotomy that has been performed. One prospective study comparing postoperative irradiation to NSAID therapy demonstrated efficacy of both approaches with slightly more success with irradiation.

When the heterotopic ossification is symptomatic the bone can be excised when it has matured. When combining surgical excision with postoperative irradiation, an average increase of 45° of flexion and 25° of abduction was obtained.

Infection

Two-stage exchange remains the standard for the treatment of any infection of total joint arthroplasty except during the first 1 to 3 months after surgery or in the presence of an acute hematogenous infection. Meticulous, extensive débridement and identification of the organism are essential for optimal results. Articulating antibiotic-impregnated spacers are being used more frequently in the interval between the removal of the infected arthroplasty and reimplantation of the new prosthesis, especially in patients with extensive bone loss. Success rates for this procedure can be as high as 95%. Recent studies also support the use of selective one-stage exchange when the organism is known, easily treatable by antibiotics, and when adequate débridement can be obtained at the time of surgery. Success rates of 92% to 100% have been obtained with this approach when it is used selectively. In addition, in the early postoperative period (preferably 1 to 2 months after surgery) *Staphylococcus* infections can be successfully treated with aggressive débridement of the joint and a combined drug regimen of rifampin and ciprofloxacin for 3 to 6 months.

Nerve Palsy

Up to 70% of patients demonstrate evidence of mild nerve damage on nerve conduction and electromyographic studies after THA. Clinical nerve palsy is uncommon, with an overall prevalence of approximately 1%. Females, patients with hip dysplasia, and those undergoing revision surgery are at greatest risk. In a majority of cases the origin is unknown. In some series leg lengthening of more than 2 to 3 cm was a common finding. Complete recovery occurs in 41% of patients; 44% have mild deficits and 15% have a poor outcome with persistent dysesthesias or weakness that limits ambulation. Prognosis is good if limited motor function is present immediately after surgery or if some motor function returns in the first 2 weeks postoperatively. Although intraoperative nerve monitoring has been suggested in high-risk cases, the occurrence of the problem has not been shown to be diminished by such monitoring in THA. When the problem is recognized postoperatively, the patient should be examined for a large hematoma causing compression (evacuate if present) and extension of the hip and flexion of the knee to relieve any tension on the nerve should be considered. No data exist to demonstrate that nerve exploration is helpful in returning function other than in patients in whom a large hematoma was present.

Limb-Length Inequality

Limb-length discrepancies have been noted in up to 18% to 32% of THA patients. Six percent to 50% of these patients find this discrepancy problematic. Techniques of accurate preoperative templating, anatomic component geometry, and intraoperative assessment (including use of outrigger jigs, center of the head to lesser trochanter distances, relationship of the knees and heels before and after reconstruction as well intraoperative radiographs in difficult cases) have diminished the prevalence of inadvertent lengthening of the limb by reproducing the normal anatomic relationships. The actual or true limb-length inequality is caused by lengthening of the prosthetic head-neck distance. The apparent or functional limb-length inequality describes the amount that is attributable to other factors such as the tightness of the anterolateral soft tissues about the hip and degenerative disease with scoliosis of the lumbar spine, causing obliquity of the pelvis. Orthopaedic surgeons have gained a better understanding of functional limb-length inequality over the last several years as well as the need for soft-tissue balancing of the hip. Identification of pelvic obliquity and degenerative spinal scoliosis on radiographs and tight hip flexor muscles and tensor fascia muscles (Ober's sign) on examination are preoperative factors, and the patient should be made aware of the potential for perceived limb-

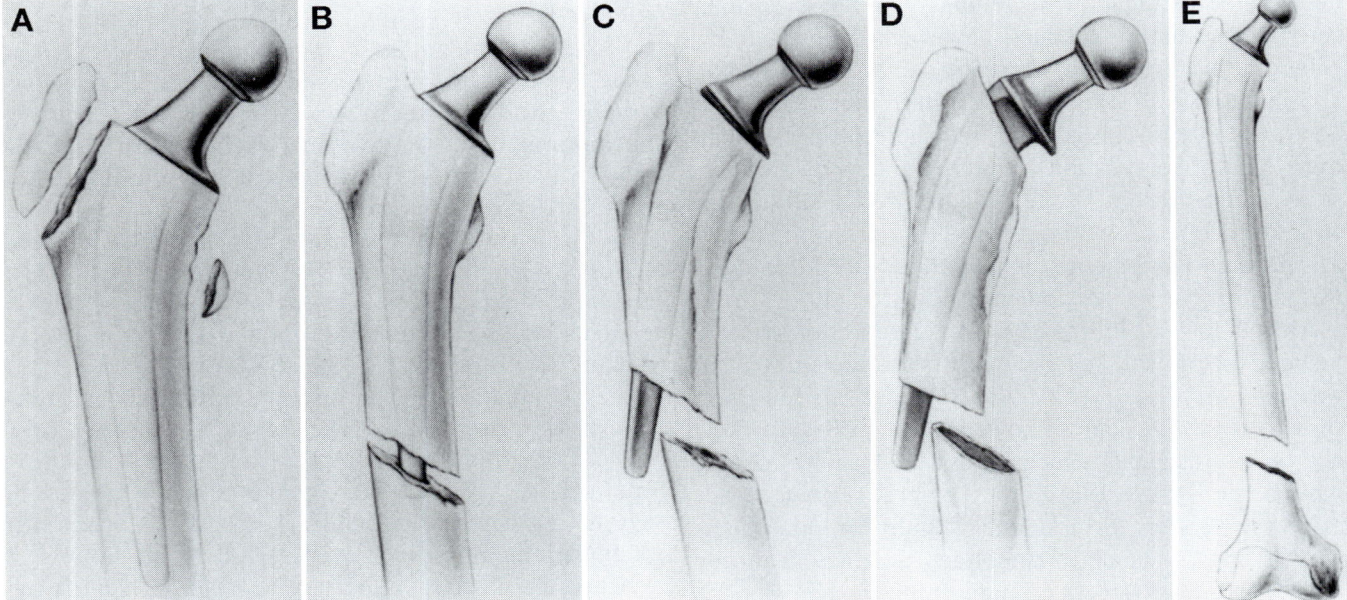

Figure 9 Vancouver classification of periprosthetic femoral fractures. **A,** Type A trochanteric fractures, lesser or greater. **B,** Type B fractures around the stem with intact femoral components. **C,** Type B2 fractures around the stem with loose femoral components. **D,** Type B3 fractures around the loose stem with severe comminution, generalized osteopenia, or severe osteolysis. **E,** Type C fractures occurring well distal to the stem. *(Reproduced with permission from Brady OH, Garbuz DS, Masri BA, Duncan CP: Classification of the hip in periprosthetic fractures after major joint replacement. Orthop Clin North Am 1999;30:217-219.)*

length inequality postoperatively, even if the hip is reconstructed to the anatomic relationship of the opposite hip. Intraoperative release of the rectus femoris, tensor fascia lata, anterior hip capsule, gluteus medius, and/or psoas tendon is a possibility to adequately flex the knee while bringing the hip to the neutral position (in abduction/adduction) and extension. Aggressive stretching (especially the hip abductors and flexors) and patient reassurance after surgery are mandatory. Reoperation with capsular and muscle release rarely is required.

Periprosthetic Fractures

Intraoperative and postoperative fractures around THAs have been on the rise over the past decade. The increase in intraoperative fractures can be attributed to the use of press-fit techniques for the insertion of cementless devices. The increase in postoperative fractures can be attributed to an increase in THAs, younger patients, increase in the length of time the hip replacement is being used in patients with aging skeletons undergoing simultaneous loss of bone mass, and loosening with associated osteolysis and bone loss that occurs in a percentage of patients.

Periprosthetic femoral fractures are more common than acetabular fractures. The Vancouver classification based on the site of the fracture, stability of the implant, and the surrounding bone stock has gained wide acceptance (Fig. 9). The fractures are divided into

A, B, or C depending on their location. Type A fractures occur proximal to the prosthesis and are trochanteric, either greater (A_G) or lesser (A_L). Type B fractures occur around or just below the stem. Type C fractures occur well below the stem tip. Type A fractures can be further subdivided into stable and unstable depending on whether surgical stabilization is necessary. Similarly, type B fractures are subdivided depending on the stability of the femoral component. Type B1 includes fractures in which the component is solidly fixed, and B2 includes fractures in which the component is loose. The quality of bone is an important subdivision within the type B group. In the B1 and B2 subgroup, the surrounding bone stock is adequate. If the femoral component is loose and there is severe bone stock loss, the fracture is classified as type B3. Type C fractures occur well below the stem tip where the fracture can be treated independently of the prosthesis. This classification has been found to be reliable and valid in psychometric testing.

Type A fractures are treated nonsurgically if stable and surgically if unstable. Type B1 fractures are treated with plating or allograft struts or a combination of the two. Type B2 fractures are treated with longer prostheses; long, curved, cementless stems with bone graft augmentation (struts and morcellized) often are necessary. Type B3 fractures can be treated similarly; however, allograft composites or tumor prostheses and cement fixation sometimes are necessary.

Acute fractures, if recognized at surgery, can be treated with cerclage wiring. If recognized postoperatively and if the posterior cortex along the linea aspera is intact, nonsurgical treatment with bracing in a compliant patient is adequate. If patients are noncompliant or if the posterior cortex is fractured, cerclage wiring should be considered.

Nonunion of periprosthetic femoral fractures can be treated by revision to a long stem or use of a proximal femoral prosthesis. Healing of the fracture site only occurred in 9 of 13 patients according to one study. Treatment is difficult, with a high rate of complication and relatively poor functional outcome. Periprosthetic fractures of the acetabulum are uncommon. The use of cementless acetabular components with press-fit fixation (underreaming the acetabulum in relationship to the size of the component) has been associated with an increased incidence of intraoperative fractures as well as fractures recognized in the early postoperative period (that probably occurred intraoperatively). These fractures are common in women with osteopenic bone. Periprosthetic acetabular fractures have been classified as radiographically stable or radiographically unstable. Radiographically stable fractures should be treated nonsurgically; however, even if the fracture heals, the component may need to be revised at a later time. Unstable components need revision and acetabular cages and plating of pelvic discontinuities may be necessary for the reconstruction. In one series, satisfactory outcomes were noted in 77% of patients with cages and 56% of patients with uncemented components and plating; no patients with cemented components had satisfactory outcomes.

Wear in Total Hip Arthroplasty

As the fixation of total joint implants has become more reliable and durable and as the technology of total joint replacement has been applied to younger and more active patients, the current limitations of total joint arthroplasty are related to the wear of the components. Wear is the removal of material, with the generation of wear particles that occurs as a result of the relative motion between two opposing surfaces under load. In complex mechanic-biological systems such as THA, there can be many types of wear. Although the mechanical consequences of wear, such as progressive thinning of polyethylene components can limit the functional life of a joint replacement, the clinical problems from wear more frequently are the result of the release of an excessive number of wear particles into a biologic environment. When particles within a certain size range are phagocytized in sufficient amounts, the macrophages enter into an activated state of metabolism, releasing cytokines that can result in periprosthetic bone resorption. Progressive loss of periprosthetic bone can necessitate a reoperation, which is the definitive measure of clinical failure of a joint arthroplasty.

Several investigators have found that capsular tissue has some capacity to transport particles through the lymphatic system by means of perivascular lymph spaces, leading to regional and systemic distribution. If the capacity for elimination by this mechanism is exceeded, then particles accumulate in the periarticular tissues. The pseudocapsule appears to be the primary location for phagocytosis of particles. This process results in the development of foreign body granulomas with areas of necrosis and fibrosis that are somewhat proportional to the amount of particles. Extension of this foreign body response into the cement-bone interface could cause loosening of the implant. Conceptually, the effective joint space includes all periprosthetic regions that are accessible to joint fluid and, thus, accessible to wear particles. This is the mechanism by which the products of wear contribute to the osteolysis and loosening process (Fig. 10).

It is important to distinguish the fundamental mechanisms of wear (adhesion, abrasion, and fatigue); the changes in the appearance or the morphologic characteristics of the bearing surfaces (wear damage); and the conditions under which the prosthesis was functioning when the wear occurred (wear modes) (Fig. 11). Adhesion involves bonding of the surfaces when they are pressed together under load. Sufficient relative motion results in material being pulled away from one or more surfaces, usually from the weaker material. Abrasion is a mechanical process wherein asperities on the harder surface cut and plow through the softer surface, resulting in removal of material. When local stresses exceed the fatigue strength of a material, that material then fails after a certain number of loading cycles, releasing material from the surface. One or more of the classic mechanisms of wear may be operating on the prosthesis in a particular wear mode, and a prosthesis may function in several wear modes over its service life in vivo. The predominant type of wear of one prosthetic joint can differ from that of another. Furthermore, in a specific joint, there may be different types of wear occurring at different times over the service life of the implant. The damage to an implant is a result of all of the mechanisms of wear that have acted on it over time, with the most recent events having the greatest influence.

Mode 1 wear results from the motion that is intended to occur between the two primary bearing surfaces, such as the motion of the prosthetic femoral head against the polyethylene acetabular bearing surface. Mode 2 wear refers to the condition of a primary

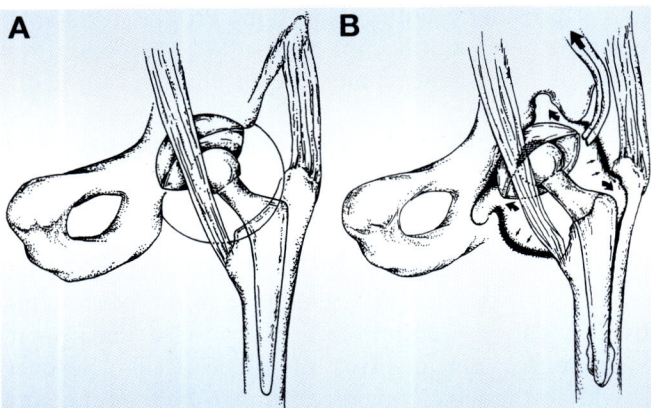

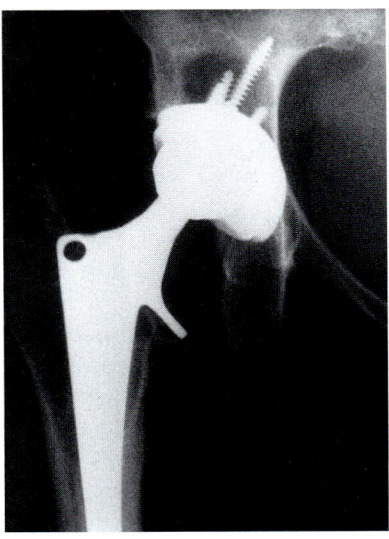

Figure 11 Expansile pelvic osteolysis associated with polyethylene wear of cementless acetabular components. Note eccentric femoral head location in relationship to the acetabular shell.

Figure 10 **A,** Diagram showing the effective joint space, which includes all periprosthetic regions that are accessible to joint fluid. The surgical implantation procedure alters the natural anatomy of a joint. In prosthetic THA and total knee arthroplasty, some bone as well as the implant-bone interfaces are exposed within the new joint space. Contraction of muscles, such as the psoas and abductor muscles, and changes in joint position (flexion, extension, abduction, adduction, and rotation) can alter the volume of the effective joint space, resulting in changes in intracapsular joint-fluid pressure. **B,** Diagram showing wear and the release of wear particles into the effective joint space. Capsular tissue has some capacity to transport particles through the lymphatic system (large straight arrow). In the effective joint space, joint fluid and wear particles follow the path of least resistance, which is dependent on the prosthetic and anatomic details of each specific reconstruction. The pseudocapsule becomes thickened (small straight arrows) because of phagocytosis of wear particles and the development of foreign-body granulomas. The effective joint space can extend along interfacial planes, expand into bone, or expand into soft tissues or a variety of combinations is possible (curved arrows). *(Reproduced with permission from Schmalzried TP, Callaghan JJ: Wear in total hip and knee replacements. J Bone Joint Surg Am 1999;81:127.)*

bearing surface that moves against a secondary surface that it is not intended to move against. Mode 3 wear refers to the condition of the primary surfaces as they move against each other but with the interposition of third-body particles. In mode 3 wear, the contaminant particles directly abrade one or both of the primary bearing surfaces. This type of wear is known as three-body abrasion or three-body wear. The primary bearing surfaces may be transiently or permanently roughened by this interaction.

Mode 4 wear refers to two secondary (nonprimary) surfaces rubbing together. Examples of mode 4 wear include impingement of the femoral neck of the prosthesis on the rim of the acetabular component; motion at the stem-cement or bone-cement interface or relative motion of a porous coating, or other metallic surface, against bone; relative motion of the external surface of a modular polyethylene component against the metal support (so-called backside wear); fretting between a metallic substrate and a fixation screw, and fretting and corrosion of modular taper connections as well as that of extra-articular sources.

Most THAs have one primary bearing surface made of ultra-high molecular weight polyethylene (referred to as polyethylene). Although there are many potential sources of wear particles, in most total hip and knee

replacements the greatest contribution of wear is from mode 1 wear—that is, polyethylene particles generated by the intended motion of the joint at the primary bearing surfaces.

Clinical rates of wear traditionally have been expressed using a denominator of time because of convenience, not accuracy. More appropriately, investigators performing in vitro studies involving laboratory wear simulators have always used the number of loading cycles as a denominator. Similar to the use of a set of automobile tires, the wear of a prosthetic hip or knee is a function of use or the number of cycles and not a function of time in situ. In addition to activity level, higher wear rates have been associated with male sex, younger age, and smaller femoral head sizes. Digital edge detection has been developed to accurately measure wear on serial radiographs. Hips with linear wear rates of more than 0.2 mm per year have been associated with an increased prevalence of osteolysis and hips with linear wear rates of less than 0.1 mm per year have infrequently been associated with osteolysis.

Acetabular Revision in Total Hip Arthroplasty
Classification Systems
Two commonly used classification systems for grading acetabular bone loss exist. The first was published by the American Academy of Orthopaedic Surgeons™ and bone defects are divided into two main types, segmental and cavitary defects (Table 3). This classification system permits interoperative classification of acetabular defect severity; however, it is less helpful in preoperative planning.

The second classification system emphasizes the presence or absence of the acetabular rim, the deficiencies of the acetabular dome and walls, and the integrity of

TABLE 3 | Classification of Acetabular Defects

Type	Description
Type I	Segmental deficiencies
	Peripheral
	Superior
	Anterior
	Posterior
	Central (medial wall absent)
Type II	Cavitary deficiencies
	Peripheral
	Superior
	Anterior
	Posterior
	Central (medial wall intact)
Type III	Combined deficiencies
Type IV	Pelvic deficiencies
Type V	Arthrodesis

the anterior and posterior column. Using this information, the amount of coverage that can be attained for cementless acetabular fixation can be determined and therefore preoperative planning for appropriate reconstruction methods can be accomplished. This classification system describes three types of defects (Table 4). In a type I defect, the rim and walls are intact and the columns are intact and supportive. More than 50% coverage can be obtained and the bony bed is cancellous. In type I defects, a simple cementless or cemented acetabular reconstruction is appropriate. In a type II defect, the rim and walls are distorted. However, the columns are intact and supportive. Generally, defects can be filled with compacted allograft bone chips and placed with a cementless acetabular reconstruction with supplemental screw fixation. In type II defects, occasionally, the acetabular component may be placed in a high hip center to obtain superior wall support.

In a type III defect, the rim is missing and the walls are severely compromised. In addition, the columns offer no support, making a structural allograft necessary. Recent trends have been to use either a distal femur or acetabular allograft instead of a femoral head because of the volume of bone available. Currently, when a structural allograft is used, most surgeons are then adding an acetabular support cage to load-share with the graft. A polyethylene cup is cemented into the cage. Previous intermediate-term results with either cementless or cemented cups into bulk structural grafts

have shown relatively high failure rates. It is hoped that the addition of a load-sharing device such as an antiprotrusio cage will improve survivorship of these difficult reconstructions. From a surgical standpoint, appropriate preoperative recognition of a type III defect will ensure that appropriate bone graft and implants are available in the operating room.

Goals of Revision Surgery

In acetabular revision, the most important goal is to obtain a rigid construct. The implant has to be inserted in such a way that it is immediately stable. The majority of reconstructions are done using porous-coated acetabular components with supplemental screw fixation. In order to obtain bone ingrowth, the constructs have to be stable, with micromotion less than approximately 50 μm. In addition, the porous-coated surface has to be in direct contact with viable host bone over a sufficient surface area to allow ingrowth and long-term stabilization. If at least 50% to 60% of the implant is not in direct contact with host bone, alternative means of reconstruction must be considered, such as the use of bone grafts and a cage.

The position of the implant also is important to avoid dislocation. With isolated acetabular revisions,

TABLE 4 | Classification of Acetabular Defects

Type of Defect	Superior Migration of Hip Center*	Osteolysis of Ischium[†]	Medial Migration of Hip Center[‡]	Osteolysis of Teardrops[§]
I	Minimum	None	None	None
IIA	Minimum	Mild	Grade I	Mild
IIB	Minimum to marked	Mild	Grade II	Mild
IIC	Minimum	Mild	Grade III	Moderate to severe
IIIA	Marked	Moderate	Grade II+ or III	Moderate
IIIB	Marked	Severe	Grade III+	Severe

*Minimum = at least 3 cm proximal to the superior transverse obturator line, and marked = more than 3 cm proximal to the superior transverse obturator line
[†]Mild = 0 to 7 mm distal to the superior transverse obturator line, moderate = 8 to 14 mm distal to the obturator line, and severe = 15 mm or more distal to obturator line
[‡]Grade I = lateral to Köhler's line, grade II = migration to Köhler's line, grade II+ = medial expansion of Köhler's line into pelvis, grade III = migration into pelvis with violation of Köhler's line, and grade III+ = marked migration into pelvis
[§]Mild = minimum loss of the lateral border, moderate = complete loss of the lateral border, and severe = loss of the lateral and medial borders

the dislocation rate can be high. Careful trial reduction is important and the use of postoperative braces is now common.

Because implant position is an important factor, revision acetabular reconstructions are often done in a slightly high hip center. Some controversy exists as to the consequences of using a high hip center from a biomechanical standpoint and therefore implant survivorship. However, in revision surgery with a porous-coated implant, as long as the hip center is high and not lateral, there does not appear to be any significant deleterious effect in terms of implant loosening. Impingement leading to dislocation may be a problem with the high hip center, and later reconstruction may be problematic because of poor bone stock. The alternative would be to use a structural graft to bring the hip center down to its normal location.

Finally, bone stock should be restored during revision surgery. This often can be done with a morcellized graft. Allograft bone chips are now commonly available and can be impacted into cavitary defects and contoured using acetabular reamers in reverse. In addition, a morcellized allograft often can be used in segmental defects of the medial wall. A soft-tissue membrane in the presence of a medial wall defect can contain the graft material. When the acetabular rim is intact, the reamers can be used to compact this graft to the medial wall. Intermediate-term results using this technique have been good with both cemented reconstructions in Europe and cementless reconstructions in North America. When there is a major defect to the superior wall or posterior column, a structural graft often is required to obtain component stability. The anterior column is not as critical in terms of providing support for acetabular reconstructions and therefore a structural graft often is not needed.

Reconstruction Methods
Porous-Coated Acetabular Reconstructions
Approximately 90% of acetabular revisions can be performed using a hemispherical porous-coated socket. The majority of intermediate- to long-term results have been reported using a socket with a titanium fiber mesh porous coating fixed with multiple screws. Screw supplementation is necessary in the majority of revision surgeries to ensure adequate implant stability. In order to use the porous-coated socket with supplemental screws, criteria include contact with at least 50% host bone and lack of coverage of no more than 30%. These criteria can be met in most patients by using hemispherical reamers to enlarge the socket protecting the posterior column and wall and superior wall and filling cavitary defects as well as segmental defects of the medial wall with morcellized graft.

Several recent reports have documented the durability of the Harris-Galante titanium fiber mesh socket (Zimmer, Inc, Warsaw, IN). At 5- to 12-years follow-up, no radiographic evidence of loosening was reported. No component was revised and no revisions were scheduled during that period. Another study reported that after 7- to 11-years follow-up, only 5% of 109 sockets had a complete radiolucent line at the metal bone interface. A radiolucent line adjacent to a screw was seen in only 2% of patients and small osteolytic lesions were noted at the margin of the cup in 4% at a mean follow-up of 98 months. There were no repeat revisions for aseptic loosening, and only one acetabular component demonstrated radiographic evidence of loosening. Revision of the acetabular component with a porous-coated hemispherical fiber metal cup with supplemental screw fixation has been associated with a low rate of radiographic loosening and reoperation at up to 12 years after revision surgery. This information represents a significant improvement over previous studies in terms of survivorship of the acetabular component when compared with cement. These results cannot be generalized to other cementless acetabular components with different fixation surfaces and different modes of fixation. When a hemispherical porous-coated socket cannot be used because of the degree of bone loss, other techniques need to be used.

Structural Allografts and Antiprotrusio Cages
There is now relatively widespread agreement that the use of structural grafts on the acetabular side is associated with a guarded long-term prognosis and should be avoided if possible. Failure rates approaching 50% at 10 years have been reported. This is true both with cemented and cementless sockets. Despite the guarded prognosis, there are clinical situations in which bulk allografts must be used in revision acetabular surgery. The structural grafts are indicated for the treatment of uncontained defects to provide bony support for the implant. If the anatomy and limb lengths are acceptable and there is adequate bone stock, using a high hip center is technically easier and probably preferred; however, lateralization of the implant should be avoided. In addition, compensation for the limb-length inequality must be accomplished by using a long neck femoral component on the femoral side. If there is a well-fixed component with a nonmodular femoral head, use of a bulk graft may be necessary to restore the normal hip center and create a stable reconstruction from the standpoint of dislocation. Recent trends for the use of antiprotusio cages include large defects treated with morcellized grafts in which there is less than 50% contact with host bone, in conjunction with bulk grafts and in cases of pelvic discontinuity (Fig 12).

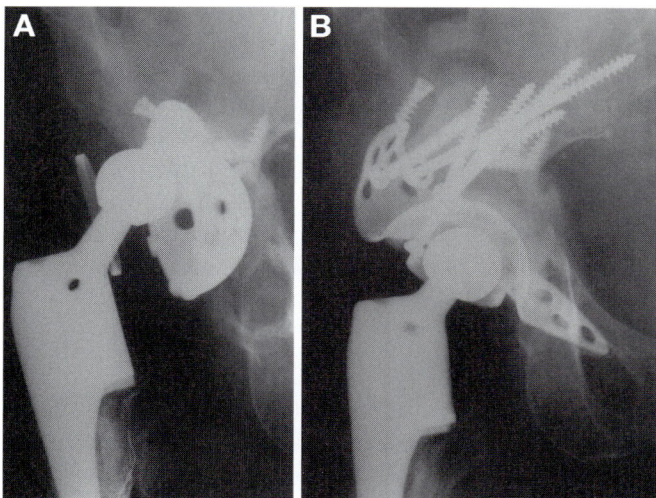

Figure 12 **A,** Failed oblong type socket. **B,** Reconstruction with structural allograft and antiprotrusio cage.

The advantages of structural grafts include restoration of normal anatomy and bone stock. Even when these grafts fail, it is now well recognized that they provide increased bone stock for the next revision. However, the disadvantages of structural grafts can be significant. With revascularization and remodeling, these grafts can collapse and weaken with time, leading to the high intermediate- and long-term failure rates previously discussed. Transmission of diseases (such as hepatitis C and B and human immunodeficiency virus (HIV) is another potential complication associated with the use of allograft bone. Deep freezing does not decrease the risk of disease transmission significantly. However, 2.5 mrads of radiation effectively eliminates bacteria as well as hepatitis B and C and significantly reduces the viral load with HIV.

In terms of available grafts, there has been a gradual increase in the number of acetabular allografts and distal femoral grafts with a concomitant decrease in the use of femoral heads. Major column defects are best restored with these large structural grafts, which can be fixed to the host bone with either large cancellous screws or screws and plates. In addition, the grafts are often protected by reconstruction rings that bridge the defect from one host bone to another. It is important to try to fix the graft both to the ilium and ischium. If inadequate bone is present in the ischium for screw fixation, the flange on the acetabular ring can be slotted into the ischium in many cases. It is hoped that the use of these load-sharing devices will improve the intermediate- to long-term results with bulk structural grafts; however, few data exist in these specific situations.

If a bulk graft provides 30% to 50% of the bony support for the acetabular component, a structural ring may not be necessary and a porous-coated socket can be used. In this case, the structural graft is contributing to implant stability to allow ingrowth in the remaining host bone. If less than 30% of a socket is noncontained, a structural graft is not necessary. In these cases either morcellized allograft packed into the defect may be as effective as a bulk graft if it can be contained.

Pelvic Discontinuity

Pelvic discontinuity should be suspected if there is significant damage to the posterior column, associated disruption of Köhler's line, or visible fracture. If a pelvic discontinuity is not recognized and treated appropriately, a high failure rate results. General treatment are to first treat the discontinuity, then treat the associated defect, and then reconstruct the acetabulum. The pelvic discontinuity is most commonly treated with a pelvic reconstruction plate on the posterior column; however, in certain circumstances, the discontinuity can be stabilized with an anti-protrusio cage or a large porous-coated socket with screws.

Bilobed Cups

The bilobed cup has been used as an alternative reconstruction method for patients whose failed hip is associated with extensive acetabular bone loss (Fig 13). The oblong or bilobed acetabular component was designed to address some of these problems associated with significant bone loss to the acetabulum. The theoretical advantage of these implants includes increased contact with viable host bone against a fixation surface, the potential to avoid structural allografts, and the possibility of returning the hip center to the normal center of rotation.

Clinical results have been variable. In one multicenter report, 38 oblong bilobed noncustom porous-coated titanium acetabular components were used to reconstruct failed THAs with large superior segmental acetabular bone deficiencies. In this group of patients, only 2 of the 38 implants migrated more than 2 mm and then stabilized.

In another report, the high potential rate of complications with this reconstruction was studied. In a series of 34 patients (37 hips) who were followed for a minimum of 2 years and a maximum of 5.5 years, only 76% of the cups were stable. Eight percent were probably unstable, and 6% were definitely unstable. Preoperative radiographic findings that were correlated with postoperative socket instability included superior migration of the socket more than 2 cm and disruption of Köhler's line. In addition, undersizing the implant identified radiographically by a failure of the component to extend distal to the inner teardrop line also was associated with migration. This group of patients had a high rate of early problems with probable or

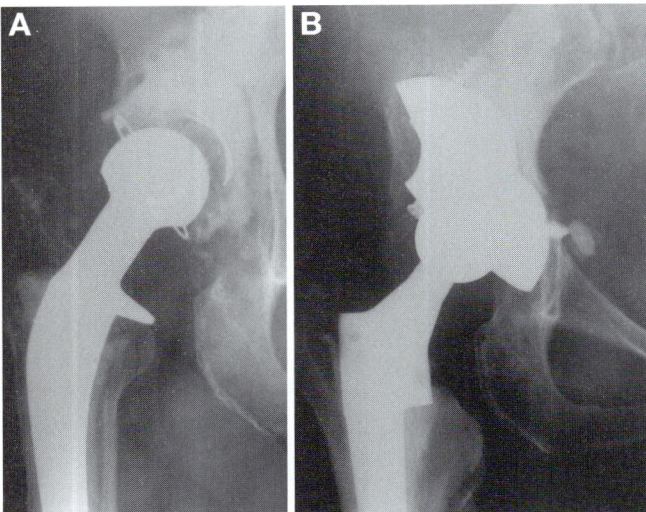

Figure 13 **A,** Failed cemented socket with large superior cement bolus. **B,** Reconstruction with oblong type socket.

definite loosening in 24%. Based on this data, it was recommended that the bilobed cups be used only when a patient has an oblong acetabular defect and the surgeon wants to correct an elevated hip center. These reconstructions can be technically difficult and it is important that the surgeon have an alternate plan in place if the implant cannot be stabilized.

Pelvic Osteolysis in the Presence of a Well-Fixed Porous-Coated Socket

Pelvic osteolysis in conjunction with porous-coated sockets when well fixed is associated with a new problem not previously encountered with failed cemented sockets. Significant osteolysis can occur in the pelvis with a porous-coated cementless socket in the absence of loosening. Removal of a well-fixed acetabular component can result in significant loss of bone, including column defects and pelvic discontinuity. A classification system has been developed in order to help direct treatment. In a type I case, the acetabular component is well fixed and the polyethylene liner is exchangeable. The lytic lesion is débrided and grafted. The liner is exchanged and results at 5 to 10 years have been excellent. In a type II case, the acetabular component is well fixed, however, the liner is not exchangeable. Relative contraindications to liner exchange include gross malposition of a component, significant damage to either the locking mechanism and/or metal shell, or an unacceptable track record. More recently, some surgeons have cemented liners into shells that are osseointegrated but damaged or no liner is available. Short-term results appear satisfactory but no intermediate-term data are available at this time. It is important when deciding whether to leave a noncemented

component in place to have some idea how that socket performs over time. Some fixation surfaces at 7 to 10 years are showing increased failure rates and in those cases the sockets probably should be removed. Removal of a well-fixed socket can be associated with significant bone loss and adequate graft, fixation plates, and implants should be in place to address these potential complications. In type III cases, the socket is loose and must be removed. The approach is similar to that used with loose cemented sockets.

Femoral Revision

Over the past 3 decades, femoral component revision surgery has advanced from a procedure with highly variable results and often limited durability to a much more sophisticated operation with more predictable early clinical results and greater long-term success. This improved success is the result of improvements in surgical techniques and from improved revision implants that provide stable long-term fixation and allow the surgeon to effectively manage femoral bone loss. Methods to remove failed implants and cement also have improved, thereby simplifying femoral revision and allowing it to be performed more efficiently.

Goals of Femoral Revision

The main goals of femoral revision are to (1) extract failed implants with minimal bone damage; (2) implant a new stem that will provide long-term stable fixation; and (3) manage bone loss and when possible augment deficient bone stock. Stable fixation is the key to a good clinical result (pain relief and function), and also is essential to halting the cycle of repetitive revisions that lead to more bone loss. Efforts to augment bone stock should not be made at the expense of long-term stable implant fixation.

Implant Removal

Most loose implants can be extracted from the femur with implant-specific or universal extraction devices. The anticipated path of the implant during removal should be cleared to prevent femoral or trochanteric fracture. Cement can be removed from the canal with hand instruments, power instruments, or ultrasonic instruments. Fluoroscopic guidance can be useful to avoid femoral perforation.

Well-fixed cemented and cementless implants can be difficult to remove, and vigorous extraction attempts that might lead to bony fracture should be avoided. The strategy for implant removal depends on implant design, the particular femoral anatomy, and the planned type of femoral reconstruction. Some well-fixed cemented stems can be extracted from the cement prior to removal of the cement from the bone. Most well-fixed cementless implants can be removed using thin power instruments to divide the areas of bone ingrowth into the implant before the implant is extracted. Thick space occupying instruments, which can cause fractures, should not be used to divide the interface of well-fixed implants.

Extended greater trochanteric osteotomies facilitate removal of well-fixed cemented and cementless stems in an efficient and bone-sparing manner (Figs. 14 and 15). The best indications for extended trochanteric osteotomies include (1) overhang of the lateral femur or greater trochanter beyond the shoulder of the failed implant, increasing the risk for fracture during implant removal; (2) well fixed or a large amount of cement in the femoral canal; (3) a well-fixed cementless femoral implant with extensive bone ingrowth; and (4) the proximal femur is remodeled with a large varus bow. In this circumstance the extended osteotomy not only facilitates removal of the failed implant but also helps facilitate placement of the new implant in optimal position. Extended trochanteric osteotomies are most compatible with femoral reconstruction, using cementless femoral stems that provide for diaphyseal fixation.

Femoral Reconstruction Options

Many different implant designs and philosophies can be used for femoral revision and each has its own advantages and disadvantages. The femoral fixation method of choice depends on the pattern of femoral bone loss, the femoral canal geometry, patient demographic characteristics, and the surgeon's philosophy. Of these, femoral bone loss pattern probably is the most important, and several useful systems of bone loss classification are available (Fig. 16).

Cemented Femoral Revision

Cemented femoral revision relies on interdigitation between the cement and bone for a mechanically durable interface. Studies have demonstrated that this interface is less strong in revision surgery because much of the cancellous bone has been lost. Modern cement technique improves the durability of cemented femoral fixation at 10 years, probably because it optimizes the cement interdigitation with remaining intramedullary cancellous bone. Several studies of cemented stems implanted with modern techniques with follow-up of at least 10 years demonstrate mechanical failure rates of approximately 15% to 20%. As cementless revision implants have improved and as the 10-year results of successful cementless implants have become available, the role of cemented femoral fixation in revision has decreased.

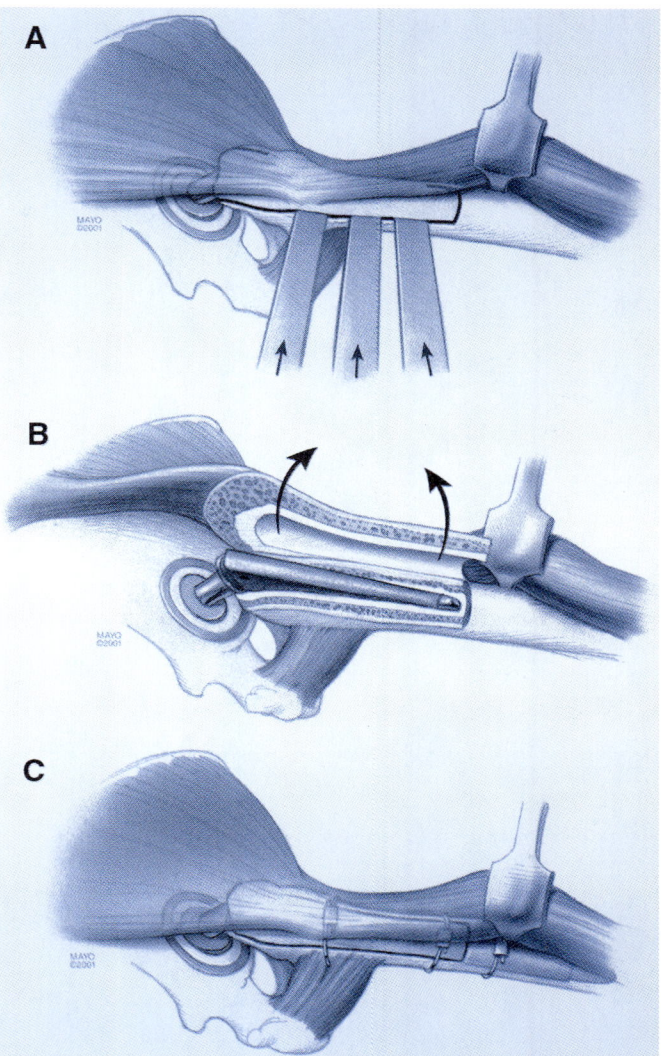

Figure 14 **A,** Extended greater trochanteric osteotomy. The medial limb of the osteotomy is complete as a controlled fracture of the femur. **B,** Extended greater trochanteric osteotomy demonstrating access to failed implant and cement. **C,** Closed extended greater trochanteric osteotomy after fixation with cables. A prophylactic cerclage cable placed prior to implantation of the new cementless stem is shown. *(Reproduced with permission from the Mayo Foundation, Rochester, MN.)*

Older patient age and better initial bone-cement interface are two main factors associated with successful cemented femoral fixation. Older age probably correlates with better durability because of lower patient activity. Better initial radiographic bone-cement interface is a sign of better cement interdigitation with bone; either because of better technique, better remaining cancellous bone, or both. When cemented revision is performed membrane and neocortex around the failed implant should be removed to expose remaining cancellous host bone. At present the most common role of cemented femoral revision in North America is revision of older patients with good remaining intramedullary cancellous bone.

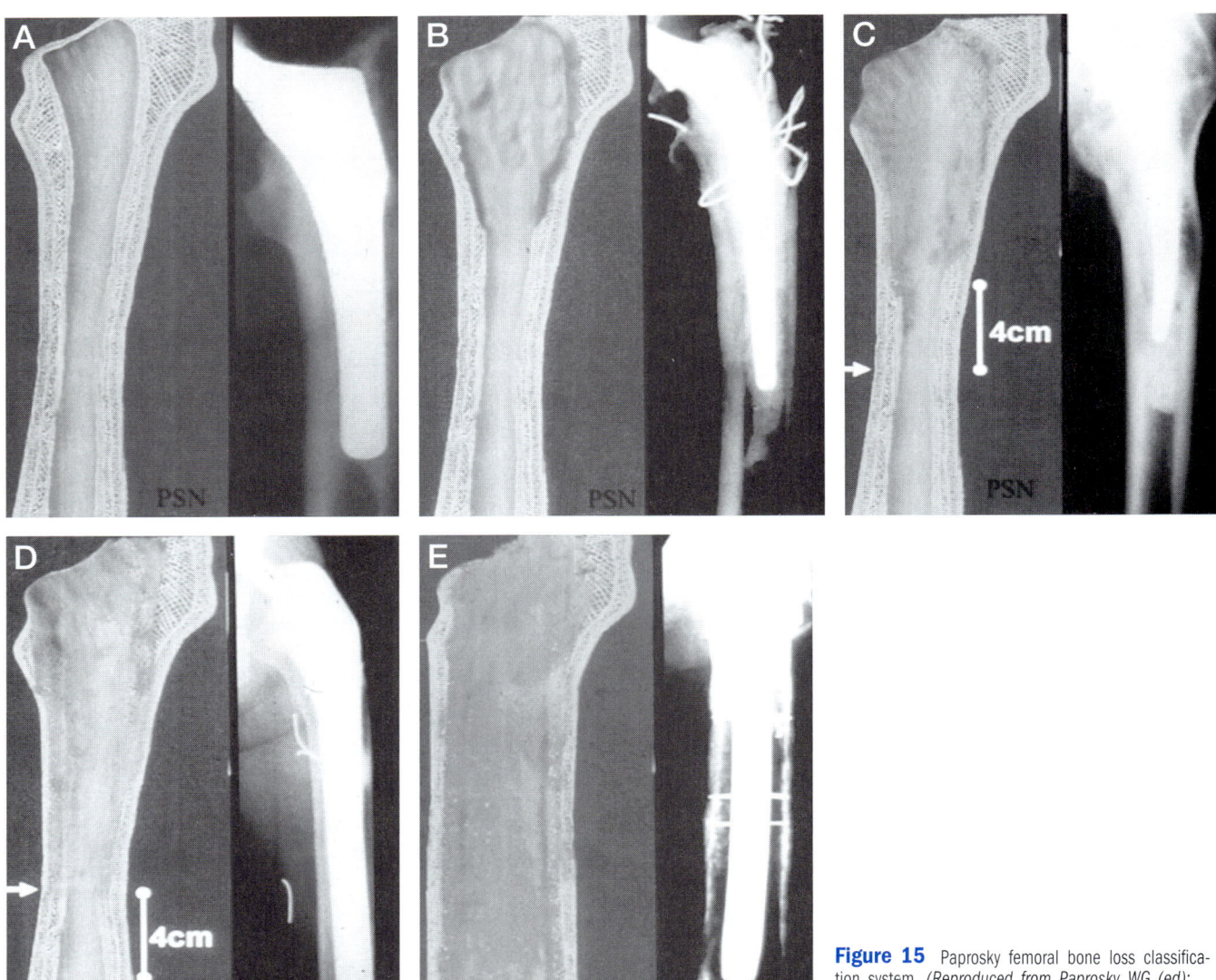

Figure 15 Paprosky femoral bone loss classification system. *(Reproduced from Paprosky WG (ed): Revision Total Hip Arthroplasty. Rosemont, IL, American Academy of Orthopaedic Surgeons, 2001, pp 33-49.)*

Cement Within Cement

A minority of cemented femoral components fail, leaving behind a well-fixed cement mantle and good underlying bone. Failure can occur when an implant without a rough surface finish debonds from the cement and becomes symptomatically loose or when a cemented stem fractures. In these circumstances, a new stem may be cemented back into the old cement mantle because the new cement can bond effectively to the old cement. Favorable results at midterm follow-up have been reported.

Cementless Revision

Cementless femoral revision has become increasingly popular several reasons. Cementless implants provide the potential for long-term biologic implant fixation. Specific methods of cementless femoral fixation have

demonstrated excellent clinical results with durable implant fixation at 10 years or more. Cementless revision techniques can be done efficiently and are easy to reproduce.

Cementless implants must gain initial rigid axial and rotational stability in the femur and in the long term they must gain biologic fixation to the femur. When the bone of the other femur is normal, many cementless implant types can provide this stability; when the proximal bone is damaged (usually the case in the revision setting), the diaphyseal bone usually provides better support for initial implant fixation and better biologic potential for bone ingrowth. Cementless femoral components used for femoral revision may be divided into three main categories: proximally porous coated implants, implants designed for diaphyseal fixation, and modular implants.

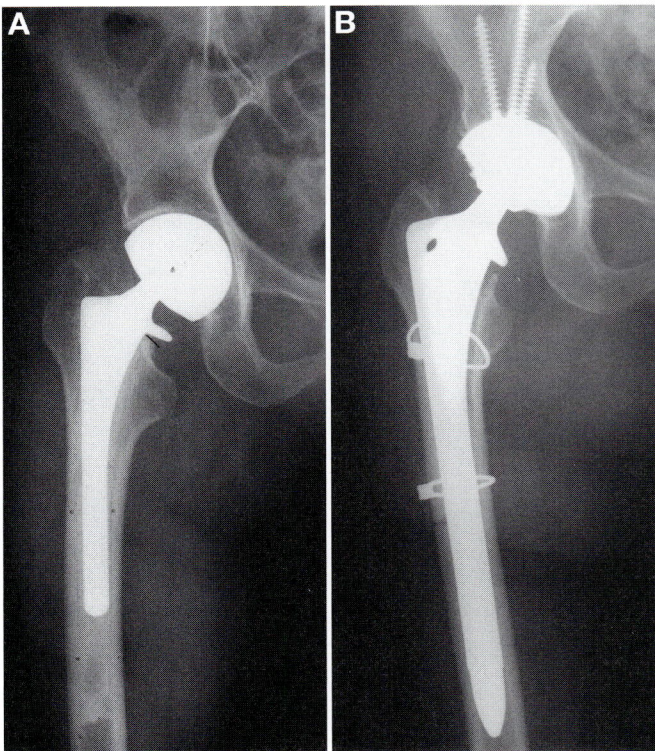

Figure 16 **A,** Preoperative radiograph of a patient with loose hip arthroplasty. The diaphyseal bone is well preserved. **B,** Postoperative radiograph after revision, extended greater trochanteric osteotomy, and extensively porous-coated stem.

Proximally Porous-Coated Implants

The theoretical advantage of proximally porous-coated devices is the potential for biologic fixation with a small amount of stress shielding. Disadvantages include the problems of obtaining short- and long-term fixation in the damaged proximal femoral bone commonly present in revision arthroplasty. Proximally porous-coated wedge-shaped implants designed for fixation in the metaphysis alone and implanted using a broach to shape the proximal femur have not worked well with revisions.

Success has been reported with one modified proximally coated stem, a calcar replacement device with proximal porous coating that extends in the upper diaphysis. These design features enhance axial and rotational implant stability even when there is moderate proximal bone loss.

Diaphyseal Fixation

The most popular method for femoral revision takes advantage of biologic fixation in the diaphysis of the femur. For femoral revision the advantages of this approach are compelling. The poor proximal bone is bypassed and fixation is gained in the diaphysis where the best preserved bone, in respect to strength and biologic activity, remains. This method is characterized by a very high likelihood of long-term biologic implant

fixation. The main disadvantages are the potential for proximal femoral stress shielding and the difficulty of implant extraction if required. Most devices designed for diaphyseal fixation are either extensively porous-coated devices with a cylindrical distal shape or grit-blasted fluted devices with a conical distal shape. Titanium stems have a lower modulus of elasticity but cannot be fully porous-coated for reasons of strength.

Extensively porous-coated devices have been most popular in North America and gain stability from a tight scratch fit of the porous implant in the diaphyseal bone. Most systems provide stems of different lengths and provide for the option of calcar augmentation; this variety of implants allows the surgeon to manage a wide spectrum of bone loss severity. These devices have provided the most durable results reported for femoral revision.

Fluted, conically-shaped devices, popularized in Europe, help achieve initial and long-term fixation in the diaphysis. The flutes provide rotational stability, the conical shape provides axial stability, and the grit-blasted titanium surface allows biologic fixation. Limited favorable information on the results of this method is also available.

Diaphyseal fixation has led to marked improvement in the durability of femoral fixation in revision surgery and has expanded markedly the range of femoral bone loss problems that can be managed with cementless implants. Additionally, implants fixed in the diaphysis work well in combination with extended greater trochanteric osteotomies that facilitate failed implant removal. The main contraindications for use of diaphyseal fixation include proximal bone loss so severe that an allograft prosthetic composite or tumor prosthesis is required; severe distal diaphyseal bone loss with no isthmus to provide for diaphyseal fixation; an extremely large femoral canal diameter that precludes prosthetic fit or that raises a strong concern that a very large diameter stiff implant will cause severe proximal stress shielding.

Modular cementless implants have gained some popularity because they provide a number of practical advantages in revision surgery. By uncoupling the fit of the stem in the diaphysis from the fit in the metaphysis, many combinations of implant geometry are achieved and leg length and soft-tissue tension can be managed effectively. A potential disadvantage of this method is the possibility of fretting or corrosion of modular interfaces, but this has not yet been demonstrated as a major clinical problem.

Impaction Grafting With Cement

Impaction grafting seeks to restore cancellous structure to the femoral canal by densely packing cancellous

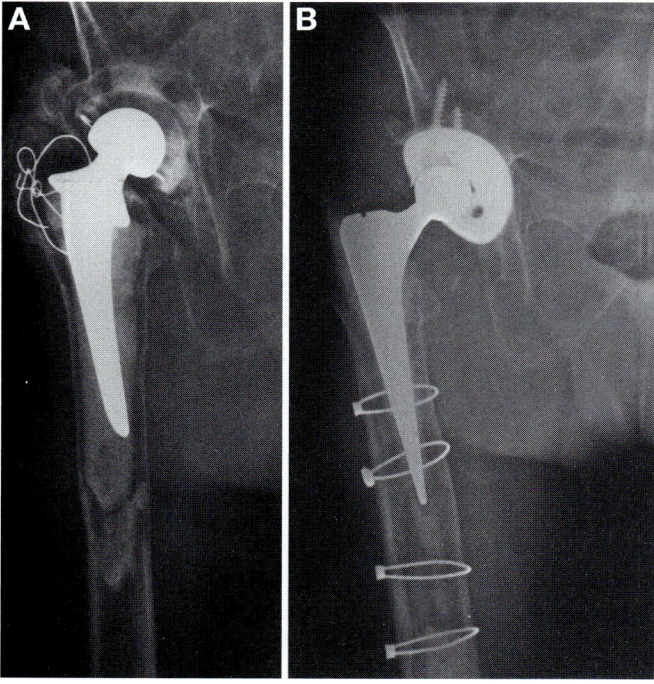

Figure 17 **A,** Preoperative radiograph of a patient with loose THA and proximal femoral bone loss. The canal diameter is over 20 mm. **B,** Postoperative radiograph after reconstruction with impaction bone grafting and cemented stem. A strut graft was placed on the femur.

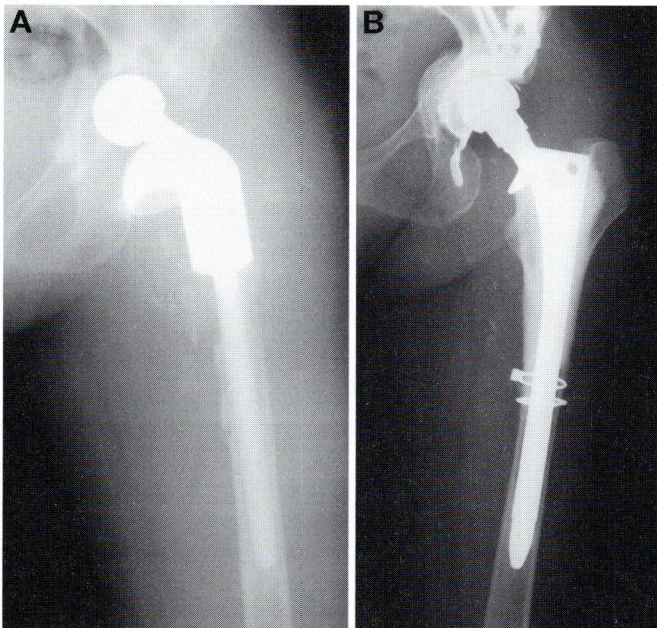

Figure 18 **A,** Preoperative radiograph of a patient with failed THA and massive bone loss. **B,** Postoperative radiograph after femoral reconstruction with allograft prosthesis composite.

bone chips into the canal (Fig. 17). A stem then is cemented into the cancellous bone, which must be packed tightly enough to provide axial and rotational implant stability. The main advantages of impaction grafting are the potential to restore bone stock to the proximal femur and its compatibility with unusual femoral canal geometries or very large femoral canal diameters. Main disadvantages include technical difficulty, the large amount of bone graft required, and unknown long-term results.

The results of impaction grafting have been mixed and its role remains controversial. Several favorable midterm reports demonstrate excellent pain relief, prosthetic stability, and some evidence of bone reconstitution of the proximal femur. However, a few studies also have reported a high rate of marked early implant subsidence, possibly partly related to inadequate density of graft packing at operation. Postoperative periprosthetic femur fractures have been one of the more common complications of the procedure because of the short stem length used in most early series. Longer stems now are available that allow the surgeon to bypass femoral defects more satisfactorily. Many issues that remain to be clarified may affect the results of impaction grafting; these include prosthetic design, bone graft particle size, and bone graft composition. The role of impaction grafting varies according to each surgeon's philosophy, but in North America the technique has been used mostly in situations

in which distorted femoral canal geometry or large femoral canal diameter make the patient a suboptimal candidate for conventional cemented or cementless femoral revision.

Allograft Prosthetic Composites and Tumor Prostheses

Allograft prosthetic composites and tumor prostheses are used when there is severe segmental proximal femoral bone loss, inadequate for support of a routine off-the-shelf revision femoral component. In most circumstances, allograft prosthetic composites are favored because they provide better soft-tissue and bone attachment potential than does a metal tumor prosthesis. Tumor prostheses usually are reserved for older, low-demand patients who need a faster operation that allows early mobilization without the early protection required of an allograft prosthetic composite.

The results of allograft prosthetic composite reconstruction have been favorable and several studies have shown significant improvements in pain and hip scores for patients with these difficult salvage problems (Fig. 18). The most common complications of allograft prosthetic composites include dislocation and infection. Healing of the allograft host-bone junction usually occurs between 3 and 6 months after operation, but junctional nonunions can occur. The segmental allograft remains mostly avascular. Greater trochanteric union to the allograft, with a stable fibrous or bony interface, can be anticipated in about 75% of cases.

Managing Femoral Bone Loss

The type of implant used for reconstruction is chosen in part based on the severity of femoral bone loss. Likewise, the means by which the femoral bone loss is managed in part is contingent on the type of implant used to reconstruct the femur. Most segmental calcar bone loss is managed by using calcar replacement type implants or standard-shaped implants with longer femoral necks. Short segment "napkin ring" allografts around the proximal femur tend to resorb and are used rarely. Full-thickness areas of diaphyseal cortical bone loss can be treated with cortical strut allografts, which have a high rate of healing and can effectively reconstitute bone. Areas of cavitary bone loss can be filled with cancellous bone or simply can be ignored and bypassed with a stem. With cementless reconstructions many of these cavitary deficiencies gradually remodel with time. When possible, significant cavitary or segmental lesions of the femur should be bypassed with a longer femoral stem by several canal diameters to reduce the risk of postoperative fracture. When bypass of the stem is not possible, cortical strut allografts over the lesions may be considered to reduce late periprosthetic fracture risk.

Annotated Bibliography

Alternatives to Total Hip Arthroplasty

Baber YF, Robinson AH, Villar RN: Is diagnostic arthroscopy of the hip worthwhile? A prospective review of 328 adults investigated for hip pain. *J Bone Joint Surg Br* 1999,81:600-603.

In this study of 328 patients undergoing arthroscopy of the hip, a new diagnosis was made in 75 patients including previously undiagnosed osteochondral defects (34), torn labra (23), synovitis (11), and loose bodies (9). Arthroscopy was found to be valuable in the assessment and treatment of patients with hip pain of uncertain cause.

Hussell JG, Rodriguez JA, Ganz R: Technical complications of the Bernese periacetabular osteotomy. *Clin Orthop* 1999;363:81-92.

This article analyzes the technical complications encountered in more than 500 periacetabular osteotomies including intra-articular and posterior column extension of the osteotomy, rare neurovascular or osteonecrotic problems, and most commonly, insufficient or excessive correction.

Ito H, Kaneda K, Matsuno T: Osteonecrosis of the femoral head: Simple varus intertrochanteric osteotomy. *J Bone Joint Surg Br* 1999;81:969-974.

Varus intertrochanteric osteotomy was done on 26 hips with osteonecrosis and the patients were followed for a mean of 12.5 years. Seventy-three percent of patients had a good or excellent result. Varus intertrochanteric osteotomy was the recommended treatment if, after correction, the medial necrotic lesion measured less than two thirds of the weight-bearing area and the superolateral bone was normal.

Krder HJ, Williams JI, Jaglal S, Axcell T, Stephen D: A population study in the Province of Ontario of the complications after conversion of hip or knee arthrodesis to total joint replacement. *Can J Surg* 1999;42: 433-439.

This study evaluated 40 patients who underwent an elective conversion of a hip fusion to a total joint arthroplasty and showed that there was a high rate of complications after the conversion.

Miyanishi K, Noguchi Y, Yamamoto T, et al: Prediction of the outcome of transtrochanteric rotational osteotomy for osteonecrosis of the femoral head. *J Bone Joint Surg Br* 2000;82:512-516.

The correlation between prevention of collapse and the ratio of intact articular femoral head cartilage after rotational osteotomy for osteonecrosis was studied. A minimum postoperative intact ratio of 34% was found to be prognostic for a good outcome.

Nakamura S, Ninomiya S, Takatori Y, Morimoto S, Umeyama T: Long-term outcome of rotational acetabular osteotomy: 145 hips followed for 10-23 years. *Acta Orthop Scand* 1998;69:259-265.

This study reviews the outcomes of rotational acetabular osteotomies in 145 dysplastic hips at an average follow-up of 13 years. Eighty percent of the 112 hips with stage 1 or 2 preoperative osteoarthritis had a good or excellent result. Only 9 of 33 hips with stage 3 or 4 preoperative osteoarthritis had a good or excellent result.

Tennant S, Kinmont C, Lamb G, Gedroyc W, Hunt DM: The use of dynamic interventional MRI in developmental dysplasia of the hip. *J Bone Joint Surg Br* 1999;81:392-397.

This article describes a new technique of dynamic MRI that allows for the assessment of hip stability.

Tonnis D, Heinecke A: Acetabular and femoral anteversion: Relationship with osteoarthritis of the hip. *J Bone Joint Surg Am* 1999;81:1747-1770.

This article outlines the developmental relationship of hip arthritis with torsional abnormalities of the acetabulum and femur. Decreased femoral anteversion was found to be more common than increased femoral anteversion. The abnormal acetabular or femoral version can be treated successfully with reorientation osteotomy of the acetabulum and/or femur.

Trumble SJ, Mayo KA, Mast JW: The periacetabular osteotomy: Minimum 2 year follow-up in more than 100 hips. *Clin Orthop* 1999;363:54-63.

This article reports on 123 periacetabular osteotomies followed for a minimum of 2 years. The average Harris Hip Score increased from 65 preoperatively, to 89 at final follow-up. Seven hips had undergone conversion to THA. The majority of complications resulted from an osteotomy performed through an ilioinguinal approach.

Osteonecrosis

Glueck CJ, Fontaine RN, Gruppo R, et al: The plasminogen activator inhibitor-1 gene, hypofibrinolysis, and osteonecrosis. *Clin Orthop* 1999;366:133-146.

In this study, 59 patients with osteonecrosis of the hip were screened with coagulation tests and studies for four genes associated with thrombophilia and hypofibrinolysis. Plasminogen activator inhibitor-1 was noted to be higher than controls, lending support that plasminogen activator inhibitor-1 gene may be a major pathoetiology in primary osteonecrosis.

Hungerford MW, Mont MA, Scott R, Fiore C, Hungerford DS, Krackow KA: Surface replacement hemiarthroplasty for the treatment of osteonecrosis of the femoral head. *J Bone Joint Surg Am* 1998;80:1656-1664.

This report reviews the results of limited femoral head resurfacing at long-term follow-up. Thirty-three femoral head resurfacing procedures (25 patients) were performed for Ficat stage II and early stage IV disease. At a mean 10.5 years follow-up (range, 4 to 14 years), a good or excellent clinical and radiographic result was noted in 20 hips.

Mont MA, Jones LC, Sotereanos DG, Amstutz HC, Hungerford DS: Understanding and treating osteonecrosis of the femoral head. *Instr Course Lect* 2000;49: 169-185.

This article provides an excellent, comprehensive, up-to-date review from pathogenesis and supposed etiology to treatment options and future directions.

Primary Total Hip Arthroplasty

Anderson MJ, Harris WH: Total hip arthroplasty with insertion of the acetabular component without cement in hips with total congenital dislocation or marked congenital dysplasia. *J Bone Joint Surg Am* 1999;81: 347-354.

Twenty-four THAs, fixed with press-fit hemispherical acetabular cups and screws, were followed for a mean of 83 months. No patient had migration, loosening, revision, or radiographic evidence of pelvic osteolysis.

Barrack RL, Paprosky W, Butler RA, Palafox A, Szuszczewicz E, Myers L: Patients' perception of pain after total hip arthroplasty. *J Arthroplasty* 2000;15: 590-596.

Pain drawings and visual analog scales were used to determine the incidence and severity of thigh pain following THA using extensively coated cylindrical stems, proximally coated cylindrical stems, and cemented stems. Patient who received proximally coated stems were found to have twice the incidence of thigh pain as those who received extensively coated stems. Patients with the extensively coated stems had an incidence of thigh pain equivalent to that of patients with cemented stems.

Bourne RB, Rorabeck CH, Skutek M, Mikkelsen S, Winemaker M, Robertson D: The Harris design-2 total hip replacement fixed with so-called second-generation cementing techniques: A ten to fifteen-year follow-up. *J Bone Joint Surg Am* 1998;80:1775-1780.

One hundred thirty-one THAs were performed in patients with a mean age of 67 years and mean follow-up of 12 years. Nine percent of acetabular and 2% of femoral components were found to be radiographically loose.

Callaghan JJ, Albright JC, Goetz DD, Olejniczak JP, Johnston RC: Charnley total hip arthroplasty with cement: Minimum twenty-five-year follow-up. *J Bone Joint Surg Am* 2000;82:487-497.

Three hundred thirty Charnley THAs were performed in 262 patients. Fifty-one patients (62 hips) were alive at least 25 years postoperatively. In these patients the prevalence of revision for acetabular loosening was 15% compared to 7% for the femoral stems.

Callaghan JJ, Forest EE, Olejniczak JP, Goetz DD, Johnston RC: Charnley total hip arthroplasty in patients less than fifty years old: A twenty to twenty-five-year follow-up note. *J Bone Joint Surg Am* 1998;82: 704-714.

Seventy hips were followed for at least 20 years; 5% of the femoral components were revised for aseptic loosening, and 8% had definite radiographic loosening at final follow-up.

Clohisy JC, Harris WH: The Harris-Galante porous-coated acetabular component with screw fixation: An average ten-year follow-up study. *J Bone Joint Surg Am* 1999;81:66-73.

One hundred ninety-six cementless Harris Galante-I acetabular components were implanted and followed for an average of 122 months. There were no revisions for aseptic loosening and a 5% incidence of periacetabular osteolysis.

Crowninshield RD, Jennings JD, Laurent ML, Maloney WJ: Cemented femoral component surface finish mechanics. *Clin Orthop* 1998;355:90-102.

Cemented stem with a rough surface finish were found to have greater cement-metal adhesion and lower interface motion. Interface motion with rough stems produced more particulate debris, however.

Iida H, Matsusue Y, Kawanabe K, Okumura H, Yamamuro T, Nakamura T: Cemented total hip arthroplasty with acetabular bone graft for developmental dysplasia: Long-term results and survivorship analysis. *J Bone Joint Surg Br* 2000;82:176-184.

A femoral head autograft of the acetabulum was performed for developmental dysplasia in 133 hips in 112 patients and followed for a mean of 12.3 years. Survival of the acetabular component at 15 years was 96% with revision for loosening as the end point and 75% for radiographic loosening as the end point.

Lavernia CJ, Hernandez RA: Abstract: Cost utility ratios in arthroplasty surgery. *J Arthroplasty* 1999;14: 249.

One hundred fifteen patients were studied using a quality of well being index and costs to calculate the cost of a QWY. The average cost of a QWY at 2 years for a THA was $7,097 which ranks as a highly cost-effective intervention.

Lehtimaki MY, Kautiainen H, Lehto UK, Hamalainen MM: Charnley low-friction arthroplasty in rheumatoid patients: A survival study up to 20 years. *J Arthroplasty* 1999;14:657-661.

One thousand five hundred fifty-three consecutive Charnley cemented stems were used in 1,086 patients with rheumatoid arthritis. The femoral component survival was 93.2% at 10 years and 89.9% at 15 years, while the acetabular component survival was 93.6% at 10 years and 87.1% at 15 years.

Maloney WJ, Galante JO, Anderson M, et al: Fixation, polyethylene wear, and pelvic osteolysis in primary total hip replacement. *Clin Orthop* 1999;369:157-164.

One thousand eighty-one cementless Harris Galante-I acetabular components were implanted with line to line reaming and screw fixation and followed for an average of 81 months. There was a 1% incidence of radiographic loosening. The incidence of acetabular osteolysis was age-related with 22% lytic lesions in patients under 50 years of age and no lytic lesions in patients more than 70 years of age.

Manley MT, Capello WN, D'Antonio JA, Edidin AA, Geesink RG: Fixation of acetabular cups without cement in total hip arthroplasty: A comparison of three different implant surfaces at a minimum duration of follow-up of five years. *J Bone Joint Surg Am* 1998;80: 1175-1185.

The results of THA in 477 patients (428 hips) are reviewed. At mean follow-up of 7.9 years, 1 of 131 (1%) hydroxyapatite threaded, 2 of 109 (2%) porous-coated, and 21 of 188 (11%) hydroxyapatite press-fit cups had been revised for aseptic loosening.

McAuley JP, Moore KD, Culpepper WJ II, Engh CA: Total hip arthroplasty with porous-coated prostheses fixed without cement in patients who are sixty-five years of age or older. *J Bone Joint Surg Am* 1998;80: 1648-1655.

Extensively coated cobalt-chrome stems were implanted in 196 hips in patients older than 65 years of age. At mean follow-up of 8.5 years only one was revised for loosening. There was a 9% incidence of pain that limited activity.

Saleh KJ, Gafni A, Saleh L, Gross AE, Schatzker J, Tile M: Economic evaluations in the hip arthroplasty literature: Lessons to be learned. *J Arthroplasty* 1999;14: 527-532.

A Medline search of articles on economic aspects of THA from 1966-1996 yielded 68 articles that met study criteria. The orthopaedic literature was found to be deficient in methodologically sound economic evaluations.

Complications After Total Hip Arthroplasty

Bartz RL, Noble PC, Kadakia NR, Tullos HS: The effect of femoral component head size on posterior dislocation of the artificial hip joint. *J Bone Joint Surg Am* 2000;82:1300-1307.

In a cadaver experimental model, increasing the femoral head size from 22 mm to 28 mm increased the flexion range by 7.6° before dislocation. Increasing head size further to 32 mm did not increase motion before dislocation. With larger head sizes, impingement between osseous femur and acetabulum was more common, whereas with smaller head sizes prosthetic femoral neck-acetabular liner impingement was more common.

Callaghan JJ, Katz RP, Johnston RC: One-stage revision surgery of the infected hip: A minimum 10-year follow-up study. *Clin Orthop* 1999;369:139-143.

Twenty-four one-stage exchange THAs were done with antibiotic-impregnated cement and followed for 10 years. Infection recurred in only 8.3% of patients.

Crockarell JR Jr, Berry DJ, Lewallen DG: Nonunion after periprosthetic femoral fracture associated with total hip arthroplasty. *J Bone Joint Surg Am* 1999;81: 1073-1079.

Twenty-three nonunions occurring after treatment of periprosthetic fractures were treated and followed for an average of 8.3 years. Union, when attempted, occurred in only 9 of 13 patients.

Dearborn JT, Harris WH: Postoperative mortality after total hip arthroplasty: An analysis of deaths after two thousand seven hundred and thirty-six procedures. *J Bone Joint Surg Am* 1998;80:1291-1294.

Eight deaths (mortality rate, 0.3%) occurred within 90 days after 2,736 THAs performed by a single surgeon. Half of the deaths occurred after discharge and five occurred 30 or more days postoperatively.

Dowd JE, Sychterz CJ, Young AM, Engh CA: Characterization of long-term femoral-head-penetration rates: Association with and prediction of osteolysis. *J Bone Joint Surg Am* 2000;82:1102-1107.

In 48 hips followed for more than 10 years, no hip with a wear rate of less than 0.1 mm per year, and 100% with a wear rate more than 0.3 mm per year developed osteolysis.

Duncan CP, Callaghan JJ (eds): Periprosthetic fractures after major joint replacement. *Orthop Clin North Am* 1999;30.

This entire volume is dedicated to the management of periprosthetic fractures around total joint replacements.

Goetz DD, Capello WN, Callaghan JJ, Brown TD, Johnston RC: Salvage of a recurrently dislocating total hip prosthesis with use of a constrained acetabular component: A reprospective analysis of fifty-six cases. *J Bone Joint Surg Am* 1998;80:502-509.

Fifty-six constrained Omnifit (Osteonics, Allendale, NJ) tripolar components were inserted for recurrent dislocation. After average follow-up of 64 months, only two components (4%) had a subsequent dislocation.

Kelley SS, Lachiewicz PF, Hickman JM, Paterno SM: Relationship of femoral head and acetabular size to the prevalence of dislocation. *Clin Orthop* 1998;355:163-170.

In a report of two series of modular components used in THA, one randomized to 22- and 28-mm heads and the other using 28-mm heads, the use of 22-mm heads and large diameter cups (56 mm and above in the randomized series and 62 mm and above in the 28 mm series) were associated with higher dislocation rates.

Longjohn D, Dorr LD: Soft tissue balance of the hip. *J Arthroplasty* 1998;13:97-100.

In patients with static and dynamic contractures around the hip, soft-tissue release accelerates postoperative rehabilitation, decreases knee and groin pain, increases range of motion, and reduces functional limb-length differences.

Neal BC, Rodgers A, Gray H, et al: No effect of low-dose aspirin for the prevention of heterotopic bone formation after total hip replacement: A randomized trial of 2,649 patients. *Acta Orthop Scand* 2000;71: 129-134.

In a prospective, randomized trial, aspirin was found to be ineffective in preventing heterotopic ossification.

Parvizi J, Holiday AD, Ereth MH, Lewallen DG: Sudden death during primary hip arthroplasty. *Clin Orthop* 1999;369:39-48.

Of 22,666 primary arthroplasties performed at one institution there were 11 intraoperative deaths (mortality rate, 0.05%). The mortality rate decreased in later years when better understanding and management of the intramedullary hypertension and hypotensive and hypovolemic effects of the procedure were realized. There were no intraoperative deaths when cementless fixation was used.

Parvizi J, Morrey BF: Bipolar hip arthroplasty as a salvage treatment for instability of the hip. *J Bone Joint Surg Am* 2000;82:1132-1139.

Twenty-seven patients underwent bipolar hip replacement for recurrent dislocation of the hip. The mean duration of follow-up was 5 years. Bipolar arthroplasty prevented dislocation in 22 hips (81%).

Pellicci PM, Bostrom M, Poss R: Posterior approach to total hip replacement using enhanced posterior soft tissue repair. *Clin Orthop* 1998;355:224-228.

In 395 cases there were no dislocations when a posterior capsule tendinous closure was performed versus a 4% rate when it was not performed.

Schmalzried TP, Callaghan JJ: Wear in total hip and knee replacements. *J Bone Joint Surg Am* 1999;81: 115-136.

An extensive review of wear and wear mechanisms in THA and total knee arthroplasty is presented.

Schmalzried TP, Shepherd EF, Dorey FJ, et al: Wear is a function of use, not time. *Clin Orthop* 2000;381:36-46.

A pedometer was used to assess patient activity, and results demonstrate a wide variability of activity in patients with THAs and that wear is most closely associated with activity and use rather than the time the prosthesis has been in place.

Schneider DJ, Moulton MJ, Singapuri K, et al: Inhibition of heterotopic ossification with radiation therapy in an animal model. *Clin Orthop* 1998;355:35-46.

Using a rabbit model, the authors demonstrated the efficacy of preoperative radiation in preventing postoperative heterotopic ossification. In a previously published clinical study, preoperative radiation prevented heterotopic ossification in 76% of cases compared with 73% of cases with postoperative radiation therapy.

Sell S, Willms R, Jany R, et al: The suppression of heterotopic ossifications: Radiation versus NSAID therapy: A prospective study. *J Arthroplasty* 1998;13: 854-859.

Diclofenac (50 mg three times a day) was compared with three 3.3 cGy doses of irradiation for prevention of heterotopic ossification after THA. Both treatments were effective, with irradiation slightly more effective than Diclofenac.

Sharkey PF, Hozack WJ, Callaghan JJ, et al: Acetabular fracture associated with cementless acetabular component insertion: A report of 13 cases. *J Arthroplasty* 1999;14:426-431.

Thirteen fractures occurred during insertion of cementless acetabular components that had underreaming of the acetabulum. Eleven of 13 were in osteopenic female patients.

Ure KJ, Amstutz HC, Nasser S, Schmalzried TP: Direct-exchange arthroplasty for the treatment of infection after total hip replacement: An average ten year follow-up. *J Bone Joint Surg Am* 1998;80:961-968.

Twenty patients with infected THAs underwent one-stage exchange with antibiotic-impregnated cement. No patient had recurrence of infection.

Zimmerli W, Widmer AF, Blatter M, Frei R, Ochsner PE: Role of rifampin for treatment of orthopedic implant-related Staphylococcal infections: A randomized controlled trial: Foreign Body Infection (FBI) Study Group. *JAMA* 1998;279:1537-1541.

Patients with implants infected with *Staphylococcus* were randomized into groups that received ciprofloxacin only versus ciprofloxacin and rifampin. The cure rate in the ciprofloxacin group was 58%, versus 100% in the combined group.

Acetabular Revision in Total Hip Arthroplasty

Berry DJ, Lewallen DG, Hanssen AD, Cabanela ME: Pelvic discontinuity in revision total hip arthroplasty. *J Bone Joint Surg Am* 1999;81:1692-1702.

Pelvic discontinuity is a special problem in revision hip replacement surgery and is associated with a high rate of complications. Appropriate treatment of these patients dictates fixation of the discontinuity, reconstruction of bone defects, and then appropriate implant choice.

Chen WM, Engh CA, Hopper RH, McAuley JP, Engh CA: Acetabular revision with use of a bilobed component inserted without cement in patients who have acetabular bone-stock deficiency. *J Bone Joint Surg Am* 2000;82:197-206.

Bilobed acetabular components can be used as an alternative reconstruction method for those patients with extensive acetabular bone loss. It may in some cases be able to obviate the need for a structural graft. However, these cases are technically challenging and a steep learning curve is likely.

Dearborn JT, Harris WH: Acetabular revision arthroplasty using so-called jumbo cementless components: An average 7-year follow-up study. *J Arthroplasty* 2000;15:8-15.

The use of jumbo cementless acetabular component revision socket surgery has shown durable results in intermediate-term follow-up and is a reasonable option when a large acetabular component can be used to bridge from the ilium to the ischium and pubis.

Gill TJ, Sledge JB, Muller ME: The Burch-Schneider anti-protrusio cage in revision total hip arthroplasty: Indications, principles and long-term results. *J Bone Joint Surg Br* 1998;80:946-953.

Anti-protrusio cages are being used with greater frequency in North America. This study reviews a minimum 5-year follow-up on 63 operations with three revisions required during that time period for aseptic loosening.

Goetz DD, Capello WN, Callaghan JJ, Brown TD, Johnston RC: Salvage of a recurrently dislocating total hip prosthesis with use of a constrained acetabular component: A retrospective analysis of fifty-six cases. *J Bone Joint Surg Am* 1998;80:502-509.

In cases of recurrent dislocation, reoperation is only successful in approximately 70%. The use of constrained acetabular components may be a reasonable alternative especially if there are additional factors relating to their dislocation, including disruption of the abductor mechanism, poor health, or neurologic compromise.

Leopold SS, Rosenberg AG, Bhatt RD, Sheinkop MB, Quigley LR, Galante JO: Cementless acetabular revision: Evaluation at an average of 10.5 years. *Clin Orthop* 1999;369:179-186.

At a mean of 10.5 years after cementless socket revision using a porous-coated implant with a titanium fiber mesh surface, Kaplan-Meier survivorship was 84% at 11.5 years when revision for any reason or aseptic loosening was used as an endpoint. When aseptic loosening alone was used as an end point, survivorship was more than 95%. Late osteolysis was associated with separation or fragmentation of the fiber metal porous pads.

Schatzker J, Wong MK: Acetabular revision: The role of rings and cages. *Clin Orthop* 1999;369:187-197.

A thorough review of the use of rings and cages in revision surgery is presented.

Femoral Revision

Bono JV, McCarthy JC, Lee J, Carangelo RJ, Turner RH: Fixation with a modular stem in revision total hip arthroplasty. *J Bone Joint Surg Am* 1999; 81:1326-1336.

The authors review the results of the use of a modular cementless femoral component for revision THA.

Haddad FS, Garbuz DS, Masri BA, Duncan CP, Hutchison CR, Gross AE: Femoral bone loss in patients managed with revision hip replacement: Results of circumferential allograft replacement. *J Bone Joint Surg Am* 1999;81:420-436.

The results of circumferential proximal femoral allografts in revision hip replacements are reviewed.

Head WC, Malinin TI: Results of onlay allografts. *Clin Orthop* 2000;371:108-112.

At 8 to 12 years, 251 patients treated with cortical strut allografts during femoral revision all demonstrated healing of the allograft struts. The authors found the grafts underwent adaptive remodeling secondary to physiologic load bearing.

Hultmark P, Kärrholm J, Strömberg C, Herberts P, Möse CH, Malchau H: Cemented first-time revisions of the femoral component: Prospective 7 to 13 years' follow-up using second-generation and third-generation technique. *J Arthroplasty* 2000;15:551-561.

The 7- to 13-year results of a prospective study of older patients (mean age, 71 years) treated with cemented femoral revision demonstrated a 10-year survivorship of 85.4%, free of mechanical implant failure. Younger age, use of a short stem nonrevision implant, and more severe prerevision bone loss all correlated with a higher risk of failure.

Leopold SS, Berger RA, Rosenberg AG, Jacobs JJ, Quigley LR, Galante JO: Impaction allografting with cement for revision of the femoral component: A minimum four-year follow-up study with use of a precoated femoral stem. *J Bone Joint Surg Am* 1999;81:1080-1092.

Twenty-nine patients were revised using impaction allografting and cement with a rough surface stem. At a minimum of 4 years the mean Harris Hip Score improved to 87 points. The Kaplan-Meier survivorship with aseptic loosening as an end point was 92% at 6 years.

Paprosky WG, Greidanus NV, Antoniou J: Minimum 10-year-results of extensively porous-coated stems in revision hip arthroplasty. *Clin Orthop* 1999;369:230-242.

According to this study, 170 femoral revisions were done with an extensively porous-coated cobalt chromium stem and followed up for 10 to 16 years (mean, 13.2 years). Eighty-two percent of the femoral stems showed radiographic evidence of bone ingrowth and only 4.1% were revised for loosening or were radiographically grossly loose. Severe stress shielding was seen in 6% of patients, all of whom had initial osteopenia.

Classic Bibliography

Amstutz HC, Fowble VA, Schmalzried TP, Dorey FJ: Short-course indomethacin prevents heterotopic ossification in a high-risk population following total hip arthroplasty. *J Arthroplasty* 1997;12:126-132.

Berry DJ, Harmsen WS, Ilstrup D, Lewallen DG, Cabanela ME: Survivorship of uncemented proximally porous-coated femoral components. *Clin Orthop* 1995;319:168-177.

Callaghan JJ, Brand RA, Pedersen DR: Hip arthrodesis: A long-term follow-up. *J Bone Joint Surg Am* 1985;67:1328-1335.

Chiari K: Medial displacement osteotomy of the pelvis. *Clin Orthop* 1974;98:55-71.

Dohmae Y, Bechtold JE, Sherman RE, Puno RM, Gustilo RB: Reduction in cement-bone interface shear strength between primary and revision arthroplasty. *Clin Orthop* 1988;236:214-220.

Elting JJ, Mikhail WE, Zicat BA, Hubbell JC, Lane LE, House B: Preliminary report of impaction grafting for exchange femoral arthroplasty. *Clin Orthop* 1995;319:159-167.

Ganz R, Klaue K, Vinh TS, Mast JW: A new periacetabular osteotomy for the treatment of hip dysplasias: Technique and preliminary results. *Clin Orthop* 1988;232:26-36.

Garbuz D, Morsi E, Gross AE: Revision of the acetabular component of a total hip arthroplasty with a massive structural allograft: Study with a minimum five-year follow-up. *J Bone Joint Surg Am* 1996;78:693-697.

Gie GA, Linder L, Ling RS, Simon JP, Slooff TJ, Timperley AJ: Impacted cancellous allografts and cement for revision total hip arthroplasty. *J Bone Joint Surg Br* 1993;75:14-21.

Girdlestone GR: Acute pyogenic arthritis of the hip: An operation giving free access and effective drainage. *Lancet* 1943;1:419-421.

Ikeda T, Awaya G, Suzuki S, Okada Y, Tada H: Torn acetabular labrum in young patients: Arthroscopic diagnosis and management. *J Bone Joint Surg Br* 1988;70:13-16.

Katz RP, Callaghan JJ, Sullivan PM, Johnston RC: Long-term results of revision total hip arthroplasty with improved cementing technique. *J Bone Joint Surg Br* 1997;79:322-326.

Lawrence JM, Engh CA, Macalino GE, Lauro GR: Outcome of revision hip arthroplasty done without cement. *J Bone Joint Surg Am* 1994;76:965-973.

Maloney WJ, Herzwurm P, Paprosky W, Rubash HE, Engh CA: Treatment of pelvic osteolysis associated with a stable acetabular component inserted without cement as part of a total hip replacement. *J Bone Joint Surg Am* 1997;79:1628-1634.

Martell JM, Berdia S: Determination of polyethylene wear in total hip replacements with use of digital radiographs. *J Bone Joint Surg Am* 1997;79:1635-1641.

McLaughlin JR, Harris WH: Revision of the femoral component of a total hip arthroplasty with the calcar-replacement femoral component: Results after a mean of 10.8 years postoperatively. *J Bone Joint Surg Am* 1996;78:331-339.

Meding JB, Ritter MA, Keating EM, Faris PM: Impaction bone-grafting before insertion of a femoral stem with cement in revision total hip arthroplasty: A minimum two-year follow-up study. *J Bone Joint Surg Am* 1997;79:1834-1841.

Mont MA, Waldman B, Banerjee C, Pacheco IH, Hungerford DS: Multiple irrigation, debridement, and retention of components in infected total knee arthroplasty. *J Arthroplasty* 1997;12:426-433.

Mulroy WF, Harris WH: Revision total hip arthroplasty with use of so-called second-generation cementing techniques for aseptic loosening of the femoral component: A fifteen-year-average-follow-up study. *J Bone Joint Surg Am* 1996;78:325-330.

Paterno SA, Lachiewicz PF, Kelley SS: The influence of patient-related factors and the position of the acetabular component on the rate of dislocation after total hip replacement. *J Bone Joint Surg Am* 1997;79: 1202-1210.

Ranawat CS, Rodriguez JA: Functional leg-length inequality following total hip arthroplasty. *J Arthroplasty* 1997;12:359-364.

Retpen JB, Varmarken JE, Jensen JS: Survivorship analysis of failure pattern after revision total hip arthroplasty. *J Arthroplasty* 1989;4:311-317.

Rosenwasser MP, Garino JP, Kiernan HA, Michelsen CB: Long-term follow-up of thorough debridement and cancellous bone grafting of the femoral head for avascular necrosis. *Clin Orthop* 1994;306:17-27.

Santore RF: Intertrochanteric osteotomy for osteonecrosis. *Semin Arthroplasty* 1991;2:208-213.

Schmalzried TP, Noordin S, Amstutz HC: Update on nerve palsy associated with total hip replacement. *Clin Orthop* 1997;344:188-206.

Shinar AA, Harris WH: Bulk structural autogenous grafts and allografts for reconstruction of the acetabulum in total hip arthroplasty: A sixteen-year-average follow-up. *J Bone Joint Surg Am* 1997;79:159-168.

Sotereanos DG, Plakseychuk AY, Rubash HE: Free vascularized fibula grafting for the treatment of osteonecrosis of the femoral head. *Clin Orthop* 1997; 344:243-256.

Steinberg ME, Hayken GD, Steinberg DR: A quantitative system for staging avascular necrosis. *J Bone Joint Surg Br* 1995;77:34-41.

Strathy GM, Fitzgerald RH Jr: Total hip arthroplasty in the ankylosed hip: A ten-year follow-up. *J Bone Joint Surg Am* 1988;70:963-966.

Trousdale RT, Ekkernkamp A, Ganz R, Wallrichs SL: Periacetabular and intertrochanteric osteotomy for the treatment of osteoarthrosis in dysplastic hips. *J Bone Joint Surg Am* 1995;77:73-85.

Urbaniak JR, Coogan PG, Gunneson EB, Nunley JA: Treatment of osteonecrosis of the femoral head with free vascularized fibular grafting: A long-term follow-up study of one hundred and three hips. *J Bone Joint Surg Am* 1995;77:681-694.

Younger TI, Bradford MS, Magnus RE, Paprosky W: Extended proximal femoral osteotomy: A new technique for femoral revision arthroplasty. *J Arthroplasty* 1995;10:329-338.

Chapter 40

Femur: Trauma

Philip R. Wolinsky, MD

Nirmal Tejwani, MD

Prior to the use of routine surgical stabilization, femoral shaft fractures were associated with a high incidence of morbidity and mortality. Antegrade reamed intramedullary nailing is the current treatment of choice. For fractures treated with this method, the rates of union are at least 95%, rate of infection less than 1%, and rates of malunion are low. Stabilization of the femoral shaft within the first 24 hours of injury in multiply injured patients (injury severity score [ISS] > 18) has decreased the incidence of pulmonary insufficiency and adult respiratory distress syndrome (ARDS), and decreased the length of stay and hospitalization costs for patients with less severe associated injuries.

Evaluation

Femoral shaft fractures, with the exception of those in the elderly, usually occur as the result of a high-energy injury mechanism. Associated injuries are common. Bilateral femur fractures in particular represent a high-energy injury pattern and are associated with a significantly higher risk of death, ARDS, and other injuries.

The initial evaluation of the involved extremity should include palpation from the pelvis to the foot, evaluation of neurologic and vascular status, and a circumferential examination of the limb for soft-tissue injury. Gross malalignment should be reduced with in-line traction, and any open wounds covered with a sterile dressing. A splint or traction splint should be applied to reduce the patient's pain, decrease muscle spasms, and prevent further soft-tissue damage. Initial radiographs should include AP and lateral views of the entire femur, pelvis (part of the Advanced Trauma Life Support protocol), and knee. The hip should be scrutinized for an ipsilateral femoral neck fracture.

Femoral shaft fractures are classified by their location (proximal third, middle third, distal third, junction of proximal and middle thirds, or junction of middle and distal thirds), geometry of the fracture line, degree of comminution, and severity of the soft-tissue injury. The Winquist and Hansen classification system is used to describe fracture comminution (Fig. 1). The AO classification system incorporates all of these factors (Fig. 2).

Timing of Fracture Stabilization

The benefits of early stabilization of femoral shaft fractures are well established. In a prospective, randomized series, early femoral shaft stabilization in patients with an ISS greater than 18 led to a decrease in the incidence of ARDS and pulmonary complications, and a decrease in the length of stay in the intensive care unit. No pulmonary complications occurred in the less severely injured group (ISS less than 18), but patients who underwent immediate stabilization spent fewer days in the hospital and incurred lower costs.

Treatment Options

Traction

Femoral shaft fractures will heal in traction but the period of bed rest associated with this method has several disadvantages. Traction is most often used as a temporizing measure until the limb is physiologically stable enough to undergo definitive surgical stabilization.

External Fixation

Frequent pin tract infections, scarring, and knee stiffness with femoral shaft external fixation pins occur as a result of the musculature surrounding the femoral shaft. The use of external fixation usually is reserved for severe open fractures, initial stabilization of fractures with associated vascular injuries, and initial stabilization in patients who cannot tolerate further blood loss. External fixation in these situations is usually converted to definitive stabilization once the patient can tolerate this surgery.

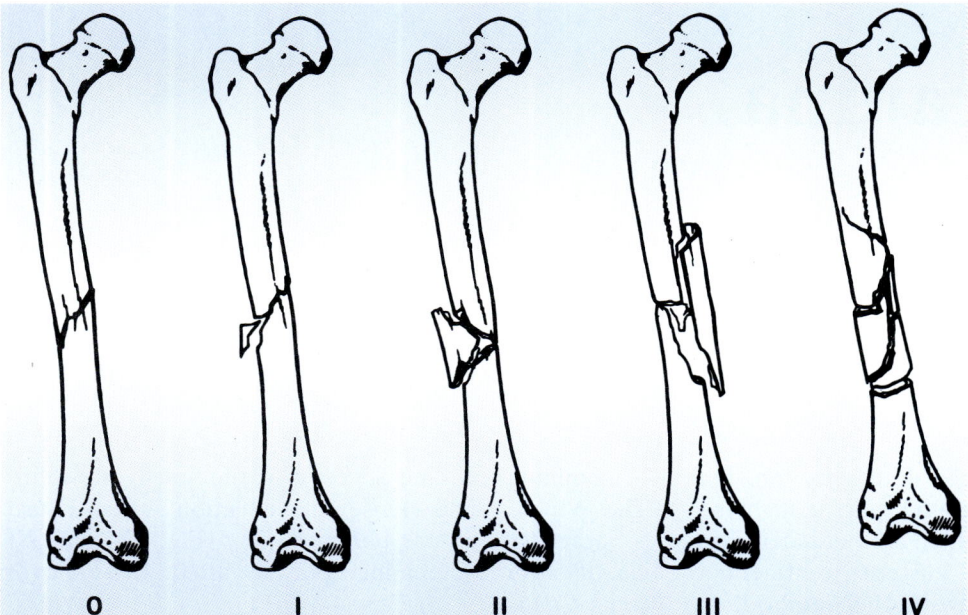

Figure 1 Winquist and Hansen classification of femoral shaft fractures. *(Reproduced from Poss R (ed): Orthopaedic Knowledge Update 3. Park Ridge. IL, American Academy of Orthopaedic Surgeons, 1990, pp 513-527.)*

O   I   II   III   IV

Plating

Open reduction and internal fixation has been successfully used for the primary treatment of femoral shaft fractures at some centers. However, because of the need for an open surgical approach, which has the potential for increased blood loss, and an increase in the complication rate compared with that associated with intramedullary nailing, plating usually is reserved for special situations. These include ipsilateral femoral neck and shaft fractures, vascular injuries, and patients with small femoral intramedullary canals. According to most surgeons, plating results in a higher incidence of infection, nonunion, and implant failure than intramedullary nailing. Current techniques of femoral plating include careful soft-tissue dissection, extraperiosteal bone exposure, indirect fracture reduction, bridge plating of comminuted segments, minimal use of lag screws, and use of longer plates with fewer screws. Bone grafting, although not done routinely, is the current recommended technique for open reduction and internal fixation of the femoral shaft.

Intramedullary Nailing

Treatment of femoral shaft fractures with closed reamed intramedullary nailing using interlocked nails offers several advantages. The nail is inserted with minimal soft-tissue dissection at a site distant from the fracture site, the fracture site is not opened, and stable fixation of the fracture is obtained. If there is cortical contact then nails are load-sharing implants, and because of their central location are subjected to less bending stresses when compared with an eccentrically placed implant such as a plate and screws. Results of numerous studies have revealed that intramedullary nailing is superior to other treatment methods for fractures of the femoral shaft. The largest series to date examined 551 fractures treated with antegrade intramedullary nailing. Fracture union was obtained in 99%, and complications were infrequent.

A statically locked antegrade intramedullary nail inserted using closed techniques is the current standard of care for the treatment of femoral shaft fractures.

It has been demonstrated that intramedullary femoral nails always should be statically interlocked. In 10% of cases when a fracture was thought to be stable enough to be treated with a dynamically locked nail, shortening or rotation occurred. Static locking does not impede fracture healing when an antegrade reamed nail is used, and routine nail dynamization is not needed to obtain fracture union.

Fracture Table Versus Radiolucent Table

Fracture tables traditionally have been used during intramedullary nailing to regain and maintain length and alignment, with excellent results. However, fracture tables prevent easy access to the remainder of the ipsilateral limb or the contralateral limb for patients with multiple fractures, are time-consuming to set up, and can make access to the starting hole difficult, particularly in obese patients.

Several studies have documented that reamed intramedullary nailing of the femoral shaft done on a radiolucent table using manual traction for reduction is fast and accurate. Fracture alignment does not differ between fractures treated with or without a fracture

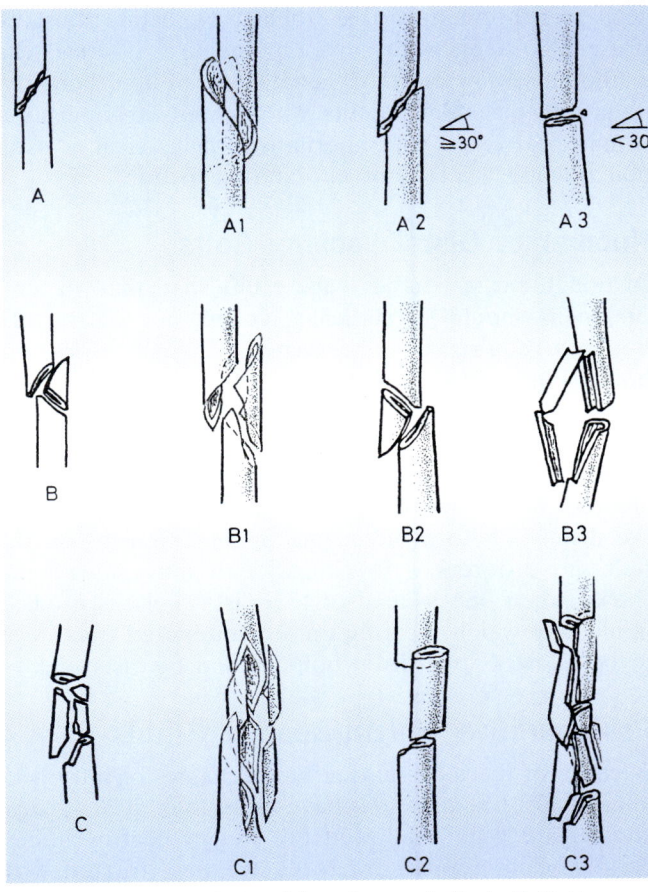

Figure 2 The AO classification of femur fractures. **A,** Simple. **B,** Wedge. **C,** Complex. *(Reproduced with permission from Müller ME, Nazarian S, Koch P, Schatzker J (eds): The Comprehensive Classification of Fractures of Long Bones. Berlin, Germany, Springer-Verlag, 1990.)*

table, and the time for surgery is reduced. This technique is particularly useful for patients with multiple fractures.

Retrograde Femoral Nails

Retrograde femoral nails are inserted through the distal femur via a starting hole placed just anterior to the cruciate ligaments. Short nails that extended to or below the isthmus were available at first; longer nails that extend to the proximal metaphysis are now available. The proximal locks of the longer nails are inserted using the freehand technique from anterior to posterior to simplify fluoroscopic imaging. A cadaver study revealed that the locking bolts should be inserted proximal to the lesser trochanter to reduce the risk of injury to the femoral artery and the femoral nerve branches.

Although the absolute indications for the use of retrograde nails are still unclear, relative indications include obesity, ipsilateral tibial shaft injuries, bilateral femur fractures, ipsilateral acetabulum fractures, ipsilateral femoral neck and shaft fractures, uncontami-

nated traumatic knee arthrotomies, through-knee amputations, pelvic ring injuries, pregnancy (to cut down on fetal radiation exposure), grossly contaminated injuries around the insertion point for antegrade nails, unstable spine injuries, patients who have not had their spine cleared, and patients with multiple fractures. A fracture table is not used during the procedure, and patients are positioned supine.

The potential complications associated with retrograde nails center around the intra-articular entry point and include intra-articular infection (particularly in the case of an open femoral shaft fracture because the fracture site now communicates with the knee joint), damage to the articular cartilage of the patellofemoral joint with the possibility of late degenerative joint disease, knee stiffness, and possible damage to the cruciates during nail insertion. A cadaver study demonstrated no increase in patellofemoral joint pressure when the nail was countersunk or placed flush with the cartilage but pressures increased significantly with even 1 mm of nail prominence. This suggests that with proper placement the nails do not alter patellofemoral joint biomechanics, but proper placement is critical. At present the long-term effects of the intra-articular entry portal on knee function are unknown.

Nonreamed Retrograde Nails

Clinical studies reviewing nonreamed retrograde femoral nails have revealed a rate of union of 85% to 95% after the initial procedure. The diameter of the nail must be matched to the diameter of the canal and not undersized. Nails should be dynamized at 6 to 12 weeks postoperatively if adequate callus is not seen, to maximize the chances of fracture union. Knee range of motion in patients without associated injuries averaged 130°, and the use of continuous passive motion during the postoperative period did not increase the ultimate knee range of motion. There have been no intra-articular infections in patients with open fractures, and no hardware failures. Alignment was satisfactory in all patients. Early nail dynamization and weight bearing are important to minimize the chance of nonunion when a nonreamed nail is used.

Reamed Retrograde Nails

A series of consecutive patients treated with a 10-mm reamed retrograde nail revealed an 85% rate of union after the initial procedure and a 98% rate of union after secondary procedures. Planned dynamization may not be needed when reamed retrograde nails are used. In more recent studies where the nail diameter was matched to the diameter of the femoral canal, rates of union have been comparable to those of antegrade reamed nails.

Reamed Versus Nonreamed Nails
Pulmonary Effects
Pulmonary embolization of fat and bone marrow content has been documented during antegrade reamed femoral intramedullary nailing. The design and sharpness of the reamer are factors that affect the degree of embolization. The use of sharp reamers, with deep flutes and small reamer shafts, and slowly advancing the reamer generates less fat embolization.

It has been suggested that the detrimental pulmonary effects of reamed intramedullary nailing of the femoral shaft might outweigh the benefits in patients with pulmonary injuries. This suggestion spurred the development of femoral nails designed to be inserted with no or minimal reaming. Clinical and animal studies performed in North America have not been able to reproduce this finding. It has been demonstrated that delayed stabilization of a femoral shaft fracture was associated with a higher pulmonary complication rate independent of blunt thoracic trauma. In a sheep model, peak intramedullary pressures of 205 mm Hg occurred in the reamed group, whereas mean pressures of 203 mm Hg occurred during insertion of the solid nonreamed nail, suggesting no advantage to the use of nonreamed nails.

In a comparison of multiply injured patients with femoral shaft fractures with and without thoracic injuries treated at two institutions, one group treated the femur fractures with reamed intramedullary nails, the other with plates. There was no difference in the incidence of pulmonary complications. According to the literature on early femoral stabilization with reamed intramedullary nails in patients with thoracic trauma, the incidence of ARDS and pulmonary failure in patients with multiple injuries, thoracic trauma, and acutely treated femur fractures is less than 3%. The morbidity associated with thoracic trauma is independent of the treatment of the femur fracture. Pulmonary failure occurs as a result of the pulmonary injury, not the method of fracture fixation.

Effects on Fracture Healing
A review of the literature concluded that reamed nailing remains the treatment of choice for femoral shaft fractures because of (1) a higher union rate; (2) a lower need for secondary procedures to obtain union; and (3) the absence of detrimental pulmonary effects when reamed nails are used.

For adequately resuscitated patients, reamed intramedullary nailing remains the treatment of choice. Coagulopathies and hypothermia must be corrected before surgery. Objective evidence of resolving shock

such as a normalizing base deficit or lactate must be present. Patients with severe pulmonary injuries who cannot be adequately oxygenated as well as hemodynamically unstable patients who remain hypoperfused should be treated with alternative means such as skeletal traction, a plate, or an external fixator.

Number of Distal Locking Bolts
Although earlier studies have established that all femoral nails should be statically locked, not all fracture patterns require the placement of two distal locking bolts. Foregoing placement of the second bolt decreases surgical time, radiation exposure, and cost. If one bolt is used it usually is placed in the more proximal of the two distal holes so that a stress riser is not created. When the fracture line is sufficiently far from the distal bolt to avoid toggle of the fragment on the bolt, no differences in clinical outcomes have been shown when one instead of two distal bolts is used. If immediate weight bearing on a comminuted fracture is to be allowed, two distal bolts should be inserted.

Postoperative Weight-Bearing Status
Because of the load-sharing biomechanics of intramedullary nails, fractures that have more than 50% cortical contact are usually allowed full weight bearing immediately. Comminuted fractures are best treated with two distal bolts to allow immediate weight bearing as demonstrated in a recent study. Constructs with one distal locking bolt instead of two bolts had decreased fatigue strength.

Functional Outcomes
Although the rate of union for femoral shaft fractures treated with a reamed intramedullary nail is high, several series have found that a significant number of patients may have persistent pain or muscle weakness after intramedullary nailing. In one study, 41% of patients complained of pain that was significant enough to interfere with their lifestyle or mobility. The pain was not found to correlate with nail prominence. Eighty-eight percent of patients with heterotopic ossification at the nail insertion site had proximal thigh pain. This pain was not consistently relieved by nail removal.

Other studies have shown a persistent decrease in quadriceps, hamstring, or hip abductor strength after femur fracture. Patients may complain of pain only after performing strenuous activity. A review of fractures treated without internal fixation revealed that initial fracture displacement was predictive of quadriceps weakness. It is possible that the muscle injury resulting from the initial injury may be responsible for quadriceps and hamstring weakness, whereas the muscle-splitting approach for nail insertion may be responsible for hip abductor weakness.

Special Situations

Open Fractures

Surgical débridement, wound irrigation, the administration of appropriate antibiotics, fracture stabilization to prevent ongoing soft-tissue damage, and delayed closure of open wounds remain the basic concepts of treatment of open fractures. Immediate reamed intramedullary nailing has been used successfully for the treatment of grades I, II, and IIIA open fractures of the femoral shaft. The treatment of grade IIIB and IIIC open fractures is still controversial. These situations may be an indication for nonreamed nails, but available data are insufficient.

Ipsilateral Femoral Neck and Shaft Fractures

Femoral neck fractures occur in combination with femoral shaft fractures in 2.5% to 5% of cases. Patients are usually young with a high-energy mechanism of injury, and associated injuries are common. These fractures occur most commonly in association with comminuted midshaft fractures, but can occur with any fracture pattern of the femoral shaft. The neck fracture is usually vertical, at the base of the femoral neck, and many have no or minimal displacement.

The femoral neck fracture may initially be missed for many reasons, including the presence of other more obvious injuries and the tendency to image the proximal femur in external rotation while the best view of the femoral neck requires an internal rotation view. Prompt recognition of this injury is key to its treatment. Therefore, the femoral shaft must be evaluated carefully in all patients with femoral neck fractures. Because of awareness of this injury pattern, standardized treatment protocols, and the development of trauma centers, the incidence of missed fractures is decreasing.

Because of the potential complications of osteonecrosis or nonunion of the femoral neck, treatment of the femoral neck fracture takes precedence. Successful treatment of the femoral neck fracture requires an anatomic reduction via a closed or open reduction and stable internal fixation. The outcome of the femoral neck fracture in combination with a femoral shaft fracture may be better than for an isolated femoral neck fracture because some of the energy of injury is dissipated at the femoral shaft fracture site, making the femoral neck fracture a lower energy injury with less vascular injury.

Many stabilization schemes have been described in the literature for this injury pattern. The goal is to obtain anatomic reduction and stable fixation of both fractures using an approach that will minimize complications. The particular technique chosen will depend on whether the femoral neck fracture is discovered prior to stabilization of the femoral shaft fracture, and the surgeon's comfort with a particular device. The most commonly used constructs include stabilization of the shaft component with either a plate or a retrograde intramedullary nail and multiple screw or sliding hip screw fixation of the femoral neck fracture; antegrade nailing of the femoral shaft combined with screw fixation of the femoral neck placed anterior to the intramedullary nail; or a second-generation interlocking nail with the proximal locks extending into the femoral neck and head.

The use of separate devices to stabilize fractures of the femoral shaft and neck is advantageous because an ideal fixation device is used for each fracture, only one fracture at a time is reduced, and there is no further disruption of the blood supply of the femoral head. This technique can only be used when the femoral neck fracture is detected prior to surgery.

Antegrade nailing with screws placed anterior to the nail can be used when the fracture is discovered either prior to or after insertion of the intramedullary nail. The screws must be placed anteriorly on the femur in order to miss the nail. The disadvantages of this technique include possible displacement of the femoral neck fracture during insertion of the intramedullary nail, difficulty in passing the screws anterior to the intramedullary nail, and possible further disruption of the blood supply to the femoral neck.

Use of a second-generation interlocking nail allows stabilization of both fractures with one device, but reduction and stabilization of two fractures at once is technically difficult.

The incidences of osteonecrosis and nonunion after ipsilateral femoral neck and shaft fractures are unclear, as many studies have only limited follow-up. Rates of osteonecrosis as high as 86% and as low as 18% have been reported. According to the literature, the osteonecrosis rate is approximately 4% and the nonunion rate 5%.

Gunshot Wounds

Fractures that result from low-velocity gunshot wounds (< 2,000 ft/s) can be safely treated with wound débridement and immediate reamed intramedullary nailing. Gunshot wounds at close range and at high velocity require more aggressive care as a result of the higher energy of injury, which causes greater soft-tissue damage. Extensive serial soft-tissue débridements are required, along with intravenous antibiotics for up to 72 hours. Alternatives for fracture stabilization include external fixation for severe type IIIC injuries or non-reamed nails for the less severe type IIIA and IIIB soft-tissue injures.

Femur Fractures and Associated Head Injuries

Although early fixation of fractures in patients with multiple injuries has been shown to be beneficial, this philosophy recently has been questioned in patients with significant head injuries. Patients who undergo early stabilization of long bone fractures may be exposed to a secondary brain injury because the auto-regulation of cerebral blood flow is altered after head injury.

To date there are studies indicating that early fixation causes further neurologic deterioration, and others indicate that neurologic complications are related to the severity of the initial head injury and not the timing of surgical fracture stabilization. In fact, early stabilization simplifies patient care and decreases respiratory complications. Patients must be adequately resuscitated before surgery because intraoperative hypotension, hypoxia, and cerebral hypoperfusion must be avoided. Invasive monitoring is required to ensure that adequate systemic resuscitation has been achieved, and may require placement of an intracranial pressure monitor to ensure that cerebral perfusion is maintained during the surgical procedure.

Complications

Infection

Infection as a result of reamed intramedullary nailing occurs in less than 1% of patients. When infection does occur, débridement of all infected soft tissue and necrotic bone in combination with intravenous antibiotics and skeletal stabilization is needed. In cases of a low virulent infection, when sufficient fracture stability to allow nail removal has not occurred, the nail can be left in place and the infection suppressed until fracture union is obtained. Then the nail can be removed, the canal overreamed, and the patient treated with intravenous antibiotics to definitively eradicate the infection. For more virulent infections, the nail must be removed, the canal overreamed, the nail replaced, and suppressive antibiotics administered until fracture healing has been achieved. At that time the nail is removed, the canal overreamed, and antibiotics again are administered to definitively treat the infection.

Nonunion/Delayed Union

Treatment options for delayed union include nail dynamization, exchange nailing with or without bone grafting, or plate fixation with bone graft.

Nail dynamization should be used only when the fracture length is stable. The problems of dynamization of potentially length unstable fractures have been discussed in the literature. According to a recent study, 5 of 24 patients (21%) had more than 2 cm of shortening after dynamization. If dynamization is unsuccessful, or if the fracture is judged to be unstable in length, reamed exchanged nailing with insertion of a larger diameter nail can be performed. Although excellent results for this procedure have been reported in the past, the results now seem to be unclear. Two recent studies demonstrated the efficacy of exchange nailing. In one, 78% of patients experienced healing after nail exchange. Eight of eight nonsmokers were healed, whereas only 10 of 15 smokers experienced healing, suggesting that smoking had a deleterious effect on nonunion healing. In contrast, the second study found that the use of tobacco had no effect on healing and that exchange nailing led to a union rate of 53%.

Malunion
Axial Malalignment

Axial malalignment rarely occurs when intramedullary nails are used. It is most common in distal third fractures where the femoral shaft flares out into the condyles. To prevent malalignment of distal third fractures the guide wire must be kept centered in the distal femur, or nail placement will cause malreduction of the fracture.

Length

When a fracture table is used, the most common error is to lengthen the femur; when manual traction on a radiolucent table is done, femur shortening is the most common error. To prevent lengthening or shortening of a comminuted fracture, the length of the contralateral femur must be known prior to nail insertion so that the nail is the appropriate length.

Rotational Malalignment

Rotational malalignment occurs frequently after intramedullary nailing, but most patients are asymptomatic. According to one study, the mean malrotation was 16°, but no patient agreed to undergo a derotation osteotomy. Patients may compensate by using pelvic rotation so that the femoral rotational deformity is not clinically significant. If gross malrotation is identified in the immediate postoperative period, it can be corrected by removal of the locking screws, derotation of the femur, and reinsertion of the locking screws. After fracture healing has occurred, malrotation can be corrected with a closed femoral osteotomy using an intramedullary saw, followed by renailing.

Compartment Syndrome

Acute compartment syndrome of the thigh after femur fracture is rare. Risk factors include vascular injury, coagulopathy, prolonged external compression, use of pneumatic antishock garments, and hypotension. In the largest series to date, 8 of 17 patients died, and infection was noted in 6 of the remaining 9 patients. Residual morbidity was common.

Neurologic Injury

Nerve injuries can occur during intramedullary nailing, usually when a fracture table is used. Pudendal or sciatic nerve injuries can occur as a result of excessive or prolonged traction on the fracture table. The development of pudendal nerve palsy is related to the magnitude, but not duration, of the traction. Therefore, efforts should be made during surgery to minimize the amount of traction used. The patient must be completely relaxed under anesthesia. Reduction does not have to be maintained during the approach and creation of the starting hole, and hip adduction should be limited to the aspect of the procedure that requires it. If nailing is delayed, the femur should be kept out to length in traction prior to the surgery.

Heterotopic Ossification

Heterotopic bone may develop in the hip abductor musculature after intramedullary nailing. Local factors such as muscle damage created during the approach, reaming debris, and systemic factors may create an environment that promotes heterotopic ossification. Severe heterotopic ossification may limit hip motion, cause pain and limp, and make nail removal more difficult.

In one study 60% of patients developed heterotopic ossification that was moderate or severe in 26% of cases. The presence or absence of a head injury and other factors such as age, sex, severity of the injury, level or type of fracture comminution, timing of nailing or type of intramedullary fixation did not correlate with the development of heterotopic ossification. Wound irrigation with pulsatile lavage to remove reaming debris had no effect on the severity or frequency.

Heterotopic ossification has been shown to develop more frequently in patients who have had a reamed nail than in those with nonreamed nails. It is unclear if this finding is related to less reaming debris or less local tissue damage because of the smaller incision and no use of reamers in the nonreamed group. Routine prophylaxis is not indicated.

Subtrochanteric Fractures

These fractures occur either as the result of high-energy injuries or, in osteopenic patients, a simple fall. There is no uniform definition of subtrochanteric fractures. A general definition of the area includes the upper border of the lesser trochanter to 5 cm distal to it.

This region of the femur is subjected to high compressive forces medially and tensile forces laterally, which can lead to fatigue fracture of implants. The area is also a transition zone from the cancellous bone of the intertrochanteric region to the cortical bone of the femoral shaft, and is slow to heal. If the medial buttress cannot be reconstructed then large bending moments are placed on implants, which can result in fatigue fracture. Therefore, the implants used must be strong enough to withstand the high compressive forces until fracture healing takes place. Because of the extensive comminution that may be present, the vascularity of fracture fragments may be compromised. Therefore, reduction and fixation techniques that do not further devascularize the fragments are needed.

Fractures of the subtrochanteric region are classified by their relation to the lesser and greater trochanter, degree of comminution, and displacement. The Russell-Taylor fracture classification system incorporates the involvement of the piriformis fossa (Fig. 3). Type I fractures do not involve the piriformis fossa, so nailing techniques are straightforward. Type II fractures extend into the fossa. Because the starting hole of the intramedullary nail is now involved, caution must be used during nailing to make sure that the nail does not fall out the back of the proximal fragment. Extension of the fracture into the piriformis fossa is best seen on

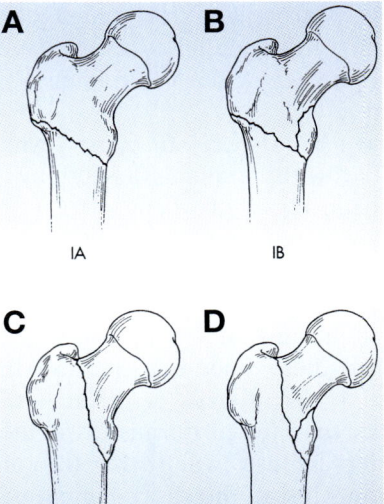

Figure 3 Russell-Taylor classification of subtrochanteric fractures. **A,** Type IA: fracture extension with any degree of comminution from below the level of the lesser trochanter to the isthmus with no extension into the piriformis fossa. **B,** Type IB: fracture extension involving the lesser trochanter to the isthmus with no extension into the piriformis fossa. **C,** Type IIA: fracture extension into the piriformis fossa. Stable medial construct. **D,** Type IIB: fracture extension into the piriformis fossa in the lesser trochanteric area with no stability of the medial femoral cortex. (Reproduced with permission from Guyton JL: Fractures of the hip, acetabulum, and pelvis, in Canale ST (ed): Campbell's Operative Orthopaedics, ed 9. St. Louis, MO, Mosby, 1998, p 2200.)

the lateral radiograph, or can be seen on the lower cuts of the trauma abdominal-pelvic CT scan, which usually includes the proximal femur.

Advantages of using an intramedullary device include preservation of the periosteal blood supply, a load-sharing implant, and the bone grafting effect of reaming with less need for supplemental bone grafting. Several series have reported high union rates for fractures treated with intramedullary nails. Fracture reduction prior to the insertion and interlocking of the nail is essential. The intramedullary nail will maintain the reduction that has been obtained, but will not reduce the fracture as a result of its insertion.

Fractures below the level of the lesser trochanter can be treated with a first-generation intramedullary nail. These fractures can be difficult to align because of the flexion, abduction, and external rotation of the proximal fragment. A small nail can be inserted into the proximal fragment and used to align the proximal fragment with the distal fragment.

Fractures that occur above the level of the lesser trochanter require treatment with either a plate device or a second-generation nail with the proximal locking screws directed into the femoral head and neck. If the fracture extends into the piriformis fossa, intramedullary nailing becomes technically difficult because the nail tends to fall out of the proximal fragment prior to the insertion of the proximal locking bolts. Close attention to detail ensuring that the nail stays contained within the proximal femur must be used if a nail is used to treat these fractures.

A biomechanical study revealed no difference in stiffness or strain for stable subtrochanteric fractures stabilized with either a reconstruction nail, short intramedullary hip screw, or a long intramedullary hip screw. However, for unstable fractures the reconstruction nail was significantly stronger. Prior studies have shown that on average intramedullary devices were twice as strong as extramedullary devices for unstable subtrochanteric fractures.

Plates and screws have been successfully used when the device was inserted with minimal dissection. A 100% union rate has been reported when 24 fractures were treated using indirect reduction, compared with a 16.6% delayed or nonunion rate when the fracture lines were under direct observation.

Long gamma nails or intramedullary hip screws can also be used to stabilize these fractures. Because the starting hole for these types of nails is through the greater trochanter rather than the piriformis fossa, they are theoretically easier to use when the fracture extends into the piriformis fossa. The short gamma nail had a high complication rate including malunion; and fractures at the distal end of the nail. More recently a

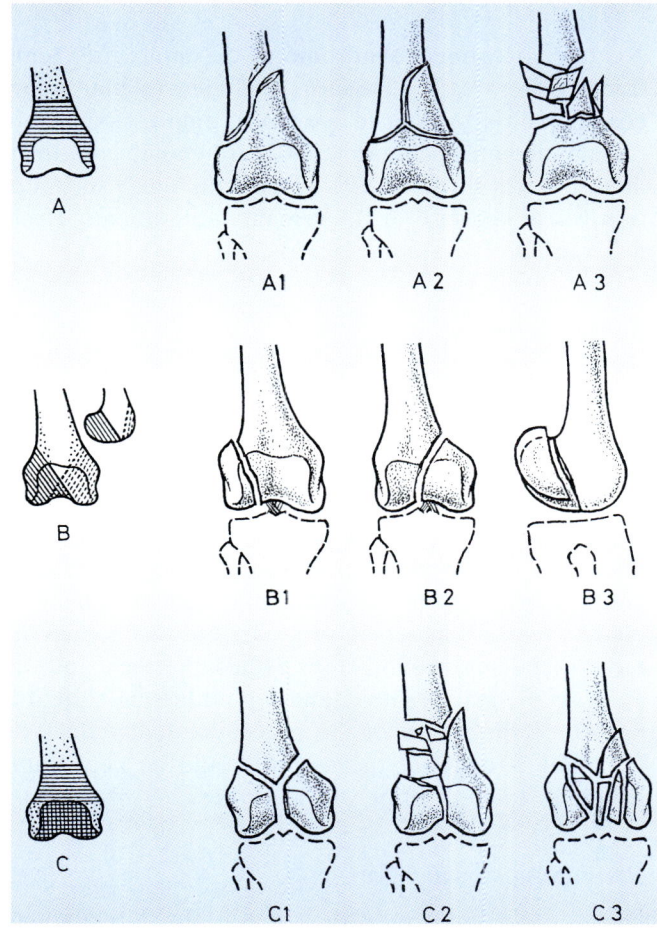

Figure 4 The Müller classification. *(Reproduced with permission from Müller ME, Nazarian S, Koch P, Schatzker J (eds): The Comprehensive Classification of Fractures of Long Bones. Berlin, Germany, Springer-Verlag, 1990.)*

longer, newer version of the gamma nail that avoids diaphyseal placement of the distal locks has been introduced. In a retrospective review of 42 fractures treated with long gamma nails, there were no implant failures or loss of fixation. In another study, the outcomes of 87 consecutive patients with subtrochanteric fractures treated with either a short gamma nail or the long intramedullary hip screw were compared. All fractures healed by 12 months but there was a higher complication (22% versus 5%) rate in the gamma nail group. These included intraoperative fractures, postoperative fractures, and fixation failures and were thought to be caused by nail design.

Distal Femur Fractures

Distal femur fractures range from small avulsion fractures to complex intra-articular fractures. These are classified according to the Müller classification (Fig. 4).

These fractures are categorized into low-energy injuries in the elderly and high-energy injuries in the young, active adult. High-energy injuries in young adults may result in significant disability, because of cartilage damage, bony comminution, and soft-tissue injury. The most common injury mechanism is a flexed knee, driven against a dashboard during a motor vehicle accident. Associated injuries including femoral neck fractures, hip dislocations, and acetabular fractures must be excluded.

The goal of treatment is to restore articular congruity, the mechanical axis of the knee joint, and allow early knee joint range of motion. The intra-articular component is first fixed anatomically, followed by stabilization of the articular block to the shaft. A variety of implants may be used, including retrograde nails, condylar blade plates, or condylar buttress plates. The Hoffa fracture, a coronal split of the femoral condyle, will necessitate AP lag screw fixation of the fragment. The presence of this coronal fracture may preclude the use of a blade plate or dynamic compression screw. Use of these implants requires expertise and familiarity with the surgical technique and instruments to achieve a satisfactory result. It is important to prevent a varus deformity or medialization of the distal fragments while using these implants.

Retrograde Nailing

Retrograde nailing is indicated in distal femur fractures with either no or minimal articular involvement amenable to lag screw fixation and a long enough distal fragment for placement of two locking bolts. The use of a nail is advantageous because the incision is small and soft-tissue stripping at the fracture site is avoided. Biomechanical studies have shown the nail to be as strong as a dynamic compression screw in varus bending, but weaker in torsion and torsion with axial load. Retrograde nailing is a good procedure in the elderly, because it avoids extensive exposure for fixation; however, the hold of the distal interlocks can be a problem because of poor bone quality. Washers or nuts may need to be used to secure the bolts to the bone. Retrograde nails are inserted using a medial parapatellar approach and the nail diameter should be matched to the canal size to maximize the rate of union. Use of the correct insertion technique will avoid damage to the patellofemoral joint and the anterior cruciate and posterior cruciate ligaments. Retrograde nailing requires an arthrotomy and an entry hole in the cartilage, and there is concern about the long-term effects in young patients and potential infection in patients with open fractures. There is also a slightly higher risk of malunion and nonunion with retrograde nails that can be minimized by matching the nail diameter to the canal size. Retrograde nails are not indicated for nonunion of the distal femur, where plating is still the gold standard. Patients with severe articular involvement or

with Hoffa fractures should not be nailed; plating is the procedure of choice.

Percutaneous Fixation

Percutaneous fixation may be attempted for certain fracture patterns using special precontoured plates, after articular reduction and fixation. Complex intra-articular fractures require a formal open reduction and internal fixation of the articular surface, though the fixation of the metaphysis/diaphysis may still be percutaneous. This technique allows maximum preservation of soft tissue and bony vascularity, while still achieving stable fixation. The basic principles are anatomic joint reduction, proximal axial and rotational alignment, combined with the use of longer plates used with fewer screws. Excellent results have been reported using this biologic or indirect reduction technique for distal femur fractures, although there is a significant learning curve.

A small lateral parapatellar incision is first made to visualize the articular surface, allowing anatomic reduction. The plate is then slid up the lateral surface of the femur submuscularly and locked with screws inserted through stab wounds. The metadiaphyseal reduction is achieved indirectly using traction and bumps placed under the thigh. A femoral distractor can also be used to regain length and alignment while inserting the plates.

The Less Invasive Skeletal Stabilization (LISS) plates are precontoured to fit the distal femur and have an external jig that allows percutaneous insertion of the proximal shaft screws. The screw heads of the system have threads that lock into the plate, creating multiple fixed-angle devices. Stable fixation of comminuted fractures is achieved without the use of double plates.

The condylar periarticular plates are also precontoured and have a low profile distally to prevent prominence where there is less soft tissue. They also can be inserted percutaneously after the initial articular fixation and the proximal part may be fixed through a small proximal incision or stab holes using fluoroscopy.

The dynamic compression screw may also be used for percutaneous fixation of distal femur fractures. A small distal incision is needed for articular reduction and insertion of the lag screw. The barrel plate is then slid up the shaft with the barrel pointing toward the surgeon. Once the plate is in, the barrel is reversed and inserted over the lag screw, guided by the insertion device. The proximal screws are then inserted using stab holes with the aid of the c-arm fluoroscopy.

The determination of appropriate length and rotation can be difficult, especially when indirect reduction techniques are used. The use of an intraoperative modified scanogram using an electrocautery cord and fluoroscopy for length, or the cortical diameter on c-arm fluoroscopy and/or comparison of hip rotations may be useful.

A joint spanning external fixator may be used for the initial treatment of high-energy injuries, open fractures, or vascular injuries. This is usually a simple anterior frame used as a temporizing measure to allow soft-tissue or wound healing. Definitive fixation can be performed at a later date when the soft-tissue envelope allows.

Periprosthetic Fractures

As the population ages and the number of knee and hip replacements increases, there is bound to be a corresponding increase in periprosthetic fractures, which are complicated by osteoporosis and the lack of endosteal blood supply secondary to internal reaming and cementing.

Fractures proximal to a knee prosthesis can be stabilized in several ways. If the prosthesis is well fixed, a retrograde nail (if the prosthesis design permits it) or a lateral plate (with or without cerclage wires) may be used. These fractures also can be fixed percutaneously with a dynamic compression screw device or the LISS plate, using the same technique as described above. For fractures distal to a well-fixed hip implant, a retrograde nail can also be used. However, a stress riser may result between the tip of the nail and the tip of the prosthesis, and fractures can occur in this area. Alternatively, a lateral plate may be used to fix these fractures. If the plate will overlap the prosthesis, a system with cerclage cable fixation should be used. If there is concern about osteoporosis or inadequate fixation, a strut graft may be used as supplemental fixation and held with cerclage wires to the bone and the lateral plate.

If either the hip or knee prosthesis is loose, revision should be done with a longer stem to bypass the fracture.

Annotated Bibliography

Bhandari M, Guyatt GH, Tong D, Adili A, Shaughnessy SG: Reamed versus nonreamed intramedullary nailing of lower extremity long bone fractures: A systematic overview and meta-analysis. *J Orthop Trauma* 2000;14:2-9.

In a meta-analysis of the literature, reamed intramedullary nailing of lower extremity long bone fractures had a lower rate of nonunion and implant failure when compared with nonreamed nailing. Reamed intramedullary nailing did not increase the risk of malunion, pulmonary emboli, compartment syndrome, or infection.

Brumback RJ, Toal TR, Murphy-Zane MS, Novak VP, Belkoff SM: Immediate weight-bearing after treatment of a comminuted fracture of the femoral shaft with a statically locked intramedullary nail. *J Bone Joint Surg Am* 1999;81:1538-1544.

In 25 skeletally mature patients younger than the age of 70 years who were allowed immediate, full weight bearing on their nailed femoral shaft fracture, all fractures healed. One patient needed dynamization at 5 months to heal and no nail or screw breakage occurred.

Clatworthy MG, Clark DI, Gray DH, Hardy AE: Reamed versus unreamed femoral nails: A randomised, prospective trial. *J Bone Joint Surg Br* 1998;80:485-489.

A randomized prospective trial comparing reamed (22 patients) to nonreamed nails (23 patients) for femoral shaft fractures is presented. The fractures in the nonreamed group took longer to heal (39.4 versus 28.5 weeks) and required 14 additional procedures in 10 patients versus 3 procedures in 3 patients in the reamed group to achieve union.

Nowotarski PJ, Turen CH, Brumback RJ, Scarboro JM: Conversion of external fixation to intramedullary nailing for fractures of the shaft of the femur in multiply injured patients. *J Bone Joint Surg Am* 2000;82:781-788.

In a retrospective review, 59 fractures of the femoral shaft were initially stabilized with external fixation followed by a planned conversion to an intramedullary nail. Of the 58 of 59 fractures that were followed until union, 56 healed within 6 months. The infection rate was 1.7%. There was an 11% incidence of unplanned surgical procedures. Knee range of motion averaged 107° (range 60° to 140°).

Ostrum RF, Agarwal A, Lakatos R, Poka A: Prospective comparison of retrograde and antegrade femoral intramedullary nailing. *J Orthop Trauma* 2000;14:496-501.

In a prospective, randomized trial, there was no difference in rate of union or knee range of motion. There was, however, an increased need for distal hardware removal and dynamization with a longer time to union for retrograde nails. Antegrade nailing had an increased incidence of hip and thigh pain.

Scalea TM, Scott JD, Brumback RJ, et al: Early fracture fixation may be "just fine" after head injury: No difference in central nervous system outcomes. *J Trauma* 1999;46:839-846.

In a retrospective analysis, 171 blunt trauma victims with an admission Glasgow Coma Scale of less than 13, and a pelvic or lower extremity fracture that required surgical fixation. The authors grouped patients into an early fixation group (≤ 24 hours after admission) or a late fixation group (> 24 hours after admission).

Tornetta P, Tiburzi D: Reamed versus nonreamed anterograde femoral nailing. *J Orthop Trauma* 2000;14: 15-19.

In a prospective randomized trial of 172 patients, time to union differed significantly between reamed (80 ± 30 days) and nonreamed (109 ± 62 days) fractures (*P* = .002). There were more technical complications in the nonreamed group.

Wolinsky PR, McCarty E, Shyr Y, Johnson K: Reamed intramedullary nailing of the femur: 551 cases. *J Trauma* 1999;46:392-399.

In 551 femur fractures stabilized with a reamed femoral nail, the union rate was 98.9% (93.6% healed after the initial procedure). There were six infections, all in closed fractures. No open fractures (n = 90) developed an infection. No fracture healed with more than 10° of angulation, 44 healed with more than 5°. Only a distal third location was found to correlate with an increased chance of angulation.

Wolinsky PR, McCarty EC, Shyr Y, Johnson KD: Length of operative procedures: Reamed femoral intramedullary nailing performed with and without a fracture table. *J Orthop Trauma* 1998;12:485-495.

In a retrospective study of consecutive femur fractures treated over a 10-year period, multivariate analysis revealed that use of a fracture table prolonged preparation and drape time by 20 minutes, surgical time by 17 minutes, and anesthesia time by 73 minutes.

Classic Bibliography

Bolhofner BR, Carmen B, Clifford P: The results of open reduction and internal fixation of distal femur fixation using a biologic (indirect) reduction technique. *J Orthop Trauma* 1996;10:372-377.

Bone LB, Johnson KD, Weigelt J, Scheinberg R: Early versus delayed stabilization of femoral fractures: A prospective randomized study. *J Bone Joint Surg Am* 1989:71:336-340.

Brumback RJ, Reilly JP, Poka A, Lakatos RP, Bathon GH, Burgess AR: Intramedullary nailing of femoral shaft fractures: Part 1. Decision-making errors with interlocking fixation. *J Bone Joint Surg Am* 1988:70: 1441-1452.

Brumback RJ, Uwagie-Ero S, Lakatos RP, Poka A, Bathon GH, Burgess AR: Intramedullary nailing of femoral shaft fractures: Part II. Fracture-healing with static interlocking fixation. *J Bone Joint Surg Am* 1988; 70:1453-1462.

Koval KJ, Kummer FJ, Bharam S, Chen D, Hadler S: Distal femoral fixation: A laboratory comparison of the 95 degrees plate, antegrade and retrograde inserted reamed intramedullary nails. *J Orthop Trauma* 1996;10: 378-382.

McKee MD, Schemitsch EH, Vincent LO, Sullivan I, Yoo D: The effect of a femoral fracture on concomitant closed head injury in patients with multiple injuries. *J Trauma* 1997;42:1041-1045.

Pape HC, Auf'm'Kolk M, Paffrath T, Regel G, Sturm JA, Tscherne H: Primary intramedullary femur fixation in multiple trauma patients with associated lung contusion: A cause of posttraumatic ARDS? *J Trauma* 1993; 34:540-548.

Riska EB, von Bonsdorff H, Hakkinen S, Jaroma H, Kiviluoto O, Paavilainen T: Prevention of fat embolism by early internal fixation of fractures in patients with multiple injuries. *Injury* 1976;8:110-116.

Schatzker J, Horne G, Waddell J: The Toronto experience with the supracondylar fracture of the femur, 1966-1972. *Injury* 1974;6:113-128.

Swiontkowski MF, Winquist RA, Hansen ST: Fractures of the femoral neck in patients between the ages of twelve and forty-nine years. *J Bone Joint Surg Am* 1984;66:837-846.

Tornetta P, Ritz G, Kantor A: Femoral torsion after interlocked nailing of unstable femoral fractures. *J Trauma* 1995;38:213-219.

Winquist RA, Hansen ST, Clawson DK: Closed intramedullary nailing of femoral fractures: A report of five hundred and twenty cases. *J Bone Joint Surg Am* 1984;66:529-539.

Chapter 41

Knee and Leg: Pediatric Aspects

Perry Schoenecker, MD

Scott Luhmann, MD

Knee

Congenital Dislocation of the Knee

Congenital dislocation of the knee is a rare deformity that can be unilateral or bilateral. Milder forms are associated with breech position in utero, whereas the more severe forms often occur in association with systemic disorders such as arthrogryposis, Larson's syndrome, or myelodysplasia. Congenital dislocation of the knee occurs in association with hip dysplasia (45% concomitant occurrence) and/or congenital foot deformities (clubfoot and/or vertical talus, 31% concomitant occurrence). Clinically, the newborn infant presents with hyperextension of the knees of varying severity and quadriceps tendon contracture. In type I deformity, the knee is hyperextended but typically can be flexed to 90° or more. In type II deformity, the tibia is anteriorly subluxated on the femur, but is reducible with variable knee flexion. In type III deformity, the hyperextended knee cannot be flexed because the tibia is irreducibly dislocated anteriorly on the femur with a severe quadriceps contracture (Fig. 1).

Treatment begins at birth with manipulative stretching combined with serial casting. Milder deformities are corrected quickly and once flexion of 60° or more is obtained, removable splints or a Pavlik harness can be used to maintain correction. If serial casting is unsuccessful, surgical reduction with or without preoperative skin traction is attempted. A percutaneous quadriceps release may be efficacious in a less severe type III deformity. Severe type III deformities typically require extensive surgery to obtain a stable reduction of the dislocated tibia on the femur. Surgical reconstruction includes extensive quadricepsplasty, anterior capsular release, variable release of collaterals (not cruciates), and occasional hamstring lengthening. Postoperatively, cast immobilization in 45° or more of flexion followed by splinting is done to maintain reduction and optimize quadriceps function and joint flexibility.

Ipsilateral hip dysplasia, which usually requires surgical treatment, is best treated after surgical correction of the knee deformity. The long-term functional outcome of surgical treatment is variable, with better outcomes for milder grades and deformity. At follow-up, range of motion is usually from near full extension to 80° to 120° flexion. Residual flexion contracture can be problematic and is more frequent in patients with more severe pathology.

Congenital Dislocation of the Patella

Congenital dislocation of the patella is an uncommon lateral patella displacement on the femur. Although it may present variably from infancy to late childhood, the predictable pathologic anatomy is that of lateral patella subluxation/dislocation that eventually becomes fixed with an associated knee flexion deformity. The resulting deformity is limited active extension of the knee and variable genu valgum with external rotation of the tibia, leading to lateral placement of the tibial tubercle. Patients with this condition must be distinguished from those with the less severe but more common recurrent dislocation of the patella. The onset of symptoms associated with recurrent dislocation of the patella is later (at age 11 to 12 years) than with congenital dislocation of the patella. In recurrent dislocation of the patella, there is lateral tracking and/or intermittent dislocation. In congenital dislocation of the patella, fixation of the patella in a laterally dislocated position is gradual.

The natural history of congenital dislocation of the patella is that of worsening symptoms of patellar pain and quadriceps weakness, as well as functional limitations caused by the deformity. Surgical correction of congenital dislocation of the patella can be done at any age and always includes an extensive lateral release, medial transfer of the patellar tendon, and lateral transfer of the medial retinaculum and the vastus medialis obliquus. In skeletally immature patients, the

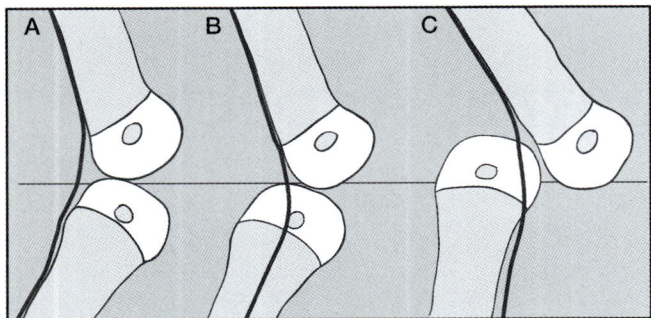

Figure 1 Three forms of congenital hyperextension of the knee. **A,** Recurvatum, **B,** subluxation, and **C,** dislocation modified from Levenf and Pais. *(Adapted with permission from Curtis BH, Fisher RL: Congenital hyperextension with anterior subluxation of the knee: Surgical treatment and long-term observations. J Bone Joint Surg Am 1969;51:255-269.)*

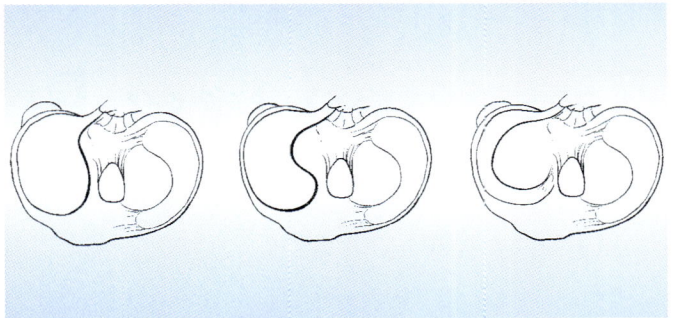

Figure 2 Classification of lateral discoid meniscus by Watanabe: 1) complete discoid meniscus (type 1); 2) incomplete discoid meniscus (type 2); 3) Wrisberg's ligament type, with no posterior capsular attachment (type 3).

patellar tendon is completely transected from the tibia and along with the attached fat pad transposed medially, effectively restoring normal patellar alignment. In a skeletally mature patient, the patellar tendon is transposed with an attached block of bone. Function is anticipated to improve after surgical reconstruction.

Quadriceps Contracture

A quadriceps contracture limits knee flexion and can occur in children after distal femoral fracture (with and without infection) or femoral lengthening, in association with congenital dislocation of the knee, and after intramuscular injection into the thigh. Idiopathic quadriceps contracture typically occurs in children of Asian ancestry. Limited improvement is expected with a circumferential release of the adherent quadriceps mechanism for a contracture after an injury. For contractures associated with a congenital dislocation of the knee joint, the quadriceps mechanism lengthening must often be accompanied by a partial release of the collateral ligaments of the knee joint. For idiopathic contractures, lengthening of the multiple contracted tendinous bands within the quadriceps muscle will improve both knee flexion and function. Postoperatively, the knee is initially splinted in flexion, and flexion is alternated with extension. Typically, there is permanent improvement in range of motion without loss of quadriceps extension power.

Discoid Meniscus

Discoid meniscus is an infrequent cause of knee pain in children and is a congenital variant of unknown etiology. The condition occurs bilaterally in 20% of patients, and the lateral meniscus, which is grossly abnormal in shape and contour, is usually involved. The Watanabe classification is the current standard (Fig. 2). The usual presentation includes a history of pain, and mechanical symptoms such as snapping, popping, or catching. Inability to achieve full knee extension and locking can also be seen. Most discoid menisci occur in childhood. Plain radiographs are usually unremarkable. The imaging study of choice is MRI, which allows identification of meniscal shape, contour, and intrasubstance tears. However, identification of the type 3 (Wrisberg) variants can be difficult because they can appear morphologically normal.

Treatment is reserved for symptomatic knees; incidental discoid menisci seen during arthroscopy typically are not treated. For discoid menisci with intact peripheral attachments (types 1 and 2), partial menisectomy or contouring of the meniscus yields excellent results. In the Wrisberg-type discoid meniscus (type 3), repairing the meniscus to its normal capsular attachment site is optimal. If reestablishment of meniscal stability is possible, then sculpting or partial menisectomy should be done. However, if repair is not possible because of meniscal shape or intrasubstance breakdown, then total menisectomy is the preferred treatment, but its long-term results raise concern for the early development of osteoarthritis.

Osgood-Schlatter Disease

Osgood-Schlatter disease is an osteochondrosis of the proximal tibial apophysis associated with the rapid growth of adolescence. The development of pain and swelling is secondary to repeated tensile forces in a susceptible knee. The disease is more common in boys than girls. Because of later ossification of the tibial tubercle in boys, they are afflicted at an older age (12 + 9 years versus 10 + 8 years in girls). Activities associated with the development of the disease include running and jumping sports such as soccer, basketball, and volleyball. Forty percent of patients present with bilateral complaints with symptoms localized to the tibial tubercle. Plain radiographs should be obtained to rule out other pathology. Patella alta, which theoretically increases the force needed from the quadriceps to achieve full extension, is associated with Osgood-Schlatter disease. MRI and ultrasound have demonstrated more signal changes in the patellar tendon and surrounding soft tissues than in the tibial tubercle physis.

Nonsurgical management is the mainstay of treatment and includes activity modification (not elimination) for up to 6 weeks, ice application, stretching, and the use of nonsteroidal anti-inflammatory drugs. A patellar tendon strap or protective brace over the tibial tubercle can help minimize symptoms. Casting and steroid injections are not recommended. Resumption of activities is possible once symptoms abate. For more than 95% of patients, pain typically lasts for 12 to 24 months with resolution of symptoms as the patient nears skeletal maturity. In 32% of patients an ossicle can develop, and, if symptomatic, excision after skeletal maturity may relieve pain. Long-term follow-up of patients with Osgood-Schlatter disease demonstrates that 60% of patients are unable to kneel without pain or discomfort and 24% have some limitation of activity.

Sinding-Larsen-Johansson Disease

Sinding-Larsen-Johansson disease occurs secondary to an overuse traction phenomenon at the inferior pole of the patella and typically occurs earlier than Osgood-Schlatter disease. Tenderness to palpation is present over the inferior pole of the patella, and patients will have decreased knee flexion because of pain. Radiographs occasionally demonstrate distal pole fragmentation or elongation of the inferior pole of the patella. Treatment is similar to that for Osgood-Schlatter disease. The patient may resume activity once symptoms resolve.

Osteochondritis Dissecans

Osteochondritis dissecans is a condition in which a portion of the subchondral bone undergoes partial or complete separation from its underlying bony bed. The overlying articular cartilage surface is initially intact but may become disrupted. Trauma and vascular causes are accepted theoretical etiologies for this condition with 21% of patients presenting with a history of trauma. Males are affected twice as often as females, and 33% of cases are bilateral. Clinical symptoms include vague activity-related pain, mechanical symptoms (catching, popping, or snapping), and an effusion (typically indicates articular surface disruption). When detachment of the lesion occurs and a loose body is present, the symptoms may additionally include sensations of locking and giving way. On physical examination an effusion, knee flexion contracture, or localized tenderness may be present.

Imaging studies include plain radiographs (especially notch or tunnel views) and MRI, which can define the size of the lesion, extent of subchondral involvement, and assess the condition of the overlying articular surface. If there is no effusion, gadolinium enhancement improves identification of the articular surface disruption. Technetium Tc99m pyrophosphate bone scans can demonstrate the progression of healing and vascular supply to the lesion. Most lesions (75% to 85%) present on the medial femoral condyle, with fewer on the lateral condyle (13% to 6%), patella (1% to 6%), trochlea (1%), or tibial plateau (less than 1%).

Skeletal maturity, age, and lesion location are important factors to be considered for successful nonsurgical management. Nonsurgical management is the initial intervention for the skeletally immature patient; surgical intervention is reserved for the presence of a loose body. Pain relief through limitation of activities, no weight bearing, and possibly brace use is the goal of nonsurgical treatment. Nonsurgical management will be more likely to succeed if more than 1 year has passed since physeal closure. MRI assessment is helpful in predicting the potential for spontaneous healing. Lesions with a diameter of less than 20 mm, no articular surface disruption, and no effusion tend to do better without surgery. Overall, spontaneous healing rates have been reported as high as 82%. Lesions in the classic lateral location on the medial femoral condyle heal only 55% of the time, whereas those located in the inferocentral location of the medial or lateral condyle have spontaneous healing rates of 89% to 100%. Healing time is greater in the classic location (mean, 18.7 months) compared with the inferocentral location (mean, 12.0 months). Atypical locations (medial side of medial femoral condyle, lateral condyle, patella, tibia) have fewer satisfactory results with closed treatment.

In skeletally mature patients, lesions 20 mm or larger with articular surface disruption and/or effusions fare better with surgical intervention. Failure of the lesion to show signs of healing by a minimum of 3 months with a cold bone scan and lesion detachment (on MRI) are indications for surgical intervention. Patients with mechanical symptoms (such as catching, locking, or popping) and effusions are more likely to have lesions with detachment and articular surface disruption. Lesions with intact articular surfaces should be drilled using either direct intra-articular visualization or through the epiphysis using a guide to prevent violation of the articular cartilage. Drilling is theorized to promote vascular ingrowth from the healthy epiphyseal bone surrounding the lesion, thereby stimulating the healing process. Drilling has been reported to be successful in 90% of skeletally immature patients.

Open or arthroscopic stabilization of in situ lesions with articular cartilage breach, and in patients in whom primary drilling is unsuccessful, can be done with Kirschner wires, Steinmann pins, Herbert screws, and bioabsorbable rods or screws. Fixation reestablishes bony stability to allow a good environment for bony healing. Studies report more than 80% good and excellent results after fixation. Loose bodies with associated comminution, those smaller than 1 cm^2, and purely cartilaginous fragments are excised with curettage and drilling of the exposed bone. Loose bodies larger than 1 cm^2 originating from the weight-bearing zone of the knee are associated with poor long-term results. Repair of acute loose bodies larger than 1 cm^2 with sufficient subchondral bone is preferable. Chronic loose bodies undergo changes in contour, making replacement into the native bed difficult. Excision of chronic loose bodies is preferable to nonanatomic repair. New surgical techniques including osteochondral autograft transfer, autologous chondrocyte culture and implantation, and chondroinductive matrices show early promising results. Osteochondral grafting as a salvage technique for lesions smaller than 2.5 cm^2 has shown early encouraging results. Osteochondral grafting of lesions larger than 2.5 cm^2 is more difficult because of the need for multiple grafts to fill the recipient site. This situation can create potential donor site morbidity and the need for larger areas of fibrocartilage proliferation between the grafts at the recipient site. Fresh osteochondral allografts (dowel or block) are reserved for large lesions of the femoral condyles in skeletally mature patients.

Lower Extremity

Varus Deformity

The normal physiologic knee alignment at birth is 10° to 15° of varus, which typically remodels to a neutral femorotibial alignment by age 18 to 24 months. If physiologic bowing persists into early childhood, it must be differentiated from the pathologic bowing in infantile tibia vara (Blount disease), metabolic bone disease, and skeletal dysplasia. Pathologic bowing will progress without treatment. Physiologic bowing and Blount disease should be perceived as two different points on the same spectrum, as the end results of persistent infantile bowing. The distinction between physiologic bowing and Blount disease may not initially be obvious because the pathologic radiographic changes of early Blount disease (maximal medial metaphyseal beaking and cystic-like changes) are often not present until 2 to 3 years of age. Although not diagnostic, the metaphyseal-diaphyseal angle can help to differentiate physiologic bowing from infantile Blount disease (Fig. 3). If the metaphyseal-diaphyseal angle is less than 10°,

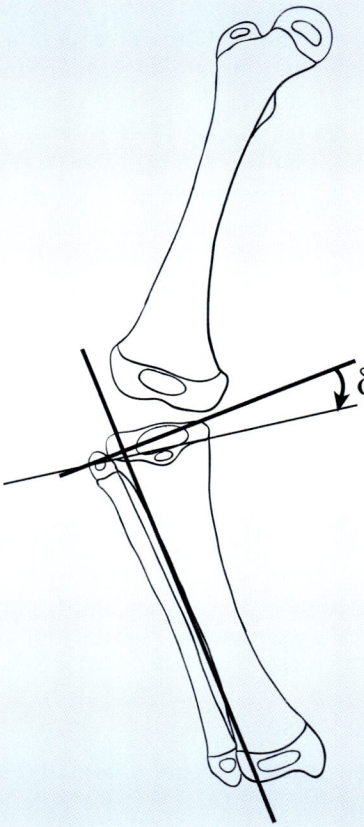

Figure 3 Illustration of the metaphyseal-diaphyseal angle described by Levine and Drennan. The angle lies between a line drawn through the most distal point on the medial and lateral beaks of the tibial metaphysis and a line perpendicular to the lateral cortex of the tibia.

there is a high probability that the diagnosis is physiologic bowing. Conversely, if the metaphyseal-diaphyseal angle is > 16°, then there is a high probability that the diagnosis is Blount disease. Sometimes physiologic bowing must also be differentiated from the pathologic bowing associated with metabolic bone disease and/or skeletal dysplasia. Rickets (either dietary or X-linked hypophosphatemic) is the most likely metabolic bone disease seen as a bowed leg deformity in the toddler. Infants with rickets are of short stature, with the measured height being less than the 10th percentile. The diagnosis of rickets is made by noting the characteristic radiographic changes as well as abnormalities in both serum and urine calcium and phosphate concentration. Patients with skeletal dysplasias occasionally have a bowing deformity of the lower extremity. Children with skeletal dysplasia also are of short stature, typically with measured height being less than the fifth percentile.

Infantile Blount disease occurs with variable severity as a resistant, typically bilateral genu varum deformity in infants and children ages 1 to 8 years. There is a distinct predilection in blacks. The genu varum deformity that occurs in infantile Blount disease is an osteochondrosis of the proximal medial tibial metaphysis. Early walking and childhood obesity are factors that contribute to the relatively excessive compression forces

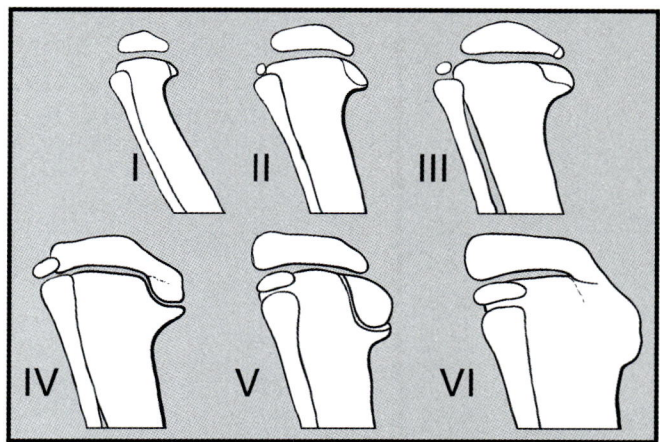

Figure 4 Diagram of the progressive radiographic changes seen in infantile tibia vara and their development with increasing age, as described by Langenskiöld.

across the medial proximal tibial physis that prevent normal medial physeal growth, with the subsequent development of pathologic genu varum. The inherent natural progression of Blount osteochondrosis through six distinct radiographic stages, as described by Langenskiöld (Fig. 4), can be altered with treatment. Bracing can be effective (using a nonarticulated knee-ankle-foot orthosis) in treating patients younger than age 3 years at Langenskiöld stage III or below or with unilateral deformity. Brace treatment will predictably fail in older patients, in those with changes at stage III or above, and/or bilateral deformity. Surgical correction (proximal tibiofibular varus-correcting osteotomy) is indicated for patients age 3 years or older and/or in those patients with changes at stage III or above. If performed prior to age 4 years and prior to progression to Langenskiöld stage IV radiographic changes, a proximal tibial varus correcting osteotomy will typically result in resolution of infantile Blount disease. Once the pathology has progressed to Langenskiöld stage IV or above, spontaneous resolution will not predictably occur after corrective osteotomy alone. Varus corrective osteotomy or proximal lateral tibial hemiepiphyseal stapling must be combined with a resection of a bony medial physeal bar for attempted restoration of symmetric growth for stage IV and V changes. For the severe changes seen with stage VI deformity, a varus correcting osteotomy and an intra-articular osteotomy to directly elevate the pathologically depressed medial-tibial plateau are necessary to restore more normal knee joint anatomy and lower extremity mechanics. Long-term follow-up is essential in all patients requiring surgical treatment for Blount disease. Recurrence of varus is possible after a varus correcting osteotomy for any Langenskiöld stage. Uni-

lateral cases must be monitored for the presence of a limb-length inequality.

In older children or adolescents with varus deformity, the most likely diagnosis is adolescent Blount disease. Patients with a normal habitus (not obese) will typically have a history of physiologic bowing persisting through early childhood. More likely, patients are variably obese with only a recent history of genu varum deformity. These patients typically have relatively wide thighs. During normal gait, floor contact is in a straight line of progression. Resultant growth inhibition produces a progressive varus and procurvatum deformity of both the proximal tibia and distal femur. Lateral knee joint laxity may occur, leading to additional varus deformity within the knee joint itself. In severe cases, compensatory distal tibial valgus occurs. The varus deformity is typically bilateral, but varies in severity. The incidence of adolescent Blount disease has increased in proportion to the alarming increase in the incidence of adolescent obesity. Adolescent Blount disease occurs in association with slipped capital femoral epiphysis. Radiographic assessment must include long cassette (36- or 51-in) views of both lower extremities with the patellae pointing straight ahead. The hips, knees, and ankles must be viewed to allow for a comprehensive assessment of any frontal plane deformity. A lateral radiograph of the tibia allows for assessment of procurvatum deformity. Because the epiphysis is almost fully ossified and much less deformable than in the younger child, the relative degree of pathologic bony changes in the proximal medial tibia in adolescent Blount disease is far less severe than the advanced pathologic changes seen in children with infantile tibia vara. Occasionally, genu varum deformity is seen in children as young as 6 to 8 years of age. Changes typical of Blount disease can occur at this age either secondary to late-presenting infantile or early-presenting adolescent Blount disease. It is important to make this differentiation to allow for the correct surgical treatment of tibia vara deformity.

Adolescent tibia vara should be treated with osteotomy or hemiepiphysiodesis. Hemiepiphysiodesis of the proximal lateral tibia and/or the distal lateral femur with Blount-type reinforced staples can be the definitive treatment if the growth plates are open (with more than 15 months of growth remaining) and the deformity is mild to moderate. Osteotomy is the mainstay of treatment. Careful preoperative planning is essential and includes preoperative radiographic assessment and comprehensive surgical correction of all aspects of the deformity. Optimal surgical technique includes the use of a circumferential and/or monolateral external fixator to obtain and maintain correction of the complex proximal tibial deformity in the patient with a very large extremity. It is essential to correct the tibial varus, recurvatum, and internal rotation through the proximal tibial osteotomy. If present, the distal femoral varus and distal tibial valgus are similarly corrected. For a lasting satisfactory outcome, the restoration must reestablish the normal anatomic relationships between the knee and ankle joint and a normal mechanical axis. Limb-length inequality must also be addressed in unilateral deformity.

Valgus Deformity

Children typically present with a knock-knee deformity between 3 and 5 years of age, when the normal femorotibial angle is at maximum valgus. The diagnosis is almost always physiologic knock-knee. Physiologic knock-knee can be categorized by the intermalleolar distance (IMD) as follows: normal if IMD < 2 cm; mild if IMD = 2 to 5 cm; moderate if IMD = 5 to 9 cm; severe if IMD > 9 cm. Physiologic valgus usually remodels by age 7 years. As pathologic conditions can lead to normal-occurring varus in early childhood, they similarly can lead to the normal valgus that occurs later in childhood. Metabolic bone disease (X-linked hypophosphatemic rickets or rickets secondary to chronic renal disease), skeletal dysplasias, and posttraumatic causes (progressive varus occurring after proximal tibial metaphyseal fracture [Cozen's fracture]) must be considered in the differential diagnosis. Idiopathic valgus deformity persisting or presenting after 8 to 9 years of age can become pathologic (genu valgum). Weight bearing may become awkward because of the knees rubbing together, and knee pain may occur with weight bearing. Long cassette radiographs of the lower extremities are essential to document and measure valgus deformity of the distal femur and proximal tibia. The degree of lateral displacement of the mechanical axis of the involved extremity is measured and used to assess response to treatment. Deviation of the mechanical axis near and beyond the lateral edge of the tibia is pathologic. Pathologic genu valgum is corrected with medial staple hemiepiphysiodesis of the distal femur, proximal tibia, or both. Hemiepiphysiodesis is ideally initiated with sufficient growth remaining to allow full correction of the deformity. Staples must be placed extraperiostally. If significant growth remains at the time of correction, staple removal will be necessary. Typically, overcorrection is desirable because a variable degree of rebound growth will occur after staple removal. Subsequent monitoring until skeletal maturity is critical. Alternatively, bilateral physiodesis can be performed when the mechanical axis has been corrected. In skeletally mature patients, problematic genu valgum usually is corrected typically with a distal femoral osteotomy.

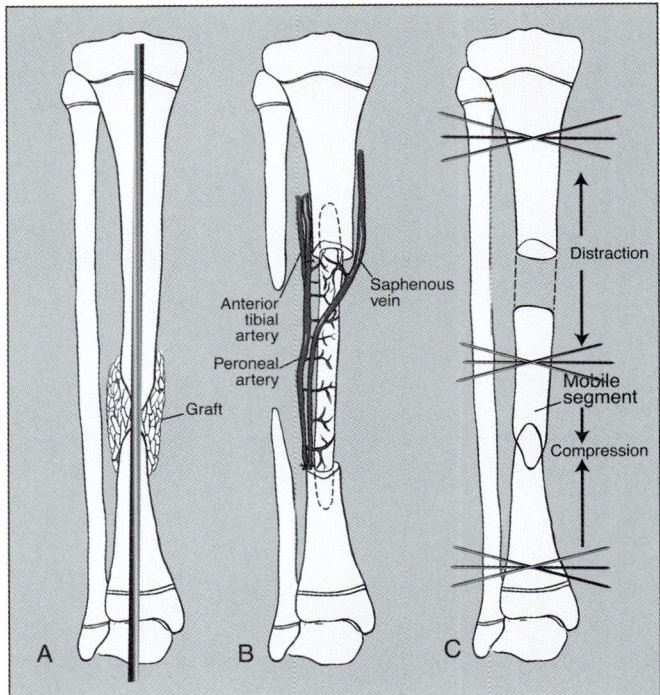

Figure 5 Surgical options for pseudarthrosis of the tibia. **A,** Coleman osteosynthesis. **B,** Vascularized fibular graft form the opposite leg. **C,** Ilizarov technique of lengthening above and compression of the pseudarthrosis to achieve union. *(Adapted with permission from Sponseller PD: Localized disorders of bone and soft tissue, in Morrissey RT, Weinstein SL (eds): Lovell and Winter's Pediatric Orthopaedics. Philadelphia, PA, Lippincott-Williams & Wilkins, 1996, pp 305-344.)*

Anterolateral Bowing

Bowing of the tibia that is present at birth typically occurs either anteriorly (in association with fibular hemimelia), anterolaterally (in association with congenital pseudarthrosis), or posteromedially (in association with calcaneovalgus foot deformity). Anterolateral bowing of the tibia is rare (occurring in 1 in 140,000), yet it is the most common type of congenital pseudarthrosis. Neurofibromatosis occurs in approximately 50% of patients with anterolateral bowing with or without pseudarthrosis of the tibia. Fracture with resultant pseudarthrosis typically occurs within the first 4 to 5 years of life. Boyd's and other classification systems have been used to assess the natural history and outcome of treatment. When anterolateral bowing occurs in association with neurofibromatosis, progression of deformity and treatment failure are more likely to occur.

Orthotic treatment is initially indicated for deformity without fracture. However, despite early orthotic treatment, anterolateral bowing typically progresses. If a pseudarthrosis does not occur, an onlay bone graft may help to improve bone quality. In past years, treatment of an established congenital pseudarthrosis of the tibia has been one of the most challenging orthopaedic surgical problems. Three different surgical approaches have evolved, which are currently used with variable success (Fig. 5). The overall good early results with these newer and/or refined surgical techniques are encouraging. However, the true success of treatment of congenital pseudarthosis of the tibia in the growing child can only be determined by follow-up of these patients until skeletal maturity. Despite technical advances, a lasting consolidation is not always possible. Amputation (Syme's or below-knee) has been and often still is a prudent alternative.

Posteromedial Bowing of the Tibia

Posteromedial bowing of the tibia is a congenital anomaly associated with calcaneovalgus foot deformity. The diagnosis is made at birth and is characterized by the extremely dorsiflexed position of the foot against the posteromedially bowed tibia. Plantar flexion is limited. Even though there is severe bowing at birth, the angulatory deformity remodels. Pseudarthrosis does not develop in posteromedial bowing. The angulation remodels to some degree with an occasional resultant distal tibial valgus deformity. The absolute limb-length inequality increases with growth as the growth inhibition rate remains constant. Initial treatment consists of primarily passive stretching of the foot. A shoe lift is necessary in early childhood, and occasionally an ankle-foot orthosis is needed for the valgus deformity. Serial scanograms will help predict limb-length inequality at maturity. An appropriately timed epiphysiodesis is the treatment of choice for limb-length discrepancies of up to 4 to 5 cm. Limb lengthening is considered for those discrepancies predicted to be 4 to 5 cm or greater and is performed through a proximal tibial osteotomy. A second distal osteotomy is indicated for correction of persistent distal valgus.

Fibular Longitudinal Deficiency

Fibular hemimelia is the most common limb deficiency and can be characterized by a marked variability of fibular deficiency (from total absence to a minimal degree of both proximal and distal fibular developmental deficiency). In a fibular-centered limb deficiency, a spectrum of musculoskeletal anomalies involving the femur, hip and knee joint, the tibia, fibula, and ankle joint, and the foot have been identified, and is termed postaxial hypoplasia of the lower extremity. The femur is variably short and externally rotated with a unique lateral femoral condylar deficiency, lateral patellar subluxation, and genu valgum deformity. The cruciates and tibial eminences are typically underdeveloped, and the knee joint is unstable. The tibia is variably shortened and in severe deficiencies bowed anteromedially. The foot is characteristically hypoplastic with lateral ray deficiency. An equinovalgus foot deformity may be present. Complete hindfoot coalition usually is present with a secondary ball-and-socket ankle joint.

The lower extremity deformities that develop in association with longitudinal deficiency of the fibula variably require surgical correction. In the mildest of the deficiencies, the leg-length discrepancy usually is definitively treated with contralateral epiphysiodesis for the predicted 3- to 5-cm discrepancy. Alternatively, ipsilateral leg lengthening is an option for predictably longer discrepancies. As the degree of anticipated shortening increases, there is increased potential for acute or chronic ankle equinus and valgus deformity occurring during the lengthening procedure. Even when surgical and prosthetic stabilization of the foot under the tibia is attempted, progressive foot valgus and equinus deformity or ankle stiffness often preclude a satisfactory long-term functional outcome. Alternatively, after a Syme's or Boyd amputation is performed, functional outcome is predictably very satisfactory.

Tibial Longitudinal Deficiencies

Tibial longitudinal deficiencies are quite rare and can be inherited. They are classified into four types, with a wide spectrum of severity. The severe deficiencies (type I) occur most often. The tibia is typically absent or rudimentally developed proximally. In type I deficiency, the entire extensor mechanism is typically absent and the deformity can occur bilaterally. The involved extremity is short with severe varus deformity centered about a nonfunctional knee and ankle joint. Frequently, there is extra ray formation. There is an associated incidence of hip dysplasia, congenital thoracolumbar function spine anomalies, and symphalangism of the hands. Given the extent of the deficiency, knee disarticulation and prosthetic fitting are the treatments of choice for type I deficiencies. For type Ib and II deficiencies, a Syme's amputation is done in the first year of life. At variable ages, the proximal tibia will have developed sufficiently to allow for a surgical synostosis of the proximal fibula to the tibia and allow subsequent fitting with a modified below-knee prosthesis (fibular centralization will predictably fail without the presence of a quadriceps mechanism and proximal tibial anlage). Knee hinges and/or thigh corset are typically necessary for stability. For the very rare type III deformity, a Syme's amputation is done and a prosthesis is used. For the patient with type IV deformity (the anatomic equivalent of congenital diastasis of the ankle joint), reconstruction of the ankle joint may be possible. Predictable leg length inequality (7 to 9 cm) must be addressed later.

Limb-Length Inequality

Limb-length inequality occurs from congenital and acquired etiologies. The latter includes developmental, traumatic, and inflammatory causes. Because the natural history of limb-length inequality varies, knowing the cause of a particular limb-length inequality is essential in predicting eventual deformity. Congenital limb deficiencies are associated with variable limb-length inequalities and typically have a rate of growth inhibition that remains constant with growth. Knowing the type of deficiency and determining the degree of inhibition in early childhood can be very helpful in estimating leg length inequality at maturity.

The simplest way to measure functional limb-length inequality is with the patient standing to allow assessment of the lower extremities, pelvis, and torso. With the patient positioned with both feet on the floor and the knees extended, the effect of any functional limb-length inequality will be reflected in an unbalanced pelvis. Leveling of the pelvis is achieved by placing blocks under the short leg. The height of the blocks is an accurate approximation of functional limb length deficiency. In patients age 7 years and older, a scanogram is a more accurate tool for measurement. A radiograph of the hand is taken with each scanogram to estimate skeletal age. A CT scanogram ideally optimizes accuracy and minimizes radiation exposure; however, CT imaging often is not available for routine use.

Prediction of the deformity at maturity can be measured by the White-Menelaus "rule of thumb" method (the assumption that the distal femur and proximal tibia grow at a fixed rate of three eighths and one fourth inch per year, respectively, and that growth in girls stops at age 14 years and growth in boys at age 16 years), the Green-Anderson tables, which predict growth remaining, and the Moseley graph. Application of the "rule of thumb" method is limited to small deformities (2 to 4 cm) in patients whose bone age hopefully is similar to the chronological age. Typically, the Moseley graph and/or the Green-Anderson tables are used in estimating the discrepancy at maturity and determining treatment strategies. Ideally, three or four sequential scanograms (with bone age noted) are obtained prior to deciding on projected discrepancy and appropriate treatment. Special problems that may need to be considered in formulating treatment plans include joint instability, fixed spinal deformity, pelvic obliquity, angular deformity, foot height discrepancy, and associated neuromuscular hemiparesis.

Treatment guidelines are as follows: Discrepancy of 0 to 2 cm—no treatment other than shoe lift; 2 to 6 cm—shortening (epiphysiodesis and/or osteotomy); 4 to 8 cm—lengthening; 8 to 15 or 20 cm—combination (shortening and/or lengthening); 15 to 20 cm or greater—consider amputation or a van Ness rotationplasty.

Epiphysiodesis is the treatment of choice for discrepancies under 4 to 6 cm. Timing of the epiphysiodesis is critical and it can be done at the distal femur, proximal tibia, and less frequently, the distal tibia. Percutaneous epiphysiodesis under image intensifier yields predictably good results. Follow-up clinical evaluation is essential to ensure that the growth plates close, angular deformity does not occur, and limb length equalizes. After skeletal maturity, shortening on the long side can be achieved with either femoral or tibial osteotomy. Proximal or distal femoral shortening osteotomy is fixed with a blade plate and diaphyseal shortening with an intramedullary rod. For the skeletally mature patient, a closed femoral shortening technique using an intramedullary saw facilitates rapid and assured union. Serious and potentially life-threatening pulmonary complications have been reported as a result of reamed marrow particulate matter entering the circulatory system as fat emboli. Tibial shortening osteotomies heal slowly and therefore are performed infrequently. The maximum extent of shortening that can be successfully achieved is less than 4 cm. A distal or proximal diaphyseal shortening with intramedullary fixation is preferred.

Limb lengthening is a treatment option for discrepancies of 4 to 6 cm or greater. Lengthening is gradually accomplished with either a monolateral or circumferential external fixator. Lengthening is ideal at the metaphyseal level, where bone formation is most active. Distraction is begun within a few days at a rate of 1 mm per day. The lengthening index is a ratio of the number of months the fixation is applied to the centimeters lengthened, typically 1 to 1.5 months/cm. Currently, hybrid circular frames optimally incorporate use of both transfixing wires and half pins. Bone grafting is typically unnecessary. Complications occur with far greater frequency if the percent of lengthening exceeds 20% of the length of the bone being lengthened. Bone formation is optimized with weight bearing. The quality of distraction callus is monitored by radiographs. Deformity of the lengthened segment can occur if the device is removed too soon. Many patients experience pin tract irritation and/or infection, a complication that must be handled on an ongoing basis. Temporary and potentially permanent loss of adjacent joint motion and/or joint subluxation can occur. Femoral lengthening has been performed over a locking intramedullary rod, which minimizes the occurrence of deformity during lengthening and also allows for fixation removal as soon as the desired length has been obtained.

For severe congenital deficiencies, usually femoral, and with more than 20 cm of predicted discrepancy and knee joint instability, a van Ness rotationplasty allows the ankle to function as a knee joint. Foot stability is essential, hip instability is not. Plantar foot flexion becomes knee extension, and dorsiflexion become knee flexion. Greater prosthetic control is noted with activities such as stepping forward and stair climbing. If lengthening is not practical and/or rotationplasty not acceptable, a Syme's amputation can be performed and the patient fitted with a below-knee prosthesis.

Traumatic Abnormalities

Meniscal Tear

Approximately one third of children with meniscal tears have no history of trauma. Fifty-three percent of preadolescents and 45% of adolescents with meniscal tears have hemarthrosis. There is a 50% prevalence of meniscal tears with anterior cruciate ligament (ACL) tears. Medial meniscal lesions are more common. MRI in children and adolescents may have a high false-positive rate; however, arthroscopy can be beneficial in diagnosis. Optimal treatment is meniscal repair if adequate tissue of good quality is present and the tear is located in the red-on-red or red-on-white zone. Complex and horizontal tears are treated with partial menisectomy, avoiding total menisectomy.

ACL Injury

An intra-articular knee injury with effusion in children and adolescents is associated with a high frequency of ACL tears (53%). Poor reliability in examination of injured knees in children, especially in those younger than age 12 years, makes diagnosis of ACL injuries difficult. Serial clinical examinations and plain radiographs allow for a diagnosis of most ACL injuries. MRI currently is the most useful noninvasive tool in diagnosing ACL tears, with a high specificity and sensitivity in detecting these injuries. Osseous contusions of the lateral femoral condyle are common (83%) as are posterolateral joint injuries (96%). Partial tears are associated with fewer associated meniscal tears in comparison to complete lesions. Nonsurgical treatment of complete tears has been unsuccessful in returning the patient to sports requiring pivoting. Patients with partial tears have greater success in returning to sports at their previous level. Patients with recurrent episodes of instability have a high incidence (60% to 90%) of new meniscal tears.

Extra-articular reconstructions have been associated with 50% to 100% incidence of recurrent instability. Primary repairs of midsubstance tears have not

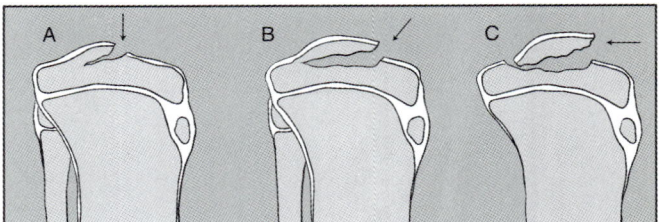

Figure 6 Meyers and McKeever classification of fractures of the anterior tibial spine. **A,** Type 1 fracture with no displacement of the fracture. **B,** Type 2 fracture with elevation of the anterior portion of the anterior tibial spine, but with the fracture posteriorly reduced. **C,** Type 3 fracture that is totally displaced.

restored stability and are not recommended. Intra-articular reconstructions are the gold standard for the symptomatic ACL-insufficient knee. Patients near the end of growth (documentation of growth spurt, Tanner stage 4 or 5, and closing physes) can be managed with bone-patellar tendon-bone autografts. Postoperatively, 95% of knees are stable and have no documentation of growth disturbances. For individuals with less than 2 cm of growth remaining at the knee, the ACL can be reconstructed with quadrupled hamstring grafts through anatomic bony tunnels. If more than 2 cm of growth is left at the knee, nonsurgical management is preferred. Indications for surgical management in individuals with open physes and significant growth remaining are recurrent instability, pain, and meniscal tear.

Fractures

Tibial Eminence Fracture

Children between the ages of 8 and 14 years are usually affected. The mechanism is forceful hyperextension or a direct blow to the distal femur with the knee in a flexed position. An axial force directed along the ACL causes an avulsion of the anterior tibial eminence. The amount of displacement is categorized according to the Meyers and McKeever classification (Fig. 6). Type 3 fractures are the most common (45%), followed by type 2 (39%) and type 1 fractures (15%). Closed treatment of type 1 fractures is with long leg casting in 10° to 15° knee flexion. Type 2 fracture reduction can be attempted with hyperextension, followed by long leg casting. Fractures treated in a closed fashion should be monitored to ensure maintenance of fracture reduction. Surgical intervention is recommended for irreducible type 2 and all type 3 fractures. A malunited fracture fragment can prevent full knee extension by blocking at the intercondylar notch. Formal open arthrotomy or arthroscopically assisted reduction and fixation techniques are appropriate for inadequately reduced type II and all type III fractures. Fixation can be achieved through cannulated screw fixation of the fracture in the epiphysis or suture stabili-

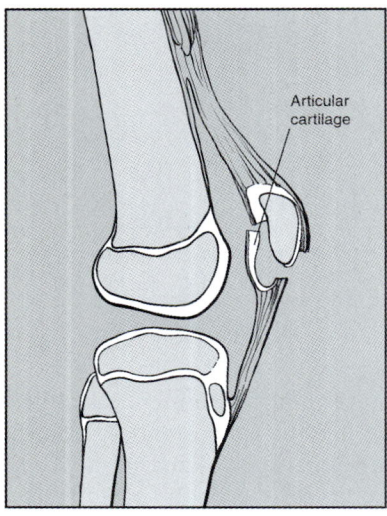

Figure 7 Sleeve fracture of the patella. A small segment of the distal pole of the patella is avulsed with a relatively large portion of the articular surface.

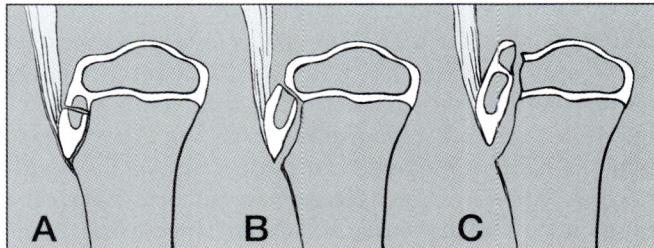

Figure 8 Watson-Jones classification of tibial tuberosity fractures. **A,** Type 1 fracture occurs before the secondary ossification center of the tuberosity has joined the epiphyseal ossification center. The fracture line runs between the ossification centers. **B,** Type II fracture occurs after the tuberosity ossification centers have joined. The fracture line divides the tuberosity from the proximal tibial plateau. **C,** Type III fracture extends from the tibial tuberosity through the primary ossification center into the point.

zation through the base of the eminence fracture, which is then secured over the anterior tibial cortex. Residual objective instability of the ACL has been documented in most series regardless of treatment technique, with type 3 fractures having the greatest degree of measured instability at follow-up. Interstitial elongation of the ACL occurs prior to avulsion of the tibial eminence. Most patients do not report subjective instability, with 84% returning to their previous level of sports participation.

Patellar Fracture
Patellar fractures typically occur in older children and are caused by sudden contraction of the extensor mechanism or by a direct blow. Patellar fractures are classified by location, type, and amount of displacement. Sleeve fractures (Fig. 7) are avulsion fractures off the patella with a large cartilaginous component and appear only as a small bony fragment on radiographs. The large cartilaginous sleeve is in continuity with the peripatellar soft tissues, such as the patellar tendon in inferior pole fractures. Most occur off the medial border (47%), followed by the inferior pole (38%) and superior pole (15%). Medial sleeve fractures are usually secondary to acute patellar dislocations. The ability to extend the knee with inferior pole fractures depends on the degree of fracture displacement and the amount of disruption of the medial and lateral retinaculum. Nonsurgical management is appropriate for fractures with less than 2 mm of displacement and an intact extensor mechanism. Open reduction and internal fixation is often necessary to reestablish extensor mechanism function. Fixation methods using tension-band techniques or screw fixation are not associated with growth disturbances. Smaller, displaced osteochondral fragments are treated with excision and soft-tissue repair. Long-term results typically are good; comminuted fractures are more likely to have poor outcomes.

Osteochondral Fracture
This fracture occurs off the femoral condyles or the patella. Medial patellar fractures are pathognomonic for acute lateral patellar dislocations. Assessment of patellar instability and positive apprehension to laterally directed pressure helps in the identification of patellar dislocation. An osteochondral fracture may become loose intra-articular fragments from the lateral femoral condyle or the patella, or remain attached to the medial retinaculum. Plain radiographs (AP, lateral, Merchant views) may underestimate the size of lesion, or fail to identify a completely cartilaginous fragment. MRI can successfully detect an osteochondral fracture in those patients with normal radiographs, especially in the presence of an effusion. Arthroscopy is indicated to extract loose bodies and to confirm diagnosis in those knees with suspected loose bodies. Small loose fragments should be removed. Lesions larger than 1 cm, in weight-bearing areas, and with an adequate bony component should be reduced and stabilized. Open arthrotomy can aid in achieving proper reduction and assuring stable fixation.

Distal Femoral Physis Fracture
Fractures about the distal femur (and proximal tibia) typically occur in older children and adolescents with a mean patient age of 14 years. These potentially serious lower extremity injuries are typically secondary to a hyperextension force. Physeal growth disturbance occurs more frequently than in any other location because of the morphology of the physis. Significant fracture energy is necessary to cause physeal failure which thereby compromises the growth capacity of the physis. Most (54%) are Salter-Harris II fractures and these occur more frequently than the other periarticular physeal fractures of the knee (proximal tibial and tibial tubercle). Careful neurovascular examination is

important and may reveal decreased pulses or abnormal function of the tibial or peroneal nerve. Plain radiography typically is adequate. Salter-Harris I and II fractures usually can be managed with closed reduction and under general anesthesia, with screw or pin fixation (crossing proximal to the fracture in the metaphysis). Percutaneous cannulated screw fixation can be placed metaphyseal, using the Thurston-Holland fragment. Fractures with unacceptable alignment should not undergo repeated manipulations, which may further damage the physis. Open reduction is indicated for inadequately reduced fractures. Salter-Harris III and IV fractures are intra-articular and require open anatomic restoration of the articular surface and physis, with fixation, to optimize long-term prognosis. Cannulated screws are placed intercondylar/epiphyseal and should not violate the physis. Anatomic restoration does not guarantee normal growth but minimizes the development of a physeal bar and its effect on growth. Greater fracture displacement at the time of injury is associated with higher incidence of growth disturbance and limb-length discrepancy. Limb-length discrepancy occurs in 32% of fractures and angular deformity in approximately 24%. Neurovascular complications are uncommon and occur in only 2% of fractures.

Tibial Tubercle Fracture

Tibial tubercle injuries occur during maximum contraction of the quadriceps muscle during sport-related activities involving jumping or landing. These injuries are common just before the completion of growth, usually appearing at around age 15 years. The Watson-Jones classification is typically used and is described in Figure 8. Symptoms include pain, swelling, and tenderness over the tibial tubercle with the knee in 20° to 40° of knee flexion. Adequate treatment of type I fractures with minimal displacement is closed reduction with a long leg cast in extension for 6 weeks. Displaced type II and III fractures generally require open reduction and internal fixation. In younger children the fracture should be stabilized with smooth pins to minimize the chance of apophyseal closure and secondary recurvatum. Adolescents with little remaining growth can have their fractures stabilized with more rigid screw fixation.

Proximal Tibial Physis Fracture

Salter-Harris II fractures are most common, followed by type III. Posterior displacement can cause vascular compression at the trifurcation because of the proximity to the proximal tibial metaphysis. Vascular compromise occurs in 5% to 7% of fractures. Prompt reduction is usually definitive; however, persistent vascular impairment requires further study, and possibly treatment. Types I and II can usually be treated with closed reduction, and may be stable in an extended long leg

cast. Fixation of unstable fractures is recommended using smooth, crossed Kirschner wires placed percutaneously using image intensifier guidance. Salter-Harris III and IV fractures are intra-articular and the articular surface and physeal alignment are important in order to minimize the development of a physeal bar and to optimize the long-term function of the articular surface. Open reduction is indicated in intra-articular fractures, to properly align the articular surface and physis, and in irreducible type I and II fractures. Angular deformity occurs in 28% of fractures.

Proximal Metaphyseal (Cozen's) Fractures

These fractures usually occur in children age 6 years or younger. Proximal fractures are associated with tibial overgrowth and a progressive valgus deformity can develop. To minimize this deformity, any acute valgus fracture deformity must be reduced with the extremity immobilized in extension. Valgus deformity noted after the fracture healing should be observed. Initial progression of deformity is typically followed by subsequent remodeling for mild to moderate deformities. A less common occurrence is progression of the valgus deformity and associated tibial overgrowth, which may eventually require surgical treatment. Correction by osteotomy or staple should be deferred as long as possible so as to minimize the potential for recurrence. Correction of a recurrence, if necessary, can be obtained with staple hemiepiphysiodesis.

Diaphyseal Fractures

In children, 30% of fractures of the diaphysis of the tibia occur as an isolated injury. If necessary, closed reduction is performed with conscious sedation or general anesthesia and the fracture immobilized in a long leg cast. Associated plastic deformation of the fibula may prevent correction of the varus deformity. Tibial fractures occurring in association with fibular fractures are potentially more unstable. Acceptable limits of reduction are 50% apposition and 1 cm or less of shortening with less than 10° angulation in the coronal, sagittal, and rotatory planes. (Varus is better tolerated than valgus, and apex anterior angulation better tolerated than apex posterior.) External rotation is better tolerated than internal rotation. If the fractures are reduced, patients are observed closely for neurovascular compromise. Subsequently, fractures are monitored frequently for loss of satisfactory reduction. After fracture consolidation, the above-knee cast is replaced with a well-contoured below-knee cast. Surgical treatment of fractures of the tibia and fibula is indicated if satisfactory alignment by closed means is not possible, or in the presence of comminuted fractures. Treatment of open fractures in children includes the same principles as for adults. Open fractures in children (types I to III) should be treated with immediate irrigation, débridement, and fracture stabilization. Internal or external stabilization can be considered, as appropriate, in fracture management. Recent technical innovations with flexible titanium intramedullary rods have allowed internal fixation of more severely unstable fractures in the skeletally immature patient. For severely comminuted unstable fractures, preferred treatment is the application of an external fixator (monolateral for diaphyseal and circumferential for more distal fractures). Ambulation is encouraged; dynamization is essential in minimizing bone atrophy and delayed consolidation.

Distal Metadiaphyseal Fractures

These fractures are unique to children age 1 to 3 years and occur as a result of tripping and/or falling. The typical scenario is a barely visible distal tibial metadiaphyseal fracture or minimal displacement on radiographs with an intact fibula. Treatment is with a long and/or short leg cast for 3 to 4 weeks. Bicycle-spoke injuries occur in children age 2 to 8 years. Severe compression and/or crushing of the soft tissue occur with the spiral fracture of the distal tibia. This "wringer" type injury should be splinted, and the child admitted for close observation. Fractures of the distal tibia and/or fibula in older children and adolescents typically involve the distal tibia and or fibular physes. Isolated nondisplaced Salter I or II fractures of the distal fibula often masquerade as an ankle sprain (an unlikely injury in this age group) and are typically difficult to see on radiographs. Rotational displacement may occur with a distal tibial Salter I or II injury and if present must be reduced. If the injury goes unrecognized, a permanent rotational deformity can result. Salter II injuries with angular and rotational deformity are more typical and should be reduced under conscious sedation or general anesthesia so as to minimize any further physeal injury. Open reduction may be necessary for the occasional fracture that cannot be reduced because of soft-tissue interposition. The reduced fracture is immobilized in a bent knee long leg cast for 3 to 4 weeks, then converted to a short leg cast for 2 to 3 more weeks. Long-term follow-up is necessary to ascertain any physeal injury affecting growth (predictable in 50% of those significantly displaced).

Annotated Bibliography

Congenital Dislocation of the Knee

Ko JY, Shih CH, Wenger DR: Congenital dislocation of the knee. *J Pediatr Orthop* 1999;19:252-259.

In a review of 24 consecutive cases treated definitively very early (often within the first few hours of life), with closed reduction with or without concomitant traction, results were better in children without associated musculoskeletal anomalies.

Congenital Dislocation of the Patella

Gordon JE, Schoenecker PL: Surgical treatment of congenital dislocation of the patella. *J Pediatr Orthop* 1999;19:260-264.

This article presents a concise review of the unique knee disorder of congenital dislocation of the patella. The surgical technique is comprehensively described and illustrated and the treatment outcomes of 11 patients are also presented.

Discoid Meniscus

Raber DA, Friederich NF, Hefti F: Discoid lateral meniscus in children: Long-term follow-up after total meniscectomy. *J Bone Joint Surg Am* 1998;80:1579-1586.

In a 20-year follow-up study of 17 knees that had undergone total meniscectomy for discoid lateral meniscus, 7 knees were normal, 6 were nearly normal, 3 were abnormal, and 1 severely abnormal. Ten of 17 knees had clinical symptoms of osteoarthritis and two thirds of the knees had radiographic osteoarthritic changes.

Osteochondritis Dissecans

Hefti F, Beguiristain J, Krauspe R, et al: Osteochondritis dissecans: A multicenter study of the European Pediatric Orthopedic Society. *J Pediatr Orthop Br* 1999;8:231-245.

In this large, multicenter retrospective study of 452 patients, better results were noted in skeletally immature patients with lesions smaller than 20 mm, no articular surface disruption, and no effusion. Patients with lesions larger than 20 mm, and knees with effusions and articular surface disruptions had better results with surgical intervention.

Sales de Gauzy J, Mansat C, Darodes PH, Cahuzac JP: Natural course of osteochondritis dissecans in children. *J Pediatr Orthop Br* 1999;8:26-28.

There were 31 cases of osteochondritis dissecans in 24 children (mean age, 11 ± 4 years). No formal treatment was prescribed except for discontinuation of sports activities until pain resolved. Thirty of the 31 cases demonstrated complete radiographic and clinical healing. Some of the lesions required 18 months to heal.

Varus Deformity

Raney EM, Topoleski TA, Yaghoubian R, Guidera KJ, Marshall JG: Orthotic treatment of infantile tibia vara. *J Pediatr Orthop* 1998;18:670-674.

Richards BS, Katz DE, Sims JB: Effectiveness of brace treatment in early infantile Blount's disease. *J Pediatr Orthop* 1998;18:374-380.

Zionts LE, Shean, CJ: Brace treatment of early infantile tibia vara. *J Pediatr Orthop* 1998:18;102-109.

These three similar studies involved a total of 89 patients with Langenskiöld stages I to III infantile Blount disease report resolution of deformity with orthotic treatment in the majority of patients. A lock-knee orthosis was used during weight bearing. Orthotic treatment was less effective in patients with bilateral deformity and not effective in Langenskiöld stage III.

Valgus Deformity

Lin CJ, Lin SC, Huang W, Ho CS, Chou YL: Physiological knock-knee in preschool children: Prevalence, correlating factors, gait analysis, and clinical significance. *J Pediatr Orthop* 1999;19:650-654.

Physiologic knock-knees in 305 preschool children were quantified by measuring the IMD and calculating the IMD index (%) (ratio of IMD to height and weight). The prevalence of physiologic knock-knees was attributed in part to use of walking chairs in infancy.

Stevens PM, Maguire M, Dales MD, Robins AJ: Physeal stapling for idiopathic genu valgum. *J Pediatr Orthop* 1999;19:645-649.

In this large series, 96 patients (152 knees) ranging in age from 6 to 15 years at time of stapling were assessed to skeletal maturity. No premature physeal closure was noted. Knee pain and gait abnormalities resolved with correction.

Fibular Longitudinal Deficiency

Stevens PM, Arms D: Postaxial hypoplasia of the lower extremity. *J Pediatr Orthop* 2000;20:166-172.

This article presents a concise yet comprehensive review of the lower extremity musculoskeletal abnormalities that occur in association with congenital deficiency of the fibula.

ACL Injury

Lee K, Siegel MJ, Lau DM, Hildebolt CF, Matava MJ: Anterior cruciate ligament tears: MR imaging-based diagnosis in a pediatric population. *Radiology* 1999;213:697-704.

Forty-three patients (ages 5 to 16 years), 19 with ACL tears and 24 intact ACLs, underwent MRI evaluation and arthroscopy. Overall sensitivity and specificity of MRI in detecting ACL tears were 95% and 88%, respectively.

Traumatic Abnormalities

Berson L, Davidson RS, Dormans JP, Drummond DS, Gregg JR: Growth disturbances after distal tibial physeal fractures. *Foot Ankle Int* 2000;21:54-58.

This article presents a review of 14 years of experience in the varied treatment of 24 patients for angulatory (average 17°) and/or limb-length discrepancy (average 48 mm) as a result of distal tibial physeal fracture deformities. Analysis of outcome suggests surgical treatment for ≥ 9° or greater of angulation and/or greater than 2 cm of limb-length discrepancy.

Mah JY, Adili A, Otsuka NY, Ogilvie R: Follow-up study of arthroscopic reduction and fixation of III tibial-eminence fractures. *J Pediatr Orthop* 1998;18:475-477.

Nine children (mean age, 13.1 years) with 10 displaced type III tibial eminence fractures underwent arthroscopically-assisted reduction and suture fixation. Ninety percent of the patients had meniscal interposition that was preventing reduction. At final follow-up excellent results were reported in all patients, with no clinical or objective evidence of knee laxity, and full range of motion.

Classic Bibliography

Achterman C, Kalamchi A: Congenital deficiency of the fibula. *J Bone Joint Surg Br* 1979;61:133-137.

Aronson J: Limb-lengthening, skeletal reconstruction, and bone transport with the Ilizarov method. *J Bone Joint Surg Am* 1997;79:1243-1258.

Boero S, Catagni M, Donzelli O, Facchini R, Frediani PV: Congenital pseudarthrosis of the tibia associated with neurofibromatosis-1: Treatment with Ilizarov's device. *J Pediatr Orthop* 1997;17:675-684.

Boyd HB: Pathology and natural history of congenital pseudarthrosis of the tibia. *Clin Orthop* 1982;166:5-13.

Davids JR, Huskamp M, Bagley AM: A dynamic biomechanical analysis of the etiology of adolescent tibia vara. *J Pediatr Orthop* 1996;16:461-468.

Drennan JC: Congenital dislocation of the knee and patella. *Instr Course Lect* 1993;42:517-524.

Gilbert A, Brockman R: Congenital pseudarthrosis of the tibia: Long-term followup of 29 cases treated by microvascular bone transfer. *Clin Orthop* 1995;314:37-44.

Graf BK, Lange RH, Fujisaki CK, Landry GL, Saluja RK: Anterior cruciate ligament tears in skeletally immature patients: Meniscal pathology at presentation and after attempted conservative treatment. *Arthroscopy* 1992;8:229-233.

Hofmann A, Wenger DR: Posteromedial bowing of the tibia: Progression of discrepancy in leg lengths. *J Bone Joint Surg Am* 1981;63:384-388.

Hughston JC, Hergenroeder PT, Courtenay BG: Osteochondritis dissecans of the femoral condyles. *J Bone Joint Surg Am* 1984;66:1340-1348.

Johnston CE II: Infantile tibia vara. *Clin Orthop* 1990;255:13-23.

Langenskiold A: Tibia vara: A critical review. *Clin Orthop* 1989;246:195-207.

Paley D, Herzenberg JE, Tetsworth K, McKie J, Bhave A: Deformity planning for frontal and sagittal plane corrective osteotomies. *Orthop Clin North Am* 1994;25:425-465.

Paley D, Herzenberg JE, Paremain G, Bhave A: Femoral lengthening over an intramedullary nail: A matched-case comparison with Ilizarov femoral lengthening. *J Bone Joint Surg Am* 1997;79:1464-1480.

Price CT, Scott DS, Greenberg DA: Dynamic axial external fixation in the surgical treatment of tibia vara. *J Pediatr Orthop* 1995;15:236-243.

Salenius P, Vankka E: The development of the tibiofemoral angle in children. *J Bone Joint Surg Am* 1975;57:259-261.

Sasaki T, Fukuhara H, Iisaka H, Monji J, Kanno Y, Yasuda K: Postoperative evaluation of quadriceps contracture in children: Comparison of three different procedures. *J Pediatr Orthop* 1985;5:702-707.

Stanitski DF, Dahl M, Louie K, Grayhack J: Management of late-onset tibia vara in the obese patient by using circular external fixation. *J Pediatr Orthop* 1997; 17:691-694.

Thompson GH, Carter JR: Late-onset tibia vara (Blount's disease): Current concepts. *Clin Orthop* 1990; 255:24-35.

Thomson JD, Stricker SJ, Williams MM: Fractures of the distal femoral epiphyseal plate. *J Pediatr Orthop* 1995;15:474-478.

Willis RB, Blokker C, Stoll TM, Paterson DC, Galpin RD: Long-term follow-up of anterior tibial eminence fractures. *J Pediatr Orthop* 1993;13:361-364.

Chapter 42

Knee and Leg: Bone Trauma

Gerald J. Lang, MD

Patella Fractures

Diagnosis

Patella fractures can be caused by direct or indirect trauma. Direct trauma is usually caused by a motor vehicle crash (the knee strikes the dashboard) or a fall. Injury to the skin and soft tissue overlying the patella often occurs with an abrasion, contusion, or even an open wound. The retinaculum is often disrupted but can remain intact in some minimally displaced patella fractures caused by direct trauma. The functional integrity of the extensor mechanism can be tested in patients with an intact retinaculum with a straight leg raise against gravity. Comminution and articular impaction of the patella can be quite severe. Ipsilateral limb injuries, such as femoral shaft fractures or posterior hip dislocations, also can occur in injuries caused by direct trauma.

Indirect trauma usually is caused by eccentric muscle contraction of the quadriceps in the face of knee flexion. This situation causes a tension fracture of the patella with disruption of the extensor mechanism, including the retinaculum. Cephalad migration of the proximal fracture fragment is common. Straight leg raising is not possible with complete extensor mechanism rupture.

Standard radiographic evaluation of a patient with a knee injury begins with AP and lateral views. Patella fractures are most easily viewed in the lateral projection. Displacement, comminution, and articular impaction are apparent. The AP view is obscured by the overlying femur but can reveal valuable information about complex fracture patterns and vertically oriented fracture lines. Occasionally the sunrise view is helpful in evaluating vertical fractures, highly comminuted fractures, and osteochondral injuries associated with patellar dislocations. CT scanning is rarely indicated in the evaluation of patella fractures. MRI has been of value in imaging the unossified portion of the patella in skeletally immature patients suspected of having patellar sleeve fractures.

Treatment Options

Nonsurgical

Minimally displaced or nondisplaced patella fractures with a functioning extensor mechanism and acceptable articular alignment ($\leq$ 2 mm of displacement) can be managed without surgery. Early weight bearing with the knee in full extension is encouraged. Early active knee range of motion can be initiated with the use of a hinged brace. The benefits of early weight bearing and early functional motion outweigh the small risk of fracture displacement. Cylinder cast application is recommended for noncompliant patients. Patients should be reevaluated both clinically and radiographically at regular intervals to detect loss of alignment and to document the integrity of the extensor mechanism function. Generally, results are good to excellent in 90% of patients. Nonsurgical treatment is sometimes appropriate in patients with displaced patellar fractures who are elderly, debilitated, have low physical demands, or have medical contraindications to surgical treatment.

Surgical

The general indications for surgical treatment are unacceptable articular alignment ($\geq$ 2 to 3 mm of fracture displacement) and/or an incompetent extensor mechanism. Open reduction and internal fixation generally is favored except in severely comminuted fractures where partial or complete patellectomy is involved. It is thought that preserving even a portion of the patella is preferable to a complete patellectomy. The minimum size of patellar fragment needed for partial patellectomy has not been determined. Complete patellectomy is rarely indicated. The importance of a meticulous repair of the retinaculum and other soft tissue cannot be overemphasized.

Modified AO techniques using Kirschner wires and a tension band wire in a figure-of-8 pattern have been used for the classic two-part transverse fracture. Many comminuted fractures have a predominant transverse component. Lag screws and Kirschner wires are used to stabilize other, often more vertically oriented, fracture lines. A moderate rate of fracture displacement (up to 22%) has been reported using modified AO techniques. Technical errors and patient noncompliance have been listed as factors contributing to displacement. One recognized technical error was the failure to establish good contact between the tension wire and the poles of the patella. This factor also has been noted in displacement demonstrated during laboratory testing of transverse patellar fracture models.

Therefore, lag screws (standard or cannulated) combined with a tension band device (wire or heavy braided suture) have been used. Heavy braided suture (No. 5) has been shown to be comparable to 18-gauge wire in laboratory testing and is advantageous because it is easier to handle. Tension band wires (or suture) through parallel-cannulated screws has been shown to be more stable than modified AO tension band wiring or lag screws alone. It is important that the threaded portions of the cannulated screws do not protrude through the end of the bone because the tension devices (suture or wire) could be weakened or ruptured by the sharp edges of the screw.

Accurate reduction and secure fixation of fracture fragments is important. Reduction should be confirmed by palpation of the articular surface through the retinacular disruption and by occasional use of fluoroscopy. Fixation strategies vary according to fracture patterns and bone quality. Lag screws, Kirschner wires, wire, and heavy suture can be used in combination for fixation of comminuted fractures. Partial patellectomy and soft-tissue repair is recommended for comminuted fractures in which accurate reduction or stable fixation is not possible. Occasionally, open reduction and internal fixation of larger fragments can be combined with partial patellectomy.

The postoperative regimen will depend on the stability of the repair. If secure fixation and retinacular repair are obtained, early weight bearing in extension and early range of motion (ROM) are recommended. If fixation is less secure, then delaying ROM may be indicated. If loss of reduction of less than 2 mm occurs during the early postoperative period, repeat open reduction and internal fixation should be considered. Overall reported rates of complication have been low, with 70% to 80% of patients reporting good to excellent results. Symptomatic hardware and loss of reduction have been the most common complications.

Tibial Plateau Fractures
Classification

The Schatzker classification is the most well recognized and is used to classify tibial plateau fractures. Types I, II, and III fractures involve only the lateral tibial plateau, whereas type IV fractures typically involve the medial tibial plateau. Types V and VI fractures involve both medial and lateral portions of the tibial plateau.

The AO/ASIF classification scheme is also well recognized and has been adopted by the Orthopaedic Trauma Association (OTA). It divides fractures into nonarticular (type A), partial articular (type B or Schatzker types I through IV) and complete articular (type C or Schatzker types V and VI). Further subcategorization is done according to the degree of articular and metaphyseal comminution. It is helpful to subdivide Schatzker type VI fractures into AO type C (1, 2, and 3) to represent a broad range of osseous injury.

Associated Injuries

It is important to evaluate the injury to the soft tissue around the tibial plateau. Soft-tissue injuries, which can range from minimal to quite severe, are manifested by generalized edema, skin contusion/abrasion, fracture blisters, compartment syndrome, and open fracture wounds. Recognizing and respecting the limitations of the injured soft tissues of the proximal tibia will help guide clinical decision-making. The more severe the soft-tissue injury, the greater the likelihood of increased operative morbidity in open procedures. Delaying fracture fixation until the soft-tissue injury evolves is gaining popularity, because this decision is believed to lead to a reduction in complications.

Injuries to other structures around the knee associated with fractures of the tibial plateau are common. The ligamentous structures all are susceptible to injury. Similarly, injuries to both the medial and lateral meniscus are often associated with fractures of the tibial plateau or fracture dislocations of the knee. Direct chondral injury is frequently seen in injuries caused by axial compression.

Injuries to the popliteal artery, peroneal nerve, and tibial nerve are rare but can be seen with severe tibial plateau fractures. Similarly, severe soft-tissue injury and swelling of the lower leg can lead to compartment syndrome. Ipsilateral limb injuries (femoral shaft, distal femur, tibial shaft, or distal tibial) can alter standard treatment plans. Careful timing and planning is needed in these situations.

Evaluation

Patient history regarding the injury is useful for predicting the degree of soft-tissue trauma and determining the

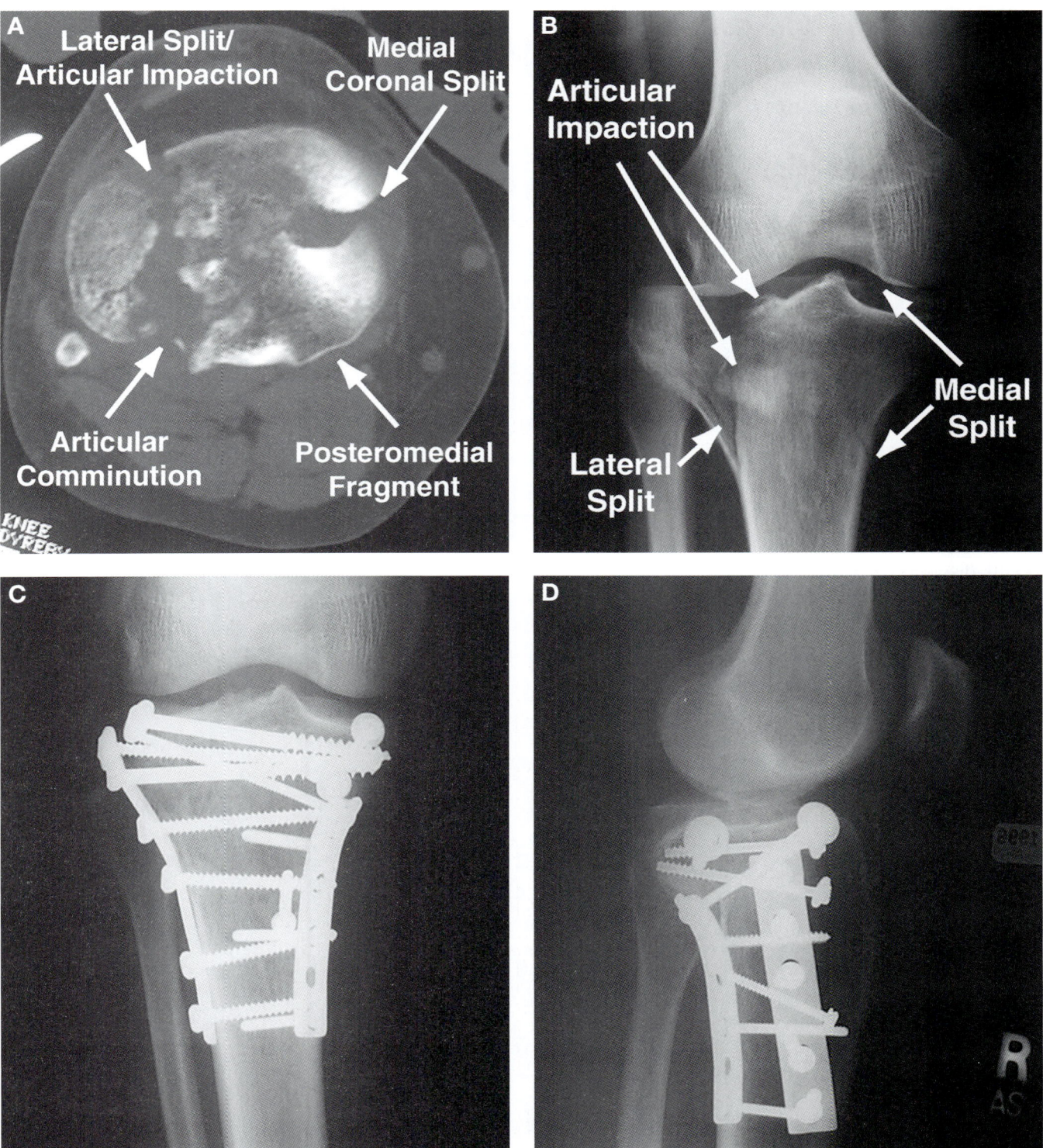

Figure 1 Extensively comminuted bicondylar tibial plateau fracture. Inspection of CT scan (**A**) and plain radiographs (**B** through **D**) reveals articular impaction of the lateral compartment and a coronal split in the medial compartment. Reduction and fixation was accomplished through simultaneous anterolateral and posteromedial incisions.

likelihood of associated injuries. A thorough physical examination of the entire limb should be done to assess neurologic and circulatory status. Significant knee effusion, deformity, and instability can be present.

The initial imaging studies in the evaluation of a tibial plateau fracture include an AP and lateral radiograph of the knee taken on long cassettes. An AP radiograph with 10° of caudal tilt can more accurately profile the posterior slope of the tibial articular surface.

CT scanning is helpful to further evaluate the osseous injuries of tibial plateau fractures. Standard axial images can be reformatted to coronal and sagittal two-dimensional reconstructions to further define the location, degree, and size of articular impaction and supply critical cross-sectional anatomy of the fracture, which is useful in planning surgical techniques, particularly those that are less invasive (Fig. 1). Three-dimensional CT scanning has not been widely used in these injuries.

MRI is useful in assessing soft-tissue injury around the knee in the presence of a tibial plateau fracture. The status of the ligamentous structures as well as the menisci can usually be determined. MRI can accurately reveal simple fracture geometry but has some limitations in detailed imaging of severely comminuted fractures.

Treatment Options

Nonsurgical

Nonsurgical treatment is indicated for low-energy, minimally displaced fractures. There should not be any significant articular offset or depression (< 3 to 5 mm) and no significant clinical instability on examination. When the relative risks of surgery become too high (severe soft-tissue damage, poor host), nonsurgical treatment is pursued. Simple immobilization with a brace or a cast is initially performed. Once acute swelling and pain diminishes, the patient should be converted to a hinged fracture brace and allowed to work on ROM. It is important to delay weight bearing until radiographic healing has occurred (generally 8 to 12 weeks).

Surgical

The main indications for surgical treatment of tibial plateau fractures are articular displacement and instability. Articular depression or fracture displacements that contribute to joint instability are also used as an indication for surgery. Absolute surgical indications include open fractures and fractures associated with an acute compartment syndrome. These indications, however, are focused on the treatment of soft-tissue components of the injury. The amount of articular depression that would warrant surgical intervention is not universally accepted. Instead of focusing on a particular amount of depression or displacement, it is more useful to combine this information with the rest of the injury pattern. Every effort should be made to preserve or repair an injured meniscus that occurs in association with a tibial plateau fracture.

In a Schatzker type I (simple split) fracture, reduction and fixation either by open or closed methods are possible and can lead to a successful outcome. Fixation with either lag screws or lag screws with a buttress plate is recommended. The quality of bone, size of the split fragment, and condition of the surrounding soft tissue help guide the degree of surgical exposure and fixation devices. Arthroscopy or fluoroscopy have been used as aids to indirect reduction techniques.

In a type II (split/depression) fracture, the emphasis is on accurate elevation of the impacted articular segments and stable fixation of the split and depressed fragments. Often severe articular impaction or displacement is associated with a peripheral lateral meniscal tear, which is driven down into the fracture site. This must be retrieved prior to the reduction of the fracture. Meniscal repair (when possible) is indicated in this situation. This fracture type often requires open reduction with the elevation of the articular fractures and filling the bone defect with either autogenous iliac crest bone graft, allograft, or bone substitute. These fractures typically are treated with a buttress plate and lag screws. More anatomically-shaped plates that allow placement of screws close to their articular surface to help support the impacted articular segments are available. These plates can be more easily applied using indirect or percutaneous methods. There has been an emphasis on minimizing surgical exposure and also on using a fluoroscope or arthroscope to assess the quality of the articular reduction.

A type III (depressed segment only) plateau fracture is relatively rare and has an intact peripheral rim of cortical bone. This variety of fracture is ideal for arthroscopic evaluation. Generally, a hole has to be drilled in the tibial metaphysis below the fracture and the articular impaction is elevated either under fluoroscopic guidance or under direct visualization through the arthroscope. Once these impacted articular segments are elevated, they are supported by subchondral screws and graft material.

Type IV fractures vary in severity. Generally the medial plateau fracture fragment maintains the normal anatomic relationship with the medial femoral condyle. The lateral articular surface and shaft are usually dislocated laterally from the lateral femoral condyle. Surgical treatment is needed to reestablish the osseous anatomy, usually with either an open or closed reduction with lag screws, which may or may not need to be augmented with a buttress plate. Once the osseous injury is repaired, the ligamentous examination should further identify lateral ligamentous injuries in need of repair. If the patient has posterolateral instability, a direct repair of the posterolateral corner is indicated. Soft-tissue trauma can be quite severe with these injuries.

Bicondylar fractures (types V and VI) are the most complex and often are associated with the most severe soft-tissue injuries. A significant amount of preoperative planning is necessary in order to understand all components of the injury and to create a strategy for repair. Direct articular exposure and reduction is needed if significant articular impaction is seen. Simple articular fractures can often be reduced with closed or minimally invasive methods and percutaneous lag screw fixation. Most metaphyseal components of type VI fractures (AO type C2 and C3 fractures) can be aligned by indirect means and stabilized in a minimally invasive manner (external fixator or bridge plate). More experience has been obtained with the use of fine wire fixators either combined with standard Ilizarov type rings distally or half pins for so-called hybrid fixators. These methods are very effective in bridging across the metaphyseal-comminuted area but cannot be considered a substitute for a satisfactory articular reduction. Soft-tissue problems have been minimized using this technique; however, placement of the fine wires near the knee joint has given rise to an occasional infection with intra-articular spread. It has been recommended that the fine wires for a circular fixator be placed no closer than 15 mm of the articular surface to minimize the problem of knee sepsis 2° to a pin tract infection. Medial and lateral plates placed through a midline incision have fallen out of favor because of the excessive soft-tissue stripping needed. Using two plates through separate soft-tissue incisions has shown improved results while minimizing complications. Often this method is combined with an anterolateral and posterior medial incision. Again, all emphasis is on maintaining the integrity of the soft tissue and minimizing soft-tissue problems, while at the same time obtaining anatomic reductions and stable fixation.

Tibial Shaft Fractures

Tibial shaft fractures run the spectrum from nondisplaced low-energy fractures that heal with immobilization and produce no disability to severe open fractures with bone and soft-tissue loss that can necessitate primary below-knee amputation. Because of their relatively superficial location and poor blood supply, tibial shaft fractures are often open injuries and healing may be slow.

Classification

Several classification schemes have been developed for both open and closed tibial shaft fractures and can be useful for comparing studies and selecting appropriate treatment for each individual patient. The goal of proper classification is to identify the fractures that have a poor prognosis for healing and leg function (generally the higher-energy fractures).

The AO/ASIF classification scheme is the most common and has been adopted by the OTA. It divides fractures into type A (simple, caused by low force or torsional indirect trauma), type B (bending wedge, intermediate force), and type C (complex, direct high-energy trauma). Soft-tissue injury surrounding comminuted fractures (type C) is generally moderate to severe. Simple fractures have the best prognosis and complex fractures have the worst.

The Tscherne classification system of soft-tissue injury associated with closed fractures is useful and can aid in the decision-making process in the management of closed tibial shaft fractures. A grade 0 injury has minimal soft-tissue damage and swelling; a grade 1 injury has some abrasion/contusion of the skin and moderate swelling; a grade 2 injury has deep abrasions/contusions with significant soft-tissue swelling to the point of an impending compartment syndrome; and a grade 3 injury is a decompensated compartment syndrome requiring fasciotomy. Grades 0 and 1 injuries are generally caused by indirect or moderate direct trauma, have simpler fracture patterns, and have soft tissue suitable for direct incisions. Grade 2 and 3 soft-tissue injuries are indicative of high-energy trauma, more fracture comminution, and skin that is less suitable for surgical incisions. These injuries generally are caused by high-energy direct trauma or crush injuries.

Open fractures are classified by the amount of damage to the soft tissue around the fracture. The Gustilo classification scheme is the most widely used. Grade I injuries are minor open fractures with a small (≤ 1 cm) skin wound likely caused by the bone poking through the skin and have simple fracture patterns. Grade II injuries have larger open wounds (1 to 10 cm) but still have simple fracture patterns with minimal periosteal stripping. Grade III injuries have severe soft-tissue damage; IIIA fractures can still be closed primarily; and IIIB wounds require a flap (local or distant) for soft-tissue coverage. Grade IIIB fractures have been further subdivided into those with significant bone loss and those without because limb reconstruction with bone loss is more difficult with a higher complication rate. Grade IIIC open fractures require repair or reconstruction of an arterial injury to maintain limb viability.

Patient Evaluation

Careful patient evaluation and history is imperative and will provide some insight into the amount of energy absorbed to cause the fracture so that appropriate treatment can be initiated. A torsional injury sustained in a sporting event versus one caused by a motor vehicle are, to most clinicians, two very distinct injuries. Focused evaluation of the limb should document the degree of soft-tissue injury visible, degree of deformity and/or instability at the fracture site, and neurovascular function. The injury is generally considered an open fracture if an open wound is present, even if it is quite distant from the fracture. Because diaphyseal and metaphyseal fracture lines can occasionally extend into the knee and ankle joints, full radiologic examination (AP and lateral) should include these joints in addition to the tibial shaft.

Treatment Options

Treatment options are quite broad when it comes to treating the full spectrum of tibial shaft fractures. In general, the higher grade the injury, whether open or closed, the more aggressive the surgical treatment needed to maximize function.

Most authors recommend ≤ 5° of angular alignment, ≤ 10° of rotation malalignment, and ≤ 12 mm of shortening as guidelines for acceptable alignment of a tibial shaft fracture after healing. Although firm evidence is lacking, it is believed that there is some threshold of malalignment that will lead to poor function of the limb.

Closed reduction and casting followed by bracing is the treatment of choice for most low-energy and many midrange-energy fractures. Plate osteosynthesis has a role in the tibial metaphyseal region whereas intramedullary nails have limitations. Interest in plating has increased as less invasive (percutaneous) methods of insertion have been developed.

External fixation is used for osseous and soft-tissue stabilization in open fractures of the tibia. The procedure is minimally invasive and can be applied as either definitive or provisional stabilization. External fixation is preferred when the injured tibia has a small canal (< 8 mm) or when an amputation is being considered.

Intramedullary (IM) nailing remains the treatment of choice for unstable and/or displaced tibial shaft fractures. Locking screws provide stability for axially unstable and metaphyseal fractures. When locking IM nails became available for the tibia, the smallest size was 12 mm in diameter, making reaming of the canal imperative for insertion. Nails are now available in diameters as small as 8 mm, which allows nails to be placed into the tibia without reaming the canal in many instances. It was believed that placing small-diameter nails without reaming caused significantly less damage to the endosteal circulation and promoted earlier healing; however, fracture stability (which is generally better with larger nails) and fatigue strength of the implants (both nails and interlocking screws) were compromised.

Reaming of the canal has been shown to damage the endosteal circulation of the tibia in an animal model. The bone injury caused by reaming, however, may have a paradoxical response on the periosteal circulation.

The benefits of the larger diameter reamed nail are better fracture stability, larger locking screws (which resist fatigue failure better), and better fatigue properties of the nail (although nail breakage has not been a significant problem with small-diameter nails). Reamings placed at the fracture site may also contribute to healing.

Proponents of the unreamed technique believe that the practice leads to less damage to the vessels providing endosteal circulation. The blood supply of the tibia is adversely affected during nail insertion, much as during the first pass with a reamer, but revascularization is much quicker in animal models. However, because the implants and locking screws are smaller, fixation is less stable and fatigue strength is diminished. The fractures most often managed with the unreamed technique are those with more severe biologic injury. These fractures take longer to heal, which makes the fatigue strength of the locking bolts an issue.

A newer concept, called limited reaming, allows the insertion of moderate-sized nails with larger locking screws so that iatrogenic damage to the endosteal circulation will be limited, while the canal will be enlarged enough to place a nail with larger cross bolts. This approach is an attempt to balance the biologic and mechanical environment most suitable for healing.

Closed Tibial Fractures

As a general rule, low-energy and minimally displaced fractures can be treated with initial reduction (if needed) and cast application, with subsequent transition to a prefabricated patellar tendon bearing fracture brace and early weight bearing. Indications for cast/brace treatment are limited to closed transverse fractures that have axial stability after reduction and to axially unstable tibial fracture patterns (spiral, oblique, or comminuted) associated with no more than 12 mm of initial shortening. Severe soft-tissue injury (Tscherne grade 2 and 3) with swelling and/or impending compartment syndrome makes casting/bracing unreasonable. If alignment is unacceptable, surgical treatment should be considered. Most indications for surgical treatment of closed tibial fractures are relative and include segmental fractures, ipsilateral limb injury (floating knee, ankle or calcaneus fracture), multiple trauma, intra-articular extension, and bilateral fractures. High-energy, unstable closed tibial fractures (AO/ASIF type B and C, or Tscherne grade 1, 2, or 3) that will take longer to heal, such as comminuted and severely displaced fractures, have less predictable results with casting and bracing and should be considered for surgical treatment.

Several prospective randomized trials of reamed versus unreamed tibial nailing for closed tibial shaft fractures revealed a slightly higher healing rate and less hardware failure (locking bolts only) for the reamed group. No difference was seen in the rate of malunion, infection, compartment syndrome, or knee pain. It appears that reamed techniques are favored in the treatment of closed fractures.

Open Tibial Fractures

Several issues must be considered when treating open fractures. These fractures are usually the result of high-energy direct trauma, with associated trauma elsewhere in the body likely. The presence of a wound over the fracture increases the likelihood of infection. The incidence of infection appears to be correlated with the degree of soft-tissue and bone injury, degree of contamination, use of antibiotics, and the timing and adequacy of débridement. The urgency and adequacy of the débridement and the timely administration of antibiotics are factors potentially controlled by the surgeon.

With the increasing ability to salvage severely traumatized limbs with open tibial fractures, an effort has been made to more clearly define which limbs can be successfully reconstructed and which should be immediately amputated. A recent study reported on the prospective application of a multiple scoring scheme to 357 type III open tibial fractures and evaluated the recommended threshold value for amputation. All of the scoring systems, including the Mangled Extremity Severity Score, the Predictive Salvage Index, the Limb Salvage Index, NISSSA (an acronym for the following variables: Nerve Injury, Ischemia, Soft-Tissue Injury, Skeletal Injury, Shock, and Age) and the Hannover Fracture Score, had relatively low sensitivity and relatively high specificity. Of all the amputations, 58% to 90% occurred above the indices' critical thresholds and 16% to 22% occurred below the thresholds. This study concluded that no current scoring system index can be used alone to decide whether limb salvage or amputation should be done.

Stabilizing the extremity can be done with a plate, an external fixator, or interlocking IM nail. On occasion, it is appropriate to place a stable low-grade open fracture into a cast.

Use of a plate to stabilize an open tibial fracture has been discouraged in the past because of the additional soft-tissue stripping needed to apply the plate. Plates still have a limited role in the treatment of open tibial diaphyseal fractures, and can be used only when minimal additional soft-tissue dissection is needed (percutaneous application) or where the use of nails is limited (proximal and distal metaphysis).

There has been concern that placing an IM nail to stabilize an open tibial fracture leads to high infection rates. In pooling data from multiple studies on open tibial fractures treated with unreamed nailing, the rate of deep infection is reported as zero for type I open fractures, 4% for type II fractures, 7% for type IIIA fractures, and 17% for grade IIIB fractures. Acceptably low infection rates are obtained when the use of aggressive wound débridements is combined with the use of nonreamed IM nails.

External fixators have been used extensively for osseous stabilization of open tibial fractures. Their main benefit has been to provide needed stability and limit any further surgical insult on the leg during the acute period. Although external fixation provided satisfactory results, the instances of nonunion and malunion were high, as were the rates of pin tract infections. With the advent of small-diameter interlocking IM nails, it became possible to stabilize these injuries without reaming.

Several studies have compared the results of external fixation and nonreamed IM nailing in the management of open tibial fractures. All studies concluded that IM nailing provided better results than external fixation. Patients with IM nailing had less deformity, improved limb function, and shorter time to weight bearing. The use of IM nailing also simplified soft-tissue coverage and subsequent bone grafting operations. Rates of infection and speed of healing were not affected by the choice of implant. It can also be concluded that the most important factor determining the occurrence of infection is not the implant selected for stabilization but rather the degree of soft-tissue damage and management of soft-tissue envelope and bony injury. Therefore, although external fixation remains a valuable adjunct in the management of open tibial fracture, it appears that the use of IM nailing is preferred in most instances.

Reamed Intramedullary Nailing With Open Fractures

The use of reamed IM nailing has generally been contraindicated in open tibial fractures because of concern over historically high infection rates and excessive damage to the endosteal blood supply caused by reaming. This hypothesis has been tested at two centers with prospective randomized trials and has not shown a significant increase in the rate of infection when comparing reamed and nonreamed nailing. Pooled data on 139 open fractures randomized either to reamed or nonreamed nailing showed an overall infection rate of only 3.5%. Five infections developed: two in the nonreamed group and three in the reamed group, one of which occurred after nail removal. At both centers, antibiotic bead pouches were routinely used after initial débridement, which may help explain the overall low rate of infection. The rate of healing was similar in both groups. A larger number of interlocking screw fatigues were present in the nonreamed group.

The risk of infection and rate of healing of open tibial fractures are both dependent on many factors. Based on these two studies, it does not appear as though the method of nail insertion had much of an effect. More recently, reaming has been done on a limited basis to minimally enlarge the canal and limit the amount of endosteal cortical necrosis. This method of limited reaming is an attempt to minimize the biologic insult of nailing yet obtain optimal mechanical stability with a slightly larger nail and larger locking screws with better fatigue properties.

Proximal Tibial Fractures

The widespread use of IM nailing has been extended to the proximal segment of the tibia. Fractures of the proximal third are relatively uncommon, representing 5% to 10% of tibial fractures in most series. Standard nailing techniques often lead to malalignment of proximal fractures. Multiple etiologies have been described and adjustments to the surgical techniques have been proposed. The tibial nail insertion point should be located on the very proximal portion of the anterior cortex. It has been pointed out that the central starting point in the proximal tibia is in line with the medial portion of the lateral tibial eminence. Improved alignment with nailing of proximal fractures has been reported with a semiextended position, the use of small temporary unicortical plating (to secure reduction prior to passing the nail), and the use of a femoral distractor for reduction. Other investigators have recognized that they are at the limits of their ability with IM nailing and have recommended alternate techniques using external fixation, plating, or a combination of the two.

Complications

Knee Pain With Intramedullary Nailing

A high incidence of knee pain (10% to 60%) has been associated with IM nailing. Nail removal as a result of knee pain ranges from 10% to 55%, depending on the duration of follow-up. However, the pain is not always completely resolved. The incidence of pain is higher when the nail was inserted by a patellar tendon-splitting approach versus a paratendon approach.

The exact cause of knee pain remains unclear. The desired staring point for tibial nail insertion has migrated proximally near the articular surface of the tibia. The medial meniscus and lateral tibial articular surface are close to the insertion point and at risk for injury.

Compartment Syndrome

Compartment syndrome is a well-recognized complication associated with open and closed fractures of the tibial shaft, with an incidence ranging from 1% to 9%. If left untreated, compartment syndrome will lead to irreversible necrosis of muscle in the lower leg and also loss of nerve function. Diagnosis and recognition of this condition can be difficult; complaints from the patient and subjective observation of the leg are diagnostic factors. Often, intracompartmental pressure monitoring is needed to diagnose compartment syndrome. In the past, absolute pressure values of 30 to 45 mm Hg inside the compartments were used as guidelines for diagnosing compartment syndrome. More recently, a relative value—the difference between the patient's diastolic blood pressure and compartment pressure—has been used as a guideline. The critical point appears to be when the compartment pressure is within 30 mm Hg of the diastolic pressure.

Iatrogenic compartment syndrome associated with tibial nailing is also cause for concern. The most important factors that increase intracompartmental pressure are longitudinal traction, placement of an IM device, and the position of the lower leg. There are peaks in the intracompartmental pressure during fracture reduction, initial reamer passage (in reamed nail insertion) and with nail passage (in nonreamed nail insertion), but these are generally not sustained and do come back down to baseline levels. Prolonged distraction or use of a countertraction device on the posterior thigh, which is common during a 90°-90° positioning on a fracture table, may also play a role in the development of compartment syndrome. The role of reaming has been a cause for concern with IM nailing in its relationship to compartment syndrome, leading to increased interest in using nonreamed techniques to stabilize fractures with Tscherne grade II and III soft-tissue injuries. However, results from two studies that compared reamed versus nonreamed nailing of closed tibial fractures in the same patient population indicated that the instance of compartment syndrome was no different in either group. Results from another recent study indicated similar compartment pressures for both reamed and nonreamed nailing of closed tibial fractures treated without the use of a fracture table.

Once the diagnosis of compartment syndrome has been made, fasciotomy should be done promptly, through a single long lateral incision based over the fibula or a more traditional two-incision technique, in which the first incision is based over the intermuscular septum between the anterior and lateral compartments, and the second posterior to the medial crest of the tibia. All four compartments should be released along the entire length. Management of the wounds includes moist dressing, elevation, and attempted closure at 2 to 7 days. If swelling remains excessive, split-thickness skin grafting is recommended.

Nonunion

Because the tibia is a commonly fractured bone and also has a relatively poor healing potential, tibial fracture nonunions are common. Contributing factors include degree of soft-tissue and bone trauma, history of an open wound, smoking, and method of initial treatment. Occult infection should be considered in a previously open fracture or a fracture treated surgically.

There are many options for treating fracture nonunion, including IM nailing, exchange nailing (recommended for previously nailed fractures), plate fixation with bone grafting (recommended for fractures previously treated with external fixators) or bone grafting alone. Exchange nailing is not recommended in nonunions with significant amounts (> 30% to 40%) of cortical bone loss. Open bone grafting is recommended. Complex nonunions with compromised soft tissue and malalignment have been managed effectively with the Ilizarov technique.

The role of nonsurgical methods, such as ultrasound or electrical stimulation, remains unclear. Bone morphogenetic protein-2 or -7 is being developed for treatment of tibial nonunions.

Annotated Bibliography

Patella Fractures

Patel VR, Parks BG, Wang Y, Ebert FR, Jinnah RH: Fixation of patella fractures with braided polyester suture: A biomechanical study. *Injury* 2000;31:1-6.

Under biomechanical testing, nonabsorbable suture (two strands of No. 5 Ethibond) performed similarly to a loop of 1.25-mm stainless steel wire in a transverse patella fracture. Displacement (greater than 1 mm) seen during mechanical testing was due to surgical error (not having close contact with the loops of sutures or wire at the poles of the patella) and not selection of material future tension band technique.

Tibia Fractures

Adams CI, Keating JF, Court-Brown CM: Cigarette smoking and open tibial fractures. *Injury* 2001;32:61-65.

This study compared two groups of patients with open tibial fractures: 140 smokers versus 133 nonsmokers. Healing was slower (32 versus 28 weeks), flap failure rate was higher (20% versus 14%) and rate of nonunion higher in the smoking group.

Bosse MJ, MacKenzie EJ, Kellam JF, et al: A prospective evaluation of the clinical utility of the lower-extremity injury-severity scores. *J Bone Joint Surg Am* 2001;83:3-14.

In 556 high-energy lower extremity injuries, each limb was assigned several widely used limb salvage injury scores. These scores did not appear to be appropriate for deciding whether to amputate, because some limbs above the thresholds were salvaged. A score below the threshold may be helpful in attempting limb salvage in certain situations.

Emami A, Petren-Mallmin M, Larsson S: No effect of low-intensity ultrasound on healing time of intramedullary fixed tibial fractures. *J Orthop Trauma* 1999;13:252-257.

Thirty-two tibial fractures were treated with reamed IM nailing supplemented with either low-intensity ultrasound or placebo. No significant difference in healing was seen between the groups.

Finkemeier CG, Schmidt AH, Kyle RF, Templeman DC, Varecka TF: A prospective, randomized study of intramedullary nails inserted with and without reaming for the treatment of open and closed fractures of the tibial shaft. *J Orthop Trauma* 2000;14:187-193.

Forty-five open (grade I-IIIA) and 49 closed fractures were randomized to either reamed or nonreamed nail insertion. Reamed nailing showed slightly faster healing in closed fractures (but not open). Nonreamed nail insertion did not protect patients from infection or compartment syndrome as these rates were similar in both groups.

Henley MB, Chapman JR, Agel J, Harvey EJ, Whorton AM, Swiontkowski MF: Treatment of type II, IIIA, and IIIB open fractures of the tibial shaft: A prospective comparison of unreamed interlocking intramedullary nails and half-pin external fixators. *J Orthop Trauma* 1998;12:1-7.

One hundred seventy-four open grade II, IIIA, and IIIB were prospectively randomized to skeletal fixation with either an external fixator (70) or an IM nail (104) placed without reaming. Malalignment was more prevalent in the external fixator group (21% versus 8%). Secondary surgery to obtain healing was less likely with IM nailing. Infection rates at the open fracture site and rate of fracture healing were similar in both groups. IM nailing also simplified soft-tissue coverage.

Karladani AH, Granhed H, Edshage B, Jerre R, Styf J: Displaced tibial shaft fractures: A prospective randomized study of closed intramedullary nailing versus cast treatment in 53 patients. *Acta Orthop Scand* 2000;71:160-167.

In a study of 53 displaced tibial shaft fractures randomized to either IM nailing (27) or cast treatment (26), delayed union, nonunion, and malunion, and restricted knee and ankle motion were all more common in the cast group. Knee pain was present in 44% of the IM nailing group and absent in the cast group.

Nassif JM, Gorczyca JT, Cole JK, Pugh KJ, Pienkowski D: Effect of acute reamed versus unreamed intramedullary nailing on compartment pressure when treating closed tibial shaft fractures: A randomized prospective study. *J Orthop Trauma* 2000;14:554-558.

In 49 closed tibia fractures undergoing IM nailing, compartment pressure transiently increased with reaming in the reamed group and with nail passage in the reamed group. Higher pressures were seen in the nonreamed groups postoperatively. No patient developed a compartment syndrome. Acute nailing (less than 3 days) proved to be safe in this study of closed fractures without a fracture tube and reaming did not show any adverse effects.

Reid JS, Van Slyke MA, Moulton MJ, Mann TA: Safe placement of proximal tibial transfixation wires with respect to intracapsular penetration. *J Orthop Trauma* 2001;15:10-17.

This anatomic and MRI study located the extent of capsular reflection below the subchondral bone of the proximal tibial. The capsular reflection was less than 14 mm below the joint and was the lowest posterior to the proximal fibula.

Classic Bibliography

Berg EE: Open reduction internal fixation of displaced transverse patella fractures with figure-eight wiring through parallel cannulated compression screws. *J Orthop Trauma* 1997;11:573-576.

Blachut PA, O'Brien PJ, Meek RN, Broekhuyse HM: Interlocking intramedullary nailing with and without reaming for the treatment of closed fractures of the tibial shaft: A prospective randomized study. *J Bone Joint Surg Am* 1997;79:640-646.

Bolhofner BR: Indirect reduction and composite fixation of extraarticular proximal tibial fractures. *Clin Orthop* 1995;315:75-83.

Bone LB, Sucato D, Stegemann PM, Rohrbacher BJ: Displaced isolated fractures of the tibial shaft treated with either a cast or intramedullary nailing: An outcome analysis of matched pairs of patients. *J Bone Joint Surg Am* 1997;79:1336-1341.

Carpenter JE, Kasman RA, Patel N, Lee ML, Goldstein SA: Biomechanical evaluation of current patella fracture fixation techniques. *J Orthop Trauma* 1997;11:351-356.

Cook SD, Ryaby JP, McCabe J, Frey JJ, Heckman JD, Kristiansen TK: Acceleration of tibia and distal radius fracture healing in patients who smoke. *Clin Orthop* 1997;337:198-207.

Duwelius PJ, Rangitsch MR, Colville MR, Woll TS: Treatment of tibial plateau fractures by limited internal fixation. *Clin Orthop* 1997;339:47-57.

Georgiadis GM: Combined anterior and posterior approaches for complex tibial plateau fractures. *J Bone Joint Surg Br* 1994;76:285-289.

Gustilo RB, Mendoza RM, Williams DM: Problems in the management of type III (severe) open fractures: A new classification of type III open fractures. *J Trauma* 1984;24:742-746.

Holt MD, Williams LA, Dent CM: MRI in the management of tibial plateau fractures. *Injury* 1995;26:595-599.

Hooper GJ, Keddell RG, Penny ID: Conservative management or closed nailing for tibial shaft fractures: A randomised prospective trial. *J Bone Joint Surg Br* 1991;73:83-85.

Keating JF, O'Brien PJ, Blachut PA, Meek RN, Broekhuyse HM: Locking intramedullary nailing with and without reaming for open fractures of the tibial shaft: A prospective, randomized study. *J Bone Joint Surg Am* 1997;79:334-341.

Keating JF, Orfaly R, O'Brien PJ: Knee pain after tibial nailing. *J Orthop Trauma* 1997;11:10-13.

Koval KJ, Sanders R, Borrelli J, Helfet D, DiPasquale T, Mast JW: Indirect reduction and percutaneous screw fixation of displaced tibial plateau fractures. *J Orthop Trauma* 1992;6:340-346.

Lang GJ, Cohen BE, Bosse MJ, Kellam JF: Proximal third tibial shaft fractures: Should they be nailed? *Clin Orthop* 1995;315:64-74.

McQueen MM, Court-Brown CM: Compartment monitoring in tibial fractures: The pressure threshold for decompression. *J Bone Joint Surg Br* 1996;78:99-104.

Oestern HJ, Tscherne H: Pathophysiology and classification of soft tissue injuries associated with fractures, in Tscherne H, Gotzen L (eds): *Fractures With Soft Tissue Injuries*. Berlin, Germany, Springer-Verlag, 1984, pp 1-9.

Saltzman CL, Goulet JA, McClellan RT, Schneider LA, Matthews LS: Results of treatment of displaced patellar fractures by partial patellectomy. *J Bone Joint Surg Am* 1990;72:1279-1285.

Sarmiento A, Sharpe FE, Ebramzadeh E, Normand P, Shankwiler J: Factors influencing the outcome of closed tibial fractures treated with functional bracing. *Clin Orthop* 1995;315:8-24.

Schandelmaier P, Krettek C, Rudolf J, Kohl A, Katz BE, Tscherne H: Superior results of tibial rodding versus external fixation in grade 3B fractures. *Clin Orthop* 1997;342:164-172.

Smith ST, Cramer KE, Karges DE, Watson JT, Moed BR: Early complications in the operative treatment of patella fractures. *J Orthop Trauma* 1997;11:183-187.

Templeman D, Thomas M, Varecka T, Kyle R: Exchange reamed intramedullary nailing for delayed union and nonunion of the tibia. *Clin Orthop* 1995;315:169-175.

Tornetta P III, Collins E: Semiextended position of intramedullary nailing of the proximal tibia. *Clin Orthop* 1996;328:185-189.

van der Schoot DK, Den Outer AJ, Bode PJ, Obermann WR, van Vugt AB: Degenerative changes at the knee and ankle related to malunion of tibial fractures. *J Bone Joint Surg Br* 1996;78:722-725.

Weiner LS, Kelley M, Yang E, et al: The use of combination internal fixation and hybrid external fixation in severe proximal tibia fractures. *J Orthop Trauma* 1995;9:244-250.

Chapter 43

Knee and Leg: Soft-Tissue Trauma

Charles Bush-Joseph, MD

Thomas R. Carter, MD

Mark D. Miller, MD

Andrew S. Rokito, MD

Michael J. Stuart, MD

Introduction

The current emphasis on health and fitness has resulted in an active population and an increased incidence of overuse and traumatic knee injuries. According to the National Center for Health Statistics, the average number of annual visits to an orthopaedic surgeon has increased by 28% over the past 20 years (from 11.3 to 14.5 per 100 persons). Greater public awareness of advances in treatment options for knee injuries has fueled a more aggressive approach in the treatment of patients with knee ligament, meniscus, and articular cartilage injuries. Current treatment philosophies include restoration of joint stability, repair or replacement of damaged menisci, and protection or restoration of articular cartilage integrity.

Advances in the treatment of knee injuries have paralleled the development of minimally invasive techniques using arthroscopy. Decreased surgical and perioperative morbidity has widened surgical indications to patients not previously considered.

Anterior Cruciate Ligament Injuries

Clinical Evaluation

The characteristic history of an anterior cruciate ligament (ACL) injury involves a rapid deceleration or rotational injury to the knee. An audible "pop" is noted in 30% to 50% of patients. Knee ligament injuries occur as a result of direct contact (30%) and noncontact (70%). Direct contact injuries typically involve at least one cruciate and one collateral ligament. Immediate on-field examination demonstrates a positive Lachman test and a hemarthrosis occurs within hours of the injury. The pivot shift test is difficult to assess in the awake patient once joint swelling (effusion) and muscle spasm have developed. Joint line tenderness may suggest meniscal or capsular injury but is not specific in the first 10 to 14 days after the injury. Collateral ligament injury is detected by varus or valgus laxity with the knee in 25° of flexion. Significant collateral ligament laxity in full extension is indicative of a more severe injury involving multiple ligaments and potentially both cruciates.

Plain radiographs are indicated to rule out fractures or physeal injuries in patients with open physes. A Segond fracture (avulsion fracture of lateral tibial plateau) is pathognomonic of an ACL injury. Although not typically needed to make the diagnosis of an ACL tear, MRI has been useful is assessing associated pathology. Bone bruising or marrow changes in the posterolateral aspect of the lateral tibial plateau and midcentral aspect of the lateral femoral condyle occur in 80% to 90% of patients with ACL injuries. Bone bruising on MRI studies may represent chondral fracturing or delamination, which has a more guarded prognosis. A recent study noted that patients with bone bruising and normal-appearing articular cartilage displayed marrow and subchondral changes on MRI studies 6 years after injury. The presence of significant meniscal or collateral ligament injury on MRI studies is useful in planning treatment.

Treatment

The early management of ACL injuries includes measures to control pain and swelling. Early resumption of weight bearing and muscle activation aid in the recovery of knee range of motion. Regaining full extension is critical in the early period after injury and is dependent on quadriceps muscle function.

Issues to be considered when determining whether surgical or nonsurgical treatment should be recommended include patient age, skeletal maturity, activity and skill level, associated meniscal and ligamentous injuries, frequency of instability, and patient compliance and motivation. The International Knee Documentation Committee (IKDC) developed a knee evaluation system that is useful in evaluating the treatment outcomes of patients with knee ligament and cartilage injuries. The IKDC defined four types of activity: level I, jumping, cutting, and pivoting sports (such as football, basketball, and soccer); level II, heavy manual labor, side-to-side sports (such as skiing and tennis); level III, light manual work, noncutting sports (such as jogging and running); and level IV, sedentary activity without sports.

The natural history of patients with ACL deficiency is linked to the integrity of the menisci and the frequency of buckling episodes. Recurrent episodes of giving way lead to meniscal and articular cartilage damage with eventual knee arthrosis and disability. Thus, patients with significant meniscal or associated ligamentous pathology, or those who participate in level I or II activities, are considered for surgical reconstruction. Functional bracing can be used in patients who wish to avoid surgery but are at risk for episodes of giving way.

Although older patient age was previously considered a relative contraindication to surgical treatment, recent reports have documented similar outcomes and levels of patient satisfaction in patients older than age 40 years when compared with younger patients.

Controversy remains, however, about children and adolescents with open physes. Activity restriction is impractical in this age group and repeated buckling events can lead to significant meniscal and articular damage. A recent study of ACL reconstructions in adolescents with a skeletal age of 14 years revealed no growth or angular complications. Transphyseal tunnels and soft-tissue grafts were used. Transphyseal metallic fixation is used with caution in patients with a skeletal age of less than 14 years because of anecdotal reports of significant growth disturbances.

Surgical Treatment

The goals of surgical treatment are to restore knee stability, protect meniscal and articular cartilage, and minimize perioperative morbidity. Early surgical intervention may minimize recurrent knee buckling and therefore avoid articular and meniscal injuries. A recent study compared the 5- to 15-year outcome of patients undergoing ACL reconstruction based on meniscal damage at the time of surgery: 87% of patients with intact menisci rated their knee as normal or nearly normal, but only 63% of those who required meniscectomy did so.

To decrease the incidence of arthrofibrosis, surgery is delayed until the immediate postinjury inflammatory phase has subsided. Joint swelling, range of motion, quadriceps function, and gait are variables that must be considered before surgical intervention is considered. Acute primary repair or extra-articular reconstructions have little chance of lasting success and generally are not indicated.

Current minimally invasive techniques allow anatomic placement of high-strength grafts through bone tunnels. Sixty percent of surgical failures are caused by technical problems, including improper tunnel placement, leading to graft impingement or graft failure. Accurate tunnel placement can be done through a miniarthrotomy, two-incision, or endoscopic technique. Endoscopic techniques allow decreased morbidity and improved cosmesis but are technically demanding.

With appropriate surgical technique and rehabilitation, a variety of graft choices are suitable for ACL reconstruction. Bone-patellar tendon-bone (BTB) autograft and four-strand hamstring autograft remain the most popular. The quadriceps tendon or allograft tendons are used by some authors in primary ACL reconstructions; however, allografts are more commonly used in revision surgery.

The BTB graft is often selected for young, high-demand athletes because BTB techniques with titanium interference screw fixation allow early range of motion, full weight bearing, and accelerated rehabilitation. Anterior knee pain and kneeling pain remain the most common complaints occurring in 14% to 31% of patients undergoing ACL reconstruction with this method. Perioperative patellar fractures and patellar tendon ruptures are rare (0.2%), but are serious complications. Longer-term (9- to 15-year) follow-up studies have confirmed this technique as a durable, reliable, and reproducible method.

The advantages of hamstring techniques include smaller incisions, theoretically less perioperative pain, and potentially decreased anterior knee pain. Current hamstring techniques emphasize larger grafts (four-strand gracilis-semitendinosus) with improved fixation and decreased donor site morbidity. Potential problems with hamstring techniques have centered on initial graft fixation. Suspension fixation techniques include use of buttons or cross pins. Cross-pin fixation methods provide initial strength and stiffness approaching that of BTB techniques. These and other methods that rely on fixation distant from the joint line can lead to a "windshield wiper effect," in which the graft moves in an anterior to posterior plane with flexion and extension of the knee, potentially leading to graft abrasion or tunnel expansion. This theoretic problem has led to advances in fixation of soft-tissue grafts at the joint line (aperture fixation) (Fig. 1). Aperture fixation using round-threaded metallic or bioabsorbable screws has been used in isolation or as a complement to suspension techniques.

Proponents of various graft sources have used donor site morbidity as a major factor in graft selection. Donor site morbidity, specifically anterior knee pain with autogenous patellar grafts, is minimized with

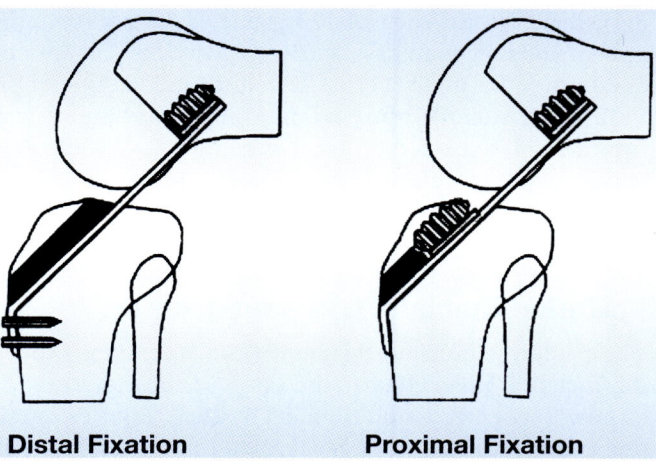

Distal Fixation   **Proximal Fixation**

Figure 1 A schematic diagram depicting distal versus proximal or aperture fixation. *(Reproduced with permission from Fu FH, Bennett CH, Ma CB, Menetrey J, Lattermann C: Current trends in anterior cruciate ligament reconstruction: Part II. Operative procedures and clinical correlations. Am J Sports Med 2000;28: 124-130.)*

immediate and aggressive rehabilitation techniques. Hamstring weakness, associated with semitendinosus/gracilis grafts, resolves within 6 to 12 months and rarely leads to lasting disability. Several follow-up studies comparing donor site morbidity among varying graft sources detected little or no significant differences in patients more than 2 years after surgery. Patients with patellar tendon grafts have a greater likelihood of kneeling problems and those with hamstring grafts have a higher incidence of tibial hardware complaints. Regardless of graft source, 85% to 95% of patients will have clinically stable knees and 80% to 94% will have a normal or nearly normal knee using the IKDC rating system.

Complications

The frequency of complications associated with ACL surgery has declined, but graft failure, hardware problems, and loss of motion persist. Reoperation rates range from 5% to 21% for subsequent meniscal tears, hardware problems, and loss of motion. Patellar fracture and patellar tendon rupture may occur after the use of patellar tendon autografts (0.2% to 0.4%). The fracture may occur intraoperatively but typically occurs 6 to 12 weeks after surgery, in conjunction with vigorous rehabilitation, including cutting and jumping. Surgical fixation with cannulated screws and immediate motion is effective. Although significant quadriceps atrophy may occur, longer-term follow-up is similar to that in uncomplicated cases.

Perioperative septic arthritis occurs in 0.5% patients after ACL reconstruction. Typical presentation includes increased pain, swelling, and erythema within 2 to 14 days after surgery. Elevated white blood cell count on joint aspiration or the presence of bacteria on Gram stain warrants immediate arthroscopic irrigation and débridement of all surgical wounds. *Staphylococcus aureus* is the most common bacteria isolated, although *S. epidermidis* has been implicated with instrument contamination. Recent reports have noted that with aggressive intervention (average 2 to 4 surgical procedures) and proper antibiotic regimens (6 to 12 weeks), the ACL graft can be salvaged and motion retained. Long-term results may be compromised because of articular cartilage damage from the infection.

Revision ACL Surgery

Revision ACL reconstruction is likely to become more common as the number of primary ACL reconstructions increase. Consideration of revision ACL surgery requires careful planning and realistic expectations for success. Patients with recurrent laxity often have significant meniscal and articular surface damage that compromises clinical outcomes. In many patients, the goal of surgery is to restore stability for activities of daily living and light recreational sports only.

Identification of the reason for failure can often guide the plan for revision. Typical causes include either anterior or central tunnel location on the femur or anterior tunnel location on the tibia. Patients with poorly located tunnels often require alternative drilling methods. Failed endoscopic reconstruction with central femoral tunnels can be revised with a two-incision rear entry femoral tunnel (Fig. 2). Plain radiographs, MRI, and CT are used to determine if properly located tunnels can be safely drilled or if bone grafting of defects is necessary. Tunnel dilation or poor bone stock occasionally requires staged procedures with bone grafting followed by delayed reconstruction after 3 to 6 months. Graft failure with properly located bone tunnels usually is due to poor graft strength, inadequate fixation, or overaggressive rehabilitation. Revision strategies include the use of high-strength grafts (quadriceps tendon, hamstring tendons, or allograft tissue) with dual fixation (suspension techniques and interference screws) on both the tibia and femur. Reharvesting a central third patellar tendon autograft is not advised unless other graft sources are unavailable. Synthetic grafts currently are of historic interest only, but may have future applications. Rehabilitation after revision surgery is more conservative than after primary ACL reconstruction. Protected weight bearing and limited knee motion may be necessary if graft fixation is of concern. The success rates of revision ACL surgery vary from 62% to 75%, although meniscal loss and articular surface damage compromise functional results.

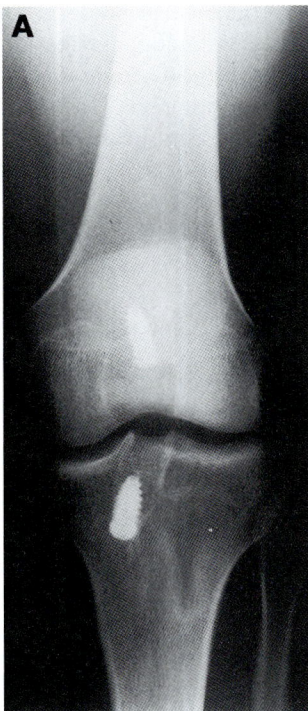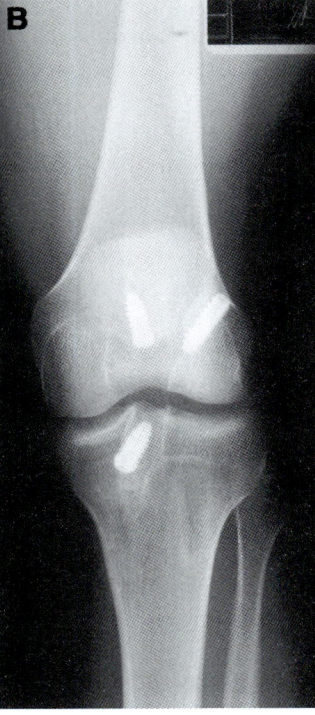

Figure 2 **A,** Central femoral tunnel leading to graft failure. **B,** Revision with outside-in femoral tunnel.

Medial Collateral Ligament Injuries

Most medial collateral ligament (MCL) injuries are caused by a laterally applied valgus force, as commonly occurs during participation in contact sports. Combined rotational forces may result in other ligamentous injuries. It is critical to examine the knee in 30° of flexion and in full extension. Isolated MCL injuries result in medial joint opening at 30° of flexion but not in full extension. Medial joint opening in full extension usually indicates a combined injury involving the cruciate ligament(s). Plain films usually are not helpful, but, in long-standing MCL injuries, calcification adjacent to the medial femoral epicondyle (Pellegrini-Stieda lesion) may be seen. MRI is quite accurate in identifying MCL injuries, but usually does not add any appreciable information beyond a careful physical examination. One recent MRI study demonstrated that most isolated MCL tears occurred on the femoral side; they were associated with lateral bone bruises (trabecular microfractures) in almost half of the cases. Nonsurgical treatment is standard. Most authors recommend treatment of MCL injuries with a hinged knee brace. Early motion and functional rehabilitation are keys to early return of athletes to previous levels of sports participation. Return to play is largely based on the existing degree of discomfort and residual instability. The average time to return to play is approximately 2 weeks for an isolated grade I injury (0 to 5 mm of medial opening), 3 weeks for an isolated grade II injury (6 to 10 mm of medial opening), and 6 to 8 weeks for an isolated grade III injury (11 to 15 mm of medial opening). Future treatment options may include administration of platelet-derived growth factor, which has been shown to improve healing in an animal model. Another recent animal study demonstrated that there was no deleterious effect of ibuprofen on MCL healing.

Posterior Cruciate Ligament Injuries

The posterior cruciate ligament (PCL) continues to be the focus of much clinical and basic science research. It is now recognized that significant PCL injuries often are combined PCL and posterolateral corner injuries, which may explain why reconstruction of so-called isolated PCL injuries has in the past not been as successful as ACL reconstructions. The mechanism of PCL injury is typically a blow to the anterior tibia (dashboard injury). Hyperflexion injuries are responsible for most PCL injuries in sports. The key examination for PCL injury is the posterior drawer test. It is essential to evaluate the position of the tibia in relation to the medial femoral condyle. Normally, the medial tibial plateau is anterior to the condyle. With PCL deficiency the tibia may be subluxated posteriorly to lie even with or posterior to the medial femoral condyle, and it can be displaced even further with a posterior drawer force. The amount of displacement is classified according to grade (Fig. 3). Plain films should be obtained, but often are not diagnostic. However, bony avulsions of the PCL should be recognized and fixed acutely. Stress radiographs have gained wider acceptance in the objective evaluation of PCL injuries and reconstructive techniques and have widely supplanted the use of knee arthrometry in the evaluation of PCL laxity. MRI is highly sensitive and specific for the diagnosis of complete PCL injuries. Recent evidence suggests that the MRI appearance of partial PCL injuries may return to normal over time.

Treatment of PCL injured knees continues to be a matter of much debate. One recent study confirms that grades I and II PCL injuries can be successfully managed nonsurgically. Nonsurgical management emphasizes quadriceps strengthening with early avoidance of hamstring exercises. Most authors recommend surgical treatment of grade III injuries, especially combined (PCL and posterolateral corner) injuries. Surgical options include traditional arthroscopic transtibial reconstruction, tibial inlay reconstruction, two-bundle reconstruction, or a combination of techniques. Transtibial reconstructions have recently been criticized because the graft has to negotiate a "killer turn" around the back of the tibia. This movement of the graft has been shown to lead to graft stretching in a

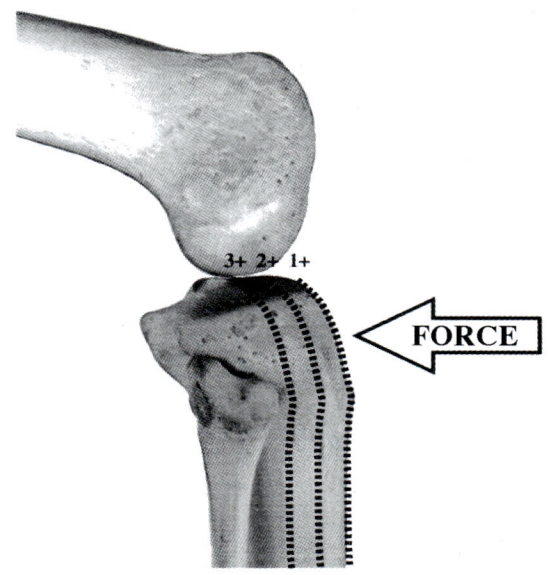

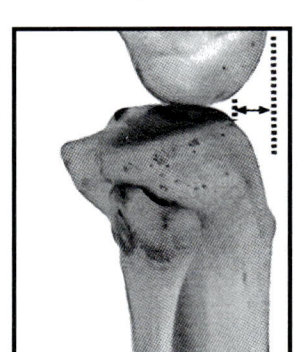
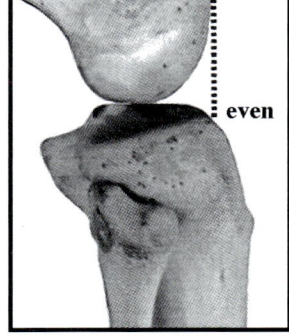
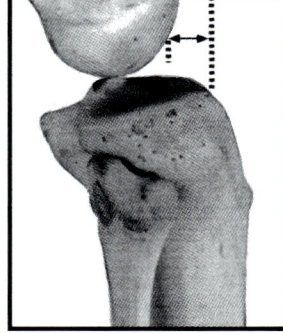

Figure 3 Diagrammatic representation of the grades of PCL injuries. Note that in grade 3 injuries, the tibia can be displaced posterior to the medial femoral condyle. *(Reproduced from Miller MD, Bergfeld JA, Fowler PJ, et al: The posterior cruciate ligament injured knee: Principles of evaluation and treatment. Instr Course Lect 1999;48: 199-207.)*

cyclically loaded cadaver model, and has been implicated as a cause of graft stretching clinically. Tibial inlay reconstruction may reduce this risk, but can be technically challenging. Two-bundle reconstructions have recently been studied in vitro and demonstrate improved biomechanical properties over single-bundle reconstructions in both extension and flexion. Clinical data are lacking regarding the most effective surgical technique. Graft options also are controversial, but include autologous bone-patellar tendon-bone, quadriceps tendon, hamstring tendons, and allograft Achilles tendon or bone-patellar tendon-bone grafts.

Rehabilitation after PCL reconstruction should be more cautious than after ACL rehabilitation. Knee extension against gravity is discouraged in the early postoperative period; assisted prone motion is helpful. Bracing in full extension, quadriceps rehabilitation, and avoidance of early hamstring rehabilitation are appropriate. Because PCL reconstruction is a relatively uncommon procedure, there are few clinical series. In general, results are satisfactory but not excellent. Improvement from grade III to grade I injury is common. Perhaps new techniques will result in improved clinical results.

Posterolateral Complex Injuries

Several recent basic science studies have provided new insight into the importance of restoring posterolateral complex structures after injury. The posterolateral structures, which include the popliteus, popliteofibular ligament, biceps tendon, iliotibial tract, and lateral collateral ligament, play an important role in knee stability. The popliteus has been shown to be an important secondary stabilizer against posterior tibial translation, especially when the PCL is absent. Other studies also have demonstrated the synergistic effect of the PCL and posterolateral corner structures. One biomechanical study demonstrated increased posterior tibial translation, external

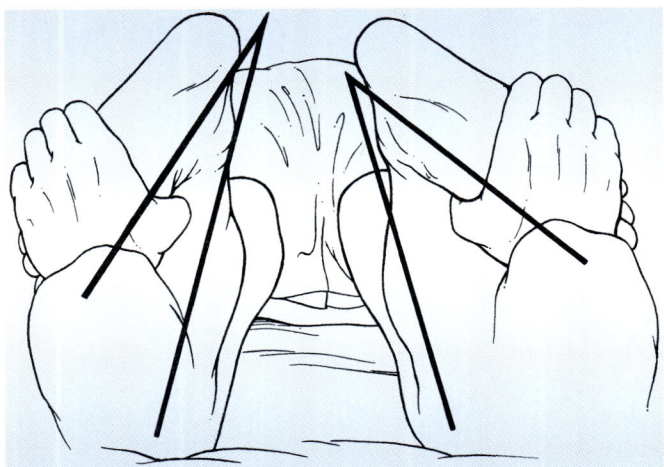

Figure 4 Prone external rotation test at 30°. External rotation of the affected (right) foot of more than 10° greater than the normal (left) side is suggestive of a posterolateral complex injury. If this difference is also present at 90° of knee flexion, a combined PCL and posterolateral complex injury must be suspected. *(Reproduced from Veltri DM, Warren RF: Isolated and combined posterior cruciate ligament injuries. J Am Acad Orthop Surg 1993;1:67-75.)*

rotation, and PCL graft stresses associated with deficiency of posterolateral structures.

The mechanism of injury for posterolateral complex injuries typically involves hyperextension with a varus moment and a twisting force. A posterolaterally-directed blow to the medial tibia with the knee in extension (resulting in hyperextension and external rotation) is the most common mechanism of injury. Combined injuries (usually PCL, but also ACL) are common. Isolated posterolateral complex injuries may result in posterolateral pain, peroneal nerve paresthesias (up to 30%), and instability with knee extension. Several physical examination tests, including the posterolateral drawer test, external rotation recurvatum test, reverse pivot shift test, and the external rotation test, depend on comparison with the contralateral (normal) knee. The most reliable test is for asymmetric tibial external rotation (Fig. 4). A difference of more than 10° compared with the contralateral limb is evidence of a pathologic condition. The test is performed at 30° and 90° of flexion. With an isolated posterolateral injury, the difference is noted only at 30°. With a combined PCL and posterolateral injury, the difference is noted at 30° and 90° of knee flexion.

MRI of the posterolateral complex has improved dramatically. Opening of the lateral joint more than 1 cm with varus stress (drive-through sign) on arthroscopy has also been described with posterolateral complex injuries.

Primary repair of posterolateral complex injuries offers the greatest chance of clinical success. These repairs may include supplementation with local autogenous tissues (biceps or iliotibial band strip) or other tissues (autogenous hamstring tendons, other autogenous tendons, or allograft tendons). Simultaneous reconstruction of other damaged structures (for example, the cruciate ligaments) is also indicated. Advancement or recession of tissues may be a reasonable procedure for chronic posterolateral corner injuries with intact but lax structures. The disadvantage of this approach is that the structures are shifted from their normal center of knee rotation, which may result in late failure. Reconstruction is recommended when the acutely injured structures are irreparable or are chronic cases. Biceps tenodesis is less often recommended, in favor of more anatomic procedures. Various techniques have been described (Fig. 5), but clinical results are largely unknown. Chronic posterolateral complex injuries with varus deformity often require a valgus osteotomy. Many surgeons prefer medial opening wedge osteotomies in this setting.

Postoperative rehabilitation depends on the extent of surgery, but generally requires protection of the graft in a hinged brace with protection from external rotation and varus stress for a minimum of 6 to 8 weeks. Return to sport may be difficult, especially at the same level, but should be delayed for 9 to 12 months.

Combined Injuries

Clinical evaluation and imaging of combined injuries require a thorough examination of all structures. Emphasis on evaluation of AP laxity, varus-valgus laxity, rotational asymmetry, and patellar instability is paramount for every acute knee injury.

For most ACL-MCL injuries, nonsurgical management of the MCL (hinged brace) and ACL reconstruction is recommended. Some authors recommend surgical repair of grade III MCL injuries at the time of ACL reconstruction when they occur together although this approach is controversial. Postoperative loss of motion can be a problem, and therefore acute surgery and prolonged immobilization should be avoided.

Combined ACL and posterolateral complex injuries require acute reconstruction of both the ACL and repair or reconstruction of the posterolateral complex. Initial rehabilitation should focus on the posterolateral complex. There is significant controversy regarding the treatment approach to PCL-MCL injuries. An initial nonsurgical approach with protection in a hinged brace may convert the injury to an isolated PCL injury, which then can be managed accordingly. Some surgeons recommend early repair of one or both ligaments. For PCL-posterolateral corner injuries, surgical intervention for both injuries is indicated. Postoperative rehabilitation must protect both the PCL and the posterolateral corner and therefore needs to be undertaken with caution.

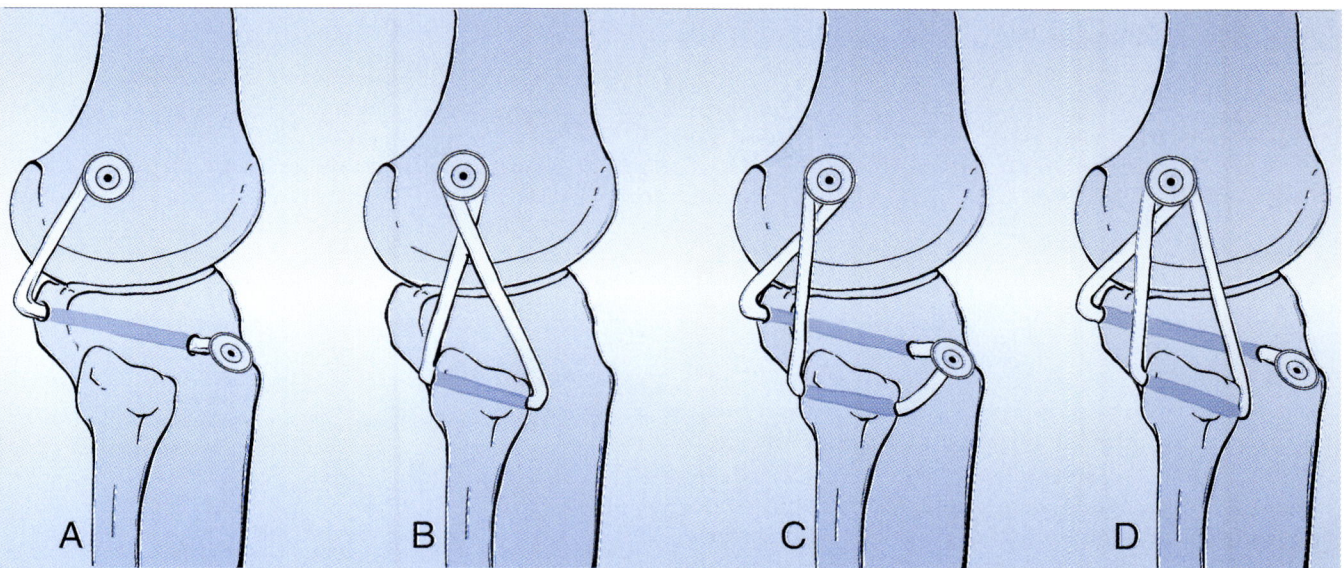

Figure 5 "Anatomic" techniques for posterolateral complex reconstruction. **A,** The popliteal bypass, originally described by Müller, is very similar to the posterolateral corner sling procedure advocated by Albright. **B,** The figure-of-8 technique, described by Larson, was developed to take advantage of isometry. **C,** The two-tailed technique, originally described by Warren, attempts to recreate both the tibial and fibular attachments of the popliteus. **D,** The modified two-tailed technique, which requires more tissue, includes an anterior arm for additional stability and/or LCL supplementation. Alternatively, the LCL can be reconstructed separately with a central biceps tendon strip or other tissue.

Knee Dislocations

Dislocation of the knee is an uncommon but potentially limb-threatening injury. Some dislocations may be unrecognized because of spontaneous relocation. The mechanism varies from low-energy athletic injuries to high-velocity motor vehicle trauma. Prompt recognition of the dislocation and identification of associated injuries are essential. Damage to the popliteal artery and the peroneal nerve is common, occurring in approximately 25% of dislocations. Approximately half of peroneal nerve injuries result in permanent neurologic deficits. Initial treatment involves immediate closed reduction and treatment of vascular compromise. Physical examination and imaging studies detect the specific anatomic structures disrupted. Surgical treatment of ligament injuries is preferred for most patients who have satisfactory vascular supply, skin coverage, rehabilitation potential, and anticipated future activity demands. The timing and extent of surgery remain controversial because of concern for knee stiffness. Improved surgical techniques, the use of allogenic graft sources, and controlled postoperative knee range of motion have reduced the risk of arthrofibrosis. Surgical repair and reconstruction of the knee ligaments and associated structures followed by early rehabilitation provide the highest level of function.

Clinical Evaluation

Clinical evaluation begins with an overall assessment of the patient and the neurovascular status of the extremity. The magnitude of force that caused the injury has prognostic significance. High-velocity trauma is associated with injuries to other organ systems, neurovascular involvement, and open dislocations and fractures. Low-velocity dislocations have a better prognosis with fewer vascular injuries, reduced meniscal damage, and fewer osteochondral fractures. Fundamental diagnostic questions that must be answered immediately include whether the injury is open or closed, whether the knee joint is dislocated, subluxated or reduced, and whether the limb is adequately perfused or not. The injured limb is initially evaluated and treated in the sequence presented in Table 1.

If the knee is dislocated, prompt closed reduction is imperative. The position of the tibia relative to the femur provides a clue to the mechanism of injury and helps guide the reduction technique. A distinct type of posterolateral knee dislocation, which cannot be reduced by closed means, is recognized by the posterolateral position of the tibia relative to the femur, puckering of the medial skin, and persistent medial joint space widening and lateral tibial subluxation after attempted closed reduction. The medial femoral condyle is buttonholed through the soft tissues and the displaced medial retinaculum in the notch blocks joint reduction. Surgical treatment is required to achieve reduction.

The neurovascular examination should be repeated after any manipulation of the extremity. The popliteal artery is at risk when the knee is dislocated because

TABLE 1 | Initial Evaluation and Treatment of Injury

Neurovascular examination

Closed reduction

Repeat neurovascular examination

Splint in extension/slight flexion

Verify intact perfusion with serial examination of pulses or angiography

Determine injury pattern (physical examination, radiographs, MRI)

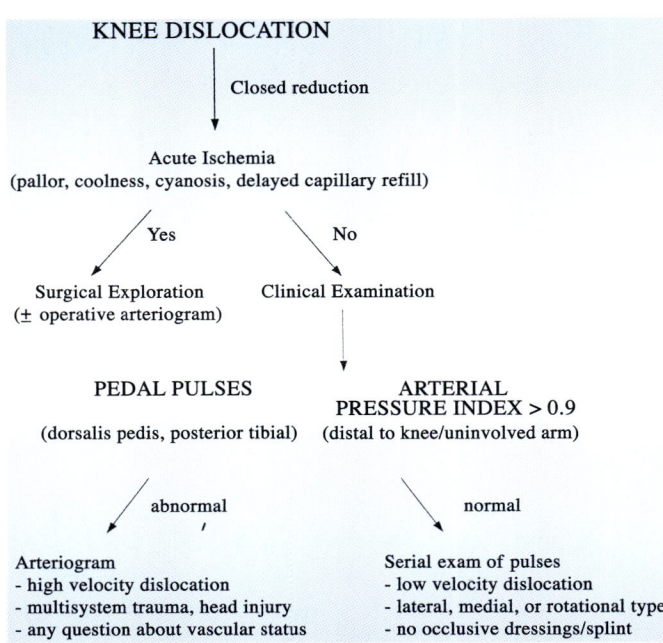

Figure 6 Algorithm for the evaluation of the vascular status in a limb with a dislocated knee.

this artery is tethered between the adductor hiatus proximally and the soleus arch distally. A delay in the diagnosis of ischemia can result in an above-knee amputation. A high index of suspicion for arterial injury necessitates careful physical examination and selective arteriography (Fig. 6). Surgical exploration (with or without arteriogram at surgery) is done immediately if there are signs of acute ischemia such as pallor, coolness, cyanosis, and delayed capillary refill. Prompt revascularization is mandatory and usually requires excision of the damaged segment and reverse saphenous vein grafting. Consultation with a vascular surgeon and an arteriogram are necessary if circulation is not normal after joint reduction. Collateral circulation can maintain tenuous limb viability and produce a detectable pedal pulse. If a Doppler examination is required to document a pulse, arteriography is mandatory. Patients with palpable, normal, symmetric pulses and an arterial pressure index of more than 0.9 (distal to the knee/uninvolved arm) can be monitored carefully without an arteriogram. Repeated examinations are required because abnormal pulses may develop as a result of vessel spasm, thrombosis, or progression of an intimal tear.

Detailed physical examination of the knee identifies the injured capsuloligamentous structures. The ability to perform a straight leg raise and extend the knee against gravity verifies continuity of the extensor mechanism. Examination under anesthesia may be helpful to further define the specific ligament involvement and the extent of the damage. The anatomic classification system is the most pragmatic because it defines the specific ligament structures involved and whether there is an associated fracture, nerve, or artery injury (Table 2).

Imaging

Radiographs
Standard radiographs include AP, lateral, oblique, and patellar views. A normal-appearing knee with slight joint space widening may be the only clue to a reduced dislocation. The radiographs must be analyzed to identify periarticular and osteochondral fractures along with ligament avulsions. Tibial plateau fractures may require restoration of articular congruity and stabilization with internal fixation. Avulsion fractures provide clues to specific ligament involvement and guide surgical technique. A fibular head avulsion fracture may include the lateral collateral ligament (LCL), popliteofibular ligament, and biceps femoris insertions. Comparison stress views may be helpful to clarify the extent of ligamentous damage or to rule out a physeal injury in a skeletally immature patient. Careful scrutiny of AP and lateral radiographs after a closed reduction is essential to verify satisfactory alignment (Fig. 7). An irreducible dislocation is recognized by lateral subluxation of the tibia caused by interposed medial retinacular tissue.

Magnetic Resonance Imaging
Physical examination can be difficult because of pain, muscle spasm, swelling, ipsilateral fractures, vascular injuries, bilateral injuries, and polytrauma. MRI helps identify meniscal tears, intraosseous contusions, occult fractures, capsular disruptions, and muscle tears. MRI helps with detailed surgical planning including the location of incisions, extent of exposures, specific procedures required (reattachment or reconstruction), number and types of grafts needed, and the order of repair and reconstruction.

Treatment

Initial Treatment
Indications for immediate surgery include arterial injury, open dislocation, irreducible dislocation, or

TABLE 2	**Anatomic Classification Scheme for the Dislocated Knee**
Class	**Injured Structures**
KD I	ACL, collateral(s); PCL intact
	PCL, collateral(s); ACL intact
KD II	ACL, PCL; PLC, MCL intact
KD III-M	ACL, PCL, MCL; PLC intact
KD III-L	ACL, PCL, PLC; MCL intact
KD IV	ACL, PCL, MCL, PLC
KD V	Associated periarticular fracture

KD = knee dislocation *(Adapted from Schenck RC Jr, Hunter RE, Ostrum RF, Perry CR: Knee dislocations.* Instr Course Lect *1999;48:515–522.)*

compartment syndrome. If an arterial injury requires treatment, ligament repair or reconstruction should not delay the vascular procedure. A four-compartment fasciotomy is done to relieve elevated pressures or as a prophylactic measure for an ischemic limb. A spanning external fixator is applied in patients with multisystem trauma, an open dislocation, or a vascular repair if joint reduction cannot be maintained in a splint. Two bicortical half-pins are placed in the mid-diaphyseal lateral femur and two in the mid-diaphyseal anteromedial tibia. Joint stabilization with a transarticular femorotibial pin or olecranization of the patella is discour-

aged. All open wounds are irrigated and débrided. Ligament surgery may be delayed for 1 to 2 weeks to allow monitoring of the vascular status and wound healing or for up to 4 to 6 weeks when the external fixator is removed. This allows for planning of the surgical procedures. Ligament repair or reconstruction can be done at the time of vascular surgery depending on the patient's health and the surgeon's experience. A tourniquet may be used during subsequent surgical procedures only if approved by the vascular surgeon.

Definitive Treatment

Surgical treatment of ligament injuries is preferred for most patients who have satisfactory vascularity, soft tissues, rehabilitation potential, and future activity demands. Improved surgical techniques, including the use of allogenic graft sources and early, controlled postoperative knee range of motion, have reduced the risk of arthrofibrosis. Surgical exploration and treatment of all involved ligaments provide the most reliable results. The injured leg is positioned very carefully during preparation for surgery to avoid additional neurovascular injury. The arthroscope is a valuable tool for diagnosis, meniscus repair, or partial meniscectomy as indicated, and preparation of bone tunnels for cruciate ligament reconstruction. Joint capsule disruption requires maintenance of adequate fluid outflow and careful monitoring for extravasation in order to prevent a compartment syndrome. The soft tissues must be handled carefully and skin flaps should be kept at full thickness to minimize any problems with wound healing. Both cruciate ligaments are reattached, aug-

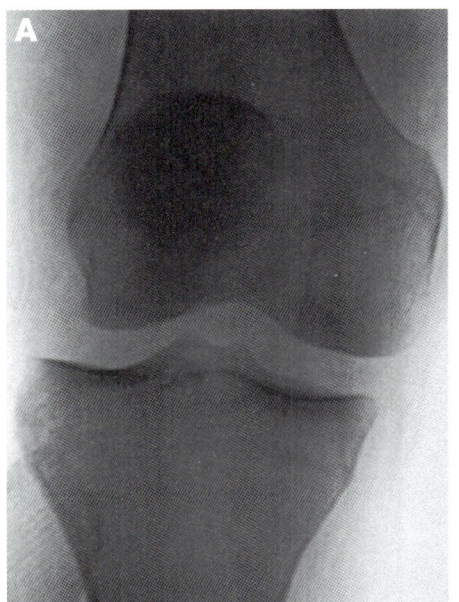
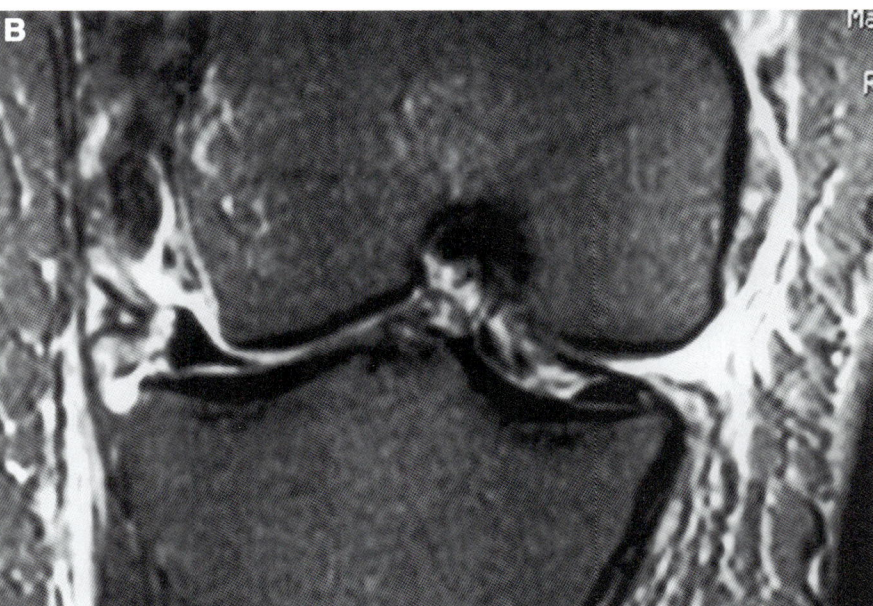

Figure 7 Irreducible dislocation. AP radiograph **(A)** and coronal MRI **(B)** following an attempted closed reduction of a posterolateral knee dislocation. Lateral subluxation of the tibia persists because of interposed medial retinacular tissue.

mented, or reconstructed as necessary (ACL reconstruction can be delayed according to surgeon preference). Intrasubstance ligament damage with attenuation typically occurs before actual rupture. Cruciate ligament anatomic reattachment may result in unacceptable ligament tension (nonfunctional ligament). Occasionally, a PCL bone or periosteal avulsion can be reattached using a screw and spiked ligament washer or nonabsorbable braided, locking whipstitch sutures pulled through drill holes. A midsubstance PCL disruption is reconstructed with a patellar tendon or Achilles tendon allograft or semitendinosus/gracilis, patellar or quadriceps tendon autograft according to the surgeon's preference. The ACL is ignored or reconstructed according to the surgeon's preference. The menisci, osteochondral fractures, and extensor mechanism are repaired as necessary. The timing of surgery is dependent on the specific structures that are disrupted.

ACL and PCL With Intact Collateral Ligaments A rehabilitation brace is locked in full extension when weight bearing, but unlocked for range of motion exercises. Arthroscopic reconstruction is done when capsular disruption has healed and full knee motion is restored (approximately 4 to 6 weeks).

ACL, PCL, and Posterolateral Complex Early surgery is advised because anatomic repair of the lateral and posterolateral structures is more difficult after retraction and scarring have occurred. Arthroscopically-assisted cruciate ligament reconstructions and lateral side anatomic repair are done within 3 to 10 days after injury. The LCL, posterolateral corner, and associated tendinous injuries (biceps, popliteus, iliotibial band) are repaired and augmented as necessary.

ACL, PCL, and MCL With Intact Posteromedial Capsule The knee is immobilized at 20° of flexion in a locked brace or cast for 2 weeks, and then range of motion is encouraged with the knee in a rehabilitation brace. Arthroscopic cruciate ligament reconstruction is done when the MCL has healed and full knee motion has been restored (approximately 6 to 8 weeks). Proximal and midsubstance MCL tears usually heal without surgery. Acute repair with capsular reefing may precipitate knee stiffness. If a distal MCL disruption does not heal satisfactorily, a repair or advancement is done at the time of cruciate ligament reconstruction along with repair of the posteromedial corner and associated tendinous injuries (medial gastrocnemius) as necessary.

Rehabilitation

General guidelines for postoperative rehabilitation are presented in Table 3. Postoperative rehabilitation is individualized according to the injured structures and the

---

TABLE 3 | Rehabilitation Protocol

0 to 4 weeks

Prone passive flexion 0° to 90°, touch weight bearing with brace locked in extension patellar mobilization, isometrics and straight leg lifts, and electrical muscle stimulation as necessary.

4 to 8 weeks

Passive and active-assisted gradual full flexion, partial weight bearing with brace locked in extension, and low resistance closed chain strengthening (mini squats and leg press).

8 to 12 weeks

Full active range of motion, full weight bearing with brace locked in extension, progressive resistance closed chain strengthening, low resistance bicycling, and swimming.

12 to 16 weeks

Full weight bearing with brace unlocked, low resistance bicycling, swimming, and hamstring strengthening.

16 to 52+ weeks

Functional brace or unloader brace (if collateral ligament repair or reconstruction performed), continued strengthening and proprioceptive training exercises.

---

procedures performed. A soft compressive dressing is placed after surgery and the knee is maintained in slight flexion for the first week. A custom polypropylene knee-ankle-foot orthosis or a rehabilitation brace with an extension lock and a 90° flexion stop is then applied. The brace is locked in extension at all times except when performing range of motion exercises.

Meniscus

The meniscus has several roles that are essential to normal knee function, including load transmission, shock absorption, joint stability, lubrication, and nutrition. Because even partial meniscectomy may predispose the knee to arthritis, meniscal tears should be repaired whenever possible.

The first step in treating meniscal pathology is knowing which tears do not require treatment. Tears that are considered stable and do not require repair or excision include full-thickness but short tears (10 mm or smaller), vertical longitudinal tears at the meniscocapsular junction, short radial tears (3 mm or smaller), and partial-thickness tears.

When deciding whether to repair or excise a tear, several variables need to be considered. Because the vascular supply of the meniscus is from the periphery inward, location of the tear has the greatest influence on healing potential. If a tear is within 3 mm of the meniscal synovial junction (red-on-red zone), it should be considered vascular. Tears in the 3- to 5-mm range (red-on-white zone) have variable vascularity but are typically sufficient to warrant repair. Tears 5 mm or more from the periphery should be considered avascular unless there is evidence to the contrary. An exception is an area anterior to the popliteus tendon where the meniscus has uniformly poor vascularity. Other factors associated with higher success rates of repair are a traumatic tear as opposed to an insidious or degenerative tear, ligamentous stable knee, or concomitant ACL reconstruction if unstable. Surgical techniques used to enhance healing include rasping of the meniscal synovial junction and the torn surfaces of the tear, use of a fibrin clot, and creation of vascular access channels by trephination.

Several different surgical techniques can be used for meniscal repair. Although open repair is still an option, three arthroscopic methods are typically used: inside-out, outside-in, and all-inside. Each method has advantages and disadvantages, and no one is superior in all situations.

The popular inside-out technique is useful for placing mattress sutures across the tear for two-point fixation and can assist in reducing unstable tears. A disadvantage is the risk of neurovascular injury. The outside-in technique is the treatment of choice for anterior horn tears. However, when used for extreme posterior tears, the obliquity of the sutures raises concern of the tear being fully apposed. The all-inside method, although initially described as a technically challenging method for repair of peripheral posterior horn tears, has been simplified by bioabsorbable devices. This technique also reduces the risk of neurovascular insult. If, however, improper length is selected, the device can penetrate the capsule and cause neurovascular injury or act as a mechanical irritant. Other reported complications include cyst formation, chondral injury, and breakage and migration of the implant. In addition, most bioabsorbable implants provide only a single fixation point and may require augmentation with other repair methods when treating complex or grossly unstable tears.

The merits of absorbable and nonabsorbable suture materials continue to be debated. Proponents of nonabsorbable sutures cite the fact that fixation is maintained longer and thus they are particularly useful in treating tears that are in areas of limited vascularity. Advocates of absorbable sutures cite the risk of entrapping tissue or puckering the meniscus, which can cause permanent deformation, as reasons to avoid nonabsorbable sutures.

There is general agreement, however, that the suturing method with the greatest strength is vertical mattress. Capturing a greater number of circumferential meniscal fibers makes the load to failure of vertical mattress sutures twice that of horizontal mattress sutures. Biodegradable devices have failure loads similar to horizontal mattress sutures, but tend to gap at the repair at lesser loads before pulling through the meniscus, while sutures typically fail by rupture of the knot.

Rehabilitation after meniscal repair is an area of debate. Historically, rehabilitation was very conservative, with early programs recommending 4 to 6 weeks of immobilization and minimal or no weight bearing. Running was restricted until 4 months, with sports typically limited from 6 to 9 months. As research found the meniscus to have little translation from 0° to 60°, many rehabilitation protocols subsequently allowed immediate motion, but limited flexion for the initial 4 weeks, and protected weight bearing. More recent accelerated protocols claim success rates similar to traditional protocols, but permit full range of motion and weight bearing with unrestricted activities at 3 to 4 months. Additional clinical studies are required before these accelerated programs are routinely implemented. Variables, including the type and location of tear and the stability of the repair, all need to be considered when determining postoperative treatment.

Depending on the many factors known to influence healing, the reported success rates of meniscal repairs have ranged from 60% to 90%. Invasive methods, such as second-look arthroscopy or arthrography, have been necessary to evaluate healing because conventional MRI studies show as much as 90% persistence of grade III signal after successful repairs. Recent specialized fast spin-echo techniques have improved the ability of MRI to detect healing at least as accurately as arthrography.

Meniscal Allografts

Because most meniscal tears are not suitable for repair, and meniscectomy is known to increase the risk of arthritis, efforts to replace or regenerate the meniscus are under intense research. Prosthetic replacements have been unsuccessful because of the inability to replicate the complex biomechanical properties of the normal meniscus. Although methods such as tissue engineering show promise, they are considered experimental at present.

Meniscal allografts have been found to be a feasible meniscal replacement. Basic science studies have found little evidence of clinical rejection and the grafts readily heal at the repair site. Biomechanical testing has found that the grafts reduce joint forces compared to meniscectomy, but do not replicate normal function. Because of the structural alterations that occur with freeze drying or sterilization with gamma irradiation, neither method should be used when processing the meniscus. The grafts need to be secured by bone at the anatomic attachment sites if they are to be functional.

Clinical studies with short to intermediate follow-up have shown that meniscal allografts can be of subjective benefit, but the procedure is technically challenging with narrow clinical indications. Early experience found that patients with significant knee arthritis had the most symptomatic improvement, but most grafts failed within 2 years. As a result, patients with grade IV chondromalacia or radiographic evidence of noticeable joint incongruity are not candidates for the procedure. Joint stability and alignment are other variables that have a direct effect on success. Although an area of controversy, it is generally believed that a patient should be symptomatic before replacing the meniscus. The durability of the allograft and its long-term ability to deter arthritis remain unanswered.

Articular Cartilage Injuries

Because of their limited healing potential, articular cartilage injuries are some of the most difficult orthopaedic injuries to treat. A number of techniques have been investigated, but an ideal method has yet to be found that can fully replicate the highly organized, complex structure and function of articular cartilage.

Before deciding on a treatment method, the correct diagnosis of a chondral injury must be made. Presenting symptoms and physical findings of a chondral lesion can range from localized pain with catching that mimicks a meniscal tear to vague aching with limited effusion. Plain radiographs can be helpful if the lesion is large and there is a bony component if degenerative changes are present or weight-bearing views, but otherwise typically are of little help. MRI has historically been of equivocal benefit, but recently described imaging sequences have to improved sensitivity and specificity in the range of 85% to 95% when evaluating chondral abnormalities.

Although a chondral lesion may produce symptoms, many are incidental findings during arthroscopy for other pathology. In one published series reviewing over 31,000 arthroscopies, the frequency of chondral abnormalities was 63%, with grade IV lesions present in 20% of all patients, and in 5% of those less than 40 years of age. With many patients never seeking treatment and the natural history of many chondral injuries unknown, opinion is mixed about treating asymptom-

atic lesions. As of yet, no independent, prospective, randomized, long-term study has compared the outcome of nonsurgical treatment to the various types of surgical treatment.

Many variables must be considered when choosing the surgical technique, including the patient's age and activity demands, size and depth of the defect, etiology of the lesion, associated pathology, and the required rehabilitation. If a patient is elderly and has low activity demands, simple débridement frequently is sufficient. If the defect is large or accompanied by significant bone loss in a young, active individual, a more aggressive approach may be indicated. Anterior cruciate insufficiency and limb alignment have a direct effect on outcome and need to be corrected during or before treatment of the defect. Lesions that are secondary to osteoarthritis or involve the femur and tibia of the same compartment, commonly termed kissing lesions, typically do poorly regardless of the treatment method.

An isolated symptomatic defect can be treated with simple débridement or one of three basic types of articular resurfacing methods: bone marrow stimulating techniques, transplantation of autologous tissues or cells, and allogeneic osteochondral grafts. The use of growth factors, cytokines, synthetic matrices, and gene therapy are a few of the methods currently under investigation.

Débridement, or chondroplasty, is the simplest treatment method. Removal of unstable flaps that may cause mechanical symptoms and induce inflammation improves symptoms in approximately two thirds of patients. The relief is temporary because the procedure does not correct the underlying pathology, and results deteriorate significantly after a few years. Recently, radiofrequency electrothermal techniques have been used in the débridement process. Because of the risk of thermal necrosis, additional study is needed to evaluate its efficacy and safety.

Bone marrow stimulation techniques encompass penetrating the subchondral bone plate to induce vascular-mediated healing of the defect. Abrasion, drilling, and microfracture are methods to achieve this goal. The response depends on the vascularity of the underlying bone and can be unpredictable. The theoretical advantage of drilling and microfracture over abrasion is the capability of evoking a greater vascular response and providing a better anchor for the healing tissue. Advocates of microfracture state avoidance of thermonecrosis and ease of access to lesions as benefits over drilling.

Rehabilitation after marrow stimulating procedures is prolonged and should be taken into consideration when choosing treatment. Patients are encouraged to immediately perform range of motion exercises, but routinely are toe-touch weight bearing for 6 to 8 weeks. Avoidance of sports for 6 to 8 months frequently is recommended.

Although there are reports of microfracture healing with hyaline-like cartilage, the consensus is that marrow stimulation methods result in predominantly fibrocartilage filling of the defect; making durability of repair a concern. Several authors have reported results similar to those after débridement, while others have reported good results at more than 5 years. Because the method is technically easy, with limited cost, and does not preclude further treatment options, it may be a reasonable first step in the management of small, previously untreated condylar defects.

Autologous transplantation procedures rely on cells or tissue from one area used to fill a defect in another. Although the category encompasses several different methods, autologous chondrocyte implantation (ACI) and osteochondral autografts are the most widely used.

ACI is a two-stage procedure in which small portions of cartilage are arthroscopically harvested and subsequently expanded in a culture medium. The cells are then implanted in the defect using a periosteal patch applied in a second procedure through an arthrotomy. If the defect is deep, bone grafting is required at the time of the initial harvesting. After the procedure, weight bearing is restricted for 6 weeks, with gradual progression to full weight bearing at 12 weeks. Because of the time required for graft maturation, high-impact activities are avoided until 9 to 12 months after surgery. Correction of instability and malalignment is vital to limit forces across the involved area during healing of the repaired tissue.

Most reports on this procedure have only short-term follow-up. The longest experience is from Sweden, with studies reporting 80% to 90% good to excellent results at 2 to 10 years after treatment of femoral condyle defects. Lesions in the patellofemoral compartment did not fare as well, with a 60% to 70% success rate. Biopsies from the repair tissue are descirbed as hyaline-like, but actually show a mixture of fibrocartilage and hyaline cartilage. Because it is not true articular cartilage, the durability of the repair has been questioned. Additional disadvantages include the cost of the procedure and reoperation rates of 5% to 10% because of arthrofibrosis/hypertrophy of the healed tissue and other complications. Although ACI has been used to treat small lesions, because of the above concerns it is typically limited to defects of 2 cm or larger (up to 10 cm^2), and where more than one lesion is present and are nonarticulating.

Osteochondral autograft transfer procedures place a cylindrical osteochondral plug(s) from a less weight-bearing region into the articular defect. Methods have been described for using a large plug to completely fill a defect or a series of small ones to match the joint contour and fill larger areas. The benefit of this technique is having true articular cartilage fill the defect, although fibrocartilage surrounds the plugs. The procedure can be done arthroscopically or open. It is technically demanding because the graft must match the joint surface height and contour to be functional. Another suggested benefit is that recovery is typically faster than with many other techniques. Full weight bearing is permitted by 6 weeks. However, stress across the patellofemoral joint is limited for the initial 8 weeks to allow donor site maturation. Activities without restriction are permitted at 3 to 4 months.

Donor site morbidity and limited donor availability are obvious drawbacks of the procedure. Although several possible donor areas have significantly less contact pressure than others, none is completely free from contact pressure (Fig. 8). With the early success rates in treating small defects, some surgeons have expanded the indications to include lesions several centimeters in size despite little knowledge of long-term donor morbidity. Until further information is gained, most authors recommend the use of osteochondral autografts for defects up to 2 to 2.5 cm.

Osteochondral allografts have the advantage of replacing a defect with fully formed hyaline cartilage without the donor site morbidity or size restrictions that exist with autogenous grafts. However, because chondrocyte viability is directly related to graft success, fresh grafts are used, which carry a risk of disease transmission and immune response. Techniques have been developed to prolong cell viability in fresh grafts to allow disease screening, but the critical level of viable cells for graft success is still unknown. As with autogenous osteochondral grafts, extreme attention to surgical detail is needed for the graft to be functional. Because of the slower healing of allografts, weight bearing is restricted for 6 to 12 weeks, depending on whether dowel or shell grafts were used. Athletic activities are generally not permitted until 6 months after a femoral condyle graft and 12 months after a tibial plateau graft.

Several authors reported success rates of 90% at 5 years and 70% at 10 years after treatment of monopolar defects due to osteochondritis dissecans or trauma. Poor results have been reported after treatment of bipolar defects or lesions caused by osteoarthritis or osteonecrosis. Because of concerns about disease transmission, possible immune response, and limited availability, allografts currently are recommended for use only in large defects (minimum of 2 cm).

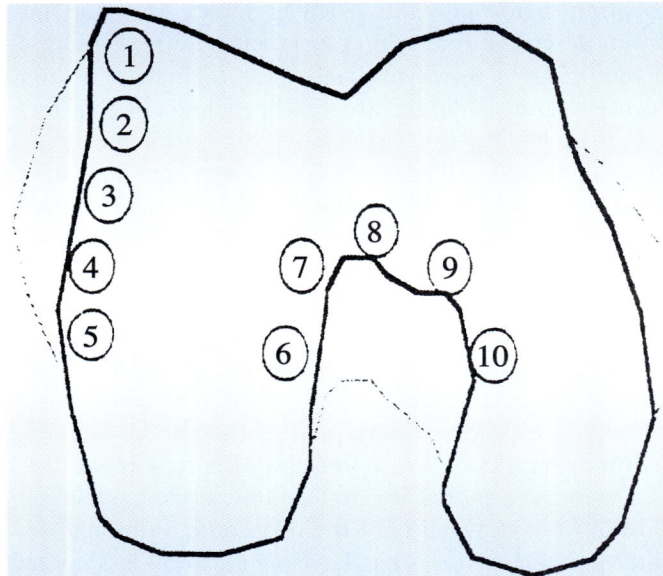

Figure 8 Numbered sites for osteochondral plug harvest with measured contact pressure. *(Reproduced with permission from Simonian PT, Sussmann PS, Wickiewicz, et al: Contact pressures at osteochondral donor sites in the knee. Am J Sports Med 1998;26:491-494.)*

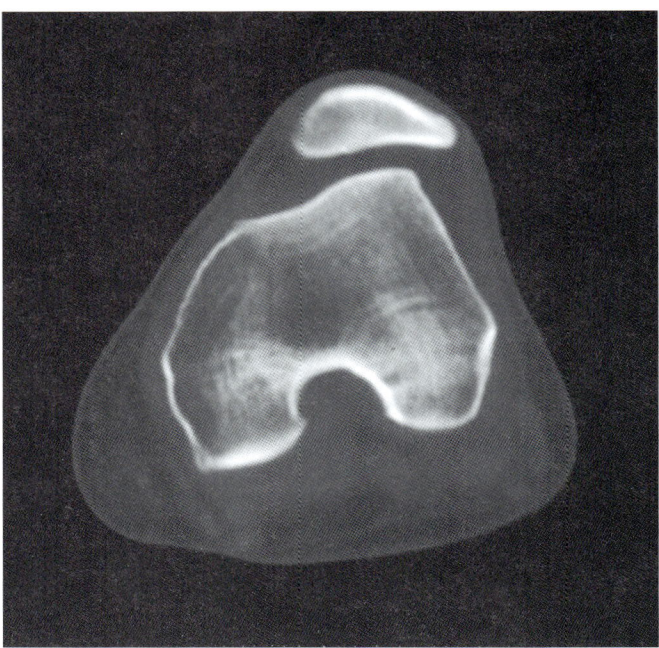

Figure 9 Midpatellar transverse CT image obtained at 45° of knee flexion demonstrating lateral patellar subluxation and trochlear hypoplasia. Normally, the patella enters and stays within the trochlea by 15° of knee flexion.

Patellofemoral Disorders

Knee pain that is patellofemoral in origin is a common condition that can be divided into three categories: soft-tissue abnormalities (patellar tilt, patellar or quadriceps tendinitis, medial plica syndrome, and reflex sympathetic dystrophy [RSD]), patellar instability, and patellofemoral degeneration. A careful, detailed history and physical examination are required for an accurate diagnosis.

The history should provide information regarding the nature of onset, quality, frequency, and location of the pain. Patellofemoral pain frequently occurs while squatting, ascending or descending stairs, or after a prolonged period of sitting. Patients should be asked whether they have experienced feelings or episodes of instability, which should not be confused with episodes of giving way during knee flexion, which may be secondary to quadriceps weakness or pain. Physical examination should include assessment of lower extremity alignment (varus, valgus, rotational), quadriceps angle, degrees of atrophy or effusion, patellar tracking and mobility, crepitus, areas of tenderness (such as the patellar facets and patellar tendon), and tightness of the lateral retinaculum. Provocative maneuvers such as patellar apprehension and grind also should be done.

In addition to AP and lateral views, standard radiographs also should include an axial view of the patella, such as a Merchant or Laurin view, to evaluate patellar subluxation and tilt and trochlear morphology. Trochlear hypoplasia is best seen with an axial view. A lateral view with the knee in 30° of flexion should be spe-cifically assessed for the presence of patella alta or baja. The normal length of the patellar tendon should be no more than 1.2 times the height of the patella on the bilateral view. CT has been recommended as a useful imaging modality for the evaluation of patellar alignment. Midpatellar transverse images are obtained at 15°, 30°, and 45° of knee flexion (Fig. 9). Patellar tilt and congruence angles can then be measured. In general, MRI is not helpful in the routine evaluation of patellofemoral pain; however, it can sometimes be useful in providing information regarding articular cartilage or intraosseous lesions as well as to rule out any meniscal or ligamentous pathology. Radionuclide scanning may be helpful in identifying occult fractures, tumors, or early RSD.

Patellofemoral disorders usually are successfully treated nonsurgically, beginning with reduction of inflammation by activity modification and administration of nonsteroidal anti-inflammatory medication and local modalities. A well-structured, well-supervised rehabilitation program that emphasizes stretching and strengthening of the quadriceps and hamstring musculature is the mainstay of treatment. In general, therapy should initially consist of closed chain exercises performed in a pain-free arc of motion. Although therapy should be individualized to the specific patient, biomechanical studies have shown patellofemoral contact pressures to be lowest within a short arc range of motion (between 0° and 30° of flexion). Open chain resistance exercises, although an effective form of strengthening, may exacerbate symptoms and should be reserved for later stages in the rehabilitation process. Therapy also should include manual stretching of the lateral retinaculum to address patellar tightness or tilt. Patellar bracing or taping can be helpful in some patients.

Acute patellar dislocations initially are treated with closed reduction, aspiration of the hemarthrosis as needed, and a short period of immobilization followed by rehabilitation. The incidence of recurrent dislocation, however, reportedly ranges from 15% to 44%, consequently treatment of these injuries remains controversial. Surgery should be considered to treat associated osteochondral lesions either by removal or internal fixation. Surgical repair of the acutely disrupted medial patellofemoral ligament has been advocated by some, especially in young, athletic individuals who have a high risk of recurrence. A recent study documented the success of immediate surgical repair of the medial patellar stabilizers for acute patellar dislocation. A tear of the medial patellofemoral ligament from the adductor tubercle and the vastus medialis obliquus muscle from the adductor magnus tendon was documented with open surgical repair.

When nonsurgical treatment is unsuccessful, surgery may then be considered. In general, however, surgery to relieve pain in the absence of identifiable and correctable pathology such as patellar tilt, instability, or patellofemoral arthrosis should be avoided. Arthroscopic evaluation should include viewing from a superomedial portal to assess tilt and tracking. By 20° to 25° of knee flexion the lateral facet should engage the trochlea, and the midpatellar ridge should align by 35° to 40°.

Surgical treatment for isolated patellar tilt is a lateral release done either open or arthroscopically. In the arthroscopic technique the release is done under direct vision approximately 5 mm lateral to the patella. Extending the release into the tendon of the vastus lateralis must be avoided because this may result in retraction, imbalance, and further destabilization of the patella. The overall success rate of arthroscopic release for isolated patellar tilt is approximately 80%.

For skeletally mature patients with extensor mechanism malalignment and recurrent patellar subluxation or dislocation despite compliance with an extensive rehabilitation program, distal patellar realignment should be considered. The goal of this procedure, which also includes a lateral release, is medial transfer of the tibial tubercle to correct the quadriceps angle. This method can be accomplished with an Elmslie-Trillat procedure in which the tibial tubercle is osteotomized and transferred medially, leaving the distal portion hinged to improve stability. Additional fix-

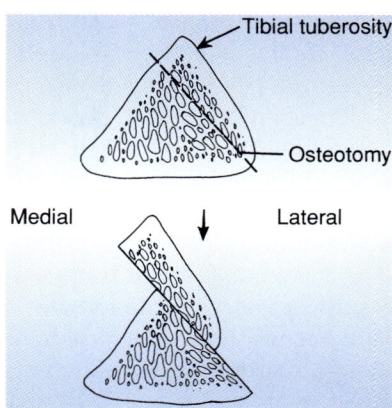

Figure 10 An oblique osteotomy angled from anteromedial to posterolateral reduces patellofemoral contact forces and realigns the extensor mechanism. (Reproduced from Fulkerson JP: Patellofemoral pain disorders: Evaluation and management. J Am Acad Orthop Surg 1994;2:124-132.)

ation with a screw allows early postoperative motion. If there is concomitant chondral degeneration, anteromedial transfer of the tibial tubercle can effectively realign the extensor mechanism and decrease patellofemoral contact forces, which is accomplished by angling the osteotomy from anteromedial to posterolateral (Fig. 10). A hinge of bone is maintained distally as the tubercle is transferred both medially and anteriorly. It is then secured into position with rigid fixation. In both procedures the degree of correction should be individualized to the patient. Complications of tibial tubercle transfer include wound healing problems, compartment syndrome, popliteal artery laceration, postoperative stiffness, persistent pain, medial patellar instability, RSD, and fracture of the proximal tibia. Postoperative rehabilitation should include an initial period of protected weight bearing. Procedures that result in posterior displacement of the tubercle (Hauser procedure) should be avoided because they will result in increased patellofemoral contact forces and predispose to degenerative changes.

Surgical management of patellofemoral arthritis is based on the patient's age and activity level, the extent and location of articular damage, and patellofemoral mechanics. For patients with lateral facet arthritis caused by long-standing patellar tilt, a lateral release may help to relieve symptoms. Lateral facet arthritis caused by subluxation, however, is better managed with anteromedial tibial tubercle transfer. The degree of anteriorization and medialization can be controlled by adjusting the angle of the osteotomy and by the addition of a bone graft. The success of this procedure, however, depends on the condition of the articular cartilage of the proximal medial patella because loads will be transferred to this region. For patients with patellofemoral arthritis without malalignment, direct anterior displacement of the tibial tubercle with bone graft (modified Maquet procedure) can be considered. This procedure, however, has been associated with less predictable outcomes and occasional problems with wound healing. In the case of extensive patellar articular cartilage degeneration unresponsive to other forms of treatment, patellectomy may be considered. Patellectomy should be regarded as a salvage procedure that will result in significant loss of strength. In addition, pain and crepitus might persist. When both the patella and trochlea are diffusely damaged and the medial and patellofemoral compartments have no evidence of arthritis, patellofemoral prosthetic arthroplasty or total knee arthroplasty are possible treatment options. The reported results of isolated patellofemoral arthroplasty, however, are inconsistent with problems of continued pain, instability, and prosthetic loosening.

Loss of Motion

Loss of motion, in particular knee extension, after ACL reconstruction should be distinguished from arthrofibrosis. Loss of knee extension typically results from insufficient notchplasty, improper tunnel placement, or prolonged immobilization. Arthrofibrosis is characterized by extensive periarticular and intra-articular scarring with restriction of both flexion and extension resulting from diffuse capsulitis. This condition represents an excessive inflammatory reaction to a stimulus such as trauma, infection, or surgery. The extensive scarring and stiffness that characterize arthrofibrosis lead to abnormal kinematics, poor function, and early arthrosis. Intra-articular, periarticular, and extra-articular processes may all be involved.

Patients with arthrofibrosis present with diffuse pain, edema, warmth, restricted patellar mobility, and limitation of both flexion and extension. As the process continues, there may be ankylosis and patellar entrapment as the capsule loses its compliance and fibrosis extends into the quadriceps muscle. Radiographs may demonstrate osteopenia secondary to disuse and a patella infera. The hallmark of treatment is prevention, which includes adherence to proper surgical technique, avoidance of prolonged immobilization with emphasis on obtaining and maintaining immediate full extension, and accelerated rehabilitation. Treatment of arthrofibrosis begins with nonsteroidal anti-inflammatory medication and physical therapy. A tapered course of methylprednisolone also can be used to reduce inflammation. If there is no improvement despite up to 12 weeks of nonsurgical treatment, and knee range of motion has reached a plateau with a firm endpoint at extremes, manipulation under anesthesia and arthroscopic débridement are indicated. For extension loss, notchplasty enlargement as needed and excision of all anterior and intercondylar notch scar tissue should be done (Fig. 11). In addition, extensor mechanism adhesions and the medial and lateral retinacula are released, and peripatellar scar tissue is excised when necessary to restore flexion and normal patellar track-

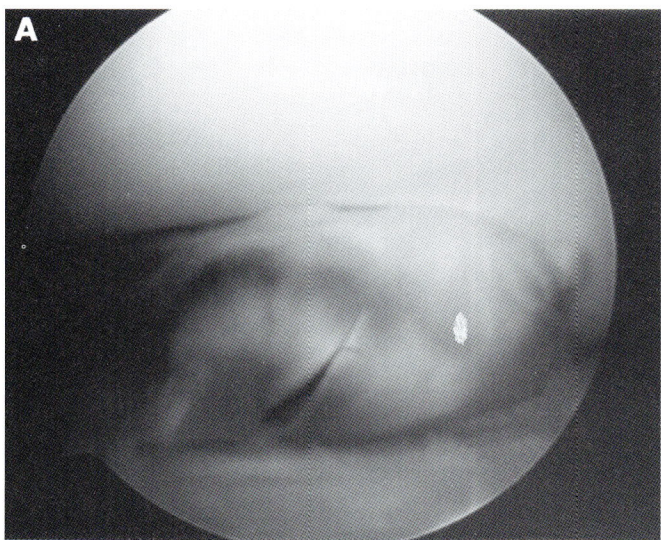

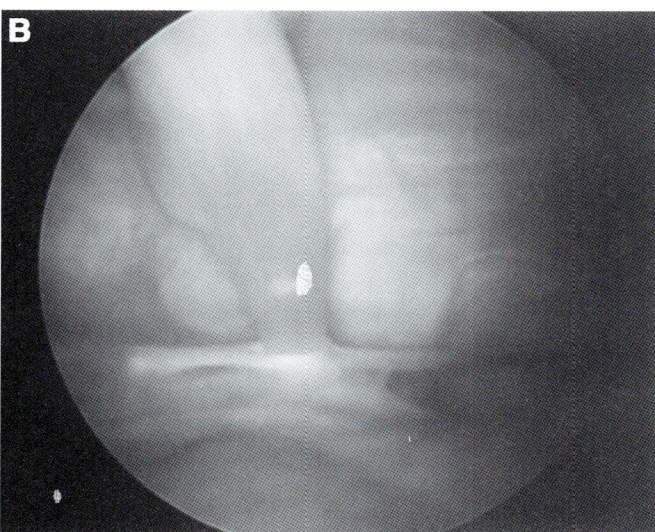

Figure 11 Arthroscopic photographs demonstrating **(A)** intercondylar notch scar tissue (cyclops lesion) and **(B)** suprapatellar adhesions associated with arthrofibrosis following ACL reconstruction.

ing. Open débridement and soft-tissue release may be necessary as a salvage procedure. Complications associated with manipulation under anesthesia include periarticular fractures and extensor mechanism disruption. The use of intravenous corticosteroids, continuous epidural anesthesia, cryotherapy, and continuous passive motion assists in maintaining range of motion achieved in the operating room. In addition, an extension cast or brace may be worn at night to maintain full extension.

Reflex Sympathetic Dystrophy (Complex Regional Pain Syndrome)

Complex regional pain syndrome (CRPS) refers to a condition characterized by intense burning pain along

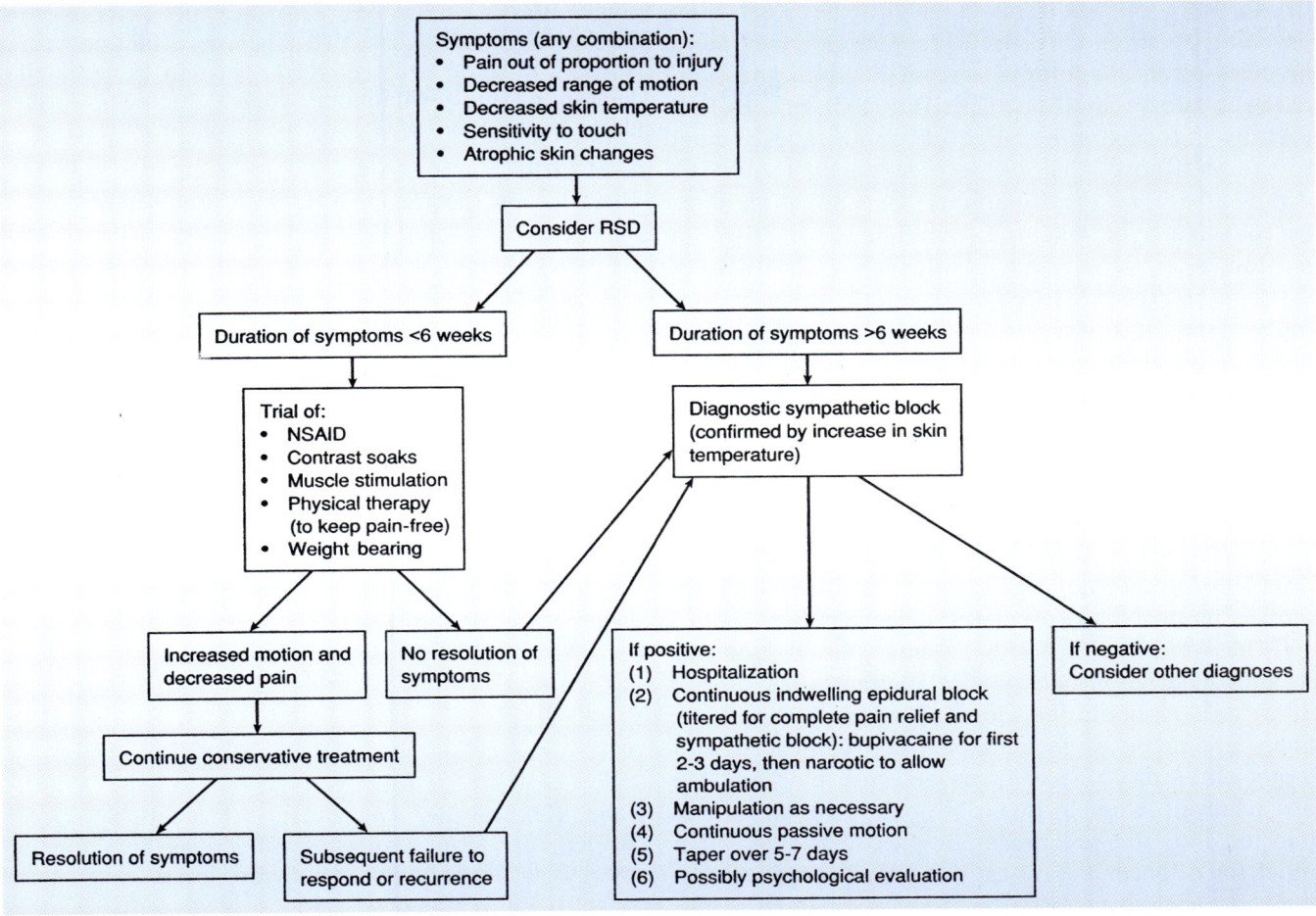

Figure 12 An algorithm for the treatment of RSD of the knee. (*Reproduced from Cooper DE, DeLee JC: Reflex sympathetic dystrophy of the knee.* J Am Acad Orthop Surg *1994;2:79-86.*)

with autonomic and tissue changes over an extremity after an injury. This group of symptoms is known as RSD, or in the case of a known nerve injury, causalgia.

Normally, the sympathetic nervous system is activated in response to injury. The initial vasoconstriction and swelling that ensue gradually decrease as sympathetic tone is reduced. In CRPS sympathetic tone persists inappropriately, and a vicious cycle is created in which tissue edema with resultant capillary collapse and ischemia causes pain that in turn restimulates the sympathetic nervous system. The successful treatment of CRPS depends on the interruption of this abnormal positive feedback loop.

The diagnosis of CRPS is based primarily on the patient's clinical presentation. There typically is a history of recent or remote trauma with pain that is out of proportion to the degree of injury. The course of CRPS has been divided into stages. It should be recognized, however, that CRPS of the knee may not follow the classic sequence of stages and the clinical presentation may be quite variable. Patellofemoral symptoms usually are present; however, early loss of

motion, in particular knee flexion, helps distinguish CRPS from other sources of patellofemoral pain. A high index of suspicion must be maintained, especially when pain appears to be out of proportion to the severity of injury.

Osteopenia of the patella is a common radiographic finding; however, this condition develops late in the disease process because calcium content must be altered 30% to 50% before becoming evident on plain radiographs. Three-phase bone scans and thermograms also have been used for the diagnosis of CRPS, with variable degrees of sensitivity and specificity reported. The most reliable diagnostic test is a successful response to a lumbar sympathetic block in which pain is significantly improved and skin temperature rises by 1°C as a result of vasodilatation. Incomplete pain relief should not rule out the diagnosis of CRPS, because some lumbar sympathetic fibers may bypass the sympathetic chain and escape being blocked.

Early detection and initiation of treatment are the most important factors in a successful outcome. A multidisciplinary approach that involves the orthopaedic surgeon, pain management specialist, and psychiatrist should be used. In general, treatment involves physical therapy, oral medication, and sympathetic blockade (Fig. 12). The goal of physical therapy is to maintain range of motion and prevent further stiffness. The use of ice packs should be avoided because these patients have an intolerance to cold. To avoid painful stimuli, passive range of motion is avoided while gentle active and active-assistive exercises are encouraged. A patient, supportive therapist is critical for the successful treatment of these often difficult patients.

Several drugs have been used to relieve the symptoms of CRPS, including alpha blocking agents, antidepressants, calcium channel blockers, anticonvulsants, nonsteroidal anti-inflammatory drugs, and oral corticosteroids. Because these drugs are associated with a number of side effects, as well as the possibility of drug interaction and dependence, they are best prescribed by physicians experienced in their use.

If the symptoms of CRPS are not relieved promptly by oral medication and physical therapy, sympathetic interruption should be done. Because sympathetic fibers are the least myelinated when compared with motor and sensory nerve fibers, selective blockade can be achieved with a low dose of local anesthetic injected into the subarachnoid space. Sustained pain relief for a longer period can be achieved by using an indwelling epidural catheter on an inpatient basis. Long-lasting anesthetic agents can be delivered directly to the sympathetic chain, providing a paravertebral block. However, this procedure is technically difficult to perform. Finally, surgical sympathectomy from the tenth thoracic to fourth lumbar vertebra should be considered as a salvage procedure because symptoms tend to recur.

Annotated Bibliography

Anterior Cruciate Ligament Injuries

Aronowitz ER, Ganley TJ, Goode JR, Gregg JR, Meyer JS: Anterior cruciate ligament reconstruction in adolescents with open physes. *Am J Sports Med* 2000;28:168-175.

In this study, 19 adolescents (age 11 to 15 years, skeletal age ≥ 14 years) undergoing ACL reconstruction were reviewed. Surgical technique included soft-tissue grafts and transphyseal tunnels. At an average 2-year follow up, all patients remained stable and 16 of 19 patients returned to sports. No limb-length discrepancies or angular deformities were detected.

Bach BR Jr, Levy ME, Bojchuk J, Tradonsky S, Bush-Joseph CA, Khan NH: Single-incision endoscopic anterior cruciate ligament reconstruction using patellar tendon autograft: Minimum two-year follow-up evaluation. *Am J Sports Med* 1998;26:30-40.

Bach BR Jr, Tradonsky S, Bojchuk J, Levy ME, Bush-Joseph CA, Khan NH: Arthroscopically assisted anterior cruciate ligament reconstruction using patellar tendon autograft: Five to nine-year follow-up evaluation. *Am J Sports Med* 1998;26:20-29.

Retrospective follow-up studies of two-incision and endoscopic ACL reconstructions using patellar techniques are presented. At 5 to 9 years, the two-incision group showed excellent stability although 12% had symptomatic flexion contractures. The endoscopic group revealed 91% with negative pivot shift with 5% undergoing reoperation for flexion contracture.

Brandsson S, Kartus J, Larsson J, Eriksson BI, Karlsson J: A comparison of results in middle-aged and young patients after anterior cruciate ligament reconstruction. *Arthroscopy* 2000;16:178-182.

This retrospective study compared the outcomes of young (age 20 to 24 years) and older (> 40 years) patients. Using the IKDC rating scale, similar outcomes were noted when comparing stability and function. Interestingly, the older patients had a higher level of subjective satisfaction.

Faber KJ, Dill JR, Amendola A, Thain L, Spouge A, Fowler PJ: Occult osteochondral lesions after anterior cruciate ligament rupture: Six-year magnetic resonance imaging follow-up study. *Am J Sports Med* 1999;27: 489-494.

The MRI appearance of occult osteochondral injuries is compared 6 years after ACL injury. All patients were noted to have a normal-appearing articular cartilage at the initial arthroscopy. At 6-year follow-up, 65% of patients displayed persistent marrow abnormalities with many patients also showing articular thinning in the involved area.

Fu FH, Bennett CH, Lattermann C, Ma CB: Current trends in anterior cruciate ligament reconstruction: Part I. Biology and biomechanics of reconstruction. *Am J Sports Med* 1999;27:821-830.

Fu FH, Bennett CH, Ma CB, Menetrey J, Lattermann C: Current trends in anterior cruciate ligament reconstruction: Part II. Operative procedures and clinical correlations. *Am J Sports Med* 2000;28:124-130.

These articles present a current concepts review of basic science and clinical trends in ACL reconstruction.

Griffin LY, Agel J, Albohm MJ, et al: Noncontact anterior cruciate ligament injuries: Risk factors and prevention strategies. *J Am Acad Orthop Surg* 2000;8: 141-150.

A review of anatomic, hormonal, biomechanical, and environmental risk factors leading to noncontact ACL injuries is presented. Risk prevention strategies are outlined and areas of future research are suggested.

Hewett TE, Lindenfeld TN, Riccobene JV, Noyes FR: The effect of neuromuscular training on the incidence of knee injury in female athletes: A prospective study. *Am J Sports Med* 1999;27:699-706.

This article presents a prospective study on the effects of neuromuscular and plyometric training in preventing knee injury in female athletes. With a minimum of 4 weeks of preseason training, a significant decrease in the incidence of serious knee injuries was demonstrated among female high-school athletes.

McAllister DR, Parker RD, Cooper AE, Recht MP, Abate J: Outcomes of postoperative septic arthritis after anterior cruciate ligament reconstruction. *Am J Sports Med* 1999;27:562-570.

The authors report on the treatment of postoperative septic arthritis after ACL reconstruction. With aggressive management, graft preservation and knee motion can be maintained. Clinical results and function outcome were compromised by articular cartilage damage.

Schappert SM (ed): Office visits to orthopaedic surgeons: United States 1995-96, in *Advance Data: Centers for Disease Control and Prevention/National Center for Health Statistics.* Hyattsville, MD, US Dept Health and Human Services, DHHS no. (PHS) 98-1250, number 302, 1998.

The most recent demographic report on the rising occurrence of knee injuries and the increasing frequency of patients with knee symptoms presenting to an orthopaedic surgeon is provided.

Shelbourne KD, Gray T: Results of anterior cruciate ligament reconstruction based on meniscus and articular cartilage status at the time of surgery: Five- to fifteen-year evaluations. *Am J Sports Med* 2000;28:446-452.

This article presents a 5- to 15-year follow-up study comparing the results of ACL reconstruction based on meniscal status at the time of surgery. Patients who maintained both menisci were found to have an 87% good to excellent IKDC score and 97% normal or near-normal radiographs. Those with loss of both menisci, despite having stable knees, fared worse.

Medial Collateral Ligament Injuries

Miller MD, Osborne JR, Gordon WT, Hinkin DT, Brinker MR: The natural history of bone bruises: A prospective study of magnetic resonance imaging-detected trabecular microfractures in patients with isolated medial collateral ligament injuries. *Am J Sports Med* 1998;26:15-19.

In 65 young patients (average age 24.8 years) who had isolated MCL injuries, MRI showed associated bone bruises (trabecular microfractures) primarily involving the lateral side of the knee in 45%. Follow-up MRI studies were accomplished at various intervals in 83% of these patients. All of these bone bruises resolved by gradual diffusion over a 2- to 4-month period.

Moorman CT III, Kukreti U, Fenton DC, Belkoff SM: The early effect of ibuprofen on the mechanical properties of healing medial collateral ligament. *Am J Sports Med* 1999;27:738-741.

In an animal study, the authors determined that there was no significant difference in the values of mechanical properties of MCLs from rabbits treated with ibuprofen versus those treated with placebo at either 14 or 28 days after injury. The findings suggest that there is no deleterious effect of a short course of ibuprofen on the mechanical behavior of injured MCLs.

Posterior Cruciate Ligament Injuries

Harner CD, Janaushek MA, Kanamori A, Yagi M, Vogrin TM, Woo SL: Biomechanical analysis of a double-bundle posterior cruciate ligament reconstruction. *Am J Sports Med* 2000;28:144-151.

This article, winner of the 1999 Cabaud award, compares the biomechanics of the single versus double bundle technique for PCL reconstruction. Ten cadavers were tested with a high-tech robotic system and comparisons were made between intact knees, single bundle reconstructed knees, and double bundle reconstructed knees. The double bundle reconstruction more closely restores the biomechanics of the knee throughout the range of motion.

Miller MD, Bergfeld JA, Fowler PJ, Harner CD, Noyes FR: The posterior cruciate ligament injured knee: Principles of evaluation and treatment. *Instr Course Lect* 1999;48:199-207.

This article presents an update of basic science and clinical applications regarding PCL injuries and reconstruction techniques.

Shelbourne KD, Davis TJ, Patel DV: The natural history of acute, isolated, nonoperatively treated posterior cruciate ligament injuries: A prospective study. *Am J Sports Med* 1999;27:276-283.

Follow-up of 133 patients with isolated grade I and II PCL injuries was accomplished at average 5.4 years after injury. Objective evaluation was completed on 68 of these patients and subjective data was collected on all patients. On objective examination, there was no change in laxity from the initial injury. Subjectively, the mean modified Noyes knee score was 84.2 and the mean Lysholm score was 83.4. One half of patients were able to return to their same sport at the same level or higher, one third returned to the same sport at a lower level, and one sixth did not return to the same sport.

Posterolateral Complex Injuries

Chen FS, Rokito AS, Pitman MI: Acute and chronic posterolateral rotatory instability of the knee. *J Am Acad Orthop Surg* 2000;8:97-110.

This review article includes surgical techniques for both acute and chronic posterolateral corner injuries. Recent research and treatment options are summarized.

Harner CD, Vogrin TM, Hoher J, Ma CB, Woo SL: Biomechanical analysis of a posterior cruciate ligament reconstruction: Deficiency of the posterolateral structures as a cause of graft failure. *Am J Sports Med* 2000;28:32-39.

Using a robotic system in cadaver knees, sectioning of the posterolateral structures increased posterior tibial translation in PCL reconstructed knees by 6 mm, external rotation by 14°, and in situ forces 22% to 150%. This study demonstrates that PCL reconstruction is ineffective if posterolateral structures are deficient.

LaPrade RF, Gilbert TJ, Bollom TS, Wentorf F, Chaljub G: The magnetic resonance imaging appearance of individual structures of the posterolateral knee: A prospective study of normal knees and knees with surgically verified grade III injuries. *Am J Sports Med* 2000;28:191-199.

This article accurately describes MRI findings of injury to individual structures of the posterolateral complex.

Knee Dislocations

Almekinders LC, Dedmond BT: Outcomes of the operatively treated knee dislocation. *Clin Sports Med* 2000;19:503-518.

Surgical outcome measures including range of motion, pain and swelling, return to work, return to athletics, subjective rating, instability, and posttraumatic arthritis are analyzed by a review of the literature.

Brautigan B, Johnson DL: The epidemiology of knee dislocations. *Clin Sports Med* 2000;19:387-397.

This article discusses the epidemiology of knee dislocations and its effect on treatment.

Hegyes MS, Richardson MW, Miller MD: Knee dislocation: Complications of nonoperative and operative management. *Clin Sports Med* 2000;19:519-543.

Potential nonsurgical complications include vascular injury, neurologic injury, delay in diagnosis, compartment syndrome, open dislocation, associated fractures, and proximal tibiofibular joint dislocation. Potential surgical complications include iatrogenic vascular injury, iatrogenic nerve injury, compartment syndrome, tourniquet problems, infection, wound healing problems, complex regional pain syndrome, loss of motion, and residual laxity.

Huang FS, Simonian PT, Chansky HA: Irreducible posterolateral dislocation of the knee. *Arthroscopy* 2000;16:323-327.

The pathoanatomy, diagnosis, and treatment of an irreducible posterolateral knee dislocation are discussed in this case report.

Klimkiewicz JJ, Petrie RS, Harner CD: Surgical treatment of combined injury to anterior cruciate ligament, posterior cruciate ligament, and medial structures. *Clin Sports Med* 2000;19:479-492.

The authors preferred surgical technique is patellar tendon allograft ACL reconstruction, Achilles tendon allograft PCL reconstruction, and medial side repair.

Mariani PP, Santoriello P, Iannone S, Condello V, Adriani E: Comparison of surgical treatments for knee dislocation. *Am J Knee Surg* 1999;12:214-221.

This retrospective review of surgical treatment methods for the dislocated knee found better range of motion and stability after combined ACL and PCL reconstruction. Direct repair of the cruciate ligaments is discouraged.

Schenck RC Jr, Hunter RE, Ostrum RF, Perry CR: Knee dislocations. *Instr Course Lect* 1999;48:515-522.

The classification, evaluation, and management of the dislocated knee are discussed.

Shelbourne KD, Klootwyk TE: Low-velocity knee dislocation with sports injuries: Treatment principles. *Clin Sports Med* 2000;19:443-456.

Treatment of the low-velocity knee dislocation is based upon the unique physiologic healing potential of each injured structure in the author's experience. MCL tears are treated nonsurgically. PCL tears are allowed to heal if laxity is 2+ or less, but reconstructed acutely if the initial posterior drawer is > 2+. ACL reconstruction is performed in a delayed manner only in symptomatic patients. Lateral side repair is performed acutely to reattach structures to their distally torn site.

Wascher DC: High-velocity knee dislocation with vascular injury: Treatment principles. *Clin Sports Med* 2000;19:457-477.

This detailed review of high velocity knee dislocations outlines the initial care, vascular repair, nerve treatment, and the author's approach for ligamentous injuries.

Wascher DC, Becker JR, Dexter JG, Blevins FT: Reconstruction of the anterior and posterior cruciate ligaments after knee dislocation: Results using fresh-frozen nonirradiated allografts. *Am J Sports Med* 1999;27:189-195.

The authors retrospectively reviewed 13 patients who underwent simultaneous ACL and PCL reconstructions using patellar and Achilles tendon allografts. At short-term follow-up (mean, 38 months), six knees were rated as nearly normal, five as abnormal, and one as grossly abnormal by the IKDC scale. Six patients returned to unrestricted sports activity and four returned to modified sports activity.

Meniscus

Boenisch UW, Faber KJ, Ciarelli M, Steadman JR, Arnoczky SP: Pull-out strength and stiffness of meniscal repair using absorbable arrows or Ti-Cron vertical and horizontal loop sutures. *Am J Sports Med* 1999;27:626-631.

The use of bioabsorbable arrows and vertical and horizontal loop sutures were compared. Results showed that vertical sutures have the highest pullout strength.

Carter TR: Meniscal allograft transplantation. *Sports Med Arthrosc Rev* 1999;7:51-62.

A review of meniscal allograft transplantation and personal experience with the procedure are presented.

DeHaven KE: Meniscus repair. *Am J Sports Med* 1999;27:242-250.

A concise yet comprehensive review of indications and techniques of meniscus repair is presented.

van Trommel MF, Potter HG, Ernberg LA, Simonian PT, Wickiewicz TL: The use of noncontrast magnetic resonance imaging in evaluating meniscal repair: Comparison with conventional arthrography. *Arthroscopy* 1998;14:2-8.

Specialized fast spin/echo MRI techniques were evaluated, revealing the need for intra-articular contrast when evaluating meniscal repair.

Articular Cartilage Injuries

Bugbee WD, Convery FR: Osteochondral allograft transplantation. *Clin Sports Med* 1999;18:67-75.

The authors present an overview of the use of osteochondral allografts in knee surgery, including their institution's experience.

O'Driscoll SW: The healing and regeneration of articular cartilage. *J Bone Joint Surg Am* 1998;80:1795-1812.

A general review of the various treatment options available for treating articular injury is given.

Potter HG, Linklater JM, Allen AA, Hannafin JA, Haas SB: Magnetic resonance imaging of articular cartilage in the knee: An evaluation with use of fast-spin-echo imaging. *J Bone Joint Surg Am* 1998;80:1276-1284.

This article presents a study on modified MRI sequences in which articular surface abnormalities were accurately assessed.

Patellofemoral Disorders

Ahmad CS, Stein BE, Matuz D, Henry JH: Immediate surgical repair of the medial patellar stabilizers for acute patellar dislocation: A review of eight cases. *Am J Sports Med* 2000;28:804-810.

Eight patients underwent open surgical repair of the injured medial patellofemoral ligament and vastus medialis obliquus after acute patellar dislocation. At an average follow-up of 3 years, no patients experienced a recurrent dislocation.

Gambardella RA: Technical pitfalls of patellofemoral surgery. *Clin Sports Med* 1999;18:897-903.

The three main areas that significantly influence outcomes from patellofemoral surgery are reviewed: misdiagnosis, miscommunication, and improper rehabilitation. By improving technical expertise in these areas, the success of patellofemoral surgery will be greatly enhanced.

Griffiths GP, Selesnick FH: Operative treatment and arthroscopic findings in chronic patellar tendinitis. *Arthroscopy* 1998;14:836-839.

Seven patients (eight knees) with chronic patellar tendinitis underwent arthroscopy and open excision of degenerated tissue and stimulation of a healing response. Fibrotendinous degeneration was consistently found. Overall, 86% of patients had an excellent result.

Millett PJ, Williams RJ, Wickiewicz TL: Open debridement and soft tissue release as a salvage procedure for the severely arthrofibrotic knee. *Am J Sports Med* 1999;27:552-561.

A retrospective study of eight patients with severe postoperative loss of motion was done. Risk factors for arthrofibrosis included multiligament injuries, acute reconstructions, and septic arthritis. Average range of motion improved from 62.5° to 124°. The authors recommend this procedure as a salvage procedure to restore motion in the profoundly arthrofibrotic knee.

Myers P, Williams A, Dodds R, Bulow J: The three-in-one proximal and distal soft tissue patellar realignment procedure: Results, and its place in the management of patellofemoral instability. *Am J Sports Med* 1999;27:575-579.

The authors reviewed the results of a three-in-one procedure that includes lateral release, vastus medialis obliquus advancement, and transfer of the medial third of the patellar tendon. Thirty-two of 42 knees with recurrent patellar dislocation had an excellent or good result. The redislocation rate was 9.5%.

Petsche TS, Hutchinson MR: Loss of extension after reconstruction of the anterior cruciate ligament. *J Am Acad Orthop Surg* 1999;7:119-127.

This review article discusses the various surgical and nonsurgical factors associated with loss of extension following ACL reconstruction. Preoperative, intraoperative, and postoperative techniques for prevention of this complication are reviewed.

Post WR: Clinical evaluation of patients with patellofemoral disorders. *Arthroscopy* 1999;15:841-851.

The author highlights the key components of the clinical evaluation (history, physical examination, imaging studies) necessary for proper diagnosis and treatment of patients with patellofemoral disorders.

Sanchis-Alfonso V, Rosello-Sastre E, Monteagudo-Castro C, Esquerdo J: Quantitative analysis of nerve changes in the lateral retinaculum in patients with isolated symptomatic patellofemoral malalignment: A preliminary study. *Am J Sports Med* 1998;26:703-709.

Histologic evaluation of 16 lateral retinacula revealed a correlation between total neural area and pain. The authors also concluded that patellofemoral malalignment can be explained in part by a loss of proprioception caused by neural damage.

Shalaby M, Almekinders LC: Patellar tendinitis: The significance of magnetic resonance imaging findings. *Am J Sports Med* 1999;27:345-349.

MRI studies of patients with clinical patellar tendinitis were evaluated and compared with those of a control group. Only stage III lesions were associated with abnormal findings on MRI, which had a sensitivity and specificity of only 75% and 29%, respectively.

Classic Bibliography

Aglietti P, Buzzi R, Insall JN: Disorders of the patellofemoral joint, in Insall JN, Windsor RE, Scott WN, Kelly MA, Aglietti P (eds): *Surgery of the Knee*, ed 2. New York, NY, Churchill Livingstone, 1993.

Barber FA, Click SD: Meniscus repair rehabilitation with concurrent anterior cruciate reconstruction. *Arthroscopy* 1997;13:433-437.

Bellemans J, Cauwenberghs F, Witvrouw E, Brys P, Victor J: Anteromedial tibial tubercle transfer in patients with chronic anterior knee pain and a subluxation-type patellar malalignment. *Am J Sports Med* 1997;25:375-381.

Bobic V: Arthroscopic osteochondral autograft transplantation in anterior cruciate ligament reconstruction: A preliminary clinical study. *Knee Surg Sports Traumatol Arthrosc* 1996;3:262-264.

Boden BP, Pearsall AW, Garrett WE, Feagin JA: Patellofemoral instability: Evaluation and management. *J Am Acad Orthop Surg* 1997;5:47-57.

Brittberg M, Lindahl A, Nilsson A, Ohlsson C, Isaksson O, Peterson L: Treatment of deep cartilage defects in the knee with autologous chondrocyte transplantation. *N Engl J Med* 1994;331:889-895.

Buckwalter JA, Mankin HJ: Articular cartilage: Part II. Degeneration and osteoarthrosis, repair, regeneration, and transplantation. *J Bone Joint Surg Am* 1997;79:612-632.

Cooper DE: Tests for posterolateral instability of the knee in normal subjects: Results of examination under anesthesia. *J Bone Joint Surg Am* 1991;73:30-36.

Cooper DE, DeLee JC: Reflex sympathetic dystrophy of the knee. *J Am Acad Orthop Surg* 1994;2:79-86.

Curl WW, Krome J, Gordon ES, Rushing J, Smith BP, Poehling GG: Cartilage injuries: A review of 31,516 knee arthroscopies. *Arthroscopy* 1997;13:456-460.

Frassica FJ, Sim FH, Staeheli JW, Pairolero PC: Dislocation of the knee. *Clin Orthop* 1991;263:200-205.

Fulkerson JP: Patellofemoral pain disorders: Evaluation and management. *J Am Acad Orthop Surg* 1994;2:124-132.

Garth WP, Pomphrey M, Merrill K: Functional treatment of patellar dislocation in an athletic population. *Am J Sports Med* 1996;24:785-791.

Gellman H, Nichols D: Reflex sympathetic dystrophy in the upper extremity. *J Am Acad Orthop Surg* 1997;5:313-322.

Ghazavi MT, Pritzker KP, Davis AM, Gross AE: Fresh osteochondral allografts for post-traumatic osteochondral defects of the knee. *J Bone Joint Surg Br* 1997;79:1008-1013.

Good L, Johnson RJ: The dislocated knee. *J Am Acad Orthop Surg* 1995;3:284-292.

Green NE, Allen BL: Vascular injuries associated with dislocation of the knee. *J Bone Joint Surg Am* 1977;59: 236-239.

Hangody L, Kish G, Karpati Z, Eberhart R: Osteochondral plugs: Autogenous osteochondral mosaicplasty for the treatment of focal chondral and osteochondral articular defects. *Op Tech Orthop* 1997;7: 312-322.

Hewett TE, Noyes FR, Lee MD: Diagnosis of complete and partial posterior cruciate ligament ruptures: Stress radiography compared with KT-1000 arthrometer and posterior drawer testing. *Am J Sports Med* 1997;25:648-655.

Indelicato PA: Non-operative treatment of complete tears of the medial collateral ligament of the knee. *J Bone Joint Surg Am* 1983;65:323-329.

Kendall RW, Taylor DC, Salvian AJ, O'Brien PJ: The role of arteriography in assessing vascular injuries associated with dislocations of the knee. *J Trauma* 1993;35: 875-878.

Lindenfeld TN, Bach BR Jr, Wojtys EM: Reflex sympathetic dystrophy and pain dysfunction in the lower extremity. *Instr Course Lect* 1997;46:261-268.

Maenpaa H, Lehto MU: Patellar dislocation: The longterm results of nonoperative management in 100 patients. *Am J Sports Med* 1997;25:213-217.

Meyers MH, Harvey JP Jr: Traumatic dislocation of the knee joint: A study of eighteen cases. *J Bone Joint Surg Am* 1971;53:16-29.

Milachowski KA, Weismeier K, Wirth CJ: Homologous meniscus transplantation: Experimental and clinical results. *Int Orthop* 1989;13:1-11.

Noyes FR, Barber-Westin SD: Reconstruction of the anterior and posterior cruciate ligaments after knee dislocation: Use of early, protected postoperative motion to decrease arthrofibrosis. *Am J Sports Med* 1997;25:769-778.

O'Brien SJ, Ngeow J, Gibney MA, Warren RF, Fealy S: Reflex sympathetic dystrophy of the knee: Causes, diagnosis, and treatment. *Am J Sports Med* 1995;23: 655-659.

Rubman MH, Noyes FR, Barber-Westin SD: Arthroscopic repair of meniscal tears that extend into the avascular zone: A review of 198 single and complex tears. *Am J Sports Med* 1998;26:87-95.

Shapiro MS, Freedman EL: Allograft reconstruction of the anterior and posterior cruciate ligaments after traumatic knee dislocation. *Am J Sports Med* 1995;23: 580-587.

Shelbourne KD, Patel DV, Adsit WS, Porter DA: Rehabilitation after meniscal repair. *Clin Sports Med* 1996;15:595-612.

Shelbourne KD, Patel DV, Martini DJ: Classification and management of arthrofibrosis of the knee after anterior cruciate ligament reconstruction. *Am J Sports Med* 1996;24:857-862.

Shelbourne KD, Porter DA: Anterior cruciate ligament-medial collateral ligament injury: Nonoperative management of medial collateral ligament tears with anterior cruciate ligament reconstruction. A preliminary report. *Am J Sports Med* 1992;20:283-286.

Sisto DJ, Warren RF: Complete knee dislocation: A follow-up study of operative treatment. *Clin Orthop* 1985;198:94-101.

Steadman JR, Rodkey WG, Singleton SB, Briggs KK: Microfracture technique for full-thickness chondral defects: Technique and clinical results. *Oper Tech Orthop* 1997;7:300-304.

Tenuta JJ, Arciero RA: Arthroscopic evaluation of meniscal repairs: Factors that effect healing. *Am J Sports Med* 1994;22:797-802.

Thompson WO, Thaete FL, Fu FH, Dye SF: Tibial meniscal dynamics using three-dimensional reconstruction of magnetic resonance images. *Am J Sports Med* 1991;19:210-216.

Treiman GS, Yellin AE, Weaver FA, et al: Examination of the patient with a knee dislocation: The case for selective arteriography. *Arch Surg* 1992;127: 1056-1063.

Veltri DM, Warren RF: Isolated and combined posterior cruciate ligament injuries. *J Am Acad Orthop Surg* 1993;1:67-75.

Veltri DM, Warren RF: Posterolateral instability of the knee. *J Bone Joint Surg Am* 1994;76:460-472.

Williams RJ, Laurencin CT, Warren RF, Speciale AC, Brause BD, O'Brien S: Septic arthritis after arthroscopic anterior cruciate ligament reconstruction: Diagnosis and management. *Am J Sports Med* 1997;25: 261-267.

Chapter 44

Knee Reconstruction

Michael J. Archibeck, MD   David C. Ayers, MD

Richard A. Berger, MD   Robert Buly, MD

Kevin L. Garvin, MD   Erik T. Otterberg, MD

Michael J. Stuart, MD   Russell E. Windsor, MD

Nonsurgical Treatment

Medical Treatment

Physical and pharmacologic therapy for osteoarthritis can modulate symptoms but do not alter the underlying biochemical abnormalities. Medical treatment involves a stepwise progression, beginning with the less invasive, less expensive, and best-tolerated options.

Nonsteroidal anti-inflammatory drugs (NSAIDs) decrease pain and inflammation by inhibiting the cyclooxygenase enzyme. Traditional NSAIDs suppress prostaglandin synthesis in both the cyclooxygenase-1 (COX-1) and cyclooxygenase-2 (COX-2) pathways. COX-1 regulates cellular function in the gastrointestinal tract, kidneys, liver, central nervous system, and platelets. Potential side effects of these drugs include gastrointestinal upset, peptic ulcer, renal impairment, liver toxicity, hemorrhage, and even death. Specific COX-2 inhibitors have been developed. There is no evidence that these selective anti-inflammatory drugs are more effective, but they are associated with a much lower incidence of dyspepsia, nausea, abdominal pain, and ulcer formation. COX-2 inhibitors are preferred for patients with a history of gastrointestinal problems or coagulopathy and with concurrent corticosteroid use or therapeutic anticoagulation. COX-2 inhibitors can be continued until surgery and also used in the immediate postoperative period because they do not affect thromboxane synthesis or platelet function. COX-2 inhibitors can decrease the efficacy of angiotension-converting enzyme inhibitors. Traditional NSAIDS and the COX-2 inhibitors should be avoided in patients with congestive heart failure, dehydration, renal disease, or advanced age.

Intra-articular injection of local anesthetic and steroid is unpredictable but often transiently effective. The potent anti-inflammatory effect of cortisone is beneficial for acute synovitis. Arthrocentesis is performed prior to the injection if an effusion is present.

Intra-articular injection of hyaluronic acid derivatives (hyaluronan) is known as viscosupplementation. Hyaluronan restores some elastic and viscous properties of synovial fluid, resulting in pain modulation and improved joint function. Hyaluronic acid is a large, linear glycosaminoglycan found in articular cartilage and synovial fluid that is composed of repeating disaccharide units of N-acetylglucosamine and glucuronic acid. In osteoarthritis, hyaluronic acid has a lower molecular weight and a reduced synovial concentration.

Short-term clinical trials have demonstrated that viscosupplementation can modulate pain and improve function in some patients with osteoarthritis of the knee; however, some clinical studies have failed to demonstrate an effect. The incidence of side effects appears small, but a local inflammatory response has been observed in 3% to 7% of knees. A severe reaction with development of a very large knee effusion mimicking septic arthritis typically occurs after the third injection in some of these patients. Multicenter double-blind clinical trials comparing hyaluronan with saline injections (in 60 knees) have documented complete or near-complete pain relief at 10 to 24 weeks in 39% to 56% of knees with hyaluronan compared with only 13% in the saline group. Hyaluronan injections were at least as good or better than NSAIDs for all outcome measures except activity restrictions.

Hyaluronan injections do not replace weight loss, muscle strengthening, and other nonsurgical treatment methods and should be avoided in patients with mechanical symptoms, varus malalignment more than 10°, valgus malalignment more than 15°, terminal extension loss more than 20°, and a history of allergy to birds or feathers.

Therapy and Orthotic Devices

Physical therapy measures such as weight loss, muscle strengthening, and low impact exercise along with shoe modifications and bracing each play an important role in the nonsurgical management of knee osteoarthritis. Lateral wedge insoles decrease the external varus moment and estimated medial compartment load, resulting in pain improvement. The resultant subtalar joint calcaneus valgus and mechanical axis change is significantly more effective for early stage arthritis. An unloader brace applies a varus or valgus moment that reduces force transmission in the most involved knee compartment. The unloader brace can be used in an active, compliant patient with isolated unicompartmental disease, pain and tenderness localized to the affected compartment, malalignment, and a correctable deformity with manual stress testing.

Arthroscopy

The published results of arthroscopic débridement are variable and the recommendations are inconsistent because of varied entrance criteria, procedures, and outcome measures. A pilot study of 10 patients with symptomatic osteoarthritis of the knee compared skin puncture wounds only (placebo), arthroscopic lavage, and "standard" arthroscopic débridement. All three groups reported similar results, and the five patients who received the skin puncture wounds reported improvement in their knee pain at 6 months after surgery. This analysis introduces some skepticism on the mechanism of pain relief after arthroscopic treatment of osteoarthritis.

Carefully selected patients with relatively acute symptoms (of less than 6 months' duration), near-normal limb alignment, and mild or moderate unicompartmental degenerative disease can be considered for arthroscopic treatment if a nonsurgical program is unsuccessful. The most important factor when considering arthroscopic intervention is axial alignment of the leg. If the mechanical axis passes through the lesion, the procedure is less likely to be effective. Indications for arthroscopic débridement, partial meniscectomy, and/or loose body removal include a discrete chief complaint, such as well-localized joint line pain, persistent effusion, catching or locking, and mild to moderate radiographic degenerative changes.

Synovectomy

Surgical removal of the hypertrophic, inflamed synovium by open or arthroscopic means has been recommended for the relief of severe pain and chronic effusions in rheumatoid arthritis, seronegative arthritis (psoriatic, Reiter's syndrome, ankylosing spondylitis), pigmented villonodular synovitis, and synovial chondromatosis. Long-term follow-up (up to 23 years) after open synovectomy reveals satisfactory results in 60% of knees. Degenerative changes progress radiographi-

cally, but the inflammatory disease is temporarily arrested in two thirds of the knees.

Potential advantages of arthroscopic synovectomy include reduced bleeding, decreased postoperative pain, easier rehabilitation, and faster return to work, along with the option to perform simultaneous bilateral surgery or repeat operations if necessary. Comparison of arthroscopic synovectomy and open synovectomy reveals the same clinical response and gradual deterioration, but worse radiographic changes in the open group. Arthroscopic synovectomy produces 80% to 96% good or excellent results in rheumatoid knees after 2 years. The satisfactory results decrease to approximately 60% after 4 years and patients with seronegative arthritis fare less well. Loss of knee motion following surgery does not appear to be a problem.

Tibial Osteotomy

The normal knee joint has a femoral-tibial angle of 5° to 7° valgus and a mechanical axis that should pass near the center of the knee joint. The normal weight-bearing distribution is 60% on the medial side and 40% on the lateral side. A knee with degenerative changes usually is associated with malalignment (varus or valgus deformity) that increases the stress on the damaged articular cartilage, leading to a progression of the degenerative changes and an accentuation of the angular deformity (Fig. 1). The goal of a realignment osteotomy about the knee is to redistribute the mechanical forces from the compartment with arthritic changes to a portion of the knee with healthy articular cartilage. The ideal patient for osteotomy to correct cartilage overload has single compartment arthritis, ligamentous stability, and is young and physically active. Absolute contraindications include: inflammatory arthritis, severe tricompartmental disease, a flexion arc of 90° or less, marked tibiofemoral subluxation, and previous meniscectomy in the contralateral compartment. Relative contraindications include: age older than 60 years, patellofemoral arthritis, collateral ligament insufficiency, lateral tibial subluxation, or a varus deformity more than 10°.

The critical aspect of osteotomy planning includes assessment of location, direction, and magnitude of alignment. Preoperative assessment includes a thorough physical examination in order to ascertain range of motion, ligament stability, angular deformity, and ipsilateral hip function. Radiographic evaluation includes weight-bearing radiographs with 30° of flexion to assess the joint space, and full-length radiographs of the leg (hip to ankle) to determine the mechanical axis and the true femoral-tibial angle. In general, varus deformities are corrected

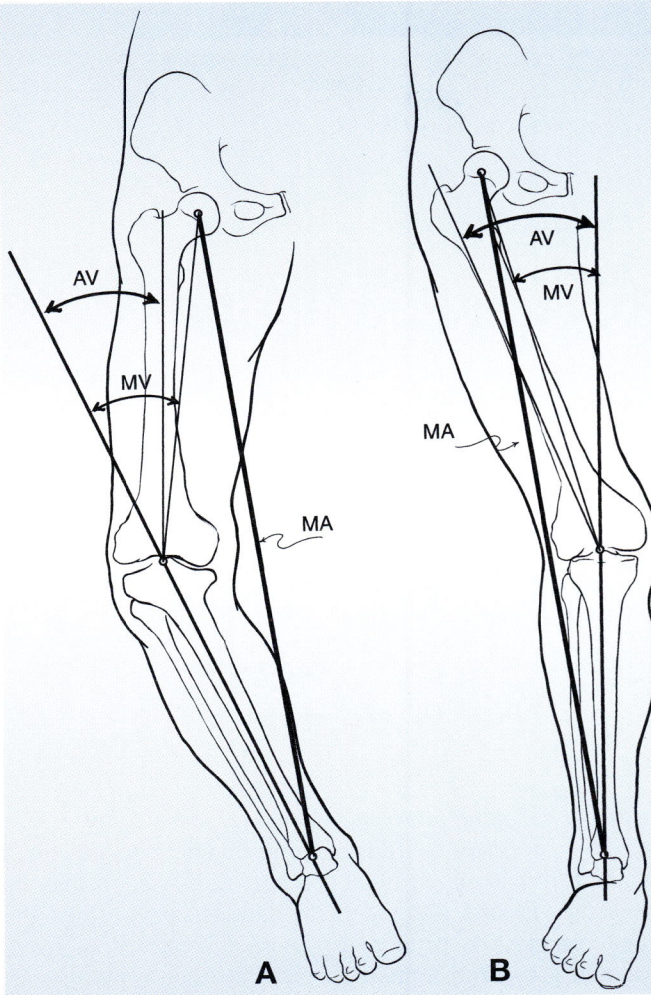

Figure 1 The effect of knee deformity on alignment and mechanical axis (MA). **A,** Varus deformity. **B,** Valgus deformity. Anatomic varus or valgus (AV) reflects the femoral-tibial angle. Mechanical varus or valgus (MV) is the total angular deviation from normal alignment.

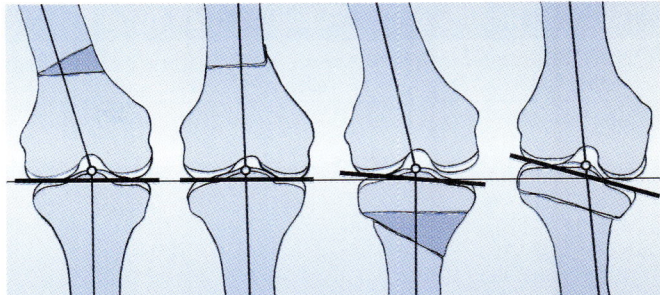

Figure 2 For most valgus deformities, an osteotomy in the distal femur will leave a horizontal joint line. A tibial osteotomy will create an oblique joint line.

with a lateral closing wedge osteotomy. For large varus deformities (greater than 12° to 15°), a dome osteotomy may be more appropriate in order to maintain joint line obliquity and to minimize the amount of bone resected.

A medial opening wedge osteotomy may be considered for either a posttraumatic deformity or concurrent anterior cruciate ligament (ACL) reconstruction. A medial closing wedge osteotomy may correct a mild valgus deformity (femoral-tibial angle less than 12° to 15°). For deformities with more valgus, a tibial osteotomy will lead to an oblique joint line and subsequent subluxation (Fig. 2). Larger valgus deformities are best handled with osteotomy of the distal femur. The opening wedge correction may be maintained with autogenous bone graft, allograft bone, or a specialized plate with a metal spacer that fills the gap. Healing may be less predictable with an opening wedge osteotomy. The

advantage of an opening wedge osteotomy is that the fibula may be left untouched.

The goal of tibial osteotomy is to correct deformity while maintaining a level joint line and minimizing the effect on ligament balance. Varus deformities should be overcorrected slightly to approximately 9° to 10° of anatomic valgus. Routine arthroscopy need not be done with osteotomy. Arthroscopy is a useful adjunct in the presence of meniscal tears, cartilage flaps, or loose bodies.

Internal fixation allows for early range of motion, which may reduce the risks of stiffness and patella baja. External fixation has the benefit of allowing further correction after performance of the osteotomy. Recently, osteotomy has been combined with hemicallotasis, which can be done with either unilateral or circular fixators. However, external fixation after osteotomy is associated with higher rates of nerve palsy, nonunion, and infection. To avoid tethering of the lateral closing wedge osteotomy by the fibula, an osteotomy of the fibular shaft, a disruption of the proximal tibiofibular syndesmosis, or fibular head excision can be done.

Complications

Complications include infection, peroneal nerve palsy, undercorrection, nonunion, and overcorrection. Osteotomies below the tibial tubercle are slower to heal, with nonunion rates three to four times higher than those done above the tubercle. Infection and nerve palsies have a higher incidence when external fixators are used. It is crucial to keep the proximal limb of the osteotomy at least 2 cm from the joint line to prevent fracture through the proximal fragment with violation of the joint space. Care must be taken during execution of the osteotomy to avoid injury to the popliteal artery and branches of the peroneal nerve. Prophylaxis for deep vein thrombosis should be used and patients monitored postoperatively for the possible development of compartment syndrome.

TABLE 1 | Results of TKA Following High Tibial Osteotomy*

Author	Year	Follow-up (Years)	TKA (No.)	Results
Katz	1987	2.9	21	Results worse than primary TKA
Staeli	1987	3.7	35	Results similar to primary TKA
Windsor	1988	4.6	45	80% had patella baja, results similar to revision TKA
Scuderi	1989	N/A	66	89% had patella baja
Amendola	1989	3.1	42	Knee scores similar, but less ROM in the HTO group
Jackson	1994		20	Worse results after HTO compared to UKR, because of complications
Mont	1994	6.1	73	Worse knee scores in HTO group
Gill	1995	3.8	30	Better results after HTO than after UKR
Bergenudd	1997	4-9	14	No difference in knee scores, more complications in HTO group
Toksvig	1998	10	40	No difference in knee scores, no difference in RSA tibial movement
Walther	2000		35	Worse knee scores in HTO group
Meding	2000	7.5	39	No difference in knee scores when compared with TKA in opposite knee

*ROM = range of motion; HTO = high tibial osteotomy; UKR = unicompartmental knee replacement; RSA = roentgen stereophotogrammetric analysis

Results

Good or excellent outcomes from multiple series are 73% to 95% at 5 years, 45% to 80% at 10 years, and 30% to 46% at around 20 years. The best results are obtained in patients with pure unicompartmental disease with less than 12° of deformity, ligamentous stability, more than 90° of flexion and age younger than 50 years. Overcorrection may be just as deleterious as undercorrection. The primary cause of poor results is undercorrection with subsequent return of the deformity. The other major cause is progressive arthritis in the unaffected compartment. Patients with a body mass index more than 1.3 times that of normal tend to have worse outcomes. Patients with ACL insufficiency complicating medial compartment arthritis may consider having both procedures done simultaneously or staged.

Tibial Osteotomy and Total Knee Arthroplasty

A review of the literature reveals conflicting reports regarding the influence of high tibial osteotomy on subsequent total knee arthroplasty (TKA) (Table 1). In the series that reported inferior results, these problems were attributed to a higher incidence of patella baja and lateral release, leading to overall lower knee scores. These changes can be minimized with the use of internal fixation and early range of motion.

However, there are potential technical pitfalls associated with TKA after tibial osteotomy. The lateral plateau may be deficient after closing wedge osteotomy and it may be necessary to add a lateral augment to the tibial plateau. If a stemmed tibial component is used, it may be necessary to offset the stem to allow passage down the canal. It may be prudent to consider removal of hardware in a separate operation prior to knee replacement.

Distal Femoral Osteotomy

Indications and Contraindications

The indications for distal femoral osteotomy are similar to those for tibial osteotomy except distal femoral osteotomy is used more frequently to correct a valgus deformity. The osteotomy is generally indicated in younger, active individuals with valgus deformity and moderate lateral compartment arthritis. Contraindications are also similar to those listed for tibial osteotomy. Relative contraindications include inflammatory arthritis, severe patellofemoral arthritis, and significant joint instability with a medial thrust on gait.

In most cases, a medially-based closing wedge osteotomy of the distal femur with stable internal fixation is the method of choice. The goal of the surgical correction is approximately 2° of anatomic valgus, with care taken to avoid extending the alignment into varus.

Complications

Prophylaxis should be used for deep vein thrombosis. Nonunion rates are much higher than those of tibial osteotomy, reported to be in the range of 4% to 19%, with rates as high as 29% with medially-based fixation. The use of stable implants that permit early range of motion can minimize stiffness and nonunion.

Results

As with tibial osteotomy, good results may be obtained that have a tendency to diminish with time. The best results have been obtained with stable internal fixation and early range of motion, leading to 90% good or excellent results at 5 years. With inadequate fixation, the incidence of good results drops to 71% at 8 years. When combined with casting, the incidence of good results may be as low as 33% over a similar period of time. The results seem to be best when the alignment is corrected to approximately 2° of anatomic valgus.

Influence of Femoral Osteotomy on Subsequent Total Knee Arthroplasty

Allthough distal femoral osteotomy certainly makes subsequent knee replacement more difficult, the osteotomy still should be performed if the correct indications are present. It may be desirable to remove the hardware as a separate procedure prior to arthroplasty. The femoral shaft may be displaced in relation to the metaphysis, which can limit the use of a conventional stemmed component. It may be necessary to use custom components. Another potential problem is soft-tissue balancing. In extension, the knee has a varus alignment, but in flexion it has the characteristics of the valgus deformity. If adequate soft-tissue balance cannot be achieved, it may be necessary to use constrained implants.

Unicompartmental Knee Replacement

Medial resurfacing is more common than lateral compartment procedures. Initial design flaws, such as thin polyethylene and metal-backed cementless tibial components, led to higher failure rates in some studies. The success rate in the initial series of unicompartmental knee replacements was usually lower than that obtained with conventional TKA. Contraindications include inflammatory arthritis, a restricted range of motion (more than 15° of flexion contracture or less than 90° of flexion), or a large angular deformity that is difficult to correct by way of unicompartmental knee replacement alone. Other contraindications include inflammatory arthritis, grade 4 articular cartilage loss in the patellofemoral joint, lateral subluxation of the tibia, or ligament instability.

Survivorship has ranged from 87% to 98% at 10 years in numerous studies. The main reasons for failure have been excessive wear of the polyethy-

lene and progression of arthritis in the unresurfaced compartment.

The conversion of a failed unicompartmental knee replacement to conventional knee replacement is technically more demanding than a primary TKA. Overall knee scores are lower in these cases. The surgeon must be prepared to use structural bone graft or implant augmentation to correct any significant bone defects noted at the time of knee replacement.

Primary Total Knee Arthroplasty

Patient Selection

Patient selection for primary TKA is based on the presence of pain, functional compromise of activities of daily living, and radiographs that demonstrate severe arthritis consistent with the patient's history. The elderly, more sedentary patient in whom nonsurgical therapy has failed is an ideal candidate. Contraindications to primary TKA include active infection (in the knee or elsewhere), an incompetent extensor mechanism, compromised vascularity to the extremity, and local neurologic disruption affecting musculature. Younger, more active patients with knee arthritis continue to be challenging to treat.

Results

Pain relief and improved function make TKA a successful procedure. The rapid introduction of new technology and designs increases the need for outcome studies. Most analyses show 90% to 95% survivorship at 10 years.

Two recent reviews of TKA in young patients show somewhat varied results. Results from one study demonstrated a 99% implant survival to revision at 10 years in patients with rheumatoid arthritis (64% of the entire group) with an average age of 43 years at the time of surgery. Results from another study of TKA in patients age 40 years or younger with osteoarthritis demonstrated an aseptic failure rate of 12.5% at 8 years, higher than that observed in most older patients. In a another study of patients older than age 85 years, preoperative cardiac comorbidity and postoperative confusion was higher than that in patients age 60 to 70 years, but knee pain, functional scores, and quality of life were significantly improved.

TKA in obese patients was associated with lower functional scores, increased patellar pain, and an increased incidence of nonprogressive radiolucent lines. Although postoperative knee scores were lower, improvement in knee scores was higher and revision rates similar in these patients compared with nonobese patients.

In workers' compensation patients, TKA resulted in a 71% fair or poor Knee Society score versus a 12%

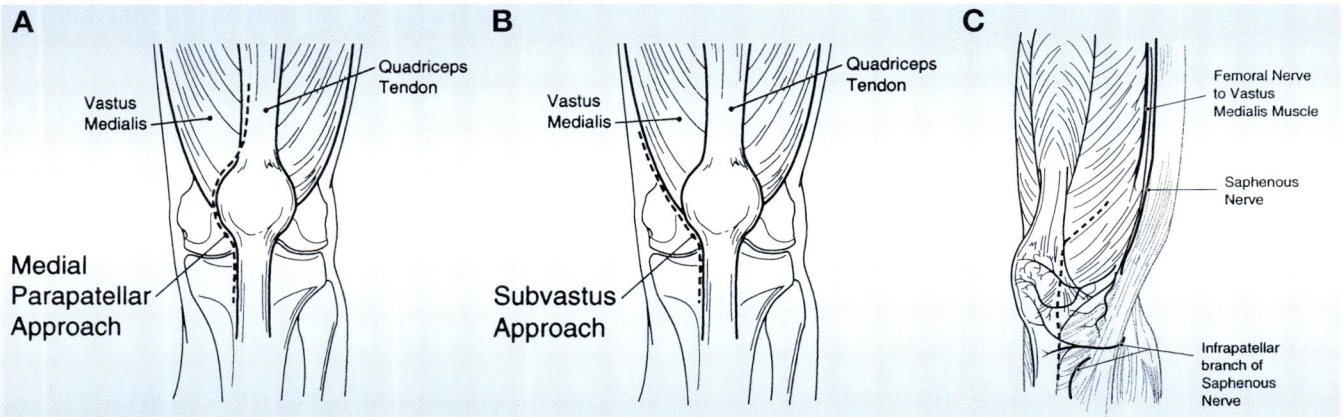

Figure 3 Diagrammatic representation of the medial parapatellar approach. **A,** Subvastus approach. **B,** Midvastus approach. **C,** (*Figs. 3A & 3B are Reproduced with permission from Matsueda M, Gustilo RB: Subvastus and medial parapatellar approaches in total knee arthroplasty. Clin Orthop 2000;371:161-168. Fig. 3C Reproduced with permission from Engh GA, Parks NL: Surgical technique of the midvastus arthrotomy. Clin Orthop 1998;351:270-274.)*

fair or poor score in the non-workers' compensation control group. Objective findings, such as range of motion, stability, radiographic alignment, or lucent lines, showed no difference.

Surgical Approaches

If a previous incision exists, it should be used for the current surgical approach provided that adequate exposure can be obtained. If multiple longitudinal incisions exist, the most lateral of these should be used if possible. Transverse incisions should be crossed at 90° angles when possible. Plastic surgery consultation is often helpful in preoperative evaluation of the multi-operated knee if the skin is compromised and at risk for healing problems.

Using the midline skin incision, a medial or lateral parapatellar arthrotomy can be done. With the more common medial arthrotomy, a small cuff of tissue just medial to the tubercle is left to protect the extensor mechanism and provide adequate tissue for closure. A lateral parapatellar incision is sometimes recommended in the valgus knee.

In the subvastus approach the integrity of the quadriceps tendon is maintained at the expense of limited exposure of the lateral compartment, particularly in the obese patient. A modification of this approach, the midvastus approach, has addressed these issues while maintaining quadriceps tendon integrity (Fig. 3).

Surgical Techniques

Soft-Tissue Balancing

Soft-tissue balancing is critical to the long-term success of TKA. The sequence for releasing soft tissues that cause deformities in TKA has been addressed in several studies. In general, release of contracted soft tissues is favored over reefing of lax tissues and struc-

tures. Varus deformity at the knee is corrected by releasing the sleeve of contracted medial structures (capsule, pes tendons, collateral ligament) in a subperiosteal fashion from the tibia. The greatest factor in restoring the gap is after the release of the sleeve, up to 8 cm from the medial joint line, although the distance of release depends on the size of the individual and degree of deformity.

There is no consensus regarding the sequence of soft-tissue release to correct a valgus knee deformity. Preserving the integrity of the lateral collateral ligament and lengthening rather than transecting the iliotibial band are thought to be important factors in preventing overcorrection and lateral soft-tissue laxity.

Flexion contractures require release of the posterior capsule and when severe, additional distal femoral bone resection may be necessary.

Limb Alignment

Restoration of anatomic limb alignment has been shown to be critical to the long-term success of TKA. The means of establishing the correct alignment is difficult. The use of intramedullary guides on the femoral side is a reliable method for assessing and restoring the anatomic position of the femoral component. Intramedullary or extramedullary devices both can be used to cut the tibia anatomically. Embolization of marrow contents may be a concern if intramedullary guides are used in individuals undergoing bilateral knee replacements with multiple canal instrumentation. Alternately, extramedullary tibial guides can be used to reliably restore alignment.

Component Rotational Position

A number of methods have been described for restoring femoral component rotation to balance the flexion space and improve patellofemoral tracking, including the transepicondylar axis, posterior condylar line, and anteroposterior line of the femoral sulcus (Fig. 4). One

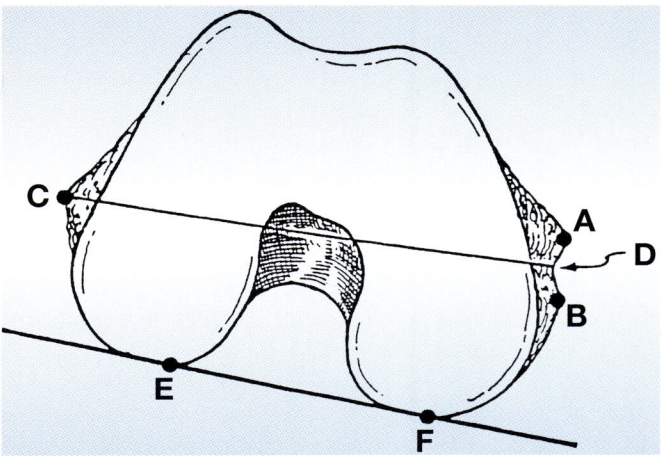

Figure 4 The transcondylar axis is drawn by connecting a line from the medial sulcus to the lateral epicondylar prominence (AB, CD). The posterior condylar line is the line connecting the posterior condyles (EF). The anteroposterior line connects the lowest point of the femoral sulcus to the center of the intercondylar notch. *(Reproduced with permission from Griffin FM, Math K, Scuderi GR, Insall JN, Poilvache PL: Anatomy of the epicondyles of the distal femur. J Arthroplasty 2000;15: 354-359.)*

study correlated patellofemoral complications with failure to reconstruct the epicondylar axis and/or the tibial rotational axis. Combined internal rotation of the femoral and tibial components is most likely to result in patellofemoral problems.

Resurfacing the Patella

Resurfacing the patella in TKA is controversial. Whether or not the patella is resurfaced, it is critical that the joint is balanced. Factors associated with a good result if the patella is not resurfaced are a congruent match with the femoral component and minimal articular damage. The advantages of not resurfacing the patella include a shorter surgery time, maintaining bone stock, and avoiding the complications associated with patellar resurfacing. Conversely, resurfacing the patella may lessen anterior knee pain and obviate the need for resurfacing in patients with recalcitrant pain after TKA who have not had the patella resurfaced during the initial surgery.

Prosthesis Design

Posterior Cruciate Ligament Sparing Versus Sacrificing

Good results can be obtained with a prosthesis that either spares or sacrifices the posterior cruciate ligament (PCL). Survival of the cemented PCL-sparing TKA is over 90% at 10 to 15 years. One study found a 97% survival rate at 13 years in patients with rheumatoid arthritis who had their knees replaced with a PCL-sparing design.

Fluoroscopic evaluation has shown that the PCL does not have normal function after TKA. The kine-

matics of the PCL-sparing designs may be different in vivo than they were designed to function.

Flexion and stability of the knee after PCL-sparing TKA are important. Instability can occur because of preoperative ligament deterioration, intraoperative injury, or postoperative injury or attenuation.

Posterior Cruciate Ligament Substitution

Long-term studies have not identified a drawback to sacrificing or substituting the PCL and neither knee stability nor range of motion is compromised. Posterior rollback is reproducible in the studies of the PCL-substituting prosthesis. Proprioception in stair climbing results is comparable for patients after PCL-substituting and PCL-sparing TKAs.

Rotating Platform

The rotating platform prosthetic knee was developed to reduce polyethylene wear and in turn reduce prosthetic loosening and prolong survival of the knee replacement. The rotating platform prosthesis was designed to reduce mechanical polyethylene contact stresses and fatigue wear by conforming surface design. In one study of 114 low contact stress total knees performed by one surgeon and followed for 9 to 12 years, none required reoperation and none of the mobile bearings dislocated. There was no evidence of osteolysis or prosthetic loosening, suggesting that backside wear of the polyethylene also was minimal. The complications of spinout, breakage, and wear must continue to be evaluated as new designs are developed.

Design and Patellofemoral Function

The primary function of the patella is to act as a fulcrum for the extensor mechanism. Anterior knee pain is the most common complaint after surgery. Several designs (for example, dome, oval, and anatomic) have been developed to help minimize postoperative symptoms. Regardless of design or whether the patella is resurfaced, stair climbing and other activities loading the patellofemoral joint can be difficult and painful for the patient.

Several factors may contribute to a good result. The patellofemoral surface should be congruent. Femoral and tibial component rotation must be appropriate and the patellofemoral joint should maintain its mechanical advantage but not be too thick or thin. This factor can be assessed by measuring the thickness of the patella before and after it is reconstructed. Additionally, the femoral component should rest on the anterior cortex of the femur as anatomically as possible. Translation of the patellar component, either medially or laterally, also should be avoided. Finally, reconstruction of the joint line is known to correlate with a successful result. Results from one study correlated worse clinical results when the joint was elevated more than 8 mm. The authors recommended that distal augments be used to lower the joint line if necessary.

Polyethylene Thickness and Wear Issues

Successful long-term results of TKA often are associated with knee designs using polyethylene with a conforming surface geometry, a minimum thickness of 6 to 8 mm, and a good locking mechanism with minimal backside wear. Additionally, this study group of patients is usually older and less active. Conversely, success is less likely if a flat-on-flat design with thin polyethylene and a poor locking mechanism allowing for backside wear is used, particularly in a young, active patient population.

Recently, the type of sterilization technique and the shelf life of the polyethylene have been noted to greatly affect wear and long-term success. In one study, 135 knees were evaluated in 105 patients who were followed for a mean of 5.8 years (range, 2.1 to 11.3 years). Six failures were identified. Prosthesis survival if the polyethylene shelf life was less than 4 years was 100%, 4 to 8 years, 88.6%, and 8 to 11 years, 79.2%. Sterilization in air also is detrimental. A study of 1,635 retrieved polyethylene knee bearings found that gamma irradiation in air resulted in a high incidence of cracking, delamination, and complete wear. Polyethylene knee bearings sterilized in ethylene oxide showed no evidence of fatigue damage.

Perioperative Issues

Tourniquet

The use of a tourniquet during TKA has been studied. Options include no tourniquet, tourniquet use for cementing only, and tourniquet use throughout the procedure. The use of tourniquets has been associated with complications including nerve palsies and vascular injuries, particularly in the presence of vascular disease. Other concerns include delays in recovery of muscle function, changes in circulating blood volume to the heart during tourniquet inflation and release, as well as an increase in the risk of deep vein thrombosis. In patients with severe vascular compromise, appropriate arterial evaluation should be obtained prior to surgery and tourniquet use may place these patients at risk for increased vascular complications. There was no change in surgical time, incidence of postoperative pain, analgesic requirements, postoperative drain output, postoperative swelling, the incidence of wound complications, or the incidence of deep vein thrombosis according to the results of a well-matched prospective study comparing TKA performed with and without the use of a tourniquet.

Drains

The role of drains after routine TKA has not been resolved despite a number of published articles. Surgeons who favor the use of drains indicate less ecchymosis, hematoma formation, and minimal wound drainage. Those who oppose drains are concerned about bacterial colonization of the drain tract and the cost of routine drain use. Studies on the topic are hampered by too few patients, which limits the studies from proving the hypothesis.

Continuous Passive Motion

Proponents of continuous passive motion (CPM) describe benefits of decreased incidence of manipulation, increased range of motion, decreased incidence of deep vein thrombosis, and a decrease in the use of analgesics. Opponents cite no significant changes in late range of motion or rates of knee manipulation, an increased need for analgesics and postoperative blood loss, and an increased incidence of wound complications. Results from a recent study demonstrated early improvement in range of motion with CPM, but no significant difference in range of motion at 1 year and no difference in the number of patients requiring manipulation. An increased need in analgesic requirements and an increase in postoperative drain output also have been reported. Results of a second study demonstrated no statistical differences in cumulative analgesic requirements, range of motion at any measured interval, no change in length of stay, or no change in Knee Society scores when comparing standard and high-flexion CPM to a group not receiving CPM.

Postoperative Pain

Pain in the early postoperative interval after TKA is unavoidable. Oral, intramuscular, and intravenous narcotics are the mainstay of postoperative pain control, but epidural and local anesthetics have all been tried with varying degrees of success. Concerns about epidural hematoma have led to the development of specific protocols to guide the use of epidural catheters with various anticoagulant agents.

Revision Total Knee Arthroplasty

As the number of primary TKAs and life expectancy of the population increase, the need for revision TKA also increases. The same basic principles that apply to primary TKA must be adhered to for revision TKA.

Preoperative Planning

The preoperative evaluation of a failed TKA should include the patient's history, physical examination, laboratory analysis, and radiographs (as discussed in evaluation of the painful TKA). Specific assessment of collateral ligament integrity, bone loss, and extensor mechanism function is necessary to select the appropriate implants and reconstruction techniques.

Bone Defect Classification

There are two classifications of bone defects in the knee. Tibial defects are classified based on the percentage of the plateau with a deficiency. This classification was meant as a guide for use of bone grafts or metal augments and acrylic cement. The defects were subclassified into contained (cortical rim intact) and noncontained defects (cortical rim deficient).

For revision TKA, the Anderson Orthopaedic Research Institute classification is used. The classification is meant as a guide to determine the need for metal augments and bone grafts and to determine the severity of bone loss that is encountered during revision surgery. A type 1 defect (intact bone) is defined as relatively healthy metaphyseal bone with good cancellous structure present at a reasonably normal joint line level. Usually, a primary style component is used in the revision of a type 1 defect. A type 2 defect (damaged bone) is defined as bone loss that includes some loss of cancellous structure for component fixation. Without repair of the bone damage, the joint line is altered. Modular and stemmed revision components are generally recommended to manage these defects. Type 2 lesions are further subdivided into 2A (one condyle is severely deficient) and 2B (both condyles are deficient). Thus, a tibial defect located entirely on the medial side would be termed a type 2A deficiency. Type 3 bone defects usually involve a large osteolytic lesion, severe component migration, a large area of bone loss filled with cement, or a failure of a hinged prosthesis. The epicondyles frequently are flared away from the femur. Type 3 defects represent severe tibial bone loss that presents as a trumpet-shaped proximal expansion of the tibia. Options for treating this type of defect include a hinged or custom-designed component, or repair of the metaphyseal segment with allograft and long-stemmed prosthesis. Femoral head allografts may fill in one condyle or plateau.

Stages

Once the cause or causes of failure are recognized, revision TKA can be done, with the surgeon aware of the challenges that accompany each stage of the operation. After adequate preoperative planning, revision TKA may be subdivided into the following surgical stages: exposure, extensor mechanism treatment, removal of the failed components, assessment of bone loss, collateral ligament, and joint line, flexion-extension space balancing, implantation of new components, and closure of the wound.

Surgical Techniques

Exposure

The previous incision should be used whenever possible. Skin flaps should be minimally undermined to preserve the skin's vascular supply, which comes from vessels perforating through the deep fascia. If patellar eversion is difficult, early lateral retinacular release may help. A nonthreaded Steinmann pin may be placed into the tibial tubercle to reinforce the distal insertion of the patellar tendon during patellar eversion. For many revision TKAs, a medial parapatellar arthrotomy provides sufficient exposure. Other secondary procedures may be done to minimize the risk of extensor mechanism disruption and facilitate exposure, including the quadriceps snip, tibial tubercle osteotomy, and V-Y quadricepsplasty. Complications of tibial tubercle osteotomy include nonunion and fracture. Complications of rectus tendon transection include extensor lag and patellar osteonecrosis of the patella.

Component Removal

Component removal must be done with the goal of minimizing further bone loss and preventing fracture. Complete cement removal is mandatory only in infected cases. Well-fixed cement may be retained in aseptic cases if there is a chance that substantial bone loss would result from its removal. Generally, 4 mm of bone is lost during removal of a well-fixed implant. For severe osteolysis, a complete synovectomy is done to minimize the osteolytic process from continuing after the revision TKA.

Soft-Tissue Balancing

The principles of collateral ligament balancing are the same in both primary and revision TKA. Collateral ligament release is rare in revision situations and disrupted or attenuated collateral ligaments are frequently encountered. Collateral ligament repair or advancement has been done but the integrity of the repair is suspect.

If flexion-extension space symmetry is obtained but collateral ligament imbalance persists, a constrained condylar unlinked implant will be required. Because of the added stresses that internal constraint places on the implants, intramedullary stems should be added to achieve greater fixation stability. Advancement or reconstruction of attenuated collateral ligaments using pants over vest repair or advancement should be protected by the use of an unlinked constrained device. Collateral ligament repair can prevent overlengthening of the limb by limiting the use of increasing thicknesses of tibial inserts to provide soft-tissue sleeve stability.

The PCL, if present, may be preserved during revision TKA. However, proper ligament balancing is

TABLE 2 | Gap Balancing Options During Revision TKA*

| | Extension Space | | |
Flexion Space	Tight	Normal	Loose
Tight	Resect additional proximal tibia	Resect additional proximal tibia, distally augment femoral component Downsize femoral component Shift femoral component anteriorly +/− offset stems	Resect more proximal tibia, distally augment femoral component Downsize femoral component, with distal augments Shift femoral component anteriorly, with distal augments +/− offset stems
Normal	Resect additional distal femur	Goal of revision surgery: Balanced collateral ligaments	Augment distal femur
Loose	Resect additional distal femur, use even thicker tibial insert until balanced	Downsize femoral component Shift femoral component anteriorly +/− offset stems	Increase tibial polyethylene insert thickness

*There are a few general rules regarding the management of flexion and extension space mismatches. Changes on the tibial side affect both flexion and extension spaces equally. Resection of femoral bone or femoral component augmentation affects the extension space balancing only. Changes in femoral component size or position affects the flexion space balancing only.

more difficult, and its function is reliable only in cases of minimal bone and soft-tissue destruction.

There are nine permutations of flexion-extension gap. The flexion and extension gaps each may be loose, tight, or normal. The goal is to achieve an equal flexion and extension space with appropriate alignment and stability. The choices available for each permutation are summarized in Table 2.

Bone Resection

In revision TKA, significant bone resection is the exception rather than the rule. In most cases, a minimal resection is performed to create a smooth bone surface for fixation of a metal wedge or augment. The purpose of bone resection is to provide a fresh cancellous bone bed for cementless fixation or for interdigitation of acrylic cement. If the new implant design will be changed from a PCL-sparing to a PCL-substituting (posterior stabilized) design, bone from the femoral intercondylar notch must be resected according to the dimensions of the implant. The notch bone may then be used as autograft for other bone defects on the femur or tibia.

Joint Line Restoration

Because a standard bone resection already has been performed during the primary TKA, allowance must be given on the femoral side to the additional bone loss that results from removing a well-fixed implant or from osteolysis in the vicinity of a grossly loose pros-

thesis. Therefore, in most situations some form of distal femoral augmentation (4 to 8 mm) is usually necessary, except in cases where a cementless fixation interface is disrupted and the bone loss is less than 4 mm.

Additional tibial bone loss occurs at the proximal tibial condyles and around the stem. In many cases, it will be necessary to choose a tibial insert thickness 2 mm or greater to account for this loss. By remembering these simple parameters, the joint line may be preserved in most instances. If soft-tissue destruction has been minimized, the peripheral meniscal scar may serve as a reference point for the joint line. Restoring the joint line will aid in preserving patellofemoral mechanics. Actual reproducible anthropomorphic dimensions from the fibular head to the proximal tibial joint line or from the insertion points of the medial and lateral collateral ligaments to the distal femoral joint line may vary with the size of the patient and are only rough estimates.

Patellofemoral Joint

Joint line restoration will preserve the proper patellofemoral relationships for optimum flexion and quadriceps muscle power. Proper patellar tracking must be restored. Three factors affect correct tracking of the patella in the anterior flange and trochlear groove of the femoral component. First, the femoral component must be placed in line with the epicondylar axis. Second, proper tibial component rotation on the tibial plateau should be obtained. Third, assuming that the first and second conditions are satisfied, the tracking of the patellar component must be assessed in the same manner as is done during a primary TKA.

Scarring is frequently seen in the patellar ligament, causing patella infera. Elevation of the height of the patella by proximal translocation of the tibial tubercle is not easily accomplished. If there is enough patellar bone stock, the patellar height can be slightly elevated by placing a smaller patellar implant more superiorly into the proximal pole of the patella.

Patellar bone stock deficiency is frequently encountered during revision TKA, and there are no good ways to augment it. Partial patellectomy with reshaping of the patella has been done with some success. Some preliminary success has been obtained by using a porous patellar implant that is coated with Hydrocel, a metal material that allows for soft-tissue and bone ingrowth. Extensor mechanism allografts (tibial tubercle-patellar ligament-patella-distal quadriceps tendon) have been used with mixed results. Soft-tissue coverage and proper tensioning of the graft is difficult to achieve. The allograft should ordinarily be placed as tight as possible, but clinical success has been quite variable depending on the surgeon's experience.

Component Selection

Level of Constraint

Nonconstrained resurfacing designs are used in the majority of revision TKA cases. PCL sparing may be accomplished during a first revision TKA with little bone loss and an intact PCL. However, in many cases, the integrity of the PCL is suspect and a change to a PCL-substituting design is warranted. This change will require additional bone resection from the intercondylar notch, which can be used as autograft to rebuild bone defects in the femoral condyles or tibial plateau.

If the collateral ligaments are damaged or attenuated, an unlinked, constrained, condylar device is required. The augmented polyethylene spine of the tibial insert will provide added constraint and preserve mediolateral stability. The best collateral ligament balance should be obtained so that the soft-tissue sleeve can contribute to stability. In some cases, both collateral ligaments are damaged and there is a danger of excessive lengthening the limb in order to obtain proper balance. A patient with low physical demands will do well with an unlinked constrained-condylar device. However, high-demand patients may develop recurrent instability and may best be served by a constrained, linked rotating hinge prosthesis.

Most total knee replacement systems provide modularity so that metal augments may be easily attached.

Intramedullary stem extensions are recommended to add further rigidity to the implant fixation.

Stems

Intramedullary stems are used when there is a need for added constraint or for enhanced rigidity of fixation when significant bone loss compromises normal fixation control of the implant. Stems are required when an unlinked or linked constrained device is implanted. The stems add further three-point fixation. Stems come in different lengths, widths, and configurations, and are of three basic stem designs: positive sharp flutes, flattened or smooth negative flutes, and clothespin.

Stems should be press fit or placed without cement in most cases. It usually is not necessary to fully cement the stem. The distal femoral or proximal tibial components are cemented with the press-fit stem extensions. It is not necessary to ream the intramedullary canals to obtain a rigid cortical stem fit, as this may contribute to postoperative stem tip pain or further compromise the cortex, leading to stem migration. Porous-coated stems are used in cases of cavitary bone loss where cement interdigitation will not be possible. Porous-coated stems, positive fluted stems, and clothespin stems should not be cemented because they would pose a substantial risk for total bone destruction if they had to be removed during a second revision TKA.

Smooth stems may be cemented when there is no other way to obtain stable stem fixation. When a long-stem total hip replacement is located above the distal femur and there is no possibility to fix the knee implant stem at the femoral isthmus or bow, complete cementing of the stem will be necessary. However, this clinical situation is rarely encountered.

Additional stem length provides greater stability of the implant at the expense of the additional metal requirement. Length above 100 mm will be needed in cases of profound bone loss where there is no possibility of substantial proximal tibial or distal femoral condylar support. For stem lengths more than 125 mm, bowed stems may be required. Offset stems minimize the likelihood of proximal tibial or distal femoral component overhang caused by distorted canal anatomy. Rarely, custom-designed stem configurations are needed in cases of severe anatomic distortion.

Bone Loss

The treatment choices for bone loss include autogenous bone graft, morcellized or bulk allograft, modular metal augments, and synthetic bone substitution. Custom-designed implants rarely are required.

Autogenous bone graft from the iliac crest is used rarely in minimal bone loss situations. Allograft is the most available and plentiful bone substitute. Synthetic bone substitution has also been used recently to add some bone-augmenting stimulus to revision surgery although it is more widely used in fracture treatment. Particulate bone graft and cement are used for contained defects although in some hands complete cementless fixation may be chosen for fixation. Metal wedges, augments, and structural allografts fill uncontained defects with the femoral head being the most prevalent bone material available to rebuild this loss. The femoral head is the most easily obtained allograft and can provide biologic augmentation for most deficiencies. Structural allografts are reserved for profound bone loss situations. Fracture or dissolution of the graft may occur in up to 45% of the procedures for which a complete distal femur or proximal tibial allograft are used. For many cases, a combination of bulk and morcellized allograft is used in addition to metal augments.

Modular revision systems provide numerous block and wedge augments of different widths and lengths to address different bone loss situations. The proximal tibia may be augmented by metal blocks and half or full wedges up to 25°. Femoral loss can be dealt with by the use of distal and proximal augments. Press-fit intramedullary stem extensions are recommended whenever large wedges, metal augments, or major allografts are used. Rarely do the stems require cement, which is used only when there is an inability to have sufficient bone length to achieve a rigid press fit. With the greater size availability and modularity of stock revision systems, custom-designed implants are rarely needed.

Resection Arthroplasty and Arthrodesis

Resection arthroplasty and arthrodesis represent salvage procedures for revision TKA. These options are mostly considered for the treatment of the infected TKA and rarely are used for the salvage of aseptic revision cases.

Resection arthroplasty is done in infected cases where the medical condition of the patient precludes reimplantation of another total knee replacement. All cement and infected material are removed and the knee joint is placed in an immobilizer or splint. An antibiotic-impregnated spacer block usually is placed into the knee. The antibiotic spacer block may be removed at a later date to prevent mechanical wearing of the acrylic over time. Occasionally, the antibiotic spacer may not be placed in the knee and the knee may simply be allowed to stiffen. Ordinarily, the patient will require a brace for walking and will have a short limb that requires a shoe lift. Patients who were severely disabled prior to the primary TKA are more satisfied with this procedure than those who did not have significant functional limitation. These latter patients may eventually require formal arthrodesis or late reimplantation of a new prosthesis.

The indications for arthrodesis of the infected TKA are patient choice, existence of increased risk of wound breakdown and subsequent reinfection, a patient who is medically immunosuppressed and at greater reinfection risk, and surgeon choice when the functional result of reimplantation of a new prosthesis will not be better than a fused joint. There are four surgical methods for arthrodesis: (1) single intramedullary rod, (2) articulating rod, (3) dual frame half-pin external fixation, and (4) plates and screws. The single intramedullary rod best achieves arthrodesis. The intramedullary rod allows easier rehabilitation and a greater incidence of fusion of the joint. The optimum position of the arthrodesis is 10° to 15° flexion, and 4° to 7° valgus. A shoe lift will be required to provide added length to the shortened limb.

Evaluation of the Painful Total Knee Arthroplasty

Patient Evaluation

In the small percentage of patients whose pain is not relieved after TKA, systematic evaluation using patient history, physical examination, and radiographic and laboratory studies is necessary. The differential diagnosis includes both extrinsic and intrinsic sources of pain (Table 3).

History

The patient's history is a critical source of information. Pain should be characterized by onset, location, severity, associated symptoms, and modifying factors, and classified as intrinsic or extrinsic. Intrinsic pain can be mechanical or nonmechanical in origin.

The history includes the patient's symptoms prior to primary TKA. If preoperative pain is unchanged in character, an erroneous preoperative diagnosis is indicated. Any history of prior knee surgery or infection should be noted. Primary wound healing difficulties or prolonged drainage at the time of TKA suggest an infectious etiology.

Well-localized pain is often indicative of etiology: anterior knee pain is generally of patellofemoral origin, pain in the region of the patellar tendon indicates tendinitis, and anteromedial tibial pain may represent pes anserinus bursitis. Diffuse pain that extends above and below the knee usually indicates a radicular etiology. Groin pain that extends to the knee could arise from the hip. Calf pain that extends up and down the leg may represent vascular claudication.

The temporal characteristics of the pain can be suggestive of its etiology. If the discomfort has been present since the index procedure, infection should be

TABLE 3 | Differential Diagnosis of the Painful TKA

Surgical Diagnosis

    Prosthetic loosening and failure

    Component wear

    Component overhang

    Patellofemoral tracking problems

    Instability

    Sepsis

    Osteolysis

    Arthrofibrosis

    Recurrent intra-articular soft-tissue impingement

    Recurrent effusion and synovitis

Nonsurgical Diagnoses

    Referred pain

      Hip

      Back

    Reflex sympathetic dystrophy

    Bursitis-tendinitis

      Pes anserine bursitis

      Patellar tendinitis

      Popliteal tendinitis

    Persistent crystalline deposition

      Gout

      Calcium pyrophosphate deposition disease

    Neurovascular problems

      Neuropathy

      Radiculopathy

      Vascular claudication

      Thrombophlebitis-deep vein thrombosis

    Fibromyalgia

    Expectation/Result mismatch

      Multiply operated knee

      Secondary gain issues

      Unrealistic expectations

    Psychiatric disorders and depression

considered a possible cause. Disability that arises after a period of good pain relief is suggestive of mechanical pain or late hematogenous infection. Aggravating and relieving factors should be identified. Pain that is present at all times, including during periods of rest, is suggestive of an inflammatory or infectious source. Start-up pain and activity-related pain is generally caused by component loosening (or failure of ingrowth in a cementless knee). Mechanical symptoms such as popping or clicking can be a patellar clunk, heard as the knee moves from flexion to extension. Pain with recurrent effusions can represent soft-tissue impingement or polyethylene synovitis. Anterior knee pain, effusions, and a sense of instability in flexion can be indicative of instability; posterior instability in a PCL-sparing knee or midflexion instability in the PCL-substituting knee.

The magnitude of the patient's current disability should be identified as well. Relevant information includes distance or duration of ambulation, the use of any assistive devices, the ability to ascend and descend stairs, and any sense of instability. Minimal disability in the face of significant patient complaints may indicate unrealistic patient expectations.

Issues related to the patient's secondary gain must be explored. The employment history and workers' compensation involvement should be questioned. Any psychiatric history may alter the patient's interpretation of pain and may require more extensive psychiatric evaluation in addition to orthopaedic evaluation. Furthermore, pain may be temporally related to discontinuation of antidepressants or psychotropic drugs in these patients.

Physical Examination

A thorough examination of the patient includes evaluation of possible intrinsic and extrinsic sources of knee pain, with careful assessment of the spine, hip, and neurovascular status.

Examination of the knee includes observation of gait and weight-bearing alignment. Antalgia, deformity, instability, or contractures should be investigated. Supine examination of the knee includes inspection of any wound abnormalities, swelling, erythema, or deformity. Range of motion measurements include both active and passive range of motion to identify any evidence of fixed contractures or extensor lag. Observation and palpation of patellar tracking can identify any subluxation or frank dislocation. Patellar clunk is generally caused by entrapment of a suprapatellar fibrotic nodule in the patellar notch at 35° to 45° of flexion. The strength of the extensor mechanism should be carefully measured; extensor mechanism weakness is one of the most common reasons for pain after a well-performed TKA. Palpation of the knee identifies the presence of an effusion or tenderness. Point tenderness is suggestive of localized pathology such as a neuroma, bursitis, tendinitis, or overhang of the prosthesis. Crepitation or squeaking with palpation of the patellofemoral articulation is suggestive of wear or delamination of a metal-backed patellar component. Coronal plane ligamentous stability is tested in full extension, 45°, and 90° of flexion. The amount and direction of the laxity should be noted, as should the quality of the end point. Laxity is suggestive of ligamentous insufficiency, component subsidence, or polyethylene wear. Posterior instability should be assessed in patients with a cruciate retaining knee.

Imaging Studies

Standard radiographs used to evaluate a painful TKA include a weight-bearing AP view, a lateral view, a Merchant view, and a full-length AP view of the entire weight-bearing extremity. Fluoroscopic images may help to improve visualization of the implant-bone interface, especially in cementless knees. Previous radiographs should be reviewed. Although partial radiolucencies are relatively common, complete or progressive radiolucencies suggest loosening. When these lines are rapidly progressive, infection should be considered. Evidence of metallic particulates, the so-called metal arthrogram, is indicative of metal-on-metal articulation. Discrete areas of heterotopic ossification may cause impingement, sites of point tenderness, or limit motion. Diffuse heterotopic ossification may indicate infection.

The AP radiograph is useful in identifying alignment of the TKA, the tibial interface, and any evidence of gross instability with weight bearing. This view should be taken tangential to the tibial component. If instability is suspected but not evident on weight-bearing views, AP stress views can be obtained. The level of the joint line can be assessed on this view as well. Excessive joint line elevation (more than 8 to 10 mm) has been shown to be associated with patellofemoral complications.

The lateral view demonstrates femoral component flexion or extension relative to the femoral diaphysis. Excessive flexion or extension of the femoral component can limit range of motion in the opposite direction. Femoral sizing can be estimated on a lateral view; an oversized femoral component can lead to limited flexion. The lateral view shows the degree of posterior slope on the tibial component. PCL-sparing TKAs generally are implanted with 7° to 10° of posterior slope, whereas PCL-substituting TKAs should have minimal posterior slope (zero to 3°). Less than this amount of slope or anterior slope can result in limited flexion. Evidence of posterior instability in a PCL-sparing knee can be identified on the lateral view as the tibiofemoral contact point is displaced anterior to the midline or, conversely, excessive PCL tightness can be identified with excessive rollback. The lateral view also demonstrates patella baja or alta, and the thickness of the patella. Patellar underresection can lead to pain, limited flexion, or both.

The full-length radiograph allows inspection of component alignment. The femoral and tibial components should be positioned perpendicular to the mechanical axes of the femur and tibia, respectively. The mechanical axis of the extremity should pass through the center of the TKA.

The Merchant view or a sunrise view is often ignored but is extremely important because it can identify patellar subluxation, dislocation, fracture, or loosening. Wear or delamination of metal-backed patellar components can be identified as direct contact between the metal surfaces; these views can be obtained at 15°, 30°, 45°, and 60° of flexion to obtain a more dynamic image of patellar tracking.

The role of CT scanning in the diagnosis of femoral or tibial rotational malalignment has been well established. Internal rotation of the femoral component relative to the epicondylar axis and/or internal rotation of the tibial component relative to the tibial tubercle usually results in patellar tracking problems. Furthermore, a mismatch between the rotations, with one component internally rotated and the other externally rotated, can cause rotational instability or impingement. CT can also be useful in quantifying osteolysis and bone defects.

Radionucleotide studies, including technetium Tc 99m (^{99m}Tc), indium In 111 (^{111}In) white blood cell (WBC), monoclonal antibody, or polyclonal antibody scans, can be of assistance in establishing the diagnosis of malalignment. If the fixation status of a total knee component remains unknown, despite thorough evaluation of serial radiographs, a bone scan should be obtained. A negative bone scan suggests that the knee is neither loose nor infected and probably not the source of pain. A positive bone scan is less diagnostic; ^{99m}Tc diphosphonate scans can remain positive for over 1 year after successful TKA especially in cementless knees. Serial bone scans are useful because they should demonstrate successively less uptake with time if the prosthesis is well fixed. In identifying infection, combining the ^{99m}Tc and ^{111}In scans has been shown to improve sensitivity up to 64% to 100% and specificity to 78% to 97%.

Other imaging studies that may provide information regarding possible extrinsic causes of knee pain in selective cases include noninvasive vascular studies of the extremities to evaluate claudication, and MRI or CT of the lumbar spine to evaluate radiculopathy.

Laboratory Analysis

Routine laboratory tests in evaluating painful TKA include a peripheral WBC count, erythrocyte sedimentation rate (ESR), and C-reactive protein (CRP). Elevated levels of WBCs can indicate acute infection, but the WBC count is rarely elevated in a chronic infection of a total joint. Although ESR is often elevated in cases of infected TKA, it may be elevated for months after implantation and can be slightly elevated with aseptic loosening; however, the CRP returns to normal

3 to 4 weeks after TKA. Elevation of CRP is consistent with infection. A negative ESR and CRP essentially rule out infection, while a positive ESR and CRP are highly suggestive of infection.

Aspiration is an important step in the evaluation of the painful total knee. The aspirate should be evaluated for cell count, crystal analysis, glucose level, Gram stain, and culture. A WBC count of more than 25,000/mm³ with a more than 75% preponderance of polymorphonuclear leukocytes is strongly suggestive of infection. With a sensitivity of 60% to 100%, and a specificity of 97% to 100%, aspiration remains one of the most valuable laboratory tools in the diagnosis of septic TKA and should be done routinely in the painful TKA. When indolent infection with a negative initial aspiration is suspected, repeat aspirations can increase sensitivity.

Patellofemoral Complications After Total Knee Arthroplasty

Early prosthetic designs for the knee did not include the option to resurface the patellofemoral joint, which resulted in persistent patellofemoral pain in up to 30% of patients. Modern prosthetic designs allow for resurfacing of the patellofemoral compartment but routine patellar resurfacing remains controversial. The incidence of patellofemoral complications after TKA ranges from 2% to 10%. Improvements in prosthetic design and surgical technique have led to a decrease in the incidence of patellofemoral complications.

Soft-Tissue Impingement

A nodule of fibrous tissue may develop on the undersurface of the distal aspect of the quadriceps tendon at the junction with the superior aspect of the patella, causing patellar clunk syndrome (Fig. 5), which occurs as the knee is actively extended from 60° to 30°. Changes in the design of the femoral component (deepening and elongating the femoral groove) and in surgical technique (excision of the soft tissue in the area where the nodule develops) has led to a reduction in the incidence of patellar clunk syndrome. Treatment consists of excision of the fibrous nodule.

Loosening of the Patellar Component

Factors that predispose to loosening of the patellar component include osteonecrosis of the patella, patellar fracture, patellar subluxation, osteoporosis, malposition of one or more components, improper patellar resection, and insufficient bone for cement fixation. Patients with minor or no symptoms may be managed with observation. Symptomatic patients typically require surgical treatment. Patellar component revision

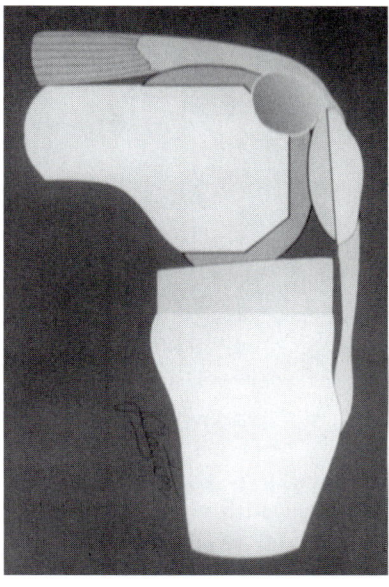

Figure 5 An example of a fibrous nodule that may form at the superior pole of the patella and lead to patellar clunk syndrome.

is indicated if adequate patellar bone is present. Patelloplasty may be performed if there is inadequate patellar bone.

Patellar Component Failure

Patellar component failures frequently have been associated with metal-backed patellar designs. In many designs, the addition of metal backing results in a reduction in the polyethylene thickness, often most pronounced at the periphery of the patellar implant. Failure modes that have been reported to occur with metal-backed patellar prostheses include poor ingrowth of bone into porous-coated designs with secondary loosening, wear and fracture; peg failure caused by high sheer stresses at the fixation peg-patellar interface; and dissociation of the polyethylene and the metal plate. Polyethylene dissociation and wear complications that expose the femoral component to the metal base plate may cause synovitis, pain, and audible grating. Metal-on-metal wear of the patellofemoral articulation affects the entire prosthetic joint and can lead to rapid failure if left untreated.

Patellar Instability

The incidence of symptomatic patellar instability after TKA varies from 1% to 20% (Fig. 6). Patellar subluxation is seen more frequently than frank dislocation. Identification of the etiology of the patellar instability following TKA is critical to successful management of the problem. Standard radiographs of the knee, including a patellar axial view, should be obtained. CT may be used to determine the rotation of the femoral component with reference to the transepicondylar axis of

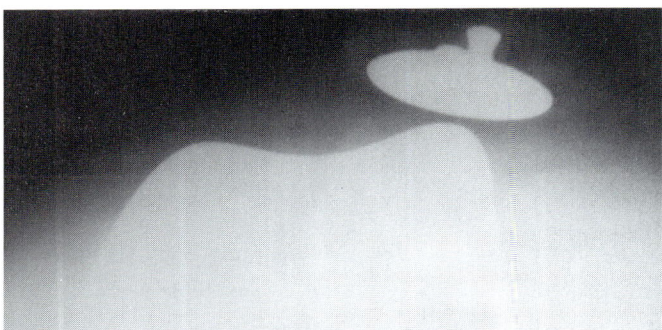

Figure 6 An example of patellar instability after TKA.

the femur and the tibial component with reference to the tibial tubercle.

An isolated lateral retinacular release may be sufficient for patellar subluxation with normally aligned components. Proximal or distal realignment procedures may be used to treat some instability problems. Rotational malalignment of the femoral or tibial component typically is corrected by revision of the component(s).

Extensor Mechanism Rupture

Extensor mechanism rupture is an infrequent but devastating complication occurring after TKA. The reported incidence of the patellar tendon rupture varies between 0.17% and 2.3%. The etiology of tendon rupture is multifactorial and includes mechanical, vascular, and surgical technique factors. Surgical repair is the treatment of choice for extensor mechanism ruptures. Reported results are superior for acute repairs in comparison with delayed repairs. Augmentation of the repair with local autogenous tissues (semitendinosus tendon) or allograft material is preferred. Clinical results after repair are often disappointing, with extensor lag and persistent tendon rupture. Chronic extensor mechanism disruption can be salvaged using extensor mechanism allografts.

Neurovascular Complications

Vascular injury during or after TKA is an uncommon complication with no reported incidence in the literature. Prompt recognition and correction of the arterial complication is extremely important. The role of the tourniquet in arterial complications related to TKA has been debated. Surgeons should consider carefully whether to use a tourniquet in patients with peripheral vascular disease.

Peroneal nerve palsy is the most common neurologic complication occurring after TKA, with a reported incidence of 0.3% to 4.0%. Peroneal nerve palsies often are associated with the correction of severe valgus and flexion deformities. The mechanism of peroneal nerve injury

has been reported to be traction of the nerve caused by realignment of the limb or direct compression. Risk factors for peroneal nerve palsy after TKA include severe preoperative valgus and/or flexion deformity, use of epidural anesthesia, previous lumbar laminectomy, and previous high tibial osteotomy.

Patients found to be at risk for peroneal palsy may benefit from preventive measures such as avoidance of compressive dressings and keeping the knee flexed until intact peroneal nerve function has been established. Should a peroneal nerve palsy occur, all dressings should be removed immediately and the knee positioned in flexion. Whether exploration of the nerve is of benefit is controversial. Partial palsies typically proceed to a full recovery, whereas complete palsies are associated with a more variable recovery.

Wound Problems

Prevention is the best treatment for wound problems after TKA. Risk factors associated with wound problems after TKA include prior incisions about the knee, conditions associated with altered microcirculation about the knee (such as diabetes mellitus and rheumatoid arthritis), history of prior infection, burn injury or radiation of the knee, obesity, and immunosuppression. Careful preoperative evaluation for risk factors is important.

If prior incisions are present about the knee, the surgical approach should be done through an existing incision if possible, and through the lateral incision if more than one incision is present. If this is not possible, skin bridges of approximately 7 cm should be maintained. Smaller strips of skin that lie between two incisions present the risk of skin necrosis. Previous transverse incisions can be crossed with a new incision that is perpendicular to the existing transverse incision. Vascular oxygen tension measurements on the edges of lateral skin flaps are lower than those measured on the medial flap. The more medial the incision, the lower the lateral flap oxygen tension.

Wound problems from multiple incisions, prior trauma, or prior infection may be averted by the use of soft-tissue reconstruction before TKA. Soft-tissue expansion of contracted tissue anterior to the knee with balloon skin expansion has been reported to be successful in preventing wound healing problems. Excision of abnormal skin and coverage with either a gastrocnemius flap or a free vascular flap have provided satisfactory soft-tissue coverage either during or after TKA.

Wound problems occurring after TKA should be treated aggressively. Persistent drainage, progressive and painful erythema, and marginal skin necrosis are often early signs of infection. The knee should be aspirated to assess the presence or absence of deep infection. Early débridement and irrigation followed by parenteral antibiotic therapy are based on deep joint cultures. Should the TKA implant become exposed as a result of soft-tissue loss, aggressive reconstructive soft-tissue techniques should be used.

Periprosthetic Fracture

Distal Femur Fracture

The incidence of fracture of the distal femur proximal to a TKA has been reported to vary between 0.3% and 2.5%. Risk factors include rheumatoid arthritis, chronic steroid use, revision TKA, neuromuscular disorders, poor flexion arc, stiff knee, osteolysis, osteoporosis, and anterior femoral notching. The goal of treatment is to achieve fracture union and return the patient to prefracture activity with a painless, stable, and mobile knee replacement. Factors to consider in choosing a method of treatment include the fracture displacement, alignment, rotation, and comminution, the integrity of fixation of the femoral component to the bone, and the design characteristics of the femoral component.

Nonsurgical treatment is indicated for nondisplaced or minimally displaced fractures with satisfactory alignment and rotation. Such fractures can be treated in a cast and/or cast brace. Surgical treatment of these fractures is indicated for displaced, malaligned, malrotated, or comminuted fractures. Surgical treatment is also indicated if the femoral component is loose. Methods of surgical treatment include internal fixation with plates, retrograde intramedullary locked rod, and external fixation. Surgical treatment also includes revision knee replacement surgery with intramedullary stems with or without allograft augmentation.

Proximal Tibia Fractures

Proximal tibia fractures below a TKA are uncommon. Treatment of these fractures depends on the fracture characteristics and the fixation of the tibial component to the tibia. When the tibial component is well fixed, typical fracture treatment can be used to restore limb alignment and knee function. When the tibial component is loose, revision knee replacement using stemmed tibial components is indicated. The stem should bypass a proximal tibial reconstruction with or without allograft augmentation and provide distal intramedullary fixation.

Patella Fractures

Patella fractures after TKA have a reported incidence that varies from 0.5% to 21%. The etiology of patella fracture includes factors such as patellar maltracking, obesity, prosthetic design, excessive knee flexion, trauma, large central fixation lugs, excessive patellar bone removal, use of an excessively large femoral component in the AP dimension, and avascularity of the patella.

Treatment of patella fractures is dependent on whether the patellar component is loose and the status of the extensor mechanism. Fractures that do not involve loosening of the patellar component or disruption of the extensor mechanism can be treated nonsurgically with good success. Loose patellar components may be removed and the patella resurfaced if 10 to 12 mm of bone remains. If less bone remains, a patelloplasty is preferred. In marked comminuted fractures, component removal with partial patellectomy and extensor mechanism repair may be the treatment of choice.

Polyethylene Wear

Polyethylene wear after TKA is multifactorial. Surgical technique, patient selection, and choice of implant design are factors that have a direct impact on the rate of polyethylene wear. Surgical technique is intimately associated with polyethylene wear, particularly the postoperative mechanical axis of the limb, the alignment of the tibial component in the coronal plane, and the thickness of the tibial insert. A minimum thickness of 8 mm of true polyethylene should be chosen for the tibial insert in TKA in order to ensure that the polyethylene functions as a

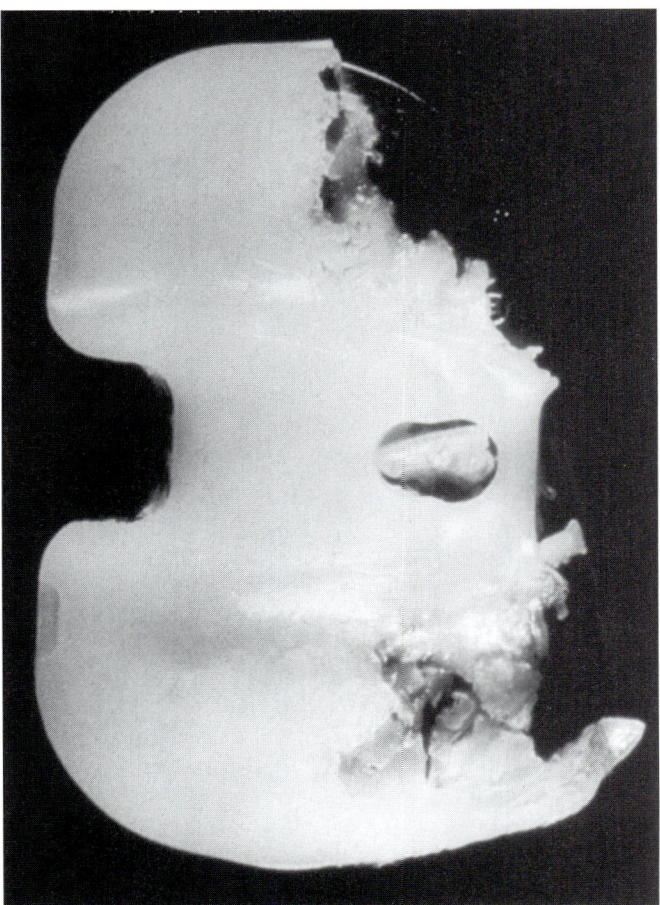

Figure 7 Catastrophic failure of a polyethylene insert less than 8 mm thick.

weight-bearing material (Fig. 7). The level of the tibial resection determines the thickness of the tibial insert that can be used. A minimum 10 mm of tibial bone must be resected from the normal tibial plateau, using a measured resection technique, in order to use a tibial prosthesis that contains 8 mm of polyethylene and 2 mm for the metal base plate.

Presenting symptoms associated with polyethylene wear include pain, swelling, progressive varus or valgus deformity, instability, and clicking or grinding. The clinical diagnosis of polyethylene wear is made with weight-bearing radiographs. Surgical treatment of patients with polyethylene wear is typical. Simple insert exchange is often unsuccessful, particularly if the polyethylene wear has occurred within 5 years of the initial knee replacement. Revision TKA is recommended for the treatment of polyethylene wear and associated loosening of the implant, prosthesis rotational or coronal malalignment, or severe scratching or burnishing of the articular surface. Recently, backside wear of the polyethylene component secondary to motion between the polyethylene insert and the tibial component has been noted. This wear mechanism may result in loosening of the tibial component secondary to generation of polyethylene wear debris and lysis.

Annotated Bibliography

Nonsurgical Treatment

Crenshaw SJ, Pollo FE, Calton EF: Effects of lateral-wedged insoles on kinetics at the knee. *Clin Orthop* 2000;375:185-192.

A motion analysis system and force plate demonstrated a reduction in external varus moment and medial compartment load in 17 healthy subjects when a lateral wedge insole was used.

Crofford LJ, Lipsky PE, Brooks P, Abramson SB, Simon LS, van de Putte LB: Basic biology and clinical application of cyclooxygenase-2 inhibitors. *Arthritis Rheum* 2000;43:4-13.

The relationship between the COX-2 isoform and prostaglandin production is reviewed. The authors point out that selective COX-2 inhibitors demonstrate reductions in gastrointestinal side effects but no definite clinical efficacy when compared to nonselective anti-inflammatory medications.

Deyle GD, Henderson NE, Matekel RL, Ryder MG, Garber MB, Allison SC: Effectiveness of manual physical therapy and exercise in osteoarthritis of the knee: A randomized, controlled trial. *Ann Intern Med* 2000;132:173-181.

A randomized, controlled clinical trial compared physical therapy (manual therapy and strengthening) to placebo (subtherapeutic ultrasound) in 83 patients with osteoarthritis of the knee. Patients in the treatment group had statistically significant gains in walking distance and Western Ontario and

McMaster University Osteoarthritis Index (WOMAC) scores at 1 year. Twenty percent of patients in the placebo group and 5% of patients in the treatment group had undergone TKA.

Kirkley A, Webster-Bogaert S, Litchfield R, et al: The effect of bracing on varus gonarthrosis. *J Bone Joint Surg Am* 1999;81:539-548.

A prospective, parallel-group randomized clinical trial compared a custom (unloader) valgus-producing brace, a neoprene sleeve, and medical treatment only (control group) in 119 patients with osteoarthritis of the knee. Patients were stratified according to age, mechanical axis, and the status of the ACL. Significant improvement was discovered in the disease-specific quality of life and in function for both the neoprene sleeve group and the unloader brace group compared with the control group at 6 months. There was a strong trend toward a significant difference between the unloader brace group and the neoprene sleeve group with regard to the WOMAC aggregate and physical function scores.

Laine L, Harper S, Simon T, et al: A randomized trial comparing the effect of rofecoxib, a cyclooxygenase-2 specific inhibitor, with that of ibuprofen on gastro-duodenal mucosa of patients with osteoarthritis. *Gastroenterology* 1999;117:776-783.

Endoscopy was repeated at 6, 12, and 24 weeks on 742 osteoarthritis patients without ulcers who were randomly assigned to receive rofecoxib, ibuprofen, or placebo. Rofecoxib, at doses two to four times the dose demonstrated to relieve symptoms of osteoarthritis, caused significantly less gastroduodenal ulceration than ibuprofen, with ulcer rates comparable to placebo.

McAlindon TE, LaValley MP, Gulin JP, Felson DT: Glucosamine and chondroitin for treatment of osteoarthritis: A systematic quality assessment and meta-analysis. *JAMA* 2000;283:1469-1475.

This meta-analysis or 15 randomized placebo-controlled trials showed that glucosamine and chondroitin sulfate demonstrate moderate to large effects on osteoarthritis symptoms.

Rosier RN, O'Keefe RJ: Hyaluronic acid therapy. *Instr Course Lect* 2000;49:495-502.

Intra-articular hyaluronate therapy is an invasive procedure that is well tolerated and probably not harmful to articular cartilage. No clinical evidence to date documents a chondroprotective effect and cost-effectiveness requires further study.

van Baar ME, Assendelft WJ, Dekker J, Oostendorp RA, Bijlsma JW: Effectiveness of exercise therapy in patients with osteoarthritis of the hip or knee: Systematic review of randomized clinical trials. *Arthritis Rheum* 1999;42:1361-1369.

In this literature review of randomized clinical trials, small to moderate effects of exercise therapy on pain, small beneficial effects on self-reported and observed disability, and moderate to great beneficial effects according to patients' global assessment are identified.

van Baar ME, Dekker J, Oostendorp RA, et al: The effectiveness of exercise therapy in patients with osteoarthritis of the hip or knee: A randomized clinical trial. *J Rheumatol* 1998;25:2432-2439.

Two hundred one patients with osteoarthritis of the hip and knee were randomized to receive education and medication only or the addition of exercise therapy for 12 weeks. Exercise therapy was effective in reducing pain and disability.

Tibial Osteotomy

Billings A, Scott DF, Camargo MP, Hofmann AA: High tibial osteotomy with a calibrated osteotomy guide, rigid internal fixation, and early motion: Long-term follow-up. *J Bone Joint Surg Am* 2000;82:70-79.

The results of 64 high tibial osteotomies were reported in 56 patients using a calibrated guide, internal fixation, and early range of motion. Twenty-one were converted to TKA at an average of 65 months. The remaining two thirds had a good or excellent knee score at an average of 8.5 years. Patella baja was not present, and conversion to TKA was not difficult.

Giagounidis EM, Sell S: High tibial osteotomy: Factors influencing the duration of satisfactory function. *Arch Orthop Trauma Surg* 1999;119:445-449.

The results of 94 knee osteotomies (71 for varus, 23 valgus) were reported at an average follow-up of 9 years (range, 2 to 21 years). Seventy-three percent had good or excellent results regarding ambulatory pain relief. Previous injury, meniscal pathology, and the degree of arthritis all had a significant effect on the outcome.

Meding JB, Keating EM, Ritter MA, Faris PM: Total knee arthroplasty after high tibial osteotomy: A comparison study in patients who had bilateral total knee replacement. *J Bone Joint Surg Am* 2000;82:1252-1259.

Thirty-nine patients underwent bilateral TKA, having previously undergone high tibial osteotomy in one knee at an average of 8.7 years earlier. The incidence of valgus alignment, diminished lateral tibial bone stock, and patella baja were all increased in the osteotomy group. At an average follow-up of 7.5 years for the osteotomy knees and 6.8 years for the contralateral knees, there were no differences in knee or function scores. Although previous osteotomy presents more of a challenge, it does not seem to jeopardize subsequent TKA.

Naudie D, Bourne RB, Rorabeck CH, Bourne TJ: Survivorship of the high tibial valgus osteotomy: A 10- to 22-year followup study. *Clin Orthop* 1999;367:18-27.

Eighty-five patients with 106 high tibial osteotomies were evaluated at a minimum 10-year follow-up. The percentage not requiring TKA was 73% at 5 years, 51% at 10 years, 39% at 15 years, and 30% at 20 years. Early failure was associated with age older than 50 years, previous arthroscopic débridement, lateral thrust, range of motion less than 120°, undercorrection, and delayed or nonunion. Survivorship was 95% at 5 years, 80% at 10 years, and 60% at 15 years in patients younger than age 50 years with a flexion arc greater than 120°.

Noyes FR, Barber-Westin SD, Hewett TE: High tibial osteotomy and ligament reconstruction for varus angulated anterior cruciate ligament-deficient knees. *Am J Sports Med* 2000;28:282-296.

Forty-one patients with varus angulation of the knee and ACL deficiency underwent high tibial osteotomy. Most had either lost the medial meniscus or sustained medial articular cartilage damage. Thirty-four patients underwent ACL reconstruction at an average of 8 months following high tibial osteotomy. Pain relief was good or very good in 71%, giving way was eliminated in 85%.

Potter HG, Linklater JM, Allen AA, Hannafin JA, Haas SB: Magnetic resonance imaging of articular cartilage in the knee: An evaluation with use of fast-spin-echo imaging. *J Bone Joint Surg Am* 1998;80:1276-1284.

This study documents the versatility of a fast-spin-echo MRI technique to assess the status of knee articular cartilage. Outerbridge ratings at surgery were compared with preoperative MRI assessments. The technique had a sensitivity of 87%, specificity of 94%, and an accuracy of 92%.

Rinonapoli E, Mancini GB, Corvaglia A, Musiello S: Tibial osteotomy for varus gonarthrosis: A 10- to 21-year followup study. *Clin Orthop* 1998;353:185-193.

Sixty high tibial osteotomies in 58 patients were reviewed an average of 15 years (range, 10 to 21 years). The 74% with a satisfactory outcome reported previously at 8-year follow-up, fell to 46% at 18 years. Fifty-five percent had a good or excellent Hospital for Special Surgery knee score. The average loss of correction was 3°, with 24% sustaining a loss of greater than 5° degrees.

Wada M, Imura S, Nagatani K, Baba H, Shimada S, Sasaki S: Relationship between gait and clinical results after high tibial osteotomy. *Clin Orthop* 1998;354:180-188.

The outcome of high tibial osteotomy was compared between 25 patients with a high preoperative adduction moment versus 7 with a low adduction moment. At 6-year follow-up, the preoperative adduction moment status did not correlate with outcome or radiographic appearance, provided that sufficient valgus correction was obtained at osteotomy.

Westrich GH, Peters LE, Haas SB, Buly RL, Windsor RE: Patella height after high tibial osteotomy with internal fixation and early motion. *Clin Orthop* 1998;354:169-174.

Thirty-two patients undergoing 34 high tibial osteotomies with cast immobilization were compared with 33 patients undergoing 35 high tibial osteotomies with internal fixation and early range of motion. Early range of motion resulted in significantly less patellar tendon shortening, despite equal amounts of angular correction in the two groups. Less patella baja should make subsequent TKA easier to perform.

Distal Femoral Osteotomy

Stahelin T, Hardegger F, Ward JC: Supracondylar osteotomy of the femur with use of compression: Osteosynthesis with a malleable implant. *J Bone Joint Surg Am* 2000;82:712-722.

Varus osteotomy of the distal femur was performed in 21 knees with valgus deformity. Nineteen (90%) had a good or excellent result at an average follow-up of five years (range, 2 to 12 years). A malleable plate was used with an oblique closing wedge osteotomy to establish medial cortical contact. There was one nonunion; none was converted to TKA.

Unicompartmental Knee Replacement

Chakrabarty G, Newman JH, Ackroyd CE: Revision of unicompartmental arthroplasty of the knee: Clinical and technical considerations. *J Arthroplasty* 1998;13:191-196.

Seventy-three unicompartmental knee replacements were converted to TKA, mostly for disease progression or implant failure at an average of 56 months. After bony preparation, bone defects were not present in 42%, were located on the tibia or femur in 23%, and were located in both in 34%. The defect required augmentation in 30%. At an average of 56 months follow-up, good and excellent results totaled 79%. The results were thought to be comparable to other series of revision TKA.

Murray DW, Goodfellow JW, O'Connor JJ: The Oxford medial unicompartmental arthroplasty: A ten-year survival study. *J Bone Joint Surg Br* 1998;80:983-989.

The results of 109 Oxford mobile bearing unicompartmental knee replacements were studied in patients with medial osteoarthritis. At an average follow-up of 7.6 years (maximum 13.8), five revisions were performed, none for polyethylene wear or tibial loosening. Survivorship at 10 years was 97%.

Newman JH, Ackroyd CE, Shah NA: Unicompartmental or total knee replacement? Five-year results of a prospective, randomised trial of 102 osteoarthritic knees with unicompartmental arthritis. *J Bone Joint Surg Br* 1998;80:862-865.

One hundred two knees deemed suitable for unicompartmental replacement were randomized at the time of surgery to receive either unicompartmental knee replacement or TKA. The average age at surgery was 69 years. At 5-year follow-up, two unicompartmental knee replacements were revised, one TKA was revised, and one was loose. Pain relief was equal in both groups; the unicompartmental knee replacement group had better range of motion, less morbidity and a faster recovery.

Squire MW, Callaghan JJ, Goetz DD, Sullivan PM, Johnston RC: Unicompartmental knee replacement: A minimum 15-year followup study. *Clin Orthop* 1999;367: 61-72.

One hundred forty Marmor unicompartmental knee replacements were performed in 103 patients. The average Hospital for Special Surgery knee score was 57 before surgery and 82 at follow-up. Fourteen knees (10%) underwent revision. Major long-term problems were disease progression (46%) and tibial subsidence with polyethylene wear (10%). The results in 34 patients (48 knees) were reported at a minimum 15-year follow-up. Six underwent revision (12.5%), five for progression of arthritis.

Primary Total Knee Arthroplasty

Akagi M, Matsusue Y, Mata T, et al: Effect of rotational alignment on patellar tracking in total knee arthroplasty. *Clin Orthop* 1999;366:155-163.

Forty-four patients (65 knees) were retrospectively evaluated to determine the effect of rotational alignment on patellar tracking in TKA. In the 22 patients (32 knees) in whom the femoral component was set parallel to the posterior condylar axis, 34% required a lateral release. In the remaining patients (33 knees), the femoral component was set in an external rotated position of 3° to 5° compared with the posterior condylar axis and 6% of patients required a lateral release.

Berger RA, Crossett LS, Jacobs JJ, Rubash HE: Malrotation causing patellofemoral complications after total knee arthroplasty. *Clin Orthop* 1998;356:144-153.

Two total knee patient groups were compared. The first patient group of 30 knees had isolated patellofemoral complications and was compared with 20 patients with well-functioning TKAs without patellofemoral complications. Femoral and tibial rotation was measured using CT. Excessive combined internal rotation of the femoral and tibial components was measured in the group with patellofemoral complications.

Bugbee WD, Ammeen DJ, Parks NL, Engh GA: 4- to 10-year results with the anatomic modular total knee. *Clin Orthop* 1998;348:158-165.

One hundred eighty-six consecutive TKAs with the anatomic modular knee design were reported. The revision rate of the femoral, tibial, and patellar components was 1.4% (2 of 142) at an average follow-up of 84 months.

Callaghan JJ, Squire MW, Goetz DD, Sullivan PM, Johnston RC: Cemented rotating-platform total knee replacement: A nine to twelve-year follow-up study. *J Bone Joint Surg Am* 2000;82:705-711.

In 119 consecutive TKAs (86 patients) with the low contact stress rotating platform femoral and tibial components at 9 to 12 years after surgery, none of the 114 knees for which the outcome was known required reoperation. Further, none of the polyethylene platforms became dislodged. There was no periprosthetic osteolysis and no evidence of loosening.

Campbell MD, Duffy GP, Trousdale RT: Femoral component failure in hybrid total knee arthroplasty. *Clin Orthop* 1998;356:58-65.

The authors reviewed 74 hybrid total knee designs (cementless femoral component, cemented tibial component) in 65 patients followed for an average of 7.4 years. Ten knees (13.8%) required revision surgery, leading to the recommendation that hybrid fixation should be abandoned.

Matsuda S, Miura H, Nagamine R, Urabe K, Matsunobu T, Iwamoto Y: Knee stability in posterior cruciate ligament retaining total knee arthroplasty. *Clin Orthop* 1999;366:169-173.

Anteroposterior knee laxity was evaluated in 14 patients (19 knees) who had a PCL-retaining Miller-Galante I prosthesis. The patients were evaluated an average of 105.9 months after surgery using a KT-2000 arthrometer. Greater anteroposterior instability was noted in knees with greater range of motion.

Matsueda M, Gustilo RB: Subvastus and medial parapatellar approaches in total knee arthroplasty. *Clin Orthop* 2000;371:161-168.

The subvastus approach was compared with the medial parapatellar approach in two consecutive groups of patients. No difference was seen in patellar subluxation or range of motion. The subvastus group showed improved patellar tracking (83% versus 63%) and less need for lateral retinacular release (37% versus 67%).

Olcott CW, Scott RD: Femoral component rotation during total knee arthroplasty. *Clin Orthop* 1999;367: 39-42.

In a series of 100 consecutive PCL-retaining TKAs, a femoral component was aligned to create a rectangular flexion gap. The flexion gap technique was compared to other techniques using the Whiteside line, the transepicondylar axis, and 3° of external rotation compared with the posterior condyles of the femur. The transepicondylar axis was the most consistent in recreating the flexion gap.

Revision Total Knee Arthroplasty

Barrack RL, Matzkin E, Ingraham R, Engh G, Rorabeck C: Revision knee arthroplasty with patella replacement versus bony shell. *Clin Orthop* 1998;356:139-143.

Revision TKAs were studied with respect to patellar replacement with salvage of the patella. Results of 123 of 130 consecutive revision TKAs were examined. In 21 knees (17%) a shell of patellar bone was left in the patellar region. This group of patients had lower knee function scores than those patients who had an intact patella with a patellar prosthesis in place.

Coyte PC, Hawker G, Croxford R, Wright JG: Rates of revision knee replacement in Ontario, Canada. *J Bone Joint Surg Am* 1999;81:773-782.

This study evaluated the incidence of revision TKA in a region of Canada between April 1, 1984, and March 31, 1991. The revision rate was 7.0% (1,301 of 18,530 TKAs). However, estimates of the proportion of knee replacements that would need to be revised within 7 years ranged from a low of 4.3%, with use of an algorithm for the longest time to revision, to a high of 8.0%, with use of an algorithm for the shortest time to revision. Patients older than 55 years, living in a rural area, or with a diagnosis of rheumatoid arthritis had a significantly longer duration before revision surgery than did other patients.

Partington PF, Sawhney J, Rorabeck CH, Barrack RL, Moore J: Joint line restoration after revision total knee arthroplasty. *Clin Orthop* 1999;367:165-171.

In this study, 107 knee revision TKAs were analyzed with respect to the postoperative joint line position that was obtained. The Knee Society scores were analyzed with respect to joint line elevation. The joint line was elevated in 79% of the cases and elevation of the joint line greater than 8 mm correlated with a lower Knee Society Clinical Rating score. The study emphasized the need to preserve joint line height by measuring the preoperative joint line position and using a greater thickness of distal femoral augment to achieve this anatomic relationship.

Schmalzried TP, Callaghan JJ: Wear in total hip and knee replacements. *J Bone Joint Surg Am* 1999;81:115-136.

The causes of wear are analyzed in depth as polyethylene wear is becoming one of the greatest concerns as a cause of TKA failure and osteolysis. The different forms of wear and types of polyethylene are discussed.

Evaluation of the Painful Total Knee Arthroplasty

Berger RA, Crossett LS, Jacobs JJ, Rubash HE: Malrotation causing patellofemoral complications after total knee arthroplasty. *Clin Orthop* 1998;356:144-153.

Patients had excessive combined (tibial plus femoral) internal component rotation that was directly proportional to the severity of the patellofemoral complication. The epicondylar axis and tibial tubercle are reproducible landmarks that can be used intraoperatively. In addition, these landmarks are visible on CT scans and can be used preoperatively to determine which component needs to be revised in a failed total knee.

Hanssen AD, Rand JA: Evaluation and treatment of infection at the site of a total hip or knee arthroplasty. *Instr Course Lect* 1999;48:111-122.

This article provides a recent review of infected total hip and knee arthroplasty.

Kersey R, Benjamin J, Marson B: White blood cell counts and differential in synovial fluid of aseptically failed total knee arthroplasty. *J Arthroplasty* 2000;15:301-304.

A cell count and differential was obtained on synovial fluid samples from 79 TKAs on which revision for aseptic failure was done over a 5-year period. In patients with osteoarthritis as a primary diagnosis, a synovial WBC count of less than 2,000/mm^3 and a differential of 50% polymorphonuclear leukocytes or less had a 98% negative predictive value for the absence of infection.

Lucas TS, DeLuca PF, Nazarian DG, Bartolozzi AR, Booth RE Jr: Arthroscopic treatment of patellar clunk. *Clin Orthop* 1999;367:226-229.

Thirty consecutive patients (32 knees) were treated arthroscopically. Knee Society scores increased from an average of 64 points preoperatively to 93 points postoperatively.

Teller RE, Christie MJ, Martin W, Nance EP, Haas DW: Sequential indium-labeled leukocyte and bone scans to diagnose prosthetic joint infection. *Clin Orthop* 2000;373:241-247.

Preoperative sequential imaging was compared to joint aspiration and clinical assessment during revision knee or hip arthroplasty. Scans were considered positive if ^{111}In leukocyte uptake was incongruent or focally more intense than ^{99m}Tc uptake. Of 166 cases, infection was noted in 22. Sequential ^{99m}Tc and ^{111}In leukocyte imaging was 64% sensitive and 78% specific. Fever, physical findings, or ESR did not identify infection reliably, and preoperative aspirate culture was only 28% sensitive in this study. The authors concluded that the routine use of sequential ^{99m}Tc and ^{111}In leukocyte imaging cannot be advocated for differentiating occult infection from mechanical failure in painful, loose total joint arthroplasties.

Patellofemoral Complications After Total Knee Arthroplasty

Kumar SN, Chapman JA, Rawlins I: Vascular injuries in total knee arthroplasty: A review of the problem with special reference to the possible effects of the tourniquet. *J Arthroplasty* 1998;13:211-216.

A survey of 147 members of the British Association for Surgery of the Knee documented 14 arterial complications following TKA. Three were caused by direct trauma and 11 were caused by thrombosis.

Classic Bibliography

Adams ME, Atkinson MH, Lussier AJ, et al: The role of viscosupplementation with hylan G-F 20 (Synvisc) in the treatment of osteoarthritis of the knee: A Canadian multicenter trial comparing hylan G-F 20 alone, hylan G-F 20 with non-steroidal anti-inflammatory drugs (NSAIDs) and NSAIDs alone. *Osteoarthritis Cartilage* 1995;3:213-225.

Aichroth PM, Patel DV, Moyes ST: A prospective review of arthroscopic debridement for degenerative joint disease of the knee. *Int Orthop* 1991;15:351-355.

Andriacchi TP, Yoder D, Conley A, Rosenberg A, Sum J, Galante JO: Patellofemoral design influences function following total knee arthroplasty. *J Arthroplasty* 1997;12:243-249.

Ayers, DC, Dennis DA, Johanson NA, Pellegrini VD Jr: Common complications of total knee arthroplasty. *J Bone Joint Surg Am* 1997;79:278-311.

Barrack RL, Wolfe MW, Waldman DA, Milicic M, Bertot AJ, Myers L: Resurfacing of the patella in total knee arthroplasty: A prospective, randomized, double-blind study. *J Bone Joint Surg Am* 1997;79:1121-1131.

Buechel FF, Pappas MJ: Long-term survivorship analysis of cruciate-sparing versus cruciate-sacrificing knee prostheses using meniscal bearings. *Clin Orthop* 1990;260:162-169.

Cartier P, Sanouiller JL, Grelsamer RP: Unicompartmental knee arthroplasty surgery: 10-year minimum follow-up period. *J Arthroplasty* 1996;11:782-788.

Caruso I, Pietrogrande V: Italian double-blind multicenter study comparing S-adenosylmethionine, naproxen, and placebo in the treatment of degenerative joint disease. *Am J Med* 1987;83:66-71.

Casha JN, Hadden WA: Suture reaction following skin closure with subcuticular polydioxanone in total knee arthroplasty. *J Arthroplasty* 1996;11:859-861.

Chandler HP, Tigges RG: The role of allografts in the treatment of periprosthetic femoral fractures. *J Bone Joint Surg Am* 1997;79:1422-1432.

Colizza WA, Insall JN, Scuderi GR: The posterior stabilized total knee prosthesis: Assessment of polyethylene damage and osteolysis after a 10-year minimum follow-up. *J Bone Joint Surg Am* 1995;77:1713-1720.

Coventry MB, Ilstrup DM, Wallrichs SL: Proximal tibial osteotomy: A critical long-term study of eighty-seven cases. *J Bone Joint Surg Am* 1993;75:196-201.

Diduch DR, Scuderi GR, Scott WN, Insall JN, Kelly MA: The efficacy of arthroscopy following total knee replacement. *Arthroscopy* 1997;13:166-171.

Doets HC, Bierman BT, von Soesbergen RM: Synovectomy of the rheumatoid knee does not prevent deterioration: 7-year follow-up of 83 cases. *Acta Orthop Scand* 1989;60:523-525.

Duff GP, Lachiewicz PF, Kelley SS: Aspiration of the knee joint before revision arthroplasty. *Clin Orthop* 1996;331:132-139.

Emerson RH Jr, Head WC, Malinin TI: Reconstruction of patellar tendon rupture after total knee arthroplasty with an extensor mechanism allograft. *Clin Orthop* 1990;260:154-161.

Engh GA: Bone defect classification, in Engh GA, Rorabeck CH (eds): *Revision Total Knee Arthroplasty.* Baltimore, MD, Williams & Wilkins, 1997, pp 63-120.

Escalante A, Beardmore TD: Risk factors for early wound complications after orthopedic surgery for rheumatoid arthritis. *J Rheumatol* 1995;22:1844-1851.

Ettinger WH Jr, Burns R, Messier SP, et al: A randomized trial comparing aerobic exercise and resistance exercise with a health education program in older adults with knee osteoarthritis: The Fitness Arthritis and Seniors Trial (FAST). *JAMA* 1997;277: 25-31.

Feinstein WK, Noble PC, Kamaric E, Tullos HS: Anatomic alignment of the patellar groove. *Clin Orthop* 1996;331:64-73.

Felix NA, Stuart MJ, Hanssen AD: Periprosthetic fractures of the tibia associated with total knee arthroplasty. *Clin Orthop* 1997;345:113-124.

Feller JA, Bartlett RJ, Lang DM: Patellar resurfacing versus retention in total knee arthroplasty. *J Bone Joint Surg Br* 1996:78:226-228.

Finkelstein JA, Gross AE, Davis A: Varus osteotomy of the distal part of the femur: A survivorship analysis. *J Bone Joint Surg Am* 1996;78:1348-1352.

Garvin KL, Scuderi G, Insall JN: Evolution of the quadriceps snip. *Clin Orthop* 1995;321:131-137.

Gibson JN, White MD, Chapman VM, Strachan RK: Arthroscopic lavage and debridement for osteoarthritis of the knee. *J Bone Joint Surg Br* 1992;74:534-537.

Gill T, Schemitsch EH, Brick GW, Thornhill TS: Revision total knee arthroplasty after failed unicompartmental knee arthroplasty or high tibial osteotomy. *Clin Orthop* 1995;321:10-18.

Gold DA, Scott SC, Scott WN: Soft tissue expansion prior to arthroplasty in the multiply-operated knee: A new method of preventing catastrophic skin problems. *J Arthroplasty* 1996;11:512-521.

Haas SB, Insall JN, Montgomery W III, Windsor RE: Revision total knee arthroplasty with use of modular components with stems inserted without cement. *J Bone Joint Surg Am* 1995;77:1700-1707.

Healy WL, Anglen JO, Wasilewski SA, Krackow KA: Distal femoral varus osteotomy. *J Bone Joint Surg Am* 1988;70:102-109.

Healy WL, Wasilewski SA, Takei R, Oberlander M: Patellofemoral complications following total knee arthroplasty: Correlation with implant design and patient risk factors. *J Arthroplasty* 1995;10:197-201.

Healy WL: Tibial fractures below total knee arthroplasty, in Insall JN, Scott WN, Scuderi GR (eds): *Current Concepts in Primary and Revision Total Knee Arthroplasty.* Philadelphia, PA, Lippincott-Raven, 1996, pp 163-167.

Hernigou P, Medevielle D, Debeyre J, Goutallier D: Proximal tibial osteotomy for osteoarthritis with varus deformity: A ten- to thirteen-year follow-up study. *J Bone Joint Surg Am* 1987;69:332-354.

Hsu HC, Luo ZP, Rand JA, An KN: Influence of patellar thickness on patellar tracking and patellofemoral contact characteristics after total knee arthroplasty. *J Arthroplasty* 1996;11:69-80.

Idusuyi OB, Morrey BF: Peroneal nerve palsy after total knee arthroplasty: Assessment of predisposing and prognostic factors. *J Bone Joint Surg Am* 1996;78: 177-184.

Insall JN, Joseph DM, Msika C: High tibial osteotomy for varus gonarthrosis: A long-term follow-up study. *J Bone Joint Surg Am* 1984;66:1040-1048.

Insall JN, Lachiewicz PF, Burstein AH: The posterior stabilized condylar prosthesis: A modification of the total condylar design: Two- to four-year clinical experience. *J Bone Joint Surg Am* 1982;64:1317-1323.

Ishikawa H, Ohno O, Hirohata K: Long-term results of synovectomy in rheumatoid patients. *J Bone Joint Surg Am* 1986;68:198-205.

Jordan LR, Olivo JL, Voorhorst PE: Survivorship analysis of cementless meniscal bearing total knee arthroplasty. *Clin Orthop* 1997;338:119-123.

Klein W, Jensen KU: Arthroscopic synovectomy of the knee joint: Indication, technique, and follow-up results. *Arthroscopy* 1988;4:63-71.

Lewonowski K, Dorr LD, McPherson EJ, Huber G, Wan Z: Medialization of the patella in total knee arthroplasty. *J Arthroplasty* 1997;12:161-167.

Lindenfeld TN, Hewett TE, Andriacchi TP: Joint loading with valgus bracing in patients with varus gonarthrosis. *Clin Orthop* 1997;344:290-297.

Maquet P: Valgus osteotomy for osteoarthritis of the knee. *Clin Orthop* 1976;120:143-148.

Merchan EC, Galindo E: Arthroscope-guided surgery versus nonoperative treatment for limited degenerative osteoarthritis of the femorotibial joint in patients over 50 years of age: A prospective comparative study. *Arthroscopy* 1993;9:663-667.

Moseley JB Jr, Wray NP, Kuykendall D, Willis K, Landon G: Arthroscopic treatment of osteoarthritis of the knee: A prospective, randomized, placebo-controlled trial: Results of a pilot study. *Am J Sports Med* 1996;24:28-34.

Muller-Fassbender H: Double blind clinical trial of S-adenosylmethionine versus ibuprofen in the treatment of osteoarthritis. *Am J Med* 1987;83:81-83.

Nagel A, Insall JN, Scuderi GR: Proximal tibial osteotomy: A subjective outcome study. *J Bone Joint Surg Am* 1996;78:1353-1358.

Odenbring S, Egund N, Knutson K, Lindstrand A, Larsen ST: Revision after osteotomy for gonarthrosis: A 10- to 19-year follow-up of 314 cases. *Acta Orthop Scand* 1990;61:128-130.

Ogilvie-Harris DJ, Weisleder L: Arthroscopic synovectomy of the knee: Is it helpful? *Arthroscopy* 1995;11:91-95.

Ranawat CS, Flynn WF Jr, Saddler S, Hansraj KK, Maynard MJ: Long-term results of the total condylar knee arthroplasty: A 15-year survivorship study. *Clin Orthop* 1993;286:94-102.

Rand JA: Role of arthroscopy in osteoarthritis of the knee. *Arthroscopy* 1991;7:358-363.

Ritter MA, Herbst SA, Keating EM, Faris PM, Meding JB: Long-term survival analysis of a posterior cruciate-retaining total condylar total knee arthroplasty. *Clin Orthop* 1994;309:136-145.

Ritter MA, Herbst SA, Keating EM, Faris PM, Meding JB: Patellofemoral complications following total knee arthroplasty: Effect of a lateral release and sacrifice of the superior lateral geniculate artery. *J Arthroplasty* 1996;11:368-372.

Rolston LR, Christ DJ, Halpern A, O'Connor PL, Ryan TG, Uggen WM: Treatment of supracondylar fractures of the femur proximal to a total knee arthroplasty: A report of four cases. *J Bone Joint Surg Am* 1995;77:924-931.

Scuderi GR, Insall JN, Windsor RE, Moran MC: Survivorship of cemented knee replacements. *J Bone Joint Surg Br* 1989;71:798-803.

Shoji H, Insall J: High tibial osteotomy for osteoarthritis of the knee with valgus deformity. *J Bone Joint Surg Am* 1973;55:963-973.

Sochart DH, Hardinge K: Nonsurgical management of supracondylar fracture above total knee arthroplasty: Still the nineties option. *J Arthroplasty* 1997;12:830-834.

Stern SH, Insall JN: Posterior stabilized prosthesis: Results after follow-up of nine to twelve years. *J Bone Joint Surg Am* 1992;74:980-986.

Stuart MJ, Grace JN, Ilstrup DM, Kelly CM, Adams RA, Morrey BF: Late recurrence of varus deformity after proximal tibial osteotomy. *Clin Orthop* 1990;260:61-65.

Wang JW, Kuo KN, Andriacchi TP, Galante JO: The influence of walking mechanics and time on the results of proximal tibial osteotomy. *J Bone Joint Surg Am* 1990;72:905-909.

Whiteside LA: Distal realignment of the patellar tendon to correct abnormal patellar tracking. *Clin Orthop* 1997;344:284-289.

Chapter 45

Ankle and Foot: Pediatric Aspects

Kristen L. Carroll, MD

Peter F. Armstrong, MD

Congenital Deformities

Metatarsus Adductus

Metatarsus adductus is a forefoot adduction deformity that is associated with a normal, plantigrade hindfoot and is believed to be a result of intrauterine positioning. Metatarsus adductus is usually classified by two different criteria: flexibility (passively correctable or rigid) and degree of deformity. The degree of deformity (mild, moderate, severe) is ascertained by the heel bisection line. Mild deformities often can be observed. Serial casts during the first 6 months of life are suggested for moderate to severe deformities and for those that appear less flexible. Below-knee casts usually are used for 6 to 12 weeks. For severe, rigid, and persistent deformities, midfoot capsulotomy and abductor hallucis lengthening can be done.

Long-term follow-up studies indicate that 90% of metatarsus adductus cases should spontaneously correct by 5 years and 95% by 16 years. Even in the presence of residual deformity and an oblique medial cuneiform, there is little sequela in adult life.

Clubfoot (Equinovarus) Deformity

There are three types of clubfoot: positional, idiopathic congenital, and teratologic.

Positional Clubfoot

The infant's foot is in equinovarus but does not have a deep posterior or plantar medial crease and is thought to be the result of intrauterine positioning of the foot. The foot can be passively brought to a plantigrade position and is amenable to cast correction. In general, 1 to 3 months of above-knee cast correction precludes surgical intervention.

Idiopathic Congenital Clubfoot

The etiology of idiopathic clubfoot is unknown and occurs in 1 out of 1,000 live births. Males are twice as likely as females to be affected. Initial treatment (birth to 6 months) is manipulation and cast correction. The Iowa casting protocol is typically used. First, the cavus is corrected by supination of the forefoot and dorsiflexion of the first metatarsal. The supinated forefoot is then abducted under the talus to an outwardly rotated position. The lateral aspect of the talar head is the fulcrum, rather than the calcaneal cuboid joint as in the Kite casting protocol. The calcaneus abducts by rotating under the talus. Once the foot is abducted under the talus to 60° outward rotation, dorsiflexion is attempted. These corrections take 6 to 8 weeks to attain. If the equinus is rigid, a percutaneous Achilles tendon lengthening is done in clinic, or as outpatient surgery with possible inclusion of a posterior capsular release. Following the conclusion of cast use, a Denis-Browne bar is worn at night for up to 3 years. The concept of correction with the forefoot supinated is constant, however. Proponents have observed that the rate of full posteromedial release has steadily decreased with experience and now falls under 10%, although up to 40% may require anterior tibialis tendon transfer for residual forefoot supination. The long-term outcome at skeletal maturity has been marked by the excellent appearance and, most importantly, suppleness of the foot. If correction is not attained by casting techniques with or without Achilles tenotomy, a full or partial posteromedial release is undertaken. The outcome of surgery is best when performed after 6 months but before 1 year of age. Through a Cincinnati incision, the Achilles, posterior tibialis, and if necessary, long toe flexor tendons are lengthened. Capsular releases include posterior ankle, talonavicular, subtalar, and posterolateral tethers of the calcaneus, and sometimes the calcaneocuboid joint. The more rigid and severe the deformity, the more complete the release must be, although this can increase the risk of overcorrection. If the talocalcaneal realignment is suboptimal despite complete subtalar release, the calcaneocuboid joint should be opened medially and laterally to enhance correction. In all studies, the rate of recurrent deformity requiring subsequent surgical intervention (anterior tibial tendon transfer) usually is between 15% and 50%.

Long-term studies show that the surgically treated foot is 1 to 1.5 cm shorter than the contralateral foot and has a smaller calf circumference. The gastrocnemius-soleus complex is only 80% as strong as that of the contralateral foot, with a 23% decrease in the plantar flexion strength. Ankle motion is decreased in 94% of surgically treated feet; ankle valgus is present in two thirds and may compensate for an undercorrected hindfoot or add to the deformity of an overcorrected one. The most common residual effects of surgical intervention are stiffness, forefoot adduction, and supination/cavus.

Teratologic Clubfoot

The most common causes of a teratologic clubfoot are either neuromuscular, such as in spina bifida, or syndromic, as in arthrogryposis or osteochondrodysplasias such as diastrophic dwarfism. The teratologic clubfoot is unlike the idiopathic clubfoot in that attempts at cast correction are unsuccessful, making surgery necessary. In patients with spina bifida, the equinovarus deformity is often present at birth and can progress over time. Radical posteromedial release (tenotomy rather than tendon lengthening) provides good results in 76% of cases. Often the anterior tibialis tendon is also lengthened. After radical release, it is essential that not only the talonavicular, but the subtalar joint be pinned in adequate position. The higher the spina bifida lesion, the worse the prognosis. Talectomy can be considered for patients with recurrence of symptoms after radical posteromedial release, and is often done in patients with high-level spina bifida lesions because of a 50% recurrence rate after soft-tissue surgery alone.

For the rigid teratologic clubfoot resulting from arthrogryposis or osteochondrodysplasia, initial casting is done prior to surgery. A radical soft-tissue release of the Achilles tendon, posterior tibialis and flexors, and capsular releases are required. These joints, narrowed by disuse and paralysis, are often difficult to identify. Many authors suggest primary talectomy and often cuboidectomy. Orthotic devices are required to maintain the position postoperatively. In patients in whom symptoms recur after soft-tissue release, talectomy appears to be the best salvage procedure, with better outcome and less complications than triple arthrodesis. In addition, talectomy is useful in a younger age group when a plantigrade foot is essential, but bone maturity precludes triple arthrodesis.

Flatfoot Deformity (Pes Planus)

The majority of babies are born with flat (or fat) feet, but an arch becomes more apparent with age. The relatively benign natural history should not overshadow the importance of accurate diagnosis. Significant ankle valgus, vertical talus, tarsal coalition, and skewfoot must be accurately differentiated from flexible pes planus.

Flexible flatfoot deformity appears to be familial, with occasional association of generalized ligamentous laxity. Careful evaluation of possible occult Achilles tendon contracture is done by holding the hindfoot in varus, and dorsiflexing the ankle. Achilles tendon contracture can signify a more severe flatfoot variant. The flexibility of the hindfoot is evaluated by having the child stand on the toes or dorsiflexing the first ray passively in the absence of weight bearing. This maneuver, the windlass mechanism, tightens the plantar fascia, reconstituting an arch and hindfoot varus if the foot is indeed flexible. If hindfoot flexibility and an underlying arch are present, then the diagnosis of flexible flatfoot is made. Recent data indicate that surgical or orthotic treatment of asymptomatic flexible flatfoot is unnecessary.

In the small subset of children with a painful flexible flatfoot, careful attention must be paid to possible Achilles tendon contracture, and the possibility of coalition or tumor must be considered. Radiographs are necessary in this population. A fibrous coalition may still retain some flexibility and require a CT scan for diagnosis. Tumors, such as solitary bone cysts, though rare, can occur. These patients are treated with shoe inserts and observation. If pain continues into adolescence, indicating that more aggressive treatment is required, calcaneal lengthening will correct the flatfoot without decreasing hindfoot motion. Arthroereisis, or placement of a Silastic plug in the subtalar joint with fusion, has been studied, but the long-term effects of indwelling Silastic within the subtalar joint are still unknown.

Tarsal Coalition

Tarsal coalition is defined as a congenital fibrous or bony bridging of two or more tarsal bones. Although it is the most common etiology of a rigid or peroneal spastic flatfoot, tarsal coalition rarely is seen with a cavovarus deformity. The exact prevalence is not known; it is estimated that 1% of the general population have a tarsal coalition, with 50% to 60% having bilateral coalitions.

The most common symptom is painful flatfoot. The age of presentation will vary depending on the type of coalition; symptoms worsen as the coalition ossifies and therefore becomes more rigid. The most common coa-

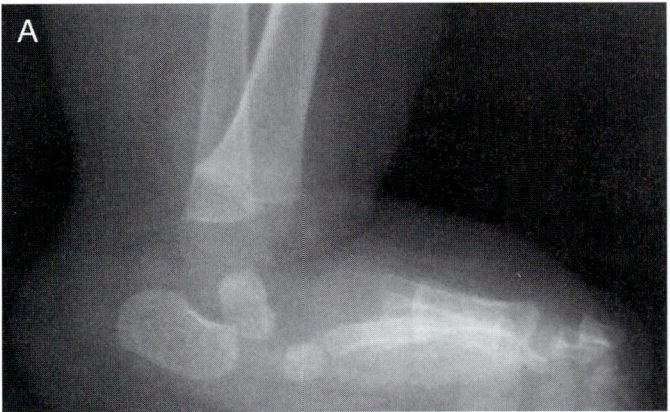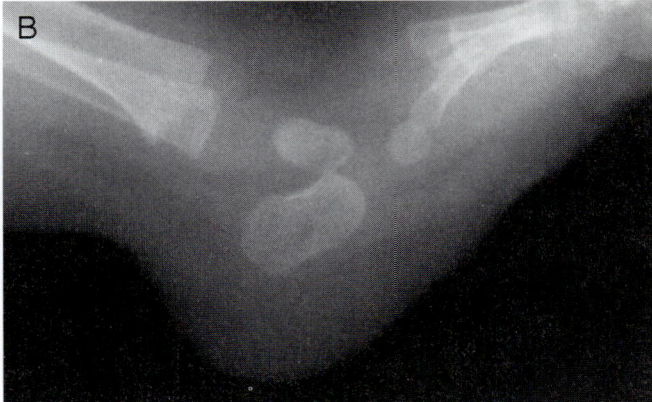

Figure 1 **A,** Lateral and **B,** forced plantar flexion lateral views of the vertical talus.

lition, calcaneonavicular, ossifies between 8 and 12 years of age, the second most common, talocalcaneal, at 12 to 16 years of age, and the least common, talonavicular, at 3 to 5 years of age. Later presentations can occur in all cases; recurrent sprains, posterior tibialis dysfunction, valgus hindfoot or a chronic ache in the hindfoot are symptoms that occur. The classic presentation is of a rigid hindfoot; when the patient attempts to stand on the toes, an arch is not reconstituted and the hindfoot remains in valgus. Peroneal spasm or contracture, if noted, also can be highly indicative of coalition. Plain radiographs are the first line of imaging. A lateral view can show talar beaking; although not regarded as a sign of degenerative arthritis, this condition indicates abnormal motion of the subtalar complex. Although calcaneonavicular coalition often can be accurately diagnosed by an oblique (or 45°) view of the foot, and a talocalcaneal coalition by a Harris view, CT and MRI are also often used. Because up to 20% of affected feet can have more than one coalition, the difficulty in seeing the accurate size of some coalitions has led most physicians to use more scans. Although CT remains the gold standard, MRI often is quite helpful, especially if other possible causes of ankle pain, such as talar dome injury, are possible. CT scans are often done on both feet because of the high incidence of bilateral coalitions.

Initial treatment, regardless of type of coalition, is nonsurgical. The patient may try activity modification, nonsteroidal anti-inflammatory drugs (NSAIDs), steroid injection, and/or orthotic devices. The goal is to reduce subtalar motion and hence inflammation. A below-knee walking cast may be tried for 3 to 6 weeks. When nonsurgical measures fail to control pain, surgical intervention is indicated. For calcaneonavicular coalition, resection is attempted with extensor digitorum brevis, fat, or bone wax placed in the excision site. An adequate amount of bone must be resected; special attention should be given to making parallel rather than trapezoidal cuts in the calcaneus and navicular. Early motion after surgery improves outcome. As long as subtalar motion can be regained, both pain and gait abnormalities are minimized. If degenerative changes are found, then an isolated subtalar fusion can be undertaken. Assuring that only one coalition is present is clearly essential to adequately treat symptoms.

Talocalcaneal coalition is more controversial. When nonsurgical treatment fails, the choice of resection versus triple arthrodesis first depends on whether degenerative changes are present. If there are no degenerative changes, resection can be attempted. In general, the coalition must be of the middle facet and less than 50% of the joint must be involved. Although degenerative changes are more likely in the older patient, age alone does not preclude an attempt at resection. Success rates are 50% to 94%, and variable. When the coalition involves less than one third of the joint, resection appears to be reasonably successful even in an older population. The rare cavovarus deformity, which can be associated with a talonavicular coalition, has a less favorable outcome after resection.

Vertical Talus

The congenital vertical talus foot is characterized by a rigid, rocker-bottom type planovalgus deformity. The extensor tendons and heel cord are both contracted, with the talar head markedly plantar flexed into the sole of the foot. Lateral radiographs show that the talus is vertical, and with forced plantar flexion of the forefoot, the talus remains vertical so as not to line up with the forefoot (Fig. 1). The navicular will often dislocate to the anterosuperior neck of the talus and the calcaneocuboid joint also may be dislocated.

In 80% to 90% of cases, the etiology of vertical talus is neuromuscular or genetic. If vertical talus is identified, a thorough neurologic examination and imaging must be undertaken. The first line of treatment for vertical talus is serial casting for 8 to 12 weeks to reduce contractures of the extensor musculature. The foot is placed in equinus, with an attempt to mold the heel in varus. It is generally accepted that in a true congenital vertical talus, casting will not correct the deformity.

Once the child reaches the age of 6 months, a surgical approach using a one-stage technique through a Cincinnati incision is done. Achilles tendon, extensor tendon, and anterior tibialis lengthening, as well as capsulotomies of the tibiotalar, subtalar, talonavicular and, if necessary, calcaneocuboid joint are essential. The talonavicular joint is reduced and pinned. The posterior tibialis is then plicated on the reduced navicular. If the hindfoot is in severe valgus, the peroneal tendons will require lengthening or tenotomy. In older children, the navicular may need to be removed to attain reduction, and/or a Grice (subtalar) arthrodesis may be required. The outcome is good in approximately 60% to 80% of patients, but the majority of these patients will have a stiff, though functional, hindfoot. Pain persists in roughly 10%.

Foot Deformities in Neuromuscular Diseases

Cerebral Palsy

Muscle imbalance resulting from cerebral palsy leads to foot deformities in 90% of patients; the type of deformity reflects the type of cerebral palsy. In the diplegic child, equinovalgus is most frequent, with equinus and calcaneus second; equinovarus is rare. The majority of this group is ambulatory. In the hemiplegic child, equinovalgus and equinovarus are equally prevalent at approximately 25%. Calcaneus, metatarsus adductus, and cavus are not as common. With whole body involvement 68% will have equinovalgus, and approximately 30% will have equinus, equinovarus, calcaneus, and hallux valgus.

Equinus often is treated with therapy and bracing until a contracture develops. At that point, botulinum toxin A injections followed by bracing can be helpful, but the results are temporary (3 to 6 months) and surgical intervention may be required. Gastrocnemius lengthening only, open Achilles tendon lengthening, and percutaneous lengthening all have proponents. Overlengthening must be avoided. A cast is used for 3 to 6 weeks after surgical intervention, often followed by a brace. Recurrence varies depending on age of the child and degree of spasticity.

Planovalgus and equinovalgus deformities are treated with a combination of heel cord lengthening and often, bony intervention. Lateral calcaneal lengthening, Grice procedures, and even subtalar arthrodesis have been used. Although not definitely proven, a subtalar fusion

may give more lasting correction in the face of severe muscle tone.

Equinovarus deformity, if flexible, is amenable to tendon transfers. With a rigid deformity, bony surgery and/or capsular release are required. Dynamic equinovarus may be caused by either excessive anterior tibialis or posterior tibialis tone. Gait laboratories are useful in differentiating which muscle is contributing to deformity. A Rancho procedure, which involves split anterior tibial transfer to the cuboid, combined with Achilles tendon and possible posterior tib lengthening, is done if anterior tibialis overpull leads to equinovarus. However, the posterior tibialis more often appears to be the deforming force. Either a split transfer to the peroneus brevis or a transfer through the interosseous membrane to the lateral cuneiform can be used for posterior tibialis overpull. When transferring the posterior tibialis anteriorly, calcaneus deformity can occur if the Achilles tendon is lengthening simultaneously. Therefore, the Achilles tendon should be balanced before anterior transfer of the split posterior tibialis tendon is done; in addition, this tendon must not be placed lateral to the third cuneiform or valgus of the heel may result. The quadriplegic child has a less favorable outcome with this technique. The entire posterior tendon transfer to the peroneus brevis may be done simultaneously with Achilles tendon lengthening because the posterior tibialis is not transformed to a dorsiflexor. Appropriate tension and adequate anchoring of the tendon are essential to success. Transfer to the peroneus brevis does not, however, enhance dorsiflexion strength.

Spina Bifida

Muscle imbalance may not play as distinct a role in the foot deformities common to myelomeningocele as once believed. In children with low level spina bifida (L5 or sacral), and therefore minimal voluntary muscle control of the foot, over 70% had foot deformity. Of those patients with thoracic to L3 lesions, 89% have deformity; L4, 88%; L5, 87%; sacral, 63%. The most common deformities in L4 lesions and below are calcaneus-equivalent (calcaneovalgus or calcaneovarus). In thoracic to L3 lesions, equinovarus or valgus is most common (51%), but even in high levels almost one third have a calcaneus-type deformity. Therefore, the etiology of spina bifida foot deformity cannot be explained solely on the basis of voluntary muscle imbalance.

Spina bifida is a common cause of both teratologic equinovarus and vertical talus. For calcaneus deformity, early soft-tissue transfer of anterior tibialis or peroneus tertius to the os calcis through the interosseous membrane is done. For a rigid deformity, osteot-

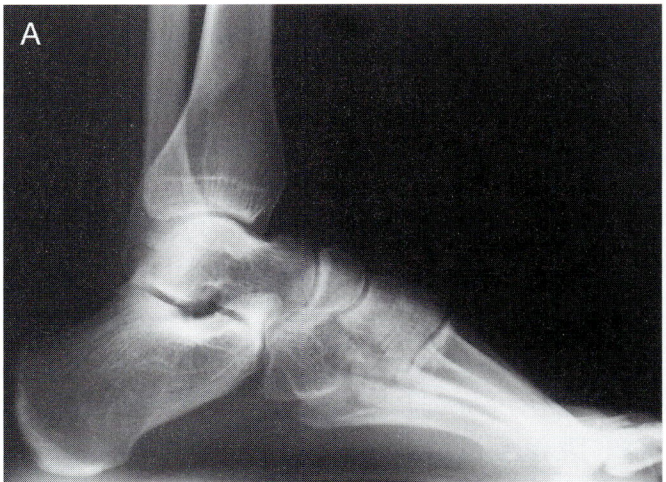
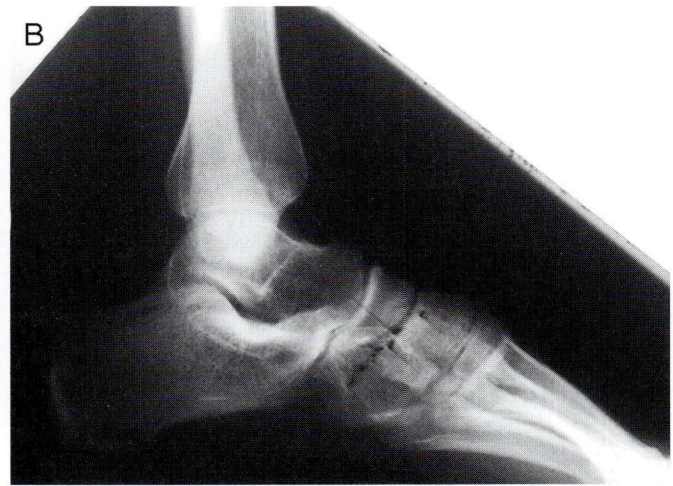

Figure 2 Cavovarus foot. **A,** Preoperative weight-bearing lateral radiograph. **B,** Weight-bearing lateral radiograph after plantar release.

omy, such as posterior displacement of the calcaneus, may be necessary. This procedure is often better tolerated than triple arthrodesis, which leads to even more rigidity of the hindfoot and increased risk of ulceration. Ankle valgus may be addressed by medial malleolar epiphysiodesis. Hindfoot valgus, if rigid, requires a displacement calcaneal osteotomy, but if flexible, calcaneal lengthening may be used.

Despite surgical treatment, many patients with myelomeningocele lose the ability to independently ambulate with age and growth. Orthotic devices can be of great assistance, not only in maintaining correction attained through surgical intervention, but also in increasing stabilization to maintain weight bearing as long as possible. The ankle-foot orthosis (AFO) stabilizes the excessive dorsiflexion, which can occur in the absence of an adequate triceps surae. With L4, L5, or S1 lesions, walking speed is faster, oxygen consumption lessened, and ankle power increased when AFOs are used. If the knee flexion contracture is less than 10°, then a floor reaction AFO can transfer excessive dorsiflexion movement at the ankle to accommodate for a weak quadriceps at the knee and assist in gait. Insensate skin must be carefully evaluated when using these orthotic devices to avoid contact pressure ulceration. Knee-ankle-foot orthosis are used if the knee flexion contracture is less than 20% to 25% and there is weakness of the quadriceps and hamstring. For patients with a high thoracic level lesion, orthotic devices that start at the hip are often needed and at times, their weight and girth preclude the very ambulation they were designed to assist.

Cavovarus Deformity

The cavovarus foot is characterized by elevation of the arch, plantar flexion of the first ray, and heel varus.

Although idiopathic cavovarus deformity exists, a thorough search for a neuromuscular cause must be undertaken. In bilateral cases, Charcot-Marie-Tooth disease (hereditary sensory motor neuropathy type I), Friedreich's ataxia, and polio are all causes of cavovarus deformity. Spinal cord abnormalities such as a syrinx, diastematomyelia, tumor, or tethered cord can cause unilateral or bilateral deformity. As noted previously, cerebral palsy and clubfoot deformity residua can lead to cavovarus. Tarsal coalition is rarely the cause of this deformity. After plain radiographs, an electromyogram and spinal MRI should be done to determine a possible neurologic etiology. Neurologic causes should be treated first if possible.

It is essential to determine before surgery whether the deformity is flexible or rigid. A Coleman block test or pressure on the lateral aspect of the forefoot with the patient prone will show if the heel can be moved from varus. If the foot is supple, a plantar release can be performed with or without tendon transfers (Fig. 2). The anterior tibialis is often weak and therefore posterior tibial tendon transfer through the interosseous membrane can be helpful. Peroneal longus lengthening or transfer has also been described to minimize plantar flexion of the first ray. As the extensor tendons compensate for weak dorsiflexion of the anterior tibialis, claw toes develop, which may be treated with resection of the proximal interphalangeal joints and transfer of the extensor tendons to the metatarsal neck (Jones procedure).

In a rigid foot, bony procedures are required. Calcaneal osteotomy (either closing wedge or calcaneal lateral shift) is needed to address varus. First metatarsal osteotomy also may be required. Triple arthrodesis is a salvage procedure for failed intervention or severe rigid deformity. Results after triple arthrodesis in patients with Charcot-Marie-Tooth disease have been discouraging.

Osteochondrosis/Apophysitis

Köhler's disease and Freiberg's infraction are rare causes of midfoot and metatarsal pain in the child/ adolescent. Sever's disease (apophysitis of the calcaneus) is another cause of foot pain in this age group.

Köhler's Disease

Köhler's disease is an osteochondrosis of the tarsal navicular bone that does not appear to be associated with Perthes' disease or Osgood-Schlatter disease. Although occasionally bilateral, the majority of cases are unilateral, affecting children 5 to 10 years of age. The child will have midfoot pain and often a flatfoot deformity due to inflammation of the posterior tibialis tendon. Treatment is supportive and ranges from rest to orthotic devices to casting. The type of intervention does not shorten the duration of the disease (8 months on average) and there appears to be no increase in osteoarthritis or flatfoot deformity even with long-term follow-up.

Freiberg's Infraction

Freiberg's infraction is rarer than Köhler's disease and occurs mostly in adolescent athletes, but can affect younger children. The condition is characterized by a unilateral (rarely bilateral) metatarsalgia most often of the second ray. Osteonecrosis is present in the head of the offending metatarsal on radiographs. The etiology appears to be repetitive trauma and microvascular changes. Arthrosis has been described in advanced cases.

Initial treatment of Freiberg's infraction is with orthotic devices and rest. If nonsurgical treatment fails, multiple surgical interventions have been described. Metatarsal head excision, although successful in removing the offending area, changes the biomechanics of the foot and can lead to pain in the adjacent metatarsal head.

Sever's Disease

Sever's disease, or calcaneal apophysitis, occurs in athletic children ages 6 to 15 years. Overuse of the powerful triceps surae muscle causes repetitive inflammation and microfracture to the calcaneal apophysis. The child has activity-related pain, a history of involvement in running sports such as soccer, and marked pain with palpation over the Achilles tendon insertion on the calcaneus. Plantar flexion against resistance can be painful as can forced extremes of dorsiflexion. Unlike Achilles tendon enthesopathy associated with autoim-

mune disorders, the pain of Sever's disease increases with activity and is relieved by rest. Radiographs are normal, as increased radiodensity and fragments of the apophysis are present in nonsymptomatic children. Treatment consists of rest, Achilles tendon stretching, and modification of activities. A heel lift can decrease apophyseal traction and therefore microfracture. NSAIDs can assist with pain and any secondary Achilles tendinitis. If the foot is still painful, immobilization in a walking cast for 1 to 3 months may be helpful. An undulating course with possible recurrences is the norm; when the apophysis closes, however, the disease will be cured.

Toe Deformities
Adolescent Bunions

The adolescent bunion is problematic, with a recurrence rate cited at close to 50%. All nonsurgical treatment should be thoroughly exhausted before surgical intervention is considered.

The medially prominent metatarsophalangeal (MTP) joint has three possible etiologies: Deviation of the MTP joint as a result of (relative primus varus) deviation of the lesser metatarsals laterally; increased angle (greater than 11°) between the metatarsals (primus varus); or true MTP joint deviation (greater than 10°) (hallux valgus interphalangeus).

The McBride procedure of soft-tissue release consists of a release of contracted lateral structures (lateral joint capsule, transverse metatarsal ligament, and adductor hallucis) with reattachment of adductor hallucis proximally. The medial bony eminence is excised and the capacious medial capsule reefed. The McBride procedure is most helpful when the intermetatarsal angle is normal or near-normal.

When the intermetatarsal angle is increased, the McBride procedure can be used alone, but appears to have best results when combined with osteotomy. Proximal metatarsal osteotomy must be used with caution so that injury to the proximal growth plate of the first metatarsal is avoided. Although excellent results have been noted with osteotomy, excessive shortening of the first ray must be avoided to prevent transfer metatarsalgia. Distal metatarsal osteotomies (Mitchell procedure) have been used most frequently. Trapezoidal step-off osteotomy can help protect against excessive shortening.

In children with a normal intermetatarsal angle but excessive MTP joint angulation, a closing wedge osteotomy of the proximal phalanx can be used in combination with soft-tissue balancing. Some children have a combination of deformity with primus varus and interphalangeal components; a closing wedge of the distal metatarsal and an opening wedge (using

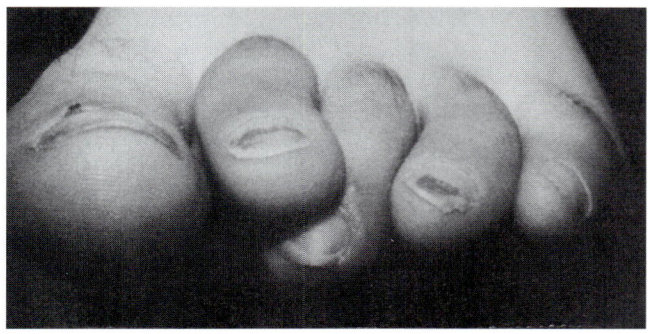

Figure 3 Curly toe deformity of the third toe showing dorsal displacement of the second toe.

resected bone from the metatarsal as graft) of the proximal phalanx can be combined. Again, soft-tissue (McBride procedure) balancing should be considered.

Curly Toe

Curly toe deformity is an autosomal dominant disorder present at birth, with the offending toe held in flexion and often medial deviation. The third, fourth, and fifth toes are most often affected. Often the parents will seek assistance because of a dorsally prominent toe, which is adjacent to the curly toe (Fig. 3). Surgical repair of the dorsally displaced toe is doomed to fail because the underlying cause, a flexion contracture of the adjacent toe, is left untreated.

Fractures of the Foot

Calcaneal Fractures

Calcaneal fractures, like cuboid fractures, are a rare cause of an otherwise benign limp in the toddler. The most common cause of limp without systemic symptoms is still a "toddler's fracture," the classic oblique fracture of the mid to distal tibia. The nondisplaced calcaneal fracture can, however, be yet another variation. In children with equinus contracture (such as cerebral palsy), overly enthusiastic stretching of the triceps surae can lead to apophyseal fracture. These fractures are often missed (up to 44%); appropriate radiographs of the foot should be carefully done.

Axial impaction injury can cause calcaneal fractures to occur; however, the pattern of the fracture is different in children than adults. In children, the majority of fractures are extra-articular and only rarely are found to be intra-articular with displacement. Displaced fractures are most often the result of a fall from a height (10 feet or more). Intra-articular fractures with displacement often need surgical treatment for the best outcome. However, casting is recommended for the majority of fractures. Outcome is better in children than in the adult population.

Triplane/Juvenile Tillaux Fractures

The triplane fracture and juvenile Tillaux fractures are uncommon but classic fractures of adolescence. At age 13 years, the distal tibial physis is closing from a medial to lateral direction. This stress riser leads to classic fracture patterns within this age group after injurious force. The majority of the fractures occur in athletes after a twisting fall.

Three fragments, the anterolateral epiphysis, medial epiphysis plus posterior distal metaphysis, and remaining metaphysis and tibial shaft are created in the triplane fracture. This fracture is usually described as a Salter IV injury, but because the physis is closing, growth plate arrest is of little concern. Instead, the intra-articular displacement is the problematic variable and may be assessed by CT scan. The medial malleolus can be involved if the epiphyseal extension passes through this region, and the fracture line may even pass completely medial to the plafond. Closed reduction can be used if there is minimal intra-articular step-off; however, with persistent intra-articular displacement open reduction and internal fixation is advised.

The juvenile Tillaux fracture also occurs most often in the adolescent age group with partial closure of the distal tibial epiphysis. These fractures are more common in athletes when a dorsiflexion and external rotation force is applied to the foot. The fracture fragment lies in the anterolateral portion of the epiphysis, which is avulsed because the medial portion is fused. Closed reduction with an internal rotation maneuver may be attempted, but open reduction may be required because of displacement. Penetration of the joint by hardware should be avoided.

Annotated Bibliography

Congenital Deformities

Comfort TK, Johnson LO: Resection for aymptomatic talocalcaneal coalition. *J Pediatr Orthop* 1998;18: 283-288.

Twenty symptomatic talocalcaneal coalitions were resected after diagnosis and evaluation by CT scan. Of resections in which the coalition was less than one third of the joint outcome was good or excellent in 77%. Increasing age was not a contraindication to resection as long as degenerative change was not present. Varus deformity had a poorer prognosis.

Emery KH, Bisset GS III, Johnson ND, Nunan PJ: Tarsal coalition: A blinded comparison of MRI and CT. *Ped Radiol* 1998;28:612-616.

In 40 feet in consecutive patients who underwent coronal and axial CT as well as MRI, MRI was found to have high correlation with CT scans can be helpful if the true etiology of ankle pain is unknown. CT was more cost effective and had slightly greater diagnostic accuracy.

Fuson S, Barrett M: Resectional arthroplasty: Treatment for calcaneonavicular coalition. *J Foot Ankle Surg* 1998;37:11-15.

A 10-year retrospective review of the results of 28 calcaneonavicular coalitions treated with resection, bone wax interposition, and early motion was done. In cases with degeneration, selective hindfoot fusion was done; three of these four patients developed reflex sympathetic dystrophy. Of the patients with resection and bone wax, 93% had excellent long term results.

Katz K, David R, Soudry M: Below-knee plaster cast for the treatment of metatarsus adductus. *J Pediatr Orthop* 1999;19:49-50.

Sixty-five infants with moderate and severe rigid metatarsus adductus were treated 6 to 8 weeks with below-knee casts. At follow-up of at least two years correction was maintained and flexibility improved.

Kodros SA, Dias LS: Single-stage surgical correction of congenital vertical talus. *J Pediatr Orthop* 1999;19:42-48.

Fifty-five feet in 41 patients with congenital vertical talus underwent single-stage surgical correction. Fewer than 10% were idiopathic. Outcome was dependent on etiology, with idiopathic feet doing the best, neuromuscular disorders doing moderately well, and malformation syndromes having only a fair result.

Kránicz J, Than P, Kustos T: Long-term results of the operative treatment of clubfoot: A representative study. *Orthopedics* 1998;2:21:669-674.

In 30 patients evaluated 20 years after posteromedial release, good results were noted in 75%. Calf and foot atrophy were visible. A higher percentage of poor results were noted if surgery occurred after 1 year of age or if multiple surgeries were required.

Kuo KN, Jansen LD: Rotatory dorsal subluxation of the navicular: A complication of clubfoot surgery. *J Pediatr Orthop* 1998;18:770-774

In this study, 168 clubfeet were retrospectively evaluated on average 7 years after index surgery; 12 (7%) showed subluxation of the navicular that appeared to be rotatory in nature.

Letts M, Davidson D: The role of bilateral talectomy in the management of bilateral rigid clubfeet. *Am J Orthop* 1999;28:106-110.

Severe bilateral equinovarus secondary to arthrogryposis, myelomeningocele, and Duchenne's muscular dystrophy underwent talectomy bilaterally. Although 10 of 14 feet had satisfactory or good results, 4 had poor outcomes. Overall low morbidity and a predictable outcome were noted.

Macnicol MF, Flocken LL: Calcaneocuboid malalignment in clubfoot. *J Pediatr Orthop* 1999;8:257-260.

In a series of 179 clubfeet in which surgical correction was done, the revision rate was 15%. Calcaneocuboid malalignment did not affect outcome unless talocalcaneal correction was doubtful.

Manzone P: Clubfoot surgical treatment: Preliminary results of a prospective comparative study of two techniques. *J Pediatr Orthop Br* 1999;8:246-250.

Thirty patients prospectively underwent two different surgical releases performed by the same surgeon. Fifteen feet had posteromedial release, 15 posteromedial with complete subtalar release. Good results were noted in 77% at an average 2-year follow-up. No significant differences were found clinically or radiographically in the short-term outcome between the two techniques.

Mountney J, Khan T, Davies AG, Smith TW: Scar quality from partial or complete wound closure using the cincinnati incision for clubfoot surgery. *J Pediatr Orthop Br* 1998;7:223-225.

A retrospective comparison of primary closure of the Cincinnati incision versus healing by secondary incision was made in 30 patients. The cosmetic result was similar in both groups and position of the foot should therefore not be compromised to attain primary closure.

Yamamoto H, Muneta T, Morita S: Nonsurgical treatment of congenital clubfoot with manipulation, cast and modified Denis-Browne splint. *J Pediatr Orthop* 1998; 18:538-542.

In 113 idiopathic clubfeet treated with manipulation and casting, 36% required posteromedial release, and at 12 years follow-up 60% had good or excellent results. The more severe the foot disorder, the more likely that surgical intervention would be required.

Foot Deformities in Neuromuscular Diseases

Blasier RD, White R: Duration of immobilization after percutaneous sliding heel-cord lengthening. *J Pediatr Orthop* 1998;18:299-303.

Thirty-one children underwent percutaneous heel cord lengthening and were immobilized for only 3 weeks. No rerupture occurred.

Corry IS, Cosgrove AP, Duffy CM, McNeill S, Taylor TC, Graham HK: Botulinum Toxin A compared with stretching casts in the treatment of spastic equinus: A randomised prospective trial. *J Pediatr Orthop* 1998;18:304-311.

In gait analysis 12 weeks after casting versus casting and botulinum toxin A, recurrence was found in the casting alone group. The botulinum toxin A group results were maintained with fewer side effects.

Duffy CM, Graham HK, Cosgrove AP: The influence of ankle-foot orthoses on gait and energy expenditure in spina bifida. *J Pediatr Orthop* 2000;20:356-361.

Gait analysis with oxygen consumption measurement was undertaken in children age 6 to 16 with spina bifida at L4 or lower. The children were studied ambulating with and without AFOs. Stride length, walking speed, and ankle power were significantly better with AFOs. With an AFO, oxygen consumption decreased as did time spent in double stance.

Frawley PA, Broughton NS, Menelaus MB: Incidence and type of hindfoot deformities in patients with low-level spina bifida. *J Pediatr Orthop* 1998;18:312-313.

In this article, 174 consecutive children with spina bifida below L4 were studied to describe their deformities and incidence. Hindfoot deformity was present in 263 of 348 feet; 64% required surgical intervention. Although calcaneus deformity due to muscle imbalance was most common in L4, both L5 and S1 lesions frequently had calcaneus deformity.

Jeray KJ, Rentz J, Ferguson RL: Local bone-graft technique for subtalar extraarticular arthrodesis in cerebral palsy. *J Pediatr Orthop* 1998;18:75-80.

Fifty-two subtalar fusions were undertaken for equinoplanovalgus in cerebral palsy using local bone graft with patient age averaging 7 years 5 months. After an average 41-month follow-up, 88% had radiographic union, and 96% had lasting correction.

O'Connell PA, D'Souza LD, Dudeney S, Stephens M: Foot deformities in children with cerebral palsy. *J Pediatr Orthop* 1998;18:743-747.

An outline of the type of cerebral palsy and the associated foot deformities is provided. Seventy-six percent of 200 children were found to have abnormalities with the incidence of mobility decreasing with severity of involvement. Equinus of some form was found in 70%, with equinovalgus being most common. Equinovarus was less common, as was hallux valgus. Calcaneus-like deformities were rare at 16%.

Torosian CM, Dias LS: Surgical treatment of severe hindfoot valgus by medial displacement osteotomy of the os calcis in children with myelomeningocele. *J Pediatr Orthop* 2000;20:226-229.

Medial sliding calcaneal osteotomy was used to control hindfoot valgus in 27 patients. After five years of follow-up, 82% were completely satisfied with the outcome. The majority of patients had marked improvement with brace and shoe wear.

Vedantam R, Capelli AM, Schoenecker PL: Subtalar arthroereisis for the correction of planovalgus foot in children with neuromuscular disorders. *J Pediatr Orthop* 1998;18:294-298.

140 STA-peg arthroereisis procedures were performed to treat planovalgus in 78 ambulatory children. Soft-tissue balancing was undertaken simultaneously. Results were satisfactory in 96.4%, at an average of 4.5 years postoperatively.

Osteochondrosis/Apophysitis

El-Tayeby HM: Freiberg's infraction: A new surgical procedure. *J Foot and Ankle Surg* 1998;37:23-27.

Thirteen patients underwent resection of the involved portion of the metatarsal head with interposition of the extensor digitorum longus. Although range of motion remained less than normal, radiographic and clinical examination at 2-year follow-up showed that 85% had good or excellent results.

Toe Deformities

de Palma L, Zanoli G: Zanoli's procedure for overlapping fifth toe: Retrospective study for 18 cases followed for 4-17 years. *Acta Orthop Scand* 1998;69:505-507.

Sixteen patients underwent Zanoli's technique (a tenodesis procedure) for varus fifth toe at an average age of 26 years. Follow-up was 8 years. Correction was successful in three patients, but all patients were satisfied with the results (100% pain relief).

Karbowski A, Schwitalle M, Eckardt A, Heine J: Long-term results after Mitchell osteotomy in children and adolescents with hallux valgus. *Acta Orthop Belg* 1998;64:263-268.

Nine patients treated with Mitchell osteotomy and soft-tissue balancing were followed 20 years. Good or satisfactory results occurred in 81%; 14% had pain, or recurrent or repeat surgery. If excessive shortening of the first ray occurred (over 3% of the length), results were poor.

Señarís-Rodríguez J, Martínez-Serrano A, Rodríguez-Durantez JA, Soleto-Martínez J, González-López JL: Surgical treatment for bunions in adolescents. *J Pediatr Orthop Br* 199B;7:210-216.

Twenty-five feet were treated with a combination of procedures depending on the underlying deformity. Good or excellent results were noted in 92% at 4 years after surgery. Proximal metatarsal osteotomy was noted to give better results than a soft-tissue procedure alone. Proximal osteotomy was used if MTP angle was over 10°.

Fractures of the Foot

Dailiana ZH, Malizos KN, Zacharis K, Mavrodontidis AN, Shiamishis GA, Soucacos PN: Distal tibial epiphyseal fractures in adolescents. *Am J Orthop* 1999;28:309-312.

Eight adolescents were surgically treated for either triplane or Tillaux fractures with no long-term sequelae.

Inokuchi S, Usami N, Hiraishi E, Hashimoto T: Calcaneal fractures in children. *J Pediatr Orthop* 1998;18:469-474.

In 18 fractures of the calcaneus, 60% were extra-articular and 20% intra-articular. Achilles tendon avulsions were often treated surgically. Diagnosis is delayed in 40% of these fractures.

Classic Bibliography

Clark MW, D'Ambrosia RD, Ferguson AB: Congenital vertical talus: Treatment by open reduction and navicular excision. *J Bone Joint Surg Am* 1977;59:816-824.

Farsetti P, Weinstein SL, Ponseti IV: The long-term functional and radiographic outcomes of untreated and non-operatively treated metatarsus adductus. *J Bone Joint Surg Am* 1994;76:257-265.

Guidera KJ, Drennan JC: Foot and ankle deformities in arthrogryposis multiplex congenita. *Clin Orthop* 1985;194:93-98.

Inglis G, Buxton RA, Macnicol MF: Symptomatic calcaneonavicular bars: The results 20 years after surgical excision. *J Bone Joint Surg Br* 1986;68:128-131.

Ippolito E, Ricciardi Pollini PT, Falez F: Kohler's disease of the tarsal navicular: Long-term follow-up of 12 cases. *J Pediatr Orthop* 1984;4:416-417.

Laaveg SJ, Ponseti IV: Long-term results of treatment of congenital clubfoot. *J Bone Joint Surg Am* 1980;62: 23-31.

Micheli LJ, Ireland ML: Prevention and management of calcaneal apophysitis in children: An overuse syndrome. *J Pediatr Orthop* 1987;7:34-38.

Turco VJ: Resistant congenital club foot: One-stage posteromedial release with internal fixation: A follow-up report of a fifteen-year experience. *J Bone Joint Surg Am* 1979;61:805-814.

Weiner BK, Weiner DS, Mirkopulos N: Mitchell osteotomy for adolescent hallux valgus. *J Pediatr Orthop* 1997;17:781-784.

Wenger DR, Mauldin D, Speck G, Morgan D, Lieber RL: Corrective shoes and inserts as treatment for flexible flatfoot in infants and children. *J Bone Joint Surg Am* 1989;71:800-810.

Chapter 46

Ankle and Foot: Trauma

Judith F. Baumhauer, MD

Mark J. Geppert, MD

James D. Michelson, MD

Arthur K. Walling, MD

Ankle and Pilon Fractures

Ankle Anatomy and Biomechanics

In a neutral position, approximately 90% of the load to the ankle is transmitted via the tibial plafond, with the remaining load borne through the lateral talofibular articulation. The talus in cross section forms a trapezoid, which is wider anteriorly than posteriorly. Consequently, during dorsiflexion of the talus, the increased talar width that is introduced into the ankle mortise forces the fibula to translate laterally and rotate externally. During weight bearing, plantar flexion is associated with internal rotation of the talus relative to the tibia. The deltoid ligament is responsible for this coupled rotation by acting as a checkrein on the talus.

The ankle is said to be stable when, under physiologic loading conditions, the talus moves in a normal pattern through the full range of motion. Injury to the ankle that results in a stable mechanical configuration therefore can be treated nonsurgically. In an unstable ankle, the joint surface contact area within the ankle is diminished, which predisposes the ankle to premature articular cartilage damage and degeneration.

The primary stabilizer of the ankle under physiologic loading conditions is the deltoid ligament, in conjunction with the deep and superficial components. If the deltoid is rendered incompetent either by direct rupture or medial malleolar fracture, the motion of the talus is markedly changed. During plantar flexion, the talus externally rotates from underneath the tibial plafond, the exact opposite of its normal pattern of movement. Stabilization of the fibula ameliorates this abnormal motion to some extent, but it is not corrected. Furthermore, in the absence of medial injury, fibular osteotomy or fracture does not result in abnormal motion of the ankle.

Radiography

The Lauge-Hansen fracture classification system is based on the mechanism of injury and may guide closed reduction. The first word (supination, pronation) denotes the position of the foot at the time of injury, and the second phrase (for example, external rotation) denotes the direction of the deforming force. The most common injury pattern is supination-external rotation, which accounts for up to 85% of all ankle fractures.

The Weber/AO classification system is based on the level of the fibular fracture: type A, below the plafond; type B, at the plafond; and type C, absent the plafond. However, Weber B ankle fractures, the most common type, do not constituent a homogeneous group of fractures because patients with medial injury benefit from surgical intervention whereas patients with isolated lateral fractures do not.

The Lauge-Hansen and Weber classification systems have poor interobserver and intraobserver reproducibility. The limitations of these classifications is a result of the uncertain link between specific fracture patterns and associated soft-tissue injuries (deltoid ligament injury) and the inherent limitations of plain radiography of ankle fractures.

The instability pattern in ankle fractures is external rotation of the talus under the plafond, not simply lateral translation. Furthermore, studies using CT have shown that the distal fibular fragment is anatomic with respect to the talus, and the apparent distal fibular external rotation is actually proximal fibular internal rotation relative to the tibia (Fig. 1). Consequently, historic radiographic criteria based on "distal fibular displacement" result from radiographic limitations and may not be adequate criteria for surgical intervention.

The complete lack of standardization for radiographic magnification renders the absolute measurement of displacement distances unreliable. The most reliable criteria for instability is a lateral talar shift on the AP or mortise view, as defined by a medial clear space that is measurably larger than the superior clear space. Three views of the ankle (AP, mortise, and lat-

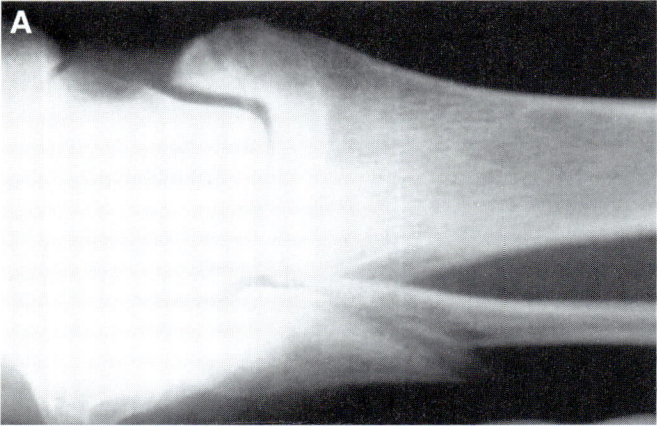

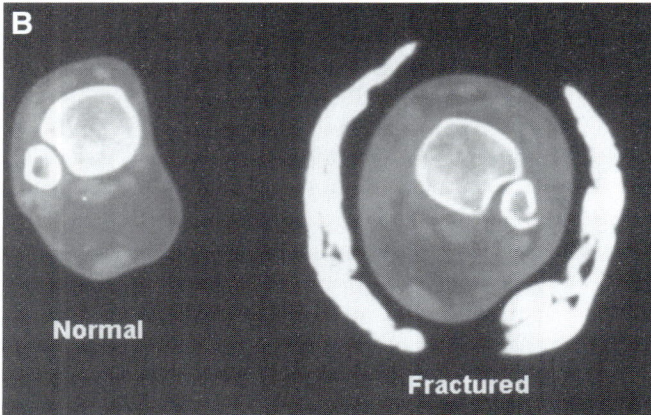

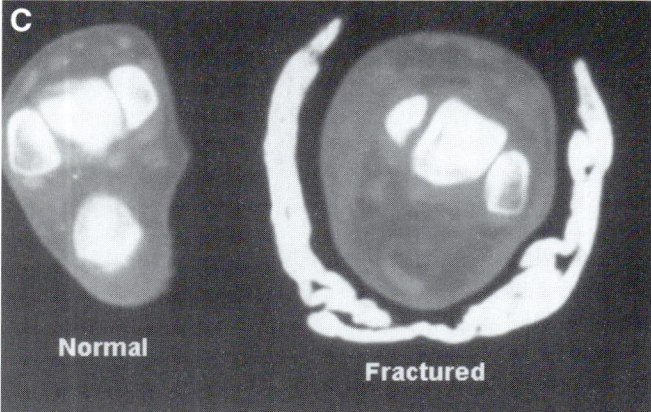

Figure 1 Demonstration of the apparent distal fibular external rotation seen on plain radiographs that actually represents internal rotation of the proximal fibula with maintenance of distal talofibular congruity. **A,** Mortise ankle radiograph showing rotation between the proximal and distal fibular segments. **B,** Transaxial CT scan proximal to the fracture showing internal rotation of the fibular shaft relative to the tibia. The space between the tibia and fibula should be even from anterior to posterior. In this image, the tibia-fibula space is larger posteriorly than anteriorly, indicating interior rotation of the fibula. **C,** Transaxial CT scan through the distal talofibular articular at the ankle joint. The fibula is anatomic relative to the talus.

eral) probably provide greater fracture detection sensitivity than two views (AP and lateral or mortise and lateral).

Treatment of Ankle Fractures

The majority of ankle fractures are stable, isolated, lateral malleolar injuries. In the absence of medial tenderness, isolated lateral malleolar fractures may be treated nonsurgically. Immobilization is primarily aimed at protecting the ankle from further injury and can consist of a short leg walking cast, a walking boot, or a high-top sneaker, all with similar satisfactory results. Surgical treatment of isolated lateral malleolar fractures carries a 1% to 3% chance of significant wound complications or infection and, on average, results in greater long-term swelling about the ankle.

Bimalleolar ankle fractures are most typically treated with open anatomic reduction and internal fixation. Although closed reduction can yield satisfactory results in up to 65% of cases, the procedure is generally reserved for patients with major associated medical problems that preclude surgical treatment. Bimalleolar fractures that are initially dislocated or significantly displaced should undergo a closed reduction and splinting at initial presentation to diminish swelling and associated soft-tissue damage. Although immediate surgical intervention prior to the onset of swelling has been advocated, it may be safer to allow the initial swelling to recede prior to surgical fixation. Surgical treatment consists of reduction and stabilization of both the medial and lateral malleoli.

For bimalleolar-equivalent fractures, in which the deltoid ligament is ruptured and the lateral malleolus is fractured, routine repair of the deltoid does not improve the clinical results and may lead to a worse long-term outcome. Medial exploration may be undertaken if the talus is not reduced anatomically underneath the plafond, in which case the deltoid ligament is extricated from between the talus and medial malleolus.

In the patient with lateral fracture and medial deltoid tenderness, any lateral talar shift signifies ankle instability and is treated accordingly. In the absence of a talar shift, individual clinical judgment dictates the treatment.

Postoperative treatment consists of initial splinting in neutral position followed by casting with progressive weight bearing and range of motion. Weight bearing may be started immediately in those patients in whom stable medial and lateral fixation has been achieved. Although there are theoretical advantages to instituting early range of motion in these patients, clinical studies have not demonstrated any major long-term benefit when compared with weight bearing in a cast or brace. After surgical treatment of a bimalleolar equivalent fracture, early range of motion should not be instituted because the long-term stability of the ankle depends on the deltoid healing at its resting length, which is with the ankle in neutral position.

Syndesmotic Injuries

Syndesmotic injuries constitute a special subgroup of fracture in which the fibular fracture is above the level of the tibial plafond and is associated with disruption of the syndesmotic ligament between the plafond and the level of fibula fracture. The contribution of the syndesmosis to ankle stability depends on the reestablishment of medial structural integrity. Provided that the fibula is anatomically reduced to the tibia, a syndesmotic screw may not be required for ankle stability as long as the deltoid is intact and the medial malleolus is either intact or surgically stabilized. In a bimalleolar-equivalent injury, where it is not possible to reestablish medial integrity, a syndesmotic screw may be placed whenever the fibular fracture is greater than 3.5 cm above the plafond. For bimalleolar-equivalent injuries with the fracture less than 3.5 cm above the plafond, as well as any syndesmotic injury in which medial integrity is restored, placement of a syndesmotic screw if the fibula is unstable to manual examination intraoperatively has been advocated. Because there are no standardized intraoperative tests for syndesmotic integrity that have been validated with follow-up clinical studies, this is an area of controversy.

When used, the syndesmotic screw is placed parallel to the tibial plafond at a distance roughly 1.5 cm proximal to the plafond. Care is taken to angle the screw 30° anteriorly from the fibula to the tibia to ensure full engagement in the tibia. The ankle is held in full dorsiflexion while the screw is placed, and lag screw technique avoided, to prevent overtightening of the syndesmosis and limitation of ankle dorsiflexion. Either 3.5-mm, 4.0-mm, or 4.5-mm screws are used that engage either three or four cortices.

Postoperatively, patients are in a cast and do not bear weight, followed by protected weight bearing. There is controversy regarding the necessity for syndesmotic screw removal prior to unprotected weight bearing. Removal before 3 months is not advised because of the risk of incomplete healing of the syndesmosis which may lead to recurrent syndesmotic widening. Weight bearing with the syndesmotic screw in place may cause fracture of the syndesmotic screw, but no major clinical consequences of such hardware failure have been reported. Initial enthusiasm for the use of biodegradable syndesmotic screws has faded because of abscess development in a sterile environment, which may require surgical débridement.

An absolute requirement for a syndesmotic screw, regardless of other considerations, is that there be persistent widening of the syndesmosis on intraoperative radiographs. The syndesmosis may be reduced using an external clamp and stabilized with screws.

Posterior malleolar fractures with more than 2 mm of displacement after fibular reduction and plating may be reduced and stabilized if they constitute more than 30% of the articular surface on a lateral radiograph, with a lag screw placed either anterior to posterior or the reverse.

Ankle fractures in patients with diabetes are associated with higher rates of complications than in nondiabetic patients. Surgical infection and would dehiscence rates are higher in diabetics than other patients. However, attempts to maintain a closed reduction in unstable fractures is associated with a high rate of skin breakdown and infection because of the high contact pressures between the skin and cast that are required to maintain the reduction. Unstable fractures, in which a reduction is difficult to achieve and maintain, may be treated surgically because this will afford greater control over the fracture and probably are associated with a lower overall complication rate. The postoperative regimen of progressive weight bearing should be markedly delayed until there is radiographic evidence of healing to minimize the risk of fixation failure and Charcot degeneration.

Pilon Fractures

The treatment of pilon fractures presents a formidable challenge to the skills of the orthopaedic surgeon. The immediate goals of pilon fracture treatment are to avoid complications, restore overall limb alignment, and reconstruct the articular surface. The ability to achieve these objectives is a function of the severity of fracture and the associated soft-tissue injuries.

Radiographic classification of pilon fractures is based on comminution (Fig. 2). A type I fracture is nondisplaced; type II has intra-articular displacement but intact metaphyseal structure; and type III has comminution and displacement at both the metaphyseal and articular regions. The degree of soft-tissue damage tends to increase with the severity of fracture type, which correlates with the force and energy that produce injury. The fracture also can be categorized as either a rotational injury or axial load injury. The former mechanism occurs during low-energy activities such as skiing, and leads to spiral or oblique fractures of the tibia and fibula with much less damage to the articular cartilage. Axial load injuries, such as from motor vehicle accidents or a fall from a height, result in burst type fractures of the plafond and tend to have greater comminution as well as more damage to the articular cartilage. The rotational injuries have a much better prognosis.

Full assessment of these injuries is aided by CT to completely define the anatomy of the fractures (Fig. 3).

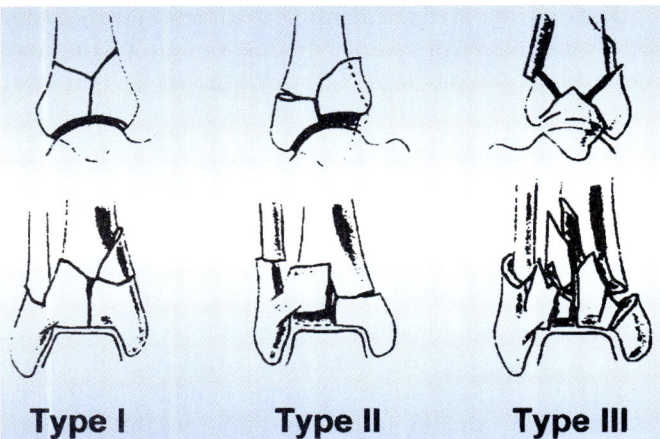

Figure 2 Diagrammatic representation of the pilon fracture classification of Ruedi and Allgower. *(Adapted with permission from Ruedi TP, Allgower M: The operative treatment of intra-articular fractures of the lower end of the tibia.* Clin Orthop *1979;138:105-110.)*

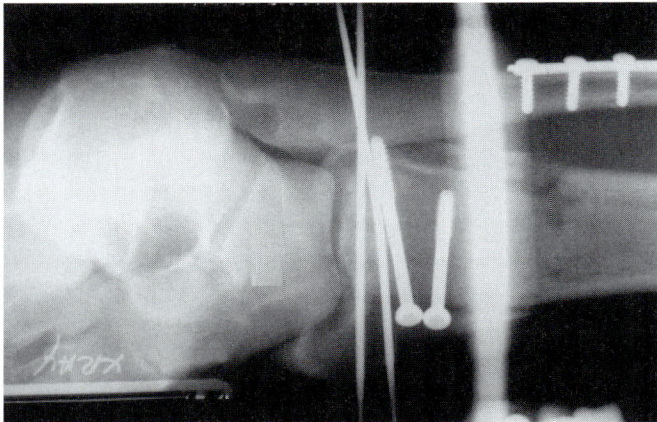

Figure 4 Example of the use of external fixation with limited internal fixation for pilon fractures. This method has been linked to a lower rate of postoperative complications than the classic technique of open reduction and internal fixation.

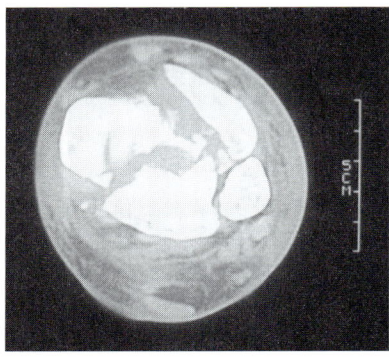

Figure 3 Transaxial CT image of a pilon fracture. This imaging is required to fully assess pilon fractures and is important in surgical planning.

Identification of anatomy is critical to planning the surgical approach because plain films are unable to provide sufficient information to guide placement of fixation devices.

The early successes in treating pilon fractures by extensive open reduction with internal fixation was directly related to the selection bias in those studies in which low-energy type I injuries were predominant. Attempts to extend the principles of anatomic reduction and rigid fixation, which entailed extensive soft-tissue dissection around the distal tibia, resulted in a major complication rate of up to 50% in patients who sustained higher energy types II and III injuries. The primary complications encountered were extensive wound dehiscence with soft-tissue loss, deep infection, nonunion, malunion, and ultimate below-knee amputation. In an attempt to head off these complications, the method of external fixation for primary stabilization accompanied by limited internal fixation for restoration of the articular surface was developed (Fig. 4). The external fixator can be uniplanar or multiplanar, can engage the tibia alone or cross the ankle and/or subtalar joints, and may or may not be reinforced by fibular plating for further stability. Small incisions (1 to 2 cm) are used to obtain articular reduction and limited interfragmentary screw fixation. Extensive dissection is avoided because an arthritic ankle with an intact soft-tissue envelope is preferable to an anatomically reduced ankle that has undergone multiple débridements for soft-tissue loss and infection.

Timing of the definitive surgery is dictated by the resolution of swelling and soft-tissue compromise around the fracture. External fixation can be applied immediately to limit additional soft-tissue damage and maintain limb length and alignment. The external fixator configuration need not be definitive, because it can be easily modified at the time of definitive surgery. There are as yet no definitive studies identifying which configuration of external fixation yields superior results.

Removal of the external fixator and the initiation of weight bearing are based on radiographic signs of healing. Weight bearing may be begun prior to the removal of external fixation if a particularly stable configuration, such as a multiplanar ring fixator, has been used. Consideration should be given to early bone grafting at 6 weeks after injury for high-energy injuries that do not demonstrate radiographic evidence of healing at the metaphyseal site. Soft-tissue defects should be expeditiously and aggressively handled by appropriate coverage techniques.

The development of arthritis in these patients is a direct consequence of the initial injury, and usually is not reflective of the surgical care rendered. Avoidance of major complications, however, is a testament to good surgical judgment and technique.

Hindfoot Trauma

Calcaneal Fractures

Calcaneal fractures account for approximately 2% of all fractures. The calcaneus is the most commonly frac-

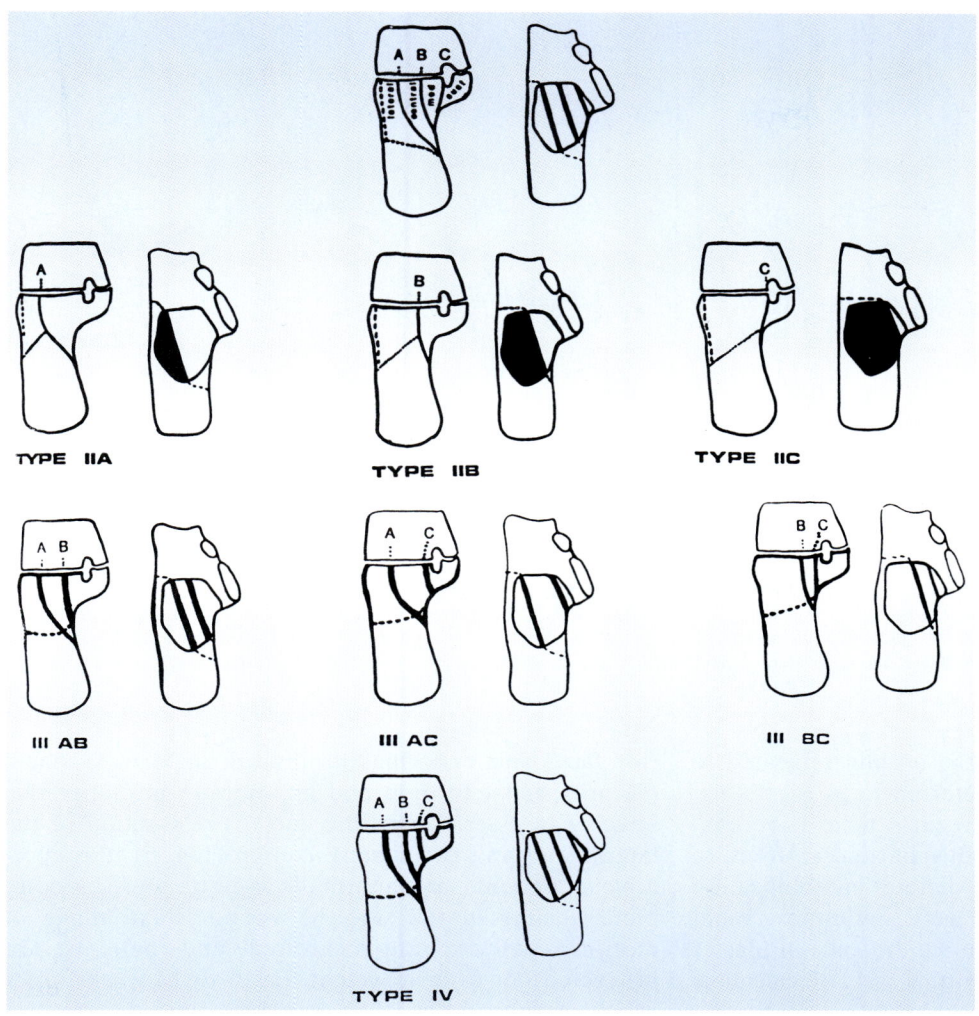

TYPE IIA
TYPE IIB
TYPE IIC
III AB
III AC
III BC
TYPE IV

Figure 5 The CT scan classification of intra-articular calcaneal fractures. *(Reproduced with permission from Benirschke SK, Sangeorzan BS: Extensive intraarticular fractures of the foot: Surgical management of calcaneal fractures. Clin Orthop 1993;292: 128-134.)*

tured tarsal bone. The majority of these fractures occur in industrial settings among males age 40 to 45 years. Associated fractures of the extremity and spine are frequent. The economic impact of these fractures is profound. Although enthusiasm for surgical treatment of calcaneal fractures has increased over the past 2 decades, there are few randomized trials on the management of calcaneal fractures.

Fracture classification is important to describe fractures, guide treatment selection, and predict outcomes. Although numerous classifications were based on standard radiographic technique, these have been largely supplemented by CT classification systems. A CT classification system has been developed based on an evaluation of 120 surgically treated calcaneal fractures (Fig. 5). This classification, based on the number and location of articular fracture fragments, has effectively suggested treatment methods and predicted outcomes.

Displaced intra-articular fractures account for 60% to 75% of all calcaneal fractures. Treatment for these fractures falls into four categories: nonsurgical; closed reduction/manipulation with or without minimal fixation; open reduction and internal fixation; and primary arthrodesis.

Indications for nonsurgical treatment include fractures where the relationship between the three facets is disrupted less than 4 mm, there is no subluxation of the subtalar joint secondary to widening (the calcaneus is widened to the extent that the two surfaces are not congruent), and there is no subfibular impingement. Shortening of the calcaneus results in an altered relationship of the facets. Treatment consists of temporary immobilization followed by the use of compression hose, early range of motion, and no weight bearing for 12 weeks. Other indications for nonsurgical treatment include severe open fractures or patients with soft-tissue compromise, such as with massive fracture blisters and prolonged edema that prevent surgery, patients with life-threatening injuries that prevent timely surgical intervention, and patients with severe peripheral vascular disease.

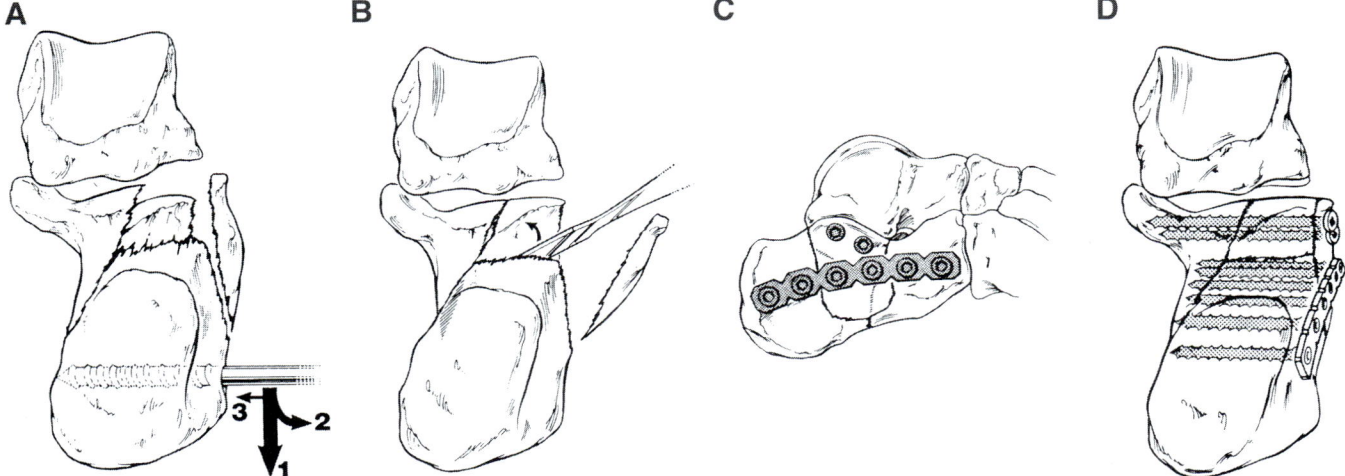

Figure 6 A reproducible approach to the internal fixation of intra-articular calcaneal fractures. **A,** A Shantz pin is placed into the tuberosity fragment. The three arrows sequentially indicate the relative motion of the pin, with the densest arrow indicating the greatest displacement. Traction on the pin brings the tuberosity fragment out to length, translated medially, and into slight valgus position. **B,** With the tuberosity fragment reduced, the posterior facet can be elevated into its native position (*arrow*). The lateral wall then can be reduced along the outer part of the posterior facet. The alignment of the tuberosity is generally maintained by Kirschner wires directed into the sustentaculum tali while the rest of the reduction is completed. **C,** Lateral view of the reduced calcaneus. **D,** Axial view of the reduced calcaneus, showing the thalamic screws crossing the posterior facet and going into the substance of the sustentaculum. The plate is straight, preventing a drifting of the calcaneus into a varus position. (*Reproduced with permission from Benirschke SK, Sangeorzan BJ: Extensive intraarticular fractures of the foot: Surgical management of calcaneal fractures. Clin Orthop 1993;292:128-134.*)

Closed reduction and pinning is usually relegated to tongue-type fractures, usually referred to as the Essex-Lopresti technique. Although recent articles have confirmed satisfactory results in this particular fracture pattern, the question remains whether immobilization and lack of early motion may negate any improvement gained by reduction. Furthermore, the pins-in-plaster technique may be associated with a risk of calcaneal osteomyelitis.

Open reduction and internal fixation usually is delayed until edema has decreased and skin lines become apparent. Ideally, surgery should be performed within 3 weeks after injury because once fracture consolidation has occurred it is much more difficult to ascertain the fracture planes. Appropriate plain radiographs and CT scans can be obtained during this initial waiting period.

The goal of open reduction and internal fixation is to restore articular integrity and height and width of the calcaneus, and correct any tuberosity malalignment. A variety of surgical approaches have been described (medial, lateral, combined); however, most studies now favor the extensile right-angled lateral incision. A full-thickness flap is created by subperiosteal dissection of all tissues off the lateral wall of the calcaneus.

The sequence of reduction varies, but basically consists of (1) opening the fracture and elevating the posterior facet that has been impacted into the body; (2) reducing the calcaneocuboid joint; (3) restoring the calcaneal height by reduction of the medial fracture fragment to the sustentaculum; (4) reducing the poste-

rior facet and restoring the crucial angle of Gissane; (5) provisional fixation and appropriate intraoperative imaging to assess reduction; and (6) restoration of the lateral wall and permanent fixation (Fig. 6). Postoperatively, patients are immobilized until there is complete healing of the surgical wound. Next, range of motion exercises are instituted and patients are instructed not to bear weight for 10 to 12 weeks, after which progressive weight bearing is allowed.

Although the use of subtalar arthrodesis for late sequelae of traumatic arthritis following calcaneal fractures is well established, the use of primary arthrodesis has been less readily accepted. Using the CT scan classification, it has been suggested that the results of open reduction and internal fixation in the highly comminuted type IV fractures remain quite poor, even in the hands of surgeons experienced in the treatment of calcaneal fractures. For this reason, it has been recommended that the shape of the calcaneus is restored first (that is, height, width, and as much articular congruity as possible); if the articular surface cannot be restored, or if alignment of the facets is not obtainable, then primary fusion should be done.

Much progress has occurred in the management of calcaneal fractures. Although anatomic reconstruction of calcaneal fractures is difficult to obtain, in two-part fractures an anatomic reduction is obtainable in more than 80% of patients. In three-part fractures, anatomic reduction is possible in approximately 60% of patients. These two subgroups account for approximately 90% of all calcaneal fractures, with 70% good to excellent clinical results obtainable with surgery. Smoking, diabetes, and open fractures are factors that increase the risk of wound complications and lead to poorer results. Cumulative risk factors further increase the likelihood of complications, and nonsurgical management should be considered.

Talar Fractures

The talus is composed of five weight-bearing articular surfaces. Articular cartilage covers 60% of these surfaces, and neither tendons nor muscles insert or originate from its surfaces. Vascular supply to the talus is limited to the nonarticular areas of the bone. Because the talus is the critical link between the subtalar, transverse tarsal, and ankle joints, injuries to the talus are serious. If the talus is damaged, the linked motions of the foot and ankle are compromised, resulting in severe disability. Fractures of the talus are classified depending on their primary location of involvement (head, neck, and body).

Fractures of the talar head are uncommon, but because they often involve the articulation between talus and navicular, treatment is necessary to avoid subsequent traumatic arthritis. Open reduction and internal fixation is indicated if there is articular step-off (more than 3 to 4 mm), talonavicular instability, and involvement of more than 50% of the articular surface.

Fractures of the talar neck are significant because of the frequency and severity of their associated complications, including malunion, nonunion, osteonecrosis, infection, and arthritis. The Hawkins classification guides treatment and addresses the increasing chance of osteonecrosis from type I to IV. Although type I fractures were considered nondisplaced, and thus could be treated nonsurgically, more recent attention has been directed toward open reduction and internal fixation to make certain that there is no subtle displacement or rotation, and to allow early range of motion by providing stable fixation. All type II through IV injuries require open reduction and internal fixation.

Surgical exposure of talar neck fractures is planned to maximize fracture and joint surface exposure, minimize soft-tissue stripping, and avoid vascular compromise. A medial approach is standard, and can be coupled with a medial malleolar osteotomy. An additional anterolateral approach is strongly recommended because it affords a better assessment of rotation and subtalar joint congruity. Occasionally, lateral malleolar osteotomy is also required. Debate exists regarding the placement of fixation from anterior to posterior or from posterior to anterior. Although posterior to anterior placement seems to offer an advantage in rigidity, an additional incision is required.

The incidence of osteonecrosis increases with the severity of injury. The appearance of Hawkins sign (radiolucent line just beneath the subchondral surface of the talar dome as seen on an anteroposterior radiograph of the ankle) at approximately 6 to 8 weeks is indicative of vascular sufficiency to the talar body. MRI can aid in determining fracture healing and vascular status. Osteonecrosis can be partial or complete, and does not always result in collapse. Prolonging nonweight bearing has not been shown to prevent collapse, and weight bearing is usually begun when fracture healing has occurred. The role of non-weight bearing or protected weight bearing to prevent further collapse is not known.

Talar body fractures encompass (1) osteochondral fractures; (2) shear, sagittal, or coronal fractures; (3) posterior process fractures; (4) lateral process fractures; and (5) crushed or compression fractures.

Osteochondral fractures are discussed elsewhere in this book. Shear, sagittal, or coronal fractures are often associated with ankle fractures. Open reduction and internal fixation is necessary for stability and early range of motion. Reductions must be anatomic, and the surgical exposure is dictated by location of the fracture.

Posterior process fractures are notable in that nonsurgical treatment fails in two thirds of these fractures. A posterior surgical approach is recommended. Open reduction and internal fixation or excision is based on the size of the fragment. These fractures are often missed or diagnosis is delayed.

Lateral process fractures are often misdiagnosed as a chronic sprain of the ankle. A high index of suspicion for this fracture is warranted. These fractures usually can be seen with conventional radiographs; additional imaging studies such as CT or MRI also can help identify these fractures. There has been increasing awareness of the lateral process fracture because of its association with snowboarding injuries. Treatment is dependent on fragment size and consists of either excision or open reduction and internal fixation.

Crush fractures are high-energy impact injuries and are usually associated with additional injury, often open, either to the talus, malleoli, or foot. The goal of treatment is to restore articular integrity and avoid infection or osteonecrosis. Primary arthrodesis or excision of involved joint surfaces or talectomy have not been shown to produce better results than restoration of bone stock.

Peritalar Dislocations

A subtalar dislocation is defined as the simultaneous dislocation of the subtalar and talonavicular joints without associated dislocation of the calcaneocuboid or tibiotalar joints, and without talar neck fracture. Medial dislocations are four times as common as lateral dislocations. High-energy injuries and sports injuries account for most of these dislocations; these injuries are often open injuries.

Prompt reduction is essential to minimize skin necrosis and circulatory compromise. Closed reduction cannot be achieved in approximately 5% to 10% of medial dislocations and 15% to 20% of lateral dislocations. Blocks to closed reduction may include the extensor digitorum brevis (medial dislocation) and the posterior tibial tendon (lateral dislocation). After either closed or open reduction, the joint is usually stable. If an unstable reduction occurs, the presence of a large intra-articular fracture must be ruled out because reduction and fixation of the fragment often will stabilize the joint. A CT scan is recommended after reduction to identify unrecognized articular fragments. Fixation or excision of displaced fragments is recommended to avoid instability or arthritis. Disagreement regarding early range of motion centers around preventing stiffness, but avoiding recurrent dislocation or instability.

Transverse Tarsal (Chopart) Dislocations

The transverse tarsal (Chopart) articulation is made up of the talonavicular and calcaneocuboid joints. Isolated dislocations of these individual articulations are rare. Transverse tarsal injuries are classified into five categories based on the direction of force and subsequent displacement. Longitudinal injuries account for approximately 40%, and often are associated with tarsometatarsal (Lisfranc) injuries because of the similar mechanism of injury. Medial stress injuries are the second most common, and lateral stress injuries are associated with compression (nutcracker) fractures of the cuboid.

Treatment options include closed reduction, open reduction and internal fixation, primary arthrodesis, or a combination of open reduction and internal fixation and limited fusion. Because of variations in the injury patterns, treatment is tailored to the specific features of the injury. Likewise, prognosis is dependent on pattern, early diagnosis, stable reduction, and articular damage.

Midfoot Trauma

The midfoot region includes the navicular, three cuneiforms, cuboid, and tarsometatarsal articulations. Because of the highly constrained joint articulations and strong plantar ligamentous support, isolated injury to one bone in this region is rare. Midfoot fractures commonly affect joint congruity, not only of the contiguous joint but also of adjacent joints that rely on coupled motion for normal function. The joints of the midfoot do not provide a significant contribution to

foot motion in any plane. Therefore, primary importance is given to the maintenance of height, width, and length of the fractured segments at the expense of contiguous joint motion (with the exception of the fourth and fifth metatarsocuboid joints) to allow for normal motion at the adjacent joints. As a result, the column theory has been discussed. The medial column of the foot consists of the medial aspect of the navicular, medial cuneiform, and first metatarsal. The middle column is made up of the middle and lateral aspect of the navicular, middle and lateral cuneiforms, and the second and third metatarsals. The cuboid and the fourth and fifth metatarsals comprise the lateral column. In comminuted segments of the midfoot or in crush injuries where articular congruity cannot be reestablished, bridging the injured column through the use of internal plating or external fixation and bone grafting may be necessary for stability and to establish appropriate column length relationships.

Injuries to the midfoot usually occur from a high-energy mechanism. A number of common fracture patterns have been described.

Navicular Fractures

Navicular fractures have been classified as avulsion, tuberosity, and body type. The avulsion fractures are characterized by capsular injuries, which commonly involve small dorsal fragments. These fractures are treated with cast immobilization and full weight bearing for 4 to 6 weeks followed by an ankle rehabilitation protocol for strengthening and proprioception. Fragments involving more than 25% of the bone may require open reduction and internal fixation to avoid dorsal subluxation of the navicular fragment.

The navicular tuberosity is the main attachment site of the posterior tibialis tendon. The posterior tibial tendon sends plantar extensions to insert on many of the tarsal and metatarsal bones. Nondisplaced fractures of the tuberosity may be treated with cast immobilization, and the patient should not bear weight for 4 to 6 weeks. It has been found that the navicular undergoes significant vertical dorsal and medial displacement with weight bearing at the stance phase of gait. Fragments displaced more than 2 to 3 mm should be reduced and stabilized with screw fixation. An accessory navicular may mistakenly be diagnosed as an acute fracture. The absence of sharp fracture lines on radiographs and the lack of clinical findings of ecchymosis, tenderness, and swelling will rule out this diagnosis. Occasionally, the synchondrosis between the accessory navicular and the main body of the bone can be injured. When clinical findings suggest a fracture of this nature, a three-phase technetium bone scan can confirm the diagnosis with increased uptake on the delayed images. If a synchon-

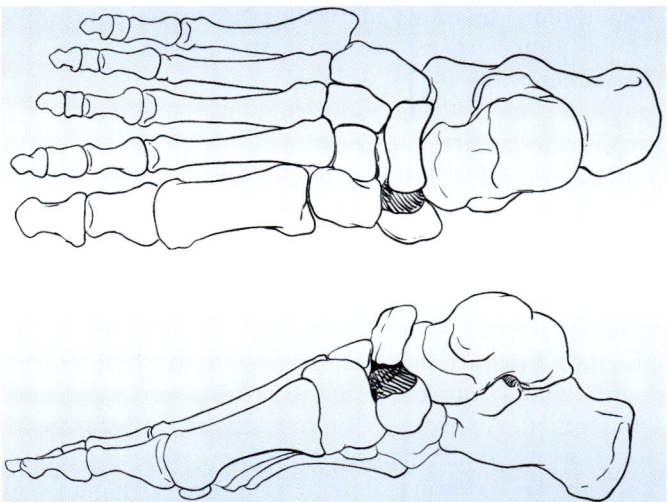

Figure 7 Type 1 body fracture of the navicular.

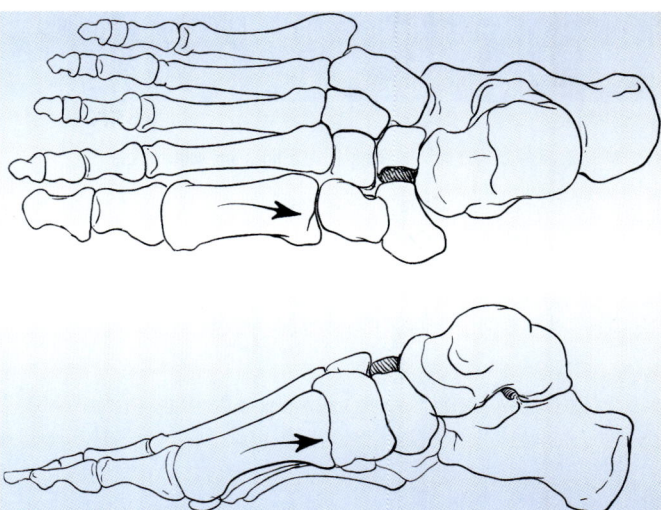

Figure 8 Type 2 body fracture of the navicular.

drosis injury is nondisplaced, it can be treated in the same manner as an acute fracture, with immobilization, if nondisplaced, in a short leg cast and no weight bearing for 4 to 6 weeks. If pain persists after immobilization and the fragment is small, resection of the ossicle with tendon reattachment (if necessary) has been successful. With a large, triangular-shaped accessory navicular (cornate tubercle), surgical stabilization with resection of the interposing cartilage may be performed after immobilization has failed.

Three types of body fractures have been described to aid in pattern recognition and treatment options. Type I is a fracture in the horizontal plane that produces dorsal and plantar fragments without forefoot angulation (Fig. 7). Interfragmentary screw fixation provides adequate stabilization through an anteromedial approach. Half pins (2 to 3 mm) placed in the talus and cuneiform can be used for temporary external fixator distraction to allow for visualization of the reduction of any type of body fracture. Type II fractures consist of a fracture in the dorsolateral to plantar-medial plane that leads to medial displacement of the major fragment and forefoot (Fig. 8). This is the most common navicular body fracture pattern. Reduction can be difficult and may require stabilization of the medial fragment to the adjacent cuneiform to maintain medial column length. Violation of the talonavicular joint is avoided because this articulation contributes significantly to coupled motion of the hindfoot. Type III navicular fractures occur from an axial load mechanism resulting in central or lateral comminution in the sagittal plane with the forefoot laterally displaced (Fig. 9). Associated injuries to the cuboid and/or anterior calcaneus are not uncommon with this fracture pattern. External fixation or bridging internal fixation across the naviculocuneiform or calcaneocuboid joints with

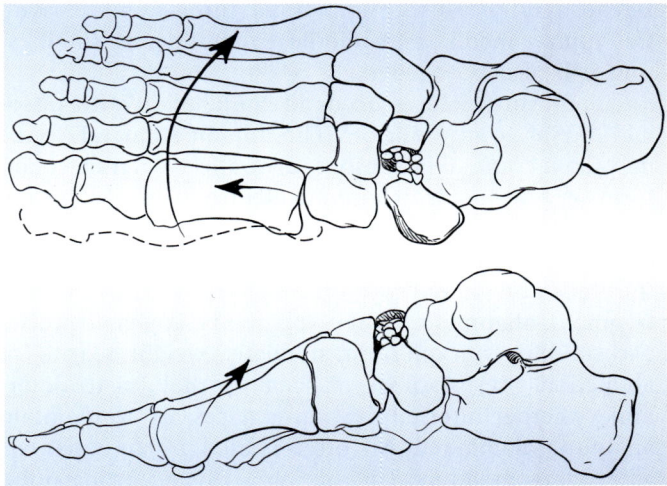

Figure 9 Type 3 body fracture of the navicular.

primary intraosseous bone grafting, or in severe cases, primary arthrodesis, may be necessary to maintain column length. Body fractures require casting without external fixation and no weight bearing for 6 to 8 weeks, followed by progressive weight bearing guided by radiographic healing.

Isolated injuries to the cuboid or cuneiforms rarely occur because of the constrained articulations and strong plantar ligaments. The nutcracker injury is a common fracture pattern involving the cuboid. The mechanism of injury is abduction of the forefoot; the cuboid is compressed as it is wedged between the fourth and fifth metatarsal bases and the anterior aspect of the calcaneus, resulting in shortening of the lateral column. The medial column injury is to the tarsometatarsal region, resulting in fractures or ligament disruptions (Lisfranc). Treatment includes the reestablishment of lateral column length with an external fix-

TABLE 1	**Normal Radiographic Findings of the Tarsometatarsal Joints on Weight-Bearing Radiographs**

Medial edge of second metatarsal base lines up with middle cuneiform (AP)

Medial aspect of fourth metatarsal lines up with medial aspect of cuboid (AP)

Notch of base of fifth metatarsal lines up with lateral aspect of cuboid

On lateral view, the metatarsals are not more dorsal than respective tarsal bones

ation or internal fixation and plate bridging of the cuboid with or without intraosseous bone grafting. Because of the disruption of all three columns with this injury, medial and middle column screw stabilization will also be needed.

Cuneiform fractures occur in conjunction with tarsometatarsal joint injuries. The tarsometatarsal joints may have pure ligamentous disruption or transcuneiform or transmetarsarsal equivalent injuries. When the tarsometatarsal or intertarsal joints appear disrupted on initial radiographs, surgical planning should address the reestablishment of joint congruity and fracture fragment alignment. When the joints appear reduced and stability is in question, simulated weight bearing or abduction stress radiographs may be helpful to determine whether internal fixation is necessary to maintain anatomic alignment. An often-missed fracture pattern with a tarsometatarsal disruption is further propagation of the injury between the medial and middle cuneiforms and exiting the medial cuneiform-navicular articulation. Failure to recognize this pattern leads to subluxation of the medial cuneiform medially and dorsally, resulting in a shortened medial column.

Nonsurgical treatment of tarsometatarsal injuries is reserved for patients with nondisplaced fracture-dislocations confirmed by CT scan or those who are medically unstable. Surgical treatment is indicated for patients with displacement of the articular surfaces of more than 1 mm. With an anatomic closed reduction, percutaneous fixation is an option in an anatomically reduced fracture; if displacement is present, open reduction is favored. Fixation consists of percutaneous screw fixation of the first, second, and potentially third tarsometatarsal joints and Kirschner wire fixation of the fourth and fifth metatarsocuboid joints is appropriate. With an inadequate closed reduction as evidenced by persistent disruption in radiographic lines (as outlined in Table 1) open reduction through one or two

longitudinal incisions allows for anatomic restoration of the joint surfaces and stabilization with screws and Kirschner wires. An additional screw placed across the navicular-medial cuneiform joint may be necessary if this injury pattern is present. The postoperative protocol consists of a non–weight-bearing cast for 8 to 12 weeks, and then progressive weight bearing and rehabilitation for ankle strengthening and proprioception. Screw removal is delayed for 4 to 6 months. Permanent screw placement has also been suggested. Posttraumatic arthritis develops in up to 50% of Lisfranc fracture/dislocations. Stiff rocker bottom shoes and nonsteroidal anti-inflammatory drugs provide some pain relief. Arthrodesis of the affected posttraumatic joints assessed through a positive response to fluoroscopy-guided lidocaine joint injection aids in pain control. The fourth and fifth tarsometatarsal joints are treated with metatarsal base resections to maintain the mobile lateral rays of the foot.

Forefoot Trauma

The forefoot consists of the metatarsals and phalanges. Fracture of the fifth metatarsal is the most common, and consists of tuberosity, metaphyseal-diaphyseal (Jones), and shaft fractures. These fractures often occur in conjunction with an inversion ankle injury and lateral ankle ligament sprain.

The fifth metatarsal base tuberosity fracture can be extra-articular or extend into the articular surface. Treatment may include a stiff-soled shoe or walking brace for comfort. Posttraumatic arthritis with this fracture is rare. Ankle rehabilitation exercises targeted at the prevention of recurrent ankle instability are implemented early and an ankle brace is used for sporting activities to avoid recurrent ankle injury.

The Jones fracture occurs at the metaphyseal/diaphyseal junction of the fifth metatarsal. This area is a watershed zone for blood flow and is particularly susceptible to delayed union or nonunion. The treatment is immobilization in a short leg cast or brace, and no weight bearing for 6 to 12 weeks until callus is seen on foot radiographs. Progressive protected weight bearing can then occur. In higher-level athletes, primary screw fixation with a 4.5-mm malleolar type screw may be undertaken. Spiral fractures of the fifth metatarsal shaft may be treated nonsurgically with weight bearing to tolerance in a stiff-soled shoe.

Metatarsal shaft fractures of the middle rays may occur with crush injuries or as a Lisfranc fracture variant. With crush injuries, additional energy is imparted to the adjacent soft tissues, which may lead to a compartment syndrome of the foot. Stiffness and neuritic pain may be the sequela of a crush injury long after the fractures have healed. Indications for surgical stabilization of metatarsal fractures include angulation of greater than 10° in the sagittal plane or displacement of more than 3 to 4 mm resulting in a prominent or unweighted metatarsal head. Attempts at open reduction of the metatarsal shafts, metatarsophalangeal joints, or phalangeal fractures leads to scarring and stiffness, adding surgical injury to the traumatic injury, and should be performed only to provide a plantigrade foot for weight bearing.

A patient history of any prodromal symptoms in the fifth metatarsal is helpful to identify a stress fracture. Clinical examination of foot and ankle alignment during weight bearing is critical to determine if there are any biomechanical issues, such as cavovarus foot malalignment, that can cause excessive forces on the fifth metatarsal. The patient's training schedule and technique should be reviewed because these, too, can lead to stress fractures. Radiographs may demonstrate sclerotic margins on the fracture fragments that are suggestive of a stress fracture. Screw fixation and potential bone grafting may be needed to facilitate healing. With a cavovarus foot malalignment, a lateral heel wedge orthosis may be helpful to alter the weight on the fifth ray and prevent recurrence of injury.

Phalangeal Fractures

Phalangeal fractures rarely require surgical intervention or stabilization, with the great toe being the rare exception. Closed reduction when possible and occasionally open reduction and Kirschner wire or minifragmentary stabilization can maintain toe alignment and function. Some phalangeal fractures can be loosely buddy taped to adjacent toes for comfort or left alone in a shoe with a wide width or stiff sole. Because of swelling, normal shoe wear may be painful. Early weight bearing in patients with phalangeal fractures has been shown to improve outcome and healing times.

Sports Injuries of the Foot and Ankle

Ankle and Subtalar Sprains/Instability

Ankle sprains are the most common athletic injury and result primarily from an inversion stress during ankle plantar flexion. The anterior talofibular ligament (ATFL), the most commonly injured ankle ligament, is intimately associated with the joint capsule and is responsible for anterior drawer stability and inversion stability during plantar flexion of the ankle. The calcaneofibular ligament (CFL) is extracapsular and is the primary restraint to inversion instability during dorsiflexion.

The most important aspect of the initial orthopaedic management of the common ankle sprain is failure to recognize an associated injury. Determination of the mechanism of force can suggest a diagnosis. External rotation is associated with syndesmotic, peroneal tendon, and deltoid injuries. Inversion stress of the dorsiflexed ankle is associated with CFL injury. Point palpation tenderness and the inability to bear weight are findings that warrant radiographic evaluation. Commonly missed diagnoses include tendon subluxation (peroneal); tendon tears (posterior tibial, Achilles); fractures (anterior process of calcaneus, lateral process of talus, fifth metatarsal, Lisfranc, navicular, calcaneocuboid); and osteochondritis dissecans of the talus. A complete radiographic examination includes three views of the foot (AP, lateral to include the ankle, and oblique) and mortise and AP views of the ankle if clinically indicated.

An emergency room evaluation occasionally reports negative ankle radiographs, whereas the pathology might have been detected with foot radiographs (for example, oblique view of the foot revealing anterior process of a calcaneus fracture). Similarly, repeat weight bearing or stress radiographs may be required to detect subtle syndesmotic or Lisfranc injuries.

Classification as grade I, II, and III ankle sprains or the high (syndesmotic) versus low (lateral collateral ligaments) sprains is important prognostically regarding time to return to sport activity.

The familiar regimen of protection, rest, ice, compression, and elevation, early weight bearing, and range of motion (alphabet) exercises form the mainstay of early rehabilitation. Functional ankle braces are used for grade I and II injuries; severely symptomatic grade III sprains may benefit from cast immobilization or removable short leg walking braces that maintain a neutral ankle position and function as a removable cast for the first few weeks after surgery. Functional rehabilitation includes isometric and resistance exercises, and proprioceptive training. Return to sport is permitted when painless cutting, running, and the ability to jump on the affected leg 10 times without pain is experienced. Protective bracing for patients with grade II and III injuries for 6 months is helpful and has not been shown to interfere with athletic performance. Several recent studies indicate extremely limited indications for acute surgical stabilization of injuries to the lateral ankle ligament.

Approximately 15% to 30% of simple sprains will result in residual symptoms with peroneal weakness; inadequate rehabilitation is indicated as the primary cause. It is important to differentiate functional instability (pain causing an ankle to give way) from mechanical instability, with attenuated restraints allowing excess motion and subsequent pain. Mechanical laxity should be clinically detectable by the standard anterior drawer test, though the reliability and specific diagnostic criteria of mechanical instability are controversial. Stress radiography can be helpful though factors such as positioning, quantity of stress applied, pain, and guarding can lead to variable results, particularly in an acute or subacute setting. Lateral radiographic stress views revealing a forward translation of 3 mm more than the contralateral limb, or an absolute value of 10 mm forward translation generally has been accepted to indicate mechanical instability.

Clinical determination of abnormal tibiotalar (inversion) instability is correlated with injury to the CFL. The CFL is a restraint to abnormal motion of both the tibiotalar and subtalar joints, and a combination of ankle/subtalar instability may exist in the unstable ankle. Abnormal tibiotalar tilt has been variably defined as 3° to 15° more than the contralateral limb, or an absolute value of 9°, limiting radiographic exposure to the symptomatic ankle. Subtalar instability is even more difficult to diagnose and its documentation more controversial than ankle instability because the recommended 40° Broden stress view demonstrated wide variability in a study of asymptomatic, uninjured patients. Loss of parallelism of the posterior facet or more than 3 mm of translation of the talus on the calcaneus on the lateral view has been defined by some authors to indicate subtalar instability. Coexistent subtalar and tibiotalar instability has been demonstrated via stress fluoroscopy in 75% of subjects with a lateral ankle sprain.

In the mechanically unstable ankle for which peroneal strengthening and proprioceptive rehabilitation fail, anatomic repair can be done using the technique originally described by Broström. The initial description emphasized repair of the ATFL in all cases, with 30% requiring repair of the CFL. The modified technique emphasizes shortening of both the ATFL and the CFL in addition to reefing of the lateral extensor retinaculum, probably accounting for the improved results noted in recent studies. The primary advantage of this technique is the preservation of dynamic stabilizers (peroneals) with the maintenance of anatomic ligament stabilizers. Variations on this technique include advancing the ligaments through drill holes and bony troughs, the use of suture anchors and resorbable sutures, or vest-over-pants suturing of the ligaments. Absolute or relative contraindications to the Broström technique include a fixed heel varus, connective tissue disorders (Ehlers-Danlos), failed prior surgery, and severely attenuated tissue (> 10 years of tibiotalar instability).

The need for revision Broström procedures with potential augmentation of a checkrein (peroneus brevis) tendon can be more difficult when a previous anterior curvilinear exposure is used as advocated in most descriptions of the Broström procedure. Inspection of the peroneal tendons and their use for a subsequent (rare) revision technique favor a longitudinal exposure during the index procedure.

Failed ankle reconstructions generally require the addition of tendon graft (half of the peroneus brevis). Numerous techniques and modifications exist, including the Evans, Watson-Jones, and Chrisman-Snook procedures. Biomechanically, the split tendon grafts are stiffer and have less strain to failure than ligaments so that nonanatomic (nonisometric) reconstructions can result in ankle stiffness or tendon graft failure. Newer augmented reconstructions emphasize drill hole placement and tendon passage in more anatomically correct positions. Excellent results have been reported with a new technique using bone anchors and passage of the tendon outside the fibula.

Reports comparing Broström anatomic reconstructions with various checkrein procedures reveal equivalent functional results but fewer complications with the anatomic reconstructions. Currently, indications and recommendations for surgical management of a clinically unstable ankle include (1) failed complete peroneal strengthening and proprioceptive training; (2) preferred anatomic reconstruction with some variation of a Broström technique if adequate tissue exists; (3) calcaneal osteotomy for excessive heel varus; (4) augmentation with a slip of peroneus brevis tendon if there is severe attenuation of tissue or ligamentous laxity, obesity, high demand, or failed prior anatomic reconstruction.

Subtalar instability is most often treated with the Chrisman-Snook procedure. Other reports indicate satisfactory results with the Broström alone, or reconstruction of the interosseous ligament. Though no consensus exists, it appears that the simple Evans procedure is not as effective because the reconstructed ligament is oriented parallel to and does not cross the subtalar joint.

Syndesmotic Injury

Injury to the ankle syndesmosis is usually associated with a combined external rotation and dorsiflexion stress. Severe injuries with associated fibular fractures and deltoid injury will be detected on radiographs, but there should be a high index of suspicion for syndesmotic injury when severe pain is associated with "normal" radiographs. If there is pain with external rotation of the ankle or when squeezing the calf several centimeters proximal to the syndesmosis, stress radiographs are warranted if the initial studies are normal. Closed treatment of syndesmotic injury without fracture is reserved for stable sprains; unstable injuries demonstrated by radiographs or stress views may be fixed with 4.5-mm cortical screws. The use of bioabsorbable fixation, weight-bearing restrictions, and the necessity of implant removal are controversial options.

Prolonged recovery time after syndesmotic injury is common and the term "high ankle sprain" can be useful in communication to trainers and coaches who quickly learn that this injury is more serious than the common ankle sprain. Protection in a functional brace and avoidance of weight bearing and functional rehabilitation until the ankle is pain-free are important to avoid prolonged recovery time.

Chronic pain after syndesmotic injury may indicate subtle instability, heterotopic ossification, or a soft-tissue impingement described in the recent arthroscopic literature. Bone scans, repeat radiographs, stress radiographs, CT scans, and selective injection can help determine a treatable cause for chronic symptoms.

Foot Sprains

Sprains of the midfoot can occur as isolated injuries but are usually associated with tarsal or tarsometatarsal (Lisfranc) fractures. Clinical examination includes provocative side-to-side midfoot compression and dorsoplantar stress of the first and second tarsometatarsal joints. Marked pain may indicate the need for weight-bearing radiographs to evaluate the alignment of the metatarsals with the respective cuneiforms and cuboid on the oblique view. Diastasis of the first or second tarsometatarsal joints of more than 2 mm should be reduced and fixed. Non–weight-bearing films might not demonstrate the instability, but excessive pain may prohibit weight-bearing radiographs from being taken. A bone scan may document a major injury to the midfoot when weight-bearing radiographs are negative. Protected weight bearing and rapidity of rehabilitation are dependent on clinical response and therefore are controversial. Medial midfoot sprains take much longer to heal than lateral sprains, and return to sports can require up to several months.

Sprains of the first metatarsophalangeal joint (turf toe) have achieved considerable attention because of the use of artificial turf on the playing surface and the involvement of well-known athletes. The mechanism of injury is an excessive dorsiflexion force frequently seen with push-off in flexible shoes while playing football. Valgus and hyperflexion injuries also have been described. Severity of injury may vary, but acute surgical treatment is rarely indicated. Radiography is necessary to rule out fractures. Treatment generally includes rest and avoidance of excessive dorsiflexion.

A thin steel prefabricated insole or a custom orthosis or orthotic insole with Morton's extension can be used for treatment. For clinically unstable or recalcitrant painful toes that require surgical treatment as a result of failed nonsurgical treatment, MRI could be used to more accurately determine the site of anatomic injury. A 50% incidence of chronic problems, including hallux valgus, hallux rigidus, and chronic pain, has been noted in the literature, reflecting the potential severity and disability resulting from this injury.

Tendon Injuries in Athletes

Achilles Tendon

Sports participation by older athletes has been associated with the increased incidence of tendon injury, including inflammation (tendinitis), degeneration (tendinosis), subluxation, and rupture. The peritenon of the Achilles tendon is frequently inflamed as an overuse injury in aging runners. Peritendinitis is commonly associated with intratendon degeneration in the hypovascular zone approximately 5 cm proximal to the calcaneal insertion. Chronic thickening usually indicates intratendon rupture.

Orthotic support of mechanical abnormalities (such as cavus feet), avoidance of training errors, and stretching exercises may diminish the frequency of this condition. Treatment includes rest, nonsteroidal anti-inflammatory drugs (NSAIDs), orthotic insoles, stretching exercises, and a gradual return to activity. Recalcitrant cases can respond to longitudinal débridement of the tendon evaluated preoperatively with MRI to identify regions of intratendinous degeneration.

Insertional Achilles calcific tendinosis is commonly associated with retrocalcaneal bursitis or Haglund's deformity, although they are distinct entities. Usual nonsurgical measures include iontophoresis, heel lifts, and cushioned heel counters. Surgical treatment includes removal of the Haglund's deformity and débridement of the calcific spur. A lateral, combined medial-lateral, or a central splitting exposure has been advised.

Rupture of the Achilles tendon is usually associated with a sudden push-off movement during sporting activity in the middle-aged athlete, but may be accompanied by antecedent symptoms. Physical examination should confirm the diagnosis without the need for ancillary tests, but lateral radiographs should be obtained to exclude an avulsion of the posterosuperior calcaneal tuberosity.

Treatment options for Achilles tendon rupture are surgical or nonsurgical. Poor results of prolonged casting in plantar flexion can be attributed to immobilization and delayed weight bearing. Nonsurgical treatment with a functional brace has produced good results. Ultrasonography can be used to monitor continued apposition of Achilles tendon ends if nonsurgical management is elected. Current postoperative rehabilitation protocols emphasize early protected range of motion and weight bearing and are probably responsible for the improved results in recent surgical studies. Athletic individuals are usually advised to undergo surgical reconstruction for improved performance, quicker return to sport activity, less atrophy, better range of motion, and fewer complaints.

There are various techniques for the surgical repair of Achilles tendon rupture, but the most important factor to consider is reproduction of the dynamic resting length of the tendon so that range of motion and push-off strength are restored. Percutaneous methods are controversial because they cannot accurately appose the tendon ends to establish an anatomic resting length, and there is a reported incidence of sural nerve injury.

Delaying surgery for 7 to 10 days and applying a plaster splint may help reduce swelling and allow some organization of the "mop-ends" of torn tendon that can facilitate a restoration of the anatomic length of the repair. Immediate surgical repair is also acceptable. The plantaris tendon may be weaved through the Achilles tendon or fanned out for use as a fascial covering to prevent skin adhesions. Bulky, retained suture material may contribute to wound complications, and some surgeons prefer smaller (No. 2), absorbable sutures. Either absorbable or nonabsorbable suture technique is justified.

Much of the favorable results of surgical treatment can be attributed to more aggressive rehabilitation emphasizing early range of motion, weight bearing, and conditioning.

Peroneal Tendons

Attritional tears of the peroneus longus and brevis tendons have been reported, but athletic injury to the tendons primarily consists of tendinitis and subluxation. Tendinitis usually responds to nonsurgical measures such as use of lateral heel wedges, peroneal strengthening, and protection with a stirrup brace. Traumatic peroneal tendon subluxation is usually associated with a forceful reflex contraction of the peroneals when the ankle is dorsiflexed and inverted. Skiing, basketball, soccer, and skating are most commonly associated with this injury.

The anatomic restraint to peroneal subluxation is the superior peroneal retinaculum. Traumatic injury involves an avulsion of this structure that may result in a rim of bone evident on plain radiographs. Nonsurgical treatment includes cast immobilization, but acute surgical stabilization of an avulsed cortical rim is another option. Symptomatic chronic peroneal tendon subluxation may be treated by reefing the superior peroneal retinaculum, fibular groove deepening, creation of soft-tissue slings, or bony block reconstruction. The simplicity and efficiency of groove deepening procedures contribute to the increasing popularity of this technique.

Chronic tendinitis or recurrent subluxation may result in attritional peroneus longus or brevis tears that are diagnosed primarily by localized physical findings in the retrofibular groove. Tears in either tendon can be found at surgery despite reports of a normal MRI study. Persistent symptoms warrant surgical intervention with resection of small longitudinal tears, and tubularization of multiple tears with an absorbable suture. Tenodesis to the adjacent tendon may be necessary if severe tendon degeneration or rupture is present.

Flexor Hallucis Longus Tendon

The flexor hallucis longus (FHL) tendon is principally injured in dancers as a result of repetitive push-off of the forefoot, particularly during en pointe and demi pointe positions. Because the tendon is constricted at the fibroosseous tunnel at the medial aspect of the calcaneus under the sustentaculum tali, this condition can be confused with either posterior tibial tendinitis or Achilles tendinitis. Diagnosis is determined clinically. With the ankle in dorsiflexion, the FHL muscle belly may be constricted by the sheath, resulting in limited dorsiflexion of the hallux (functional hallux rigidus). Increased dorsiflexion of the hallux and lessened pain are experienced during ankle plantar flexion. Treatment is with medial surgical release for refractory cases.

Impingement Syndromes in the Athlete

The tibiotalar joint is a frequent site of anterior impingement for dancers, basketball players, runners, catchers, and aging "weekend warriors" with a history of recurrent ankle sprains. Osteophytes on the anterior tibial lip are classified as type I; talar osteophyte as type II; and type III is a combination of talar and tibial osteophytes. Diagnosis is confirmed with limited dorsiflexion, pain with forced dorsiflexion, and radiographic imaging of spur formation. Heel lifts, NSAIDs, and avoidance of excessive dorsiflexion constitute nonsurgical treatment. Surgical treatment involves either arthroscopic or open débridement. Inadequate débridement is the primary cause of failed surgical treatment.

Anterolateral soft-tissue impingement of the ankle is commonly seen as a result of repetitive ankle injury. A hyalinized connective tissue lesion in the anterolateral gutter has been referred to as the meniscoid lesion. Three primary sites of origin of soft-tissue impingement of the anterolateral gutter are the superior portion of the anteroinferior tibiofibular ligament (AITF); distal AITF including a separate slip (Basset's ligament); and the ATFL. A high success rate has been reported for arthroscopic treatment of anterolateral impingement of the ankle.

Posterior impingement syndrome involves impaction of the os trigonum and/or posterior capsular structures between the tibia and calcaneus. This condition is most commonly seen in ballet dancers (nutcracker effect), but also is seen in kickers and soccer players. The potential association of FHL tendinitis with posterior impingement syndrome may alter surgical treatment. Surgical resection of the os trigonum can be performed by the medial or lateral approach whereas release of the FHL tendon can only be performed from the medial approach. An os trigonum can be excised via subtalar arthroscopy or an open medial or lateral approach.

Annotated Bibliography

Ankle and Pilon Fractures

Barrett JA, Baron JA, Karagas MR, Beach ML: Fracture risk in the U.S. Medicare population. *J Clin Epidemiol* 1999;52:243-249.

Using Medicare data of people between 65 and 90 years old in the United States, this study demonstrated that ankle fractures were the fourth most common fracture in this population. Between the ages of 65 and 90 years, the actuarial risk for ankle fracture was 3.9% for white women, 1.3% for white men, 2.4% for African-American women, and 0.9% for African-American men.

Blotter RH, Connolly E, Wasan A, Chapman MW: Acute complications in the operative treatment of isolated ankle fractures in patients with diabetes mellitus. *Foot Ankle Int* 1999;20:687-694.

Surgical treatment of 21 ankle fractures in diabetic patients resulted in a 43% complication rate compared with a 15% complication rate in a control group of nondiabetic patients ($P < 0.05$). The complications in diabetic patients were more severe, including seven infections, three fixation failures, and two below-knee amputations.

Flynn JM, Rodriguez-del Rio F, Piza PA: Closed ankle fractures in the diabetic patient. *Foot Ankle Int* 2000;21: 311-319.

In a comparative study of ankle fracture treatment complications in 25 diabetic and 73 nondiabetic patients, the rate of infection after surgery was two times higher in the diabetic patients (21% vs. 9%), but the risk of infection in diabetic patients was even higher with nonsurgical treatment. Overall, the major risk factor for infection in diabetic patients was closed reduction and immobilization, both when compared with nondiabetic patients treated surgically or nonsurgically, and to diabetic patients treated surgically.

Hintermann B, Regazzoni P, Lampert C, Stutz G, Gachter A: Arthroscopic findings in acute fractures of the ankle. *J Bone Joint Surg Br* 2000;82:345-351.

In 288 surgically treated ankle fractures, initial arthroscopy was used to determine the existence of cartilage injury. Although most ankles demonstrated some cartilage damage (70% of tali, 40% to 45% of plafonds/malleoli), less than 10% had injury extending beyond 50% of the cartilage thickness, and none had full-thickness losses.

Jensen SL, Andresen BK, Mencke S, Nielsen PT: Epidemiology of ankle fractures: A prospective population-based study of 212 cases in Aalborg, Denmark. *Acta Orthop Scand* 1998;69:48-50.

In a 1-year prospective study in Denmark, the incidence of ankle fracture was 107 per 10^5 person-years. At age 40 years or younger, men were twice as likely to have a fracture as women, but the fracture incidence in women equaled or exceeded that of men after age 45 years.

Kennedy JG, Johnson SM, Collins AL, et al: An evaluation of the Weber classification of ankle fractures. *Injury* 1998;29:577-580.

In a retrospective study of 96 patients with a minimum of 3 years follow-up, the Weber classification system for ankle fractures was not prognostic for the ultimate clinical results. The most significant predictors of a poor outcome were severe initial displacement, inadequate reduction, and more than one fractured malleolus.

Hindfoot Trauma

Flemister AS Jr, Infante AF, Sanders RW, Walling AK: Subtalar arthrodesis for complications of intra-articular calcaneal fractures. *Foot Ankle Int* 2000;21:392.

A comparison between patients with calcaneal malunion, failed open reduction and internal fixation, and primary fusion in 86 subtalar fusions is presented.

Folk JW, Starr AJ, Early JS: Early wound complications of operative treatment of calcaneus fractures: Analysis of 190 fractures. *J Orthop Trauma* 1999;13: 369-372.

Smoking, diabetes, and open fractures all increase the risk of wound complications after surgical treatment of calcaneal fractures. Risk factors are cumulative.

Metzger MJ, Levin JS, Clancy JT: Talar neck fractures and rates of avascular necrosis. *J Foot Ankle Surg* 1999;38:154-162.

An extensive literature review on talar neck fractures and rates of avascular necrosis is presented.

Sanders R: Displaced intra-articular fractures of the calcaneus. *J Bone Joint Surg Am* 2000;82:225-250.

This article presents a current concepts review of calcaneal fractures.

Thermann H, Krettek C, Hufner T, Schratt HE, Albrecht K, Tscherne H: Management of calcaneal fractures in adults: Conservative versus operative treatment. *Clin Orthop* 1998;353:107-124.

The best surgical results occur with anatomic reconstruction and function-directed postoperative management.

Tornetta P III: The Essex-Lopresti reduction for calcaneal fractures revisited. *J Orthop Trauma* 1998;12:469-473.

The Essex-Lopresti spike reduction is a useful method for the treatment of tongue-type Sanders IIC fractures of the calcaneus. Results are superior to those in previous series of intra-articular fractures treated with open reduction and internal fixation.

Tucker DJ, Feder JM, Boylan JP: Fractures of the lateral process of the talus: Two case reports and a comprehensive literature review. *Foot Ankle Int* 1998; 19:641-646.

To achieve the best possible result, early diagnosis and treatment are emphasized.

Midfoot and Forefoot Trauma

Berlet G, Anderson R, Davis WH: Tendon arthroplasty for basal 4th and 5th metatarsal arthritis. *67th Annual Meeting Proceedings*. Rosemont, IL, American Academy of Orthopaedic Surgeons, 2000, p 489.

Coss HS, Manos RE, Buoncristiani A, Mills WJ: Abduction stress and AP weightbearing radiography of purely ligamentous injury in the tarsometatarsal joint. *Foot Ankle Int* 1998;19:537-541.

This article presents a study of Lisfranc joint stability with abduction stress and simulated weight-bearing radiographs in cadavers before and after Lisfranc ligament sectioning compared with healthy volunteer controls.

Dhillon MS, Nagi ON: Total dislocations of the navicular: Are they ever isolated injuries? *J Bone Joint Surg Br* 1999;81:881-885.

This article presents a study of six cases of navicular dislocation without fracture but with complex ligamentous disruption. Instability of the medial and lateral columns of the foot were found, with a navicular dislocation necessitating stabilization of both columns.

Sports Injuries of the Foot and Ankle

Angermann P, Hovgaard D: Chronic Achilles tendinopathy in athletic individuals: Results of nonsurgical treatment. *Foot Ankle Int* 1999;20:304-306.

Two thirds of athletes were improved or cured with long-term follow-up after nonsurgical treatment of chronic Achilles tendinopathy.

Dixon DJ, Monroe MT, Gabel SJ, Manoli A II: Excrescent lesion: A diagnosis of lateral talar exostosis in chronically symptomatic sprained ankles. *Foot Ankle Int* 1999;20:331-336.

The authors describe an anterolateral exostosis at the insertion of the ATFL in stable ankles with chronic pain. Diagnosis was confirmed with CT scan. Surgical excision resulted in laxity of the ATFL, which required a Brostöm reconstruction.

Frey C, Feder KS, DiGiovanni C: Arthroscopic evaluation of the subtalar joint: Does sinus tarsi syndrome exist? *Foot Ankle Int* 1999;20:185-191.

The authors' preoperative diagnosis of sinus tarsi syndrome was changed in all cases; 10 of 14 patients had interosseous ligament tears. Arthroscopy led to a more accurate diagnosis, and good to excellent results were reported in 94% of cases.

Gerber JP, Williams GN, Scoville CR, Arciero RA, Taylor DC: Persistent disability associated with ankle sprains: A prospective examination of an athletic population. *Foot Ankle Int* 1998;19:653-660.

Early return to sports following ankle sprains is common, but approximately 40% of patients have dysfunction at 6 months. Syndesmosis sprains are more common than previously appreciated and this is the factor most predictive of residual symptoms.

Girard P, Anderson RB, Davis WH, Isear JA, Kiebzak GM: Clinical evaluation of the modified Broström-Evans procedure to restore ankle stability. *Foot Ankle Int* 1999;20:246-252.

Simple augmentation of the Broström repair with a portion of the peroneus brevis tendon is advised in overweight, hyperflexible patients or those involved in strenuous or athletic activity. Postoperatively, the average American Orthopaedic Foot and Ankle Association hindfoot score was 98 points, with no complications reported.

Hertel J, Denegar CR, Monroe MM, Stokes WL: Talocrural and subtalar joint instability after lateral ankle sprain. *Med Sci Sports Exerc* 1999;31:1501-1508.

This article discusses the coexistence of subtalar and tibiotalar instability following lateral ankle sprains. A good discussion of the evaluation of subtalar instability is provided.

Lahm A, Erggelet C, Reichelt A: Ankle joint arthroscopy for meniscoid lesions in athletes. *Arthroscopy* 1998;14:572-575.

The meniscoid lesion may be underdiagnosed, but is effectively treated with early arthroscopic resection.

Mortensen HM, Skov O, Jensen PE: Early motion of the ankle after operative treatment of a rupture of the Achilles tendon: A prospective, randomized clinical and radiographic study. *J Bone Joint Surg Am* 1999;81:983-990.

Early restricted motion shortens the time for rehabilitation and was not associated with tendon elongation or an increased incidence of complications.

Povacz P, Unger SF, Miller WK, Tockner R, Resch H: A randomized, prospective study of operative and non-operative treatment of injuries of the fibular collateral ligaments of the ankle. *J Bone Joint Surg Am* 1998;80:345-351.

Nonsurgical treatment of ankle sprains yielded results similar to surgical repair, and is associated with a shorter period of recovery. Therefore, nonsurgical treatment was advised for all patients, including athletes.

Sammarco GJ, Idusuyi OB: Reconstruction of the lateral ankle ligaments using a split peroneus brevis tendon graft. *Foot Ankle Int* 1999;20:97-103.

Bone anchors are used for a simpler, more anatomic reconstruction with a split peroneus brevis tendon. Results were 94% good to excellent, with 97% mechanical stability.

Thacker SB, Stroup DF, Branche CM, Gilchrist J, Goodman RA, Weitman EA: The prevention of ankle sprains in sports: A systematic review of the literature. *Am J Sports Med* 1999;27:753-760.

The most common risk factor for ankle sprains in sports is a history of prior sprains. Braces do not interfere with athletic performance, and a moderate or severe sprain may be braced for at least 6 months for athletic participation.

Classic Bibliography

Adelaar RS: The treatment of complex fractures of the talus. *Orthop Clin North Am* 1989;20:691-707.

Baird RA, Jackson ST: Fractures of the distal part of the fibula with associated disruption of the deltoid ligament: Treatment without repair of the deltoid ligament. *J Bone Joint Surg Am* 1987;69:1346-1352.

Bauer M, Jonsson K, Nilsson B: Thirty-year follow-up of ankle fractures. *Acta Orthop Scand* 1985;56:103-106.

Benirschke SK, Sangeorzan BJ: Extensive intraarticular fractures of the foot: Surgical management of calcaneal fractures. *Clin Orthop* 1993;292:128-134.

Bennell KL, Brukner PD: Epidemiology and site specificity of stress fractures. *Clin Sports Med* 1997;16:179-196.

Boden SD, Labropoulos PA, McCowin P, Lestini WF, Hurwitz SR: Mechanical considerations for the syndesmosis screw: A cadaver study. *J Bone Joint Surg Am* 1989;71:1548-1555.

Böhler L: Diagnosis, pathology, and treatment of fractures of the os calcis. *J Bone Joint Surg* 1931;13:75-89.

Canale ST, Kelly FB Jr: Fractures of the neck of the talus: Long-term evaluation of seventy-one cases. *J Bone Joint Surg Am* 1978;60:143-156.

Clanton TO, Ford JJ: Turf toe injury. *Clin Sports Med* 1994;13:731-741.

Colville MR: Surgical treatment of the unstable ankle. *J Am Acad Orthop Surg* 1998;6:368-377.

DeBerardino TM, Arciero RA, Taylor DC: Arthroscopic treatment of soft-tissue impingement of the ankle in athletes. *Arthroscopy* 1997;13:492-498.

DeLee JC, Curtis R: Subtalar dislocation of the foot. *J Bone Joint Surg Am* 1982;64:433-437.

Ebraheim NA, Mekhail AO, Gargasz SS: Ankle fractures involving the fibula proximal to the distal tibiofibular syndesmosis. *Foot Ankle Int* 1997;18:513-521.

Essex-Lopresti P: The mechanism, reduction technique, and results in fractures of the os calcis. *Br J Surg* 1952;39:395-419.

Glasgow MT, Naranja RJ Jr, Glasgow SG, Torg JS: Analysis of failed surgical management of fractures of the base of the fifth metatarsal distal to the tuberosity: The Jones fracture. *Foot Ankle Int* 1996;17:449-457.

Hangody L, Kish G, Kárpáti Z, Szerb I, Eberhardt R: Treatment of osteochondritis dissecans of the talus: Use of the mosaicplasty technique: A preliminary report. *Foot Ankle Int* 1997;18:628-634.

Hawkins LG: Fractures of the neck of the talus. *J Bone Joint Surg Am* 1970;52:991-1002.

Hovis WD, Bucholz RW: Polyglycolide bioabsorbable screws in the treatment of ankle fractures. *Foot Ankle Int* 1997;18:128-131.

Karlsson J, Eriksson BI, Renstrom PA: Subtalar ankle instability: A review. *Sports Med* 1997;24:337-346.

Kitaoka HB, Luo ZP, An KN: Three-dimensional analysis of normal ankle and foot mobility. *Am J Sports Med* 1997;25:238-242.

Kollias SL, Ferkel RD: Fibular grooving for recurrent peroneal tendon subluxation. *Am J Sports Med* 1997;25:329-335.

Lauge-Hansen N: Fractures of the ankle: II. Combined experimental-surgical and experimental-roentgenologic investigations. *Arch Surg* 1950;60:957-985.

Letournel E: Open treatment of acute calcaneal fractures. *Clin Orthop* 1993;290:60-67.

Lu J, Ebraheim NA, Skie M, Porshinsky B, Yeasting RA: Radiographic and computed tomographic evaluation of Lisfranc dislocation: A cadaver study. *Foot Ankle Int* 1997;18:351-355.

Mandelbaum BR, Myerson MS, Forster R: Achilles tendon ruptures: A new method of repair, early range of motion, and functional rehabilitation. *Am J Sports Med* 1995;23:392-395.

Michelson JD, Ahn U, Magid D: Economic analysis of roentgenogram use in the closed treatment of stable ankle fractures. *J Trauma* 1995;39:1119-1122.

Michelson JD, Ahn UM, Helgemo SL: Motion of the ankle in a simulated supination-external rotation fracture model. *J Bone Joint Surg Am* 1996;78:1024-1031.

Michelson JD, Magid D, Ney DR, Fishman EK: Examination of the pathologic anatomy of ankle fractures. *J Trauma* 1992;32:65-70.

Motta P, Errichiello C, Pontini I: Achilles tendon rupture: A new technique for easy surgical repair and immediate movement of the ankle and foot. *Am J Sports Med* 1997;25:172-176.

Ogilvie-Harris DJ, Gilbart MK, Chorney K: Chronic pain following ankle sprains in athletes: The role of arthroscopic surgery. *Arthroscopy* 1997;13:564-574.

Palmer I: The mechanism and treatment of fractures of the calcaneus: Open reduction with the use of cancellous grafts. *J Bone Joint Surg Am* 1948;30:2-8.

Phillips WA, Schwartz HS, Keller CS, et al: A prospective, randomized study of the management of severe ankle fractures. *J Bone Joint Surg Am* 1985;67:67-78.

Ramsey PL, Hamilton W: Changes in tibiotalar area of contact caused by lateral talar shift. *J Bone Joint Surg Am* 1976;58:356-357.

Ruedi TP, Allgower M: The operative treatment of intra-articular fractures of the lower end of the tibia. *Clin Orthop* 1979;138:105-110.

Sanders R, Fortin P, DiPasquale T, Walling A: Operative treatment in 120 displaced intra-articular calcaneal fractures: Results using a prognostic computed tomography scan classification. *Clin Orthop* 1993;290:87-95.

Schaffer JJ, Manoli A: The antiglide plate for distal fibular fixation: A biomechanical comparison with fixation with a lateral plate. *J Bone Joint Surg Am* 1987;69:596-604.

Swanson TV, Bray TJ, Holmes GB Jr: Fractures of the talar neck: A mechanical study of fixation. *J Bone Joint Surg Am* 1992;74:544-551.

Teeny SM, Wiss DA: Open reduction and internal fixation of tibial plafond fractures: Variables contributing to poor results and complications. *Clin Orthop* 1993;292:108-117.

Thermann H, Zwipp H, Tscherne H: Treatment algorithm of chronic ankle and subtalar instability. *Foot Ankle Int* 1997;18:163-169.

Thomsen NO, Overgaard S, Olsen LH, Hansen H, Nielsen ST: Observer variation in the radiographic classification of ankle fractures. *J Bone Joint Surg Br* 1991;73:676-678.

Thordarson DB, Krieger LE: Operative vs. nonoperative treatment of intra-articular fractures of the calcaneus: A prospective randomized trial. *Foot Ankle Int* 1996;17:2-9.

Thordarson DB, Motamed S, Hedman T, Ebramzadeh E, Bakshian S: The effect of fibular malreduction on contact pressures in an ankle fracture malunion model. *J Bone Joint Surg Am* 1997;79:1809-1815.

Vander Griend R, Michelson JD, Bone LB: Fractures of the ankle and the distal part of the tibia. *Instr Course Lect* 1997;46:311-321.

Wiener BD, Linder JF, Giattini JF: Treatment of fractures of the fifth metatarsal: A prospective study. *Foot Ankle Int* 1997;18:267-269.

Wuest TK: Injuries to the distal lower extremity syndesmosis. *J Am Acad Orthop Surg* 1997;5:172-181.

Wyrsch B, McFerran MA, McAndrew M, et al: Operative treatment of fractures of the tibial plafond: A randomized, prospective study. *J Bone Joint Surg Am* 1996;78:1646-1657.

Yablon IG, Heller FG, Shouse L: The key role of the lateral malleolus in displaced fractures of the ankle. *J Bone Joint Surg Am* 1977;59:169-173.

Yablon IG, Leach RE: Reconstruction of malunited fractures of the lateral malleolus. *J Bone Joint Surg Am* 1989;71:521-527.

Chapter 47

Ankle and Foot Reconstruction

Linda R. Ferris, MBBS, BSc, FRACS

Michael S. Pinzur, MD

Steven Weinfeld, MD

Hindfoot and Ankle Reconstruction

The subtalar joint is responsible for inversion and eversion of the hindfoot, whereas the ankle allows for 90% of plantar flexion and dorsiflexion of the foot. When the hindfoot is in varus position, the transverse tarsal joints are rigid, allowing for stability during toe-off. With the heel in valgus position, the foot is more supple, allowing for better shock absorption and accommodation on uneven surfaces. With the hindfoot fixed in varus position, the foot is stiff and transfers increased stresses to the midfoot and ankle during gait. Equinus contracture also alters the mechanics of the foot and may contribute to many deformities seen throughout the foot and ankle.

Adult Acquired Flatfoot

The painful flatfoot deformity may be caused by rupture of the posterior tibial tendon, degenerative arthritis of the midfoot or hindfoot, diabetic Charcot neuroarthropathy, or inflammatory arthritis of the hindfoot. Posterior tibial tendon insufficiency, the most frequent cause of flatfoot deformity, leads to attenuation of the medial supporting structures of the foot, lowering of the longitudinal arch, heel valgus alignment, and ultimately hindfoot and ankle arthritis. Stage I is characterized by pain and swelling of the medial ankle region, with pain then progressing into the arch. Stage II is characterized by dynamic hindfoot valgus deformity, attenuation of the spring ligament, and progressive flattening of the longitudinal arch. Stage III includes a fixed hindfoot valgus deformity. Stage IV exhibits secondary changes of the ankle joint and stretching of the deltoid ligament.

Physical examination reveals the inability to perform a single leg heel rise with the affected limb. Late symptoms include lateral calcaneofibular impingement with collapse of the arch and difficulty with ambulation. Variable amounts of forefoot abduction occur, leading to the "too many toes" sign. Weight-bearing radio-

graphs show lowering of the longitudinal arch, decrease in calcaneal pitch, increase of the talometatarsal angle, and uncovering of the talonavicular joint with increasing forefoot abduction. In advanced cases, attenuation of the deltoid ligament leads to valgus tilting of the ankle mortise. Etiology is related to obesity, diabetes, accessory navicular, inflammatory arthritis, and steroid injections.

Treatment of posterior tibial tendon insufficiency consists of immobilization and nonsteroidal anti-inflammatory drugs (NSAIDs) for the stage I patient who has pain but no deformity. Custom-molded orthotic insoles or a University of California Biomechanics Laboratory type orthosis also may be useful. Surgical treatment is indicated if nonsurgical measures have failed. There may be a limited role for posterior tibial tendon débridement or flexor digitorum longus transfer alone in patients with tenosynovitis and preserved architecture of the hindfoot. Once the heel has progressed into valgus deformity, a flexor digitorum tendon transfer to the navicular along with a medial calcaneal slide osteotomy to shift the axis of the Achilles tendon medially may be performed. Repair of the attenuated spring ligament and deltoid ligament may be useful in correction of hindfoot alignment, but this method is controversial. A lengthening of the Achilles tendon may be indicated if contracture is present. In patients with a rigid deformity and arthritis of the hindfoot, arthrodesis is often necessary. Fusion of the subtalar, talonavicular, calcaneocuboid joints, or combinations of these are used to stabilize the hindfoot. Lateral column lengthening through an osteotomy of the calcaneal neck or calcaneocuboid fusion may also be useful in conjunction with flexor digitorum longus tendon transfer.

Ankle Arthritis

Ankle arthritis may be seen secondary to ankle or pilon fracture, long-standing ankle instability, osteonecrosis of the talus, and inflammatory or other degenerative conditions. The diagnosis is usually confirmed with radiographic narrowing of the tibiotalar joint. Nonsurgical treatment consists of NSAIDs, external support such as with an ankle-foot orthosis (such as the Arizona brace), physical therapy, and corticosteroid injections. The severity of radiographic findings may not necessarily correlate with the patient's symptoms, so treatment should be focused in relation to the level of dysfunction.

In some cases of ankle arthritis, the osteophytes are seen anteriorly at the tibiotalar articulation. These patients may achieve symptomatic improvement with anterior cheilectomy and resection of a portion of the anterior tibia and osteophytes from the talus. With diffuse arthritis, ankle arthrodesis remains the procedure of choice for pain relief and restoration of stability of the lower limb. Arthrodesis may be performed with a limited open or arthroscopic technique using internal fixation with 6.5- or 7.3-mm compression screws. Open transfibular ankle arthrodesis may be required for correction of major deformity. The optimal position for ankle fusion is 0° to 5° of heel valgus alignment, neutral rotation, and neutral dorsiflexion-plantar flexion. This position aids in ambulation and decreases stress placed on adjacent joints of the midfoot and hindfoot.

Recently, total ankle replacement has been under renewed investigation as an alternative to arthrodesis. Early results have been encouraging, but patients should be carefully counseled about the risks because failure of this procedure may lead to amputation.

Rheumatoid Arthritis

Rheumatoid arthritis often affects the hindfoot and forefoot, and less commonly the midfoot and ankle. In the hindfoot, the talonavicular joint is most often affected. The hindfoot is warm and swollen, with limited inversion and eversion associated with pain, and there may be varying degrees of deformity. Nonsurgical treatment consists of bracing, NSAIDs, and judicious use of corticosteroid injections. Synovitis of the ankle should be differentiated from arthritis of the talonavicular joint. Synovitis may be treated with appropriate medical therapy and selective corticosteroid injections. Immobilization may be necessary to decrease the inflammation. Synovectomy may be useful if medical treatment fails in a joint with well-preserved architecture. Selective arthrodesis remains the mainstay of surgical treatment of hindfoot arthritis, attempting to preserve as many hindfoot joints as possible. Angular deformities of the hindfoot should be corrected at the time of arthrodesis to decrease shear forces transmitted to the ankle.

Cavus Foot

In cavus foot deformity, the forefoot is in equinus position in relation to the hindfoot and there is forefoot valgus deformity leading to an abnormally high arched foot. Clawing of the toes often accompanies this condition. The cavus foot may be seen in a variety of disorders such as Charcot-Marie-Tooth disease, cerebral palsy, myelomeningocele, poliomyelitis, and residual clubfoot. Weight bearing distribution may be altered in the cavus foot, with high pressures seen at the first and fifth metatarsals and the heel.

A neurologic evaluation may be helpful in patients presenting with a cavus foot. Muscle imbalance is usually present regardless of etiology, with the extrinsic muscles overpowering the dysfunctional intrinsic muscles. Overpull of the anterior and posterior tibial muscles, along with weakness of the peroneus brevis, leads to varus alignment of the hindfoot. The peroneus longus acts to cause plantar flexion of the first ray, increasing the lateral first metatarsocalcaneal angle. Dysfunction of the intrinsic musculature also contributes to the development of claw toes.

Evaluation of the patient with a painful cavus foot should include assessment of hindfoot and forefoot flexibility manually and with the Coleman block test. The patient is examined for muscle strength, balance, and sensory nerve function. Electrodiagnostic studies may be helpful in determination of muscle function. Weight-bearing AP and lateral radiographs should be obtained.

Treatment of the painful cavus foot consists of both nonsurgical and surgical reconstructive measures. Nonsurgical treatment includes a custom-molded orthosis to support the arch with a metatarsal pad proximal to the metatarsal heads to relieve pressure in this area. Lateral posting of the orthosis may help control excessive supination of the hindfoot. Shoe wear modifications are helpful in cushioning the foot at heel strike and stabilizing the foot at toe-off. In cases associated with a foot drop, an ankle-foot orthosis may be useful.

Reconstruction of the painful cavus foot is a challenging endeavor. Surgical treatment may require a combination of soft-tissue releases, osteotomies, and arthrodeses. Soft-tissue releases include division of the plantar fascia, short flexor origin, abductor hallucis, and long and short plantar ligaments from the calcaneus. Lengthening of the posterior tibial tendon, extensor hallucis longus, and Achilles tendon may be necessary. In the cavus foot, overpull of the peroneus longus may be neutralized by lengthening of this tendon or transfer to the peroneus brevis tendon. Either the tibialis posterior or tibialis anterior tendon may be subcutaneously transferred laterally to the cuboid to aid in soft-tissue balancing of the hindfoot and midfoot.

Transfer of the extensor hallucis longus to the first metatarsal neck with hallux interphalangeal fusion (Jones procedure) corrects clawing of the hallux and facilitates dorsiflexion of the first ray. Bony procedures include a lateral closing wedge osteotomy of the calcaneus (Dwyer osteotomy) to correct hindfoot varus deformity and dorsiflexion osteotomy of the first metatarsal to decrease the forefoot equinus deformity. Triple arthrodesis may be useful in patients with fixed deformities of the hindfoot associated with arthritic changes on radiographic evaluation.

Plantar Fasciitis

Plantar fasciitis is characterized by insidious onset of medial plantar heel pain that is worse upon arising out of bed or after sitting for a period of time. Patients often state the pain decreases after the first few steps of the day and returns later in the evening. The etiology is frequently unknown, but a careful history may reveal increased activity levels, weight gain, or changes in shoe wear as the inciting factor. Physical examination shows point tenderness at the medial origin of the plantar fascia or distally along the plantar fascia. Some patients also exhibit sensitivity of the first branch of the lateral plantar nerve. Nonsurgical treatment is successful in almost all cases, although patient frustration level may be high. A regimen of Achilles tendon and plantar fascia stretching combined with activity modification, NSAIDs, heel cushions or arch supports, a dorsiflexion night splint, and corticosteroid injections may be successful in the majority of patients. Corticosteroid injections should be used with caution because atrophy of the plantar fat pad and frank rupture of the plantar fascia have been reported. Recalcitrant cases may benefit from cast immobilization for several weeks. Surgical treatment is indicated in those rare patients with persistent pain despite at least 6 to 9 months of appropriate nonsurgical treatment. Shock wave therapy, used for several years in Europe to treat plantar fasciitis, is currently being evaluated in experimental trials in the United States. Surgical release of the medial plantar fascia is performed through a medial incision with release of up to 50% of the plantar fascia, and the abductor hallucis fascia is divided to decompress the lateral plantar nerve. Endoscopic release of the plantar fascia has been recently advocated, but complications, including nerve laceration, may limit its usefulness.

Forefoot and Midfoot Reconstruction

Hallux Valgus

Hallux valgus deformity affects women more frequently than men. The deformity consists of a lateral

TABLE 1 | Etiology of Hallux Valgus Deformity

Shoe wear

Genetic predisposition

Trauma

Rheumatoid arthritis

Neuromuscular conditions

Diabetes mellitus

Pes planus/pronation

Metatarsus primus varus

Developmental bony deformity

    Increased distal metatarsal articular angle

Collagen disorders

    Marfan syndrome

    Ehlers-Danlos syndrome

Disorders of the first metatarsocuneiform joint

    Lisfranc injury

    Degenerative joint disease

    Hypermobility

Lesser toe deformity

    Second metatarsophalangeal joint dislocation

    Crossover toe deformity

    Amputation of the second toe

Cystic degeneration of the medial capsule of the first metatarsophalangeal joint

deviation of the toe with pronation and is usually associated with metatarsus primus varus deformity and prominence of the medial eminence. The problem is caused or aggravated by modern shoes, especially the narrow toe box of many women's shoes. Other etiologic factors may predispose to hallux valgus deformity (Table 1).

The patient presents with pain at the medial eminence of the first metatarsal head associated with mechanical irritation from shoe wear. In some cases, medial eminence bursitis or skin ulceration may be present. Occasionally there is no pain but the deformity may be clinically relevant because of the association with a crossover toe deformity. Physical examination includes assessment of deformity severity, range of motion of the first metatarsophalangeal joint, prominence and tenderness of the medial eminence, reducibility of the deformity, presence of hallux valgus interphalangeus (valgus alignment of the proximal phalanx or interphalangeal joint), excessive mobility of the first metatarsocuneiform joint, and associated deformities

TABLE 2	**Radiographic Information for Assessment of Hallux Valgus Deformity**

First and second intermetatarsal angle

Hallux valgus angle

Relative first and second metatarsal length

Sesamoid position

Medial eminence

Arthrosis

    First metatarsophalangeal joint

    First metatarsocuneiform joint

Distal metatarsal articular angle

Congruency of first metatarsophalangeal joint

Alignment of first metatarsocuneiform joint

Lesser toe deformity

    Second metatarsophalangeal joint dislocation

    Hammer toe

    Crossover second toe

Hallux valgus interphalangeus

    Deformity of hallux proximal phalanx

    Hallux proximal-distal phalanx angle

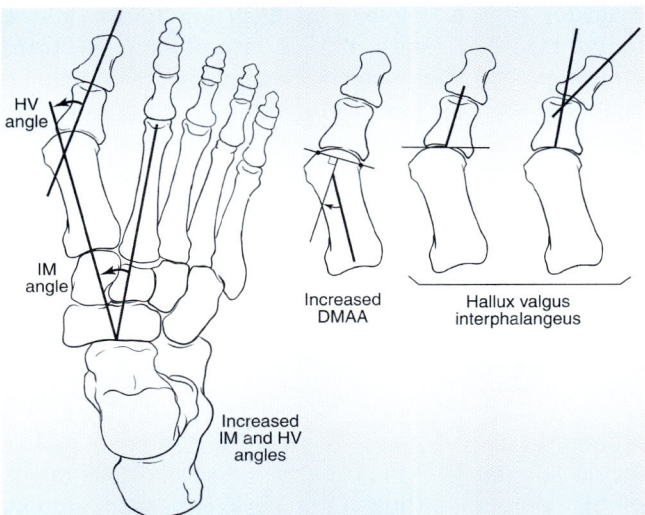

Figure 1 Quantitative assessment of hallux valgus deformity. HV = hallux valgus; IM = intermetatarsal; DMMA = distal metatarsal articular angle

betic neuropathy. Cosmesis alone is not an indication for surgery in the asymptomatic patient because residual pain or stiffness resulting from surgery may be worse than the preoperative status of the foot.

Several surgical procedures can be considered, based on magnitude and features of the deformity and the experience and judgment of the surgeon (Table 3). Among the most common procedures are the distal first metatarsal osteotomies, such as the chevron procedure for mild deformity, and the distal soft-tissue procedure (modified McBride) with or without proximal first metatarsal osteotomy. Proximal first metatarsal osteotomies include the crescentic, closing or opening wedge, proximal chevron, or proximal oblique osteotomies. A medial-based closing wedge osteotomy of the proximal phalanx (Akin) may be added for treatment of hallux valgus interphalangeus. The distal soft-tissue procedure with first metatarsocuneiform arthrodesis (Lapidus procedure) is used if an associated disorder (hypermobility, arthrosis, varus malalignment) of the first metatarsocuneiform joint is present.

Complications associated with hallux valgus surgery include pain, joint stiffness (scarring or joint incongruence), residual swelling, sensitive scar tissue, inadequate correction, hallux varus deformity, recurrent deformity, infection, degenerative arthrosis, cutaneous neuroma or nerve entrapment, nonunion or malunion of an osteotomy, shortening of the first metatarsal, and transfer metatarsalgia. The potential risk of osteonecrosis of the first metatarsal head after the chevron osteotomy may be decreased by avoiding lateral soft-tissue dissection. The risk of postoperative displacement of a chevron osteotomy may be decreased with internal fixation (screw, wire, or absorbable pin) or postoperative casting. The proximal osteotomy may be

such as lesser toe deformity. Weight-bearing radiographs of the foot may reveal bony malalignment, prominent medial eminence, arthrosis, metatarsosesamoid subluxation, and other factors important in considering treatment options (Table 2) (Fig. 1).

Nonsurgical symptomatic treatment includes shoes with a wide, soft toe box, avoidance of seams at the bunion, and stretching of the toe box at the bony prominence with a shoemaker's shoe stretcher. If there is pes planus, hallux pronation, and plantar medial callus of the hallux, an orthotic device with a medial forefoot post may provide pain relief. However, there is no evidence that orthotic insoles prevent progression of the deformity.

Surgery is considered primarily for treatment of pain and difficulty with shoe wear refractory to nonsurgical treatment. Surgery for an asymptomatic bunion may be considered in the very limited cases where shoe irritation is caused by an associated crossover second toe deformity, in which the hallux tip impinges near the third toe because of dorsal subluxation and instability of the second toe. Another indication for surgery is ulceration at the bony prominence, especially in the patient with dia-

TABLE 3 | Guidelines for Surgical Procedures for Hallux Valgus Deformity*

Procedure	Indications[†]
Silver exostectomy	Localized prominence with little hallux valgus
	Bedridden patient
	Ulceration
Distal first metatarsal osteotomy (chevron)	Mild deformity (IM < 13°; HV < 30°)
Distal soft-tissue procedure (modified McBride) with or without proximal first metatarsal osteotomy (crescentic, opening or closing wedge, proximal chevron, other), or midshaft osteotomy (Mitchell)	Moderate to severe deformity (IM > 13°; HV > 30°)
Distal soft-tissue procedure (modified McBride) with first metatarsocuneiform arthrodesis (Lapidus)	First metatarsocuneiform joint problems (hypermobility, arthrosis, varus orientation)
Proximal phalanx osteotomy (Akin)	Hallux valgus interphalangeus
Biplanar chevron osteotomy	Mild hallux valgus with increased DMAA
Resection arthroplasty (Keller)	Household ambulator or bedridden patient
Arthrodesis	Arthritis, neuromuscular disease, salvage if other failed bunion procedures

*Combined procedures (such as Chevron-Akin or triple osteotomy) may be indicated in special situations
[†]IM = first and second intermetatarsal angle; HV = hallux valgus angle; DMAA = distal metatarsal articular angle

complicated by metatarsus primus elevatus and transfer metatarsalgia. Hallux varus deformity may be caused by excessive resection of the medial first metatarsal head or fibular sesamoidectomy.

Salvage of the painful, stiff, or recurrent deformity may consist of arthodesis of the first metatarsophalangeal joint. Cutaneous neuromas may be excised and the proximal stump buried in bone. Postoperative hallux varus deformity may be corrected with medial release and split extensor hallucis longus tendon transfer.

Failed implant or resection (Keller) arthroplasty may be managed with arthodesis of the first metatarsophalangeal joint. This procedure may be done by direct apposition of the short proximal phalanx to the metatarsal without an interposition graft, leaving the foot with a functional albeit cosmetically short first ray. An alternate method that may maintain length is the use of an interposition tricortical iliac crest bone graft, but there may be a potentially greater risk of nonunion, delayed union, or postoperative infection. Implant arthroplasty for treatment of hallux valgus deformity is not usually advised because of potential complications, including implant loosening and failure. Silastic implants are most commonly used but are associated with silicone synovitis and fracture or dislocation of the prosthesis.

Hallux Rigidus

Hallux rigidus is a progressive degenerative disorder of the first metatarsophalangeal joint associated with localized pain, limited motion, and prominent dorsal osteophytes that may cause pain in the toe box. The etiology may include trauma, developmental abnormality, or genetic predisposition. The pain is dorsal or deep at the first metatarsophalangeal joint, and is aggravated during heel rise or in closed shoes. Some patients may develop lateral weight shifting and metatarsalgia or lateral rolloff that may result in peroneal tendinitis. Physical examination of the first metatarsophalangeal joint may reveal tenderness, dorsal prominence, and pain with limited motion (plantar flexion and dorsiflexion). Radiographs may show a flat first metatarsal head with lateral squaring or osteophytes, dorsal osteophytes, and narrowing of the first metatarsophalangeal joint space.

Goals of treatment include pain relief so the patient can perform activities of daily living. Nonsurgical treatment may include activity modification, such as use of an exercise bicycle with the pedal under the midfoot instead of walking for fitness. A carbon foot plate insert or shoe modification with a rocker bottom sole may limit painful motion of the first metatarsophalangeal joint. Stretching the toe box and avoiding a seam at the dorsal osteophytes may be helpful.

Surgical options include cheilectomy. The dorsal osteophytes and up to 30% of the dorsal part of the first metatarsal head are excised, and the lateral osteophytes are débrided. Furthermore, dorsal osteophytes are excised from the base of the proximal phalanx. Intraoperative assessment of an adequate cheilectomy may include achievement of adequate dorsiflexion (70° to 90° between the proximal phalanx and first metatarsal) and relief of palpable impingement during dorsiflexion. Approximately half of the intraoperative motion may be lost during the recovery. The success rate for pain relief with cheilectomy is approximately 70% to 80%, but progressive degenerative arthritis may be anticipated. Other procedures used for hallux rigidus, especially in more advanced cases with residual limitation of motion, include a dorsal closing wedge osteotomy of the proximal phalanx (Moberg procedure). Advanced cases of hallux rigidus may be primarily treated with arthrodesis of the first metatarsophalangeal joint, but women may elect cheilectomy over an arthrodesis to enable broader selection of shoes with low heels. Salvage of failed cheilectomy may include revision cheilectomy or arthrodesis of the first metatarsophalangeal joint.

The role of resection (Keller), interposition, and implant arthroplasty in hallux rigidus remains controversial. Resection arthroplasty may destabilize the hallux, and may be complicated by cockup deformity of the hallux, transfer metatarsalgia, and hallux valgus deformity. Interposition of the extensor hallucis brevis by suturing this tendon to the flexor hallucis brevis may stabilize the toe and prevent these complications. Implant arthroplasty of the first metatarsophalangeal joint has very limited indications because of complications including synovitis, osteolysis, and the complications associated with resection arthroplasty (cock-up deformity of the hallux with transfer metatarsalgia) regardless of implant type (silicone implant, grommets, titanium hemiarthroplasty, or total toe implant).

Arthrodesis of the First Metatarsophalangeal Joint

Arthrodesis of the first metatarsophalangeal joint is the most effective procedure for long-term pain relief of arthritis. For patients with rheumatoid arthritis, in which soft-tissue healing may be impaired, arthrodesis of the first metatarsophalangeal joint is the primary procedure for surgical management of hallux valgus deformity and is a primary component of reconstruction for rheumatoid forefoot deformity.

Several techniques are available for arthrodesis of the first metatarsophalangeal joint. Preparation of the arthrodesis surfaces may be done with a flat-cut joint resection or dome-reaming technique. Fixation may be done with screws, Kirschner wires, threaded Steinmann

pins, or a screw-plate construct. A low-profile mandibular plate has become available in recent years, with perhaps fewer postoperative symptoms necessitating hardware removal than previously.

The position of arthrodesis is important, but not universally agreed upon. The optimal position of the hallux includes neutral rotation, 10° to 15° of valgus, and 10° to 15° of dorsiflexion relative to the long axis of the foot. This position should allow the hallux to fit comfortably in the toe box parallel to the second toe and provide some rolloff during heel rise. Excessive dorsiflexion may cause painful impingement of the toe against the toe box, and excessive plantar flexion may cause interphalangeal joint arthrosis and lateral weight shifting during heel rise. At surgery, the plantar aspect of the foot is held against a flat surface to simulate the floor, with the ankle in neutral position, and approximately 1 cm of space will be present between the hallux toe pad and the flat surface.

Complications include nonunion and malunion. A painless fibrous union may be managed with observation. Depending on symptoms, malunion may be managed with a rocker bottom sole shoe modification or osteotomy and realignment.

Rheumatoid Forefoot Deformity

This deformity consists of a combination of hallux valgus deformity, hammer toe deformity, lesser metatarsophalangeal joint synovitis and dislocation, and crossover lesser toe deformity. The lesser toe dislocations are associated with distal migration of the plantar fat pad and plantar prominence of the lesser metatarsal heads. This condition may cause metatarsalgia (the sensation of "walking on stones") and occasionally plantar ulceration.

Nonsurgical treatment may include a rocker bottom sole shoe, extra depth toe box, and a full-length Plastazote or padded custom-molded insole. Surgical management includes arthrodesis of the first metatarsophalangeal joint combined with lesser metatarsal head resection arthroplasty and hammer toe repair. Complications include wound dehiscence that can usually be managed with dressing changes and antibiotics.

Lesser Toe Problems

Deformities of the lesser toes include hammer toe (flexion at the proximal interphalangeal [PIP] joint), mallet toe (flexion of the distal interphalangeal [DIP] joint), and claw toe (flexion of the PIP and DIP joints and extension contracture of the metatarsophalangeal joint). The deformities may be flexible or fixed.

Contributing causes to hammer toe may include a long second or third ray and small toe box. Mallet toes are often a result of arthritis of the DIP joint such as from osteoarthritis with a long toe or psoriatic arthritis. Claw toes may be associated with diabetic neuropathy, rheumatoid arthritis, compartment syndrome, and cavus foot deformity. Synovitis of the second metatarsophalangeal joint may cause joint laxity progressing to dislocation and crossover toe deformity (varus second toe dorsal to a hallux valgus deformity).

Pain from these conditions may be a result of dorsal irritation of the PIP or DIP joint on the dorsum of the toe box, irritation of the tip of the toe, or metatarsalgia associated with distal migration of the plantar fat pad and intractable plantar keratosis. Examination includes assessment of the flexibility or rigidity of the deformity.

Nonsurgical treatment may include use of a wide toe box or stretching the toe box, toe props, and pads. Synovitis may be treated with an intra-articular corticosteroid injection and use of a shoe with a rocker bottom sole. Surgical treatment may include a combination of procedures to address different components of the deformity. Extensor contracture may be improved with extensor tenotomies (extensor longus and brevis) and metatarsophalangeal joint capsulotomy. Fixed deformity may be managed with resection arthroplasty (DuVries) of the PIP or DIP joint. Flexible deformity may be corrected with a Girdlestone-Taylor flexor to extensor tendon transfer. Synovitis may be managed with synovectomy. Intractable plantar keratosis may be improved with a DuVries metatarsophalangeal arthroplasty. Crossover toe deformity may require a lesser metatarsophalangeal DuVries arthroplasty with or without lateral capsule reefing and correction of the hallux valgus deformity.

Several types of metatarsal osteotomy have been used for the treatment of metatarsalgia resulting from a prominent second metatarsal head or an intractable plantar keratosis. The distal metatarsal neck or midshaft (long oblique) osteotomies with dorsal displacement of the metatarsal head may be complicated by malunion, nonunion, and persistent keratosis. The Helal sliding osteotomy has a high complication rate due mainly to uncontrolled shortening and displacement and is not recommended. The distal metatarsal osteotomy done in the plane of the foot, with proximal translation of the distal fragment (Weil osteotomy), has been the subject of study in recent years. Proximal translation of the distal fragment may be associated with plantar translation of the metatarsal head, which may aggravate the metatarsalgia. Furthermore, the relative dorsal shift of the intrinsic tendons may cause an extension deformity at the metatarsophalangeal joint and predispose to claw toe deformity. However, some surgeons have found this procedure helpful in the treatment of metatarsalgia.

Interdigital Neuroma

Interdigital neuroma is a potential cause of forefoot pain. The condition is more common in women because of the narrow toe box of many women's shoes. The third and second interspaces are most commonly involved, and concurrent involvement of two interspaces in the same foot is uncommon. It has been hypothesized that the interdigital nerve may be irritated, compressed, or bowstrung under the intermetatarsal ligament from overuse or while wearing shoes with high heels.

In addition to forefoot pain, the patient may experience paresthesias or numbness at the involved web space and adjacent toes. Examination reveals tenderness isolated to the involved interspace, and occasionally a mechanical click (Mulder sign) is felt with mediolateral metatarsal head compression as the neuroma slides between the metatarsal heads and under the intermetatarsal ligament.

Nonsurgical treatment may include a wide toe box, metatarsal pad, interdigital corticosteroid injection, shoe with a rocker bottom sole, and avoidance of high-heeled shoes. Surgical excision may be done for persistent pain. The failure rate of surgical treatment is approximately 20%, and may be associated with incomplete neurectomy, recurrent neuroma, rheumatoid arthritis, or diagnostic error. The differential diagnosis may include other causes of metatarsalgia such as metatarsophalangeal synovitis, metatarsophalangeal instability, Freiberg's infraction, and stress fracture. Recurrent pain after primary neurectomy may be caused by a stump neuroma that may be managed by revision neurectomy, with excision of a greater length of nerve. A dorsal or plantar approach may be used for both primary and revision neurectomy, but the plantar approach may be complicated by a painful scar in a weight-bearing region. In diagnostically difficult cases, local anesthetic injection, ultrasonography, or MRI may be helpful. In the rare cases in which simultaneous resection of two interdigital neuromas in one foot is done, the number of patients who have pain relief is similar to that achieved when a single neuroma is excised.

Midfoot Problems

The differential diagnosis of midfoot pain includes tarsometatarsal (Lisfranc) injury, degenerative arthritis, rheumatoid arthritis, stress fracture, infection plantar fascia rupture or release, and Charcot arthropathy. In addition, medial midfoot pain may be caused by accessory navicular syndrome or posterior tibial tendinopathy, and lateral midfoot pain may be a result of peroneal tendinopathy, painful os peroneum syndrome, or cuboid subluxation.

Degenerative arthritis of the midfoot may be caused by Lisfranc fracture-dislocation, plantar ligament rupture, pes planus, or cavus foot. Nonsurgical treatment may include activity modification, custom orthotic insoles, and full-length rocker bottom sole shoe modification. Surgical treatment may depend on the site of arthritis. Use of selective injection of local anesthetic may help to determine which joints contribute to pain. Pain relief from tarsometatarsal and naviculocuneiform arthritis may be achieved with arthrodesis, usually accomplished with internal screw fixation. Realignment may be required if deformity is present. In the fourth and fifth metatarsocuboid joints, arthrodesis may be complicated by a higher incidence of postoperative stiffness and nonunion. Resection arthroplasty of the fourth and fifth metatarsocuboid joints, with interposition of a soft-tissue spacer made from the peroneus tertius tendon, may provide good pain relief with minimal midfoot stiffness.

Diabetic Foot and Ankle

Diabetic foot ulcers precede 85% of nontraumatic lower extremity amputations. Diabetic foot infection is the ninth most common hospital discharge diagnosis in the United States. At any point in time, 3% to 4% of patients with diabetes have a foot ulcer or deep infection, and 15% develop a foot ulcer during their lifetime. Once a foot ulcer or infection develops, the likelihood of these patients to undergo lower extremity amputation increases eightfold. Two years after transtibial amputation for diabetes or peripheral vascular disease, 36% of subjects will have died.

Risk Factors

Loss of protective sensation from peripheral neuropathy is the primary risk factor for the development of diabetic foot ulcers or deep infection. The second important risk factor is peripheral vascular disease. Further complicating wound healing is the malnutrition related to chronic renal disease.

Diabetic Neuropathy/Peripheral Neuropathy

Diabetic neuropathy affects the sensory, motor, and autonomic pathways. This neuropathy appears in a stocking-glove distribution, with affected individuals complaining of burning or searing pain. Motor neuropathy leads to muscle weakness and intrinsic muscle atrophy in both the hands and feet. These individuals have severe impairments in hand grip strength, and are susceptible to bunion, claw toe, and hammer toe defor-

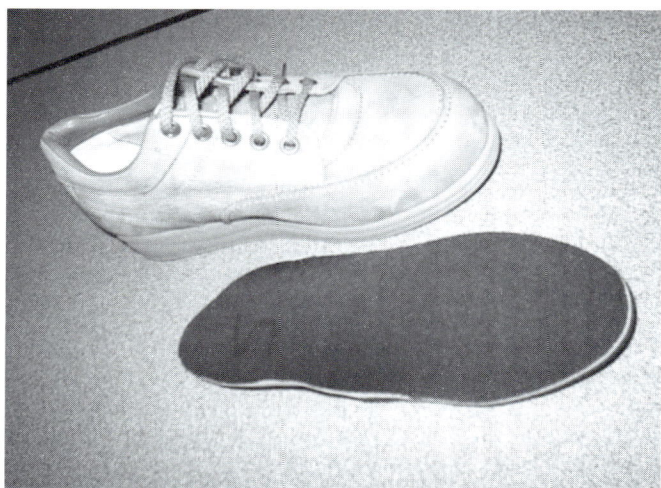

Figure 2 Depth-inlay soft leather laced shoe with custom accommodative pressure-dissipating foot orthotic device.

mities from muscle imbalance. Patients with diabetes will often have increased venous swelling that can only be managed with compression hose. The swelling may become pathogenic because the swollen tissues are less able to tolerate the stresses of weight bearing. Autonomic dysfunction causes loss of skin sweating, leading to dry and scaly foot skin. This dry skin is susceptible to cracks, allowing the entry of bacteria. Nail deformity or pathologic proliferation may make the areas adjacent to the nails foci for skin breaks or infection.

Each of these potential abnormalities make the diabetic foot susceptible to abnormal mechanical stresses that can lead to a break in the normal soft-tissue envelope and initiate a foot infection that cannot easily be resolved. Peripheral neuropathy needs to be monitored, because of its 25% incidence in diabetic patients. Once present, neuropathy is progressive with time.

Preventive Strategies

Preventive strategies combine foot-specific patient education, prophylactic skin and nail care, and protective footwear. Individualized foot-specific patient education is the most important element of a comprehensive diabetic foot program. Soft leather or athletic footwear decreases the risk of tissue breakdown from direct pressure (Fig. 2). Cushioned stockings are helpful. White socks make identification of skin breakdown easier, especially in individuals with impaired vision. Nails should be cut transversely to decrease the risk of an ingrown toenail. Once a problem arises, the patient is instructed to seek medical attention immediately. Often, the earliest sign of infection is volatility in maintaining blood sugars with slowly increasing insulin requirement. When applied to diabetic populations, these preventive programs have been shown to mark-

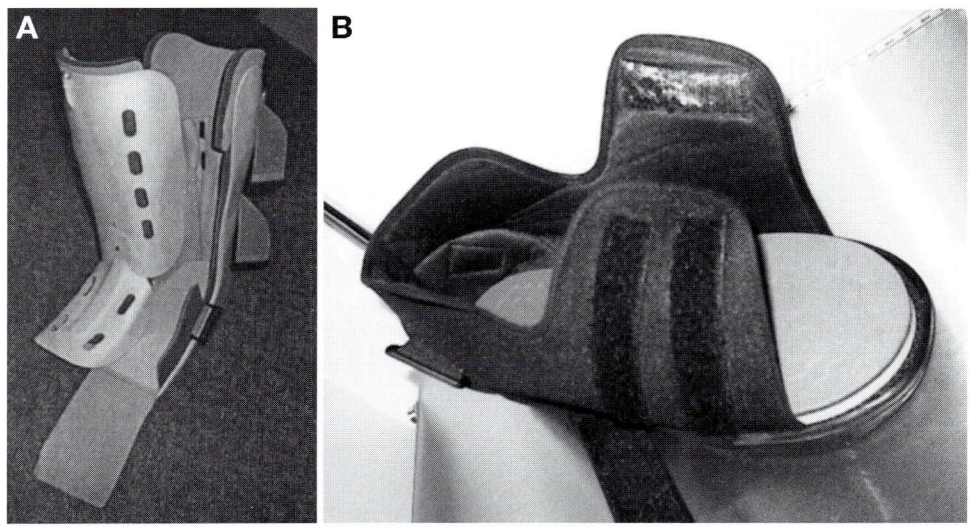

Figure 3 **A,** Removable walking boot with Plastazote lined weight-bearing surface. **B,** "Healing shoe".

edly decrease the risk of diabetic foot ulcers and lower extremity amputation.

When individuals progress to a higher degree of risk, accommodative footwear and prophylactic skin and nail care are required. Depth-inlay soft leather laced oxford shoes with accommodative pressure and shear-dissipating custom foot orthoses (insoles) have been shown to appreciably decrease the development of diabetic foot ulcers. Calluses should be cut to decrease the incidence of shear-mediated ulcer formation. Skin and nail care in these individuals should be performed by a trained professional.

Ulcer Treatment

The first step in the treatment of a diabetic foot ulcer is optimal medical management of the systemic diabetes. All ulcers should be probed with a sterile probe. If the probe comes into direct contact with bone, the presence of osteomyelitis should be assumed. Ulcers can be neuropathic or ischemic. Neuropathic ulcers are caused by pressure or shear. Once the ulcer is unroofed and the necrotic tissue is débrided, the soft-tissue base may reveal healthy granulation tissue. Neuropathic ulcers require débridement of nonviable or infected tissue, combined with local wound care and offloading. If the ulcer is unroofed, and the tissue at the base is necrotic, the ulcer is likely to be ischemic. Patients with ischemic ulcers should be evaluated by a vascular surgeon to determine whether the limb can be salvaged. A risk-benefit analysis can then be done to determine whether treatment should consist of limb salvage, amputation, or a combination of both (partial foot amputation combined with vascular bypass surgery). If the ulcer is neuropathic, noninvasive vascular testing is in order if pedal pulses are not palpable. From a practical standpoint, vascular surgery consulta-

tion is not imperative unless the patient is symptomatic with ischemic pain or a nonhealing ulcer. Ischemic ulcers generally require angioplasty or vascular bypass surgery to achieve wound healing.

Wet-to-dry wound care may promote granulation, but dry wounds may lead to desiccation and death of wound-healing cells. Dry wounds may be kept moist with either saline-soaked dressings or hydrocolloid gels. Wounds that produce massive quantities of exudate may be treated with absorbant materials (calcium alginate) and dressings, while keeping the wound moist. Growth factor gels have been shown to promote wound healing in wounds with reasonable wound-healing potential. Hyperbaric oxygen therapy is controversial, but has been shown to promote wound healing in individuals who exhibit a positive oxygen challenge (increased local transcutaneous oxygen tension when breathing 100% oxygen).

Off-loading distributes weight-bearing pressure over a larger surface area and provides an interface to decrease shear forces. Elimination of weight bearing is generally not required. The optimal off-loading device is the total contact cast, which dissipates weight bearing and shearing loads by the elimination of foot or ankle motion, using an interface material to distribute pressure and shear. Venous swelling is lessened by the compression effect of the cast. When the ulcer shows appreciable improvement, care can be simplified with prefabricated walking braces that have a plantar weight-bearing surface lined with Plastazote or other pressure-dissipating materials. When the swelling decreases, or ankle immobilization is not necessary, "healing" shoes can be used (Fig. 3). A grading system based on the depth of the ulcer that was very useful in directing treatment was updated to include an appre-

TABLE 4 | Depth-Ischemia Classification of Diabetic Foot Lesions

	Definition	Treatment
Depth Classification		
0	"At-risk" foot, no ulceration	Patient education, accommodative footwear, regular clinical examination
1	Superficial ulceration, not infected	Off-loading with total contact cast, walking brace, or special footwear
2	Deep ulceration exposing tendons or joints	Surgical débridement, wound care, off-loading, culture-specific antibiotics
3	Extensive ulceration or abscess	Débridement or partial amputation, offloading, culture-specific antibiotics
Ischemia Classification		
A	Not ischemic	
B	Ischemia without gangrene	Noninvasive vascular testing, vascular consultation if symptomatic
C	Partial (forefoot) gangrene	Vascular consultation
D	Complete foot gangrene	Major extremity amputation, vascular consultation

(Adapted with permission from Brodsky J: The diabetic foot, in Coughlin MJ, Mann RA (eds): *Surgery of the Foot and Ankle.* St Louis, MO, Mosby, 1999, p 911.)

ciation of the often associated peripheral vascular disease (Table 4).

After wound healing has occurred, off-loading should be implemented permanently. The plantigrade foot can be managed with depth-inlay soft leather oxford laced shoes and custom accommodative foot orthoses. When plantigrade alignment cannot be obtained, an ankle-foot orthosis or surgical reconstruction/stabilization is necessary.

Persistent or Recurrent Ulceration

Ulcers that do not heal, or recur in appropriate footwear, require careful evaluation. Recurrent ulceration is caused by persistent infection, failure to relieve localized pressure, or ischemia. Heel impact or increased forefoot loading can be lessened with a cushioned heel and/or rocker bottom sole modification of the shoe. Surgery should be considered when accommodative methods are unsuccessful. Increased forefoot loading, or ankle equinus (static or dynamic), can be treated with percutaneous Achilles tendon lengthening followed by immobilization in a below-knee walking cast for 4 to 6 weeks. Plastic surgery intervention with rotational flaps or free tissue transfer is occasionally indicated. The key to success in the face of recurrent ulceration is patient education, accommodative pedorthic footwear, and careful monitoring.

Prescription Writing

The Medicare Therapeutic Shoe Bill of 1993 provides financial support for one pair of appropriate inlay depth shoes and three pairs of custom foot orthoses yearly for individuals with diabetes. Most insurance carriers have developed similar guidelines; preventive strategies are cost-effective. The certified pedorthist is an essential consultant in providing these devices. The Bill requires that the prescription be signed by both the physician treating the diabetes and the orthopaedic surgeon or podiatrist treating the foot.

Charcot Foot

Charcot foot is a hypertrophic osteoarthropathy currently seen primarily in diabetic patients with peripheral neuropathy. The etiology is neurotraumatic or neurovascular. The traumatic etiology implies fracture or stress fracture without protective sensation. The hypertrophic response is caused by the inherent motion applied to a nonimmobilized fracture. The vascular etiology implies an abnormal vascular inflow, producing bony resorption, bony weakening, and a similar end result.

Stage I is the development phase of the disease. The foot is very swollen. Radiographs may reveal soft-tissue swelling early, or an acute fracture or dislocation. Stage II is the proliferative period, combining local bony destruction with the periarticular fracture or dislocation. Stage III is the phase of consolidation, or "healing", where patients are left with mechanical deformities.

Treatment has historically been anecdotal with only recent attempts at a scientific approach. The foot with active disease is immobilized in a total contact cast

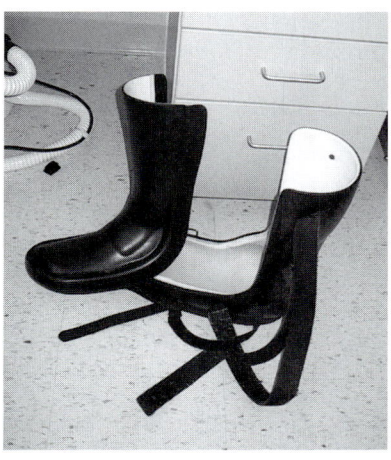

Figure 4 Charcot Restraining Orthotic Walker (CROW). *(Reproduced with permission from Morgan JM, Biehl WC III, Wagner FWW Jr: Management of neuropathic arthropathy with the Charcot Restraint Orthotic Walker. Clin Orthop 1993;296: 58-63.)*

or a prefabricated device. Weight-bearing status is controversial. At stage III, treatment has historically been accommodative, most recently with a specialized type of ankle-foot orthosis, the Charcot Restraining Orthotic Walker (CROW) (Fig. 4). If plantigrade alignment cannot be maintained, or if deformity begins to develop, early surgical stabilization/reconstruction to achieve plantigrade alignment has been recommended. Surgery is advised for bony infection, nonhealing ulcers, or deformity that cannot be accommodated with a custom orthosis.

Amputation

Any discussion about the diabetic foot requires introduction of the concept of function-preserving amputation surgery. Partial and whole foot amputations are frequently necessary as a treatment for infection or gangrene. The goal of treatment is not only preservation of tissue but preservation of function. Amputation surgery should be the first step in the rehabilitation of the patient. Because most of these individuals are ambulatory, surgical planning should be directed at creating a terminal end organ of load bearing that can most easily interface with accommodative shoe wear, prosthesis, or a combination (prosthosis). The principles that direct construction of a residual limb for weight bearing with a prosthesis should be used when performing débridement or partial foot amputation.

The major value of partial foot amputation is the potential for retention of plantar load-bearing tissues that are uniquely capable of tolerating the forces involved in weight bearing. The soft-tissue envelope should be capable of minimizing these forces. Split-thickness skin grafts should be avoided in load-bearing areas. Deformity should be avoided as much as possible. Achilles tendon lengthening should be used liberally to avoid both dynamic and static equinus deformity in partial foot amputations. Retention of a deformed foot with exposed

bony prominence will only lead to decreased walking ability and recurrent ulceration.

Annotated Bibliography

Hindfoot and Ankle Reconstruction

Acevedo JI, Beskin JL: Complications of plantar fascia rupture associated with corticosteroid injection. *Foot Ankle Int* 1998;19:91-97.
Complications suffered by 44 patients with plantar fascia rupture following corticosteroid injection were reviewed. Multiple problems presented with 26 of 44 patients remaining symptomatic at 1 year after rupture.

Easley ME, Trnka HJ, Schon LC, Myerson MS: Isolated subtalar arthrodesis. *J Bone Joint Surg Am* 2000;82:613-624.
A retrospective review of 184 isolated subtalar arthrodeses with compression screw fixation is presented. The rate of union was 92% for nonsmokers and 73% for smokers. Avascular bone and previous attempts at fusion negatively affected outcome and union rate.

Felix NA, Kitaoka HB: Ankle arthrodesis in patients with rheumatoid arthritis. *Clin Orthop* 1998;349:58-64.
Twenty-six ankle arthrodeses performed in patients with rheumatoid arthritis using both external and internal fixation were followed for 5 years. Union and complication rates were comparable to those of patients with degenerative arthritis.

Hintermann B, Valderrabano V, Kundert HP: Lengthening of the lateral column and reconstruction of the medial soft tissue for treatment of acquired flatfoot deformity associated with insufficiency of the posterior tibial tendon. *Foot Ankle Int* 1999;20:622-629.
A review of 19 patients treated with lateral column lengthening and medial soft-tissue repair is presented. All patients had satisfactory alignment and restoration of arch following surgery for stage II and stage III posterior tibial tendon insufficiency, but routine use in stage III deformity is controversial.

Horton GA, Myerson MS, Parks BG, Park YW: Effect of calcaneal osteotomy and lateral column lengthening on the plantar fascia: A biomechanical investigation. *Foot Ankle Int* 1998;19:370-373.
This cadaver study measured strain on plantar fascia after sectioning of posterior tibial tendon and spring ligament and performance of either lateral column lengthening or medial slide calcaneal osteotomy. Study results showed decrease in strain on plantar fascia after both procedures.

Johnson JE, Cohen BE, DiGiovanni BF, Lamdan R: Subtalar arthrodesis with flexor digitorum longus transfer and spring ligament repair for treatment of posterior tibial tendon insufficiency. *Foot Ankle Int* 2000;21:722-729.
Sixteen patients were retrospectively reviewed following subtalar fusion and spring ligament repair with flexor digitorum longus transfer. There was good correction of hindfoot valgus deformity and forefoot abduction, along with increase in arch height.

Kitaoka HB, Luo ZP, An KN: Reconstruction operations for acquired flatfoot: Biomechanical evaluation. *Foot Ankle Int* 1998;19:203-207.

This cadaver study showed that deltoid ligament repair was more effective than flexor tendon transfer at restoration of arch alignment.

Kofoed H, Lundberg-Jensen A: Ankle arthroplasty in patients younger and older than 50 years: A prospective series with long-term follow-up. *Foot Ankle Int* 1999;20: 501-506.

One hundred patients with total ankle replacements were followed for 15 years. There was no significant difference in outcome in patients older than age 50 years compared with patients younger than age 50 years at time of surgery.

Maier M, Steinborn M, Schmitz C, et al: Extracorporeal shock wave application for chronic plantar fasciitis associated with heel spurs: Prediction of outcome by magnetic resonance imaging. *J Rheumatol* 2000;27: 2455-2462.

Forty-three patients with chronic plantar fasciitis were treated with shock wave application. Successful clinical outcome was predicted by the presence preoperatively of calcaneal bone marrow edema.

Monroe MT, Beals TC, Manoli A II: Clinical outcome of arthrodesis of the ankle using rigid internal fixation with cancellous screws. *Foot Ankle Int* 1999;20:227-231.

Thirty patients underwent ankle arthrodesis with internal fixation with average time to union of 9 weeks. Twenty-five patients were evaluated 24 months after surgery. All stated they would undergo the procedure again. Associated workers' compensation claims negatively affected results.

O'Brien TS, Hart TS, Shereff MJ, Stone J, Johnson J: Open versus arthroscopic ankle arthrodesis: A comparative study. *Foot Ankle Int* 1999;20:368-374.

A retrospective review of 36 patients undergoing ankle arthrodesis is presented. Arthroscopic technique was recommended when little or no deformity was present. Decreased blood loss, shorter tourniquet time, and shorter hospital stays were found with arthroscopic ankle fusion.

O'Malley MJ, Page A, Cook R: Endoscopic plantar fasciotomy for chronic heel pain. *Foot Ankle Int* 2000; 21:505-510.

Twenty feet in 16 patients with chronic heel pain were treated with endoscopic plantar fasciotomy. Nine patients had complete relief, with nine others reporting satisfactory results. In one patient (treated for bilateral feet) no pain relief was experienced. No iatrogenic nerve injuries were reported in this series.

Pell RF IV, Myerson MS, Schon LC: Clinical outcome after primary triple arthrodesis. *J Bone Joint Surg Am* 2000;82:47-57.

One hundred sixty patients underwent triple arthrodesis; 111 were available for follow-up. Ninety-one percent were satisfied with the procedure at 5 years. There was a high incidence of ankle arthritis on radiographs, although it was not often clinically relevant.

Pfeffer G, Bacchetti P, Deland J, et al: Comparison of custom and prefabricated orthoses in the initial treatment of proximal plantar fasciitis. *Foot Ankle Int* 1999; 20:214-221.

Two hundred thirty-six patients from a multicenter study showed that when used in conjunction with a stretching protocol, a prefabricated shoe insert was more effective than a custom-made orthosis in relieving pain in plantar fasciitis.

Pyevich MT, Saltzman CL, Callaghan JJ, Alvine FG: Total ankle arthroplasty: A unique design. Two to twelve-year follow-up. *J Bone Joint Surg Am* 1998;80: 1410-1420.

Eighty-six patients undergoing total ankle arthroplasty were followed for an average of 4.8 years. Five ankles required revision, with delayed union and nonunion of the syndesmosis an important factor in development of lysis and migration of the tibial component. Overall, patients had a 93% satisfaction rate.

Toolan BC, Sangeorzan BJ, Hansen ST Jr: Complex reconstruction for the treatment of dorsolateral peritalar subluxation of the foot: Early results after distraction arthrodesis of the calcaneocuboid joint in conjunction with stabilization of, and transfer of the flexor digitorum longus tendon to, the midfoot to treat acquired pes planovalgus in adults. *J Bone Joint Surg Am* 1999;81:1545-1560.

Of 36 patients studied, 85% had satisfactory results after reconstruction of painful pes planus combining lateral column lengthening, cuneiform osteotomy, and advancement of posterior tibial tendon. Major complication rate was 71%; complications included nonunion and sural nerve injury. Reoperation for hardware removal or bone grafting also occurred.

Forefoot and Midfoot Reconstruction

Berlet GC, Anderson RA, Davis H: Abstract: Tendon arthroplasty for basal 4th and 5th metatarsal arthritis. *67th Annual Meeting Proceedings*. Rosemont, IL, American Academy of Orthopaedic Surgeons, 2000, p 489.

In a study of 11 patients with cuboid-metatarsal arthrosis, resection arthroplasty of the fifth metatarsal base, with or without resection of the fourth metatarsal base, with tendon interposition, resulted in an improvement in pain relief of 50% and an improvement in disability of 40%.

Chou LB, Mann RA, Casillas MM: Biplanar chevron osteotomy. *Foot Ankle Int* 1998;19:579-584.

Biplanar chevron osteotomy was performed in 14 patients (17 feet) with increased distal metatarsal articular angle (DMAA). Evaluation at an average of 33 months after surgery showed that the average American Orthopaedic Foot and Ankle Society Metatarsophalangeal-Interphalangeal Score was 91 of 100 points.

Coughlin MJ: Common causes of pain in the forefoot in adults. *J Bone Joint Surg Br* 2000;82:781-790.

A review of the diagnosis and treatment of common forefoot conditions.

Coughlin MJ: Rheumatoid forefoot reconstruction: A long-term follow-up study. *J Bone Joint Surg Am* 2000;82:322-341.

A retrospective study of 32 patients (47 feet) with severe rheumatoid deformity was done at an average of 6 years after surgical treatment with first metatarsophalangeal joint arthrodesis, resection arthroplasty of the lesser metatarsal heads, and hammer toe repair. All first metatarsophalangeal joints were fused successfully, and the results were rated as excellent in 23 feet (49%), good in 22 feet (47%), and fair in 2 feet (4%).

Gazdag A, Cracchiolo A III: Surgical treatment of patients with painful instability of the second metatarsophalangeal joint. *Foot Ankle Int* 1998;19:137-143.

In 18 patients (20 feet), instability of the second metatarsophalangeal joint was managed with flexor digitorum longus transfer to the extensor side of the base of the proximal phalanx. Excellent results were achieved in 13 feet (65%).

Mulier T, Steenwerckx A, Thienpont E, et al: Results after cheilectomy in athletes with hallux rigidus. *Foot Ankle Int* 1999;20:232-237.

Cheilectomy was performed on 20 athletes (22 feet) with hallux rigidus. At a mean of 5 years after surgery, clinical results were rated as excellent or good in 21 (96%) feet.

Thomas PJ, Smith RW: Proximal phalanx osteotomy for the surgical treatment of hallux rigidus. *Foot Ankle Int* 1999;20:3-12.

In 17 patients (24 feet), hallux rigidus was managed with cheilectomy and a dorsal closing wedge osteotomy of the proximal phalanx. All patients had subjective pain improvement, but restriction of footwear was common.

Vandeputte G, Dereymaeker G, Steenwerckx A, Peeraer L: The Weil osteotomy of the lesser metatarsals: A clinical and pedobarographic follow-up study. *Foot Ankle Int* 2000;21:370-374.

In 32 patients (59 metatarsals in 37 feet), distal metatarsal shortening (Weil) osteotomy was done to treat intractable plantar keratosis or dislocation of the lesser metatarsophalangeal joint. Clinical results at an average of 30 months after surgery were good or excellent in 32 of the 37 feet (86%). Complete disappearance of the callus was noted under 44 metatarsals (75%) and partial disappearance under 12 metatarsals (20%).

Diabetic Foot and Ankle

Brodsky JW: The diabetic foot, in Coughlin MJ, Mann RA (eds): *Surgery of the Foot and Ankle*, ed 7. St Louis, MO, Mosby-Year Book, 1999, vol 2, pp 895-969.

This textbook chapter provides a comprehensive resource for the treatment of the diabetic foot.

Pinzur MS, Slovenkai MP, Trepman E: Guidelines for diabetic foot care: The Diabetes Committee of the American Orthopaedic Foot and Ankle Society. *Foot Ankle Int* 1999;20:695-702.

This American Orthopaedic Foot and Ankle Society Diabetes Committee project describes the health system approach to the problem of the diabetic foot.

Reiber GE, Lipsky BA, Gibbons GW: The burden of diabetic foot ulcers. *Am J Surg* 1998;176(suppl 2A): 5S-10S.

A current review of the health systems impact of the diabetic foot is presented.

Classic Bibliography

Beskin JL, Baxter DE: Recurrent pain following interdigital neurectomy: A plantar approach. *Foot Ankle* 1988;9:34-39.

Coughlin MJ, Abdo RV: Arthrodesis of the first metatarsophalangeal joint with Vitallium plate fixation. *Foot Ankle Int* 1994;15:18-28.

Coughlin MJ: Crossover second toe deformity. *Foot Ankle* 1987;8:29-39.

Coughlin MJ: Juvenile hallux valgus: Etiology and treatment. *Foot Ankle Int* 1995;16:682-697.

Coughlin MJ: Hallux valgus in men: Effect of the distal metatarsal articular angle on hallux valgus correction. *Foot Ankle Int* 1997;18:463-470.

Early JS, Hansen ST: Surgical reconstruction of the diabetic foot: A salvage approach for midfoot collapse. *Foot Ankle Int* 1996;17:325-330.

Hamilton WG, O'Malley MJ, Thompson FM, Kovatis PE: Roger Mann Award 1995: Capsular interposition arthroplasty for severe hallux rigidus. *Foot Ankle Int* 1997;18:68-70.

Mann RA, Clanton TO: Hallux rigidus: Treatment by cheilectomy. *J Bone Joint Surg Am* 1988;70:400-406.

Mann RA, Prieskorn D, Sobel M: Mid-tarsal and tarsometatarsal arthrodesis for primary degenerative osteoarthrosis or osteoarthrosis after trauma. *J Bone Joint Surg Am* 1996;78:1376-1385.

Mann RA, Thompson FM: Arthrodesis of the first metatarsophalangeal joint for hallux valgus in rheumatoid arthritis. *J Bone Joint Surg Am* 1984;66:687-692.

Mann RA: Charcot-Marie-Tooth disease, in Gould JS (ed): *Operative Foot Surgery*. Philadelphia, PA, WB Saunders, 1994, pp 177-183.

McDermott JE, Conti SF (eds): *The Diabetic Foot*. Rosemont, IL, American Academy of Orthopaedic Surgeons, 1995.

Myerson M, Papa J, Eaton K, Wilson K: The total-contact cast for management of neuropathic plantar ulceration of the foot. *J Bone Joint Surg Am* 1992;74: 261-269.

Myerson MS, Henderson MR, Saxby T, Short KW: Management of midfoot diabetic neuroarthropathy. *Foot Ankle Int* 1994;15:233-241.

Pecoraro RE, Reiber GE, Burgess EM: Pathways to diabetic limb amputation: Basis for prevention. *Diabetes Care* 1990;13:513-521.

Sangeorzan BJ, Veith RG, Hansen ST Jr: Salvage of Lisfranc's tarsometatarsal joint by arthrodesis. *Foot Ankle* 1990;10:193-200.

Taylor RG: The treatment of claw toes by multiple transfers of flexor into extensor tendons. *J Bone Joint Surg Br* 1951;33:539-542.

The Diabetes Control and Complications Trial Research Group: The effect of intensive treatment of diabetes on the development and progression of long-term complications in insulin-dependent diabetes mellitus. *N Engl J Med* 1993;329:977-986.

Wagner FW Jr: Management of the diabetic neurotrophic foot: Part II. A classification and treatment program for diabetic, neuropathic, and dysvascular foot problems. *Instr Course Lect* 1979;28:143-165.

ate documentation of their effectiveness is not yet available.

Surgical Treatment

The goal of surgery is to obtain adequate 3-D correction of the deformity and maintain frontal and sagittal balance of the trunk, while fusing and instrumenting the fewest vertebrae. Surgery should be considered in skeletally immature patients with failed brace treatment and curves greater than 40° and in mature patients with curves greater than 50°, especially those with significant frontal or coronal trunk imbalance. Levels of instrumentation and fusion are selected after careful analysis of the standing PA and lateral radiographs and with either the bending, traction, push-prone, or fulcrum-bending flexibility radiographs. The concept of selective thoracic fusion in the King-Moe type II curve pattern has been validated and arthrodesis of the lumbar spine is avoided, provided that this pattern is appropriately diagnosed and that the lumbar curve is not severe. The King-Moe type V double thoracic pattern should be treated with instrumentation and fusion of both curves in the presence of a high left shoulder, a positive T1 tilt greater than 5°, or a rigid, high thoracic curve greater than 40°. Many surgical techniques and instrumentation systems are now available to correct idiopathic scoliosis. The standard approach is a posterior spinal fusion and instrumentation with a multi-rod, hook, and screw system from a neutral vertebra above to the stable vertebra (or one above) level below. The correction technique chosen, that is, rod rotation or translation, does not appear to change the outcome. Single rod constructs have no advantage over double rod constructs and are more prone to implant failure. Pedicle screws achieve slightly greater correction than hooks, but their use remains controversial, especially in the thoracic area. Anterior diskectomy and fusion is used for severe and rigid curves or for patients with open triradiate cartilage to avoid a crankshaft phenomenon.

Video-assisted thoracoscopic surgery (VATS) has emerged in recent years as an alternative to open thoracotomy. VATS allows release of the anulus fibrosus and multiple diskectomies, rib resection for costoplasty, rib harvesting for intervertebral fusion and most recently, insertion of corrective instrumentation. Although the learning curve is substantial, the technique has proved safe and effective. More follow-up reports are needed to determine its long-term benefits. Anterior instrumentation and fusion of thoracolumbar lumbar curve patterns is a well-established technique that can save fusion levels; in addition, there has been recent interest in the use of anterior instrumentation and fusion for thoracic curve patterns. On the average,

anterior instrumentation systems provide a higher coronal plane correction than posterior systems, and demonstrate a more consistent ability to restore a normal thoracic kyphosis. Fusion levels can be saved by an anterior approach, at the expense of a higher rate of pseudarthrosis, rod breakage, and loss of correction, when single rod constructs are used. The exact indications of anterior instrumentation for thoracic curves await further studies.

Regardless of the instrumentation system chosen, fusion should be done in all cases. Autogenous bone grafting with the iliac crest is the gold standard for posterior fusions with synthetic porous ceramic bone substitutes recently comparing favorably with autograft in two prospective and randomized studies on posterior instrumentation and fusion. The indications for thoracoplasty remain controversial. Spinal cord monitoring with somatosensory- and/or motor-evoked potentials, and/or Stagnara wake-up test are always indicated intraoperatively. One study suggests that combined somatosensory- and motor-evoked potentials represent a standard of care that obviates the need for an intraoperative wake-up test. Because radiographic measurements do not necessarily correlate with clinical outcomes, the recently developed and validated Scoliosis Research Society instrument for evaluation of surgical outcome should be used for outcome assessment after surgery.

Spinal cord or nerve root injury, infection, pseudarthrosis, crankshaft phenomenon, and implant failure are infrequent but well-documented complications. Late-appearing infection with posterior spinal instrumentation may occur in less than 2% of patients and usually affects soft tissue, not the bone. Late-appearing drainage may be either from infection or fretting corrosion. If the culture period is extended to 7 days, low virulence skin organisms are frequently found. This condition can be treated with device removal, primary skin closure, and short-term (6 to 10 days) intravenous and oral antibiotics.

Infantile and Juvenile Idiopathic Scoliosis

Traditionally, idiopathic scoliosis has been categorized based on the age when the scoliosis was first identified. Infantile scoliosis presents from birth through age 2 years, whereas juvenile scoliosis occurs between the ages of 3 and 10 years. Infantile scoliosis accounts for less than 1% of cases of idiopathic scoliosis in North America but is more common in Europe. The curves are generally thoracic or thoracolumbar, convex to the left, may resolve spontaneously in up to 74% of cases, and are more frequent in males. MRI of the brain and spinal cord should be obtained because of a high incidence of underlying neural axis abnormalities. The rib-vertebra angle difference (RVAD) on frontal radiographs is useful for prognosis. Curves with a RVAD greater than 20° carry a high risk of progression and should be treated aggressively.

Juvenile idiopathic scoliosis is more closely related to adolescent idiopathic scoliosis. It is more common in girls, with a female:male ratio of 2:1 to 4:1, and curve patterns are mostly right thoracic, or right thoracic and left lumbar. MRI is also indicated, but the RVAD is not as useful for prognosis. Approximately 70% of curves progress and require some form of treatment. The indication for treatment is a progressive curve 25° or greater. The treatment of choice for infantile and juvenile idiopathic scoliosis is serial casting followed by a CTLSO or TLSO in appropriately sized children to maintain correction. Surgery is indicated for patients with progressive curves greater than 60° despite proper casting and/or bracing. Spinal stabilization without fusion with a subcutaneous distraction rod or a Luque trolley followed by bracing may be used as a temporary treatment in children younger than 8 years old, but carries a high risk of crankshaft phenomenon. Anterior release and fusion combined with a posterior instrumentation and fusion is one alternative and will prevent crankshaft phenomenon, but will result in some trunk shortening.

Neuromuscular Scoliosis

Neuromuscular scoliosis can be caused by a variety of disorders and is classified as neuropathic or myopathic. Cerebral palsy is the most frequent upper motor neuron lesion and best represents the neuropathic group, while Duchenne muscular dystrophy is the most frequent myopathic disorder and represents the principles and recommended treatment for this category of curves. Myelomeningocele is a combination of a lower motor neuron disease with frequently associated congenital vertebral anomalies. The treatment of neuromuscular scoliosis is a challenge because, in general, bracing is ineffective or poorly tolerated, and surgery is associated with a high rate of complications, ranging from 44% to 62% in the recent literature.

Cerebral Palsy

The incidence of scoliosis is higher in children with cerebral palsy and increases with the severity of neurologic involvement, reaching up to 76% in bedridden and institutionalized patients with total body involvement. Curve progression is variable but there is a strong tendency toward deformity progression in more severely involved patients, creating poor sitting balance, decreased sitting tolerance, and pressure sores secondary to pelvic obliquity. Other risk factors are

thoracolumbar curves, being bedridden, and having a curve 40° or greater before age 15 years. Curve progression has also been documented after skeletal maturity. Curve patterns can be divided into two types. Group 1 curves are single thoracic or double thoracic and lumbar curves similar to those seen in idiopathic scoliosis. These curves are more frequent in ambulatory and less severely involved patients. Group 2 curves occur most often in nonambulatory patients and are long thoracolumbar or lumbar "C" shaped curves with pelvic obliquity, the high side of the pelvis usually being on the concavity of the curve.

Nonsurgical treatment depends on the severity of the curve. Small nonprogressive deformities do not impair function and require observation alone. A TLSO may be useful for ambulating patients with progressive group 1 curves measuring 40° or less. There is also evidence that nonambulating patients with short lumbar curves may respond to brace treatment. For nonambulatory children or adolescents with group 2 curves, brace treatment cannot be expected to have a lasting corrective effect, although it can be used as sitting support or in an attempt to delay progression in children 10 years old or younger.

Surgical indications revolve around radiographic progress and clinical features such as poor sitting balance. The indications for surgery include curves greater than 50° with a documented progression of greater than 10° in subjects 10 years of age or older. Skeletally mature patients with good curve flexibility can be treated with posterior segmental instrumentation and fusion only. Instrumentation should include the pelvis in group 2 curves and should extend high in the thoracic area (T2 or T3) for all patients to prevent high thoracic kyphosis. To avoid late progression of trunk deformity in skeletally immature patients, anterior spinal release and fusion combined with posterior instrumentation, preferably in a one-stage procedure, are recommended. Skeletally mature patients with large fixed curves benefit from an anterior-posterior procedure for better correction of the scoliosis and pelvic obliquity. Controversy exists about the indications of surgery for severely disabled individuals with total body involvement. Factors that lead to a greater rate of complications are the severity of neurologic involvement, the severity of recent medical problems (gastroesophageal reflux disease, poor nutritional status, respiratory infections) and the severity of scoliosis. In this group of children, the decision for surgery is based on the particular needs and presenting problems of each individual with guidance from the caregivers who best know the patient. Despite the surgical complexity and increased risks, the overall satisfactory results and high patient and caregiver satisfaction confirm that spinal surgery is beneficial for most patients with total body involvement.

Duchenne Muscular Dystrophy

The incidence of progressive scoliosis is very high in this disorder and becomes more evident and rapid (greater than 10° per year) once ambulation is lost, coinciding with a progressive loss of pulmonary function and a tendency toward obesity. The majority of curves are C-shaped lumbar or thoracolumbar with pelvic obliquity. Bracing is not useful and may interfere with respiratory function. Surgery is indicated early for patients with progressive curves greater than 30° and a forced vital capacity of 30% or more. Achievement of a well-balanced spine coupled with a solid fusion has been shown to improve sitting balance and quality of life. Posterior segmental instrumentation and fusion from T2 or T3 to the sacrum is recommended for most patients, especially those with curves with an apex below L1 and who are more at risk of progression of pelvic obliquity. Limiting the fusion to L5 appears satisfactory for subjects with less than 10° of pelvic obliquity.

Myelomeningocele

Scoliotic deformities are frequent and are a combination of neuromuscular and congenital curves. The higher the neurologic level, the higher the incidence, reaching almost 100% in subjects with thoracic level paraplegia. Any type of congenital scoliosis or kyphosis can be found in addition to central nervous system abnormalities such as hydrocephaly, cord tethering, syringomyelia, or Chiari malformations. The majority of curves are progressive, especially in nonambulatory patients.

Bracing is of limited value but may be used to delay curve progression and surgery in immature patients. The poor skin quality over the lumbar spine complicates proper brace fitting. Surgical treatment needs to be individualized according to each patient's particular deformity, neurologic level of involvement, and associated medical problems. Whatever the technique chosen, the complication rate is high, particularly the rate of infection. The congenital component of a deformity is treated with the same principles as for isolated congenital scoliosis. Progressive neuromuscular curves greater than 50° should be considered for spinal fusion. The lack of posterior elements leads to an increase in the risk of pseudarthrosis if posterior instrumentation and fusion alone are done. A combined anterior and posterior instrumentation and fusion achieve the best rate of correction and fusion. Anterior-only fusion and instrumentation may be preferable for selected patients

with thoracolumbar curves less than 75°, compensatory curves less than 40°, no increased kyphosis, and no syrinx.

Congenital Scoliosis

Congenital spine deformities are caused by a nonhereditary abnormal vertebral development process present at birth that results in asymmetric growth and is usually noted earlier in life than for patients with idiopathic scoliosis. Congenital scoliosis is classified as either a defect of segmentation (unilateral bar or bilateral bar), a defect of formation (hemivertebra, wedge vertebra), or a mixed defect (unilateral bar with hemivertebra). Each defect can be isolated or can involve multiple segments, some of the more complex deformities being unclassifiable. Curve progression is highly variable but is directly related to the growth potential and location of the anomaly around each vertebral segment, creating a 3-D deformity ranging from kyphoscoliosis to lordoscoliosis. A unilateral unsegmented bar is one of the most common types and is consistently associated with progression, creating a lack of growth on the concave side of the curve while growth continues on the convex side. Mixed defects are frequently associated with rib anomalies in the thoracic area. Bilateral bars (block vertebra) will stunt the growth of the spine, but will not create a significant scoliosis. Hemivertebrae may be single or multiple, balanced by a contralateral hemivertebra or unbalanced, and incarcerated (tucked into the spine and not changing the contour of the spine) or nonincarcerated. Curves with unbalanced and/or nonincarcerated hemivertebrae are more prone to progression. The growth potential of the growth plates above and below the hemivertebra determines the potential for curve progression: a fully segmented hemivertebra carries a high risk of progression whereas a nonsegmented or fused hemivertebra carries a low risk. The combination of a unilateral unsegmented bar with a contralateral hemivertebra are the most rapidly progressive and severely deforming of all types of congenital scoliosis, with thoracolumbar curves carrying the worst prognosis. Congenital anomalies involving other systems are frequent, including the genitourinary tract (20%), the heart (10% to 15%), the neural canal (20%) and the cervical spine (33%). Appropriate imaging of the spine includes plain radiographs, tomograms, and 3-D CT. MRI before surgery is mandatory to rule out spinal dysraphism.

The earlier detection of congenital scoliosis may result in a tendency to adopt a "wait and see" attitude when confronted with a very young child. The goal of treatment is early detection of progression and correction of the asymmetric growth before the development of a significant deformity. Observation is indicated only in cases for which the natural history is not known. Congenital curves tend to be rigid; therefore, brace treatment is contraindicated. Bracing may be used to control associated compensatory noncongenital curves, but surgery remains the only effective treatment for progressive congenital scoliosis. The surgical regimen needs to be individualized according to the patient's age, curve pattern, natural history, and type of deformity. There are four basic procedures for the surgical management of congenital scoliosis: convex growth arrest (anterior epiphysiodesis and posterior hemiarthrodesis), posterior fusion, combined anterior and posterior fusion with or without instrumentation, and hemivertebra excision. The fusion can be in situ, or with correction by traction, casting, bracing, or instrumentation. Congenital scoliosis caused by a unilateral failure of vertebral segmentation with a contralateral hemivertebra requires early prophylactic surgical treatment by anterior and posterior arthrodesis, preferably in the first 1 to 2 years of life. Hemivertebrae may be treated by in situ epiphysiodesis or in situ fusion when the deformity is small. For larger curves with decompensation, hemivertebra excision is preferred but carries a higher risk of neurologic complications. Simultaneous anterior and posterior resection of a hemivertebra and correction of the deformity with posterior instrumentation has recently been reported with success and may be the preferred treatment for this condition.

Rotational Dislocation

Congenital dislocation of the spine is a recently recognized condition characterized by a sharp kyphosis at the junction of two lordoscoliotic curvatures with bayonetting of the frontal plane alignment. This condition is associated with various dysplastic conditions such as congenital vertebral defects or neurofibromatosis. The basic feature is a lack of continuity of the spinal column. Progression can be rapid and a neurologic deficit is not rare. Early detection of this condition may prevent the development of neurologic compromise. The deformity is most commonly seen in the thoracolumbar junction. Kyphosis at the time of the diagnosis is usually severe (greater than 80°), short, and angular. Surgical treatment with early circumferential spinal fusion is recommended. To ensure a higher rate of fusion, the use of multiple anterior strut grafts in compression from the concavity is suggested. The fusion must encompass the entire kyphosis.

Kyphosis

Congenital Kyphosis

Congenital kyphosis and kyphoscoliosis are uncommon deformities with the potential to progress rapidly,

resulting in severe deformity and possible neurologic deficits (Fig. 2). Type I kyphosis is the most frequent and is caused by anterior failure of vertebral body formation, whereas type II results from a defect of segmentation. Type III consists of mixed anomalies, and type IV is unclassifiable because of its complexity. The apex of the kyphosis is usually located between T10 and L1. Curve progression is most rapid during the adolescent growth spurt and stops at skeletal maturity. Progression and curve magnitude are greatest in type III kyphosis, followed by type I. The prognosis for type II is variable, but kyphoscoliotic deformities are more progressive than pure kyphotic defects of segmentation. Neurologic deterioration caused by compression of the spinal cord can be seen in type I deformities and less frequently in type IV.

Treatment is surgical. Posterior fusion with autologous bone graft is indicated for progressive type I and II kyphosis less than 60°, and should include one level above and below the defect. Gradual correction of type I curves can be expected in young children following posterior fusion. For kyphosis greater than 60°, an anterior release and fusion followed by a posterior compression instrumentation and fusion is necessary. Traction carries a high risk of paraplegia and is not recommended. Congenital kyphosis with a neurologic deficit should be treated with bed rest followed by anterior spinal cord decompression with posterior instrumentation and fusion.

Scheuermann's Disease

This disease represents the most common cause of structural kyphosis. Although there is no consensus on the definition, the classic (type 1) disease is a rigid kyphosis with an anterior wedging of 5° or more of at least three adjacent vertebral bodies. The disease is generally localized in the thoracic area but can occur at the thoracolumbar level. The reported prevalence ranges between 0.4% to 8% of the general population. Boys and girls appear to be equally affected. Most investigators agree that mechanical factors play a significant role in the pathogenesis of the disorder. The mode of inheritance is likely autosomal dominant with high penetrance but variable expression.

Clinically, adolescents seek medical attention for cosmetic or postural complaints and/or pain. Pain is typically localized just distal to the apex of the deformity. Neurologic and cardiopulmonary complaints are rare and associated with severe kyphosis (curve greater than 95°). On physical examination, the sagittal deformity is fairly rigid on hyperextension as opposed to the more supple deformity found in postural kyphosis. Cervical and lumbar lordosis are increased and shoulder girdles are rotated anteriorly. The forward bending

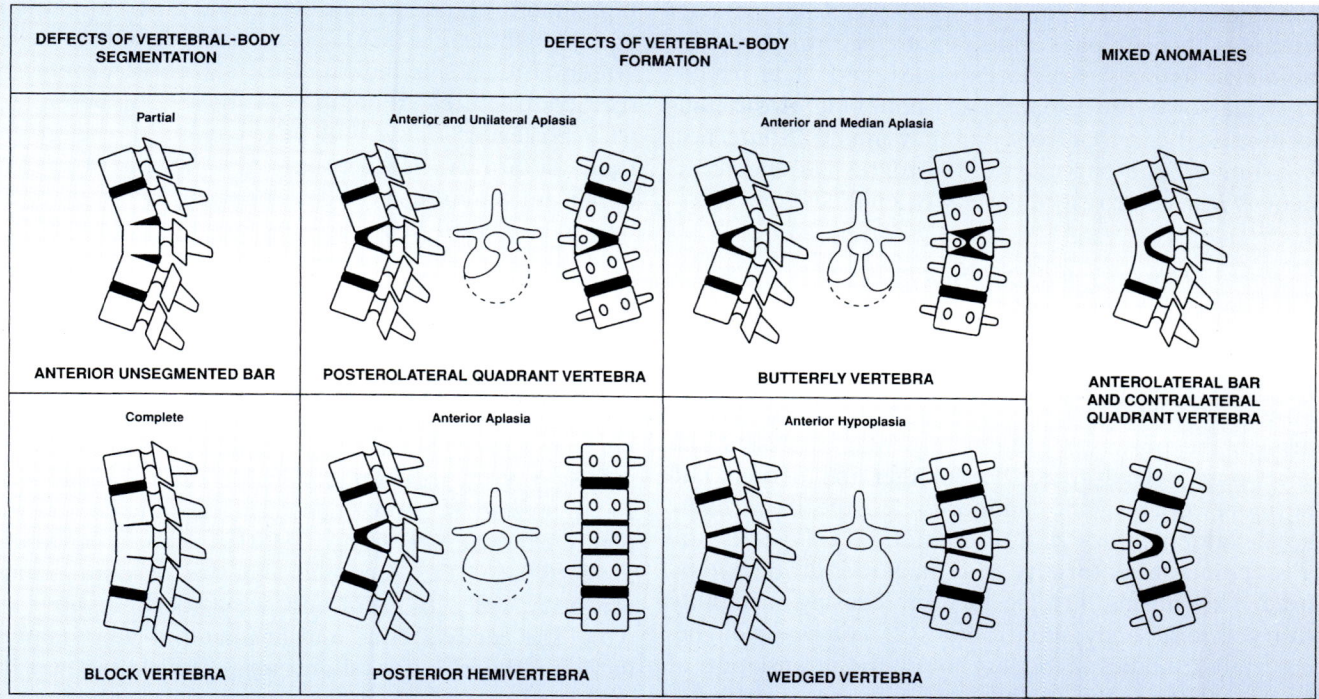

Figure 2 Drawing showing the different types of vertebral anomalies that produce a congenital kyphosis or kyphoscoliosis. *(Reproduced with permission from McMaster MJ, Singh H: Natural history of congenital kyphosis and kyphoscoliosis: A study of one hundred and twelve patients. J Bone Joint Surg Am 1999;81:1367-1383.)*

test shows a sharply angulated deformity. The hamstrings and iliopsoas muscles are often tight.

The radiologic evaluation should include standing posteroanterior and lateral radiographs of the entire spine. The classic changes include the presence of Schmorl's nodes, disk space narrowing, vertebral wedging, and irregular end plates. Associated findings are hyperlordosis of the lumbar spine, spondylolisthesis, degenerative changes, and scoliosis, which is present in about a third of the cases. A lateral radiograph in hyperextension to assess curve flexibility is obtained when treatment is considered. The differential diagnosis includes postural kyphosis, congenital kyphosis, ankylosing spondylitis, multiple compression fractures, tumor, infection, and postlaminectomy kyphosis.

The natural history of Scheuermann's disease remains controversial. The majority of patients will not seek medical attention. In general, pain tends to decrease with skeletal maturation. The likelihood of kyphotic curve progression is unknown. Although the scientific validity of the available literature is questionable, the following few guidelines can be drawn regarding the management of this condition. Initial management includes physical therapy for postural improvement, focusing on hamstring stretching and trunk extensor strengthening. Short-term anti-inflammatory medication can be used as an adjunct to nonsurgical care. The value of bracing is controversial. Current indications for bracing include a kyphosis greater than 50° in a skeletally immature patient with significant pain, a cosmetically unacceptable deformity, or documented progression. Curves with an apex above T7 are best managed with a Milwaukee brace whereas low thoracic or thoracolumbar kyphosis can usually be managed with a hyperextension TLSO. The brace should be worn for a minimum of 1 year but it is not known if full-time wear is superior to part-time. Surgical treatment should be reserved for adolescents with a rigid kyphosis greater than 75° who do not respond to nonsurgical management and have persistent pain or an unacceptable cosmetic deformity. Anterior spinal release, disk excision, and fusion in conjunction with posterior spine instrumentation and fusion are most frequently recommended. The amount of correction should be limited to 50% of the initial deformity, to minimize the development of junctional kyphosis. Recent developments in surgical techniques and instrumentation include thoracoscopic anterior release and fusion, and use of pedicle screw fixation at the distal aspect of the fusion. Further studies are required to assess the long-term benefits of these technical innovations.

Type II disease, also described as pseudo-Scheuermann, involves the lumbar spine and presents a distinct clinical entity. The condition generally is seen in active adolescent males involved in sports or heavy physical activities. The etiology is unknown but there is a strong association with repetitive activities involving axial loading of the immature spine. Typically, patients present with back pain and kyphotic deformation. The radiologic findings (Schmorl's nodes, end plate irregularity, narrowed disk spaces, and flattening of the lumbar lordosis) can be severe and may mimic an infection or a tumor. The curves are nonprogressive and treatment is based on rest and activity modification.

Postlaminectomy Spine Deformity

The incidence of postlaminectomy instability is unknown. Children are more vulnerable to develop spinal deformity after multilevel laminectomy, and two thirds of the load transmission at the cervical level is through the posterior column (articular processes and facet joints). Therefore, the younger the patient and the more cephalad the laminectomies, the more likely the development of a deformation. Kyphosis is the most common deformity and may be produced by three mechanisms: (1) facetectomy causing instability with vertebral body subluxation, (2) anterior wedging of vertebral bodies secondary to anterior translation of the weight load, and (3) hypermobility between vertebral bodies. Plain radiographs including flexion-extension views are necessary to measure and assess reducibility of the deformation. MRI should be obtained before surgery to rule out cord changes such as myelomalacia, syrinx formation, or cord atrophy. The value of bracing is unknown. Early anterior and/or posterior fusion, depending on the localization of the deformation and the bone deficit, is recommended as soon as the deformity is recognized. The best treatment is prevention by avoiding facetectomies as much as possible. Although laminoplasties seem promising in preventing the occurrence of kyphosis, addition of long-term studies are needed.

Postirradiation Spinal Deformity

The development of a spinal deformity after irradiation is related to the age of the patient and the radiation dosage, with the most severe changes occurring in subjects 2 years of age or younger. The most common side effect of abdominal irradiation is spinal deformity, with a prevalence as high as 50% after treatment for Wilms' tumor. The pattern of deformation is related to the portion of the vertebrae irradiated, with scoliosis being more common than kyphosis. Postirradiation deformations tend to progress rapidly during the growth spurt, and may continue to progress even after skeletal maturity. Usually, the initial vertebral changes occur 6 months to 2 years after irradiation. Brace treatment should be attempted for progressive scoliosis, but bracing for kyphosis is reported to be ineffective. Spinal fusion with or without instrumentation should be undertaken irrespective of the patient's age if significant curve progression is documented. Anterior release is indicated for severe deformity and scar contracture. A flexible kyphosis can be treated with posterior fusion and instrumentation whereas a rigid deformity requires a combined approach to obtain maximum correction. Postoperative immobilization is suggested to reduce the risk of pseudarthrosis.

Miscellaneous Spine Problems

Marfan Syndrome

Musculoskeletal findings in Marfan syndrome include arachnodactily, dolichostenomelia, ligamentous laxity, anterior chest wall deformities, and scoliosis (75% of subjects). Widening of the spinal canal with dural ectasia is present in more than 60% of patients and is a highly characteristic sign of Marfan syndrome, even at an early age. The presence and size of dural ectasia can be assessed by MRI and are associated with back pain. The cervical bony and ligamentous abnormalities increase the risk for atlantoaxial translation, basilar invagination, and atlantoaxial rotatory instability. Scoliosis curves are similar to adolescent idiopathic scoliosis curves in many respects, but may present at a younger age, have less female predominance, and tend to be more progressive and rigid despite the ligamentous laxity associated with the condition. Patients younger than 3 years of age had an average progression of 19° per year in one report.

The value of bracing in Marfan syndrome is controversial because of conflicting reports. In most patients, brace treatment will fail, but it may be used in younger patients to delay curve progression until they reach an appropriate age for surgery. A preoperative work-up is mandatory because of the high incidence of cardiac anomalies. The indications for surgery are similar to those for idiopathic scoliosis: posterior spinal instrumentation and fusion with autogenous bone grafting can effectively manage most scoliotic curves, but anterior diskectomy and vertebral fusion should be considered for rigid curves and for curves associated with thoracic hypokyphosis or thoracolumbar kyposis. Revision surgery may be necessary because of a higher rate of pseudarthrosis.

Neurofibromatosis

Scoliosis is seen in 10% to 30% of patients with type 1 neurofibromatosis. Two curve patterns are recognized: an idiopathic-like and a dystrophic type with a short, sharply angulated kyphoscoliosis. Dystrophic features include rib pencilling, vertebral rotation, anterior, posterior or lateral vertebral scalloping, vertebral wedging, spindling of the transverse process, widened interpedicular distance, and enlarged intervertebral foramina. Spinal deformities with seemingly few initial dystrophic features have shown a tendency to acquire dystrophic changes during long-term follow-up periods. Similarly, deformities with dystrophic changes can acquire further dystrophic features. These dystrophic changes may evolve slowly or aggressively, and may spread to other regions as well. This phenomenon is known as modulation, a feature unique to spinal deformities in neurofibromatosis that is most frequently observed in patients with spinal deformity diagnosed before 7 years of age. In these children, when a curve acquires either three pencilled ribs or a combination of three dystrophic features, clinical progression is almost a certainty.

Idiopathic-like curve patterns are managed similar to idiopathic scoliosis. Management of dystrophic curves depends on the importance of dystrophic changes and on the patient's age. Brace treatment is usually ineffective, even in young children. The most effective management for dystrophic curves is early and circumferential surgery. Posterior spinal instrumentation and fusion with autogenous bone grafting can be used for curves with minor dystrophic changes. The severe dystrophic curves always require combined anterior and posterior stabilization, particularly in younger patients, even if the sagittal curves have not become pathologic by the time of presentation. The incidence of pseudarthrosis is high, especially with posterior instrumentation fusion alone.

Spine Tumors

Benign tumors of the spine are more frequently localized in the lumbar and thoracic area, with a predilection for the vertebral arch. The most frequent histologic types are eosinophilic granuloma, osteoid osteoma, osteoblastoma, and aneurysmal bone cyst. Eosinophilic granuloma usually presents as back pain in a child younger than 10 years of age. Lesions are most commonly isolated, but may be multiple. The radiologic appearance of a vertebra plana is characteristic of this disorder, but on occasion, a biopsy may be necessary for the diagnosis of a lesion with an unusual radiologic appearance. Symptomatic treatment with temporary spine immobilization by a cast or a brace is indicated for most patients. Surgery may be necessary for the occasional patient with an associated neurologic deficit.

Painful scoliosis is a well recognized and frequent (greater than 60% of patients) presentation of spinal osteoid osteoma and osteoblastoma, and is considered to be secondary to pain-provoked muscle spasm on the side of the lesion. Scoliosis is more frequent in cases of osteoid osteoma and typically is present in the concave aspect of the curve. Night pain, relieved by nonster-

oidal anti-inflammatory drugs, may be present. Diagnosis is made with either a bone scan or CT scan. Surgical resection of the nidus is the traditional method of treatment but may be difficult, depending on the location. Percutaneous CT-guided burring or thermocoagulation of the nidus are minimally invasive techniques reported with increasing frequency as alternatives to open resection. Because of their larger size and tendency to extend in the vertebral body, osteoblastomas are best treated with open surgical excision.

Aneurysmal bone cysts of the spine comprise from 3% to 20% of all benign spinal lesions. Located in the posterior elements, aneurysmal bone cysts are expansive and destructive, and may undermine the structural integrity of the spine with secondary neurologic compromise. Extension to the vertebral body is frequent, with occasional extension to an adjacent vertebra. Current treatment recommendations involve preoperative selective arterial embolization to prevent excessive intraoperative bleeding, and intralesional curettage. The status of the structural integrity of the spine must be assessed before initiating treatment. If instability or deformity or both are already present, or if the amount of bony tissue to be resected may render the spine unstable, then instrumentation and fusion should be performed at the time of surgical resection. Percutaneous embolization has been reported to be successful and may be an alternative to surgery.

Spine Trauma

Spine injury in children is a rare event, accounting for less than 1% of all fractures, and most injuries are localized to the thoracolumbar area. Thoracic and lumbar spine injuries should be assessed and treated according to the same principles as for adult injuries. Cervical spine injuries represent only 1.5% to 3% of all spinal injuries but are more commonly associated with a neurologic compromise. Motor vehicle accidents are responsible for the majority of injuries that occur before the age of 10 years, after which sport-related accidents become frequent. In children older than age 10 years, the assessment, type of fractures, treatment, and prognosis are very similar to that of adult injuries.

For younger children, many differences need to be recognized. The level of pediatric cervical spine injury varies according to the age of the patient. Prior to the age of 10 years, cervical injuries are more frequently localized above C4, whereas after age 9 years the lower spine is more commonly involved. Because of the relatively large size of the head in children, the horizontal orientation of the facets, the ligamentous laxity, and the immature musculature providing less resistance to displacement forces, the most mobile segment of the spine moves progressively from C3-4 before age 8 years to C5-6 after age 12 years. In addition, transportation on a board equipped with a recessed area for the skull or a mattress under the thoracic area is recommended to avoid flexion of the cervical spine. Until proven otherwise a child with head or facial injuries is presumed to have a spinal injury. A complete neurologic examination should be performed, assessing spinal tenderness, widening of intervertebral space, torticollis, muscle spasm, or rigidity. Clinical examination of the neck can reliably rule out acute cervical injury in the awake and alert blunt trauma patient.

Knowledge of the normal shape and development of the spine is critical in avoiding misinterpretation of radiographic films, for example, synchondrosis of C1 and dens, and C2-3 pseudosubluxation. There is some controversy regarding the usefulness of the open mouth view in the initial cervical series of radiographs. A recent study indicates that flexion-extension radiographs for pediatric acute trauma patients are not useful if the static cervical spine radiographs are normal. A screening MRI study within 48 hours of trauma may be helpful in the comatose patient if the initial radiographic studies are normal and a cervical spine injury cannot be excluded.

Occipitoatlantal dislocation is a common cause of fatal injury. The mechanism of action usually involves a sudden acceleration-deceleration force on the head. Recently, this injury has been associated with airbag deployment systems in front seat child passengers, thereby supporting the recommendation that children younger than age 12 years should be seated in the back of cars equipped with dual airbags. In patients with a suspected occipitoatlantoaxial injury, the interspinous C1-2:C2-3 ratio was a good predictor of a rupture of the tectorial membrane. Odontoid fractures occur most commonly through the dentocentral synchrondrosis. These fractures are often associated with a neurologic deficit. For undisplaced fractures, nonsurgical treatment should be used. Surgical management is recommended for patients with neurologic deficit or instability, instability being defined as an atlanto-dens interval greater than 5 or 10 mm. The classic treatment consists of a posterior fusion but recently, screw fixation through an anterior approach has been reported as a safe procedure in children as young as 3 years old. The spinal cord injury without radiologic abnormalities syndrome is a traumatic myelopathy in children who show no radiographic evidence of skeletal injury or subluxation by radiologic investigation. It accounts for 20% to 30% of traumatic injuries of the spine in children and is caused by a self-reducing transient intervertebral subluxation of the spine. The diagnosis can be established only after a careful radiologic evaluation

has excluded any bony or ligamentous abnormalities. MRI may reveal evidence of spinal cord contusion or hemorrhage. Treatment consists of adequate immobilization by a rigid cervical collar or TLSO and restriction of physical activities for 3 months. The prognosis for recovery of the neurologic injury is good in mild cases but poor in severe cases, and serious injuries are more frequent in children younger than age 8 years.

Annotated Bibliography

Adolescent Idiopathic Scoliosis

Betz RR, Harms J, Clements DH III, et al: Comparison of anterior and posterior instrumentation for correction of adolescent thoracic idiopathic scoliosis. *Spine* 1999; 24:225-239.

In a multicenter, prospective study of two cohort groups of patients with thoracic idiopathic scoliosis, coronal correction and balance were equal in both groups. In the anterior group, there was a better correction of sagittal profiles in those with a preoperative hypokyphosis. An average of 2.5 lumbar levels were saved from fusion in the anterior group, but the use of a 3.2-mm flexible rod resulted in an unacceptable rate of rod breakage, pseudarthrosis, and loss of correction.

Coonrad RW, Murrell GA, Motley G, Lytle E, Hey LA: A logical coronal pattern classification of 2,000 consecutive idiopathic scoliosis cases based on the Scoliosis Research Society-defined apical vertebra. *Spine* 1998;23:1380-1391.

Two thousand consecutive idiopathic scoliosis records and radiographs were reviewed for coronal pattern typing and categorization. They were classified into 11 readily identifiable types incorporating the widely referenced five Moe-King types, simplifying recognition of curve patterns for purposes of identification and communication.

Crawford AH, Wall EJ, Wolf R: Video-assisted thoracoscopy. *Orthop Clin North Am* 1999;30:367-385.

A state of the art review of this new therapeutic modality for disorders of the pediatric spine is presented.

Little DG, Song KM, Katz D, Herring JA: Relationship of peak height velocity to other maturity indicators in idiopathic scoliosis in girls. *J Bone Joint Surg Am* 2000;82:685-693.

The height velocities of 121 girls with adolescent idiopathic scoliosis managed with a brace were generated from serial clinical height measurements. Most of the curves progressed at peak height velocity, which was found superior to chronologic age, age at menarche, and Risser grade to predict progression. Knowing the timing of the growth peak provides valuable information on the likelihood of progression to a magnitude requiring spinal arthrodesis.

Lowe TG, Edgar M, Margulies JY, et al: Etiology of idiopathic scoliosis: Current trends in research. *J Bone Joint Surg Am* 2000;82:1157-1168.

This article is a current concepts review on the etiology of idiopathic scoliosis. The true etiology of idiopathic scoliosis remains unknown; however, it appears to be multifactorial.

Neuromuscular Scoliosis

Alman BA, Kim HK: Pelvic obliquity after fusion of the spine in Duchenne muscular dystrophy. *J Bone Joint Surg Br* 1999;81:821-824.

A review of 48 subjects who underwent surgical treatment for this condition indicates that spinal fusion to the sacrum is preferred to ending caudally at L5, especially for patients with an apex below L1.

Comstock CP, Leach J, Wenger DR: Scoliosis in total-body-involvement cerebral palsy: Analysis of surgical treatment and patient and caregiver satisfaction. *Spine* 1998;23:1412-1425.

A nonrandomized descriptive case series of 100 patients with total-body involvement spastic cerebral palsy is presented to determine early and late outcomes, including caregiver satisfaction. Despite the surgical complexity and expected complications, spinal surgery is indicated and is beneficial for most patients.

Lipton GE, Miller F, Dabney KW, Altiok H, Bachrach SJ: Factors predicting postoperative complications following spinal fusions in children with cerebral palsy. *J Spinal Disord* 1999;12:197-205.

A retrospective review of 107 patients with cerebral palsy who had undergone posterior spine fusion with unit rod instrumentation was done to determine what factors cause complications that lead to delayed recovery time and a longer than average hospital stay.

Olafsson Y, Saraste H, Al-Dabbagh Z: Brace treatment in neuromuscular spine deformity. *J Pediatr Orthop* 1999;19:376-379.

In this review, 90 consecutive adolescents with various neuromuscular scoliotic deformities were treated with a Boston brace. Brace treatment was successful in only 23 patients. A successful outcome was seen in ambulating patients with muscle hypotonia and short curves less than 40° as well as in nonambulating patients with spastic short lumbar curves.

Congenital Scoliosis

Lazar RD, Hall JE: Simultaneous anterior and posterior hemivertebra excision. *Clin Orthop* 1999;364:76-84.

This report of 11 patients describes the resection technique, degree of deformity correction, and complications encountered with this approach to a very difficult clinical problem. The technique has evolved from many different surgical methods used in the past.

McMaster MJ: Congenital scoliosis caused by a unilateral failure of vertebral segmentation with contralateral hemivertebrae. *Spine* 1998;23:998-1005.

A retrospective analysis of 59 consecutive patients with this deformity demonstrated that these patients have the most rapidly progressive and severely deforming of all types of congenital scoliosis. All midthoracic, thoracolumbar, and lumbar curves require immediate prophylactic surgical treatment by anterior and posterior arthrodesis, preferably in the first year of life.

Kyphosis

Albert TJ, Vacarro A: Post laminectomy kyphosis. *Spine* 1998;23:2738-2745.

This review article focuses on the pathomechanics, assessment, and treatment of subjects with this condition.

Lowe TG: Scheuermann's disease. *Orthop Clin North* 1999;30:475-487.

Tribus CB: Scheuermann's kyphosis in adolescents and adults: Diagnosis and management. *J Am Acad Orthop Surg* 1998;6:36-43.

Wenger DR, Frick SL: Scheuermann kyphosis. *Spine* 1999;24:2630-2639.

These three complementary review articles provide a critical and complete analysis of this disease.

McMaster MJ, Singh H: Natural history of congenital kyphosis and kyphoscoliosis: A study of one hundred and twelve patients. *J Bone Joint Surg Am* 1999;81: 1367-1383.

This is a review of 112 consecutive patients that demonstrates that a thorough knowledge of the natural history is essential in the planning of appropriate and timely treatment to prevent progression of the deformity and neurologic complications.

Zeller RD, Dubousset J: Progressive rotational dislocation in kyphoscoliotic deformities: Presentation and treatment. *Spine* 2000;25:1092-1097.

This retrospective case study of 11 cases reviews the French experience with this recently recognized condition.

Miscellaneous Spine Problems

Ahn NU, Sponseller PD, Ahn UM, Nallamshetty L, Kuszyk BS, Zinreich SJ: Dural ectasia is associated with back pain in Marfan syndrome. *Spine* 2000;25:1562-1568.

A cross-sectional age and sex-matched study compared the prevalence and size of dural ectasia in two groups of patients with Marfan syndrome. The presence and size of dural ectasia are associated with back pain in Marfan's syndrome.

Cove JA, Taminiau AH, Obermann WR, Vanders-chueren GM: Osteoid osteoma of the spine treated with percutaneous computed tomography-guided thermoco-agulation. *Spine* 2000;25:1283-1286.

Two cases are reported in which an osteoid osteoma of the lumbar spine was treated with CT-guided thermocoagulation, an alternative and minimally invasive treatment for spinal osteoid osteomas.

Durrani AA, Crawford AH, Chouhdry SN, Saifuddin A, Morley TR: Modulation of spinal deformities in patients with neurofibromatosis Type 1. *Spine* 2000;25:69-75.

A consecutive case retrospective chart and radiographic review of 457 patients with neurofibromatosis type 1 is presented. Spinal deformities were noted in 128 patients and should be regarded as deformities in evolution. A spinal deformity that develops before 7 years of age should be followed closely for evolving dystrophic features. A curve acquiring either three pencilled ribs or a combination of three dystrophic features carries a greater than 85% risk of progression.

Papagelopoulos PJ, Currier BL, Shaughnessy WJ, et al: Aneurysmal bone cyst of the spine: Management and outcome. *Spine* 1998;23:621-628.

A review of 52 consecutive patients with an aneurysmal bone cyst of the spine is conducted to define the incidence, clinical presentation, diagnostic and therapeutic options, and prognosis of patients with this disorder.

Parisini P, Di Silvestre M, Greggi T, Paderni S, Cervellati S, Savini R: Surgical correction of dystrophic spinal curves in neurofibromatosis: A review of 56 patients. *Spine* 1999;24:2247-2253.

A review of 56 patients with dystrophic curves treated surgically between 1971 and 1992 is presented. The most effective form of treatment for dystrophic curves was early and aggressive treatment with combined anterior and posterior stabilization, particularly in younger patients.

Spine Trauma

Akbarnia BA: Pediatric spine fractures. *Orthop Clin North Am* 1999;30:521-536.

This review article discusses the pathomechanics, clinical presentation, and treatment of thoracolumbar spine fractures in children.

Eleraky MA, Theodore N, Adams M, Rekate HL, Sonntag VK: Pediatric cervical spine injuries: Report of 102 cases and review of the literature. *J Neurosurg* 2000;92(suppl 1):12-17.

A retrospective study of pediatric cervical spine injuries treated in the past decade is presented.

Odent T, Langlais, J, Glorion C, Kassis B, Bataille J, Pouliquen JC: Fractures of the odontoid process: A report of 15 cases in children younger than 6 years. *J Pediatr Orthop* 1999;19:51-54.

The authors review their experience with this rare fracture. Fusion was obtained in all cases treated conservatively.

Sun PP, Poffenbarger GJ, Durham S, Zimmerman RA: Spectrum of occipitoatlantoaxial injury in young children. *J Neurosurg* 2000;93(suppl 1):28-39.

The authors report a novel interspinous ratio criteria to predict a tectorial membrane abnormality based on the comparison of 71 cases of injury. The correlation was established by comparing MRI to plain radiographic films.

Classic Bibliography

Blount WP, Schmidt AC: Abstract: The Milwaukee brace in the treatment of scoliosis. *J Bone Joint Surg Am* 1957;39:693.

Bradford DS, Moe JH, Montalvo FJ, Winter RB: Scheuermann's kyphosis and roundback deformity: Results of Milwaukee brace treatment. *J Bone Joint Surg Am* 1974;56:740-758.

Carr WA, Moe JH, Winter RB, Lonstein JE: Treatment of idiopathic scoliosis in the Milwaukee brace. *J Bone Joint Surg Am* 1980;62:599-612.

Emans JB, Kaelin A, Bancel P, Hall JE, Miller ME: The Boston bracing system for idiopathic scoliosis: Follow-up results in 295 patients. *Spine* 1986;11:792-801.

Machida M, Dubousset J, Imamura Y, Miyashita Y, Yamada T, Kimura J: Melatonin: A possible role in pathogenesis of adolescent idiopathic scoliosis. *Spine* 1996;21:1147-1152.

McMaster MJ, David CV: Hemivertebra as a cause of scoliosis: A study of 104 patients. *J Bone Joint Surg Br* 1986;68:588-595.

Murray PM, Weinstein SL, Spratt KF: The natural history and long-term follow-up of Scheuermann kyphosis. *J Bone Joint Surg Am* 1993;75:236-248.

Nachemson AL, Peterson L-E: Effectiveness of treatment with a brace in girls who have adolescent idiopathic scoliosis: A prospective, controlled study based on data from the Brace Study of the Scoliosis Research Society. *J Bone Joint Surg Am* 1995;77:815-822.

Rowe DE, Bernstein SM, Riddick MF, Adler F, Emans JB, Gardner-Bonneau D: A meta-analysis of the efficacy of non-operative treatments for idiopathic scoliosis. *J Bone Joint Surg* 1997;79:664-674.

Winter RB, Moe JH, Lonstein JE: The surgical treatment of congenital kyphosis: A review of 94 patients age 5 years or older, with 2 years or more follow-up in 77 patients. *Spine* 1985;10:224-231.

Chapter 49

Adult Spine Trauma

Alexander R. Vaccaro, MD

Oren G. Blam, MD

Introduction

Traumatic injury to the adult spine is often the result of a motor vehicle accident or fall from a height. There is a bimodal age distribution for patients who incur a spinal injury. Most patients are between the ages of 15 and 24 years, with a secondary peak incidence occurring in people age 55 years or older. An estimated 50,000 new cases of spinal injury occur each year in North America. Of those patients surviving a cervical spine injury, up to 40% have a neurologic deficit. Ten percent to 38% of adults with thoracolumbar spine injuries have neurologic injury to the spinal cord or cauda equina.

Early recognition of spinal injury and proper initial management can have a dramatic effect on a patient's functional outcome. After trauma, a potential spinal injury must be suspected in patients with altered consciousness, complaints of neck or back pain, injuries above the level of the clavicles, or extremity weakness or altered sensation on a careful neurologic examination. Neurologic status should be documented at the scene of injury and on presentation to the hospital. A neurologic deficit may be described as complete, where there is total loss of motor and sensory function below the level of injury, or incomplete. Incomplete neurologic deficits tend to fall into one of four patterns: central cord, anterior cord, posterior cord, or Brown-Séquard syndromes. The presence of spinal shock, in which there is an absence of all distal motor and sensory function as well as loss of sacral spinal reflexes (for example, the anal wink or bulbocavernosus reflexes), precludes the diagnosis of a complete spinal cord injury. A patient's neurologic status may also be documented by the Frankel scale (Table 1) and the American Spinal Injury Association (ASIA) score, a motor and sensory grading system useful for following improvement or deterioration in neurologic status (Fig. 1).

When spinal injury is suspected, a hard cervical collar should be applied and the patient placed on a back board for transportation. Transfers from stretcher to stretcher are done with in-line manual cervical immobilization, keeping the shoulders and hips aligned at all times. Signs of neurogenic shock, including persistent hypotension despite initial volume repletion, should be recognized early and treated with further fluid infusion and judicious use of vasopressors.

Optimal spinal cord perfusion helps minimize the sequelae of the secondary cascade of cellular dysfunction after an acute spinal cord injury. These secondary mechanisms include inflammation, edema, hemorrhage, free radical formation, lipid peroxidation, electrolyte imbalance, cell breakdown, and apoptosis. The only pharmacologic means demonstrated to alter these pathways in large, multicenter, prospective, randomized clinical trials is treatment with methylprednisolone. In patients presenting within 8 hours of a spinal cord injury with no contraindications to steroid use, methylprednisolone should be administered in a bolus of 30 mg/kg, followed by a continuous infusion at a rate of 5.4 mg/kg/h. The steroid drip is continued for 24 hours if started within 3 hours of injury; otherwise it is continued for 48 hours. Relative contraindications to high-dose corticosteroid treatment of spinal cord injury include pregnancy, age younger than 13 years, concomitant infection, penetrating spinal wounds, and uncontrolled diabetes. Because of the risk of gastric bleeding from stress ulcerations in cases of acute, severe trauma and concomitantly administered high-dose corticosteroids, treatment with acid suppressors such as proton pump inhibitors is recommended.

Patients with a spinal injury at one level may have another noncontiguous traumatic spinal injury 5% to 20% of the time. A full radiographic spinal survey including cervical, thoracic, and lumbosacral views is therefore warranted in all patients suspected of having spinal injury. Upper cervical spine injuries (especially

	Modified Frankel Classification/ASIA Impairment Scale of Neurologic Deficit Following Spinal Cord Injury
TABLE 1	

Grade	Characteristics
A	Absent motor and sensory function below level of injury
B	Absent motor function below level of injury; sensation intact
C	Very weak (grade 1/5 to 2/5) motor function below level of injury; sensation intact
D	Weak (grade 3/5 to 4/5) motor function below level of injury; sensation intact
E	Normal motor and sensory function

(Reproduced with permission from the American Spinal Injury Association, International Standards for Neurological and Functional Classification, revised 1996.)

fractures of the occipital condyle, atlas, odontoid process, and axis body) have a high incidence of additional cervical spine injuries.

Upper Cervical Spine Trauma

Occipital Condyle Fractures

Injury to the occipital condyles is rare but the incidence of injury may be higher than documented because 93% of fatal motor vehicle accidents involve injury to the upper cervical spine. An occipital condyle fracture may occur as a sole injury, although 33% are associated with atlanto-occipital subluxation or other cervical spine fractures. Suboccipital tenderness and a slight head tilt are frequently noted findings on patient examination. Palsies of cranial nerves IX, X, XI, or XII and less commonly of cranial nerves VI or VII may be observed. Plain radiographic findings are usually difficult to discern, so CT is the imaging modality of choice when occipital condyle fracture is suspected.

Occipital condyle fractures are currently classified into three types. Type I fractures result from an axial load and produce no gross displacement of the fracture fragments. Type II fractures extend into the foramen magnum and are considered part of a basilar skull fracture. Type III fractures represent a displaced alar ligament avulsion fracture resulting from shear, lateral bending, or rotational force. There is variable disruption of the tectorial membrane as well. Type III fractures are considered unstable and are managed with halo immobilization or surgical stabilization. Type I and II fractures may be managed with a hard cervical collar for 2 to 3 months. Occipitocervical arthrodesis is reserved for persistent instability or for patients with another associated cervical spine injury requiring surgical management.

An alternative classification of occipital condyle fractures uses information derived from radiographs, CT, and MRI regarding condylar displacement and ligamentous injury. Type I injuries are nondisplaced and stable. Type IIa injuries are displaced but stable, whereas type IIb injuries are displaced and unstable.

Atlanto-Occipital Dislocation

Osseoligamentous separation of the skull from the cervical spine often results in severe neurologic deficit or death. Deficits at cranial nerves VII, VIII, IX, and X as well as brainstem dysfunction may be observed. The hyperextension, distraction, and rotational forces that cause atlanto-occipital dislocation may also result in submental laceration, mandibular fracture, and posterior pharyngeal wall injury. These injuries are twice as common in children than adults possibly because the immature atlanto-occipital joint is more horizontally oriented in children.

Various radiographic measures have been described to detect subtle atlanto-occipital subluxation (Fig. 2). The Powers ratio is a useful calculation derived from a lateral projection of the cervical spine on radiograph, tomogram, or CT sagittal reconstruction. The distance from the basion to the anterior edge of the posterior C1 arch is divided by the distance from the opisthion to the posterior edge of the anterior C1 arch; a value greater than 1.0 suggests pathologic displacement of the occiput relative to the atlas. Further indicators of pathologic displacement of the craniocervical articulation include displacement of the Wackenheim line (an imaginary line running along the posterior edge of the clivus and normally intersecting the posterior tip of the odontoid process) as well as a basion to odontoid tip distance greater than 10 mm in children or 5 mm in adults. Also, MRI evidence of subarachnoid hemorrhage at the craniocervical junction is suggestive of atlanto-occipital dislocation.

Atlanto-occipital dislocation is classified by the direction of displacement (Fig. 3). Type I injuries represent pure longitudinal distraction, whereas type II and III injuries are characterized by displacement of the occiput relative to C1 anteriorly or posteriorly, respectively. Type II injuries are most common. Because of the significant loss of ligamentous stabilizers, traction is contraindicated in type I dislocations and is usually limited to 2 lb to 5 lb in a gentle reduction maneuver for type II and III injuries. Treatment is with initial halo immobilization followed by a posterior occipital-cervical fusion. Delayed stabilization can lead to worsening neurologic status and may make a later reduction and decompression procedure difficult, possibly necessitating a transoral osteoligamentous or

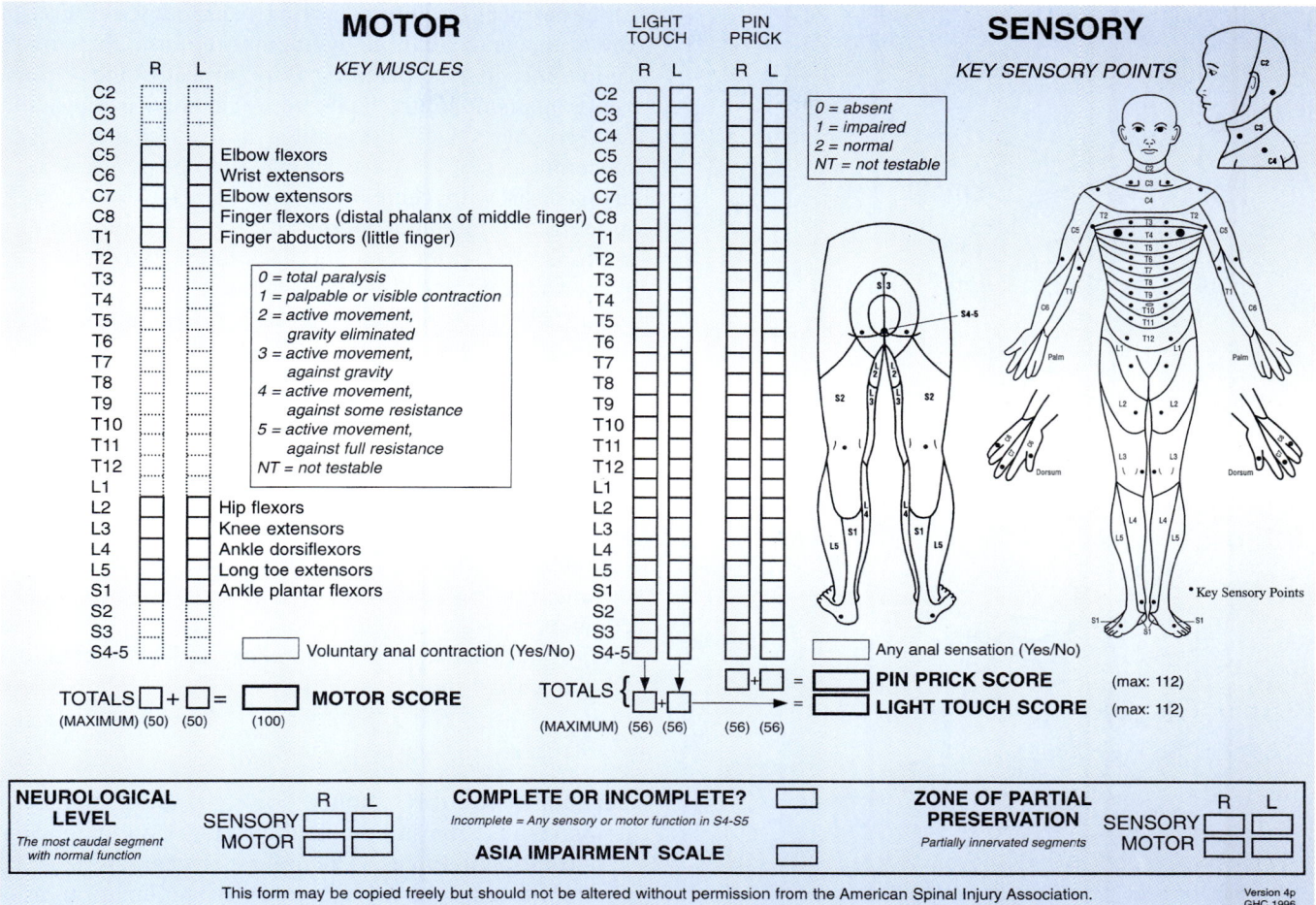

Figure 1 The full worksheet for determining a numeric grade for motor and sensory function following spinal cord injury. Motor function in 10 directed actions is assessed on a 0 to 5 scale, while sensory function to both light touch and pin prick is assessed on a 0 to 2 scale. *(Reproduced with permission from the American Spinal Injury Association, International Standards for Neurological and Functional Classification, Revised 1996.)*

upper retropharyngeal release followed by a posterior arthrodesis.

Atlas Fractures

Injury to the C1 ring usually is thought to occur from axial compression and a variable degree of hyperextension, hyperflexion, or lateral bending. Laterally directed tensile forces may also produce such fractures. Solitary atlas fractures usually result in no neurologic deficit because of the relatively larger space available for the cord at the C1 level and because these fractures tend to displace centrifugally, thereby decompressing the vertebral canal. Fifty percent of them, however, are associated with other cervical spine fractures that may result in spinal cord injury. Suboccipital pain with occasional lower cranial nerve, suboccipital nerve, or greater occipital nerve injury may occur.

An AP plain radiograph may reveal lateral displacement of the C1 lateral masses if disruption of the transverse ligamentous complex is present. CT imaging in the axial plane delineates this injury well. The C1 ring may be disrupted anteriorly, posteriorly, or through the articulating lateral masses (Fig. 4). Disruption of the C1 ring in three or four quadrants is called a Jefferson fracture. Avulsion fractures of the longus coli muscle at the anterior tubercle or a solitary C1 transverse process fracture represent low-energy injuries caused by a hyperextension moment or a laterally applied axial load, respectively.

Instability associated with C1 fractures depends on the integrity of the transverse atlantal ligament. The atlanto-dens interval (ADI) measured on a lateral radiographic projection of the cervical spine may indicate disruption of this ligament when its value is greater than 3.5 to 4 mm in an adult. On the AP radiographic projection, total combined lateral overhang of both C1 lateral masses over C2 may indicate transverse ligament failure when greater than 8 mm. CT scan evidence of bony avulsion of the transverse atlantal liga-

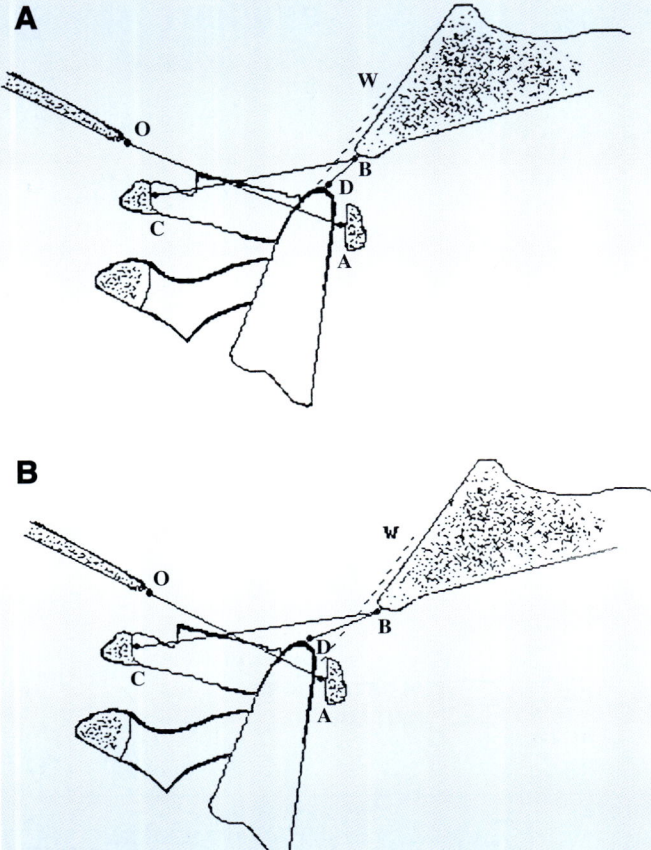

Figure 2 Measures of atlanto-occipital dislocation. **A,** Normal relationships on a lateral projection of the O-C1-C2 complex. Line O-A is longer than line B-C, yielding a Power's ratio (BC/OA) of less than 1.0. The distance from B to D is less than 5 mm in the adult, and Wackenheim's line intersects the tip of the dens. **B,** With anterior atlanto-occipital dislocation, O-A shortens and B-C lengthens; B-D lengthens beyond 5 mm in the adult; and Wackenheim's line no longer intersects the tip of the dens. (A) anterior rim of C1; (B) tip of basion; (C) posterior rim of C1; (O) tip of opisthion; (D) tip of dens; (W) imaginary (dotted) Wackenheim's line.

ment also suggests the potential for C1-C2 instability. Alternatively, MRI can directly demonstrate intrasubstance tears of the transverse ligament. Late instability after a course of nonsurgical external immobilization may be diagnosed by evaluation of the ADI on dynamic flexion and extension cervical spine radiographs.

Treatment of isolated, stable C1 ring fractures usually is with hard collar immobilization. Associated atlantoaxial instability occurring from bony avulsion of the transverse atlantal ligament often requires more rigid halo immobilization. Pure midsubstance transverse ligament injury heals unpredictably in the adult, and primary C1-C2 arthrodesis is recommended. Biomechanical studies have shown that posterior C1-C2 arthrodesis with cables and bone graft provides only moderate immediate stabilization, so supplementary postoperative external immobilization is recommended. Posterior transarticular screw fixation of the atlantoaxial articulation presents a more rigid internal fixation alternative in clinical situations of a pure midsubstance transverse ligament injury. Some situations in which a posterior approach for an atlantoaxial fusion is undesirable may be addressed with an anterior C1-C2 screw fixation and fusion or a bilateral lateral to medial C1-C2 screw fixation and fusion procedure. Unilateral anatomic anomalies such as a high-riding C2 transverse foramen that may place the vertebral artery at risk during transarticular screw placement can also be circumvented with placement of a solitary contralateral C1-2 transarticular screw supplemented by sublaminar C1-C2 wiring and bone grafting.

Atlantoaxial Rotatory Subluxation

Traumatic rotatory subluxation of the C1-C2 facet joints results from a combination of flexion, extension, and rotational forces. The injury is characterized by similar findings of C1-C2 rotatory subluxation as a result of other causes (such as infection, congenital malformation, tumors, and inflammatory conditions). A patient typically presents with suboccipital pain and decreased cervical rotation on examination. An associated head tilt in the direction of the subluxated joint with the chin rotated in the opposite direction, the so-called cock-robin position, may be noticeable.

An AP radiograph will demonstrate an asymmetric relationship of the odontoid to the lateral masses of C1 when an atlantoaxial rotatory subluxation is present. The C1 lateral mass that is rotated anteriorly appears more midline and broader on this view while the contralateral lateral mass displays overlapping of the C1 and C2 articular facets. CT imaging with three-dimen-

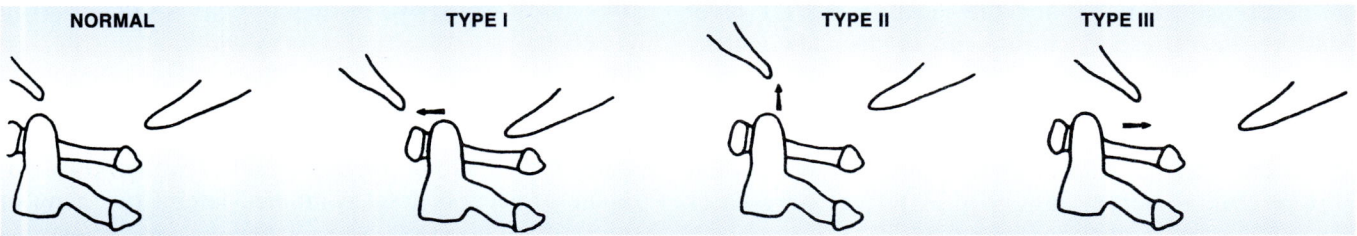

Figure 3 Diagrams demonstrating the normal atlanto-occipital relationship and three types of atlanto-occipital dislocation. Type I involves anterior displacement of the occiput with respect to the atlas. Type II is primarily a longitudinal dislocation. Type III atlanto-occipital dislocation results when there is posterior displacement of the occiput on the atlas. (Reproduced with permission from Traynelis VC, Marano GD, Dunker RO, Kaufman HH: Traumatic atlanto-occipital dislocation. J Neurosurg 1986;65:863-870.)

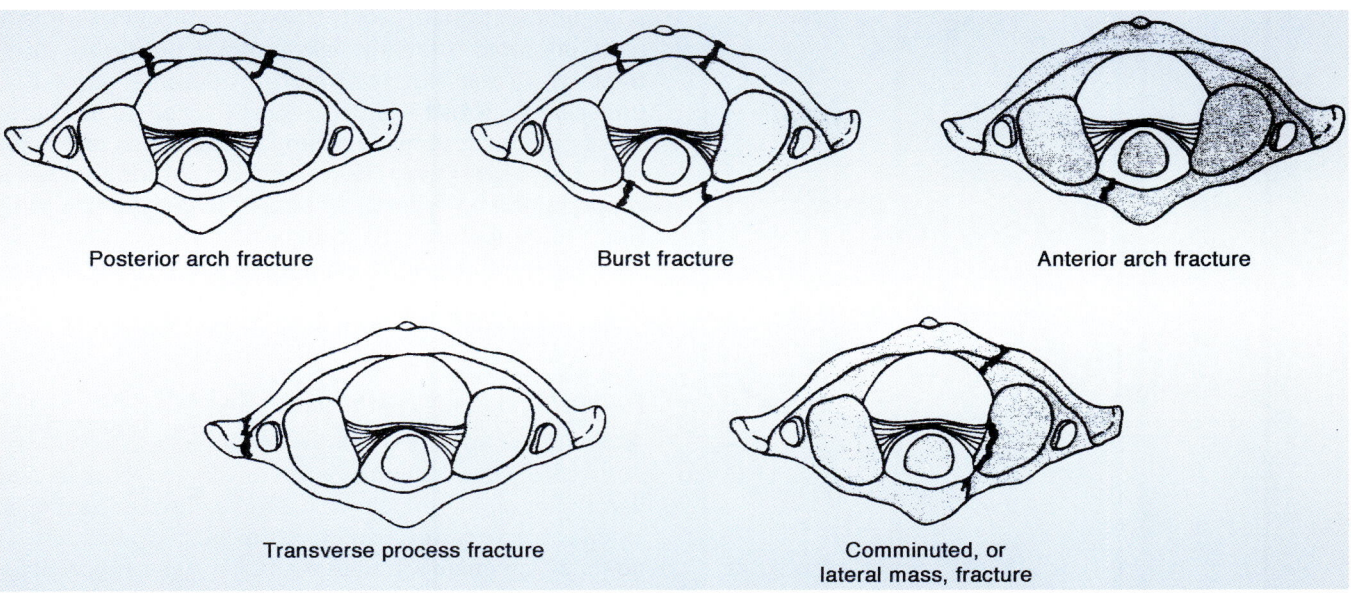

Figure 4 Types of atlas fractures. *(Reproduced with permission from Silcox DH III, Whitesides TE Jr: Injuries of the cervicocranium, in Browner BD, Jupiter JB, Levine AM, Trafton PG, Lampert R (eds): Skeletal Trauma: Fractures, Dislocations, Ligamentous Injuries, ed 2. Philadelphia, PA, WB Saunders, 1997, pp 861-893.)*

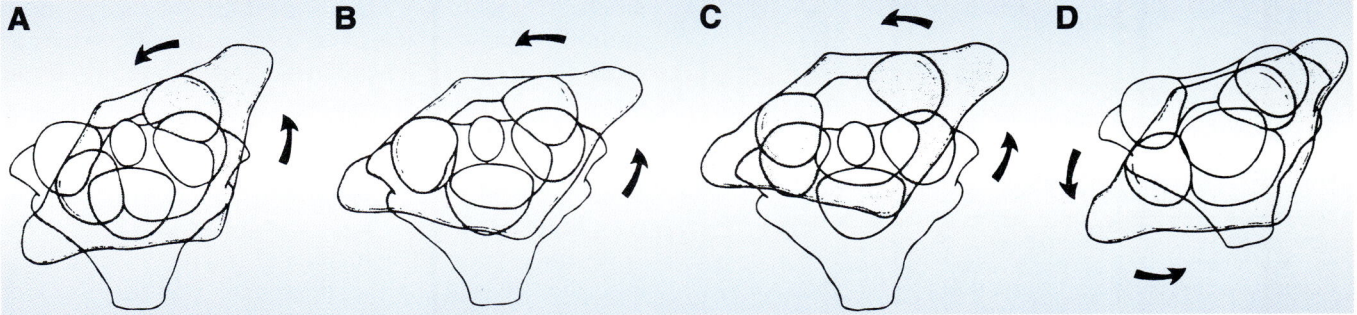

Figure 5 Drawings showing the four types of rotatory fixation. **A,** Type I, rotatory fixation with no anterior displacement and the odontoid acting as the pivot. **B,** Type II, rotatory fixation with anterior displacement of 3 to 5 mm, one lateral articular process acting as the pivot. **C,** Type III, rotatory fixation with anterior displacement of more than 5 mm. **D,** Type IV, rotatory fixation with posterior displacement. *(Reproduced with permission from Silcox DH III, Whitesides TE Jr: Injuries of the cervicocranium, in Browner BD, Jupiter JB, Levine AM, Trafton PG, Lampert R (eds): Skeletal Trauma: Fractures, Dislocations, Ligamentous Injuries, ed 2. Philadelphia, PA, WB Saunders, 1997, pp 861-893.)*

sional reconstruction can be helpful in diagnosing the injury.

Rotatory fixation has been classified into four types according to the degree of anterior translation of the atlas on the axis (Fig. 5). In type I injuries, the rotation occurs about an intact transverse atlantal ligament, so there is less than 3 mm of anterior translation as measured by the ADI. Rupture of this ligament in type II injuries allows rotation to occur about one facet joint with 3 to 5 mm of anterior displacement of C1 on C2. Greater than 5 mm of anterior displacement is indicative of a type 3 rotatory fixation, which may occur with a C1-C2 bilateral facet joint dislocation. Type IV rotatory fixation is characterized by posterior subluxation of C1 on C2, which may occur in the setting of an odontoid fracture or with odontoid hypoplasia.

Treatment of a traumatic C1-C2 rotatory subluxation usually involves attempted skeletal traction reduction and halo immobilization, although open reduction may be necessary if closed reduction fails. Rupture of the transverse atlantal ligament in types II through IV injuries often manifests as chronic atlantoaxial instability, for which atlantoaxial arthrodesis is the treatment of choice.

Odontoid Fractures

Fractures of the odontoid process result from flexion, extension, and rotational forces and are associated with a neurologic deficit in up to 25% of cases. Odontoid fractures are classified into three types (Fig. 6). Type I fractures are characterized by an oblique fracture at the tip of the dens as a result of an avulsion of the alar ligament. Occipitocervical dissociation must be ruled out in these injuries. Type II fractures occur at the base of the dens, while type III fractures extend into

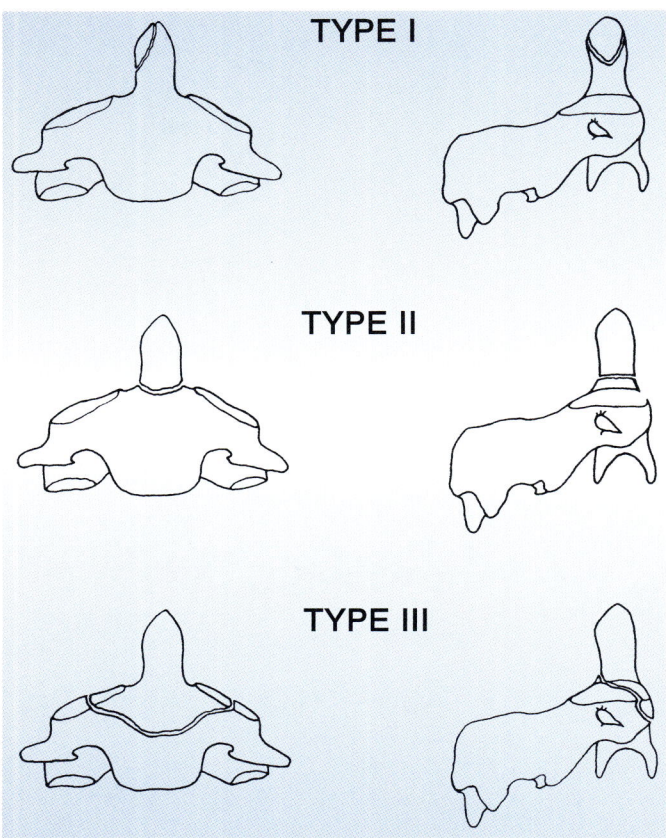

TYPE I

TYPE II

TYPE III

Figure 6 Frontal and side views of nondisplaced odontoid fractures according to the Anderson and D'Alonzo classification. Oblique fractures through the tip of the dens comprise type I fractures. Type II fractures are through the odontoid waist. Transverse plane C2 body fractures that include the odontoid in one fragment comprise type III fractures. *(Reproduced from Anderson LD, D'Alonzo RT: Fractures of the odontoid process of the axis. J Bone Joint Surg Am 1974;52:1663-1674.)*

the C2 body. Type II fractures are the most common of the odontoid fractures. Type IIa fractures have been described and represent cortical comminution at the odontoid base.

The rare type I fracture with a stable occipitocervical ligamentous complex can be treated with 3 months of external immobilization followed by flexion and extension cervical spine radiographs to rule out persistent instability. Type II fractures with less than 6 mm of displacement may achieve union in 80% of nonelderly patients following traction reduction and halo immobilization. Nonunion of these fractures is more likely in patients older than age 40 years, in fractures with more than 6 mm of displacement or 10° of angulation, and with failure to maintain reduction. Type III fractures treated nonsurgically have an 87% union rate. Halo immobilization may improve the chance for bony union over hard collar immobilization in type III odontoid fractures in the younger patient. The morbidity associated with wearing a halo for 3 months in an elderly patient as well as the high nonunion rate in nonsurgically treated elderly patients have led to the

recommendation of acute C1-C2 arthrodesis or primary odontoid osteosynthesis in the majority of type II fractures in the elderly. Anterior odontoid screw fixation has an 81% to 96% fusion rate and theoretically avoids the compromised postoperative range of motion occurring after a posterior atlantoaxial fusion. Cortical comminution in type IIa fractures may preclude anterior odontoid screw fixation. Furthermore, combined C1 ring fractures and odontoid fractures may require C1-C2 arthrodesis if incompetency of the transverse atlantal ligament is detected.

Traumatic Spondylolisthesis of the Axis

A traumatic spondylolisthesis of the axis is commonly referred to as a hangman's fracture because of its similar radiographic appearance to the distraction hyperextension injury that occurred in judicial hangings. In nonfatal hangman's fractures after a high impact loading to the cervical spine, such as may happen in a motor vehicle accident, a fracture line propagates through the C2 pars interarticularis resulting in anterolisthesis of the C2 body on C3. The force mechanism is characterized as a combination of extension, axial compression, and then flexion. Bilateral C2 pars fractures inherently decompress the spinal cord, so traumatic spondylolisthesis of the axis alone is not usually associated with a neurologic deficit. Concomitant upper cervical spine injuries and cranial nerve injuries may occur, however.

Several types of hangman's fractures have been described, based on the degree of fracture displacement (Fig. 7). Type I fractures have less than 3 mm of displacement of the C2 body on C3 and no angulation. Type II fractures have more than 3 mm of anterolisthesis and angulation. A secondary wedge compression fracture of the underlying C3 superior end plate may occur as well. Type IIa injuries demonstrate no anterolisthesis but significant angulation, signifying a disruption of the posterior longitudinal ligament and the C2-C3 disk from a distraction-flexion force. Unilateral or bilateral facet dislocation allowing further anterolisthesis occurs in type III injuries.

Type I pars fractures of the axis are stable injuries that displace minimally on flexion and extension cervical spine radiographs. This fracture subtype can be treated with collar external immobilization. Traction reduction followed by halo immobilization is the usual treatment for type II fractures, but anterolisthesis of less than 6 mm may often be treated with external immobilization without a traction reduction maneuver. Because of ligamentous disruption in type IIa hangman's fractures, traction is contraindicated. Gentle manipulation with extension and neutralization in a halo device is the treatment of choice. Type III frac-

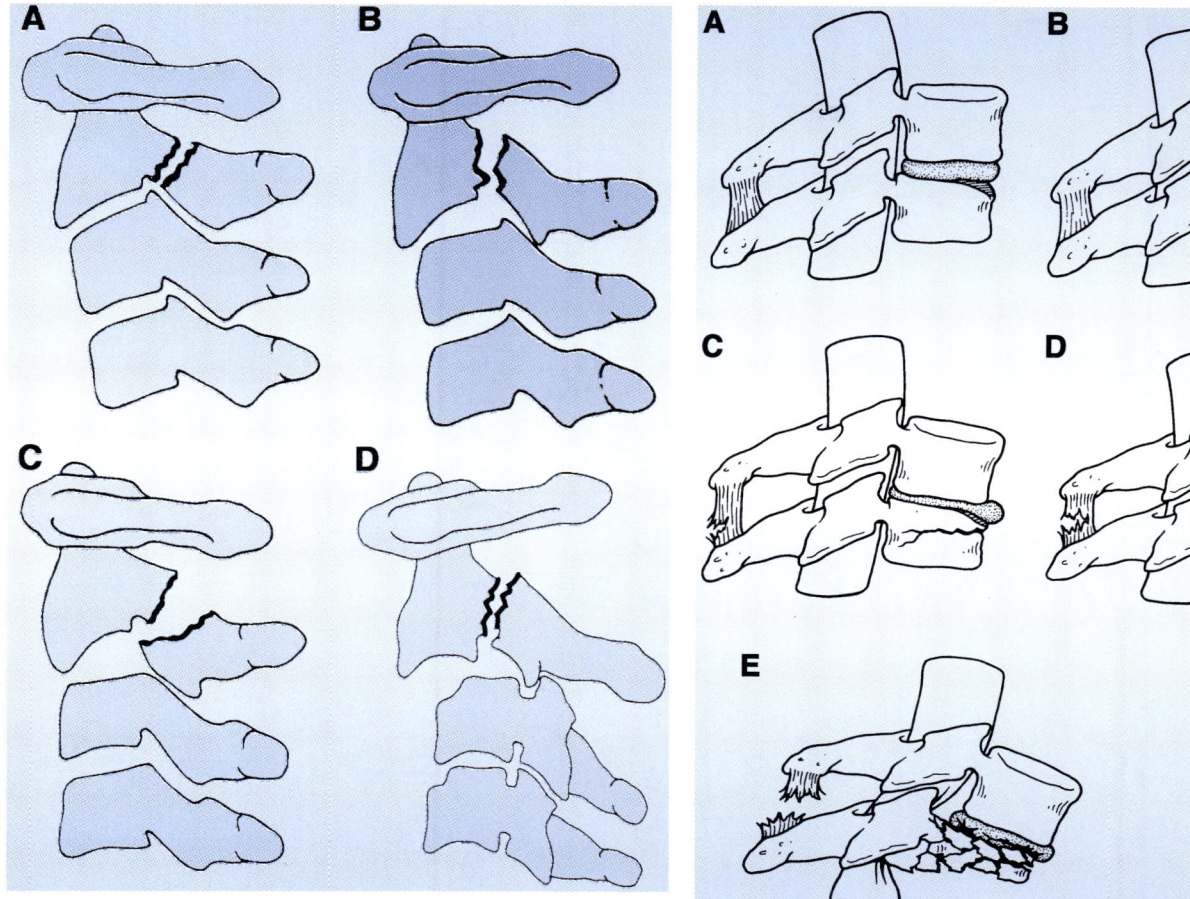

Figure 7 Classification of traumatic spondylolisthesis of the axis. **A,** Type I injuries have a fracture through the neural arch with no angulation and as much as 3 mm of displacement. **B,** Type II fractures have both significant angulation and displacement. **C,** Type IIA fractures have shown minimal displacement, but there is severe angulation. **D,** Type III axial fractures combine bilateral facet dislocation between C2 and C3 with a fracture of the neural arch of the axis. *(Reproduced from Silcox DH III, Whitesides TE Jr: Injuries of the cervicocranium, in Browner BD, Jupiter JB, Levine, AM, Trafton PG, Lampert R (eds): Skeletal Trauma: Fractures, Dislocations, Ligamentous Injuries, ed 2. Philadelphia, PA, WB Saunders, 1997, pp 861-893.)*

Figure 8 Allen and Fergusson classification of subaxial cervical spine fractures. Compression-flexion injuries are divided into 5 stages. **A,** Stage I demonstrates a rounding of the anterior-anterosuperior portion of the vertebral body. **B,** Stage II demonstrates an increasing compression of the anterosuperior portion of the vertebral body. **C,** A significant change from stages I and II, stage III progresses with a fracture line through the vertebral body, with or without posterior ligamentous injury. **D,** Stage IV is marked by comminution and depression of the vertebral body, with mild (3 mm) posterior displacement into the spinal canal and posterior ligamentous injury. **E,** Stage V progression exhibits more than 5 mm of posterior displacement of the vertebral body with posterior ligamentous disruption.

tures often require open reduction of the facet dislocation and posterior C2-C3 fusion; closed reduction usually fails because of distraction through the pars fracture. An anterior C2-C3 arthrodesis is useful to avoid extending the fusion mass cephalad to C1 in cases of symptomatic nonhealed hangman's injuries.

Axis Body Fractures

Fractures extending into the body of C2 may occur in the coronal, sagittal, or horizontal planes. Coronal plane fractures that involve the pars interarticularis are often referred to as atypical hangman's fractures. The resulting anterolisthesis may drape the spinal cord over the posterior vertebral body cortical fragment; one third of these atypical hangman's fractures are associated with a neurologic deficit. Avulsion of the anterior

longitudinal ligament may result in another type of C2 body fracture; an oblique axis body fracture recently has been described in which a fragment containing the odontoid process and one superior articular process displaces anterocaudally. Surgical stabilization may be necessary for certain coronal plane atypical hangman's fractures or sagittal plane burst fractures. Horizontal plane axis fractures are equivalent to type III odontoid fractures and are usually treated nonsurgically, as are anterior avulsion fractures.

Subaxial Cervical Spine Injuries

Lower cervical spine fractures are frequently categorized into six mechanistic types and further subdivided into stages of injury (Figs. 8 through 11). The position of the neck at the time of injury (either flexion, exten-

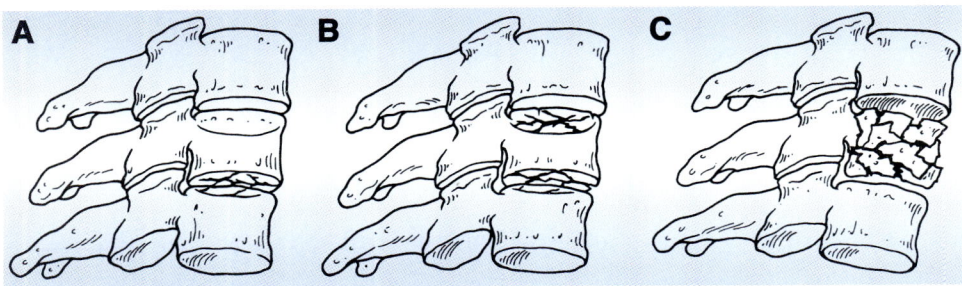

Figure 9 Three stages of vertical compression fractures. **A,** Stage 1: fracture through one end plate. **B,** Stage 2: fracture through both end plates. **C,** Stage 3: burst fracture.

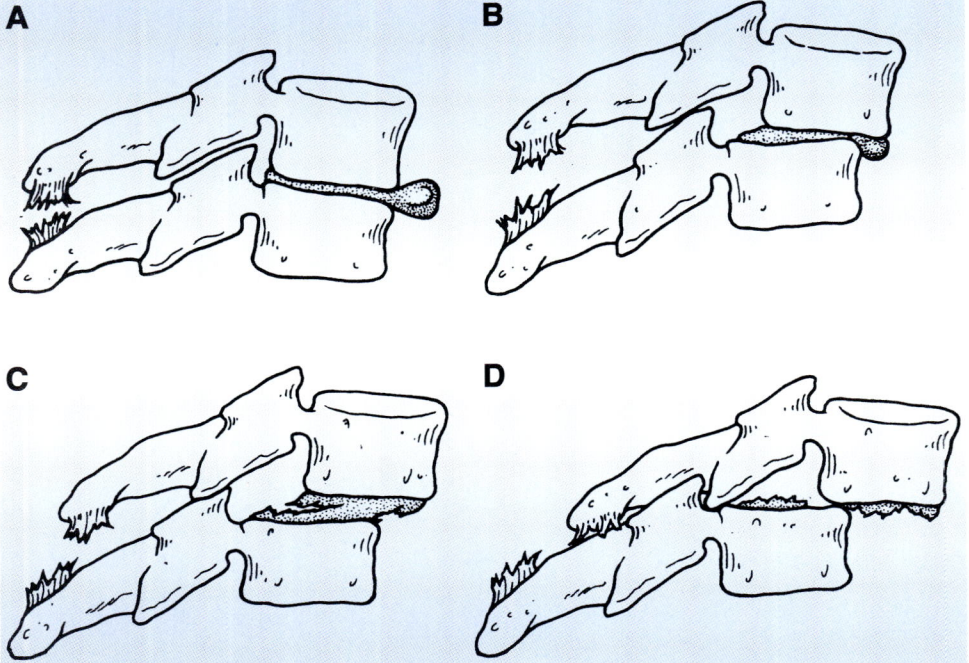

Figure 10 Distraction-flexion injuries are divided into four stages. **A,** Stage 1: flexion sprain. **B,** Stage 2: anterior subluxation with 25% anterior translation of the superior vertebral body. **C,** Stage 3: 50% translation or displacement the superior vertebral body. **D,** Stage 4: complete dislocation of the superior vertebral body.

sion, or neutral) and the direction of force (either compression, distraction, or lateral bending) are the determinants of injury patterns. Other important factors that influence fracture kinematics of the subaxial cervical spine include vertebral body mass, loading rate, and energy of injury. Classifying the injury pattern may require careful evaluation of all imaging modalities, including plain radiographs, CT, and MRI.

Compression-Flexion Injuries

Compression-flexion injuries account for 20% of subaxial cervical spine fractures and are most common at the C4, C5, and C6 levels. The pathomechanics of this injury subtype are characterized by anterior vertebral body compression with posterior element distraction. In stage 1 injuries, blunting of the anterosuperior corner of the vertebral body may progress to anterior wedging or beaking with loss of vertebral height in stage 2 injuries. Hard collar immobilization of these injuries is necessary to prevent progressive collapse and late deformity. In stage 3 injuries, a fracture line

extends from the anterosuperior vertebral body end plate posteriorly through the inferior end plate. In stage 4 fractures, less than 3 mm of retropulsion of the posterior vertebral body fragment into the spinal canal is present. Halo immobilization may be sufficient for stages 3 and 4 compression-flexion subaxial cervical spine fractures if significant posterior ligamentous incompetency is not present; otherwise an anterior cervical corpectomy and strut graft placement with instrumentation is appropriate to prevent late kyphotic deformity. With stage 5 fractures, more than 3 mm of fracture fragment retropulsion into the vertebral canal usually occurs along with posterior ligamentous compromise. In this fracture subtype, anterior decompression and fusion with instrumentation supplemented in some cases by a posterior arthrodesis is often required.

Vertical Compression Injuries

Vertical compression injuries comprise 15% of subaxial cervical spine fractures and are most common at the C6 and C7 levels. Stage 1 injuries form a cupping

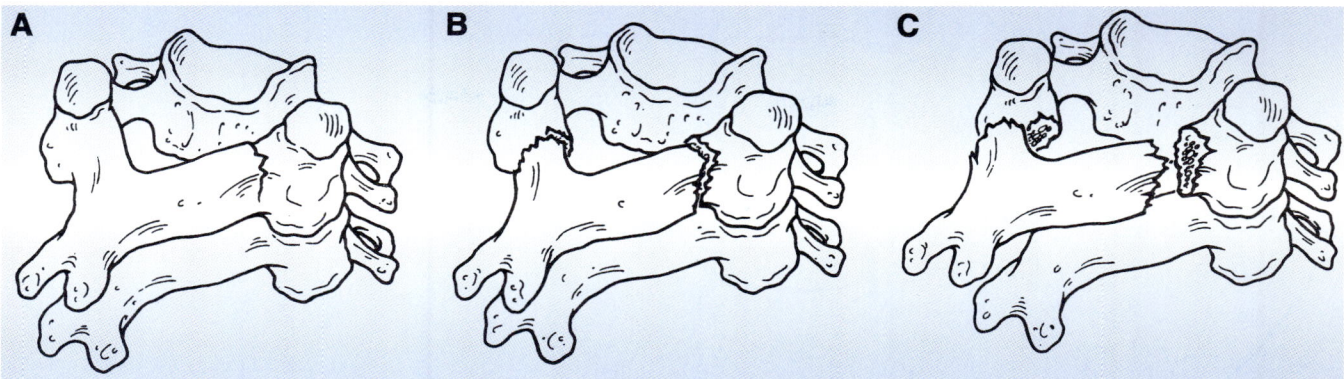

Figure 11 Three stages of compression-extension injuries. **A,** Stage 1: nondisplaced fracture of the posterior elements. **B,** Stage 2: moderately displaced fracture of the posterior elements. **C,** Stage 3: completely displaced fracture of the posterior elements. *(Note: distraction-extension and lateral flexion injuries are not shown.)* (Reproduced with permission from Clark CR: The Cervical Spine, ed 3. Philadelphia, PA, Lippincott-Raven, 1998, pp 451-454.)

deformity of the superior or inferior end plates and are usually treated with hard collar immobilization. End plate fracture without significant displacement occurs in stage 2 injuries, and stage 3 injuries involve displacement of the fracture fragments into the vertebral canal. Minimally displaced injuries without neurologic compromise are often treated with halo immobilization; otherwise an anterior corpectomy and fusion is the preferred management.

Distraction-Flexion Injuries

Distraction-flexion injuries comprise 10% of all subaxial cervical spine injuries. With stage 1 injuries, there is unilateral facet subluxation and by interspinous process widening and posterior vertebral cortical margin incongruity on a lateral plain radiographic projection. A stage 2 injury is a unilateral facet joint dislocation and appears as a 25% anterolisthesis of the cephalad vertebral body on the caudal body on a lateral radiograph. A stage 3 bilateral facet joint dislocation appears as 50% or more anterolisthesis of the cephalad on caudal vertebral body; and a stage 4 injury appears as 100% anterolisthesis or complete vertebral translation on lateral radiographs.

A traumatic disk herniation may occur in up to 54% of cervical facet dislocations. This concern for coincident herniated disk has led some physicians to conclude that prereduction MRI is necessary to identify such patients, in which case diskectomy prior to spinal reduction could avoid iatrogenic neurologic deterioration from retropulsion of the disk herniation during reduction. Nevertheless, in an awake, alert, and cooperative patient, closed reduction with skeletal traction and serial neurologic examinations has proved in repeated studies to be safe and effective in the reduction of these injuries prior to spinal canal imaging. Neurologic deterioration during closed reduction of cervical facet dislocations is actually rare and has been reported only

in intubated, anesthetized patients. Prereduction MRI may therefore not be necessary in awake, alert, and cooperative patients.

Because of ligamentous insufficiency following these distraction-flexion injuries, surgical stabilization is indicated. Preoperative MRI following a successful closed reduction should be performed prior to surgical stabilization to evaluate for the presence of a herniated disk. A posterior cervical fusion, anterior cervical diskectomy and fusion, or anterior cervical diskectomy and circumferential fusion is then indicated depending on whether or not the closed reduction was successful and whether or not a herniated disk is present.

Compression-Extension Injuries

Compression-extension injuries of the subaxial cervical spine manifest initially as failure of the posterior elements followed by injury to the vertebral body. Stage 1 and 2 injuries describe nondisplaced unilateral and bilateral posterior arch fractures, both of which are treated with hard collar immobilization. Stages 3, 4, and 5 injuries involve progressive anterolisthesis of the cephalad, injured spinal segment and variable injury to the caudal anterior vertebral body. These higher energy injuries often require posterior reduction and fusion.

Distraction-Extension Injuries

Distraction-extension injuries account for more than 20% of subaxial cervical spine injuries and are more common in patients with ankylosing spondylitis or diffuse idiopathic skeletal hyperostosis. Disk space widening in stage 1 injuries results from anterior ligamentous failure. Alternatively, this injury may present as a nondisplaced transverse fracture of the vertebral body. Stage 2 injuries involve posterior ligamentous failure with associated retrolisthesis of the cephalad on caudal vertebral segment. Stage 1 fractures without diskal disruption may be treated with halo immobilization. Dis-

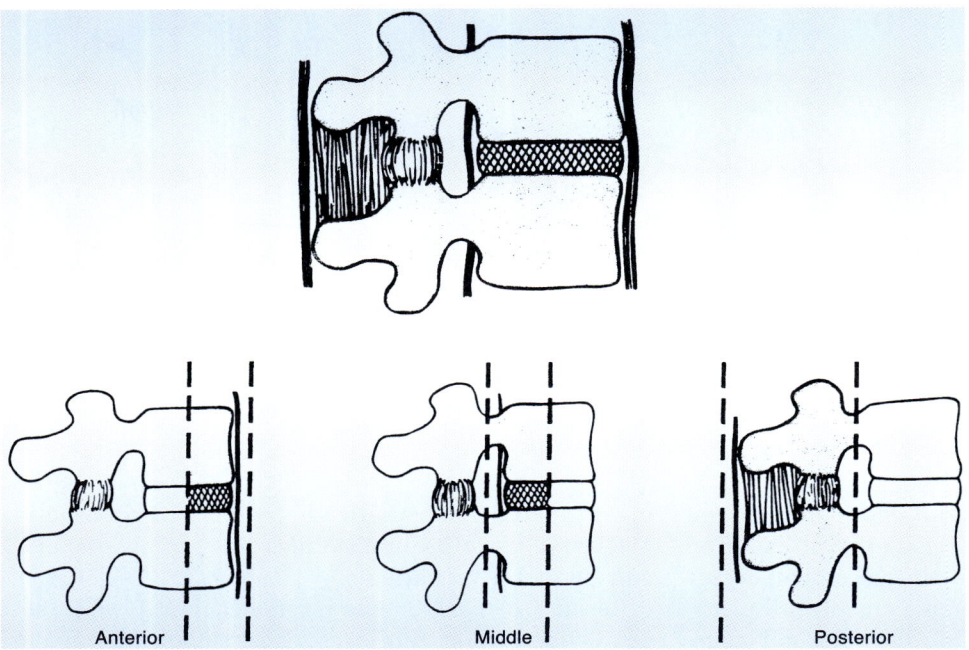

Figure 12 Denis' three-column model of the spine. The middle column is made up of the posterior longitudinal ligament, the posterior anulus fibrosus, and the posterior aspect of the vertebral body and disk. *(Reproduced with permission from Garfin SR, Blair B, Eismont FJ, Abitol JJ: Thoracic and upper lumbar spine injuries, in Browner BD, Jupiter JB, Levine AM, Trafton PG, Lampert R (eds): Skeletal Trauma: Fractures, Dislocations, Ligamentous Injuries, ed 2. Philadelphia, PA, WB Saunders, 1997, pp 947-1034.)*

Anterior   Middle   Posterior

kal disruption in the adult patient has less predictable healing, so diskectomy and fusion with anterior tension plating is often indicated. Stage 2 injuries also are best managed with skeletal traction reduction and surgical stabilization.

Lateral Flexion Injuries

Lateral flexion injuries comprise 20% of subaxial cervical spine injuries. Stage 1 injuries represent ipsilateral bony failure of the vertebral body and posterior arch. The posterior element fracture may involve the pedicle, lamina, lateral mass, or superior or inferior articulating process. These fractures are often missed on plain radiography and require CT imaging for adequate characterization. MRI evidence of accompanying ligamentous injury may provide information regarding fracture stability, especially in the presence of fracture-subluxation. External immobilization is usually sufficient for minimally displaced injuries. Articular process fractures, however, may allow a rotational displacement of the vertebral body, appearing as a lengthened vertebral body on lateral plain radiograph. This fracture variant may require surgical reduction and fixation. In stage 2 injuries, contralateral bony or ligamentous structures fail in tension with obvious vertebral displacement. This fracture often requires closed skeletal traction reduction and operative stabilization.

Thoracic Spine Injuries

Spinal stability in the upper thoracic region is augmented by the ribs, sternum, and costotransverse ligaments. Injury to this region, therefore, usually re-

quires high-energy trauma and is less common than injury elsewhere in the spine. Fractures or fracture-dislocations between T1 and T10 represent 16% of all thoracic and lumbar spine injuries. Upper thoracic fractures are usually stable injuries unless accompanied by sternal and rib injuries, in which case they may be unstable and predisposed to late collapse and kyphotic deformity. The thoracolumbar junction, however, lacks the reinforcement of the rib cage and represents an area of inflection from thoracic kyphosis to lumbar lordosis. Therefore, injuries from T11 to L1 account for 52% of all thoracic and lumbar spine injuries.

Consideration of spinal stability forms the basis of thoracolumbar injury classification and management. Studies suggest that the spine consists of three columns, each contributing variably to overall stability depending on the spinal segment level (Fig. 12). The anterior longitudinal ligament, anterior anulus fibrosus, and anterior two thirds of the vertebral body and intervertebral disk form the anterior column. The posterior third of the vertebral body, the intervertebral disk, the posterior anulus fibrosus, and the posterior longitudinal ligament form the middle column. The neural arch including the pedicles and lamina, the transverse process, the articulating facets with their surrounding joint capsule, the spinous process, the ligamentum flavum, the interspinous ligaments, and the supraspinous ligament all form the posterior column. Disruption of all three columns at a single level strongly suggests the presence of biomechanical instability at that functional spinal unit. Because of physiologic thoracic kyphosis, the posterior column in the thoracic spine is under tension and (when intact) acts as a tension band, conferring stability. Thoracic spine instability may thus depend mostly on disruption of this posterior tension band.

With the three-column concept of fracture stability, the Denis classification system for thoracolumbar fractures describes the structural characteristics and mechanism of injury for four types of injury patterns. Isolated minimally displaced fractures of the spinous process, transverse process, pars interarticularis, and facet joint are grouped as minor injuries. These minor injuries are usually managed symptomatically as long as occult instability is ruled out by dynamic flexion and extension radiography once acute pain and muscular spasm has resolved. Isolated pars fractures, however, may require external bracing with a thoracolumbosacral orthosis (TLSO). Major injuries include compression fractures, burst fractures, fracture-dislocations, and flexion-distraction injuries.

Compression Fractures

Compression injuries are characterized by failure of the anterior column without middle column involvement. An anterior wedge fracture of the vertebral body results from a flexion force vector with a variable amount of lateral flexion. Greater degrees of injury may also cause the posterior column to fail in tension. Posterior ligamentous disruption in compression fractures must be suspected when loss of anterior vertebral height approaches or exceeds 50%.

Because the middle column is intact, retropulsion of bony fragments into the spinal canal does not occur, and neurologic dysfunction is unlikely. Acute or delayed kyphotic deformity is a concern in combined anterior and posterior column failure, however. To avoid this complication, compression fractures with 50% or more collapse in anterior vertebral height or evidence of posterior ligamentous disruption are treated with a hyperextension orthosis (TLSO) or body cast. For thoracic fractures above T7, a cervical extension to the orthosis often is required for proper immobilization. Close radiographic follow-up is mandatory, as progressive loss of sagittal plane alignment or neurologic deterioration is often managed with surgical reduction, decompression, and stabilization.

Burst Fractures

Burst fractures are defined as disruption of both the anterior and middle columns from an axial load with or without a flexion moment. Posterior ligamentous injury may be present depending on the spinal level and severity and direction of the imparted force vector

loads. Biomechanical studies have shown that the initial disruption of bony integrity begins at the base of the pedicle in the middle column and at the superior end plate in the anterior column. A sagittal plane vertebral body fracture with centrifugal displacement and retropulsion of bony fragments into the canal, along with a widened interpedicular width, is often noted on radiographic and CT imaging. Because of the normal thoracic kyphotic alignment at the T1 through T10 levels, axial compression results mostly in anterior or middle column failure. In the lower thoracic levels where there is a transition toward lumbar lordosis, burst fractures in these areas tend to involve all three columns.

Thoracic burst fracture stability is directly related to the competency of the posterior ligamentous structures. Failure of the posterior ligamentous structures is inferred radiographically by widening of the interspinous process distance. A localized kyphotic deformity of 20° to 30° or more on plain radiographs often portends a poor outcome with nonsurgical management, so surgical stabilization should be considered.

Nonsurgical management consists of immobilization in a TLSO or hyperextension body cast with or without a cervical extension for a minimum of 3 months, depending on the stability of the fracture. Stable thoracic burst fractures without posterior column disruption have equivalent radiographic and clinical outcomes following surgical and nonsurgical treatment. Unstable thoracic burst fractures, however, often require surgical reduction and stabilization. Anterior, posterior, or circumferential fusion is chosen depending on the level of injury and degree of neurologic and osteoligamentous instability. The posterior approach is used most often. In a neurologically intact patient, a three- or four-point fixation bending moment strategy using cantilever forces to restore sagittal alignment is often used. Care must be taken to avoid retropulsion of vertebral bone fragments into the spinal canal, and distraction should be minimized in the setting of posterior column disruption to avoid tension on the neural elements. Electrophysiologic monitoring is a helpful adjunct in this clinical setting.

Incomplete neurologic dysfunction in the presence of thecal sac compression in thoracic burst fractures often requires surgical decompression in addition to spinal stabilization. This procedure may be performed through an anterior (preferred) or posterolateral approach. Anterior procedures require a structural graft or implant reconstruction augmented with anterior instrumentation. In addition to standard open anterior approaches, several small case series recently have reported successful use of a videoscopic technique for fracture corpectomy, grafting, and instrumentation.

Fracture-Dislocations

A fracture-dislocation of the thoracic spine is a high-energy injury that results in a neurologic deficit in over 70% of cases. All three spinal columns are disrupted following a distraction and rotational load application. Gross malalignment of the spine occurs from anterior, posterior, or rotational listhesis of the injured vertebral body. Early surgical reduction and stabilization allows for prompt patient mobilization regardless of neurologic status, thereby decreasing overall morbidity and mortality. Decompression of the spinal cord in this injury subtype is often achieved by realignment of the spine through a posterior approach. A subsequent anterior decompression and reconstruction may be necessary in the setting of residual thecal sac compression and incomplete neurologic deficit.

Flexion-Distraction Injuries

A flexion-distraction injury results in tension failure of the posterior and middle columns with compression or tension failure of the anterior column depending on whether the traumatic axis of rotation is anterior or posterior to the anterior longitudinal ligament. Spinal column failure may occur entirely through bone as in a Chance fracture; entirely through the soft-tissue diskal and ligamentous structures; or through a combination of both bony and soft-tissue elements. Because injured bony spinal elements have a more predictable healing potential than do diskal or ligamentous disruption, Chance fractures may be treated nonsurgically with closed reduction in extension and external immobilization. Adults, however, have not enjoyed the same healing success as the bony Chance fracture in children; some physicians have recommended posterior surgical stabilization in all flexion-distraction injuries. In all other flexion-distraction injury variants, a posterior reduction and fusion with compressive segmental fixation one level above and one level below the injury is often undertaken. Care must be taken to avoid significant posterior compression in patients with a comminuted posterior vertebral body to prevent iatrogenic bony fragment retropulsion into the spinal canal.

Lumbar Spine Injuries

The three-column concept of spinal stability helps guide the classification and management of spinal injuries from L1 to L5. Flexible lumbar lordosis tends to dampen the magnitude of flexion forces before bony or ligamentous failure occurs, so axial loading injuries resulting in burst fractures are more common than other types of injuries in the lumbar spine. Thoracic and lumbar burst fractures occur most commonly in the T12-L1 region. Three-column involvement with centrifugal fragment displacement and spinal canal encroachment often occurs with evidence of a greenstick fracture of the lamina on a transaxial CT. Biomechanical investigations have suggested the amount of canal encroachment in lumbar burst fractures is related to the rate of impact loading. Injuries resulting from a significant flexion-compression force vector may result in localized kyphosis with wedging of the superior end plate. This fracture type often has significant associated posterior ligamentous disruption. A high suspicion for dural laceration and nerve root entrapment should be given to any burst fracture with posterior element disruption in the setting of a neurologic deficit. If surgical intervention is selected in this situation, gentle dissection in the area of the involved posterior elements should be performed to avoid iatrogenic neural injury.

Flexion-distraction injuries in the lumbar spine are less common, comprising less than 10% of all lumbar spine injuries. Bony Chance fractures occur 50% of the time at levels L2, L3, or L4. These fractures often are minimally displaced and infrequently associated with neurologic injury. Alternatively, flexion-distraction injuries with diskal or ligamentous disruption are more prone to neurologic deficit and long-term instability if treated nonsurgically. A flexion-distraction lumbar spine injury with bilateral facet dislocation often results in significant thecal sac encroachment. Nevertheless, the degree of neurologic deficit is often less severe than in similar injuries to the thoracic spine, probably related to the presence of the cauda equina rather than spinal cord in this region as well as the larger canal diameter of the lumbar spine as compared with the thoracic region.

Avulsion injuries in the lumbar spine, including isolated spinous process or transverse process fractures, are often minor injuries in regard to spinal stability. These injuries may, however, be consequences of significant trauma such as an L5 transverse process fracture in the setting of an unstable pelvic fracture. Eleven percent of patients with a seemingly solitary lumbar transverse process fracture on plain radiography were found to have a more significant lumbar spine fracture on CT imaging in one study. Nerve root avulsion and visceral injury must also be excluded in the trauma assessment.

Stable lumbar injuries, including isolated avulsion fractures, flexion-compression fractures with less than 50% anterior vertebral body collapse, and bony Chance fractures may be managed nonsurgically in an extension orthosis or body cast. For fractures below L2, immobilization of the pelvis with a single hip spica extension attached to the orthosis or cast is often beneficial for improved spinal stabilization. Nonsurgical management of low lumbar burst fractures without neurologic deficit yields good to excellent results in the majority of cases. Canal encroachment in these fractures in the absence of a neurologic deficit is not an indication for surgery because significant remodeling and bony fragment resorption occur in the first year after injury that help reconstitute the canal's preinjury sagittal diameter.

Unstable lumbar injuries are usually characterized by three-column spinal failure with tensile disruption of the posterior ligamentous complex and sagittal or rotational plane malalignment. Surgical intervention in this patient subgroup allows for early mobilization and rehabilitation regardless of the neurologic status. Surgical intervention may be through an anterior, posterior, or combined approach. Patients with an incomplete neurologic deficit are candidates for a decompression procedure. Decompression may be achieved via a posterior, posterolateral (extracavitary or transpedicular), or anterior approach. Initial posterior surgery is useful in fracture-dislocations, flexion-distraction, and distraction-extension injuries to obtain appropriate spinal alignment. A secondary assessment of canal patency should then be performed to determine the necessity of an anterior decompressive procedure in the setting of a neurologic deficit. Burst fractures down to the L3 level may be approached anteriorly (with a corpectomy), but caution should be taken when placing anterior short instrumentation at L4 and below because of the close proximity of the great vessels.

Posterior pedicle fixation without additional anterior column support may be useful for surgical management of L4 and L5 burst fractures, yet pedicle screw failure is a potential problem without supplemental anterior column reconstruction. Posterior reduction and stabilization of thoracolumbar junction injuries using a distraction hook and rod system (two to three segments above and one to two below the level of injury) can adequately reestablish anterior vertebral body height. The potential for iatrogenic flatback deformity with hook placement below the L2 level is a concern, however, because of applied distraction forces and collapse of spanned injured disk spaces. Combined anterior and posterior procedures may avoid some of these problems.

Sacral Fractures

Fractures of the sacrum are difficult to discern on plain radiographs; 70% may be missed with radiography alone. A CT scan better delineates these injuries. In addition to avulsion injuries, the pattern of sacral fracture may be vertical, oblique, or transverse; most are vertical. According to the Denis classification system (Fig. 13), sacral fractures may occur lateral to the neu-

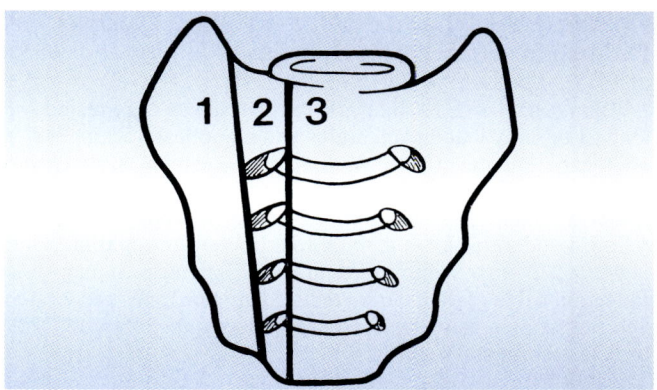

Figure 13 Denis classification of sacral fractures. Neurologic findings are most common with zone 2 and 3 fractures, which may violate the sacral neural foramina or central sacral canal, respectively, *(Reproduced with permission from Denis F, Davis S, Comfort T: Sacral fractures: An important problem: Retrospective analysis of 236 cases. Clin Orthop 1988;227:67-81.)*

ral foramina (zone 1), through the foramina (zone 2), or medial to the foramina (zone 3). Zone 3 fractures involve the central sacral canal, and more than half of these injuries occur with neurologic impairment. Zone 2 injuries are associated with neurologic deficits in over 25% of cases, usually from nerve root injury. Zone 1 sacral ala fractures may result in sciatic nerve or L5 nerve root injury in approximately 6% of cases. Transverse sacral fractures are less common and are high-energy injuries. Neurologic deficit, dural tear, and rectal perforation are commonly associated with this fracture pattern.

Displaced sacral fractures should be assessed for potential instability. These injuries are usually managed with closed or surgical reduction and stabilization with a variety of fixation strategies such as sacroiliac screws, transiliac bars, or plate and screw fixation. Closed reduction and percutaneous screw fixation for displaced longitudinal sacral fractures is an option, and refinement of screw localization techniques may make this procedure less technically demanding in the future. A neurologic deficit in the setting of a sacral fracture should lower the threshold to perform a laminectomy and exploration of the involved nerve roots at the time of surgical stabilization.

Annotated Bibliography

Amar AP, Levy ML: Pathogenesis and pharmacological strategies for mitigating secondary damage in acute spinal cord injury. *Neurosurgery* 1999;44:1027-1040.

This article presents a discussion of the pathogenesis of spinal cord injury, primary and secondary phases of injury and experimental agents used to interrupt secondary mechanisms of injury. There seems to be a narrow window of opportunity for such pharmacologic agents to be effective.

Crawford NR, Hurlbert RJ, Choi WG, Dickman CA: Differential biomechanical effects of injury and wiring at C1-2. *Spine* 1999;24:1894-1902.

　　Biomechanics of 10 cadaveric cervical spines were tested with a quasistatically loading apparatus and an optical tracking system after experimental transverse-alar-apical ligament sectioning or odontoid fracture, after odontoidectomy, and then following posterior cable-graft fixation. Greatest instability was noted following odontoidectomy. Odontoid fracture resulted in slightly higher C1-2 angular motion than did ligamentous injury alone. Posterior cable-graft fixation reduced motion only moderately, and this fixation was subject to fatigue loosening after any of the three experimental injuries.

de Klerk LW, Fontijne WP, Stijnen T, Braakman R, Tanghe HL, van Linge B: Spontaneous remodeling of the spinal canal after conservative management of thoracolumbar burst fractures. *Spine* 1998;23:1057-1060.

　　Despite greater than 25% spinal canal encroachment in 42 consecutive thoracolumbar burst fractures treated nonsurgically, significant remodeling occurred after a mean of approximately 3.5 years. The mean of 50% spinal stenosis at the time of injury decreased to a mean of 25% stenosis at the time of follow-up as measured by sagittal spinal canal diameter. The greater the initial stenosis, the greater the amount of remodeling observed. Older age correlated with a lower degree of remodeling. Neurologic deficit did not appear to influence spinal canal remodelling.

Jenkins JD, Coric D, Branch CL Jr: A clinical comparison of one- and two-screw odontoid fixation. *J Neurosurg* 1998;89:366-370.

　　This article presents a retrospective review of 42 consecutive type II odontoid fracture stabilizations determined equivalent union rates with use of one or two anterior odontoid screws. The choice to use one or two depended on the size of the dens and the ability to fit a second screw. Union occurred in 81% of the 20 patients treated with one screw, and in 85% of those treated with two screws.

Lee TT, Green BA, Petrin DR: Treatment of stable burst fracture of the atlas (Jefferson fracture) with rigid cervical collar. *Spine* 1998;23:1963-1967.

　　Twelve stable burst fractures of the atlas without evidence of C1-C2 subluxation, transverse ligament avulsion, or type II odontoid fracture were treated 10 to 12 weeks in a rigid cervical collar. No instability was noted in 10- to 12-week follow-up flexion-extension cervical radiographs, and no neurologic deterioration was noted in 1- to 2-year clinical follow-up.

Rabinovici R, Ovadia P, Mathiak G, Abdullah F: Abdominal injuries associated with lumbar spine fractures in blunt trauma. *Injury* 1999;30:471-474.

　　Lumbar spine fracture following blunt trauma in 258 patients over 7 years was associated with significant intra-abdominal injury in 26. Splenic, renal, hepatic, and small bowel injuries were noted in these 26 patients. Multilevel spinal fractures were more likely to be associated with organ injury than single level fracture, though specific spinal fracture level or type of fracture were not significantly associated with intra-abdominal injury.

Rechtine GR II, Cahill D, Chrin AM: Treatment of thoracolumbar trauma: Comparison of complications of operative versus nonoperative treatment. *J Spinal Disord* 1999;12:406-409.

　　Of 235 unstable traumatic thoracolumbar spinal injuries, 117 were treated with surgical fixation and 118 were treated nonsurgically for 6 weeks on a kinetic bed. No significant difference was noted between the two groups in the occurrence of decubitus ulcer, deep vein thrombosis, pulmonary embolus, or death. The surgical fixation group had an 8% rate of deep wound infection. Hospital stay was 24 days longer in the nonsurgical group.

Seybold EA, Sweeney CA, Fredrickson BE, Warhold LG, Bernini PM: Functional outcome of low lumbar burst fractures: A multicenter review of operative and nonoperative treatment of L3-L5. *Spine* 1999;24:2154-2161.

　　Low lumbar fractures from L3 to L5 were treated in 42 patients over a 17-year period, with 20 patients being managed nonsurgically and 22 patients undergoing surgery. After a mean of almost 4 years follow-up, there was no significant difference in functional outcome or ability to return to work, and no patient showed neurologic deterioration. Reoperation for hardware removal, kyphotic collapse, or loss of fixation was required in 41% of those being managed surgically.

Classic Bibliography

Allen BL Jr, Ferguson RL, Lehmann TR, O'Brien RP: A mechanistic classification of closed, indirect fractures and dislocations of the lower cervical spine. *Spine* 1982;7:1-27.

Anderson LD, D'Alonzo RT: Fractures of the odontoid process of the axis. *J Bone Joint Surg Am* 1974; 56:1663-1674.

Benzel EC, Hart BL, Ball PA, Baldwin NG, Orrison WW, Espinosa M: Fractures of the C-2 vertebral body. *J Neurosurg* 1994;81:206-212.

Bracken MB, Shepard MJ, Holford TR, et al: Administration of methylprednisolone for 24 or 48 hours or tirilazad mesylate for 48 hours in the treatment of acute spinal cord injury: Results of the Third National Acute Spinal Cord Injury Randomized Control Trial: National Acute Spinal Cord Injury Study. *JAMA* 1997; 277:1597-1604.

Coric D, Wilson JA, Kelly DL Jr: Treatment of traumatic spondylolisthesis of the axis with nonrigid immobilization: A review of 64 cases. *J Neurosurg* 1996;85: 550-554.

Cotler JM, Herbison GJ, Nasuti JF, Ditunno JF Jr, An H, Wolff BE: Closed reduction of traumatic cervical spine dislocation using traction weights up to 140 pounds. *Spine* 1993;18:386-390.

Denis F, Davis S, Comfort T: Sacral fractures: An important problem: Retrospective analysis of 236 cases. *Clin Orthop* 1988;227:67-81.

Denis F: Spinal instability as defined by the three-column spine concept in acute spinal trauma. *Clin Orthop* 1984;189:65-76.

Effendi B, Roy D, Cornish B, Dussault RG, Laurin CA: Fractures of the ring of the axis: A classification based on the analysis of 131 cases. *J Bone Joint Surg Br* 1981;63:319-327.

Fielding JW, Hawkins RJ: Atlanto-axial rotatory fixation (fixed rotatory subluxation of the atlanto-axial joint). *J Bone Joint Surg Am* 1977;59:37-44.

Gertzbein SD, Court-Brown CM: Flexion-distraction injuries of the lumbar spine: Mechanisms of injury and classification. *Clin Orthop* 1988;227:52-60.

Greene KA, Dickman CA, Marciano FF, Drabier JB, Hadley MN, Sonntag VK: Acute axis fractures: Analysis of management and outcome in 340 consecutive cases. *Spine* 1997;22:1843-1852.

Harris JH Jr, Carson GC, Wagner LK, Kerr N: Radiologic diagnosis of traumatic occipitovertebral dissociation: Part 2. Comparison of three methods of detecting occipitovertebral relationships on lateral radiographs of supine subjects. *AJR Am J Roentgenol* 1994;162:887-892.

Levine AM, Edwards CC: Traumatic lesions of the occipitoatlantoaxial complex. *Clin Orthop* 1989;239: 53-68.

Levine AM, Edwards CC: Fractures of the atlas. *J Bone Joint Surg Am* 1991;73:680-691.

Levine AM, Edwards CC: The management of traumatic spondylolisthesis of the axis. *J Bone Joint Surg Am* 1985;67:217-226.

Levine AM, Bosse M, Edwards CC: Bilateral facet dislocations in the thoracolumbar spine. *Spine* 1988;13: 630-640.

Przybylski GJ, Clyde BL, Fitz CR: Craniocervical junction subarachnoid hemorrhage associated with atlanto-occipital dislocation. *Spine* 1996;21:1761-1768.

Rushton SA, Vaccaro AR, Levine MJ, Smith M, Balderston RA, Cotler JM: Bivector traction for unstable cervical spine fractures: A description of its application and preliminary results. *J Spinal Disord* 1997;10:436-440.

Saboe LA, Reid DC, Davis LA, Warren SA, Grace MG: Spine trauma and associated injuries. *J Trauma* 1991;31:43-48.

Starr JK, Eismont FJ: Atypical hangman's fractures. *Spine* 1993;18:1954-1957.

Chapter 50

Cervical Degenerative Disk Disorders

K. Daniel Riew, MD

John M. Rhee, MD

Axial Neck Pain Without Radiculopathy or Myelopathy

Clinical Presentation

The spondylotic pain associated with degenerative disk disorders is typically episodic, with the acute pain improving over days to weeks. Sources of spondylotic pain include disks, facets, extensor muscles, and the greater occipital nerve. Symptoms are often exacerbated with range of motion (particularly extension) and may be associated with crepitus. Occipital headaches also may be present. The pain can vary in location and may be present centrally, laterally, over the trapezius, or in the interscapular region. A well described but frequently missed cause of axial neck pain is atlantoaxial osteoarthrosis. Patients with symptomatic atlantoaxial rather than subaxial osteoarthrosis are typically in their 70s or older and may present with pain localized to the occipitocervical junction. In these patients, rotation (to one side if the arthrosis is unilateral, or to both sides if bilateral) exacerbates the pain, but motion in the sagittal plane typically does not.

Physical examination of all patients should assess active flexion, extension, lateral flexion, and rotation of the neck. A thorough neurologic examination with provocative tests is performed to rule out radiculopathy or myelopathy. Indications for obtaining radiographs include a history of trauma, prolonged duration of symptoms (1 month or longer), presence of constitutional symptoms, known systemic disease (such as cancer or inflammatory arthritis), radiculopathy, or myelopathy. Degenerative changes in the uncovertebral joints can be identified on the AP radiograph. Lateral radiographs demonstrate overall alignment (lordosis, kyphosis), disk space narrowing, vertebral body osteophytes, and olistheses. Oblique radiographs can be helpful in identifying the presence of neuroforaminal stenosis or facet arthrosis. Flexion-extension views can be helpful if there is a history of instability or trauma, or to investigate the presence of postoperative pseudarthrosis. An open mouth odontoid view can identify odontoid fractures as well as the presence of atlantoaxial arthritis. CT scans with appropriate sagittal and coronal reconstructions may help delineate the bony anatomy associated with fractures, foraminal stenosis, facet arthritis, and the presence of ossification of the posterior longitudinal ligament. Infections and neoplasms can be further studied with MRI. MRI or CT myelograms are useful in ruling out neural compression.

In addition to degenerative cervical spine etiologies, the differential diagnosis of isolated axial neck pain includes fractures, dislocations, inflammatory arthritides (such as rheumatoid arthritis and ankylosing spondylitis), infections (such as diskitis, osteomyelitis, or epidural abscess), tumors (intradural, extradural), and nonspine sources. These causes of neck pain must be ruled out before treatment of cervical spondylosis is begun. A detailed patient history will provide essential information. Constant, unremitting pain that interrupts sleep and is associated with constitutional symptoms such as fever, malaise, and weight loss are suggestive of tumor or infection. A history of injury should be obtained to rule out traumatic etiologies, and to evaluate nonspine causes of neck and shoulder pain, such as gallbladder, coronary, rotator cuff, or brachial plexus-related pathologies. Work-up of patients with neck pain may frequently reveal a diagnosis of diffuse idiopathic skeletal hyperostosis (DISH), also known as Forestier's disease. DISH is an ossifying diathesis of unknown cause that has been reported to occur in 5% to 10% of the population over age 65 years. Radiographically, DISH is characterized by anterolateral ossification along at least four continuous vertebral bodies with relatively normal disk spaces and no facet ankylosis. Patients may be asymptomatic or have neck pain, dysphagia, or cervical myelopathy. DISH can be differentiated from ankylosing spondylitis by the

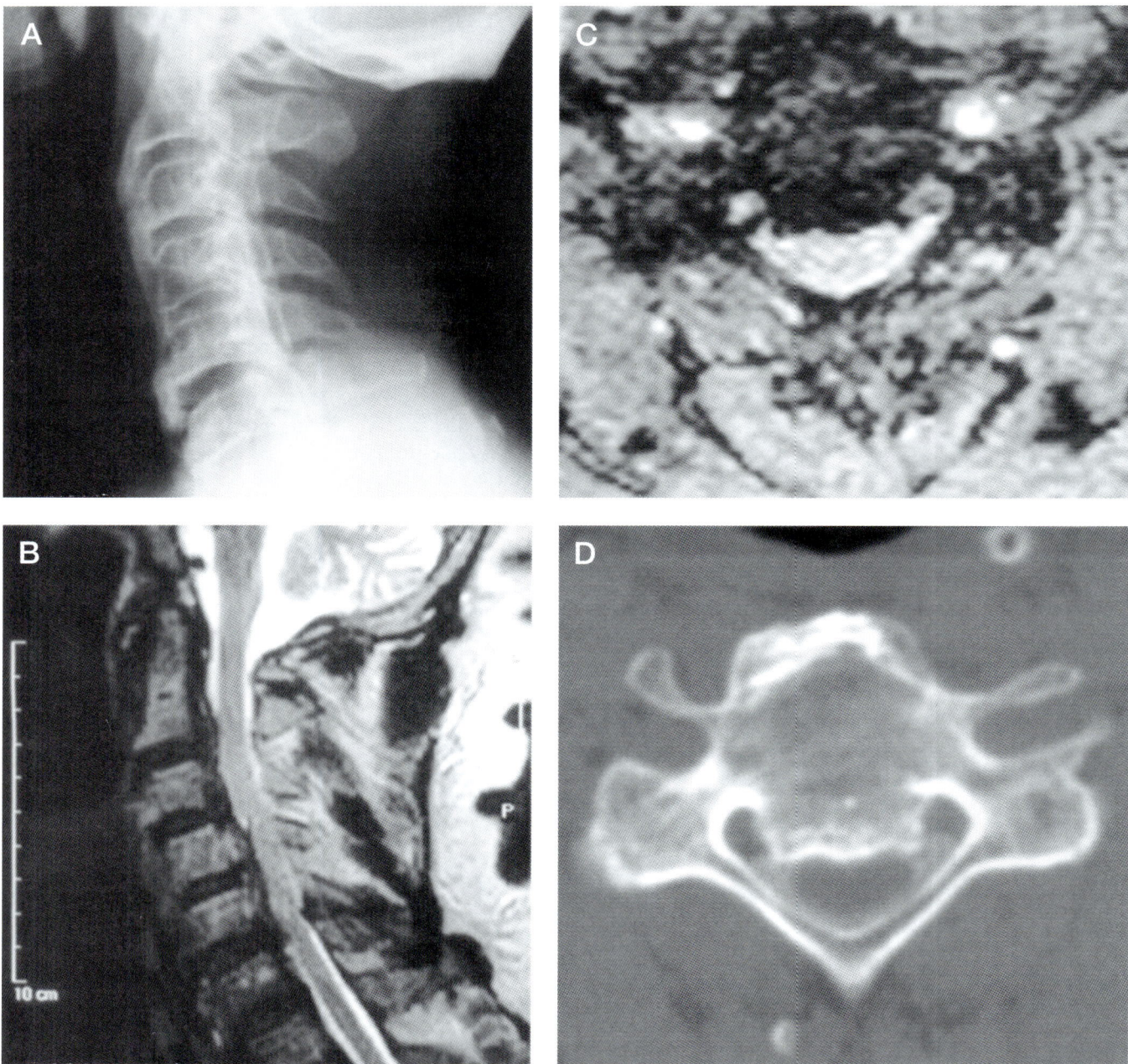

Figure 1 **A,** Lateral radiograph of a patient with DISH as well as ossification of the posterior longitudinal ligament. The ossification of the posterior longitudinal ligament is not so evident here. **B,** T2-weighted sagittal MRI of the same patient. Note the increase in the signal where the posterior longitudinal ligament lies. There is narrowing of the spinal canal secondary to this thickened posterior longitudinal ligament, indicating that extra calcium or ossification may be present in the posterior longitudinal ligament. **C,** Axial image of the same patient. It is difficult to tell from this image if the compression of the cord is due to soft disk or bone. **D,** CT scan obtained after myelogram demonstrating ossification of the posterior longitudinal ligament. If it were simply an osteophyte, it would be present mainly at the disk levels and not in the mid vertebral body, as this ossified mass is.

absence of both sacroiliitis and apophyseal joint ankylosis. Management of patients with DISH is not necessarily different than that of other patients with neck pain. However, it should be noted that cervical trauma in these patients may carry a relatively poor prognosis, with high rates of neurologic deficit and a paradoxical propensity to nonunion if diagnosis and stabilization are not achieved early. A high incidence of ossification of the posterior longitudinal ligament has also been demonstrated in non-Asian patients with DISH, and may be the cause of myelopathy in these patients (Fig. 1).

Treatment

Nonsurgical treatment is favored for the majority of patients with isolated axial neck pain caused by cervical spondylosis. Nonsteroidal anti-inflammatory medi-

TABLE 1 | Common Cervical Radiculopathy Patterns

Root	Symptoms	Motor	Reflex
C2	Posterior occipital headaches, temporal pain	–	–
C3	Occipital headache, retro-orbital or retroauricular pain	–	–
C4	Base of neck, trapezial pain	–	–
C5	Lateral arm	Deltoid	Biceps
C6	Radial forearm, thumb and index fingers	Biceps, wrist extension	Brachioradialis
C7	Middle finger	Triceps, wrist flexion	Triceps
C8	Ring and little fingers	Finger flexors	–
T1	Ulnar forearm	Hand intrinsics	–

cations are favored over narcotic-based medications. Isometric cervical muscle strengthening, the use of heat or ice massage, and short-term immobilization in a soft collar can be considered. In general, performing surgical fusion for isolated axial neck pain is controversial. Favorable results have been reported with posterior arthrodesis in selected patients with atlantoaxial osteoarthrosis in whom nonsurgical treatment is unsuccessful, demonstrate secondary C1-C2 instability, or have neurologic compromise.

Cervical Spondylotic Radiculopathy

Clinical Presentation

Patients with cervical spondylotic radiculopathy complain of pain and neurologic dysfunction along a nerve root distribution. The proportion of weakness, numbness, and pain is quite variable from patient to patient. In general, arm pain is worse than neck pain and is often exacerbated by motion of the neck. However, the exact location of pain depends on the nerve root level involved. High cervical radiculopathies are associated with unilateral upper trapezial pain, neck pain, and headaches. Patients with instability at C1 through C2 may have headaches in the C2 distribution along with retro-orbital and temporal pain. Associated kinking of the vertebrobasilar vessels can result in syncope and vertigo. Table 1 lists the most common pain and neurologic patterns associated with radiculopathies of the cervical nerve roots. Occipital headaches are common with herniations or osteophytes that broadly indent the thecal sac or cord, regardless of the level involved. Upper trapezial and interscapular pain are also common regardless of the level involved.

A careful physical examination should be performed to identify the nerve root involved, with the caveat that crossover within myotomes and dermatomes may

be present. Cervical nerve roots 1 through 7 exit above their correspondingly numbered pedicles (for example, the C6 root exits between C5 and C6). Disk herniations and foraminal stenosis in the cervical spine tend to produce radiculopathy of the nerve root exiting at the same level. Thus, both a C5-6 disk herniation and C5-6 foraminal stenosis typically produce a C6 radiculopathy. A large central to midlateral disk herniation or stenosis may, however, cause a radiculopathy of the next lower nerve root. Motor strength is graded on a scale of 0 to 5 points. Sensory testing should include at least one function from the dorsal columns (such as joint position sense, light touch) and the spinothalamic tract (such as pain and temperature sensation). If more than one root level appears to be involved, the presence of myelopathy should be considered and ruled out. The presence of long tract signs (clonus, Babinski, Hoffman) also suggests myelopathy.

A Spurling's maneuver may reproduce the radicular symptoms in a patient with a foraminal disk or stenosis. The neck is maximally extended and rotated to the side of the pathology. Adduction of the shoulder with extension of the elbow and wrist may accentuate the Spurling's sign. The maneuver narrows the foramen and stretches the nerve across it. The symptoms will disappear during maximal flexion and rotation of the neck to the other side and raising of the symptomatic arm to place the hand behind the neck, thereby opening the foramen and relaxing the nerve.

In addition to standard radiographs, MRI is helpful in demonstrating herniated disks as well as central and foraminal stenosis. CT myelography is a dynamic test that demonstrates mechanical blocks to the flow of cerebrospinal fluid. Neither study is clearly superior in demonstrating all cervical pathology. MRI may be better at identifying disk herniations, stenosis, and cord lesions, whereas CT myelography may be better at detecting foraminal stenosis and differentiating bony from soft-tissue pathology. MRI is advantageous because it is noninvasive. When interpreting a radiographic study, it is important to keep in mind that the position of the neck at the time of the study can affect the result. Conventional myelograms are obtained with the patient's neck in an extended position to prevent the flow of dye into the brain. Because the neuroforamina are narrow in extension, this position increases the likelihood of diagnosing mild to moderate foraminal stenosis. Because MRI and postmyelogram CT are most commonly performed with the patient supine with the neck in a neutral position, conditions that are symptomatic with the patient's neck in the extremes of flexion (mild disk herniations) or extension (mild foraminal stenosis) may be underdiagnosed.

The two most common causes of cervical spondylotic radiculopathy are disk herniations and foraminal stenosis. The differential diagnoses of cervical spondylotic radiculopathy are similar to those for axial neck pain. In addition, peripheral nerve entrapment syndromes (for example, carpal or cubital tunnel syndromes) and tendinopathies of the shoulder, elbow, and wrist must be considered. Selective cervical nerve root injections can be useful in confirming the source of symptoms and also may be therapeutic. Electromyographic and nerve conduction tests may help differentiate radiculopathy from peripheral entrapment neuropathies. However, false-positive and false-negative electrodiagnostic studies may be common, and these studies tend to be observer-dependent.

Treatment

The natural history of cervical spondylotic radiculopathy generally is favorable. In patients with disk herniations, symptoms resolve over time without surgical intervention. Furthermore, it is not common for patients with radiculopathy to progress to myelopathy. Thus, the initial management of cervical spondylotic radiculopathy should be nonsurgical and may include anti-inflammatory medications, physical therapy, nerve root injections, and steroid dose packs.

Indications for surgery include severe or progressive neurologic deficit (weakness or numbness) or failure to respond to conservative treatment. Depending on the pathology, cervical spondylotic radiculopathy may be surgically addressed with an anterior or posterior approach. In general, an anterior cervical diskectomy and fusion (ACDF) is preferred for most cases, because the offending pathology tends to be predominantly anterior to the cord (for example, disk or osteophytes arising from the posterior vertebral body) and thus can be removed without manipulation of the spi-

nal cord. For this reason, the anterior approach can be performed for both central and anterolateral disk herniations, whereas a posterior approach cannot be safely used for central disk herniations. Another advantage of the ACDF is that placement of an anterior bone graft in the disk space opens up the neuroforamen and thereby decompresses the nerve root. Direct nerve root decompression can also be performed by resecting the posterior aspect of the uncovertebral joint. Regaining the height of the disk space with an anterior graft also diminishes infolding of the posterior longitudinal ligament and ligamentum flavum, which may improve nerve root or cord impingement posteriorly. The major disadvantage of the anterior approach is the potential for graft-related complications (such as pseudarthrosis). Meticulous attention to fusion technique is therefore mandatory. Another potential problem is accelerated adjacent segment degeneration after fusion, but its clinical significance is not well known.

During ACDF, disk resection is carried out to the posterior longitudinal ligament. If a disk fragment is extruded posterior to the posterior longitudinal ligament, then resection of the posterior longitudinal ligament may be necessary. Uncovertebral spurs are generally removed if present, although they have been demonstrated to resorb and satisfactory results can be achieved without resecting them if a solid arthrodesis is achieved. A Smith-Robinson horseshoe-shaped graft is favored because it is stronger in compression than other graft configurations such as the Cloward graft. The use of autograft versus allograft is controversial. Autograft proponents believe that autografts increase the speed and percentage of fusion. Allograft proponents counter that the nonunion rate for a single-level arthrodesis is no different with allograft, but the morbidity associated with graft harvesting is avoided. Plating of single-level ACDFs, although controversial, is probably not necessary. Plating does not appear to decrease the rate of nonunion, but it may slightly diminish the amount of kyphosis that develops over the fused level. Furthermore, proponents state that plating obviates the need for a postoperative cervical orthosis and allows a faster return to activities and work. The nonunion rate of a single-level ACDF varies but is approximately 4%. Symptomatic nonunions have been successfully treated with repeat Smith-Robinson ACDF, or with corpectomy, strut grafting, and correction of deformity if kyphosis is present. Another alternative is a posterior fusion across the area of nonunion.

Posterior approaches to cervical spondylotic radiculopathy can be considered for unilateral or bilateral radiculopathy at one or more levels. The keyhole foraminotomy can be used to decompress the nerve root without significantly destabilizing the spine in patients with anterolateral disk herniation or foraminal stenosis without significant neck pain. The offending disk or anterior osteophyte does not necessarily need to be removed if an adequate decompression is achieved and the nerve root is freed posteriorly. The posterior foraminotomy can be particularly effective for treating high cervical radiculopathies (C2 through C3 or C3 through C4) because, unlike in the lower levels of the cervical spine, foraminal stenosis at C2 through C3 or C3 through C4 can often be caused by facet arthrosis. A major advantage of the posterior foraminotomy is that it can be performed with minimal patient morbidity. However, because the procedure does not attempt to restore disk height at the diseased level, a disadvantage is a tendency for deterioration of results with time as the degenerative disk process continues at that level.

Although fusion is not routinely necessary with a posterior foraminotomy, if more than 50% of both facet joints are resected to adequately decompress the nerve root, posterior fusion with lateral mass plates or spinous process cables should be considered.

Cervical Spondylotic Myelopathy

Clinical Presentation

Cervical spondylotic myelopathy is caused by spinal cord impingement by bone, osteophytes, disk, and other tissues arising from the degenerative disk process, often in the setting of a congenitally stenotic canal. In patients older than age 50 years, cervical spondylosis is the most common cause of myelopathy. Many patients complain of axial neck and radicular pain, but up to 20% do not. Because the majority of the compressive pathology tends to be anterior to the cord, most patients with cervical spondylotic myelopathy have an anterior cord syndrome, with greater motor involvement in the lower extremities than the upper extremities. Less commonly, a central cord syndrome is seen. Patients demonstrate a wide-based gait and have problems with balance. The fine motor function, grasp, and sensation of the upper extremities is impaired, leading to a complaint of "clumsiness." Bowel and bladder or dorsal column dysfunction occur with advanced disease, and prognosis is poor.

On neurologic examination, a combination of upper motor neuron findings in the lower extremities and either upper or lower motor neuron findings in the upper extremities can be observed. Provocative signs, including the Lhermitte's sign, may be elicited, in which neck flexion produces an electric shock-like sensation down the arms and legs, and dysdiadochokinesia (inability to perform rapid alternating movements).

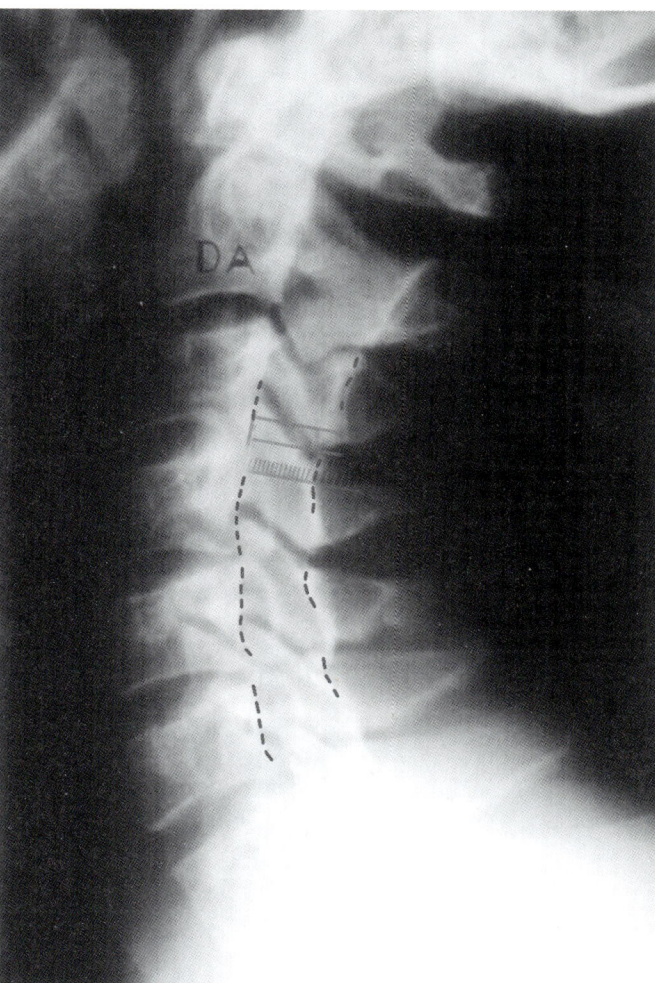

Figure 2 Lateral radiograph of a patient with congenital cervical stenosis. The superimposed ruler indicates that the space available for the cord is only 11 mm at C4. The dotted lines represent the posterior vertebral and the spinolaminar lines.

Long tract signs are often positive in myelopathic patients. The Babinski response may be positive and is a poor prognostic indicator. The Hoffman's sign occurs when flicking the volar surface of the flexed middle finger distal phalanx results in pathologic flexion of the thumb and index finger. The finger escape sign is the inability to maintain the ulnar digits in an extended and adducted position. An inverted radial reflex is seen when the brachioradialis reflex itself is diminished but causes spastic contraction of the finger flexors instead. Patients with high cervical cord compression may demonstrate the scapulohumeral reflex, in which tapping the tip of the scapula results in brisk scapular elevation and humeral abduction. Clonus and hyperreflexia of the lower extremities are also seen in myelopathic patients. However, the presence of a positive jaw jerk (opening of the mouth with tapping of the lower jaw) suggests that the upper motor neuron findings may originate in the brain rather than the spinal cord.

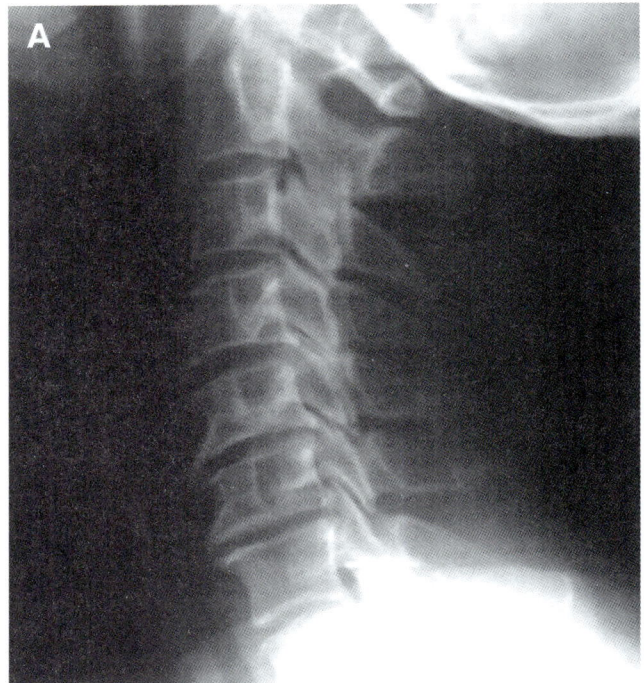

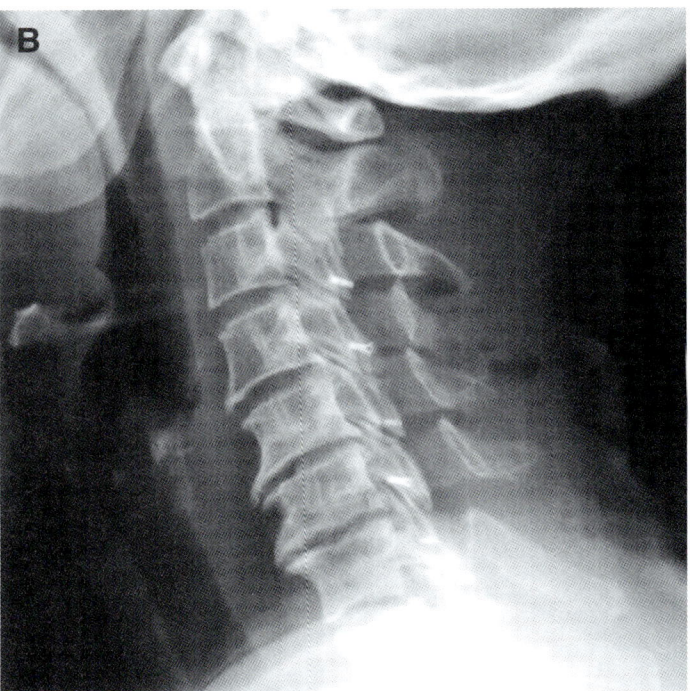

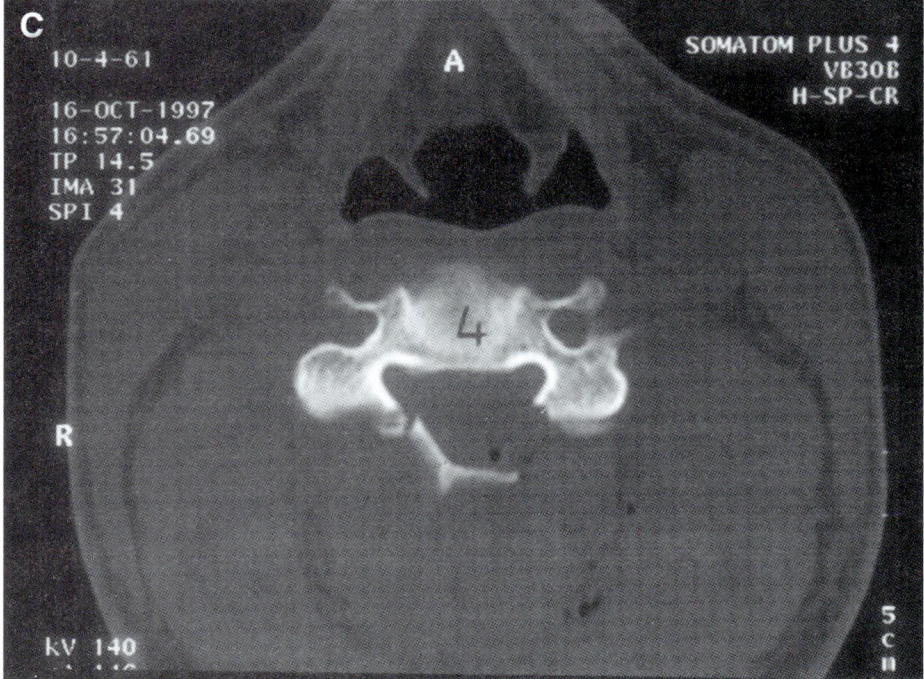

Figure 3 Lateral radiographs of a patient with congenital cervical stenosis and myelopathy. **A,** Before laminoplasty. **B,** After laminoplasty. Mini Mitek suture anchors have been placed into the lateral masses and are used to keep the laminoplasty open. Notice that the space available for the cord has significantly increased compared with the preoperative lateral radiograph. **C,** CT scan of another patient after an open door laminoplasty procedure demonstrating enlargement of the cervical spinal canal.

Peripheral nerves must be in proper working order to transmit the hyperreflexia of myelopathy. Therefore, patients with concomitant myelopathy and peripheral nerve disease from conditions such as diabetes, peripheral neuropathy, or severe multilevel foraminal stenosis can have diminished or absent reflexes. In addition, cervical myelopathy with severe lumbar spinal stenosis can result in brisk upper extremity reflexes with diminished lower extremity reflexes.

The lateral radiograph can be used to determine the degree of congenital cervical stenosis present (Fig. 2). A Pavlov ratio (AP diameter of canal/AP diameter of vertebral body) of less than 0.8 suggests congenital stenosis. A space available for the cord of 13 mm or less also suggests a narrow sagittal diameter of the spinal canal and has been shown to correlate with neurologic injury after trauma. Imaging studies that should be obtained in addition to radio-

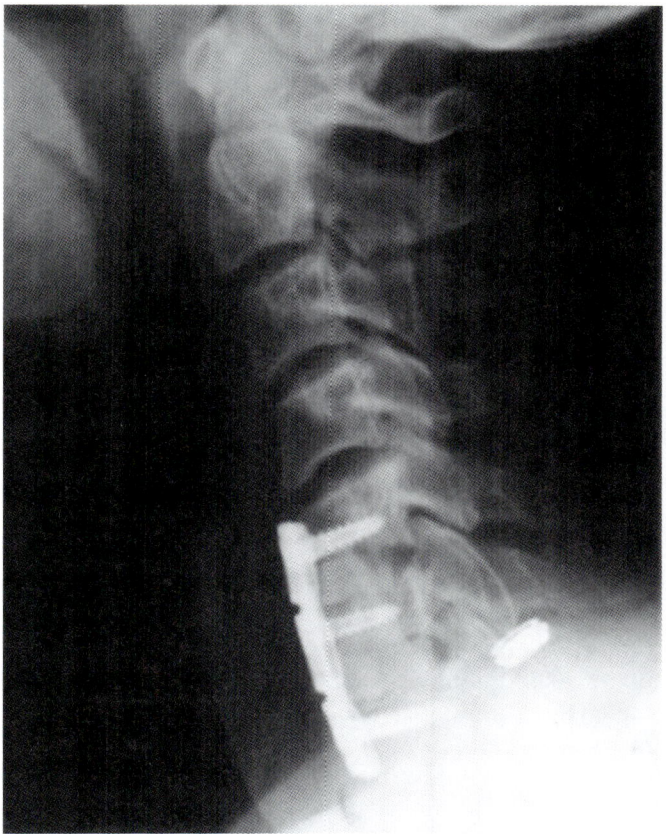

Figure 4 Radiograph obtained after a two-level anterior cervical diskectomy and fusion stabilized with an anterior cervical plate.

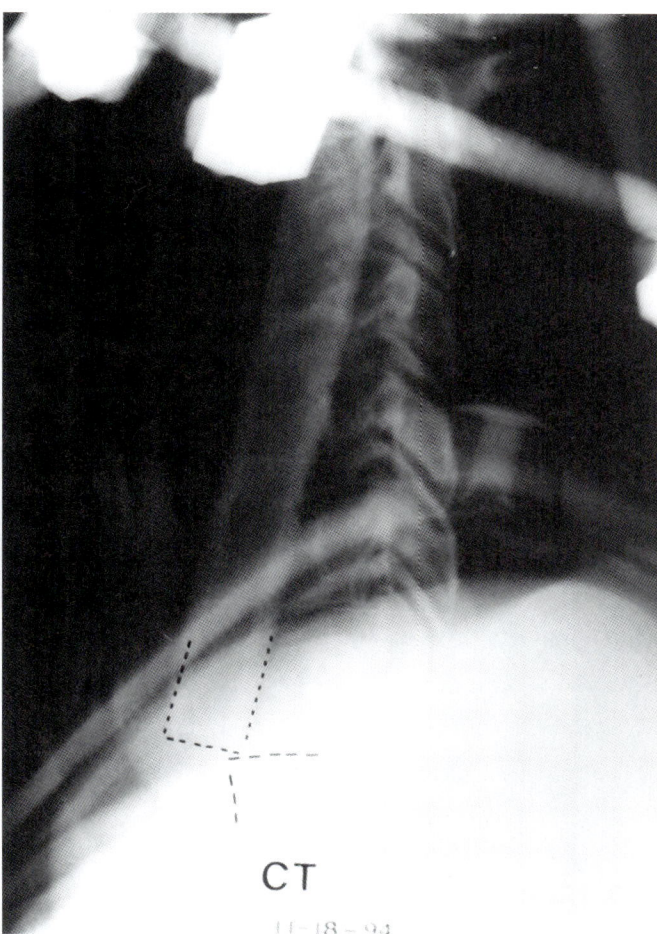

Figure 5 Radiograph showing a four-level corpectomy for postlaminectomy kyphosis and myelopathy. Despite the use of a halo vest, the fibular strut graft dislodged 1 week after surgery. Posterior fixation at the time of the initial operation most likely would have prevented this complication.

graphs include MRI and/or CT myelography. Signal changes within the cord demonstrated on MRI portend a poor prognosis. Another radiologic finding carrying a poor prognosis is a compression ratio of less than 0.4 (measured as the ratio of the smallest sagittal cord diameter to the largest transverse cord diameter at the same level). Conversely, expansion of the compression ratio to greater than 0.4 postoperatively correlates with clinical recovery.

Treatment

Unlike cervical spondylotic radiculopathy, cervical spondylotic myelopathy can be progressive and rarely improves over time without surgical management. Continued impingement by the spondylotic spine results in cord ischemia by compression of the anterior spinal artery, and there also may be a direct mechanical effect on the cord. Surgical management has been shown to improve functional outcomes, pain, and neurologic status in a recent prospective series of patients with cervical spondylotic myelopathy. It has also been demonstrated that early intervention improves prognosis before permanent destructive changes occur in the spinal cord. Therefore, nonsurgical management should be reserved only

for patients with mild cases or those who pose a prohibitive surgical risk. If conservative care is elected, careful and frequent follow-up is mandatory. A firm orthosis, anti-inflammatory medications, isometric exercises, and epidural steroids can be considered. However, traction and manipulation must be avoided because they can result in permanent quadriplegia.

There remains considerable debate regarding the optimal surgical approach for treating cervical spondylotic myelopathy. Both anterior and posterior approaches are reported to improve neurologic function, and each approach has its advantages and disadvantages. Anterior procedures such as ACDF or corpectomy with strut grafting directly remove the major offending structures impinging on the spinal cord, such as herniated disks and spondylotic vertebral body osteophytes. Kyphosis, which in many cases contributes to the myelopathy as the cord is draped over the involved levels, is often better corrected anteriorly. Correction of kyphosis enables indirect cord decompression during anterior surgery. In addition,

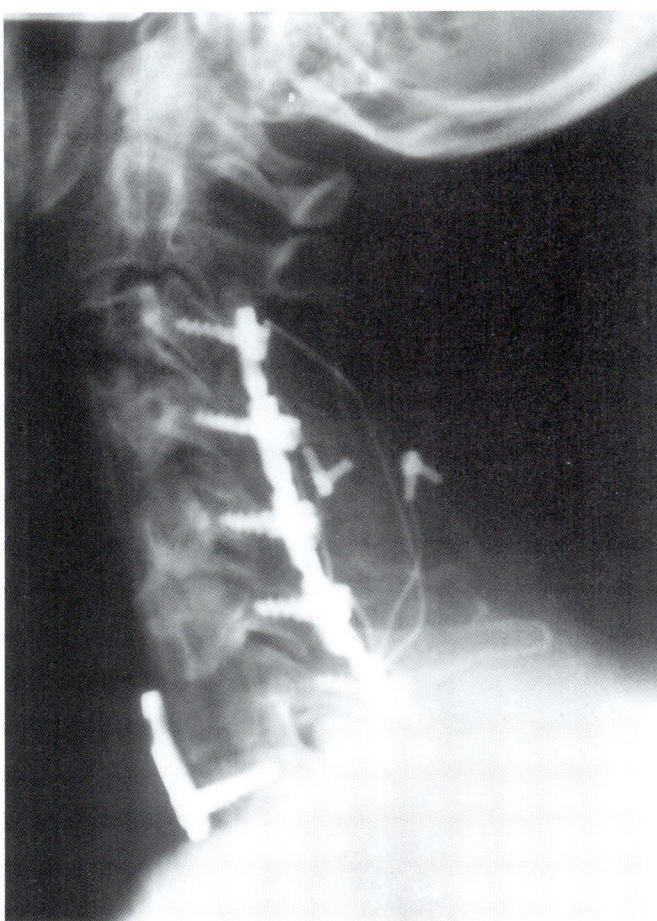

Figure 6 Lateral radiograph of a patient who underwent an anterior three-level corpectomy with strut grafting and placement of a buttress plate. Posteriorly, lateral mass plates and spinous process cables were used to lock in the strut graft and provide a more stable overall construct. *(Reproduced with permission from Riew KD, Sethi NS, Devney J, Goette K, Choi K: Complications of buttress plate stabilization of cervical corpectomy. Spine 1999;24:2404-2410.)*

decompression, in general, is preferably performed from the side with the predominant pathology, which can be assessed on MRI or CT myelogram. If the neck is kyphotic, then anterior surgery is recommended, as laminoplasty cannot undrape the cord over a kyphos. The occipitocervical junction is best approached posteriorly. In general, performing a laminectomy that compromises the facet joints without fusion is not recommended because of the substantial risk of instability and postlaminectomy kyphosis. Neurologic function typically improves early on after laminectomy but can deteriorate over time if the neck becomes kyphotic.

When cord compromise is primarily the result of disk impingement at two consecutive levels, surgical options include double ACDF versus single-level corpectomy. Although both have been used successfully, the latter may be preferred in patients at risk for pseudarthrosis (such as smokers, diabetics, and those who have had revision surgery) because healing occurs at only two sites versus four sites with double diskectomies. If double ACDF is selected, however, anterior plating should be considered because it appears to increase fusion rates and diminish kyphosis without increasing plate-related complications (Fig. 4). For disk-based disease at more than two levels, corpectomy is generally preferred over multilevel diskectomy because it carries less risk of pseudarthrosis.

Anterior plates, which are used to stabilize multilevel corpectomies, can be associated with significant complications. Meticulous attention to proper placement is crucial. If the plate is too long, the screws may injure adjacent disk spaces. If not properly contoured, the plate can act as a distraction device, prevent intimate bony contact between the graft and vertebral end plate, and inhibit healing. Other plate-related problems include implant breakage, screw migration, implant pullout, and pseudarthrosis (which reportedly is as high as 40%). Buttress plates have been advocated as a means of avoiding some of the problems associated with long cervical plates. These plates are short and are fixed to the inferior vertebra in order to prevent graft dislodgement, which typically occurs at the inferior end of the construct. Because they are short, implantation is easier, there is less risk of adjacent disk injury, and the plates do not act as a distraction device. However, plate dislodgement can result in airway obstruction and death. Based on these and other observations, buttress plating alone is not recommended for patients who undergo multilevel corpectomy for cervical spondylotic myelopathy. Anterior and posterior fusion should be considered in these patients.

Anterior and posterior fusion should also be considered in the treatment of postlaminectomy kyphosis if more than a single-level corpectomy is required (Fig. 5). Because of the previous laminectomy, performing an

the stabilizing effect of fusion is thought to allow the spinal cord the best chance for recovery from repeated trauma. On the other hand, posterior procedures such as laminoplasty also achieve a direct decompression by lifting away posterior impinging structures (Fig. 3). Laminoplasty also achieves an indirect decompression as the cord floats away posteriorly from the anterior impinging structures. Furthermore, laminoplasty can reduce neck range of motion nearly as much as fusion and thereby also provides some spinal stability needed for function to recover in the decompressed cord. A fusion procedure is not performed, thereby avoiding graft-related complications, which are the most common complications associated with anterior cervical fusions. However, radiculopathies can occur as the cord migrates posteriorly, most commonly at C5. Although usually transient, deltoid weakness or even paralysis can result.

Despite the controversy, there are some general principles in selecting the appropriate approach. The anterior corpectomy in these patients renders the spine markedly unstable. As a result, graft dislodgement is common even if a halo vest is used postoperatively. The addition of posterior lateral mass fixation or spinous process cabling may help lock in the strut graft and provide a more stable overall construct (Fig. 6).

Ossification of the Posterior Longitudinal Ligament

Ossification of the posterior longitudinal ligament is a disorder of unknown etiology that most commonly affects Asians, although it has been described in whites and blacks as well. With continued ossification, the space available for the spinal cord narrows. Patients may present with no symptoms or have neck pain, radiculopathy, or myelopathy. Several types of ossification have been described, including continuous, segmental (localized to the posterior vertebral bodies), mixed continuous and segmental, and circumscribed (localized to the posterior disk space). Although the metaplastic ossification can be seen on lateral radiographs, CT scans most reliably demonstrate the pathology.

Initial treatment is nonsurgical. Studies indicate that up to 70% of patients with neurologic dysfunction secondary to ossification of the posterior longitudinal ligament improve with skull traction in a position of mild flexion, bed rest, and application of a cervical orthosis. Extension is to be avoided. Immobilization is thought to allow the irritated spinal cord to recover from repeated episodes of injury by the ossified ligament with motion of the neck. However, when patients with severe myelopathy do not respond to conservative management, surgery is indicated.

As in the treatment of cervical spondylitic myelopathy, anterior versus posterior approaches have been advocated. In general, anterior decompression and fusion are recommended when three levels or less are involved, or in the presence of cervical kyphosis. The decompression can be performed by completely removing the ossified ligament with a diamond burr or, alternatively, by allowing a thin layer of ossified ligament to float anteriorly along with the spinal cord after resection of the vertebral body. The anterior approach provides the most direct decompression and is preferred in patients who present with significant clumsiness of the fingers or intrinsic muscle atrophy because it best decompresses the anterior horn motor cells. However, because the anterior dura is often involved in the pathologic process, anterior decompression is technically difficult and potentially dangerous. Also, anterior surgery requiresexacting technique to avoid further injury to an already compromised spinal cord during the decompression itself.

A posterior procedure such as laminoplasty is advantageous because it is safer and easier to perform than anterior decompression in patients with ossification of the posterior longitudinal ligament. However, posterior procedures rely on a posterior shift of the spinal cord to complete the decompressive effect, which may not occur to a sufficient degree in severe cases of ossification of the posterior longitudinal ligament. Furthermore, as noted previously, laminoplasty fails to decompress the cord adequately in the presence of cervical kyphosis. Nevertheless, most authors recommend laminoplasty in patients with continuous ossification of the posterior longitudinal ligament and preserved lordosis. If necessary, a staged anterior decompression and fusion can be performed 3 to 6 weeks later at the levels that have not been adequately decompressed by the laminoplasty.

Annotated Bibliography

Emery SE, Bohlman HH, Bolesta MJ, Jones PK: Anterior cervical decompression and arthrodesis for the treatment of cervical spondylotic myelopathy: Two to seventeen-year follow-up. *J Bone Joint Surg Am* 1998; 80:941-951.

The authors reported on 108 patients with cervical spondylotic myelopathy treated with ACDF (single or multilevel) and iliac crest autograft or corpectomy (subtotal, total, or multilevel) and iliac crest/fibular autograft. Seventy-one of 82 patients had improvement in gait abnormality postoperatively, and 80 of 86 patients had improvement in motor function (average Nurick score decreased from 2.4 to 1.2). Sixteen patients developed nonunion; 13 had undergone multilevel ACDF and 1 had received a fibular autograft. Patients with better preoperative neurologic function had the best postoperative recovery from myelopathy, suggesting that early intervention is desirable before the onset of irreversible cord damage. The authors concluded that anterior decompression and fusion are effective in the treatment of cervical spondylotic myelopathy.

Hilibrand AS, Carlson GD, Palumbo MA, Jones PK, Bohlman HH: Radiculopathy and myelopathy at segments adjacent to the site of a previous anterior cervical arthrodesis. *J Bone Joint Surg Am* 1999;81:519-528.

The authors reported on 374 patients who had undergone anterior cervical fusion for the treatment of cervical spondylotic radiculopathy or myelopathy. Symptomatic adjacent segment degeneration developed in 25% of the patients within 10 years. Risk factors for adjacent segment disease were a fusion at C5-6 and preoperative evidence of disk degeneration at adjacent levels. The risk of new adjacent segment disease was significantly greater for single-level versus multilevel fusion. Therefore, the authors suggest that all degenerated segments causing radiculopathy or myelopathy be included in the initial arthrodesis.

Riew KD, Hilibrand AS, Palumbo MA, Bohlman HH: Anterior cervical corpectomy in patients previously managed with a laminectomy: Short-term complications. *J Bone Joint Surg Am* 1999;81:950-957.

Eighteen patients were followed for an average of 2.7 years after anterior corpectomy and fusion. All patients had undergone previous cervical laminectomy. Plates were not used, but all patients were immobilized in a halo vest postoperatively. The most frequent complications were graft-related, and included graft extrusion and pseudarthrosis. Based on this study, the authors now recommend circumferential fusion in this patient population, as the previous laminectomy combined with an anterior decompression renders the spine markedly unstable despite the use of a halo vest.

Riew KD, Sethi NS, Devney J, Goette K, Choi K: Complications of buttress plate stabilization of cervical corpectomy. *Spine* 1999;24:2404-2410.

Complications occurring in 14 patients who underwent buttress plate fixation of the strut graft following multiple level corpectomies were reviewed. Two patients had graft extrusion leading to death in one of the patients, and three patients had pseudarthroses. The authors discourage the use of buttress plates alone to stabilize multilevel corpectomies and recommend supplementation with posterior fusion in these patients.

Sampath P, Bendebba M, Davis JD, Ducker TB: Outcome of patients treated for cervical myelopathy: A prospective, multicenter study with independent clinical review. *Spine* 2000;25:670-676.

This is a prospective, multicenter, nonrandomized study of patients with cervical spondylotic myelopathy conducted by the Cervical Spine Research Society. When compared with patients treated nonsurgically, surgically treated patients had better outcomes and significant improvement in functional status, pain, and neurologic function despite having had worse disease preoperatively.

Seybold EA, Baker JA, Criscitiello AA, Ordway NR, Park CK, Connolly PJ: Characteristics of unicortical and bicortical lateral mass screws in the cervical spine. *Spine* 1999;24:2397-2403.

This biomechanical study examined the safety and pullout strength of lateral mass screws in the cervical spine. In 21 cadavers, 3.5 mm × 14 mm lateral mass screws were placed from C3-C6 using a modified Magerl technique in a unicortical or bicortical fashion. Unicortical screws demonstrated nearly equivalent pullout strength but less injury to nerve roots and the vertebral artery.

Shafaie FF, Wippold FJ II, Gado M, Pilgram TK, Riew KD: Comparison of computed tomography myelography and magnetic resonance imaging in the evaluation of cervical spondylotic myelopathy and radiculopathy. *Spine* 1999;24:1781-1785.

The authors examined the MRI studies and CT myelograms of 20 patients with cervical spondylotic radiculopathy or myelopathy in a blinded fashion to determine the concordance between the two studies. The uncovertebral joints, facet joints, lateral recesses, cord size, spinal canal, and neural foramina were evaluated with graded scales. For most of these parameters, MRI and CT myelogram had only moderate concordance. The authors concluded that MRI and CT myelogram should be viewed as complementary rather than mutually exclusive studies in the analysis of patients with cervical spondylosis.

Wang JC, McDonough PW, Endow KK, Delamarter RB: Increased fusion rates with cervical plating for two-level anterior cervical discectomy and fusion. *Spine* 2000;25:41-45.

In this retrospective review, 32 patients who underwent two-level ACDF with plating were compared with 28 patients who were not plated. The pseudarthrosis rate was 0% in plated patients versus 25% in nonplated patients. Significantly less disk space collapse and kyphosis were also found in plated patients. The complication rate did not differ between the two groups.

Classic Bibliography

Bernard TN Jr, Whitecloud TS III: Cervical spondylotic myelopathy and myeloradiculopathy: Anterior decompression and stabilization with autogenous fibula strut graft. *Clin Orthop* 1987;221:149-160.

Bohlman HH: Cervical spondylosis with moderate to severe myelopathy: A report of seventeen cases treated by Robinson anterior cervical discectomy and fusion. *Spine* 1977;2:151-162.

Bohlman HH, Emery SE, Goodfellow DB, Jones PK: Robinson anterior cervical discectomy and arthrodesis for cervical radiculopathy: Long-term follow-up of one hundred and twenty-two patients. *J Bone Joint Surg Am* 1993;75:1298-1307.

Emery SE, Smith MD, Bohlman HH: Upper-airway obstruction after multilevel cervical corpectomy for myelopathy. *J Bone Joint Surg Am* 1991;73:544-551.

Ghanayem AJ, Leventhal M, Bohlman HH: Osteoarthrosis of the atlanto-axial joints: Long-term follow-up after treatment with arthrodesis. *J Bone Joint Surg Am* 1996;78:1300-1307.

Herkowitz HN: A comparison of anterior cervical fusion, cervical laminectomy, and cervical laminoplasty for the surgical management of multiple level spondylotic radiculopathy. *Spine* 1988;13:774-780.

Herkowitz HN, Kurz LT, Overholt DP: Surgical management of cervical soft disc herniation: A comparison between the anterior and posterior approach. *Spine* 1990;15:1026-1030.

Hirabayashi K, Watanabe K, Wakano K, Suzuki N, Satomi K, Ishii Y: Expansive open-door laminoplasty for cervical spinal stenotic myelopathy. *Spine* 1983;8:693-699.

Lees F, Aldren-Turner JW: Natural history and prognosis of cervical spondylosis. *Br Med J* 1963;5373: 1607-1610.

Nurick S: The natural history and the results of surgical treatment of the spinal cord disorder associated with cervical spondylosis. *Brain* 1972;95:101-108.

Smith GW, Robinson RA: The treatment of certain cervical-spine disorders by anterior removal of the intervertebral disc and interbody fusion. *J Bone Joint Surg Am* 1958;40:607-624.

Tsuyama N: Ossification of the posterior longitudinal ligament of the spine. *Clin Orthop* 1984;184:71-84.

Zdeblick TA, Hughes SS, Riew KD, Bohlman HH: Failed anterior cervical discectomy and arthrodesis: Analysis and treatment of thirty-five patients. *J Bone Joint Surg Am* 1997;79:523-532.

Chapter 51

Thoracic Disk Herniation

Kirkham B. Wood, MD

Amir Mehbod, MD

Introduction

Thoracic disk herniations are relatively rare compared with those of the cervical or lumbar spine. An incidence of 1 in 10,000 to 1 in one million has been estimated, which represents 0.25% to 0.75% of all symptomatic spinal disk herniations. More than 75% occur below the level of T8 and most commonly occur during the third, fourth, and fifth decades of life. Multiple herniations have been reported as comprising 5% to 15% of most series of symptomatic individuals.

The prevalence and natural history of asymptomatic thoracic disk herniations has been well documented. In an MRI study of asymptomatic individuals, 73% had positive degenerative findings at one or more levels, which included 37% with disk herniations (50% multiple) and 40% with annular tears, Scheuermann's changes, or deformity of the spinal cord. In a follow-up study more than 26 months later, none of these individuals became symptomatic.

Classification

Thoracic disk herniations are classified according to spinal level and position. They are most often mediolateral, (70% to 94% in most series) (Fig. 1), and rarely, intradural (5% to 12%) (Fig. 2). There is no strong association between the position, level, composition, or size of a thoracic disk herniation and the symptoms it may produce. For instance, a central herniation may typically cause myelopathy but can produce radicular pain, referred discomfort, or no symptoms at all. Lateral disk herniations are more likely to produce an ipsilateral radiculopathy, but a traction phenomenon can lead to radicular symptoms on the contralateral side.

Etiology

The mechanical etiologies for thoracic disk herniations are diverse and have included torsion, repetitive twisting, athletic activity, sneezing, and coughing. Thirty-three percent to 50% of patients with symptomatic thoracic disk herniations will report a history of trauma, but the actual role trauma plays in the production of these herniations is controversial and poorly defined.

Biomechanical tests have shown the most common mechanism for thoracic disk herniations to be a combination of torsion and bending load, whether flexion, extension, or lateral. The unique anatomy of the thoracic spine decreases the risk of intervertebral disk injury by the splinting effect of the thoracic rib cage and the resistance of the thoracic facets to flexion loads. The decreased height of the thoracic disk compared with that of the lumbar spine may also contribute to the low incidence of disk protrusions.

Other conditions that may be associated with a thoracic disk herniation include ossification of the posterior longitudinal ligament or the ligamentum flavum, and thoracic spinal stenosis. When present, such conditions can increase the symptomatology in even minor disk protrusions. Degeneration of the involved disks is commonly associated with thoracic disk herniations, especially in the older population, which tends to have calcification of the disks. Calcification can increase adhesions between the disk protrusion and the adjacent dura. The natural kyphosis of the thoracic spine places the spinal cord next to the posterior longitudinal ligament and disk and even a small disk herniation may then compress the cord and cause symptoms. Lumbar and cervical disk herniations have less calcification in comparison.

Clinical Presentation

The diagnosis of thoracic disk herniations can be difficult because of the relative paucity of classic findings. Because of the extreme variations in presentation, diagnosis is often delayed. Symptoms can be vague and often mimic other pathologic conditions including not

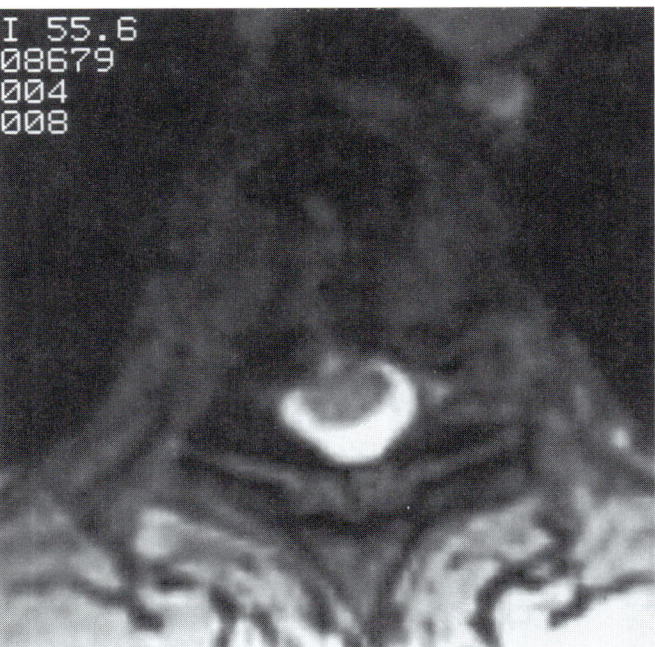

Figure 1 Mediolateral disk herniation with deformation of the spinal cord.

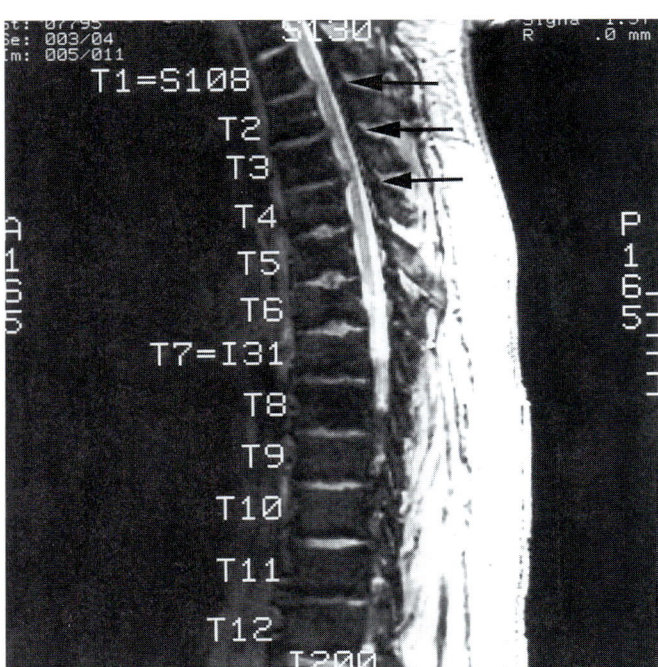

Figure 2 Sagittal MRI study demonstrating multiple disk herniations in the upper thoracic spine (*arrows*).

only lumbar disk disease and neurogenic claudication, but also cardiac, abdominal (gallbladder), and intrathoracic maladies, and even multiple sclerosis. Pain is the principal initial symptom and can be localized or circumferential, often aggravated by coughing, sneezing, and Valsalva-like maneuvers. Numbness in a dermatomal pattern is also common. Progressive levels of neurologic embarrassment can eventually lead to motor weakness, bladder dysfunction, and rarely, paralysis.

The clinical presentation of symptomatic thoracic disk herniations can be divided into three categories: mechanical, radicular, and myelopathic. Mechanical axial back pain can occur secondary to the derangement of the intervertebral disk itself, typically resulting in localized pain into the mid or lower thoracic region. Mechanical features include improvement of symptoms with rest and exacerbation by activity or prolonged sitting.

Radicular pain can arise as a result of impingement of disk material on or traction of exiting nerve roots. The nerve corresponding to the more caudal vertebral body is the root typically involved; for example, an anterolateral T8-9 disk herniation will produce a T9 radiculopathy. Patients may complain of pain in the anterior chest wall in a band-like dermatomal distribution. A differential diagnosis is the pain from herpes zoster (shingles). Axial pain also can be a component of the complaint. Radicular pain is more common with herniations of the upper thoracic spine, especially lateral protrusions, wherein they may cause symptoms

similar to a cervical disk herniation such as upper arm pain, radiculopathy, and paresthesias.

Myelopathic symptoms can occur when the disk material impinges significantly on the spinal cord. Symptomatology can range from subtle pain and sensory changes to motor disturbances or frank paraparesis. Bowel and bladder changes can be seen in 10% to 20% of symptomatic thoracic disk herniations.

During the physical examination the patient's posture is noted in both sagittal and coronal planes. Gait disturbances such as a wide base ataxic gait or foot drop should be noted. The Romberg sign is a useful tool for detecting changes in proprioception. A careful sensory examination may reveal a clear level of demarcation corresponding to the level of impingement. Upper motor neuron signs, such as hyperreflexia, clonus, and Babinski, may be present.

The differential diagnosis is expansive given the wide range of symptoms. Spinal and nonspinal pathology should be considered. Spine-related diagnoses include degenerative spondylosis, spinal and spinal cord tumors, multiple sclerosis, and transverse myelitis. Nonspinal pain origins include pancreatitis, aneurysms, and retroperitoneal neoplasms.

Diagnostic Imaging

Upright AP and lateral radiographs of the thoracic spine should be obtained first to rule out obvious fractures and/or tumors. The degree of kyphosis, osteophytes, and vertebral wedging can be noted. Thirty percent to 70% of symptomatic thoracic disk herniations have calcified disk material, as opposed to less than 10% without herniation. MRI is the neuroradiographic study of choice (Fig. 2) and should be interpreted with a heightened awareness because of the high prevalence of asymptomatic herniations. In patients for whom MRI is not an option, myelography with CT can evaluate for spinal cord encroachment on axial views with sagittal reconstructions. The procedure is invasive, but its sensitivity and specificity are comparable to that of MRI. A CT scan is also excellent for identifying disk calcifications.

A common error in the surgical treatment of thoracic disk herniation is misidentifying the level of injury. The thoracic anatomy can be more variable than in the lumbar or cervical spine, with a different number of vertebrae and ribs. A chest radiograph is important in the preoperative work-up to count the number of ribs to verify the proper level. A myelogram can also be helpful in describing the protrusion and allowing accurate identification of the pathologic level.

In instances of unclear presentation, thoracic diskography can be performed safely by experienced and skilled physicians as a provocative diagnostic test to determine the presence and location of axial thoracic pain. The procedure can be very useful in situations of multiple levels of thoracic pathology with varying grades of herniation. A large herniation with spinal cord deformation is a strict contraindication to diskography because the installation of the saline contrast runs a risk of further cord compression.

Nonsurgical Treatment

Most patients with thoracic disk herniations do not need surgical intervention, especially in the absence of neurologic findings. Only 0.2% to 2.0% of thoracic disk herniations are treated surgically each year. Symptoms will usually resolve as the natural history dictates. In a review of 55 patients with 72 symptomatic disk herniations, 73% did not require surgery and were able to return to work and vigorous sports activities.

Nonsurgical treatment consists of activity modification, low-impact aerobic exercises, and bracing. Anti-inflammatory medications and the judicious use of mild narcotics can help provide symptomatic relief. In addition, patients with radicular symptoms can be treated with a course of oral steroids or corticosteroid injections of the intercostal nerves.

Surgical Treatment

Indications for surgical intervention include myelopathy, progressive neurologic deficit, or pain at an unac-

ceptable level in those in whom a minimum of 6 months of adequate nonsurgical treatment has failed. Multiple surgical approaches have been described for thoracic diskectomy, depending on the level of involvement, relationship to the spinal cord, and consistency of the disk herniation.

The strict posterior approach via laminectomy can alleviate compressive forces from the ligamentum flavum and lamina, but does not specifically address the anterior compression. The potential for trauma to the spinal cord during this mobilization for exposure of the disk makes this approach unattractive and therefore it should be avoided.

The transpedicular approach is another posterior approach in which exposure is provided by limited excision of the posterior lamina, facet joints, and the pedicle caudal to the disk (Fig. 3, A), allowing for excision of lateral and paramedian disk material. Advantages include less dissection and less cord retraction; however, visualization can be somewhat limited. Excessive bone removal may also destabilize the spine.

A lateral extracavitary exposure is performed via an extrapleural resection of the medial portion of the rib costotransverse joint, facet, and pedicle in the superior aspect of the vertebral body inferior to the disk herniation (Fig. 3, B). This approach provides good exposure for central-lateral and lateral disk herniations at any level; however, disruption of the paraspinal muscles and the degree of bone resection are points of concern.

A costotransversectomy is a posterolateral extrapleural approach first used in the early 20th century for the treatment of tuberculosis. Exposure is provided by resection of medial ribs costotransverse joint, facet, and pedicle (Fig. 3, C). The posterior medial portion of the rib and its articulation with the transverse process and the superior aspect of the vertebral body inferior to the disk herniation is resected. This approach provides exposure of multiple levels, including the uppermost thoracic disks, and is especially useful for lateral herniations. Similar to the lateral extracavitary approach, it has the disadvantage of disrupting the paraspinal muscles in addition to large amounts of bone resection. Costotransversectomy should not be used for large central calcified herniations when large osteophytes are present, where an anterior approach is safer.

An anterior transthoracic approach allows excellent anterior exposure of T5-12 for most lateral and anterior disk herniations. The use of strut grafts or anterior instrumentation is facilitated by this direct approach. The base of the rib articulating with the vertebral body just caudal to the disk herniation is typically removed. The inferior pedicle is partially or completely removed.

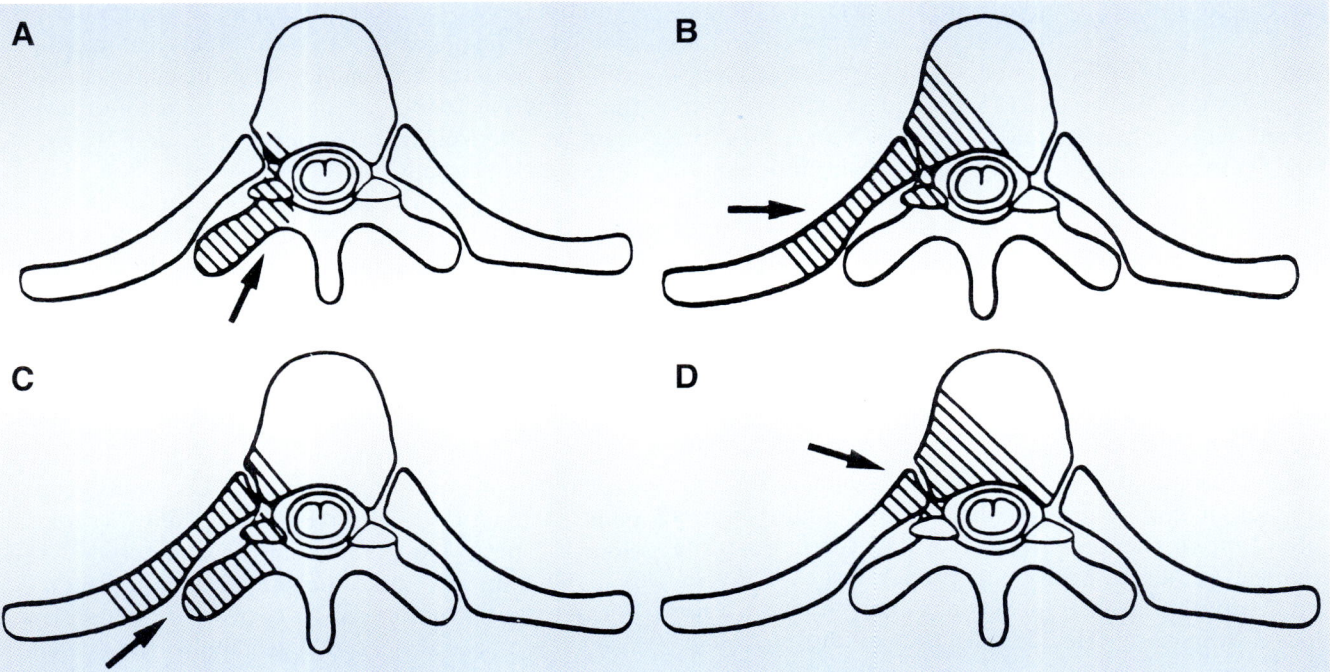

Figure 3 Approach (*arrow*) and bony resection (cross-hatched lines) in the transpedicular (**A**), extracavitary (**B**), costotransversectomy (**C**), and transthoracic (**D**) approaches. (*Reproduced with permission from Cybulski G: Thoracic disc herniation: Surgical technique.* Contemp Neurosurg *1992;14:1-6.*)

A partial diskectomy is performed, using a burr, and a trough can be created in the posterior vertebral body and the remaining disk material brought through (Fig. 3, *D*). The disadvantages of this approach include the need for a thoracotomy and the possibility of pneumothorax, pulmonary contusion, pneumonia, effusion, and atelectasis all adding to the potential morbidity of the operation.

Thoracoscopy is an emerging technology that allows thoracic diskectomy, fusion with bone graft, and possible instrumentation over a wide range of the anterior thoracic spine. Thoracoscopy is probably best suited for noncalcified herniations. Calcified protrusions are likely to have dural adherence and should be treated with an anterolateral approach.

Fusion and instrumentation are controversial topics. Although some surgeons perform fusions after diskectomy, others routinely do not. In general, fusion is an accepted part of treatment in cases that involve multiple levels of diskectomy, Scheuermann's disease, or excessive resection of bone leading to potential instability. For diskectomies over a few levels (less than three) cancellous autograft can be harvested from adjacent ribs near the costovertebral junction, an especially attractive option in thoracoscopy. Small fibular allograft rings can be packed with local autograft and provide increased structural stability. For longer fusions, especially those with instrumentation, standard bone grafting harvesting techniques (for example, iliac crest) are recommended. Because of the inherent stability of

the thoracic spine, however, instrumentation is not routinely used for fusions, except in cases of multilevel diskectomy at the thoracolumbar junction.

Annotated Bibliography

Fessler RG, Sturgill M: Review: Complications of surgery for thoracic disc disease. *Surg Neurol* 1998;49: 609-618.

A good review of peer-reviewed publications reporting clinical data relating to thoracic diskectomy and the potential complications associated with various surgical approaches.

Regan JJ, Ben-Yishay A, Mack MJ: Video-assisted thoracoscopic excision of herniated thoracic disc: Description of technique and preliminary experience in the first 29 cases. *J Spinal Disord* 1998;11:183-191.

An excellent review of the techniques of and avoidance of pitfalls with the thoracoscopic treatment of disk herniations.

Wood KB, Schellhas KP, Garvey TA, Aeppli D: Thoracic discography in healthy individuals: A controlled prospective study of magnetic resonance imaging and discography in asymptomatic and symptomatic individuals. *Spine* 1999;24:1548-1555.

Thoracic diskography was performed in 10 healthy individuals without thoracic pain. Findings showed that prominent Schmorl's nodes may be intensely painful even in life-long asymptomatic individuals. Thoracic diskography also was found to demonstrate disk pathology not readily apparent on MRI.

Classic Bibliography

Arce CA, Dohrmann GJ: Herniated thoracic disks. *Neurol Clin* 1985;3:383-392.

Awwad EE, Martin DS, Smith KR Jr, Baker BK: Asymptomatic versus symptomatic herniated thoracic discs: Their frequency and characteristics as detected by computed tomography after myelography. *Neurosurgery* 1991;28:180-186.

Brown CW, Deffer PA Jr, Akmakjian J, Donaldson DH, Brugman JL: The natural history of thoracic disc herniation. *Spine* 1992;17(suppl 6):S97-S102.

Schellhas KP, Pollei SR, Dorwart RH: Thoracic diskography: A safe and reliable technique. *Spine* 1994; 19:2103-2109.

Wood KB, Blair JM, Aepple DM, et al: The natural history of asymptomatic thoracic disc herniations. *Spine* 1997;22:525-530.

Wood KB, Garvey TA, Gundry C, Heithoff KB: Magnetic resonance imaging of the thoracic spine: Evaluation of asymptomatic individuals. *J Bone Joint Surg Am* 1995;77:1631-1638.

Chapter 52

Lumbar Degenerative Disorders

Jeffrey M. Spivak, MD

John A. Bendo, MD

Epidemiology of Lumbar Degenerative Disease

Earlier studies have suggested a genetic predisposition to the development of juvenile disk disease and disk herniation. Although it has long been believed that genetic factors play a role in adult lumbar degenerative disk disease and disk herniation, recent evidence supports this concept. In an MRI study of same-sex monozygotic and dizygotic twins unselected for back pain or disk disease, heritable factors of disk degeneration included loss of disk height and structural changes. Disk signal intensity had no apparent genetic influence, and appeared to be related more to environmental factors, such as age-related changes in disk hydration. In another study, back pain patients with a family history of surgical lumbar disk herniation had a similar incidence of low lumbar disk degeneration compared with case-matched controls with back pain and no known family history of lumbar herniated disks. However, the severity of the degenerative process was significantly higher in the patients with a family history of surgical disk herniation.

Complaints of low back pain in adolescence do not appear to predict the development of chronic pain into early adulthood. Recurrent low back pain was found in almost 8% of 14-year-olds in one study, with 35% of these patients reporting persistent pain over the 9 years of the study. In a Finnish population study of incidence of hospital admissions for low back disease in patients up to age 28 years, male patients had a 2.6 times greater incidence than females. The incidence of admissions for lumbar disk disease was 12.8 per 1,000 for males and 6.6 per 1,000 for females. Herniated disk incidence was 9.1 per 1,000 for males and 4.2 per 1,000 for females.

Pathophysiology of Lumbar Degenerative Disease

The degenerative process of the spine occurs at the level of the functional spinal unit, or motion segment.

A motion segment consists of two adjacent vertebral bodies, the intervening intervertebral disk and facet joints, and the ligamentous supports including the ligamentum flavum, interspinous, supraspinous, and intertransverse ligaments, and the facet joint capsule.

The Kirkaldy-Willis classification describes three stages of the degenerative process of the motion segment. The first stage involves dysfunction of the support tissues of the motion segment, with facet joint synovitis, annular and ligament stretching and minor tearing, and minor reducible subluxations. During the second, or unstable stage, progressive annular and ligament tearing and laxity promote hypermobility. Within the intervertebral disk, a decrease in the proteoglycan and water content of the nucleus pulposus further alters the kinematics of the motion segment. The abnormal motion also results in altered facet joint forces and mobility, with secondary productive degenerative bone formation and facet enlargement.

The third phase describes motion segment stabilization, resulting from disk height loss and osteophyte formation along the vertebral end plates. The disk space narrowing results in overriding of the facet joints, restricting but not eliminating segmental motion, and narrowing the lateral portion of the spinal canal and foramen.

As the degenerative process proceeds, a number of ensuing pathoanatomic events of clinical significance can occur. The anulus fibrosus may undergo progressive radial tearing of its concentric lamallae. On sagittal MRI evaluation, a 'high intensity zone' may be seen on the T2-weighted sequences within the posterior anulus; this finding has been associated with symptomatically painful disks. These radial tears may accumulate and a focal defect may allow for extrusion of inner disk material, resulting in a true disk herniation. Segmental spinal instability may develop as a result of progressive incompetence of the disk and facet joints to oppose the shear, bending, torsional, and axial forces that occur with activities of daily living. Spondylolisthesis may occur, with secondary lateral recess and then central canal stenosis caused by the intact posterior neural arch. Degenerative scoliosis may result, with unilateral lateral collapse and true rotatory deformity. Stenosis with degenerative scoliosis is common, and is often dynamic because of collapse in the concavity of the curve with upright posture. The resulting narrowing of the foramina and lateral recesses within the concavity of the curve causes mid or upper lumbar lower extremity symptoms on the side of the concavity. Fractional curve stenosis, with low lumbar extremity pain on the side of the convexity of the main curve, is commonly seen.

Biochemistry of Pain in Disk Degeneration and Disk Herniation

Over the past decade, much of the basic science research in degenerative disease of the lumbar spine has centered on the biochemical mechanisms and mediators of pain in the degenerative process of the intervertebral disk and in the spinal nerve root associated with disk herniation.

The process of disk degeneration is believed to have a biochemical basis, with inhibition of nuclear proteoglycan synthesis and enhanced matrix degradation caused by chemical mediators that may include interleukin (IL)-1, IL-6, nitric oxide (NO), prostaglandin E-2 (PGE-2), and matrix metalloproteinases (MMPs). Herniated and degenerated disk tissue in culture spontaneously produces increased amounts of these chemical mediators versus normal disk tissue. Both normal and herniated disk tissue in culture respond to an IL-1β stimulus with an increased production of MMPs, NO, PGE-2, and IL-6. Autocrine mechanisms may play a role as well, with local production of one cytokine affecting production of others.

These same chemical mediators responsible for proteoglycan loss leading to progressive disk degeneration may also have a direct role in the pain associated with degeneration and disk herniation by stimulation and sensitization of the afferent nerve endings in the outer anulus and other innervated structures surrounding the spinal canal. They may also have direct effects on the spinal nerve root and dorsal root ganglion, leading to radicular pain.

Phospholipase A-2 (PLA-2) also has been found in high concentrations in degenerated disks and herniated disk tissue. PLA-2 can act as an inflammatory mediator, and may act as well by sensitizing nociceptors. PLA-2 has recently been shown to cause demyelination of spinal nerve roots, which may result in regions of hypersensitivity to mechanical stimulation and sciatica.

Herniated disk material has been shown to elicit a foreign body-type macrophage inflammatory response as well as a neovascularization, which may be an integral part of both the pain-generating process and the removal of the displaced disk material commonly seen. Studies of surgical specimens have identified significant differences in the inflammatory response to contained and noncontained disk herniations. No significant differences in the cellular response is seen when comparing acute and chronic disk herniations. Experimental annular injury in an animal model produces an inflammatory response; the response to a partial-thickness injury is T cell-based, but the response to a full-thickness injury with disk herniation is macrophage-based, as is seen in humans clinically. Epidural injection of basic fibroblast growth factor facilitates resorption of disk material experimentally placed in the epidural space in animals, but epidural injection of high-dose steroids suppresses disk resorption.

Displaced disk material also has direct neurotoxic and vascular effects on the spinal nerve roots unrelated to compressive effects. Cellular effects include myelin sheath and axonal injury. Vascular effects include diminished radicular blood flow, thrombus formation, and increased permeability of intraneural microvessels.

In addition to biochemical and cellular pain mediators, a number of pathoanatomic changes have been observed that may contribute to the development of pain in lumbar disk degeneration and herniation. Degenerated lumbar disks have a much more extensive network of innervation than normal disks, including innervation of the inner anulus; immunoreactivity of many of these nerves to substance P suggests a nociceptive role. A proliferation of blood vessels and accompanying nerve fibers has been identified in the end plate region of the vertebral bodies surrounding degenerated disks in patients with severe back pain, implicating the end plate as another possible source of pain generation in degenerated disks.

Lumbosacral Back Pain

Population studies have estimated that 60% to 80% of adults in the United States will experience low back pain some time during their life. Significant low back pain episodes lasting more than 2 weeks occur in 14% of the adult population. Low back pain continues to be one of the most common causes of disability in the industrialized world. Chronic physical impairments of the back and spine are the most common cause of activity limitation in all people younger than 45 years of age. Even within the age group from 45 to 64 years, back and spine impairments rank third most common after cardiac conditions and arthritis/rheumatism. Studies have revealed that the longer patients are absent from work, the greater the likelihood that they will never return to gainful employment. Absence from work for a 1-year period secondary to a low back condition reduces the probability of returning to work to only 25%.

The majority of new episodes of low back or back-related leg pain are considered soft-tissue strains and sprains and are generally self-limited, lasting a few days to a few weeks. Chronic mechanical low back pain is defined as activity-related pain persisting for more than 3 months. The National Center for Health Statistics reports that there are over 13 million annual doctor visits for chronic low back pain. Approximately 50 million annual visits to chiropractors are for chronic low back pain. Although only 20% of afflicted persons seek medical attention, the economic consequences are overwhelming. Including both medical care costs and the costs related to disability, the current estimation of annual expenditure on this problem exceeds $50 billion.

Sciatica is not as prevalent as low back pain. The prevalence of low back pain with symptoms of sciatica persisting at least 2 weeks is 1.6%. A common clinical history for patients with sciatica includes a prodromal period of back pain that resolves or dramatically improves with the onset of the leg pain. The average age of onset of the first attack of sciatica is in the early part of the third decade of life. Even with radicular leg pain, the natural history is quite favorable, with 80% of patients having significant symptomatic improvement within 1 month. Rates of symptom recurrence are high, even after a complete clinical recovery; in the occupational setting, up to 60% of patients will suffer a recurrence within 1 year.

Known risk factors for low back pain based on large population studies include lifestyle factors (poor physical fitness, smoking, anxiety, depression, stress), recreational activities (golf, tennis, gymnastics), occupational factors (bending, stooping, twisting, heavy lifting, prolonged sitting, vibration exposure), and radiographic factors (spondyloarthropathy, severe spinal deformity, segmental spinal instability, lumbar stenosis). Factors not definitively associated with low back pain include sex, weight, and radiographic evidence of vertebral osteophytes, transitional vertebral anomalies, spina bifida occulta, and facet trophism.

The cornerstone of clinical diagnosis when treating low back pain remains an accurate and detailed history and physical examination. Full definition of the nature of both back and lower extremity pain should be determined. The relative amounts of back and lower extremity pain are assessed. Patterns of radiation are explored, and a determination of referred pain (sclerotomal in origin) or radicular pain (dermatomal in ori-

gin) should be made. The character and location of the pain should be clearly defined, and both provocative and pain-relieving positions and maneuvers, such as sitting, standing, walking, coughing, and sneezing, should be assessed. Important points in the discussion of the symptom onset include the acute or insidious nature of onset and any temporally related new physical activities or injuries. A history of any previous similar symptoms is obtained, as well as any prior treatments and diagnostic tests.

A detailed physical examination includes inspection and palpation of the back, assessing for the presence of muscle spasm, tenderness, and deformity. Gait is observed and noted, along with lumbar range of motion. Neurologic evaluation includes testing for the presence of any focal neurologic deficits of motor strength, sensation, and reflexes, examination for signs of myelopathy, and assessing for signs of nerve root tension.

Waddell's nonorganic physical signs are abnormal tenderness (superficial, nonanatomic), a positive stimulation test (pain with axial loading or whole body rotation), loss of positive findings with distraction, nonanatomic regional sensory or motor disturbances, and overreaction. The presence of three out of five of these signs correlates with a poor clinical outcome with surgery, even in the presence of true structural abnormalities consistent with the patient's complaints and physical examination.

The differential diagnosis of both back and radiating lower extremity pain must be kept in mind when evaluating these patients. Nonspinal causes of back pain include abdominal and pelvic visceral pathology, aortic aneurysm, sacroiliac joint dysfunction, and hip pathology.

During physical examination, abdominal and pelvic masses and tenderness must be assessed, and the sacroiliac and hip joints ranged and stressed. The differential diagnosis of lower extremity pain includes peripheral neuropathy, compressive neuropathy, and vascular insufficiency. Examination of the lower extremities for pulses and the possible skin changes of chronic vascular disorders must be included in the complete physical examination.

The Agency for Health Care Policy and Research, in 1994, published a Clinical Practice Guideline entitled "Acute Low Back Pain Problems in Adults". This guideline was the result of a detailed review of the relevant literature by a multidisciplinary panel of spine care specialists. A key concept from this guideline was a listing of specific aspects of the history and physical examination, labeled "red flags", which suggest the possibility of a serious underlying disorder as the cause of the patient's back pain. Historic "red flags" include constitutional symptoms (weight loss, fevers, chills, fatigue, night sweats), pain worse at night or while supine, and history of recent infection, immunosuppression, trauma, or cancer. Physical examination "red flags" include severe tenderness, bilateral neurologic deficits, saddle anesthesia, and pain out of proportion to physical findings. The severe underlying disorders to be identified early in the course of an episode of back pain include spinal infection, spinal tumors, fractures, and cauda equina syndrome. Suspicion of any of the above disorders should prompt immediate diagnostic testing to rule out the condition.

In the absence of any "red flags" on initial evaluation, treatment may be instituted without any further diagnostic testing. Plain radiographs are obtained initially only if a "red flag" is identified or in patients at extremes of age (older than 60 years or younger than 15 years) or if symptoms have been present for 4 to 6 weeks or longer.

The goals of treatment of acute low back pain include a prompt return to normal function and pain relief through the efficient and effective use of diagnostic tests and efficacious treatments. Secondary goals include limiting the cost of back pain evaluation, treatment, and disability to society and limiting the use of ineffective treatments, including inappropriate surgery. In 80% of patients with acute low back pain, no obvious cause of the pain can be found, even after a thorough evaluation. Patients must be educated about the favorable natural history and outcome of their acute lumbosacral pain.

Initial treatment consists of reassurance, medications, and activity modification. Nonsteroidal anti-inflammatory drugs (NSAIDs) and acetaminophen are the recommended oral agents. Short-term, low-dose steroid is generally reserved for those patients unresponsive to NSAIDs and with predominantly sciatic type symptoms. Opiates may be concomitantly prescribed for severe breakthrough pain. Bed rest for patients with acute pain for 1 or 2 days may be considered. Prolonged bed rest (longer than 4 days) has been shown to be detrimental in the overall recovery from low back pain as well as sciatica. Aerobic conditioning, including abdominal and low back strengthening exercises, is encouraged. Chiropractic manipulation can be considered because it has been shown to be helpful within the first 4 weeks of acute back pain symptoms, but has not been shown effective for chronic low back pain. Known significant neural compression is a relative contraindication to manipulative therapy. Other commonly used modalities for the treatment of acute back pain include the application of heat, ice, transcutaneous electrical nerve stimulation, ultrasound, massage therapy, and traction. The efficacy of these modalities has never been scientifically validated, but

they may play a role in pain relief to allow a more active exercise program for recovery.

If symptoms do not improve over 4 to 6 weeks, a reevaluation with radiographs is done. Routine laboratory work can be considered to rule out any occult infectious or neoplastic process, including a complete blood count, erythrocyte sedimentation rate, and C-reactive protein. Advanced spinal imaging with MRI is considered depending on symptoms, signs, and the degree of suspicion of underlying structural problems. Changing medications and the addition of physical therapy should be considered. Lumbar epidural steroid injections remain an option, but generally are more effective for sciatica rather than isolated low back pain. Studies have shown a high rate of misapplication of epidural injections outside the true epidural space without the use of fluoroscopic guidance and visualization. Therefore, fluoroscopic localization is recommended.

Persistent pain despite nonsurgical treatment, in the absence of an obvious disk herniation or segmental instability, may prompt the search for a specific 'pain generator' not obviously identifiable on diagnostic tests. In some cases, multiple abnormalities on scans may prompt a search for a more localized cause of the pain. The low back pain may originate from pain fibers located in tissue sites such as the anulus fibrosus, facet joint capsule, vertebral periosteum, ligamentum flavum, posterior spinal musculature, and fascia. Pain may also originate from irritation from the surrounding neural structures. Diagnostic injection tests can help define the specific origin of low back pain. Temporary pain relief via a diagnostic fluoroscopically-guided xylocaine intra-articular facet joint injection may confirm that the source of pain is from a particular arthritic facet joint. Some physicians believe that denervation of the facet joint via a percutaneous radiofrequency rhizotomy can help to diminish facet-induced low back pain. However, there are no controlled studies demonstrating any long-term benefit of this procedure.

Herniated Lumbar Disk

A herniation of a disk refers to a displacement of inner disk material, creating a focal asymmetry in the outer circumference of the anulus fibrosus. The distinction between disk bulge and herniation is that a disk bulge is a generalized outpouching of the peripheral margin of the anulus caused by early disk degeneration with loss of height, without any focal displacement of inner disk material. These terms have no implications with respect to clinical significance. A disk bulge may contribute significantly to symptomatic neural compression, and a true focal disk herniation may be asymptomatic.

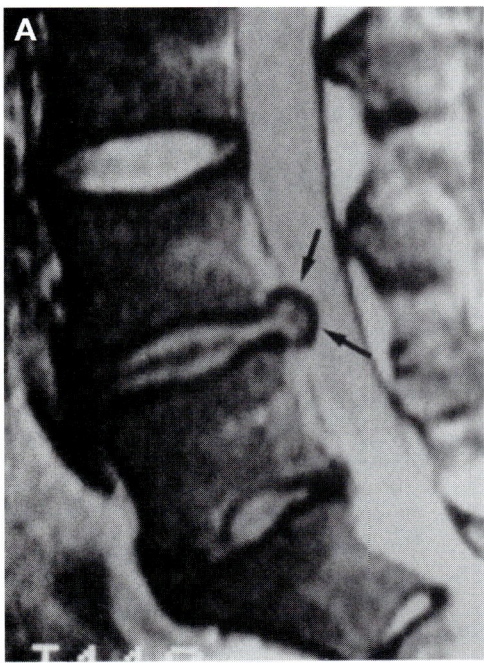

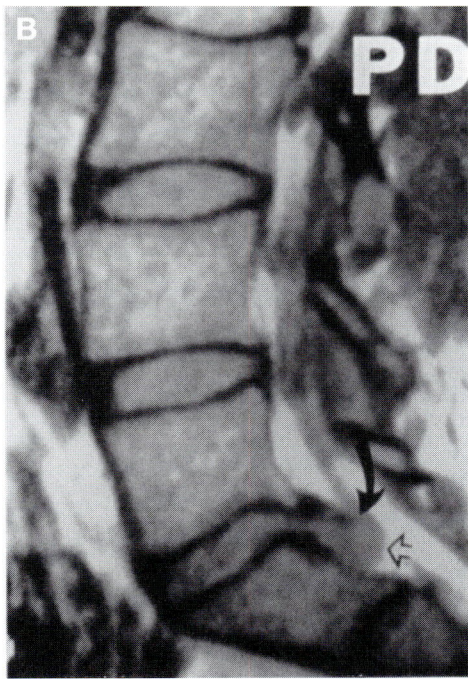

Figure 1 Sagittal MRI studies of the lumbar spine showing **(A)** a contained disk herniation (protrusion) with the outer annular fibers (dark band, arrows) intact, and **(B)** a noncontained disk herniation (extrusion) with displaced disk material (open arrow) penetrating through a complete defect of the posterior anulus fibrosus, displacing the traversing S1 nerve root (curved arrow).

A number of descriptive terms are commonly used to describe the degree and location of disk fragment displacement in herniated disks. Protrusion refers to a focal outpouching of the anulus with displacement of inner disk material within a partially torn or thinned anulus. Because the anulus is not completely disrupted, protrusions are considered contained disk herniations. In a noncontained disk herniation, the inner disk material is displaced through a complete defect of the anulus (Fig. 1). Generally, the circumference of the displaced disk material is larger than the actual defect in the anulus. Two types of noncontained disk herniation exist. In an extrusion, the displaced disk material remains in continuity with the inner disk through the annular defect. An extruded disk herniation may be described as subligamentous if the disk fragment extends completely through the anulus but remains under an intact posterior longitudinal ligament. A sequestration refers to displaced disk material no longer in direct continuity with the inner disk space of origin. In a sequestrated disk herniation, the displaced disk material may be migrated a distance from the parent disk or nearby, and the annular defect may still exist or be sealed after a reparative process.

Lumbar disk herniations can also be classified by their anatomic location within zones along the circumference of the anulus fibrosus (Fig. 2). When in the midline posteriorly, the herniation is in the central zone. A large central herniation may affect the traversing nerve roots bilaterally as well as all the roots caudad to the herniation. Toward one side but medial to the pedicle, the herniation is in the posterolateral or

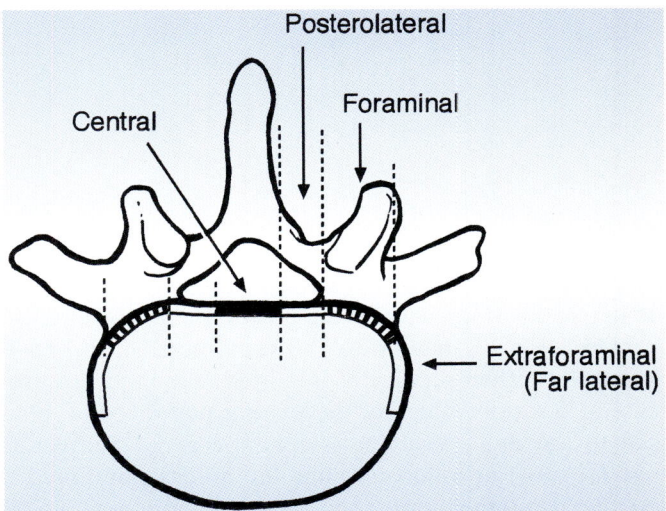

Figure 2 Axial view of the disk depicting types of disk herniations in relation to the radial zones along the circumference.

subarticular zone. This is the most common location, and here the displaced disk material generally impinges on the anterior and lateral aspect of the traversing nerve root (Fig. 3). Within the medial and lateral borders of the pedicle (within the intervertebral foramen), a herniation is in the foraminal zone, and lateral to the foramen is the extraforaminal or far lateral zone. Herniations in these locations impinge on the exiting nerve root. Commonly, a disk herniation may be large or broad enough to affect more than one of these anatomic zones. Another anatomic term used to describe the location of a disk herniation is in the

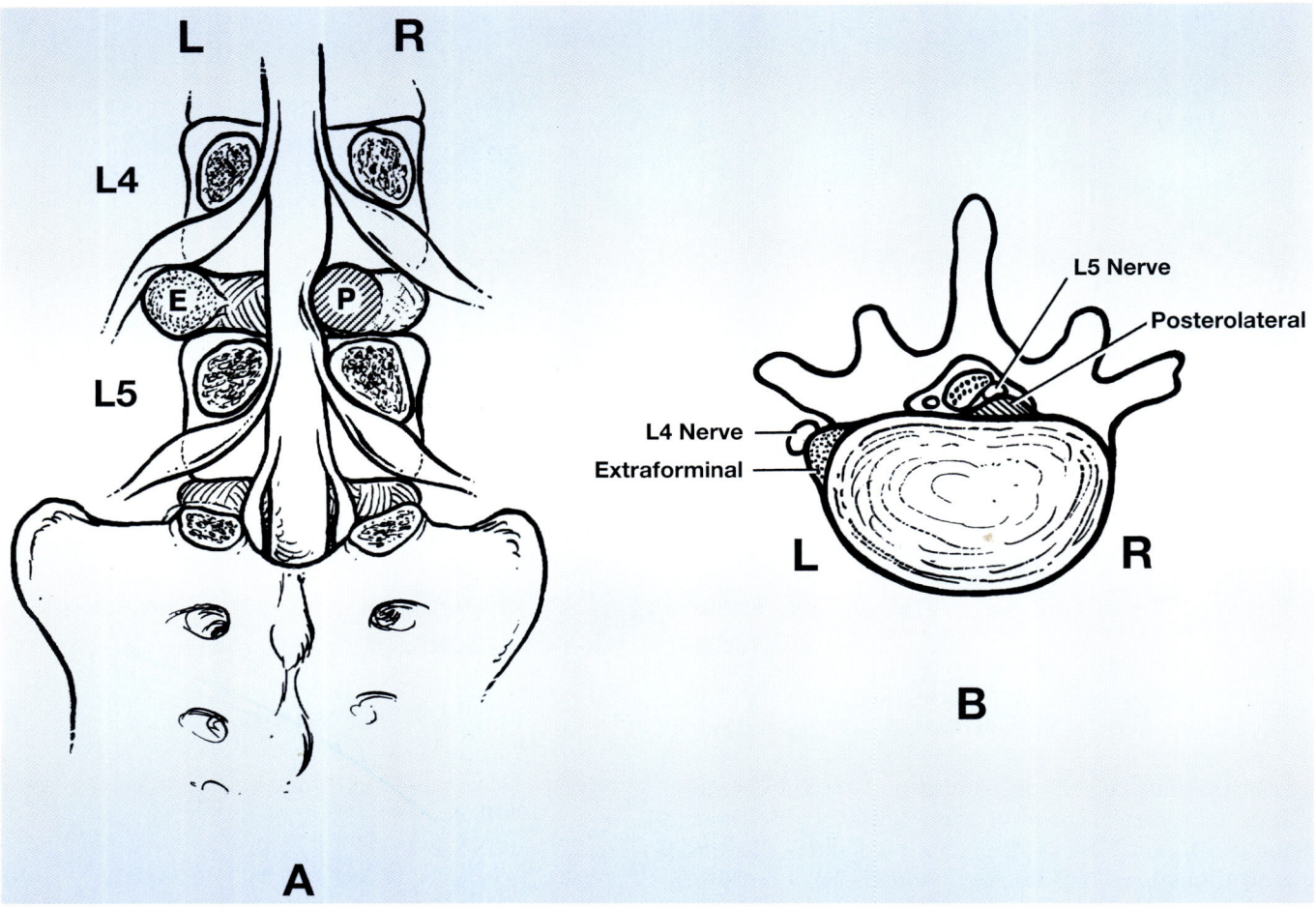

Figure 3 **A,** Posterior cutaway view and **B,** axial view of two herniated disks at the L4-5 level. (P = posterolateral, affecting the traversing L5 nerve, and E = extraforaminal, affecting the exiting L4 nerve).

axillary position. This term refers to displaced disk material located medial to the compressed nerve root, generally either superiorly migrated from the posterolateral position affecting the exiting nerve root cephalad to the disk space (most common at L4-5 affecting the L4 root) or inferiorly migrated anterior and medial to the traversing nerve root (most common at L5-S1 affecting the S1 root).

Most lumbar disk herniations occur in patients between 30 to 50 years of age and are characterized by varying amounts of back and/or leg pain; the leg pain commonly follows the dermatomal path of the compressed nerve roots. Lumbar disk herniations presenting prior to age 30 years tend to be of strong hereditary predisposition. Herniations in older patients may be particularly painful if concomitant spinal stenosis exists. The sudden onset of back pain often coincides with tearing of the highly innervated outer annular fibers. The back pain will often abate shortly after herniation occurs, with depressurization of the intervertebral space and relief of annular tension, concomitant with the onset of radicular pain. However, the back

pain may persist with a large central disk herniation secondary to irritation of the highly innervated posterior longitudinal ligament. The L5 and S1 dermatomes are often involved, signifying that most herniations occur at the L4-5 and L5-S1 interspaces. An S1 radiculopathy may less commonly present as isolated buttock or posterolateral hamstring pain, and L5 can present as lateral hip pain. The typical radicular pain may be accompanied by paresthesias as well as varying degrees of motor, sensory, and reflex loss. Activities that increase intraspinal and intradiskal pressure such as coughing, sneezing, and the Valsalva maneuver often accentuate pain. Acute onset of bowel and bladder incontinence, bilateral lower extremity neurologic motor weakness, and saddle anesthesia are the typical signs and symptoms (triad) associated with cauda equina syndrome.

The physical examination of the patient with a lumbar herniated disk often reveals an antalgic gait pattern as well as a "sciatic list". The patient will commonly lean to the opposite side of the herniation, thereby bringing the compressed nerve root away from the posterolateral herniation. Leaning toward the side of the leg pain may indicate medial nerve compression from an axillary disk herniation. Recent studies have shown that the direction of the list may not always be related to the anatomy or location of the disk. Palpation and percussion of the lumbar spine often reveals significant muscle spasm in the paraspinal region. Palpation should be continued along the course of the sciatic nerve, including the sciatic notch which may be painful. A meticulous neurologic examination including deep tendon reflexes and sensory and motor testing often reveals evidence of nerve root dysfunction. With prolonged neural compression, loss of muscle tone and atrophy may be observed.

Foot drop is a condition most commonly associated with an L5 radiculopathy. However, it may also be a manifestation of a more distal neuropathy such as a peripheral neuropathy secondary to diabetes or a compressive neuropathy of the peroneal nerve at the fibular head. Differentiation of a radiculopathic process from a neuropathic one is done with careful examination. A Trendelenburg sign due to gluteus medius denervation from an L5 radiculopathy is not present with a more distal peripheral neuropathy. Sensory examination with monofilaments may reveal a stocking glove distribution of sensory dysfunction, and motor testing of the foot everters (primarily S1) will be normal with an L5 radiculopathy but may be abnormal with common peroneal nerve dysfunction.

Nerve root tension signs are very common in the presence of a low lumbar disk herniation. The overall excursion of the L5 and S1 spinal nerves is 2 to 6 mm at the level of the foramen. The L4 root moves a lesser distance, and the more proximal lumbar roots show little motion with lower extremity motion. The supine straight leg raising test, also known as the Lasègue's sign, is performed when the examiner slowly elevates the affected lower extremity by the heel with the knee fully extended. In a positive test, clinical symptoms of radicular lower extremity pain are reproduced with between 35° to 70° of extremity elevation; this is generally indicative of L5 or S1 compression. Reproduction of low back or buttock pain without radicular pain is not considered a positive test. The sensitivity of the straight leg raising test has been found to be age dependent. A positive straight leg raising test is seen in nearly all patients younger than age 30 years with a symptomatic disk herniation. After age 30 years, however, the straight leg raising test may be negative even in the presence of a true symptomatic disk herniation. The test also can be done in the sitting position by extending the flexed knee with the hip already flexed; when the patient leans back during this maneuver to avoid pain, this is called a positive flip test. The contralateral straight leg raising test (ipsilateral radicular pain with elevation of the contralateral asymptomatic lower extremity) is exceptionally specific for a herniated disk, particularly one with axillary migration. The bowstring sign and sciatic notch tenderness are less specific signs of low lumbar nerve root tension. The femoral stretch test (anterior lower extremity pain with hyperextension of the hip and flexion of the knee) is useful for evaluating nerve root tension in the upper lumbar roots (L2, L3, and L4).

Upright lumbar radiographs are not helpful for the diagnosis of a herniated disk, but are indicated in patients with more than 6 weeks of back pain and in those with a clinical history of significant trauma, constitutional symptoms, and previous cancers. MRI is the imaging test of choice to confirm the clinical suspicion of a lumbar disk herniation when surgical intervention is contemplated. MRI is also useful in differentiating between a postoperative scar and a recurrent disk herniation in a patient with a prior history of disk surgery.

For up to 90% of patients, the natural history associated with radiculopathy secondary to a documented lumbar herniated disk is gradual and progressive resolution of symptoms without the need for surgical intervention within 3 months of the onset of symptoms. The majority of herniations, particularly large, noncontained disk fragments, will reduce in size over time. Possible mechanisms for reduction in disk fragment size include loss of initial water content, reduction of associated inflammatory mass, and macrophage removal of disk material by the incited inflammatory response. This reduction of fragment size and inflammatory response typically leads to relief of symptoms.

Because of the excellent natural history of symptomatic lumbar disk herniation, the initial treatment is typically nonsurgical, and includes medication, activity modification, and possibly a short period of bed rest, a regimen similar to that for the nonsurgical treatment for low back pain.

The use of steroid injections is becoming more common for treatment of lumbar radicular pain caused by a herniated disk. Epidural steroids can be applied via an interlaminar or a transforaminal route; both methods should be performed under fluoroscopic guidance to assure application of the steroid to the epidural space at the appropriate spinal level and prevent intravascular penetration. The efficacy of injection treatment may be only temporary, because the underlying anatomic abnormalities are not affected. A recent prospective, randomized study of a series of up to four selective nerve-root injections in patients with lumbar radicular pain, however, showed significant improvement in symptoms and a decrease in the need for surgical decompression at a mean of 23 months after the first injection. Complications associated with steroid injections in the lumbar spine are extremely uncommon, but serious complications that have been reported include transient paresis and paralysis, epidural hematoma, infection, chemical meningitis, and arachnoiditis.

Emergent and relative indications exist for decompression of a lumbar disk herniation. Emergent surgical indications include a progressive neurologic deficit or the presence of a cauda equina syndrome. A static neurologic deficit without profound functional impairment does not require immediate surgical intervention. Relative surgical indications in lumbar disk herniation include persistent radiculopathy despite an adequate trial of nonsurgical treatment (generally a minimum of 6 weeks), recurrent episodes of incapacitating sciatica, a significant motor deficit with persistent tension signs and pain, and pseudoclaudication (activity-related leg pain) caused by canal stenosis resulting from a disk herniation. Failure of nonsurgical treatment with persistent sciatica remains the most common reason for surgical intervention.

The main goal of surgical intervention is to alleviate the neural compression without further injury to the affected nerve root(s). Secondary goals are the minimal disruption of surrounding normal tissues and the maintenance of spinal stability. The surgical gold standard remains a limited open lumbar laminotomy and diskectomy, generally with magnification of the surgical field using surgical loupes or the operating microscope.

The patient is positioned in the kneeling position with the abdomen free, facilitating ventilation and decreasing epidural venous pressure and bleeding. A limited diskectomy with removal of only the displaced fragment and nearby loose intradiskal fragments is advised. No reduction in the rate of reherniation has been found with more radical disk material excision. In general, the risk of reherniation at the same level on the same side is in the range of 5%. If opposite side and adjacent levels are included, the rate of symptom recurrence caused by additional disk herniations may be as high as 20%.

Unilateral partial medial facetectomy along with removal of the lateral ligamentum flavum is often necessitated by preexisting stenosis of the lateral recess. Foraminal and far lateral herniations may be particularly painful secondary to their proximity to the sensitive dorsal root ganglion. They are often best approached more laterally using a muscle-splitting approach and dissection through the intertransverse membrane. Techniques of combined laminotomy and intertransverse approaches have been described as well, in order to avoid facetectomy for more broad

disk herniations that may have components both within the spinal canal and more laterally.

The success of limited open microdiskectomy for relief of sciatica is greater than 90% in most clinical series. Proper patient selection is the key to a successful outcome. Patients should have predominant lower extremity symptoms, and imaging studies must be concordant with any focal neurologic findings. The presence of preoperative tension signs along with the degree of herniation documented intraoperatively correlate positively with a successful outcome. Isolated back pain in the absence of any radicular symptoms is a relative contraindication to this procedure, because the relief of back pain via diskectomy is less predictable. Large central disk herniations with predominant back pain may be the one disk herniation type that may respond to diskectomy, but even in this case many surgeons would recommend a spinal fusion. Despite the high early success rate after diskectomy is performed, recent studies have revealed that these optimistic short-term results begin to decline over time secondary to the persistently advancing degenerative condition. Recent studies have indicated that early institution of an active aerobic postoperative exercise protocol and encouraging patients to return to normal activities as soon as they feel able may be beneficial in clinical outcome and accelerate overall recovery.

Perioperative complications of lumbar disk herniation surgery include incidental durotomy, wrong-level and wrong-sided surgery, retained disk fragments with persistent radiculopathy, and acute wound infections. Successful primary intraoperative repair of a durotomy may or may not be treated by a period of postoperative bed rest, but it generally does not alter the long-term surgical outcome. Wrong-level and wrong-sided surgery should be avoided by adequate intraoperative radiographic localization of spinal level and surgical confirmation of the expected pathology. Preoperative radiographs should be obtained to assess for unusual transitional anatomy, which may make intraoperative localization more difficult. Wound infections generally respond to a short course of intravenous antibiotics, although deep wound infections may require surgical débridement.

Late complications include disk space infection, recurrent disk herniation, and postoperative instability. Disk space infections usually result in worsening back pain 3 to 6 weeks after the index procedure, although occasionally an infection may appear many weeks, months, or even years after diskectomy. Erythrocyte sedimentation rate and C-reactive protein is almost always elevated, although the white blood cell count may not be elevated. MRI is used to confirm the diagnosis, followed by percutaneous cultures under radiographic guidance. Once an organism is identified, most patients respond to intravenous antibiotic administration. If antibiotic therapy is unsuccessful, treatment may consist of surgical débridement (usually done anteriorly) and fusion with autologous bone grafting.

Recurrent disk herniation is evident on repeat MRI scan and is shown as a focal mass lesion in the region of the diskectomy that does not enhance centrally after intravenous contrast administration. Rim enhancement of the surrounding inflammatory response is typically seen. Symptomatic recurrent herniations generally respond less favorably to nonsurgical treatment than primary disk herniations, with a larger percentage going on to surgical treatment to achieve relief of symptoms. Patients with predominant leg symptoms are candidates for revision diskectomy. Patients with excessive back pain should be worked up for segmental instability and/or a fracture of the pars interarticularis with standing AP and lateral radiographs, lateral flexion/extension views, and oblique views to show the pars interarticularis. CT scanning may also be useful to define the integrity of the pars interarticularis and facet joints. If significant instability exists, revision decompression with concomitant instrumented spinal fusion should be performed. Surgical outcome is expected to provide significant relief of back and leg pain in 75% to 80% of cases. Spinal fusion should be considered, even without documented instability, in the presence of excessive back pain with recurrent leg symptoms.

Lumbar Spinal Stenosis

Lumbar spinal stenosis is a narrowing of the spinal canal that results in compression of the neural elements before their exit from the neural foramen. This narrowing may involve a single motion segment, or it may span two or more motion segments. This type of stenosis can be classified according to etiology or anatomy. In the original etiologic classification, congenital or developmental stenosis is distinguished from acquired or degenerative spinal stenosis (Table 1). Congenital lumbar spinal stenosis is seen either in patients of normal stature with congenitally short pedicles or in those with a bone dysplasia, such as achondroplasia. Other rare disorders associated with congenital stenosis include hypochondroplasia, diastrophic dwarfism, Morquio's syndrome, hereditary exostosis, and cheirolumbar dystosis. Patients with congenital lumbar stenosis often first experience symptoms earlier, typically in the third or fourth decade of life. Acquired stenosis is most commonly degenerative, usually presenting with symptoms later, in the sixth or seventh decade of life.

TABLE 1	Classification of Lumbar Spinal Stenosis
Congenital/Developmental
Idiopathic
Achondroplastic
Acquired
Degenerative
Central
Lateral recess and foraminal
Iatrogenic
Postlaminectomy
Postdiskectomy
Postfusion
Miscellaneous
Paget's disease
Fluorosis
Acromegaly
Posttraumatic
Combined (acquired and congenital)

Anatomic classifications of lumbar spinal stenosis help identify specific areas of narrowing of the spinal canal and are used as guides for surgical decompression. A clearer understanding of the anatomy of the spinal canal at each vertebral segment is obtained by dividing the canal into a series of transverse regions (three levels from cephalad to caudad) and sagittal regions (three zones from midline laterally) (Fig. 4). The three transverse levels are the pedicle, intermediate (vertebral body), and disk levels. The pedicle level extends from the superior to the inferior cortical margin of the pedicle, including the flare of the pedicle at its base. The intermediate level begins at the inferior border of the pedicle and extends caudally to the inferior end plate of the vertebrae. The disk level begins at the inferior end plate and extends caudally to the superior border of the next pedicle. The three sagittal zones are the central, the lateral recess, and pedicle zones. The central zone is the area between the normal lateral borders of the noncompressed dural sac. The lateral recess zone is the area between the lateral border of the dural sac medially and a longitudinal line connecting the medial edges of the pedicles laterally. The pedicle zone is the area between the medial and lateral borders of the pedicle.

Lumbar spinal stenosis may be subclassified into central and lateral stenosis. Central stenosis commonly occurs at the disk level as a result of a bulging disk,

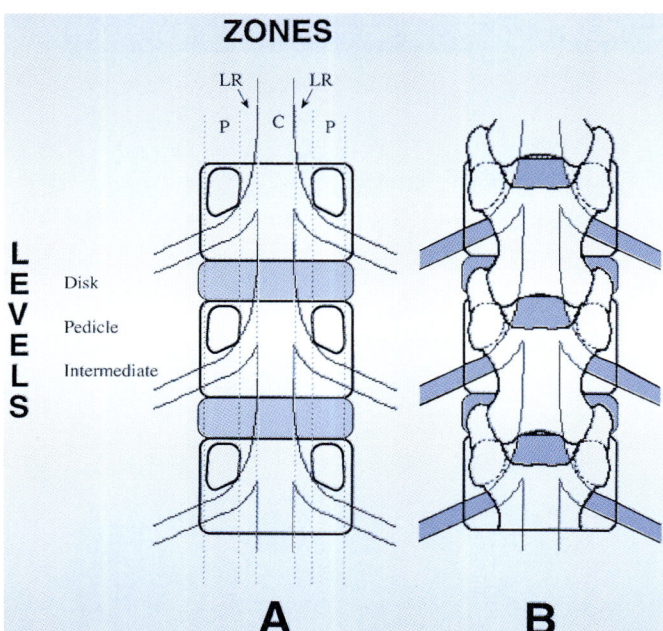

ZONES

L
E
V
E
L
S

Disk

Pedicle

Intermediate

A   **B**

Figure 4 Anatomic grid pattern used to evaluate lumbar stenosis. **A,** Posterior cutaway view showing the relationship of the neural elements to the five sagittal zones (P = pedicle, LR = lateral recess, C = central) and three axial levels. **B,** Posterior view with posterior elements intact showing the relationship of the facet joints and pars interarticularis to the neural elements and anatomic grid pattern. *(Reproduced with permission from Spivak JM: Degenerative lumbar spinal stenosis.* J Bone Joint Surg Am 1998;80:1053-1066.)

facet joint overgrowth (mainly from the inferior articular process of the cephalad vertebrae), and thickening and redundancy of the ligamentum flavum. Preexisting short pedicle length is often seen. Lateral stenosis includes both lateral recess and foraminal stenosis. Lateral recess stenosis, also known as subarticular stenosis, occurs as a result of the degenerative changes similar to those associated with central spinal stenosis and affects the spinal nerve root canal at the disk level and the superior aspect of the pedicle level. Lateral recess stenosis is uncommon at the inferior aspect of the pedicle, but may exist with hypertrophic granulation tissue from the posteriorly located pars interarticularis in patients with spondylolytic defects. Foraminal stenosis usually involves the disk level but may ascend to include the intermediate level where the nerve root must pass to exit the spine. The exiting nerve root may be compressed by bulging or herniated disk material, osteophytes arising from the inferior aspect of the cephalad vertebrae, or from the cephalad migration or hypertrophy of the superior articular process of the caudad vertebrae.

The symptoms created by degenerative lumbar stenosis usually have an insidious onset and a slow rate of progression. Vague complaints of low backache and stiffness are typical and are more related to degenerative disk disease than to nerve compression. There are two categories of leg pain symptoms seen in lumbar

spinal stenosis. One presentation is unilateral leg pain along with numbness, burning, and paresthesias radiating in a dermatomal distribution. This radicular type of presentation is present in less than 20% of symptomatic stenosis patients, and is more often seen with severe foraminal or lateral recess stenosis. Motor strength and reflex changes specific to one nerve root may be seen but are uncommon. Compression of the fifth lumbar nerve root creating weakness of the extensor hallucis longus and tibialis anterior may be encountered. Reduced reflexes in the knee and the ankle are more common in patients who have central spinal stenosis than in those who have lateral spinal stenosis. However, a symmetric loss of reflexes in the lower extremities is commonly seen secondary to the normal aging process.

More commonly, patients will present with neurogenic claudication defined as the onset of lower extremity pain, paresthesias, or motor symptoms upon walking. Symptoms typically are bilateral and consist of an aching, cramping, or burning sensation in the legs. The discomfort starts in the buttocks and often progresses to the thighs, calves, and feet. These symptoms are often exacerbated by standing or exercising in an erect or extended posture, and relieved by sitting and forward flexion. Patients will often assume a hunched or simian posture when walking, because of the variation in size of the spinal canal with different postures. Cadaveric studies have demonstrated that both central canal and foraminal dimensions increase in flexion and decrease in extension. Men often experience great difficulty shaving while standing erect. Supermarket shopping is often poorly tolerated unless the patient can lean forward on the shopping cart (positive grocery cart sign).

The findings on physical examination usually are limited. Lumbar lordosis is often reduced as is lumbar range of motion, particularly extension. Signs of nerve root tension including the straight leg raising test are usually negative. However, lumbar extension may exacerbate the lower extremity symptoms. Evaluation of the hips and knees should always be performed to rule out degenerative joint disease as a cause of leg pain. Groin pain is not characteristic of lumbar spinal stenosis and should alert the examiner to the possibility of hip arthritis or dysfunction of the sacroiliac joint. An abdominal examination, especially in the elderly, should be performed to rule out an aortic aneurysm. Palpation of the distal pulses are necessary to evaluate the possibility of peripheral vascular disease. Several maneuvers are helpful when attempting to differentiate neurogenic claudication from vascular claudication (Table 2).

TABLE 2	Differentiating Neurogenic From Vascular Claudication	
	Neurogenic	**Vascular**
Pain	Proximal to distal	Distal to proximal
	Relieved bending/sitting	Relieved by standing
	Exacerbated with lumbar extension	Not positional
	Better with stairs/incline	Worse with stairs/incline
Pulses	Present	Absent
Skin loss	Normal	Thin, shiny, hair
Neurologic deficits	May be present	Absent

Neurologic examination is often normal unless advanced lumbar stenosis has been present for an extended period. Weakness of the extensor hallucis longus is the most common motor deficit. Calf and thigh atrophy may be present with long-standing, severe lateral stenosis. A herniated disk superimposed on already advanced stenosis is a common scenario for motor deficit. Neurologic examination following ambulation-induced symptoms may be helpful to elicit objective findings as compared with the resting asymptomatic state. Loss of light touch and pin prick sensation is unusual. Asymmetric lower extremity reflexes may suggest spinal stenosis, as opposed to symmetric, age-related changes. The possibility of concomitant cervical myelopathy or an intracranial disorder should be considered with an abnormal gait pattern and any long tract findings.

Radiographic examination of a patient in whom lumbar spinal stenosis is suspected often demonstrates multilevel spondylosis, which may not be associated with stenosis of the spinal canal. Degenerative spondylolisthesis and degenerative lumbar scoliosis are radiographic findings that are more suggestive of lumbar spinal stenosis. AP and lateral radiographs should be taken in the standing position, whereas dynamic lateral radiographs in maximal flexion and extension taken in the recumbent position are useful for determining whether there is abnormal motion or instability at any level. For those patients who have associated degenerative scoliosis, weight-bearing AP and lateral radiographs taken on a 36-in cassette are particularly helpful for assessing curve magnitude as well as the overall balance of the entire spine in the coronal and sagittal planes. An AP radiograph taken with the patient supine can be helpful as a comparison to assess the collapse of the spine in the erect position.

CT scan is the most cost-effective single test for establishing the diagnosis of lumbar spinal stenosis. However, many believe that MRI is the best anatomic screening test for patients with symptomatic spinal stenosis. The diagnostic accuracy of MRI is superior to that of myelography and plain CT scanning, and it is as accurate and sensitive as myelography followed by CT scanning. The combination of axial and sagittal images allows for complete evaluation of the central spinal canal and the neural foramen. Regions of very low signal intensity on T2-weighted images caused by sclerotic osteophytes can lead to overestimation of the amount of true osseous stenosis. MRI of the scoliotic lumbar spine often is suboptimal because axial images are often not made in the proper plane parallel to the involved disk spaces. The combination of high-quality MRI and plain CT can provide complete evaluation of the spinal canal and often obviates the need for preoperative myelography.

Lumbar myelography with subsequent CT scan provides the most complete anatomic evaluation of compression of the neural elements within the lumbar spine. Myelography also allows for a dynamic assessment of stenosis by examination of lateral views made with the spine in maximal flexion and extension; this may reveal a dynamic component of the stenosis that may be the result of segmental instability or encroachment on the spinal canal by disk bulging and ligamentum flavum infolding in extension. The main disadvantage of myelography is the need for an invasive spinal tap, and so the procedure generally is used as a preoperative test when more anatomic information is needed. Recent studies have suggested that MRI and CT provide complementary information; however, postmyelographic CT is superior to MRI as a single study for the preoperative planning of decompression for lumbar spinal stenosis.

Early surgical treatment has been recommended for the treatment of symptomatic lumbar stenosis because it was thought that this disorder was always progressive. However, more recent information has suggested a more favorable natural history. The disease has been shown to be relatively stable for 70% of patients with symptomatic spinal stenosis. Long-term follow-up has indicated a 15% incidence of worsening symptoms and a 15% incidence of improvement of symptoms.

The mainstays of nonsurgical treatment include oral medications, activity modification, physical therapy and exercise, and steroid injections. None of these methods has been demonstrated to be efficacious as a sole treatment. Salicylates and NSAIDs are most often prescribed in the treatment of pain associated with lumbar spinal stenosis. Patients should be alerted to the potential gastrointestinal side effects associated with these drugs and hepatic and renal function should be monitored periodically with prolonged use. If severe radiculopathy persists, a short course of oral corticosteroids should be considered.

The most useful forms of physical therapy in the treatment of lumbar spinal stenosis are therapeutic stretching and strengthening exercises for the abdominal and spinal extensor muscles, and aerobic fitness training. Williams flexion exercises are preferred to McKenzie hyperextension exercises considering the pathoanatomy of this disease. Aquatic therapy may also be useful, limiting the demands of patient weight in exercising. Physical therapy modalities designed for the localized treatment of soft tissues, including application of ice, heat, ultrasound, transcutaneous electrical stimulation, and traction are commonly used but have not yet proved to be effective for any disorder of the lumbar spine.

The use of external lumbosacral supports in the management of lumbar spinal stenosis remains controversial. There is a paucity of clinical data to support its routine use; however, a rigid brace to maintain the spine in neutral or flexion has been useful in relief of initial symptoms. Long-term brace wear may lead to truncal deconditioning and should be discouraged.

The use of steroid injections to treat disorders of the lumbar spine, including spinal stenosis, remains controversial. Studies have shown the clinical effects of epidurally-applied steroids to be variable and unpredictable. Newer studies have shown more uniform success when the injections are radiographically guided. The efficacy of steroid injections may be temporary, because the underlying anatomic abnormalities are not affected. Longer term studies are needed. According to a recent prospective randomized study of a series of up to four selective nerve root injections in patients with lumbar radicular pain, there was a significant improvement in symptoms and a decrease in the need for surgical decompression at a mean of 23 months after the first injection. Treatment with epidural steroid injections and selective nerve root injections should be reserved for those patients with a predominance of lower extremity symptoms. An advanced radiographic study of the spinal canal is prerequisite to determine the anatomic pathology and localize the spinal level for injection. All injections should be done under radiographic guidance. Contrast instillation is recommended, especially in transforaminal epidural injections for which the incidence of intravascular penetration has recently been noted to be over 11%. Complications associated with steroid injections in the lumbar spine are extremely uncommon, but serious complications include transient paresis and paralysis, epidural hematoma, infection, chemical-induced meningitis, and arachnoiditis.

Lumbar spinal stenosis is not life-threatening and rapid catastrophic neurologic deterioration is rare; therefore, the decision to perform an operation should be made after nonsurgical treatment has failed. The presence of a nonprogressive neurologic deficit has been shown to correlate poorly with physical function and so is not an absolute surgical indication. Progression of a functionally disabling neurologic deficit or cauda equina syndrome, although rarely associated with lumbar spinal stenosis, are two indications for urgent surgical intervention. Surgery should be reserved for those patients who have evidence of severe spinal stenosis on imaging studies and have a preponderance of lower extremity symptoms. Decompression of stenosis in patients with predominant back pain has a poorer outcome than that of patients with mainly leg pain symptoms. Patients' expectations should be thoroughly discussed prior to surgery. The goals of surgery are to decrease pain and improve function.

Several techniques have been described for decompression of the degenerative stenotic lumbar spine. The standard wide decompressive laminectomy involves removal of the lamina and ligamentum flavum from the lateral border of one lateral recess to that of the other at all involved intervertebral levels. Compressed nerve roots are then decompressed from their origin at the thecal sac and throughout their course as they exit the neural foramen. All lateral recesses in which nerve roots may be entrapped should be decompressed. During the laminectomy, the patient should be prone, in the kneeling position with the abdomen hanging free. This position is associated with lower central venous pressures and so decreases the incidence of intraoperative bleeding. The more lordotic position achieved when the hips are positioned unflexed is preferred when internal fixation is planned.

Alternative techniques of decompression for the treatment of degenerative central and lateral recess stenosis have been designed in an attempt to preserve more of the osteoligamentous arch, theoretically diminishing the problem of postoperative instability. These techniques include a beveled laminectomy with angular resection of only the anterior portion of the lateral aspect of the lamina, selective single or multiple unilateral or bilateral laminotomy (fenestration procedure), multiple partial laminectomy, and lumbar laminaplasty. The early clinical results of each of these techniques have been satisfactory, but reports of long-term outcome are lacking. The problem of regrowth of bone with clinically important recurrent stenosis may be more frequent in association with methods of decompression involving limited resection of bone.

The results of surgical decompression for lumbar spinal stenosis have been good in general. According to a recent study, functional evaluation by treadmill walking was more reliable than testing using a stationary bicycle. Using this functional evaluation as well as a visual analog pain scale, decompression for lumbar stenosis provided significant clinical improvement at a minimum 2-year follow-up. However, other recent studies have suggested that the long-term outcome may not be as good as originally thought. Initial favorable clinical outcomes seem to deteriorate over time. Factors associated with a poorer outcome include multiple comorbidities, single-level decompressions, a predominance of low back pain, diabetes with neuropathy, osteoarthrosis of the hip, and preoperative degenerative scoliosis. There is a 5% incidence of symptomatic degeneration at levels adjacent to the decompression. Recurrent symptoms may be caused by recurrence of stenosis at a level that was previously decompressed, progression of stenosis at an adjacent level, or mechanical back pain with instability.

The role of arthrodesis in the surgical treatment of lumbar spinal stenosis has been the subject of much debate in the recent literature. After routine decompression is done in the absence of spinal deformity or instability, concomitant spinal arthrodesis generally does not provide additional clinical benefit and does increase perioperative morbidity. Instability created by resection of the facet joints at the time of operation is an indication for concomitant arthrodesis to prevent postoperative instability and pain. It is generally accepted that stability will be maintained if more than 50% of each facet joint is left intact. However, biomechanical evidence has suggested that instability may occur after unilateral total facetectomy, even if the remaining facet has been left completely intact.

The role of arthrodesis in the surgical treatment of lumbar spinal stenosis with associated degenerative spondylolisthesis has also been studied extensively. Most studies indicate an improvement in clinical outcome in these patients when an arthrodesis is performed at the time of initial decompression, along with a greater chance of recurrence of spinal stenosis, and instability following laminectomy without fusion in patients with spondylolisthesis. Preoperative radiographic and anatomic risk factors associated with the postoperative development or progression of spondylolisthesis at the level of the fourth and fifth lumbar vertebrae include a well maintained disk height, the absence of degenerative osteophytes, and a smaller, sagittally oriented facet joint.

The surgical management of spinal stenosis in association with degenerative scoliosis is even less clear-cut than for degenerative spondylolisthesis. Not all patients with surgically significant spinal stenosis within a lumbar scoliosis require a simultaneous spinal fusion procedure. A flexible curve that lacks osteophytes may require arthodesis to avoid postoperative progression following laminectomy. In some instances, a single symptomatic nerve root can be isolated by means of selective diagnostic injections, allowing for a more limited decompression.

Patients who are undergoing a revision lumbar laminectomy for spinal stenosis are also good candidates for concomitant arthrodesis. In this circumstance, excessive removal of the facet joints to ensure adequate decompression may lead to postoperative instability in the absence of an arthrodesis. If a patient develops stenosis adjacent to a previous fusion, decompression alone is recommended if no preoperative instability exists and no significant facet joint compromise occurs at surgery.

Simultaneous diskectomy and laminectomy raises some concerns. When combined with a laminectomy, "radical" disk excision may lead to iatrogenic spondylolisthesis because the procedure potentially destabilizes the anterior column. A unilateral diskectomy performed in addition to a total laminectomy is not likely to lead to postoperative instability when the spine is stable preoperatively. However, if bilateral diskectomy is performed along with laminectomy, consideration should be given to concomitant arthrodesis to prevent postoperative instability.

The use of spinal instrumentation with arthrodesis for lumbar spinal stenosis remains controversial. Earlier studies suggested superior clinical results and improved fusion rates when instrumentation was used. Rigid constructs have been associated with a better clinical result than semirigid constructs, which allow more motion between the fixation screws and the rod or plate. More recent studies suggest that adding instrumentation improves the fusion rate but does not result in significant improvement in clinical outcome. In a long-term (5- to 10-year) follow-up study of decompression and noninstrumented fusion for degenerative spondylolisthesis, clinical results were superior when fusion was achieved as compared to patients whose fusion surgery resulted in pseudarthrosis. Spinal instrumentation, achieving a higher fusion rate, may therefore have a positive long-term benefit. Long-term results of instrumented fusions have yet to be reported.

Degenerative Segmental Instability

Motion segment instability has been divided into subtypes. Type I is axial rotatory instability, which usually involves a fixed rotatory deformity along with occasional translatory malalignment. The spinous processes are usually malaligned on AP radiographs of the lumbar spine. Type II, or translational instability, is anterior displacement of one vertebral body on another, and traction spur formation without pedicular rotation. Type III is retrolisthetic instability, most commonly seen at the L5-S1 level. Type IV, or iatrogenic, postsurgical instability may be seen after extensive surgical removal of the posterior osteoligamentous supports.

Conflicting opinions exist regarding the definition of segmental instability in the clinical setting. Symptoms of clinical instability may include standing intolerance, giving way of the lower back, and frequent attacks of low back pain. The patient may have referred pain in the buttocks and thighs. Physical examination may reveal an extension "catch," indicated by cogwheeling or a ratchet-like motion of the spine when a patient is asked to go from a forward bending position to a fully erect position. Other signs indicative of potential instability are the presence of a palpable posterior spinous process step-off indicating a spondylolisthesis, as well as lateral deviation of the spinous process indicative of scoliosis.

Several radiographic signs may be indicative of segmental instability. Static radiograph signs best evaluated on standing AP and lateral radiographs include traction osteophytes, narrowing of the intervertebral disk space, retrolisthesis, anterolisthesis, lateral listhesis, vacuum disk sign, and malalignment of the spinous processes. Dynamic instability is best evaluated with recumbent lateral radiographs obtained during maximal flexion and extension. Radiographic criteria for dynamic segmental instability include greater than 4 mm of translational difference and/or 10° of angular difference as measured on the lateral flexion and extension radiographs.

The surgical treatment of degenerative segmental instability is spinal fusion. Exact indications are controversial, but fusion is generally reserved for persistent back pain despite nonsurgical treatment with medications and exercise. It is difficult to quantify instability and relate it directly to surgical outcome. Attempts to do so via clinical, biomechanical, and radiographic classifications have been unsuccessful. Nevertheless, it is believed that there are patients with clinically relevant instabilities that are amenable to surgical stabilization. Preoperative testing including a bracing trial, lumbar facet blocks, and provocative diskography have all been used to try to better predict which patients will respond favorably to surgical arthrodesis. No method of preoperative evaluation has proved to be regularly reliable.

Surgical options include anterior interbody fusion, posterolateral fusion with and without instrumentation, posterior interbody fusion, and combined interbody and posterolateral fusion. Fusion rates in cases of documented segmental instability are higher with the use of posterior pedicle instrumentation, but improvements in clinical outcome have not been shown to be similarly improved. Even in the best of circumstances, surgical outcomes in these patients are quite variable, with success ranging from 40% to 90%.

Discogenic Back Pain

Discogenic pain syndrome including internal disk disruption (acute traumatic annular tear) and degenerative disk disease is another frequent cause of lumbosacral pain. The diagnosis of discogenic pain is one of exclusion, considered only after other anatomic causes of back pain are ruled out. This is because the presence of a degenerated lumbar disk on radiographic or MRI examination is very common, even in asymptomatic controls.

In the absence of neural impingement, deformity, or instability this process is often referred to as "black disk disease," seen as a loss of signal intensity on T2-weighted sagittal MRI. This loss of signal intensity is considered by many as equivalent to degenerative disk disease, but may only represent a very small, clinically insignificant decrease in disk hydration. Annular tears, with fluid seen within the posterior anulus, may be more indicative of a painful disk. This so-called "high intensity zone", seen on T2-weighted images, has been shown to correlate with positive pain provocation on diskography. Intervertebral provocative diskography is considered by some the single most important test in diagnosing painful internal disk disruption. A diskogram has two components, both of which must be positive for a truly positive test. Provocation of the patient's typical pain with a pressurized contrast injection is believed to be the most important part of the test. A suspected negative level also should be investigated as a control. After the injection, the disks are imaged by radiographs and CT scan. Morphologic abnormalities must be seen in a painful disk for the test to be considered positive. The use of post-diskography CT scanning is known to increase the ability to diagnose radial tears of the anulus not seen on MRI.

Discogenic pain usually has the mechanical quality of being accentuated with prolonged sitting and standing. The pain may be intermittently sharp or knifelike when turning or changing position. Most patients with discogenic low back pain do not require surgical treatment. Most patients with back pain believed to be disk-related are successfully treated with aggressive nonsurgical management including active rehabilitation, medication, and other aspects of pain management. Surgery should be reserved as a last resort for those individuals who are highly motivated, carefully selected (preferably with one level disease), and without significant psychosocial magnification of their symptoms. There is no prospective randomized study indicating superior clinical results of arthrodesis for discogenic chronic low back pain over nonsurgical treatment to date. When indicated, surgical intervention usually involves a spinal fusion. Surgical options include anterior interbody fusion, posterior interbody fusion, posterolateral fusion with or without instrumentation, or combined interbody and posterolateral fusion. The use of concomitant segmental spinal instrumentation as well as stand-alone interbody threaded fusion cages, known to distract the disk space and provide initial stability, have recently increased. New types of interbody fusion cages are currently under investigation.

The recently described technique of intradiskal electrothermal coagulation is an alternative method to avoid fusion for degenerative lumbar disk disease. With this technique, a thermal electrode is introduced percutaneously with the active portion of the coil positioned fluoroscopically along the posterior annular pathology. Thermal energy is applied in an attempt to denervate the posterior anulus and cause thermal shrinkage of lax annular tissue. Neither response has been demonstrated experimentally; a recent study found little temperature change in tissues more than 1 to 2 mm from the electrode. Indications for intradiskal electrothermal coagulation include diskogram-positive degenerative disk disease with annular tears unresponsive to nonsurgical care for a minimum of 6 months. The presence of a focal disk herniation is a contraindication to this procedure. Longer term studies and controlled data are needed prior to validating this technique.

Failed Lumbar Surgery

Continued or recurrent pain following lumbar spine surgery remains a difficult and challenging problem. A complete evaluation (with knowledge of the initial symptoms, signs, and treatment) is necessary in order to determine if any additional structural spinal surgery may be of benefit, and to assess the chances of improvement with surgical treatment.

A thorough history includes not only all aspects of the current pain complaint, but also the initial symptoms before surgery and the effect of the surgery on the symptoms over time. The ways in which current symptoms are similar or different from the initial symptoms may help identify recurrent nerve compression, adjacent level compression, or the development of painful degenerative disease or instability. Assessment of initial relief of symptoms after surgery is important. A significant period of symptom relief after

surgery before the onset of new or recurrent symptoms portends a much better prognosis than no relief of symptoms following the initial operation.

Physical examination must include palpation of the spine for areas of tenderness, and inspection of the incision. Evidence of spondylolisthesis or degenerative scoliosis may be visible or palpable. Also important is assessment of lumbar range of motion and a detailed neurologic examination to assess focal deficits, myelopathy, and nerve root tension signs. The presence of Waddell's nonorganic physical signs and other chronic pain behaviors such as slowed gait, depressed effect, diffuse tenderness even to light touch, and giving way weakness or poor effort with motor testing are commonly found in cases of failed lumbar surgery.

Additional evaluation with diagnostic testing is based on the initial evaluation and the results of prior surgery. In patients who have had decompressive surgery alone, initial radiographic evaluation should include standing AP and lateral radiographs and lateral flexion/extension views to assess for any subluxation, severe or asymmetric disk space narrowing, or instability. Additional oblique radiographs may help to assess the integrity of the pars interarticularis. MRI is the most useful test to assess for recurrent or adjacent neural compression. Use of an intravenous contrast agent is necessary for complete evaluation, especially for differentiating between scar tissue and a recurrent disk herniation. MRI also facilitates direct evaluation of the degree and activity of disk degeneration. CT scanning may be needed for definitive assessment of the integrity of the pars interarticularis, and is also best for assessing the facet joints, sacroiliac joints, and the bony lateral recess. In patients with low back pain and radiographic evidence of severe disk degeneration, evaluation with lumbar diskography may be appropriate.

In patients who have had spinal fusion surgery, a similar initial radiographic evaluation is in order, assessing the fusion mass and any instrumentation present as well as any motion in the fused region on the bending films. The adjacent levels also are assessed for evidence of progressive degeneration and/or instability. MRI can be done in the presence of spinal instrumentation, and can be quite useful in the evaluation of segments adjacent to spinal fusion, but may provide little or no information at the fusion level if instrumentation has been used. Titanium rather than stainless steel implants are easier to see around. CT is the best imaging test to assess spinal fusion. Sagittal and coronal reconstructions of thin sections are best for assessing the intactness of a fusion, even in patients with indwelling spinal instrumentation. CT myelography is best for observation of the neural elements to check for continued or recurrent compression in the region of the instrumentation. Localized back pain and tenderness after instrumental fusion may be caused by painful implants. Injection of lidocaine into the hardware prominences under fluoroscopic control may help to confirm whether the hardware is the source of pain. Concomitant use of a steroid preparation may be therapeutic, even if only temporarily.

The initial treatment of recurrent disk herniation or spinal stenosis is nonsurgical. Translaminar epidural steroid injections can be attempted adjacent to the operated segments, but are less likely to be successful in recurrent conditions. Transforaminal epidural injection may be a better route in cases of unilateral focal recurrent compression.

Surgical indications in recurrent disk herniation or stenosis are similar to those associated with initial herniation or stenosis, including failure of nonsurgical treatment, progressive motor weakness, uncontrollable pain, and the presentation of a cauda equina syndrome. Revision decompression/diskectomy alone is considered in the absence of severe chronic midline back pain and if no postoperative instability or deformity is identified. Fusion should be considered if instability or deformity is identified, if back pain is a major complaint, and significant disk degeneration is found, or if it is a second recurrence of a disk herniation. Nerve compression resulting from herniation or stenosis at levels adjacent to the previously operated segments should be considered and treated as if they were primary problems. Disabling back pain after decompressive surgery, even in the absence of instability, may be discogenic in nature. Positive diskography and limitation of disease to one or two levels may make the patient a candidate for interbody spine fusion surgery in the setting of failure of extensive nonsurgical treatment.

In patients with previous spinal fusions, structural problems identified on the evaluation for which additional further spinal surgery may be beneficial include painful implants, adjacent level stenosis with or without degeneration or instability, and pseudarthrosis. In patients with painful implants, partial or total removal of the instrumentation can be considered depending on the focality of symptoms and the progression of the fusion. Surgery for adjacent level stenosis unresponsive to nonsurgical treatment should include complete decompression and extension of the fusion to include the new level or decompression. All documented pseudarthroses are amenable to repair, and in general refusion should be recommended. Circumferential fusion with instrumentation has the best results, although excellent or good results in general can be expected in only 50% to 60% of cases. Examination of the original preoperative scans may show a poor sur-

gical indication in the first place, so that adequate repair of pseudarthrosis and fusion is still unlikely to provide significant pain relief.

Annotated Bibliography

Ahn UM, Ahn NU, Buchowski JM, Garrett ES, Sieber AN, Kostuik JP: Cauda equina syndrome secondary to lumbar disc herniation: A meta-analysis of surgical outcomes. *Spine* 2000;25:1515-1522.

Significant improvement in motor and sensory deficits as well as urinary and rectal function occurred in patients who underwent emergent decompression within 48 hours versus after 48 hours for cauda equina syndrome secondary to lumbar disk herniation.

Booth KC, Bridwell KH, Eisenberg BA, Baldus CR, Lenke LG: Minimum 5-year results of degenerative spondylolisthesis treated with decompression and instrumented posterior fusion. *Spine* 1999;24:1721-1727.

This study evaluated outcome and complication rate in 49 patients who had undergone no prior surgery for degenerative spondylolisthesis. Eight-three percent reported satisfaction with the procedure. Radiographic transition syndromes were common (12 patients) with 5 of 12 patients being symptomatic. Major complications (2%), implant failures (2%), and symptomatic pseudarthroses (0) were low.

Cherkin DC, Deyo RA, Battie M, Street J, Barlow W: A comparison of physical therapy, chiropractic manipulation, and provision of an educational booklet for the treatment of patients with low back pain. *N Engl J Med* 1998;339:1021-1029.

Results from a prospective, randomized study of 321 adults with acute low back pain showed equal effectiveness and cost of the McKenzie method of physical therapy and chiropractic manipulation, and only minimally less favorable outcomes for patients receiving an education booklet with no other additional treatment, a much less expensive alternative.

Dolan P, Greenfield K, Nelson RJ, Nelson IW: Can exercise therapy improve the outcome of microdiscectomy? *Spine* 2000;25:1523-1532.

Twenty patients who underwent lumbar microdiskectomy were randomized into either a postoperative exercise program or control group. A 4-week postoperative exercise program can improve pain, disability, and function in patients 12 months after microdiskectomy surgery.

Gordon SL, Weinstein JN: A review of basic science issues in low back pain. *Phys Med Rehabil Clin North Am* 1998;9:323-342.

A comprehensive, well-referenced review of the current state of knowledge of the science of back pain and future directions of research is presented.

Herno A, Airaksinen O, Saari T, Pitkanen M, Manninen H, Suomalainen O: Computed tomography findings 4 years after surgical management of lumbar spinal stenosis: No correlation with clinical outcome. *Spine* 1999;24:2234-2239.

Postoperative radiologic stenosis was common in patients operated on for lumbar spinal stenosis; this factor did not correlate with clinical outcome. Caution is recommended when reconciling clinical symptoms and signs with postoperative CT findings in patients operated on for lumbar spinal stenosis.

Katz JN, Stucki G, Lipson SJ, Fossel AH, Grobler LJ, Weinstein JN: Predictors of surgical outcome in degenerative lumbar spinal stenosis. *Spine* 1999;24:2229-2233.

This prospective study evaluated predictors of outcome, including sociodemographic factors, physical examination, radiographic, psychological, social, and clinical history variables. The patients' assessments of their own health and comorbidity are the most important outcome predictors of surgery for spinal stenosis.

Loupasis GA, Stamos K, Katonis PG, Sapkas G, Korres DS, Hartofilakidis G: Seven- to 20-year outcome of lumbar discectomy. *Spine* 1999;24:2313-2317.

The long-term result of standard lumbar diskectomy is not very satisfying. More than one third of the patients had unsatisfactory results and more than one fourth complained of significant residual pain. Heavy manual work, particularly agricultural work, and low educational level were negative predictors of a good outcome.

Regan JJ, Yuan H, McAfee PC: Laparoscopic fusion of the lumbar spine: Minimally invasive spine surgery: A prospective multicenter study evaluating open and laparoscopic lumbar fusion. *Spine* 1999;24:402-411.

The perioperative morbidity of laparoscopic fusion of the lumbar spine was compared with that of open lumbar fusion. Although there appears to be a significant learning curve associated with laparoscopic fusion, once the technique is mastered its effectiveness and safety are comparable to that of open lumbar fusion.

Riew KD, Yin Y, Gilula L, et al: The effect of nerve-root injections on the need for operative treatment of lumbar radicular pain: A prospective, randomized, controlled, double-blind study. *J Bone Joint Surg Am* 2000;82:1589-1593.

This article presents an excellent prospective, randomized trial of selective nerve root injections with anesthetic alone or anesthetic plus steroid for patients with persistent lumbar radicular pain referred for decompressive surgery. Twenty-nine of 55 patients decided not to have surgery at a mean of 23 months after injection treatment. Significantly more of these (20 of 29) had received steroid in the injection.

Classic Bibliography

Boden SD, Davis DO, Dina TS, Patronas NJ, Wiesel SW: Abnormal magnetic-resonance scans of the lumbar spine in asymptomatic subjects: A prospective investigation. *J Bone Joint Surg Am* 1990;72:403-408.

Deyo RA, Diehl AK, Rosenthal M: How many days of bed rest for acute low back pain? A randomized clinical trial. *N Engl J Med* 1986;315:1064-1070.

Fischgrund JS, Mackay M, Herkowitz HN, Brower R, Montgomery DM, Kurz LT: Degenerative lumbar spondylolisthesis with spinal stenosis: A prospective, randomized study comparing decompressive laminectomy and arthrodesis with and without spinal instrumentation. *Spine* 1997;22:2807-2812.

Herkowitz HN, Kurz LT: Degenerative lumbar spondylolisthesis with spinal stenosis: A prospective study comparing decompression with decompression and intertransverse process arthrodesis. *J Bone Joint Surg Am* 1991;73:802-808.

Johnsson KE, Rosen I, Uden A: The natural course of lumbar spinal stenosis. *Clin Orthop* 1992;279:82-86.

Katz JN, Lipson SJ, Chang LC, Levine SA, Fossel AH, Liang MH: Seven- to 10-year outcome of decompressive surgery for degenerative lumbar spinal stenosis. *Spine* 1996;21:92-98.

Kirkaldy-Willis WH, Wedge JH, Yong-Hing K, Reilly J: Pathology and pathogenesis of lumbar spondylosis and stenosis. *Spine* 1978;3:319-328.

Postacchini F: Management of lumbar spinal stenosis. *J Bone Joint Surg Br* 1996;78:154-164.

Spivak JM: Degenerative lumbar spinal stenosis. *J Bone Joint Surg Am* 1998;80:1053-1066.

Waddell G, McCulloch JA, Kummel E, Venner RM: Nonorganic physical signs in low-back pain. *Spine* 1980;5:117-125.

Weber H: Lumbar disc herniation: A controlled, prospective study with ten years of observation. *Spine* 1983;8:131-140.

Chapter 53

Spondylolysis and Spondylolisthesis

Christopher Hamill, MD

Joseph M. Kowalski, MD

Introduction

Spondylolisthesis is the displacement of a cephalad vertebra on the adjacent caudal vertebra. The slippage can be anterior, posterior, or lateral. A defect in the pars interarticularis is termed spondylolysis and can occur independently or be a cause of spondylolisthesis. Spondylolisthesis is most common at the lumbosacral junction.

Wiltse Classification and Anatomic Description

The Wiltse classification system of spondylolisthesis is anatomically based and is characterized by six types: dysplastic (congenital), isthmic, degenerative, traumatic, pathologic, and postsurgical.

Type I (Dysplastic [Congenital])

The anatomic defect is a failure of formation of the anatomic elements of the lumbosacral facet joint. The facet joints may be axially oriented with dysplasia of the superior end plate of the sacrum and spina bifida occulta. Sagittally oriented facets may also predispose to slippage as can congenital kyphosis. The term congenital may be misleading as there have been no cases of spondylolisthesis observed in either a stillborn or newborn.

An intact pars interarticularis usually limits slippage to less than 30% to 35% of the vertebral body dimension. However, patients with type I spondylolisthesis may develop instability and must be followed closely until skeletal maturation. Progressive slippage to complete spondyloptosis has been reported and can cause compression of the cauda equina and neurologic symptomatology.

Type II (Isthmic)

The hallmark of this type is the presence of a defect in the pars interarticularis (isthmus). The classic radio-graphic appearance is an outline resembling a collar on a scottish terrier (scotty dog sign) (Fig. 1). The precise etiology of the lesion remains unknown, but is thought to be secondary to repetitive microtrauma or a single traumatic episode. There are three subtypes; A is a defect in the pars, B has an elongated pars, and C is thought to be an acute fracture of the pars.

Epidemiologic studies have shown a higher frequency of type II in Alaskan Eskimos (26%); the reported frequency in the general American population is 6%. The presence of an isthmic spondylolisthesis is higher in first-degree relatives of children with this condition. Upright posture may also play a role in the development of spondylolysis, suggested by the facts that defects have not been reported in newborns, have a prevalence of 4% at age six years, and reach adult prevalence rates by age 14 years. Theories regarding this lesion have concentrated on bipedal locomotion along with the upright lordotic sagittal alignment of the lumbar spine. Spondylolysis has been reported only in humans.

The reported incidence of type II is 6.4% in white men, 2.8% in black men, 2.3% in white women, and 1.1% in black women. Pars interarticularis defects are half as common in girls as in boys; however, high-grade slips are four times more common in girls.

Environmental factors may also play a role in the development of spondylolysis. Gymnasts, football players (interior lineman) and certain other athletes have a higher incidence of isthmic spondylolisthesis that is thought to be secondary to the hyperextension forces concentrated at the pars interarticularis. The end result is a fracture through the area (spondylolysis) and possibly spondylolisthesis with minimal slippage and slip angle as the facet complex remains near normal.

Type III (Degenerative)

Osteoarthritis of the facet joints and intervertebral disk is associated with degenerative spondylolisthesis, and is discussed in detail in chapter 52.

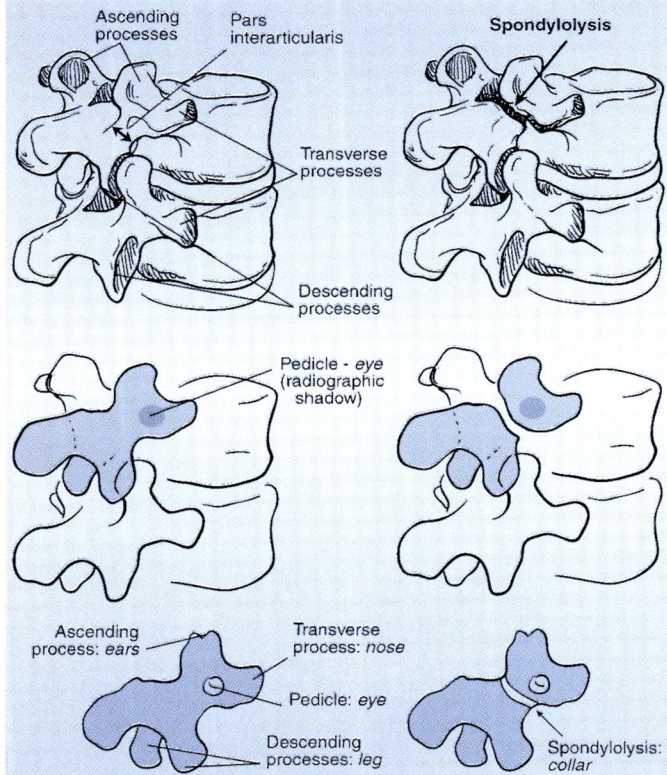

Figure 1 A schematic of an oblique radiograph of the lumbosacral spine, showing the characteristic scotty dog sign of its posterior elements. Note that the pars interarticularis appears to be a collar around the dog's neck. *(Reproduced with permission from Hoppenfeld S: Evaluation of nerve root lesions, in Hoppenfeld S (ed): Orthopaedic Neurology: A Diagnostic Guide to Neurologic Levels. Philadelphia, PA, JB Lippincott, 1977, pp 45-74.)*

Type IV (Posttraumatic)

Type IV is associated with traumatic events that disrupt the posterior arch and its articulations in areas other than the pars interarticularis. Trauma to the spine can result in fracture of the pedicles or articular facets and may cause disruption of the facet joints. These injuries may produce instability and on rare occasions may result in significant spondylolisthesis, and therefore must be considered when there is a history of trauma.

Type V (Pathologic)

Systemic diseases such as osteogenesis imperfecta, osteopetrosis, arthrogryposis, and syphilis have been associated with spondylolisthesis. Localized processes such as infection or neoplasm may also lead to potential instability and spondylolisthesis.

Type VI (Postsurgical)

Patients undergoing decompressive laminectomy for degenerative lumbar spine disease may develop instability if more than the sum of one facet joint is removed at a single level; this has been reported to occur in 3% to 5%, with most cases showing that subtle instability was present prior to the decompressive laminectomy. In these instances a bilateral posterolateral fusion is required at the index procedure.

Postsurgical spondylolisthesis can occur via two methods: direct disruption of the facet joint complex or pars interarticularis. The condition is a classic example of unisegmental instability and treatment is primarily surgical. Most biomechanical studies indicate that if removal of more than 50% of the posterior facet joint complex (the sum total of one facet) will produce an unstable situation, and fusion should be performed. Indirect postsurgical spondylolisthesis occurs secondary to the transition above or below a previously fused segment. The transition syndrome is a result of increased stress at the adjacent motion segment and can lead to premature degeneration of the disk and motion segment with subsequent instability.

Marchetti and Bartolozzi Classification

The recently developed Marchetti and Bartolozzi classification system, widely used in Europe and now gaining acceptance in North America, is based on purported etiology, which serves as a guideline for prognosis and treatment. Developmental spondylolisthesis is divided into two major types; high dysplastic and low dysplastic. Both groups are further subdivided into forms with lysis and elongation. The presence of a pars interarticularis defect or fracture is of secondary importance in this classification system.

High Dysplastic Spondylolisthesis

This type of spondylolisthesis is characterized by developmental deformity apparent in the first decade of life that is caused by underlying deficiencies of the bony hook of L5 or superior facets of the sacrum. The posterior complex may be elongated, deficient, or have a spondylolysis. The alterations in the lumbosacral disk and vertebral body growth plates result in a deformation of the adjacent vertebra. The vertebral body of L5 is typically trapezoidal and facing toward the ground whereas the upper end of the sacrum is rounded and vertically oriented. This conditon results in progressive deformity at the lumbosacral junction. Children with extensive alterations in the posterior elements are highly dysplastic and are considered at high risk for malignant progression. The posterior elements can be dragged into the spinal canal in high-grade slips and act as a pincer, causing severe spinal stenosis.

Low Dysplastic Spondylolisthesis

This type may be characterized by features of the high dysplastic group and/or the acquired group. The pars interarticularis abnormalities may be classified as elongated, fracture, or any combination. There are definite forms of lysis that are acquired (acute traumatic or stress lysis) and others that occur secondary to developmental deficiencies. Patients with low dysplastic spondylolisthesis are at relatively low risk for progression and therefore the shape of the vertebrae is maintained and the deformity is mainly a translation of one vertebra on its caudal segment. The vertebral end plates of the involved vertebra remain parallel.

Acquired Spondylolisthesis

This type includes spondylolisthesis occurring after trauma, surgery, or related to pathologic and degenerative processes. The traumatic group can be further broken down into acute versus chronic repetitive stress. The anatomic stability afforded to the lumbosacral junction via the iliolumbar ligament and the intervertebral disk make the occurrence of posttraumatic spondylolisthesis rare. The energy needed to create a traumatic spondylolisthesis must be quite severe to overcome these stabilizing factors. The bony lesions commonly involve the articular masses and not the area of the pars interarticularis. Surgical stabilization is almost always required. Repetitive microtrauma to the pars area has also been attributed to causing the lesion. The hyperextension causes a pinching effect between the lower and upper articular apophysis, resulting in a guillotine effect on the pars interarticularis. These lesions are most commonly seen in the growing athlete.

Presentation and Evaluation

Symptoms are relatively uncommon in the majority of cases in children and the lesion may be an incidental finding on radiographs following workup for gastrointestinal, genitourinary, or traumatic concerns. If pain is the predominant symptom, it is typically localized to the lumbosacral junction but may radiate to the buttocks and posterior thighs. Back pain is mechanical in nature and relieved by activity modification and nonsteroidal anti-inflammatory medications. Radicular pain may occur; however, symptoms below the knee to the feet are rare. The magnitude of deformity does not coincide with the degree and location of pain.

The physical findings range from none to severe. The patient usually has restricted motion of the lumbar spine and an inability to bend at the hips with the knees fully extended because of hamstring tightness. With severe deformity a palpable step-off may be felt at the lumbosacral junction. The prominence results from the posterior elements of L5 resting on top of the vertical sacrum and the buttocks appear heart-shaped.

The L5 vertebra and superincumbent spine have slipped anteriorly, causing focal kyphosis at the lumbosacral junction that may result in compensatory lordosis into the thoracic spine. The presence of neurologic deficits although infrequent, needs to be documented.

Diagnostic Imaging

Radiographs of the upright spine should be the first imaging study and should include AP and lateral lumbosacral views. A spot lateral of the lumbosacral junction may also be helpful. If spondylolysis is suspected but not seen on these studies, then oblique views may reveal this lesion. Standing 3-ft AP and lateral radiographs are essential in the evaluation in any patient with a spinal deformity. It is important that radiographs exclude the hips and pelvis as causes of spinal imbalance or gait disturbance (Fig. 2).

The Meyerding classification measures the anterior translation as a percentage of vertebral body dimension on the lateral radiograph. This classification system is the most widely accepted method of determining the grade of slip: grade I, 25% or less; grade II,

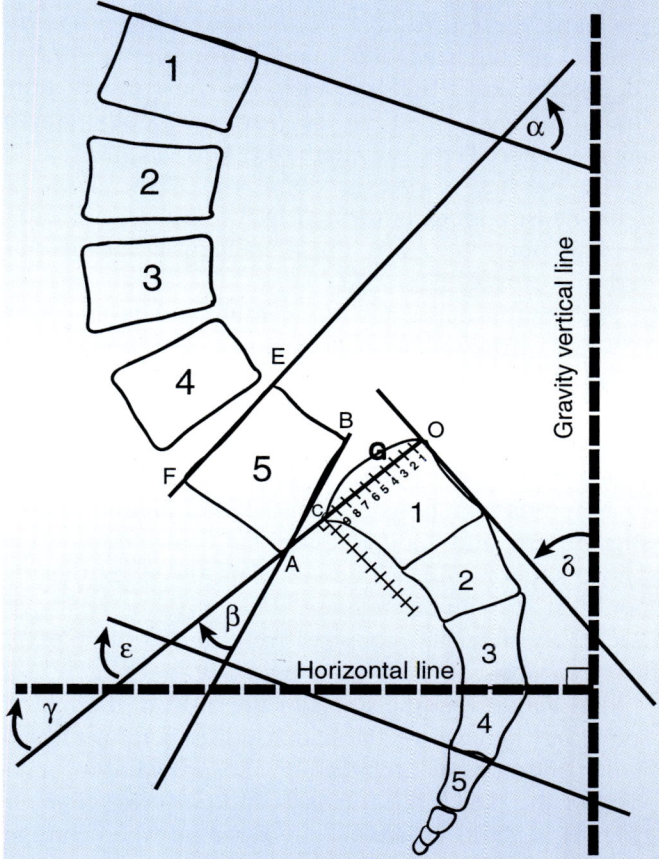

Figure 2 Radiographic measurements of spondylolisthesis. *(Reproduced with permission from Antoniades SB, Hammerberg KW, DeWald RL: Sagittal plane configuration of the sacrum in spondylolisthesis. Spine 2000;25:1085-1091.)*

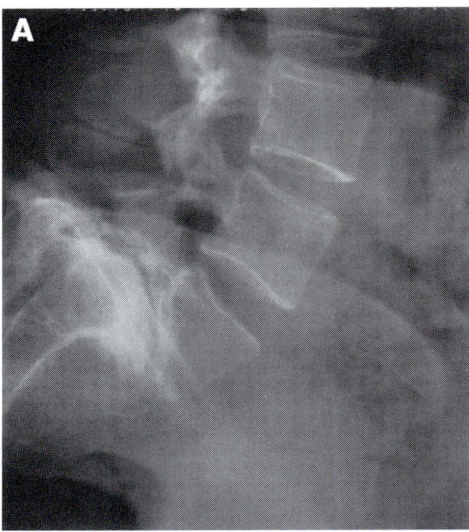
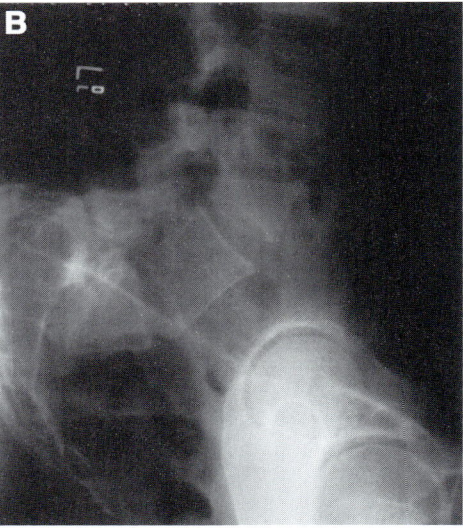

Figure 3 Lateral radiographs of the lumbosacral spine. **A,** Meyerding grade IV slip. **B,** Spondyloptosis of L5 on S1 (Meyerding grade V).

26% to 50%; grade III, 51% to 75%; grade IV, 75% to 100% (Fig. 3, *A*); and grade V (spondyloptosis), greater than 100% (Fig. 3, *B*). The slip angle is an important factor in high-grade spondylolisthesis because it is a measure of lumbosacral kyphosis. This angle is constructed by lines projecting from the superior end plates of the two adjacent vertebrae. The superior end plate is often obscured by the sacrum and the line may be constructed along the posterior aspect of the vertebral body. Sacral inclination reflects the increased vertical orientation of the sacrum as the grade of olisthesis increases. This measurement is formed by the intersection of a vertical line and a line drawn tangential to the posterior cortex of S1.

The sagittal pelvic tilt index is another radiographic criterion proposed to help identify the likelihood of progression; this is an attempt to describe the sagittal offset of L5 with respect to the acetabulum correlated with slip progression and symptoms (Fig. 4). Patients with a decreased (< 0.70) sagittal pelvic tilt index tend to be more symptomatic, demonstrate higher rates of slip progression, and require surgical intervention. Those patients with a sagittal pelvic tilt index that did not decrease and remained greater than 0.85 were effectively managed conservatively and had an excellent prognosis.

MRI may reveal the status of the disks in the lumbar spine and patency of the canal. CT is helpful in evaluating the osseous architecture and providing a better view of the pars interarticularis and posterior elements (Fig. 5). Both MRI and CT are essential when contemplating surgical treatment. A technetium bone scan may reveal increased uptake, suggesting a recent or unhealed fracture.

Natural History

The incidence of spondylolysis is low and most reports are retrospective and not uniform. The exact cause of spondylolisthesis remains unclear. It is believed that the etiology is multifactorial, making presentation and risk of progression difficult to predict.

In a study of adult patients with spondylolisthesis, 91% of those who were not treated had low back pain. Fifty-five percent of these patients had sciatica and 18% had some form of neurologic deficit. Risk factors for low back pain include slippage greater than 25% spondylolysis at L4 and early disk degeneration. Progression of the slip has been reported at 5% and is more common in adolescence and associated with the growth spurt. Progression is less common but does

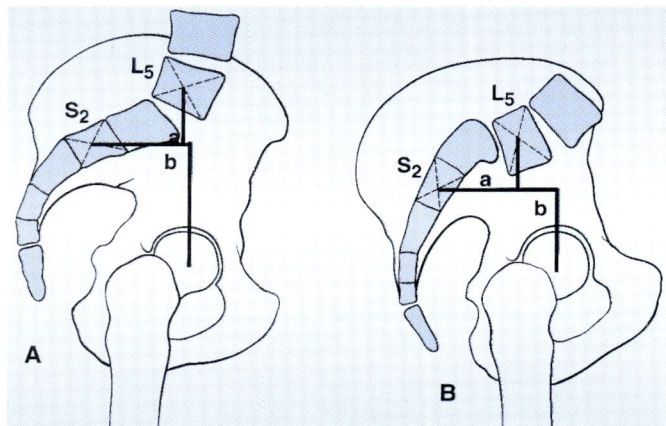

Figure 4 A schematic of a standing lateral radiograph of the lumbosacral spine. A horizontal line is drawn from the center of S2 forward to intersect a vertical line drawn from the center of the femoral head. A vertical line is dropped from the center of L5. The vertical line from the center of L5 should approximate that of the femoral head (see text for details). *(Reproduced with permission from Schwab FJ, Farcy JP, Roye DP Jr: The sagittal pelvic tilt index as a criterion in the evaluation of spondylolisthesis: Preliminary observations. Spine 1997;22:1661-1667.)*

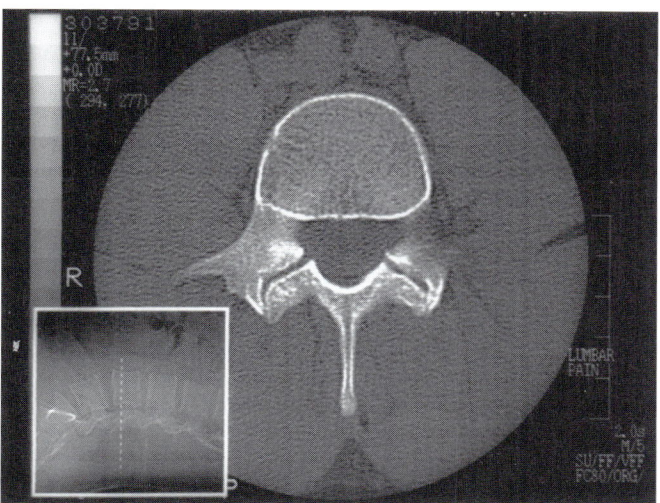

Figure 5 Axial CT scan of lumbar spine. Note bilateral pars defects with sclerotic margins.

occur in adults and is thought to be caused by degenerative changes in the intervertebral disk and facet joints.

Low back pain has been attributed to the lesion in 19% of patients studied who were younger than 25 years of age and presenting with a pars defect. However, this percentage decreased with age so that the lesion was responsible for pain in 7.6% of patients between 26 to 40 years of age, and in only 5.2% of patients older than 40 years.

Nonsurgical Management

Nonsurgical management remains the mainstay of treatment in patients with less than 50% slip progression. Most adult patients with spondylolisthesis of any kind and a chief complaint of back pain can be successfully managed with nonsurgical treatment, which includes a combination of activity modification, trunk strengthening, and bracing.

Children with high-grade spondylolisthesis (> 50% slip progression) need careful observation and are at risk for increased slip progression. Therefore, these patients are usually candidates for surgery, regardless of symptoms, to prevent progression. The younger, symptomatic patient with minimal or no spondylolisthesis can be more difficult to manage. The goal of bracing in these patients is to reduce hyperlordosis in an attempt to stabilize the motion segment. However, to immobilize the lumbosacral junction, the orthosis must include the hip joint and therefore incorporate at least one thigh.

Patients who demonstrate focal increased uptake on a technetium Tc 99m bone scan may respond to a trial of bracing in an effort to unite the pars defect and subsequently alleviate their pain. However, the absence of increased uptake may make bracing ineffective. Physiotherapy management of patients with back pain has taken on a new focus. Traditional treatment focused on flexion strengthening exercises. The new focus involves specific training of muscles surrounding the spine (deep abdominal muscles and lumbar multifidi), which are considered to provide dynamic stability and fine control of the lumbar spine. This specific exercise program has been found to be more effective than the commonly prescribed conservative treatment programs in patients with chronically symptomatic spondylolysis or spondylolisthesis.

Surgical Management

Children

Surgical stabilization of spondylolisthesis should be considered for the symptomatic child whose condition does not respond to nonsurgical management and when participation in normal activities is not tolerated. The indications for surgery may include (1) documented slip progression beyond 25% to 33%; (2) presentation with slippage greater than 50%; (3) persistence of mechanical or neurologic symptoms despite significant appropriate nonsurgical management; and (4) progressive postural deformity or gait abnormality.

Twenty percent of par defects may be unilateral. There may be evidence of reactive bone changes at the pars on radiographs or CT scan. Hypertrophy of the contralateral pedicle and posterior elements may occur to accommodate the additional forces. If nonsurgical management is unsuccessful in these patients, bone grafting and internal fixation with compression across the defect may be beneficial.

The progression of slippage from 25% to 50% requires a single-level bilateral posterolateral fusion. The low incidence of neurologic deficits in children makes the need for decompression rare. However, if leg pain is significant, then decompression is warranted. The need to rule out other causes of low back discomfort, such as disk herniation, bone or spinal cord tumors, or disk space infection is crucial to the treatment of patients with low-grade spondylolisthesis. A degenerative L4-L5 disk may be a source of pain in the presence of an L5-S1 spondylolisthesis. Surgical treatment is indicated if the slip is greater than 50% in a growing child or greater than 75% in a skeletally mature adolescent.

Two factors must be taken into account when considering surgical treatment in children: the amount of slippage or translation (Meyerding classification) and the lumbosacral kyphosis as expressed as a slip angle of L5 on the sacrum. Lumbosacral kyphosis is more important than the amount of anterior translation. The surgical approach most appropriate for adolescents requiring an in situ fusion is a bilateral posterolateral arthrodesis without midline exposure (Wiltse procedure). The patients with high-grade spondylolisthesis and small L5 transverse processes are not suitable candidates for in situ fusion secondary to the high rate of pseudarthrosis. Laminectomy alone is contraindicated in the skeletally immature child because of the increased risk for additional slippage. For those patients with a slip greater than 50%, the results of isolated posterolateral arthrodesis are not as good. Therefore, the current recommendation is to add an additional anterior column support.

A variety of reduction techniques have been described for the treatment of high-grade spondylolisthesis. Techniques for reduction include femoral traction, cast reduction, instrumented reduction, and the combined anterior-posterior approach. The most significant complication of this maneuver is traction on the L5 nerve root. The stretch injury of the L5 nerve root with reduction of the high-grade spondylolisthesis is not linear. Seventy-one percent of the total L5 nerve strain occurs during the second half of a reduction maneuver, that is, from grade II to complete reduction. Therefore, partial reduction may be significantly safer in treating high-grade spondylolisthesis. The correction of lumbosacral kyphosis may also protect the L5 nerve root during this reduction maneuver. Proponents of reduction and reconstruction cite the following pitfalls of fusion in situ: (1) high pseudarthrosis rate; (2) risk of postoperative slip progression secondary to the bending or shear forces on the fusion mass; (3) loss of motion segments; (4) residual deformity; and (5) neurologic deficit. Therefore, the potential advantages of reduction are a decreased pseudarthrosis rate, stabilization of the deformity, minimization of the length of the fusion, improved cosmesis, and prevention of acute postoperative cauda equina syndrome. However, there is little or no evidence in the literature to support these advantages in patients undergoing reduction of their spondylolisthesis.

Spondyloptosis presents additional problems because of the poor sagittal alignment. Although fusion in situ may provide adequate stabilization, patients with high-grade spondylolisthesis or spondyloptosis may require resection of the L5 vertebral body and reconstruction with placement of L4 onto the sacrum. This procedure requires extensive surgical skill and experience and poses an increased risk of complications.

Adults

The adult patient with persistent symptoms affecting quality of life may be a candidate for surgical intervention if nonsurgical care has failed. The outcomes of arthrodesis for the treatment of low back pain remain poorer than the outcomes of decompression and stabilization in the patient with radicular complaints. The adult patient requiring surgery for spondylolisthesis often has low dysplastic or degenerative types of olisthesis. The likelihood of progression of lumbosacral low dysplastic spondylolisthesis in the adult population is very low. The preoperative assessment should include an MRI study to rule out the possibility of other etiologies as a source of pain. The judicious use of diskography may be warranted to rule out other spinal levels that could be causing concordant symptomatology. Traditional treatment for patients with low-grade dysplastic spondylolisthesis with lysis (isthmic spondylolisthesis type 2A) has been decompression and concomitant fusion. The procedure involves removal of the offending lamina with foraminotomies to decompress the exiting nerve root. Recent studies have shown that patients with low-grade dysplastic spondylolisthesis with lysis may have better clinical results with arthrodesis alone versus decompression and fusion. The addition of segmental spinal instrumentation has been shown to increase radiographic rate of fusion but the clinical outcomes may be no different.

Patients with high-grade slips may have significant low back pain. Fusion in situ has been reported to provide good long-term results. Mechanical constructs need to provide for multiple points of fixation above and below the deformity, with ample sacral fixation. Circumferential fusion, which includes anterior column support, in addition to posterior segmental fixation, provides the greatest rate of fusion and long-term outcomes. Adding anterior support to a failed arthrodesis is commonly required in salvage procedures. The passage of a fibular dowel graft between the S1 and L5 vertebral bodies has also been shown to increase fusion rates in primary and revision surgery. Reconstruction with reduction and/or vertebral resection may be beneficial in young adults but is less so in the adult with significant long-standing degenerative changes.

Annotated Bibliography

Molinari RW, Bridwell KH, Lenke LG, Ungacta FF, Riew KD: Complications in the surgical treatment of pediatric high-grade, isthmic dysplastic spondylolisthesis: A comparison of three surgical approaches. *Spine* 1999;24:1701-1711.

In situ fusion results in a high rate of nonunion if the cross-sectional area of the L5 transverse processes is small (< 2 cm^2). Circumferential arthrodesis provides for the best fusion rates and clinical outcome as a primary or salvage procedure.

Moller H, Hedlund R: Surgery versus conservative management in adult isthmic spondylolisthesis: A prospective randomized study. Part 1. *Spine* 2000;25:1711-1715.
   This study suggests that once symptoms occur, surgical treatment provides better relief than an exercise program.

Moller H, Hedlund R: Instrumented and noninstrumented posterolateral fusion in adult spondylolisthesis: A prospective randomized study. Part 2. *Spine* 2000;25:1716-1721.
   This study suggests that the addition of instrumentation does not improve the fusion rate, nor does it affect the clinical outcome.

Classic Bibliography

Bradford DS: Treatment of severe spondylolisthesis: A combined approach for reduction and stabilization. *Spine* 1979;4:423-429.

Bradford DS, Boachie-Adjei O: Treatment of severe spondylolisthesis by anterior and posterior reduction and stabilization: A long-term follow-up study. *J Bone Joint Surg Am* 1990;72:1060-1066.

Carragee EJ: Single-level posterolateral arthrodesis, with or without posterior decompression, for the treatment of isthmic spondylolisthesis in adults: A prospective randomized study. *J Bone Joint Surg Am* 1997;79:1175-1180.

Fredrickson BE, Baker D, McHolick WJ, Yuan HA, Lubicky JP: The natural history of spondylolysis and spondylolisthesis. *J Bone Joint Surg Am* 1984;66:699-707.

Harris IE, Weinstein SL: Long-term follow-up of patients with grade-III and IV spondylolisthesis: Treatment with and without posterior fusion. *J Bone Joint Surg Am* 1987;69:960-969.

Johnson JR, Kirwan EO: The long-term results of fusion in situ for severe spondylolisthesis. *J Bone Joint Surg Br* 1983;65:43-46.

Johnson GV, Thompson AG: The Scott wiring technique for direct repair of lumbar spondylolysis. *J Bone Joint Surg Br* 1992;74:426-430.

Kakiuchi M: Repair of the defect in spondylolysis: Durable fixation with pedicle screws and laminar hooks. *J Bone Joint Surg Am* 1997;79:818-825.

Lehmer SM, Steffee AD, Gaines RW Jr: Treatment of L5-S1 spondyloptosis by staged L5 resection with reduction and fusion of L4 onto S1 (Gaines procedure). *Spine* 1994;19:1916-1925.

Macnab I, McCulloch JA (eds): *Backache*, ed 2. Baltimore, MD, Williams & Wilkins, 1990, pp 84-103.

Saraste H: Long-term clinical and radiological follow-up of spondylolysis and spondylolisthesis. *J Pediatr Orthop* 1987;7:631-638.

Schwab FJ, Farcy JP, Roye DP Jr: The sagittal pelvic tilt index as a criterion in the evaluation of spondylolisthesis: Preliminary observations. *Spine* 1997;22:1661-1667.

Wiltse LL, Newman PH, Macnab I: Classification of spondylolysis and spondylolisthesis. *Clin Orthop* 1976;117:23-29.

Chapter 54

Adult Scoliosis

Lawrence G. Lenke, MD

Introduction

Adult scoliosis is defined as the presentation of a scoliosis deformity after skeletal maturity. According to the Scoliosis Research Society, a patient must be at least 18 years of age upon first presentation for the treatment of the deformity. Pathophysiologic descriptions of adult scoliosis are (1) curves that start before skeletal maturity, although the patient does not seek treatment until after skeletal maturity; or (2) a deformity that arises de novo after skeletal maturity, with the patient seeking evaluation and potential treatment at that time.

The etiologic classification of adult scoliosis can be divided into idiopathic, congenital, paralytic, adolescent/adult postspinal fusion scoliosis (occurring later in life), and degenerative (de novo) scoliosis.

Idiopathic Scoliosis

Idiopathic scoliosis, the most common form of adult scoliosis, has a prevalence of approximately 5%. Deformity and pain are the main complaints. Compared with adolescents, adult scoliosis patients are usually less concerned with cosmesis. However, adults do notice increased waistline asymmetry present in thoracolumbar and lumbar curvatures, changes in the way clothes fit, gradual loss of height that occurs with a progressive scoliosis in any region of the thoracic or lumbar spine, especially if associated with a significant kyphosis. A large thoracic rib prominence may also be bothersome when sitting in hard-backed chairs.

The primary reason for both evaluation and selection of surgical treatment in adult patients is axial or occasionally appendicular pain. The first major diagnostic assessment must be to determine the exact cause of the pain. A percentage assessment of axial versus lower extremity complaints should be noted, because these patients can have lumbar radiculopathies from herniated disks and other degenerative conditions that are separate from the structural deformity. For typical axial back pain, the specific location of the pain is important to document. In patients with thoracic scoliosis and a significant rib hump, convex scapular pain caused by prominence and irritation of the posterior shoulder girdle may be present. Axial pain can occur as a result of degenerative changes that occur primarily on the concavity of curves because of facet arthrosis in any region of the thoracic and lumbar spine. Patients with thoracolumbar- or lumbar-based pain often have complaints similar to those of patients with chronic degenerative spine conditions, with axial lumbar pain emanating from degenerative disks and/or facets. Spinal fatigue, muscle-based pain can also occur in the area of the scoliosis and is often vague, and only fully appreciated after a successful spinal fusion when the fatigue pain subsides. Spinal fatigue pain seems to be most correlated with the patient age, degree of curvature, and most importantly, the overall coronal and sagittal plane global alignments.

Physical examination of these patients focuses on overall spinal alignment, mobility, and neurologic status. Coronal alignment must be evaluated with respect to shoulder balance, any deviation of the plumb line (suggesting overall coronal imbalance), trunk shift or waistline asymmetry, and rib and/or lumbar prominences evaluated by an Adam's forward bend test and quantified by a scoliometer measurement. Sagittal alignment and posture should be carefully evaluated as well. The sagittal alignment and posture of adult scoliosis patients is as important, if not more so, than the coronal alignment and balance with respect to the long-term pain patterns and function of the patient. Spinal mobility is assessed via trunk flexion, extension, and right and left side bending. Assessment of the degree of flexibility of the spine and trunk is done with the patient prone on an examination table. A thorough upper and lower extremity neurologic examination should be performed, and in idiopathic scoliosis this examination should be normal in the absence of any cervical or lumbar degenerative radiculiitides.

Upright PA and lateral long cassette (36-in) radiographs of the entire spinal axis should be performed. It is important to compare any previously obtained spinal radiographs; curve progression can be documented by comparing Cobb measurements on serial radiographs. Overall spinal balance, degenerative changes such as facet arthropathy, bony spurring, and degenerative disk changes with loss of disk height and any coronal and/or lateral vertebral subluxations are also assessed radiographically. Regional alignment and global spinal balance in the sagittal plane are important factors to evaluate as well. Regional lumbar lordosis is measured from the superior end plate of T12 to the superior end plate of S1, and should be in the range of $-55°$ to $-65°$. Two thirds of normal lumbar lordosis occurs at L4-L5 and L5-S1 with successively less degrees of lordosis present at each of the remaining lumbar levels. A coronal and sagittal plumb line from the center of the C7 vertebral body is constructed from the PA and lateral long cassette radiographs, respectively. A normal coronal plumb line should bisect the sacrum, and a normal sagittal plumb line should be at or just posterior to the back edge of the lumbosacral disk.

A total spine and pelvis bone scan is often quite helpful in noting any areas of degenerative uptake and also in ruling out other less common conditions causing axial spine pain such as sacroiliitis, spinal tumor, or infection. A lumbar MRI study provides information on the status of lumbar disk hydration and the cauda equina/lumbar nerve roots. Although somewhat controversial, diskography can be used to determine disk morphology and also quantify pain reproduction in the mid to lower lumbar disks to assess symptomatic disk degeneration.

According to natural history studies, idiopathic scoliosis can progress after skeletal maturity. Several indications of curve progression are listed in Table 1. Adult scoliosis will usually progress an average of 1° to 2° per year. In patients with accelerated degenerative changes, curves will progress more rapidly. Superimposition of degenerative changes within the disks and facets without stabilizing osteophytes can lead to rotatory subluxations in the mid to lower lumbar spine, often at the L3-L4 and L4-L5 levels. This is a much more common scenario in female patients. Superimposition of degenerative changes may produce not only degenerative instability with axial pain but also lumbosacral radiculopathies from various types of spinal stenosis caused by the spinal subluxation, resulting in central or lateral recess, or foraminal stenosis, conditions that are more commonly seen in de novo degenerative scoliosis. Follow-up every 3 to 5 years is the only way to confirm

TABLE 1	Risk Factors for Curve Progression
Most curves greater than 50°
Thoracic curves greater than 60°*
Lumbar curves greater than 50°*
Lumbar portions of double major curves (greater than 60°)*
L5 segment located at or above the intercrestal line
Significant apical rotation
Right convex deformity
Pregnancy
*Indication for surgery

progression of adult idiopathic scoliosis and assess concomitant symptomatology.

Cardiopulmonary symptoms are more common in those rare patients with curves greater than 90° to 100°. Progressive deterioration of pulmonary function in these patients may result in pulmonary hypertension and cor pulmonale. Pulmonary function tests are seldom abnormal in thoracic deformities less than 60°. Large thoracic curves are associated with decreased vital capacity and oxygen transport; subjective dyspnea is experienced only by those patients with greater than 90° to 100° of scoliosis. Loss of normal thoracic kyphosis (especially severe lordosis in the thoracic spine), and deformity in the coronal plane are implicated in declining pulmonary function. Smoking, asthma, chronic obstructive pulmonary disease, or occupational lung disease are other factors that cause cardiorespiratory compromise in the adult patient with scoliosis.

Conservative Treatment

There are a variety of nonsurgical treatment methods for symptomatic adult scoliosis, though few are universally agreed upon. Currently acceptable treatments include intermittent nonsteroidal anti-inflammatory medications or muscle relaxants for acute symptomatic musculoskeletal pain syndromes. Long-lasting therapeutic benefits may be derived from active physical therapy exercise programs designed to improve spinal extensor as well as abdominal muscle strength, and increase flexibility of the trunk and torso. Aerobic activities are especially important in these individuals to maintain overall physical and psychological well-being. A spinal orthosis may provide temporary symptomatic relief in some elderly patients; however, caution should be exercised because long-term usage and dependence on orthotic devices may promote further

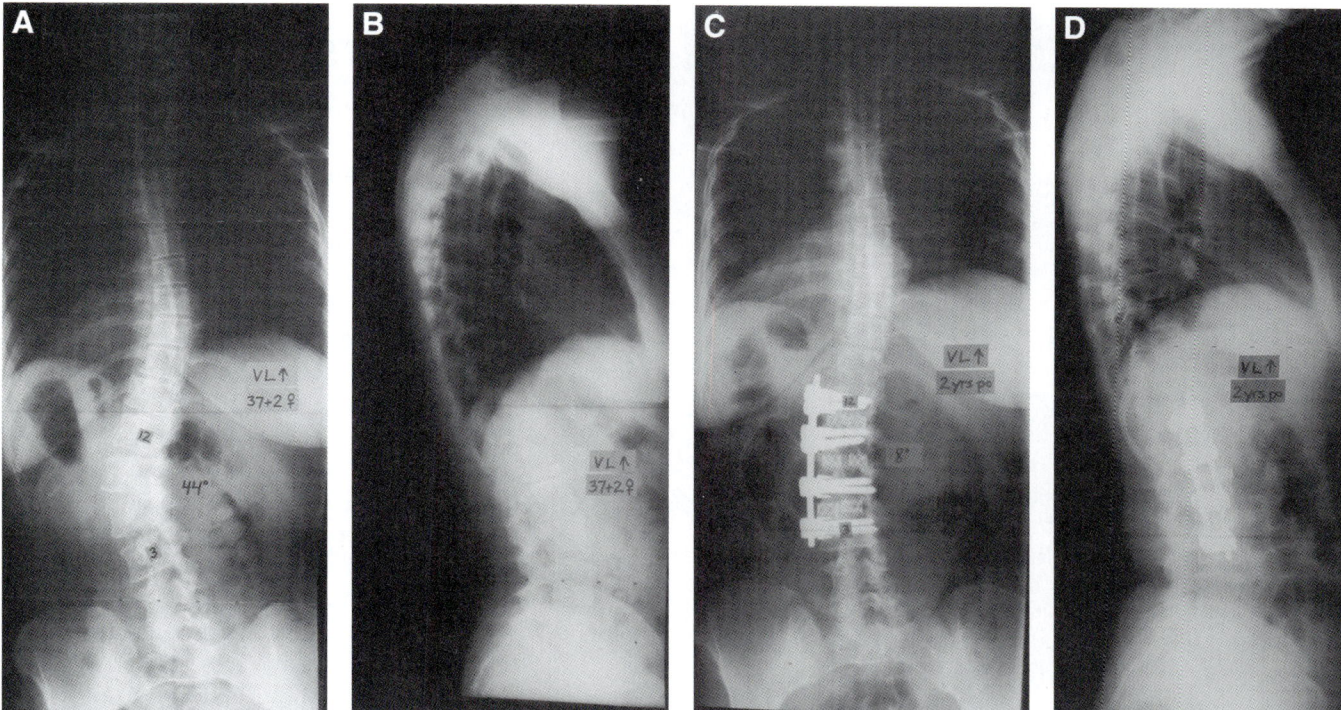

Figure 1 **A,** Standing long cassette coronal radiograph showing idiopathic left lumbar scoliosis measuring 44° with increased radioisotope activity at the L1-L2 level. **B,** Long cassette sagittal radiograph demonstrates osteophytic lipping at L1-L2 with fairly normal sagittal alignment. **C,** Anterior instrumented spinal fusion from T12-L3 with correction of the coronal curve to 8° with horizontalization of the L3 lowest instrumented vertebra. **D,** Sagittal plane alignment is unchanged after the anterior instrumented fusion, with maintained lordosis over the instrumented/fused levels.

muscle wasting. In female patients in particular, the main focus should be the prevention and treatment of osteoporosis. Thus, proper nutrition, exercise with weight-bearing activities that appropriately increase the load on the spine, and pharmacologic treatment in postmenopausal females should be considered. In addition, cigarette smoking, which is known to accelerate degenerative disk disease, should be avoided. Overall, the efficacy of each of these various treatments and preventions is largely unknown, and thus the natural history of symptomatic conservatively treated adult scoliosis is not well established.

Surgical Treatment

Surgical treatment for adult idiopathic scoliosis is performed only after appropriate counseling and assessment of various quality of life issues. The primary reason to perform surgery is to halt progression of the deformity. In addition, pain relief coincident with stabilization of the deformity may occur but cannot be guaranteed. Success rates as low as 40% to 50% in achieving adequate pain relief following spinal fusion have been reported. It is important to try to quantify and localize the patient's pain generator(s) before spinal fusion is performed.

A thorough arthrodesis with autogenous bone graft and a rigidly immobilized spine secured with segmental

spinal instrumentation are essential components of a successful surgery. The majority of adult scoliosis instrumentation and fusion procedures are performed via an isolated posterior procedure, although some younger adult patients with isolated major thoracic, thoracolumbar, or lumbar curve patterns can be successfully treated with anterior instrumentation and fusion alone (Fig. 1). Most single or double thoracic curves ending in the upper lumbar spine can be treated with an isolated posterior approach. When the scoliosis extends into the lower lumbar region, often a combined anterior and posterior fusion of the lumbar spine to optimize both correction of the deformity and fusion consolidation is the best approach. Possible indications for these circumferential fusions include: a large scoliotic curve (> 60°); any kyphotic component to the lumbar regional alignment; advanced age or spinal osteoporosis; and when fusion to the sacrum is required. If an anterior and posterior fusion is planned, the anterior fusion requires thorough diskectomies and autograft (usually rib graft from the approach) for fusion. All periapical segments should be included in the anterior fusion; for lumbar curves, as many segments as possible that will be treated posteriorly should be fused anteriorly. Consideration should be given to placing structural allograft bone or mesh cages filled with autograft bone in the mid to lower lumbar

TABLE 2	Complications Associated With Scoliosis Surgery in Adults

Complication	Rate
Neurologic deficit	< 1% to 5%
Infection	0.5% to 5%
Pseudarthrosis	5% to 27%
Residual pain	5% to 15%
Pulmonary embolism	1% to 20%
Mortality	< 1% to 5%

disks to maintain support for lumbar lordosis and also load share the posterior instrumentation during the healing process.

With the posterior procedure, rigid segmental spinal instrumentation is applied and a combination of either hooks or screws in the thoracic spine and screws are placed in the lumbar and lumbosacral spine. The posterior fusion should extend from a neutral vertebra proximal to a (ideally) neutral, horizontal, and centered vertebra distally. In addition, it is important before surgery to confirm the absence of significant degenerative changes below the distal fusion level. Therefore, careful review of the radiographs, MRI scan, and even diskography is required.

Autogenous bone graft is harvested from the posterior iliac crest. Rigid immobilization of the instrumented segments is important to increase the fusion rate and place less emphasis on external immobilization. In patients with a cosmetically unacceptable rib prominence, a convex rib thoracoplasty should be considered. However, preoperative pulmonary function values should be checked because rib harvest in adults appears to have a detrimental effect on pulmonary function in adults, even at 2 years after the procedure.

The surgical treatment of scoliosis in adults is difficult, with a much higher complication rate than similar types of deformity corrections in adolescents. Reported complications and rates are shown in Table 2. Increased blood loss due to more difficult subperiosteal stripping of the posterior musculature off the spine; less rigid attachment of instrumentation as a result of osteoporotic bone stock; lower fusion rates due to the older age of these patients; and higher perioperative and postoperative medical complication rates as a result of longer length of surgery, a higher risk of

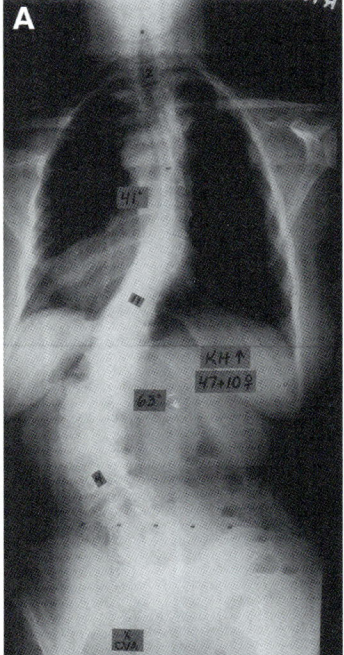 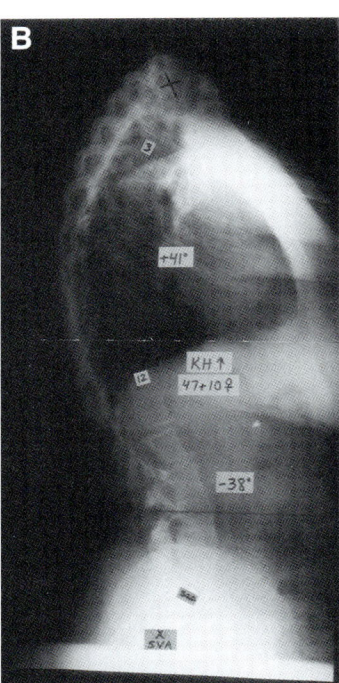 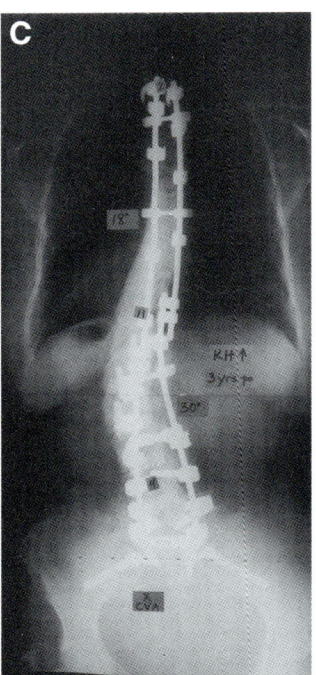 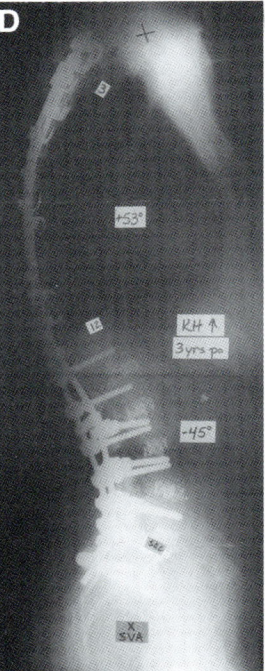

Figure 2 **A,** Standing long cassette coronal radiograph showing adult lumbar scoliosis and a compensatory structural thoracic curve. Although the L5 segment is below the intercrestal line, it has a fixed obliquity and degenerative arthritis of the left L5-S1 facet. The patient has complained of increasing truncal imbalance and lumbosacral back pain. **B,** Long cassette sagittal radiograph demonstrates lumbar hypolordosis with moderate degeneration of the L5-S1 segment that was painful on preoperative diskography. Sagittal vertical alignment is positioned well, just behind the back edge of the L5-S1 disk. **C,** Two-stage anterior and posterior spinal fusion. Anterior fusion with structural support was performed at each level from L1 to the sacrum. Posteriorly, instrumentation and fusion from T3 to the sacrum was performed, with multiple fixation points and bilateral iliac wing screws. Coronal balance is acceptable. **D,** Long cassette sagittal radiograph demonstrates excellent regional lumbar and global sagittal alignment 3 years after surgery.

infection, deep vein thrombosis, and pulmonary sequelae are factors that contribute to increased complication rates. Obviously, patients who have undergone circumferential fusion to the sacrum have an increased risk of perioperative complications. Some of these complications appear to result from nutritional depletion that occurs following these extensive spinal reconstructions. Therefore, nutritional status should be optomized both preoperatively and perioperatively in the adult patient with idiopathic scoliosis who is undergoing an extensive spinal fusion. The return to normal nutritional status usually takes more than 6 weeks in those patients with at least 10 fusion levels performed. Also, staging circumferential fusions has a detrimental effect on the nutritional status of these patients and hyperalimentation between the first and second procedures and after the second stage of combined procedures may be advantageous. It appears beneficial to perform circumferential anterior and posterior fusions on the same day under a single anesthetic if possible. However, in patients treated anteriorly over the entire lumbar spine and posteriorly from the upper thoracic spine to the sacrum, two separate anesthetics with intervening hyperalimentation may be required.

Fusion to the sacrum is sometimes indicated in the adult with primary lumbar scoliosis, and should occur in patients with fixed lumbar curvatures with L5 lumbosacral obliquity; those patients with severe loss of coronal and/or sagittal balance; and those patients with severe degenerative changes at the L4-L5 and L5-S1 segments. It is essential to structurally graft as much segmental lordosis as possible, into the L4-L5 and L5-S1 segments during instrumentation and fusion of the entire spine to the pelvis. In addition, secure lumbosacral fixation consisting of bilateral S1 and bilateral iliac screws will minimize instrument-related complications with these long fusions (Fig. 2). Optimal coronal and sagittal global spinal balance are key parameters in performing this type of surgery.

It is becoming increasingly apparent that clinical outcome studies must complement radiographic data in patients undergoing these complex spinal deformity reconstructions. Currently, there does appear to be improved quality of life following these surgeries on outcome measures that are not disease-specific, such as the SF-36. However, it will be important to show that disease-specific outcome data can document short-term clinical success and long-term consequences of adult scoliosis surgery.

Revision Scoliosis Surgery

The use of Harrington instrumentation was a significant development in scoliosis surgery that resulted in improved fusion rates and a considerable increase in the degree of coronal plane correction. Results in the thoracic plane were quite good; however, Harrington instrumentation extending into the mid and lower lumbar spine has often produced residual problems, such as loss of lumbar lordosis caused by flattening of the lumbar sagittal plane (flatback syndrome). This fixed sagittal imbalance syndrome is characterized by progressive lumbosacral pain and mild to marked forward sagittal imbalance, caused by progressive disk and facet degeneration below the previous fusion.

Long-term studies of young patients who have undergone a posterior instrumentation and fusion for scoliosis have shown no increase in overall disability, as long as the distal fusion ends in the upper lumbar spine. When the fusion extends below L3, the tendency toward lumbar spine disability and pain is significant, with 62% of patients with fusion to L4 and 82% of patients with fusion to L5 having significant clinical complaints. Many of these patients have needed revision surgery for a more distal fusion, often to the sacrum. In addition, some of these patients require extension lumbar osteotomies to improve lordosis, and thus, global sagittal balance. Thus, prevention and avoidance of flatback syndrome (loss of normal lumbar lordosis) appears to be an important component in the management of these difficult spinal reconstructions (Fig. 3). Midterm (5- to 10-year) follow-up of patients with adolescent idiopathic scoliosis treated with newer

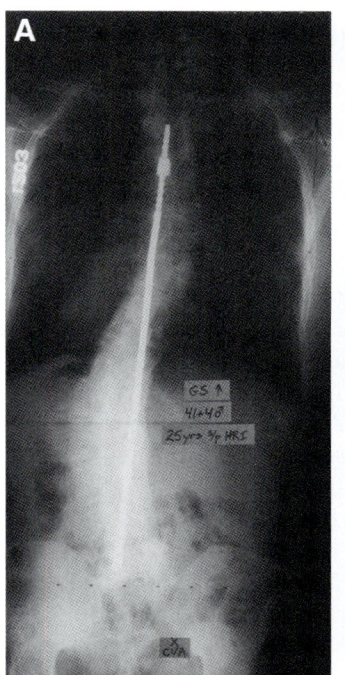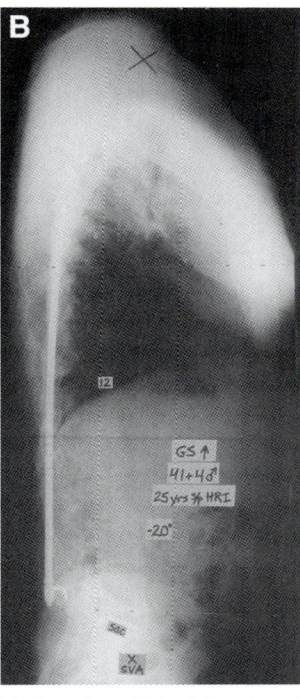

Figure 3 **A,** Flatback syndrome. The sagittal plane shows flattened thoracic and lumbar regional alignment with degeneration of the L5-S1 segment with slight forward sagittal imbalance. **B,** Extension of the fusion circumferentially to the sacrum with concomitant posterior osteotomies and reinstrumentation improved lumbar lordosis and overall sagittal balance.

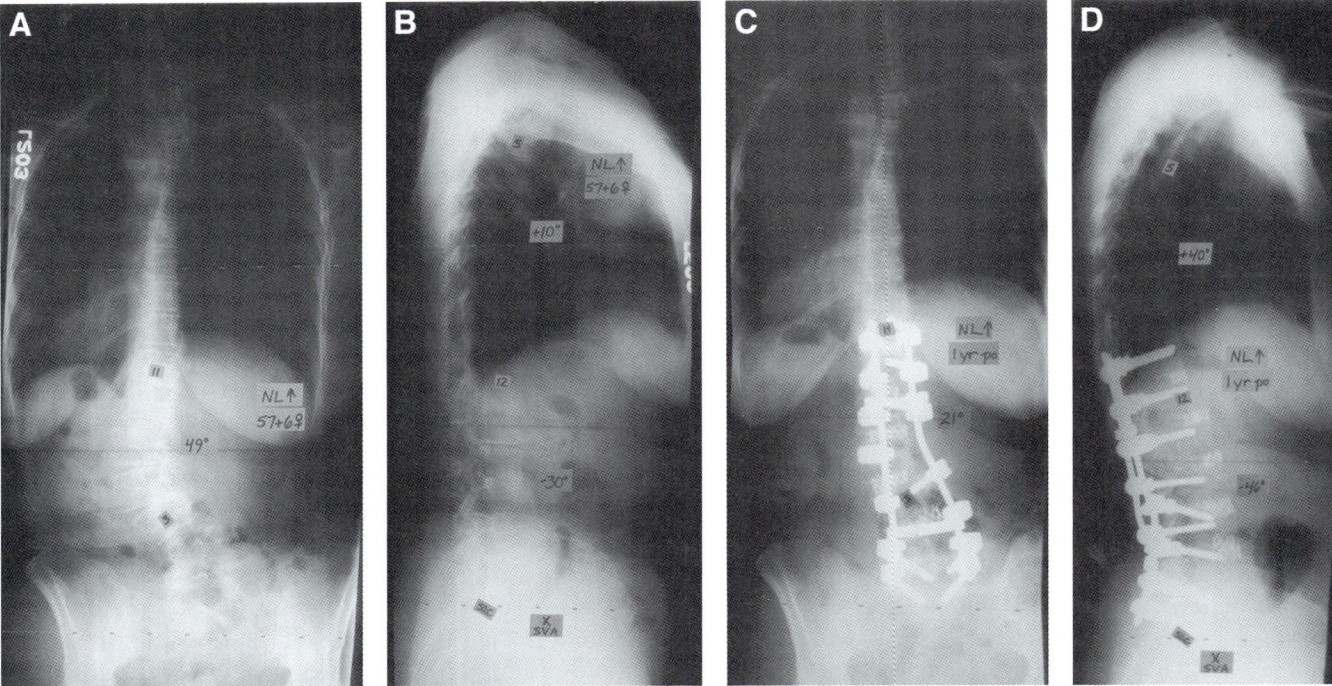

Figure 4 **A,** Standing long cassette coronal radiograph showing adult degenerative de novo scoliosis. There is marked rotatory subluxation present at T12-L1, L2-L3, and L3-L4. **B,** Sagittal plane radiographic alignment shows thoracic hypokyphosis, and lumbar hypolordosis with a slightly anterior sagittal vertical alignment while standing. **C,** Anterior and posterior spinal infusion from T11 to the sacrum was performed. Postoperative coronal view shows improved alignment of the lumbar spine with good overall balance. **D,** Postoperative sagittal view shows marked improvement of the lumbar lordosis with acceptable global sagittal alignment and balance.

segmental instrumentation systems providing normalized lumbar lordosis have not noted these problems. However, long-term (minimum 20 to 30 years and beyond) follow-up will be required to document the efficacy of these new treatments, not only in avoiding flatback syndrome but also distal spinal degeneration.

Degenerative (de novo) Scoliosis

Degenerative lumbar scoliosis is seen in patients age 60 years and older and is characterized by either lumbosacral back pain and/or leg pain. The axial pain is normally degenerative and mechanical in nature, whereas the leg pain is usually the result of spinal stenosis. Therefore, symptoms of neurogenic claudication must be fully evaluated. Also, lumbar radiculopathies from isolated lateral recess or foraminal stenosis may be the presenting complaint. Disk degeneration, facet arthropathy, ligamentous laxity, and osteoporosis are factors related to etiology.

Upright PA and lateral lumbar spine radiographs are used in the initial radiographic assessment. The presence and degree of rotatory subluxations most commonly seen at L3-L4 and L4-L5 are important factors in diagnosis. Pathophysiologically, disk degeneration and ligamentous laxity overwhelm the body's ability to autostabilize these lumbar spinal segments by either facet hypertrophy posteriorly or vertebral osteophyte formation anteriorly. In

the sagittal plane, multilevel disk degeneration with varying degrees of loss of lumbar lordosis or absolute kyphosis is apparent (Fig. 4). Rates of annual progression range from 1° to more than 10°. The main thoracolumbar or lumbar curves can range up to 50° to 60°, with a concomitant contralateral fractional lumbosacral curve. MRI often reveals spinal stenosis with associated lower extremity claudication and/or radicular complaints, but a CT myelogram provides the most accurate neuroradiographic information.

Physical therapy programs help to strengthen and maintain flexibility of the spinal musculature and increase aerobic fitness. Patients should be instructed to maintain as active a lifestyle as possible to avoid the detrimental physical and emotional effects of disuse musculoskeletal atrophy. Focal nerve root injections or epidural steroid injections can help both diagnostically and therapeutically in those patients with radiculopathies and/or stenosis.

There are three types of surgical treatments for these patients, depending on the amount of coronal deformity with vertebral rotatory subluxations, the lumbar sagittal alignment, and the amount and location of spinal stenosis. Decompression alone is reserved for patients who have spinal stenosis assessed by MRI but no major coronal or sagittal deformities or significant rotatory subluxations. Flexion/extension as well as side bending radiographs reveal minimal detectable motion. Destabilization of the spine should not occur with a midline and lateral recess decompression that spares the majority of the facet joints, as long as this procedure is not done at the concave apex of the curve where a rotatory subluxation exists.

Posterior decompression along with a posterior fusion and instrumentation is indicated in patients who have a greater degree of spinal deformity with mild to moderate rotatory subluxations present in regions that require a decompression. Overall alignment in the sagittal plane demonstrates acceptable lumbar lordosis (greater than $-40°$). After the appropriate decompression(s) has been performed, the posterior instrumentation and fusion is performed extending from the neutral vertebra of the thoracolumbar junction down to L5. It is best to avoid fusion across the lumbosacral junction if possible because of the associated high complication rates. Sometimes it is acceptable to only stabilize with instrumentation and fusion those levels with rotatory subluxations that are being decompressed, thus leaving levels above and below uninstrumented and unfused. Care should be taken to avoid transition syndromes or subluxations that occur in the coronal and sagittal planes, either above (most common) or below a short lumbar fusion.

Decompression with anterior and posterior fusion and posterior instrumentation (with placement of structural grafts or cages in the disk spaces to recreate lumbar lordosis) is highly advantageous in patients with more severe deformities in both the coronal and sagittal planes with marked hypolordosis or frank kyphosis of the lumbar spine, severe stenosis, and rotatory subluxations greater than 5 mm. In these patients, coronal and sagittal imbalances usually are not correctable on side bending or hyperextension lateral radiographs. The placement of structural graft or cage with anterior distraction creates a ligamentotaxis effect that helps reduce rotatory subluxations and increases cross-sectional diameter of the corresponding foramen. The posterior procedure is then done, with the appropriate stenosis decompressions, posterior instrumentation and fusion, and posterior convex compression forces applied for further lordosis of the spine and reduction of the curve. The fusion should begin and end at both a neutral and stable vertebra. As with any significant spinal reconstruction, the physiologic age of the patient is important as a guideline for surgical indications. Because more surgery often is needed to treat this condition, outcome is somewhat less predictable than for spinal stenosis without any deformity.

Annotated Bibliography

Bradford DS, Tay BK, Hu SS: Adult scoliosis: Surgical indications, operative management, complications, and outcomes. *Spine* 1999;24:2617-2629.
The evaluation and treatment of adult scoliosis patients is discussed. Information is provided on who is a candidate for surgery, appropriate surgical techniques, surgical risks, and well clinical outcomes.

Bridwell KH, Lenke LG, Baldus C, Blanke K: Major intraoperative neurologic deficits in pediatric and adult spinal deformity patients: Incidence and etiology at one institution. *Spine* 1998;23:324-331.
Risk factors include same-day circumferential surgery, anterior ligation of segmental vessels, preoperative thoracic hyperkyphosis, previous spinal surgery, and induced hypotension. Perioperative monitoring is important.

Linville DA, Bridwell KH, Lenke LG, Vedantam R, Leicht P: Complications in the adult spinal deformity patient having combined surgery: Does revision increase the risk? *Spine* 1999;24:355-363.
Revision surgery had complication rates similar to those of primary cases, although the surgeries tended to take longer. Perioperative hyperalimentation was strongly recommended to minimize complications.

Padberg AM, Wilson-Holden TJ, Lenke LG, Bridwell KH: Somatosensory- and motor-evoked potential monitoring without a wake-up test during idiopathic scoliosis surgery: An accepted standard of care. *Spine* 1998;23:1392-1400.
The usefulness of performing combined somatosensory- and motor-evoked potential monitoring during idiopathic scoliosis surgery is discussed.

Vedantam R, Lenke LG, Keeney JA, Bridwell KH: Comparison of standing sagittal spinal alignment in asymptomatic adolescents and adults. *Spine* 1998;23: 211-215.
Data from 88 asymptomatic adolescents without spinal deformity were compared to previously established data for asymptomatic adults. Both groups showed similar regional values of thoracic kyphosis and lumbar lordosis. However, the adolescents had a significantly more negative sagittal vertical axis than the adults. Unlike in the adults, the sagittal vertical axis in the adolescents was not significantly correlated with distal segmental lumbar lordosis.

Classic Bibliography

Albert TJ, Balderston RA: Treatment of adult scoliosis. *J South Orthop Assoc* 1996;5:229-237.

Albert TJ, Purtill J, Mesa J, McIntosh T, Balderston RA: Health outcome assessment before and after adult deformity surgery: A prospective study. *Spine* 1995;20: 2002-2005.

Ascani E, Bartolozzi P, Logroscino CA, et al: Natural history of untreated idiopathic scoliosis after skeletal maturity. *Spine* 1986;11:784-789.

Balderston RA: Adult scoliosis: The thoracic spine, in Bridwell KH, DeWald RL (eds): *The Textbook of Spinal Surgery*, ed 2. Philadelphia, PA, Lippincott-Raven, 1997, pp 715-731.

Bradford DS, Tribus CB: Vertebral column resection for the treatment of rigid coronal decompensation. *Spine* 1997;22:1590-1599.

Bradford DS: Adult scoliosis, in Moe JH, Lonstein JE, Bradford DS, Winter RB, Ogilvie JW (eds): *Moe's Textbook of Scoliosis and Other Spinal Deformities*, ed 3. Philadelphia, PA, WB Saunders, 1995, pp 369-386.

Bridwell KH: Where to stop the fusion distally in adult scoliosis: L4, L5, or the sacrum? *Instr Course Lect* 1996;45:101-107.

Cordover AM, Betz RR, Clements DH, Bosacco SJ: Natural history of adolescent thoracolumbar and lumbar idiopathic scoliosis into adulthood. *J Spinal Disord* 1997;10:193-196.

Dick J, Boachie-Adjei O, Wilson M: One-stage versus two-stage anterior and posterior spinal reconstruction in adults: Comparison of outcomes including nutritional status, complications rates, hospital costs, and other factors. *Spine* 1992;17(suppl 8): S310-S316.

Dickson JH, Mirkovic S, Noble PC, Nalty T, Erwin WD: Results of operative treatment of idiopathic scoliosis in adults. *J Bone Joint Surg Am* 1995;77:513-523.

Edgar MA, Mehta MH: Long-term follow-up of fused and unfused idiopathic scoliosis. *J Bone Joint Surg Br* 1988;70:712-716.

Grubb SA, Lipscomb HJ: Diagnostic findings in painful adult scoliosis. *Spine* 1992;17:518-527.

Grubb SA, Lipscomb HJ, Coonrad RW: Degenerative adult onset scoliosis. *Spine* 1988;13:241-245.

Grubb SA, Lipscomb HJ, Suh PB: Results of surgical treatment of painful adult scoliosis. *Spine* 1994;19: 1619-1627.

Horton WC, Holt RT, Muldowny DS: Controversy: Fusion of L5-S1 in adult scoliosis. *Spine* 1996;21: 2520-2522.

Jackson RP, Simmons EH, Stripinis D: Coronal and sagittal plane spinal deformities correlating with back pain and pulmonary function in adult idiopathic scoliosis. *Spine* 1989;14:1391-1397.

Kostuik JP: Adult scoliosis: The lumbar spine, in Bridwell KH, DeWald RL (eds): *The Textbook of Spinal Surgery,* ed 2. Philadelphia, PA, Lippincott-Raven, 1997, pp 733-775.

Kostuik JP: Operative treatment of idiopathic scoliosis. *J Bone Joint Surg Am* 1990;72:1108-1113.

Lenke LG, Bridwell KH, Blanke K, Baldus C: Prospective analysis of nutritional status normalization after spinal reconstructive surgery. *Spine* 1995;20:1359-1367.

Mandelbaum BR, Tolo VT, McAfee PC, Burest P: Nutritional deficiencies after staged anterior and posterior spinal reconstructive surgery. *Clin Orthop* 1988;234:5-11.

Ogilvie JW: Adult scoliosis: Evaluation and nonsurgical treatment. *Instr Course Lect* 1992;41:251-255.

Simmons ED Jr, Kowalski JM, Simmons EH: The results of surgical treatment for adult scoliosis. *Spine* 1993;18:718-724.

Weinstein SL, Ponseti IV: Curve progression in idiopathic scoliosis. *J Bone Joint Surg Am* 1983;65:447-455.

Weinstein SL, Zavala DC, Ponseti IV: Idiopathic scoliosis: Long-term follow-up and prognosis in untreated patients. *J Bone Joint Surg Am* 1981;63:702-712.

Chapter 55

Spinal Infections

Alan S. Hilibrand, MD

Louis G. Quartararo, MD

Mark J.R. Moulton, MD

Several factors have contributed to the increasing incidence of spinal infections, including the prolonged life expectancy of the adult population and associated medical comorbidities, increasing rates of spinal surgery and instrumentation, and improvements in early detection of vertebral osteomyelitis and diskitis.

Pyogenic Vertebral Osteomyelitis

Epidemiology and Etiology

Pyogenic vertebral osteomyelitis has been described as a disease more common in younger, male individuals, although several recent studies have noted a majority of patients over age 50 years. Other risk factors for the development of pyogenic vertebral osteomyelitis include chronic corticosteroid treatment, chemotherapy for malignancy, rheumatoid arthritis, malnutrition, and intravenous drug abuse.

Pyogenic vertebral osteomyelitis may develop as a result of hematogenous spread, contiguous involvement, iatrogenic causes, or posttraumatic inoculation. Hematogenous spread is most common, and the disease may be caused by any infection leading to bacteremia. The genitourinary tract, subcutaneous tissues, and respiratory system are often remote sites of infection. Contiguous spread of infection leading to osteomyelitis has been reported from retropharyngeal and retroperitoneal abscesses. Iatrogenic causes include invasive spinal procedures such as diskography and chemonucleolysis, as well as open surgical procedures, especially the use of internal fixation. Although rare, posttraumatic inoculation has been reported with penetrating trauma as well as with open fractures of the spine. In addition, patients with a psoas, retropharyngeal, or epidural abscess should be strongly suspected of harboring an underlying pyogenic vertebral osteomyelitis or diskitis as the initiating nidus of infection.

Traditionally, the most common pathogen associated with pyogenic vertebral osteomyelitis has been *Staph-ylococcus aureus*, which has been identified in more than 50% of all spinal infections and 75% of all positive cultures. In cases caused by intravenous drug use, the most common pathogens include *Pseudomonas*, *Escherichia coli*, and *Proteus* species. In addition, patients with sickle cell anemia have a predisposition for infection with *Salmonella*. Pathogens are believed to reach the vertebral body via embolic spread from the remote sources outlined earlier. The emboli are deposited in the metaphyseal regions adjacent to the vertebral end plates, which contain end arterioles with numerous anastomoses. From this location, the bacteria may break through the adjacent end plate into the contiguous disk space and into the adjacent vertebral body. Indeed, whether pyogenic vertebral osteomyelitis, diskitis, and spondylodiskitis represent different etiologic entities or merely a continuum of the same underlying disorder is controversial. For this reason some authors have recently recommended the use of the term "spondylodiskitis" in reference to any of these three pathologies.

Clinical Presentation

Approximately half of all cases of pyogenic vertebral osteomyelitis are found within the lumbar spine, although neurologic deficits caused by pyogenic infection are most common with cervical spine involvement. The alert, cooperative patient will usually complain of back pain. In some patients, the back pain may develop in association with fever, chills, sweats, or other constitutional complaints. The presence of constitutional symptoms as well as the progressive, unrelenting nature of the pain, which is usually not relieved with rest, helps distinguish a spinal infection from an acute lumbar sprain or strain. Radicular complaints are present in only a minority of patients. Isolated motor root findings, paresis, and even paralysis may be seen, especially with cervical or thoracic level infections. Neurologic deficits are associated with the presence of a concomitant epidural abscess, increased age, and an immunocompromised status.

Serologic analysis of patients who present with low back pain that is acute and progressive may be helpful in differentiating pyogenic vertebral osteomyelitis from the mechanical low back pain associated with a lumbar strain. Identification of the infecting pathogen through blood culture is possible in the setting of significant bacteremia, but blood culture is generally not a sensitive method of diagnosing pyogenic vertebral osteomyelitis. Similarly, an elevated leukocyte count also has a poor diagnostic sensitivity, and has been reported to be elevated in less than half of all patients with pyogenic vertebral osteomyelitis. In contrast, an elevated erythrocyte sedimentation rate (ESR) may be identified in approximately 90% of these patients regardless of immune system function. In the setting of an elevated leukocyte count and ESR, the presence of an epidural abscess or more advanced infection should be suspected. C-reactive protein (CRP), an acute phase reactant, may be more sensitive to the presence of an underlying infection than the ESR, and will normalize more rapidly in the setting of successful treatment.

Radiographic Assessment

The development of radiographic findings consistent with pyogenic vertebral osteomyelitis typically lags behind the clinical course of the disease. Radiographic changes usually develop from 2 to 4 weeks after the onset of symptoms, often in conjunction with the onset of low back pain. Early findings on spinal radiographs include disk space collapse and vertebral end plate mottling, which is often present at the end plates cephalad and caudad to a particular intervertebral disk. This radiographic feature helps distinguish spinal infections from malignancies, which are confined to the vertebral body and do not "cross" the intervertebral disk. Later in the disease process, radiographs may demonstrate anterior vertebral body destruction and collapse with a soft-tissue mass and progressive kyphosis.

MRI remains the principal imaging modality used for diagnosis. In a recent retrospective review of patients with pyogenic vertebral osteomyelitis, MRI was reported to be diagnostic in more than half of all cases within 2 weeks of clinical symptom onset, and was considered "suggestive" of the diagnosis in nearly all remaining patients. MRI was used to assess patients through their course of treatment, and these patients were found to have initial neuroradiographic progression of their disease despite early clinical symptom resolution.

Characteristic changes are seen on MRI studies in pyogenic vertebral osteomyelitis. Inflammation and edema within the vertebral marrow produce a decreased fat content and decreased T1 signal intensity. Conversely, the increase in water content (inflammation and edema) leads to an increased T2 intensity. In addition, the involved vertebral marrow and intervertebral disk should be enhanced with gadolinium contrast. Furthermore, a soft-tissue or epidural mass may be readily identified on any of these sequences, with anterior subligamentous spread across the disk space also characteristic of pyogenic vertebral osteomyelitis (Fig. 1).

Nuclear medicine studies may also be useful in the diagnosis of pyogenic vertebral osteomyelitis in patients in whom MRI is not possible, especially those with stainless steel implants or claustrophobia. These include the three-phase technetium and gallium scans, which may be combined for greater sensitivity and specificity. Either isotope can indicate the presence of an infection prior to the development of radiographic changes. A recent report comparing these modalities with MRI noted that MRI had greater sensitivity and specificity, although gallium scans were capable of identifying unsuspected remote sites of infection such as endocarditis and remote soft-tissue abscesses. In addition, gallium combined with single photon emission CT has been noted to correlate with the histologic severity of the infection. Indium-labeled white blood cell scans have been found to have a high rate of false negative results in the setting of spinal infections and are not recommended as a screening test for pyogenic vertebral osteomyelitis.

Management Considerations

Under optimal circumstances, the treatment of pyogenic vertebral osteomyelitis is nonsurgical. This route is usually taken with a younger patient with normal immune function in whom a definitive tissue diagnosis of the offending pathogen has been made through percutaneous biopsy. Care must be taken to avoid administering any antibiotic therapy until biopsy from the site of the infection has been attempted, because administration of antibiotic at this point has been shown to decrease the likelihood of identifying a causative organism. Biopsy is usually performed after localization of the nidus with MRI, and may proceed most effectively under CT guidance. After successful biopsy, the patient is usually treated with a 6-week course of intravenous antibiotics determined by the organism's sensitivity profile. For most patients, the application of a rigid brace or halo vest is necessary for immobilization and pain relief. Clinical follow-up in conjunction with serial serologic tests (ESR and CRP) should be obtained to document resolution of the infection. An MRI study may also be obtained after completion of the first 6-week course of antibiotics, although MRI

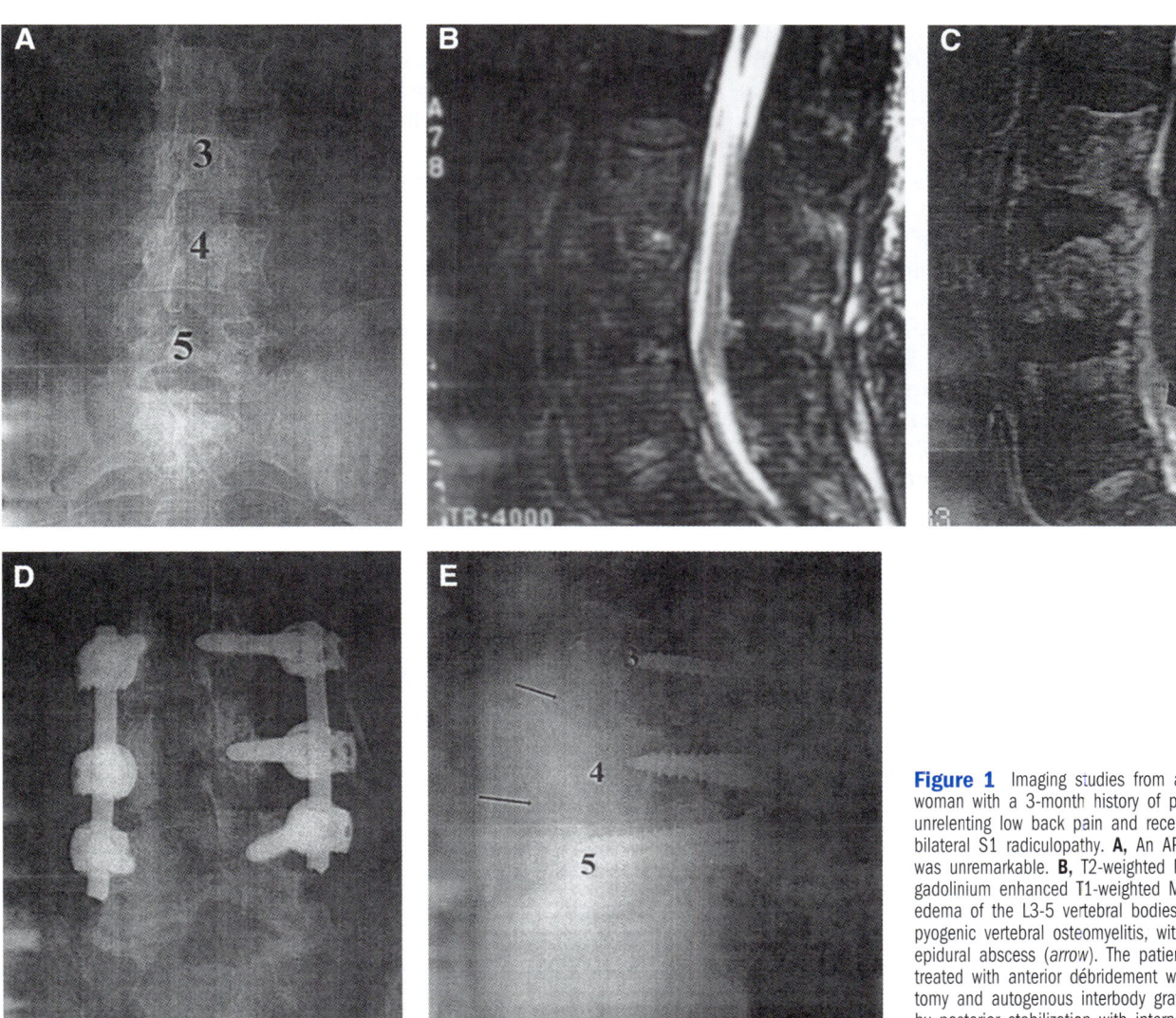

Figure 1 Imaging studies from a 64-year-old woman with a 3-month history of progressive, unrelenting low back pain and recent onset bilateral S1 radiculopathy. **A,** An AP radiograph was unremarkable. **B,** T2-weighted MRI and **(C)** gadolinium enhanced T1-weighted MRI showed edema of the L3-5 vertebral bodies secondary to pyogenic vertebral osteomyelitis, with evidence of epidural abscess (*arrow*). The patient was treated with anterior débridement with diskectomy and autogenous interbody grafting followed by posterior stabilization with internal fixation and autogenous bone grafting **(D and E)**.

findings tend to lag behind the clinical course of the infection.

Several circumstances may necessitate surgical management with débridement and stabilization. In the healthy host with a normal neurologic examination, surgery is indicated following failure of the initial 6-week course of parenteral antibiotics. Progressive vertebral body collapse and the development of symptomatic deformity may also necessitate surgical management in spite of the apparent success of antibiotic treatment. On the other hand, the development of neurologic deficits, especially in conjunction with an epidural abscess, represents an indication for urgent surgical treatment. Elderly patients, especially those with poor immune system function and multiple comorbidities, are more likely to require surgical intervention.

Appropriate surgical treatment should identify the underlying pathogen, decompress the neural elements, and drain any epidural process, débride necrotic bone and infected tissue, and stabilize the intervening spinal segments. In pyogenic vertebral osteomyelitis, the initial operation should proceed via an anterior approach, allowing direct decompression of the neural elements and drainage of any epidural process that may arise from the vertebral body or intervertebral disk anterior to the spinal cord. In addition, reconstruction of the anterior column with autogenous bone graft provides a degree of stability to the affected region. The anterior application of internal fixation in the face of pyogenic vertebral osteomyelitis is not recommended, as this may provide a "protected" environment for persistent bacterial incubation. However, because of the need for rigid stabilization in order to facilitate rehabilitation and pain control, many surgeons advocate a concomitant or "staged" posterior stabilization with internal fixation applied via a "clean" posterior spinal wound with autogenous bone grafting (Fig. 1).

A recent retrospective study at a single institution reported the diagnostic workup and treatment of a large series of patients treated for pyogenic vertebral osteomyelitis. Over half of the patients were successfully treated nonsurgically. Surgical treatment included anterior débridement and arthrodesis in most cases, with the application of internal fixation in one third of cases with neither recurrent infection nor failure of the instrumentation. In patients (89 of 111) who returned for 2-year follow-up, there was no recurrence of infection.

In another recent retrospective analysis, approximately half of all patients who presented with pyogenic vertebral osteomyelitis underwent surgical management. A variety of surgical approaches, including transpedicular diskectomies, laminectomies, anterior decompression and fusion, and combined anterior/posterior decompression and stabilization, were used. Patients treated through a combined approach had the best outcomes, whereas those undergoing laminectomy alone had poor results. The outcomes were better following surgical treatment with regard to pain, although fewer than 20% of patients with an epidural abscess had complete neurologic recovery despite surgical decompression.

Epidural Abscess

Epidemiology and Etiology

Over the past decade there has been an increased incidence of epidural abscess. Overall, most cases of epidural abscess occur in adults, with the majority occurring during the fifth and sixth decades of life and distributed equally among males and females. The incidence of epidural abscesses has been reported to be 1.96 patients per 10,000 admissions. The relative increase in the incidence of epidural abscess has been attributed to many factors, including the increase in intravenous drug use, increasing rates of epidural anesthesia, the increased rates of spine surgery and invasive spinal procedures and the growing number of cases of acquired immunodeficiency syndrome (AIDS).

A 3% overall incidence of epidural abscess after epidural analgesia has recently been reported among a group of patients with long-term epidural treatment for chronic pain. However, subsequent studies of patients with long-term indwelling epidural catheters have reported an incidence of 0.6% to 0.77% per 1,000 catheter days. The majority of epidural catheters are inserted for relatively short-term use associated with surgical procedures. A study from Denmark reported a total of 17,372 epidural catheters used during a 1-year period. The incidence of epidural abscess in this population was approximately 0.05%. There was a statistically significant discrepancy in the incidence of epidural abscesses in the university setting (0.02%) versus that of the nonuniversity setting or community hospitals (0.12%) ($P = 0.001$). Seven of the nine patients who had developed an epidural abscess in this study had neurologic deficits that required decompression of the spinal cord within 24 hours of the verification of its diagnosis. Of the seven with neurologic deficits who underwent surgery, four had persistent neurologic deficits.

Hematogenous spread of bacteria can cause epidural abscess, as well as a contiguous spread of pathogens from vertebral osteomyelitis or diskitis. Hematogenous spread may be caused by a traumatic injury such as open fracture or severe burns. Recent increases in the prevalence of epidural abscess have also been associated with an increasing frequency of provocative diskography, epidural steroid injections, and facet/nerve root blocks. Other risk factors associated with epidural abscess include intravenous drug use, diabetes, indwelling catheters, and immunocompromised conditions (such as AIDS, cancer, or poor nutritional status).

Pathogenesis

The pathogenesis of epidural abscess formation is debatable. In a meta-analysis, thoracic involvement was related to epidural abscess formation in approximately 50% of cases, lumbar involvement in 35%, and cervical spine disease in 15%. A more recent retrospective study of 41 patients demonstrated an equal incidence of cervical and thoracic epidural abscess formation at 37% each, with only 12% of patients with lumbar epidural abscesses and 16% with lumbosacral abscesses. Because the spread of the abscess longitudinally along the spinal axis is not impeded, several levels are frequently involved. On average, there are three to four segments per epidural abscess involved. The abscesses may be unifocal or have multifocal characteristics (Fig. 2).

The etiology for the neurologic sequelae of an epidural abscess is also a focus of considerable debate. Two hypotheses have been proposed: direct compression of the neural elements versus thrombosis of feeder arterioles and subsequent ischemia of the spinal cord. In a rabbit model of epidural abscess, 90% of the study animals developed acute paralysis following inoculation of *Staphylococcus* into the epidural space. Microangiographic studies demonstrated patency of the anterior spinal artery and the paired dorsal arteries to the spinal cord despite near-complete obliteration of the spinal canal itself. Ischemic injury to the spinal

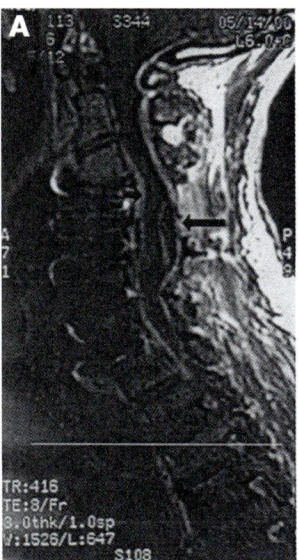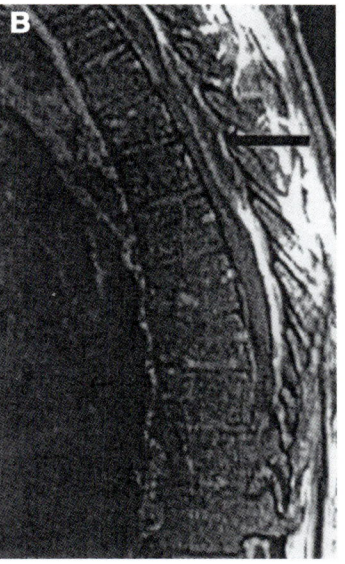

Figure 2 Sagittal MRI study of a 58-year-old woman who developed a cervical epidural abscess following anterior cervical surgery with internal fixation. Multiple foci of infection are evident in the cervical **(A)** and thoracic **(B)** spinal canal.

cord may exist with epidural abscess, but direct compression of the spinal cord appears to cause the majority of neurologic sequelae of an epidural abscess.

The clinical sequelae of epidural abscess formation typically follow four stages. The first stage involves the initial symptoms of local pain, which is followed by the onset of radicular symptoms in the second stage. The third stage is heralded by the onset of weakness with subsequent paralysis occurring in the final stage. The stage of disease generally correlates with the amount of canal compromise and has been demonstrated to correlate with long-term neurologic outcome.

Diagnostic Evaluation

The clinical presentation of a patient with an epidural abscess is variable and as many as 50% of patients may be misdiagnosed upon initial presentation. Patients may appear to have sepsis in acute phases of the disease process and typically have spinal tenderness and pain localized in the area of the infection. A recent study demonstrated that the most prevalent laboratory findings early in the process were leukocytosis followed by elevated ESR and CRP levels.

Spinal radiographs may be used to identify diskitis or vertebral osteomyelitis that may spread and subsequently cause an epidural abscess. However, the usefulness of radiographs in delineating epidural abscesses is limited if there is no associated bony destruction or loss of disk height. One study suggests that the best diagnostic imaging sequence for the detection of epidural abscess formation is MRI with T1-weighed imaging before and after the administration of gadolinium

contrast. T2-weighted MRI of the spine may also be helpful to identify early signs of diskitis or lesions involving the spinal cord itself. A recent study using an animal model of epidural abscess formation with MRI suggested that postcontrast T1 images were superior to T2 images alone for the detection of epidural abscess formation. Other studies have described the ability of gallium 67 to identify spinal abscesses that is compared to that of MRI. When MRI is not possible, such as with obscuring implants or lack of facilities, gallium 67 scintigraphy may be a satisfactory method of investigating for the presence of a spinal abscess.

Management

Successful nonsurgical treatment of epidural abscesses with immobilization and intravenous antibiotics has been reported, but with catastrophic complications of paralysis and sepsis in a subset of these patients. A recent retrospective review of nonsurgical treatment outcomes demonstrated a 20% incidence of progressive neurologic deficits despite appropriate antibiotic treatment. A univariate analysis in the study revealed that age and degree of thecal sac compression were the only significant factors influencing outcome. Patients who are neurologically stable with minimal neurologic abnormalities may be candidates for nonsurgical management, although identification of the causative organism and its antibiotic susceptibilities should be accomplished either through needle biopsy or blood cultures. An urgent change from nonsurgical to surgical treatment is warranted in any patient who has progressive neurologic compromise or new onset of neurologic deficits despite "appropriate" nonsurgical management.

In general, the optimal management of epidural abscess is via anterior or posterior débridement with the appropriate antibiotic therapy. Few authors have successfully treated epidural abscesses by drainage alone with percutaneous catheters. In the lumbar spine, where nearly 75% of abscesses develop posteriorly in the spine canal, laminectomy is generally the treatment of choice. Wide facetectomy generally is not necessary for adequate decompression of epidural abscesses, and care should be taken not to create instability by facetectomy. Should facetectomy or wide decompression be necessary, posterolateral fusion with segmental instrumentation is needed to restore spinal stability. These patients require long-term follow-up to determine whether adequate fusion and healing have occurred. In those patients in whom vertebral osteomyelitis or diskitis is present with concomitant anterior thecal sac compression, anterior decompression may be warranted. With significant bony destruction, anterior column support and reconstruction may be necessary, although supplemental posterior segmental fixation may be preferable to the use of anterior instrumentation in the face of infection.

The duration of postoperative antibiotic therapy is controversial. Following adequate decompression and débridement, appropriate antibiotic use should be based on culture and sensitivity results. While final sensitivities are pending, initial antibiotic treatment can be directed based on intraoperative Gram stain results. In cases of epidural abscess associated with invasive procedures such as diskography or indwelling epidural catheter placement, *Staphylococcus* species, including *S. aureus* and *S. epidermidis*, should be covered. In those patients with a history of intravenous drug use, gram-negative species should be covered. With no evidence of bony destruction, antibiotics are typically administered for approximately 2 to 6 weeks. In those patients with vertebral osteomyelitis, intravenous antibiotic treatment may be required for approximately 6 weeks or longer, depending upon the patient's immune status.

Tuberculous and Fungal Infections of the Spine

Since 1986, there has been an increase in the prevalence of tuberculosis (TB) in the United States. In 1987, the nationwide incidence of TB was 9.3 per 100,000. In 1991, the incidence in the state of New York was 17.3 per 100,000, with higher rates in urban areas. The reasons for this increase include factors such as poor public health, increased homelessness, increase in elderly population in nursing homes, and a rise in immigrants from Southeast Asia and Central America. The growing population with human immunodeficiency virus (HIV) in the United States and the recent development of drug-resistant strains of TB have also been contributing factors. Approximately 15% of cases of TB are extrapulmonary, and only 10% of these cases are skeletal. However, half of all skeletal TB cases involve the spinal column, with the thoracolumbar spine most commonly affected. The incidence of fungal infections is also increasing in the United States. Cases of fungal osteomyelitis have been attributed to immunosuppression (both iatrogenic and HIV-induced), hyperalimentation, and lengthened life expectancy in chronic diseases secondary to medical advances.

Pathogenesis

Mycobacteria typically infect bone via hematogenous dissemination or through the lymphatic system, draining the lung or pleural space. The acid-fast bacilli stimulate an immune response with the formation of tubercles composed of monocytes and epitheloid cells, Langerhans giant cells, and central caseation. These masses expand following the path of least resistance. The infection may spare the disk space, and spread along the anterior or posterior longitudinal ligament.

Assessment

Patients usually present with constitutional symptoms, including weakness, malaise, night sweats, fever, and weight loss. Back pain is a late symptom associated with bony collapse, and often is accompanied by neurologic compromise. Important factors in the patient's history include HIV status, intravenous drug abuse, previous infections or malignancy, and recent travel.

Laboratory studies are often nonspecific. Findings include anemia, hypoproteinemia, and mild elevation in white blood cell count and ESR. Marked elevation in white blood cell count or ESR (> 50 mm/hr) suggests pyogenic rather than mycobacterial infection. Serologic testing with enzyme-linked immunosorbent assay has been shown to have a sensitivity of 60% to 80%. Mantoux skin testing may be helpful but is not diagnostic, because it may be positive in atypical mycobacterial infections. This test also may be falsely negative in the face of anergy, which could result from immunosuppression, malnutrition, old age, renal failure, or overwhelming TB.

Radiographic studies are useful in diagnosis. By 2 to 4 weeks following infection, vertebral end plate lucency and loss of cortical margins occur. Paravertebral swelling soon follows, classically involving soft-tissue expansion across two to three spinal segments. The disk space may also become involved, with a subtle decrease in disk space height. With time, the classic pattern of disk space destruction with rarefaction of adjacent bodies and paravertebral abscess develops, with vertebral collapse into a kyphotic gibbus deformity. This pattern, although classic for TB, is mimicked by *Brucella*, *Aspergillus*, and several fungal infections.

Nuclear medicine studies are useful in diagnosis. A sensitivity of 95% has been reported for technetium bone scans, although they lack specificity. Adjunctive gallium scans may improve the specificity of the bone scan, especially in postoperative or posttraumatic cases. The combination of both studies has also been reported to increase sensitivity.

CT is excellent for delineation of bony destruction, abscess formation, and extension into the spinal canal. This imaging modality may also help determine the extent of posterior element involvement, although its principal use is for surgical planning. Currently, MRI is considered the preferred imaging modality for diagnosing tuberculous and fungal infections. MRI is valuable for differentiating between metastatic disease and vertebral osteomyelitis based on the lack of disk space involvement seen with metastatic disease. MRI with gadolinium is helpful in delineation of the disease process, discerns between new TB foci and old reactivated foci, and may have value in monitoring the response to treatment.

Despite improvements in radiographic assessment, most cases of osteomyelitis suspected secondary to TB or fungus require a histologic and microbiologic confirmation. Exceptions to this rule include adults with pyogenic osteomyelitis and a positive blood culture, and children with classic diskitis with or without a positive blood culture. The differential diagnosis includes pyogenic or fungal infections, metastatic disease, primary bone tumors, and sarcoidosis. For this reason, both cultures and biopsy specimens should be obtained.

Treatment

Chemotherapy is the mainstay of treatment of patients with spinal TB. Current drugs available for treatment include isoniazid, rifampin, and pyrazinamide, which are oral, bactericidal medications; streptomycin, which is an intramuscular, bactericidal agent; and ethambutol, which is an oral bacteriostatic agent. Other drugs that can be used in treatment include p-aminosalicylic acid, ethionamide, cycloserine, thioacetazone, kanamycin, capreomycin, and viomycin. Infectious disease consultation is recommended prior to initiating treatment because of changing regional resistance patterns.

Surgical indications include neurologic deficit, spinal instability, or advanced disease in which caseation, fibrosis, and relative avascularity result in poor antibiotic penetration. Progressive neurologic deficits require urgent surgical intervention. The choice of approach varies with the clinical scenario. Generally, thoracic lesions require transthoracic decompression, whereas thoracolumbar lesions may be approached via a retroperitoneal thoracoabdominal approach. Lumbar lesions are best approached retroperitoneally. In addition, video-assisted thoracoscopic surgery has recently shown to be valuable in the biopsy and treatment of thoracic TB. The surgical procedure should include débridement of diseased tissue and uninstrumented anterior reconstruction with autogenous bone graft. Supplemental posterior instrumentation may also be appropriate, especially for multilevel disease and other scenarios with instability. However, recent literature has suggested that anterior instrumentation may reduce kyphotic deformity without increasing the risk of disease recurrence.

Fungal and Nontuberculous Granulomatous Diseases

The incidence of fungal and other granulomatous infections is also increasing in association with an increase in the number of immunosuppressed patients. The diagnostic workup and surgical management of fungal and other granulomatous diseases is similar to that of TB. Atypical mycobacteria are acid-fast bacilli that are difficult to isolate and may be particularly virulent, requiring prolonged antimicrobial therapy and surgical débridement. Brucellosis is a gram-negative, capnophilic coccobacillus infection that is seen in areas without pasteurization of milk. Nonsurgical management is typically with tetracycline and streptomycin or cotrimoxazole and rifampin. Spinal involvement should be suspected in an individual with back pain and systemic candidiasis. Elevated serum D-arabinitol/L-arabinitol ratios may assist in making this difficult diagnosis. Amphotericin B and 5-fluorocytocine can successfully treat early infection, whereas advanced disease usually requires adjuvant surgical extirpation. Aspergillosis is a saphrophytic fungal infection diagnosed by tissue potassium hydroxide preparation. Classic radiographic presentation shows dense new bone formation with small lytic lesions and no sequestration. Initial treatment is usually nonsurgical, with amphotericin B and rifampin. When nonsurgical management is unsuccessful, surgery is required (Fig. 3). Coccidioidomycosis is a dimorphic fungus, endemic in the southwestern United States, Central America, and South America. Serum complement fixation antibodies aid in diagnosis and treatment. Medical treatment typically includes ketoconazole and amphotericin B. Blastomycosis is a broad-based budding yeast endemic in the southeastern and midwestern United States. The treatment is the same as for coccidioidomycosis.

Postoperative Spinal Infections
Epidemiology and Etiology

Infection rates in spinal surgery vary considerably, depending on the length and complexity of the surgical procedure. Simple diskectomy has the lowest rate of infection when compared with other posterior spinal procedures. Without prophylactic antibiotics, the rate of infection with a unilateral laminotomy and herniated disk removal was approximately 4%. With the addition of prophylactic antibiotics, the infection rate for lumbar diskectomy falls to less than 1%. However, a twofold increase in the infection rate has been reported when simple diskectomy is performed with the operating microscope. When a posterior fusion is added to a lumbar decompressive procedure, the incidence of infection rose from 0.9% to 6.2% in one series. In another series, the incidence of deep wound infections associated with noninstrumented scoliosis cases was approximately 2%, versus 6% when instrumentation was used. Others have reported a 4.2% rate of deep wound infections associated with pedicle screw

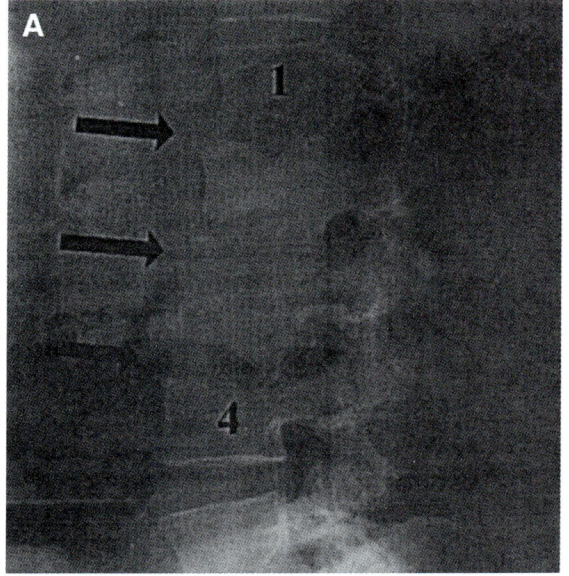

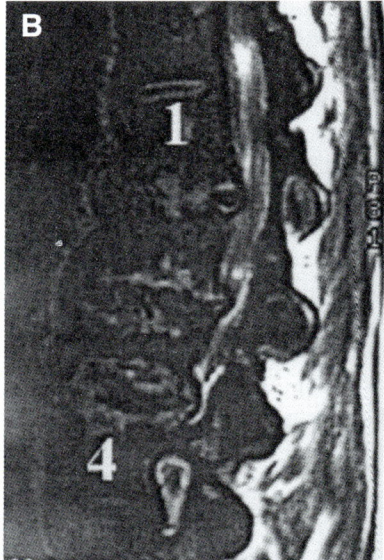

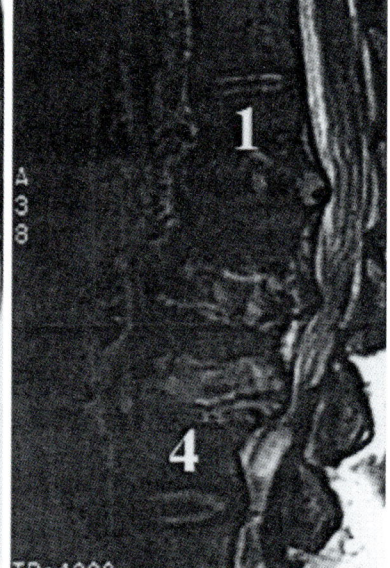

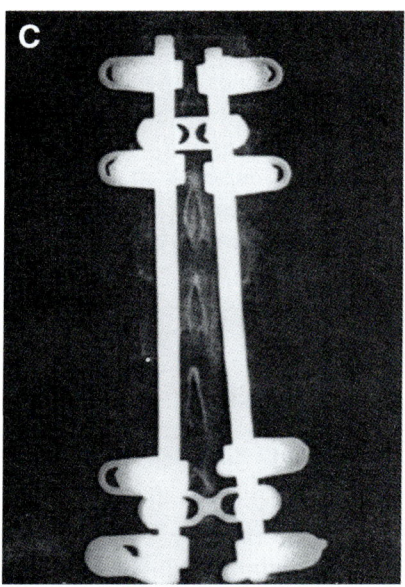

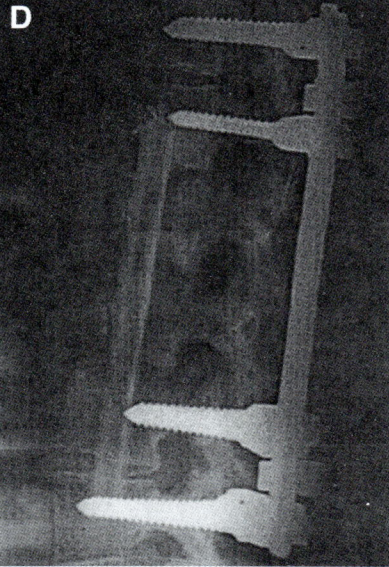

Figure 3 A 42-year-old patient with a 3-month history of incapacitating back pain and neurogenic claudication with multiple lytic lesions surrounding the end plates of L1-2 through L3-4 secondary to aspergillus infection (**A**). T2-weighted MRI study demonstrates destruction of the intervertebral disks and adjacent end plates at multiple levels (**B**). The patient underwent anterior corpectomies of L2 through L4 with autogenous fibular strut grafting from L1 to L5, followed by posterior instrumentation from T12 to L5 (**C** and **D**).

instrumentation and lumbar decompression. One study reviewed complications of spinal fusion in adults older than age 60 years. There was a reported incidence of deep wound infection of 2.4% and superficial wound infection of 4.7% in thoracolumbar fusions. There were no cervical deep wound infections in this small study. Postoperative infections involving anterior approaches to the cervical spine occur with a very low frequency, and generally are associated with injury to the esophagus.

Prophylactic Antibiotics

Prophylactic antibiotics have proved to decrease the rest of iatrogenic infection from orthopaedic surgery. A recent double-blind, placebo-controlled trial was performed with cefazolin administered 2 hours prior to primary spinal surgery. In patients receiving the placebo, 12.7% developed postoperative wound infections, versus 4.3% of patients who received 1 g of cefazolin. The authors also noted that 21 of the 71 patients who received placebo developed urinary tract infections versus 9 of 70 who received cefazolin intravenously. In addition, patients who received placebo developed infections from organisms sensitive to cefazolin. However, among patients who received cefazolin prophylactically, 43% of the organisms isolated were resistant to cefazolin or had some reduced sensitivity to the drug. General recommendations are that cefazolin or a first-generation cephalosporin should be administered 20 to 30 minutes prior to making the skin incision, with continued dosing during the perioperative period for 24 to 48 hours. If dosing is continued beyond 48 hours, there has been some suggestion that resistance to antibiotics may occur.

Ideally, prophylactic antibiotics should cover *Staphylococcus* species, *S. aureus* and *S. epidermidis,* and should reach peak concentrations after the first dose. Cefazolin shows the greatest peak serum levels of any first-generation cephalosporin, which is achieved within 20 minutes of administration. Cefazolin also has a relatively long half-life of 1.9 hours when compared with other first-generation cephalosporins.

Clinical Presentation

Most superficial wound infections that occur in the immediate postoperative period are associated with pain, tenderness, erythema, induration, drainage, and fever. Leukocytosis and elevated ESR and CRP levels are also common. Superficial infections generally occur within the first 7 to 10 days after surgery, and should be suspected in the setting of prolonged wound drainage.

The diagnosis of a deep wound infection may be difficult. Infections may occur during the immediate postoperative period or later. The physician must have a high index of suspicion for infection in order to make a timely diagnosis. Constitutional symptoms may be present, but are nonspecific. Most patients have increased pain at the site of surgery. Wound drainage is frequently present, but not necessary to qualify as a late infection. Many wounds may appear well healed, with no erythema or drainage. If infection is suspected, a leukocyte count should be done, along with assessment of ESR and CRP. It is important to note, however, that the normal response to surgical intervention is an elevation of acute phase reactants, including ESR and CRP. It has been reported that ESR remains elevated up to 42 days following an uncomplicated, noninfected spinal surgery while CRP levels usually normalize within 2 weeks following surgery.

Organisms cultured from wound infections in one series demonstrated that 59% of deep wound infections had two or more organisms present. *S. aureus* was the most common organism isolated at a rate of 56%, followed by *S. epidermidis* at 18%. Deep wound sepsis involving gram-negative bacteria developed in 40% of the patients. Although *S. epidermidis* is a low virulence bacterium, its eradication may be difficult because of the secretion of a glycocalyx, which adheres to metal surfaces and is difficult to penetrate with antibiotics.

TABLE 1	Risk Factors Indicative of Postoperative Infections
Posterior approach	
Extended length of surgery	
Presence of spinal instrumentation	
Revision surgery	
Increased blood loss	
Arthrodesis	
Morbid obesity	
Diabetes	
Congenital deformity	
Malnutrition	
Rheumatoid arthritis	
Trauma	
Advanced patient age	
Immunocompromised host	

Risk Factors for Postoperative Infections

Several comorbidities and risk factors are important predictors for postoperative infections and are listed in Table 1. Optimization of the patient's ability to heal after spinal surgery is one of the few variables that can be altered to diminish the incidence of postoperative infections. Preoperative nutritional evaluation should be performed among patients at risk for poor healing. Total lymphocyte count of less than 1,500 cell/mm^3 and an albumin level of less than 3.4 g/dL are indicators of malnutrition. Elective procedures should be postponed until nutritional improvement has been documented. Retractors should be repositioned in 45-minute intervals in order to permit soft-tissue reperfusion and to limit muscle necrosis from stationary retractors. At the time of closure, all necrotic tissue should be débrided back to healthy muscle tissue.

Management

Once the diagnosis of a wound infection has been made, management should consist of prompt aggressive débridement. Irrigation should be delivered via pulsatile lavage provided that exposed dura is not present. Antibiotics should not be administered until adequate intraoperative superficial and deep cultures are obtained. Aggressive surgical débridement includes removing all devitalized tissue or necrotic bone graft. Sharp débridement should be continued until viable, bleeding tissue is identified. Among patients with known *S. epidermidis* infections, manual scrubbing of the internal fixation device or exchanging the instrumentation may be necessary to remove potential glycocalyx. In deep infections involving implants, instrumentation should be left in place, unless it appears grossly unstable. The wound should be packed open if repeat débridement is necessary; otherwise, it should be closed over large suction drains. Serial débridement may be necessary until the infection is completely eradicated. Several articles have described the use of inflow-outflow tubes allowing for continuous irrigation with fluid, although most authors still recommend closed suction drains instead of the inflow-outflow system. Implantation of antibiotic-impregnated beads has also been advocated.

For patients who have had skin necrosis and/or wound dehiscence, surgical mobilization of muscle and skin may be necessary for closure. Occasionally, plastic surgical techniques including tissue expanders, local tissue flaps, or free flaps are helpful to manage large tissue defects. General considerations of muscle flaps should be evaluated prior to surgery, including the muscle recipient site and that of the donor muscle itself. Local flaps in the thoracic spine include the trapezius flaps, which also may be used for inferior cervical wounds. A rotational latissimus dorsi flap may be used for defects involving the midthoracic region. In lower lumbar and posterior spinal wounds, as well as sacral lesions, a gluteus maximus flap has been described. A free flap of latissimus dorsi has also been reported. Tissue expanders may be used in patients who have poor tissue compliance from multiple surgeries, radiation, and/or a myelomeningocele. Tissue expanders offer greater skin compliance without the loss of potential donor site function and morbidity.

Postoperative Diskitis

Diskitis results from inflammation of tissues in the disk space and often presents in conjunction with involvement of the surrounding soft tissue and/or bone. The incidence of postoperative diskitis has been reported to range from less than 1% to 5%. The important role of perioperative antibiotics in avoiding this complication was demonstrated by a recent study in which a postoperative spondylodiskitis was observed among 3.7% of 508 patients who did not receive prophylactic antibiotics. By comparison, there were no infections among another 1,134 patients who had an intraoperative antibiotic sponge applied at surgery. Other risk factors for a postoperative diskitis include obesity, immunosuppression, poor nutrition, and diabetes mellitus.

The clinical presentation of postoperative lumbar diskitis is fairly typical. Patients will usually experience complete relief of preoperative leg and back pain.

However, the initial pain relief is followed by progressive low back pain with loss of motion, especially flexion. Patients with diskitis typically develop these symptoms between the third and fifth weeks following surgery. At first, these symptoms may be difficult to differentiate from low back pain caused by degenerative changes that many patients experience following lumbar diskectomy, and this may delay the diagnosis of an underlying inflammatory or infectious process. The presence of increasing radicular pain, especially in conjunction with a neurologic deficit, should alert the physician to the possibility of a coexistent epidural abscess.

As with most postoperative spinal infections, elevation of ESR and CRP are common, although the most specific findings that confirm the diagnosis of postoperative diskitis may be found on MRI. Typically, there is decreased signal in the disk space and adjacent marrow on T1 images, and increased signal in these same locations on T2-weighted images. The addition of gadolinium should enhance the disk space and surrounding marrow. These findings are illustrated in Figure 3. However, MRI studies obtained within the immediate postoperative period must be interpreted with caution because of the high incidence of nonspecific postoperative changes.

In the absence of an epidural abscess or wound infection, patients with a postoperative diskitis may be treated nonsurgically. However, attempts should be made to identify the offending organism through CT-guided biopsy in order to direct antibiotic treatment. As with most spinal infections, a 6-week course of intravenous antibiotics is generally recommended, followed by a variable course of an oral antibiotic, based on the patient's response to treatment and the offending pathogen. In addition, these patients also benefit from immobilization in a thoracolumbosacral orthosis for pain control in the early stages of treatment.

Monitoring the resolution of a disk space infection involves serial evaluation of clinical, serologic, and radiologic parameters. Patients should experience progressive improvement in low back pain with improved mobility within the first month of treatment. The ESR and CRP usually return to near-normal levels by 1 month after initiation of antibiotic treatment. Radiographs may be unremarkable at the time of presentation, and destructive end plate changes are often seen only after the initiation of treatment. Most patients with postoperative diskitis will not develop plain radiographic changes until an average of 2 months after the index procedure, with the greatest degree of destructive change evident 4 months following surgery. A similar delay in resolution of inflammatory changes may be seen on follow-up MRI studies.

There are several complications that may develop in the patient with postoperative diskitis and require early recognition. The most serious is the development of an epidural abscess, which requires emergent surgical drainage. Another is the risk of meningitis, especially in the setting of an intraoperative dural tear. If suspected, coverage with an antibiotic with good cerebrospinal fluid penetration such as vancomycin is essential. Other adverse sequelae of postoperative diskitis include the development of spinal instability at the level of the infected disk space, pyogenic vertebral osteomyelitis of the surrounding vertebral bodies, sepsis, and distant infections caused by hematogenous spread of the infecting organism. In addition, between 12% and 61% of these patients may have persistent back pain that prevents return to work.

Open débridement and reconstruction for a disk space infection may be necessary in the face of failure of initial treatment, especially if there is neural element compression or progressive spinal instability. An anterior approach is preferable if there is evidence of ongoing disk space infection, in order to facilitate débridement of the infecting nidus. Spinal instability may be addressed from either an anterior or posterior approach. Bone grafting across the disk space should be autogenous, and the use of metal should be avoided in the vicinity of an active infectious process. However, a separately staged anterior débridement and autogenous grafting may be followed by a posterior stabilization procedure.

Annotated Bibliography

Carragee EJ: Instrumentation of the infected and unstable spine: A review of 17 cases from the thoracic and lumbar spine with pyogenic infections. *J Spinal Disord* 1997;10:317-324.

Despite a relatively high rate of postoperative complications, instrumentation in conjunction with débridement of the spinal infection allowed more rapid patient mobilization and did not appear to compromise the ability to eradicate the infection, based on serial clinical and serologic data.

Carragee EJ: Pyogenic vertebral osteomyelitis. *J Bone Joint Surg Am* 1997;79:874-880.

This article presents a retrospective review of the epidemiology and clinical presentation of patients with pyogenic vertebral osteomyelitis. Although less than half of the patients underwent surgical treatment, there were no late recurrences of infection and less than 10% of patients complained of chronic back pain.

Fujita T, Kostuik JP, Huckell CB, Sieber AN: Complications of spinal fusion in adult patients more than 60 years of age. *Orthop Clin North Am* 1998;29:669-678.

The authors report an incidence of postoperative spinal infection that is not substantially different than has been reported for younger patients undergoing thoracolumbar spinal fusion. Risk factors for postoperative spinal infection among elderly patients are identified.

Hadjipavlou AG, Mader JT, Necessary JT, Muffoletto AJ: Hematogenous pyogenic spinal infections and their surgical management. *Spine* 2000;25:1668-1679.

In patients undergoing surgical management, the best outcomes were achieved through a combined anterior/posterior approach, with less chronic pain among the surgically than nonsurgically treated patients. Poor neurologic recovery was reported among patients with "frank" epidural abscesses despite "immediate" surgery.

Rohde V, Meyer B, Schaller C, Hassler WE: Spondylodiscitis after lumbar discectomy: Incidence and a proposal for prophylaxis. *Spine* 1998;23:615-620.

The authors report elimination of postoperative lumbar diskitis with the application of an antibiotic "sponge" at the time of lumbar diskectomy. Risk factors for this complication are also discussed.

Yilmaz C, Selek HY, Gurkan I, Erdemli B, Korkusuz Z: Anterior instrumentation for the treatment of spinal tuberculosis. *J Bone Joint Surg Am* 1999;81:1261-1267.

The authors successfully treated a large group of patients with anterior débridement and reconstruction with grafting and internal fixation. Supplemental posterior stabilization was not performed. They report significant deformity correction without recurrence of infection with long-term follow-up.

Classic Bibliography

An HS, Vaccaro AR, Dolinskas CA, Cotler JM, Balderston RA, Bauerle WB: Differentiation between spinal tumors and infections with magnetic resonance imaging. *Spine* 1991;16(suppl 8):S334-S338.

Angtuaco EJ, McConnell JR, Chadduck WM, Flanigan S: MR imaging of spinal epidural sepsis. *AJR Am J Roentgenol* 1987;149:1249-1253.

Arnold PM, Baek PN, Bernardi RJ, Luck EA, Larson SJ: Surgical management of nontuberculous thoracic and lumbar vertebral osteomyelitis: Report of 33 cases. *Surg Neurol* 1997;47:551-561.

Eismont FJ, Bohlman HH, Soni PL, Goldberg VM, Freehafer AA: Pyogenic and fungal vertebral osteomyelitis with paralysis. *J Bone Joint Surg Am* 1983;65:19-29.

Emery SE, Chan DP, Woodward HR: Treatment of hematogenous pyogenic vertebral osteomyelitis with anterior debridement and primary bone grafting. *Spine* 1989;14:284-291.

Heller JG: Infection of the cervical spine, in An HS, Simpson JM (eds): *Surgery of the Cervical Spine*. London, England, Martin Dunitz, 1994, pp 335-356.

Hodgson AR, Skinsnes OK, Leong CY: The pathogenesis of Pott's paraplegia. *J Bone Joint Surg Am* 1967;49:1147-1156.

Hsu LC, Cheng CL, Leong JC: Pott's paraplegia of late onset: The cause of compression and results after anterior decompression. *J Bone Joint Surg Br* 1988;70: 534-538.

Kuker W, Mull M, Mayfrank L, Topper R, Thron A: Epidural spinal infection: Variability of clinical and magnetic resonance imaging findings. *Spine* 1997;22: 544-551.

Licina P, Benson S, Askin G, Whitby M: Abstract: Spinal epidural abscess: A review of fifty cases. *J Bone Joint Surg Br* 1997;79(suppl 3):286.

Loke TK, Ma HT, Chan CS: Magnetic resonance imaging of tuberculous spinal infection. *Australas Radiol* 1997;41:7-12.

Modic MT, Feiglin DH, Piraino DW, et al: Vertebral osteomyelitis: Assessment using MR. *Radiology* 1985; 157:157-166.

Post MJ, Sze G, Quencer RM, Eismont FJ, Green BA, Gahbauer H: Gadolinium-enhanced MR in spinal infection. *J Comput Assist Tomogr* 1990;14:721-729.

Rajasekaran S, Shanmugasundaram TK, Prabhakar R, Dheenadhayalan J, Shetty AP, Shetty DK: Tuberculous lesions of the lumbosacral region: A 15-year follow-up of patients treated by ambulant chemotherapy. *Spine* 1998;23:1163-1167.

Rubinstein E, Findler G, Amit P, Shaked I: Perioperative prophylactic cephazolin in spinal surgery: A double-blind placebo-controlled trial. *J Bone Joint Surg Br* 1994;76:99-102.

Whalen JL, Brown ML, McLeod R, Fitzgerald RH: Limitations of indium leukocyte imaging for the diagnosis of spine infections. *Spine* 1991;16:193-197.

Chapter 56

Tumors of the Spine

David B. Cohen, MD, MPH

Classification and Epidemiology

Tumors of the spinal column can be classified by either their tissue of origin or their biologic properties. Primary tumors can arise from any of the osseous, ligamentous, or cartilaginous tissues of the spinal column. The biologic activity of these tumors can be characterized as either benign or malignant. Secondary tumors can result from direct tumor extension into the spinal column from adjacent tissues or via metastatic spread through lymphatic or hematogenous routes. Because secondary tumors represent an extrinsic invasion of tumor into the spinal column, they normally represent malignant lesions.

Although certain primary tumors (chordoma, osteoblastoma, and plasmacytoma) tend to occur most frequently in the spinal column, they represent less than 2% of all spinal lesions. Metastatic adenocarcinoma from the lungs, prostate, breasts, kidneys, thyroid, and gastrointestinal tract account for the majority of spinal column tumors. Because of the age-related increase in the incidence of adenocarcinoma, as well as similar increases in systemic diseases such as myeloma and lymphoma, most primary and secondary spinal column tumors in adults are likely to be malignant. Conversely, in children and adolescents, only 30% of primary spinal column tumors are malignant; secondary tumors are extremely rare. Because malignant lesions are often spread or seeded via lymphatic or vascular channels, they tend to involve the vertebral body and pedicles. Most tumors of the posterior elements demonstrate a more benign biology.

Skeletal metastases can develop with virtually every type of neoplasm; however, because of vascular and lymphatic drainage patterns and bioactivity, certain tumors demonstrate a predilection for the vertebral column. Carcinoma of the breast accounts for 21% of all spinal metastases, followed by lung (14%) and prostate (8%), with renal, gastrointestinal, thyroid, and other assorted carcinoma accounting for the remainder of lesions. When lymphoma and myeloma are included with the three most common metastatic carcinomas, these tumors account for more than 60% of all spinal column lesions requiring treatment. Hence, in any patient with a personal history of previous malignancy and a current history of persistent back pain, a metastatic spinal lesion should be suspected.

Diagnosis

History

Back pain is the initial complaint in 85% of patients with a spinal column tumor. Although a vague traumatic episode may be linked with the onset of symptoms, certain features and characteristics may be more suggestive of a neoplasm. Back pain associated with spinal column tumor most typically is progressive and persistent, not relieved by rest, and more severe and disturbing at night. The rapid onset or progression of pain may suggest an advancing malignant process, and symptoms that progress more slowly may be indicative of a slower growing malignant or benign process. Severe mechanical pain occurs when a tumor causes a pathologic fracture or destroys the periosteum. Direct tumor compression or invasion of neural structures can cause neural symptoms ranging from a focal radiculitis to quadriplegia.

Pain in the extremities will often accompany axial pain from a spinal tumor. In some instances the extremity pain can simulate the radiculopathy from a herniated disk. However, similar to the axial component of the pain, the radicular pain is not relieved by rest. Although weakness is rarely the first symptom of a spinal column tumor, it can be detected on examination in 50% of patients who seek medical attention and in 70% of patients at the time of diagnosis.

Because the majority of adult spinal tumors represent metastatic adenocarcinoma, myeloma, or lymphoma, a careful review of symptoms and history is important. Constitutional symptoms such as fatigue, fever, or unexpected weight loss may suggest the presence of a tumor. A personal history of a carcinoma or a family history of certain familial syndromes may suggest a metastatic lesion. The response of the pain to various treatment modalities may suggest a certain type of tumor (for example, the pain relief with nonsteroidal anti-inflammatory drug use is associated with osteoid osteoma).

Physical Examination

A complete musculoskeletal and neurologic examination should be performed on all patients suspected of having a spinal column tumor. A careful motor and sensory examination of all dermatomes and motor groups of the upper and lower extremities is imperative. Reflexes should be carefully assessed for any evidence of myelopathy, including such findings as hyperreflexia and clonus, and Babinski and Hoffman testing should be done. In any patient with complaints of sphincter dysfunction or the presence of another deficit, a careful rectal examination including sensory, motor, and reflex function must be performed. The prostate should be palpated in male patients.

Range of motion should be assessed, and the spine examined for the presence of muscle spasm or deformity. Palpation may reveal extreme tenderness over the involved spinous process. A bony prominence, kyphotic deformity, or acute angular scoliosis can be observed after vertebral collapse. A painful and acutely progressing scoliosis in an adolescent may be suggestive of an osteoid osteoma or osteoblastoma. Soft-tissue masses are rarely palpable because of the extensive tissue and muscle layers covering the spinal column.

In addition to musculoskeletal, neurologic, and spinal examinations, the diagnostic work-up of a patient with a spinal column tumor should include a more extensive physical examination. A careful examination including the breasts, abdomen, lungs, neck, and prostate can often reveal a potential source for a metastatic spinal lesion. Palpation of the cervical, axillary, and inguinal lymph node chains can identify signs of lymphadenopathy suggestive of leukemia, lymphoma, or metastatic disease. Careful palpation of the extremities, rib cage, and iliac crests for painful areas can identify secondary sites of disease that may suggest a metastatic source of tumor and potentially provide a site more accessible for diagnostic biopsy.

Laboratory Studies

A complete blood cell count and erythrocyte sedimentation rate are sensitive screening tests for systemic disease, tumor, or infection. Serum and urine chemistry analysis, including protein electrophoresis, should be performed to identify cases of myeloma. Specific serum antigens and tumor markers such as prostate specific antigen can reveal the primary source of a spinal lesion. Stool, urine, and sputum can be examined for occult blood or cells suggestive of a primary carcinoma. These studies usually precede a more extensive imaging work-up.

Imaging Studies
Spinal Radiographs
Radiographs of the spine will demonstrate abnormalities in 80% to 90% of all spinal tumors. Loss of cortical bone at the level of the pedicle will result in a "winking owl sign" that is suggestive of an erosive tumor. Although radiographs cannot be used to accurately identify the type of tumor present, the pattern of bone destruction seen in the vertebral body will often imply a malignant process. Once sufficient bony destruction has occurred, resulting in a pathologic fracture, radiographs cannot distinguish a benign compression fracture from metastatic disease unless pedicle erosions can be seen at other vertebral levels, nor can radiographs adequately detect small tumor foci in early stages of the disease process.

Bone Scintigraphy
Compared with radiographs, technetium bone scans can serve as a more sensitive indicator of tumor involving the vertebral body. However, bone scans only identify areas of increased metabolic activity and thus have very poor specificity in determining the cause of this activity. Isolated "hot spots" can be seen in sites of arthritis, traumatic injuries, or infection and may not represent a tumor. However, multiple "hot spots" are more suggestive of a diffuse disease process that is often seen in cases of metastatic carcinoma, and can help target areas for more specific imaging modalities as well as identify areas that can be more safely biopsied to obtain diagnostic tissue. False negative bone scans can occur in cases of widespread metastatic disease, causing a diffuse uniform increased tracer uptake, multiple myeloma, or neoplasms that invade the bone so rapidly that the metabolic activity of the bone does not have a chance to change. When laboratory studies suggest multiple myeloma, secondary lesions can be identified with radiographic skeletal surveys.

Computed Tomography
CT is the optimal method of imaging intraosseous lesions when attempting to assess bony architecture and destruction, allowing accurate determination of bony cortical destruction, optimal imaging of osseous tumors, and localization of CT intracortical lesions

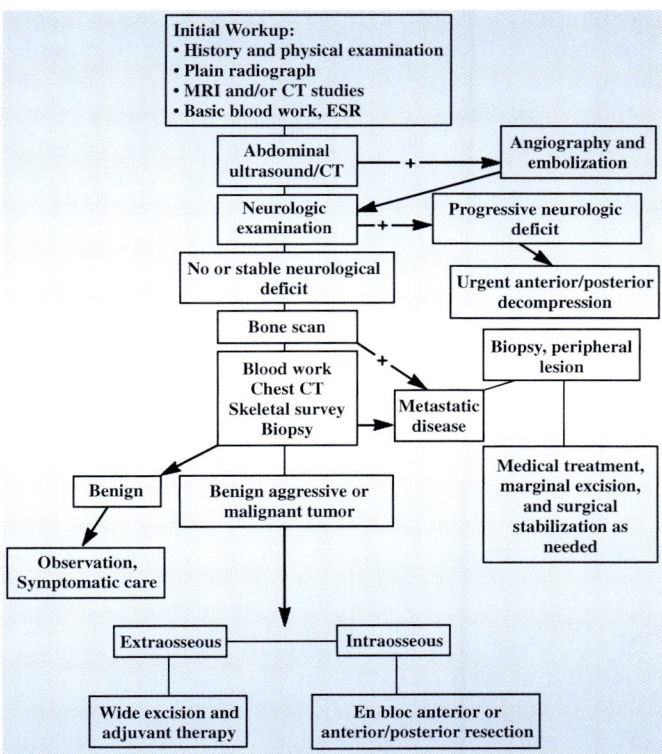

Figure 1 Algorithm for a diagnostic evaluation of spine tumor. ESR = erythrocyte sedimentation rate. (Reproduced from Beaty JH (ed): Orthopaedic Knowledge Update 6. Rosemont, IL, American Academy of Orthopaedic Surgeons, 1999, pp 723-736.)

such as osteoid osteoma. However, the usefulness of CT scans in assessing soft tissues is limited and the test is not suitable for screening large segments of the spinal column because of the amount of radiation exposure required.

Magnetic Resonance Imaging

MRI is the imaging modality of choice in assessing spinal column tumors. Large areas of the spine can be screened on sagittal and coronal images to detect the presence of disseminated disease. MRI provides direct imaging of the spinal cord, cauda equina, and nerve roots without the need for intrathecal contrast and its inherent risks. Extension of lesions into contiguous paravertebral structures can be seen better than with CT or myelography. With the use of intravenous gadolinium enhancement, MRI can accurately differentiate tumor from infection, compression fracture, hematoma, edema, and inflammation. The individual MRI signal characteristics of certain tumor types can vary; however, common features are low-intensity T1 signal, high-intensity or inhomogeneous T2 signal, gadolinium enhancement, and epidural tissue mass.

Myelography

Myelography has been replaced by MRI in the assessment of spinal tumors. However, when MRI is not an option because of the presence of certain implants (such as pacemakers or spinal stimulators), or because of patient claustrophobia, myelography and postmyelogram CT can provide much of the information gained through MRI.

Principles of Treatment

The treatment of patients with spinal tumors begins from the time of the initial evaluation. A careful and systematic workup can help differentiate most cases of metastatic carcinoma, myeloma, or lymphoma from primary spinal tumors before any invasive procedure is undertaken (Fig. 1). Knowledge of potential risks and benefits of treatment is paramount. The overall health of the patient, neurologic function, tumor type and behavior, life expectancy, length of recovery, chance of improvement with the treatment options available, and the wishes of the patient must be carefully weighed before a decision about treatment course is made. This decision is best made in conjunction with the patient, the patient's family, and primary physician. In order to make these decisions, additional work-up to identify any extraspinal disease often follows the biopsy procedure, which allows better understanding of the local and systemic behavior of a specific tumor.

Biopsy

The goal of biopsy is to provide sufficient tissue for diagnosis while minimizing the associated complications and any effect on future patient care. To achieve these goals, it is important that the most accessible lesion is biopsied in all cases (for example, an iliac crest lesion versus a C2 vertebral body lesion). All areas of the spine can be safely biopsied. Percutaneous core needle biopsy is possible for most portions of the vertebral body. Open biopsy can allow access to the entire vertebral body by using either an anterior or posterior approach, depending on the location of the lesion.

The type of biopsy can significantly affect the likelihood of positive results. Percutaneous core needle biopsy yields a positive result in 65% of osteolytic lesions and only 20% to 25% of osteoblastic metastasis. Open biopsy has a yield of 85% regardless of lesion type. Specimens for culture and Gram stain should also be obtained at the time of biopsy. Care must be taken in the appropriate planning of any open or percutaneous biopsy procedure so as not to preclude possible surgical treatment if a primary spinal carcinoma is discovered. Ideally, steroid therapy should not be begun until after biopsy is performed because the lytic effect of steroids on certain types of leukemia can lead to nondiagnostic biopsies.

Lesions involving the posterior elements of the cervical spine are readily accessible through the percutaneous approach. CT or fluoroscopic guidance should be used. Vertebral body lesions, which constitute the majority of metastases to the cervical spine, are more difficult to biopsy with a percutaneous approach. These regions are usually more easily biopsied and treated using an open anterior cervical approach. Percutaneous biopsy of the upper cervical spine is performed using a transoral approach. This approach can be used to biopsy the C1 vertebra by retracting the soft palate upward through the C3 vertebra by depressing the tongue. The body of C2 lies directly behind the mouth, with the C3 body at the level of the epiglottis. Broad-spectrum antibiotics that cover the oral flora should be administered in the perioperative period. Complications of this approach include nondiagnosed biopsy, pharyngeal edema, infection, retropharyngeal swelling, venous bleeding, vertebral body injury, dural puncture, and meningitis. All patients should be observed for pharyngeal edema and respiratory difficulties in the postoperative period.

Biopsy of the cervical spine is performed through an approach anterior to the sternocleidomastoid muscle or posterior to the sternocleidomastoid muscle. CT and MRI axial images should be used to determine the most effective approach for each particular lesion. CT guidance is mandatory in these instances. In either approach the needle should not extend too far medial in order to avoid injury to the esophagus. The lateral approach requires that the needle be inserted posterior to the sternocleidomastoid muscle and the vertebral body from the lateral aspect. The approach anterior to the sternocleidomastoid muscle requires that this muscle and carotid contents be retracted laterally to allow introduction of the needle into the anterior aterolateral aspect of the vertebral body. The carotid contents, recurrent laryngeal nerve, thyroid muscles, esophagus, nerve root, and spinal cord all are at risk for injury during this procedure.

Percutaneous biopsy of the thoracic spine can be done using either fluoroscopic or CT guidance. A transpedicular or posterolateral approach that enters the vertebral body lateral to the pedicle can be used. Craig needles are sometimes too large to be safely used in the thoracic spine, and smaller bore needles are often necessary. Because pneumothorax is the most common complication associated with percutaneous biopsy of the thoracic spine, a chest radiograph should be obtained following this procedure. Bleeding can also occur in cases of segmental vessel injury.

Lumbar vertebral body lesions are more amenable to the percutaneous approach because of their larger size (Fig. 2). Fluoroscopic or CT guidance can be used.

Posterolateral approaches are used within an entry position 6 to 7 cm lateral to the midline with a medial angulation of approximately 45°. If a transpedicular approach is planned, a more medial starting point and vertically directed needle are required. The patient is awake and in the prone position. Local anesthetic is used through a 20- or 22-gauge spinal needle. Once proper position of the spinal needle is confirmed it is replaced with a Craig needle along the same path. The Craig trocar position needs to be confirmed with biplanar fluoroscopy or by CT scanning. A report of radicular pain or sensations during the needle insertion requires the redirection of the instrument to avoid spinal nerve root injury. Sacral lesions normally require CT guidance to see the tissue of interest.

Incisional biopsy is used as the last step in tumor diagnosis only when attempts at percutaneous methods have failed to produce diagnostic tissue. Small longitudinal incisions should be used because the entire biopsy site may need to be excised if a primary malignant tumor is discovered. Careful dissection and tissue handling, as well as meticulous hemostasis, are important to avoid wound complications that can have disastrous results. An adequate amount of tissue for histologic, immunologic, and ultrastructural analysis should be sharply excised. Electrocautery should be used sparingly when removing the pathologic specimen. If possible, a frozen section should be obtained to assess the adequacy of the specimen prior to wound closure. The wound should be drained to avoid excessive soft-tissue seeding with a postoperative hematoma.

Some smaller posterior element tumors may be treated with an en bloc excision as the primary procedure, but a wide margin of resection must be obtained with ease so that patient survival is not jeopardized.

Chemotherapy

The use of primary chemotherapy for the treatment of a spinal column tumor can be extremely useful in some cases of systemic disease such as myeloma and lymphoma. As long as there is no evidence of symptomatic neurologic compression or pending pathologic fracture, treatment of the systemic disease can result in shrinkage of the spinal lesion and obviate the potential need for surgery. Adjuvant chemotherapy in both the preoperative and postoperative setting plays an important role in the treatment of certain high-grade primary malignancies such as osteosarcoma, Ewing's sarcoma, and lymphoma. Recent advances in the use of stem cell and bone marrow transplantation have led to the expanded use of more aggressive chemotherapeutic and radiation regimens for metastatic carcinomas and myelomas, followed by stem cell or bone marrow salvage.

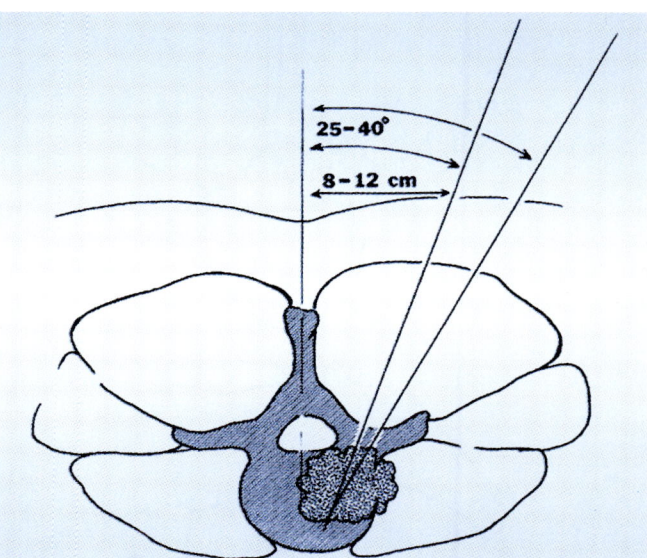

Figure 2 Approach for percutaneous needle biopsy of the lumbar spine. *(Reproduced from Beaty JH (ed): Orthopaedic Knowledge Update 6. Rosemont, IL, American Academy of Orthopaedic Surgeons, 1999, pp 723-736.)*

Radiation Therapy

Radiation therapy can be used as either a primary or an adjuvant therapy depending on the biologic properties of the tumor as well as the degree of spinal stability and neural compression. Radiation therapy is the treatment of choice for most patients with pain or early neurologic symptoms from metastatic tumors. For primary breast, lung, prostate, and lymphoreticular neoplasms, radiation therapy can provide local tumor control; however, gastrointestinal and renal neoplasms usually are unresponsive. Radiation therapy can be delivered by several modes, all of which assist in gaining local control of either a primary or metastatic tumor in the surgical bed following resection. Preoperative external beam irradiation can help shrink certain tumors, making then more amenable to resection. Similarly, postoperative external beam irradiation can assist in gaining local tumor control following intralesional excision for radiosensitive metastatic lesions. Intraoperative or perioperative brachytherapy can deliver higher local radiation doses while minimizing the risk of postirradiation myelitis. In a few centers, proton beam irradiation can deliver very high doses of radiation to exact locations, which can aid in gaining local control of previously untreatable radioinsensitive tumors such as recurrent chordoma or marginally resectable sarcomas.

Surgical Treatment

The objectives of surgical treatment for spinal tumors include decreasing patient pain, decompression of the neural elements, mechanical stabilization of the spine, and wide surgical resection to gain local control of certain primary tumors. In order to achieve these objectives as well as the overall goal of preserving the patient's quality of life, the most likely outcomes of the various potential interventions must be understood.

Surgical decompression of the spinal canal must be tailored to the individual patient. Anterior decompression is often most effective for anterior-based compression whereas posterior decompression can be effective for posterior-based tumors. Early studies on the results of laminectomy for anterior tumor compression indicated a worse outcome when laminectomy was combined with radiation therapy than radiation therapy alone, allowing fewer than 40% of patients to maintain neural function. In contrast, anterior decompression of these same lesions can result in satisfactory outcomes in 80% of patients.

In patients who cannot tolerate an anterior procedure or who have circumferential tumors, posterolateral decompression can be performed via either a costotransversectomy or a transpedicular technique to access the anterior compression in either the thoracic or lumbar spine. Bilateral transpedicular approaches may allow full visualization of the anterior dura in cases of metastatic disease, myeloma, and lymphoma. These intralesional techniques are not designed for the treatment of primary spinal tumors.

Radiation therapy can affect neural decompression when radiosensitive soft-tissue masses are the source of compression. Approximately 95% of patients who are ambulatory at the start of radiation therapy will maintain ambulation. Patients who start with a limited ambulatory function have a 60% chance of improvement after radiation therapy, and those who have lost sphincter function have at best a 40% chance to regain function.

Resection

A wide margin of excision offers improved patient survival. Many structures, including the anterior and posterior longitudinal ligaments, vertebral body, adjacent disks, and even local dura and nerve roots may need to be excised to provide a wide margin of excision. When tumors have begun to invade the dura, a true wide surgical margin is not possible because it would require spinal cord resection would be required. Recent reports suggest that this type of complete resection with wide margins can improve the survival and quality of life of patients with isolated metastatic lesions. Sometimes a better option can be to perform a marginal or intralesional resection and supplement the local treatment with intraoperative and/or postoperative adjuvant radiation, chemotherapy, or cryotherapy in order to avoid possible vascular or neurologic injury.

A staging system that divides the vertebrae into four anatomic zones and three degrees of tumor extension (intraosseous, extraosseous, and metastatic) is used to plan the surgical method and resection margins for spinal tumors (Fig. 3). Zones 1 and 2 make up the posterior spinal elements, transverse process, and pedicle to the level of the vertebral body, while zone 3 comprises the anterior vertebral body. Zone 4 is the transition area between the anterior and posterior vertebrae.

A posterior midline incision is used to approach zone 1 lesions, with the extent of incision dependent on the extent of the posterior soft-tissue mass. Bilateral en bloc resection of the lamina can be performed to remove the overlying soft tissue and spinous process. Tumors that involve the lamina can be resected en bloc by osteotomy of the transverse process and pedicle on the involved side and resection of the lamina on the contralateral side. If a facet joint is not excised in the resection, then spinal reconstruction usually is not required.

A posterolateral incision is used for zone 2 lesions. Cutting the lamina on the uninvolved side as well as partial resection into zone 4 is often necessary to obtain a wide margin. For tumors that have an extraosseous component, resection of the exiting nerve root is normally required for a wide surgical margin. Because this resection includes the superior and inferior facets, the resulting segmental instability requires posterior instrumentation and fusion. Because most of the posterior structures are resected, anterior interbody fusion is sometimes needed to ensure bony union.

An anterior approach is used for zone 3 lesions. The resection will extend from end plate to end plate for smaller lesions. If more than 50% of the vertebral body is resected or the resection extends into one of the adjacent disks, most surgeons will reconstruct the defect following the resection.

A combined anterior and posterior approach is used for zone 4 lesions. Total vertebrectomy is normally required to gain a clear margin in these transition zone tumors. Posterior resection is begun by cutting through the transverse processes and pedicles bilaterally. Following the en bloc resection of the posterior elements, a posterior stabilization is then performed. A second anterior spinal approach is then used to perform an en bloc resection of the anterior spine from the level of the disk above to the disk below. An anterior reconstruction is then added to stabilize the spine. A total en bloc spondylectomy is sometimes performed through a single posterior approach. Following the posterior element resection, blunt dissection of the area around the vertebral body is performed posterolaterally. Retractors are placed that protect structures anterior to the vertebrae and the ante-

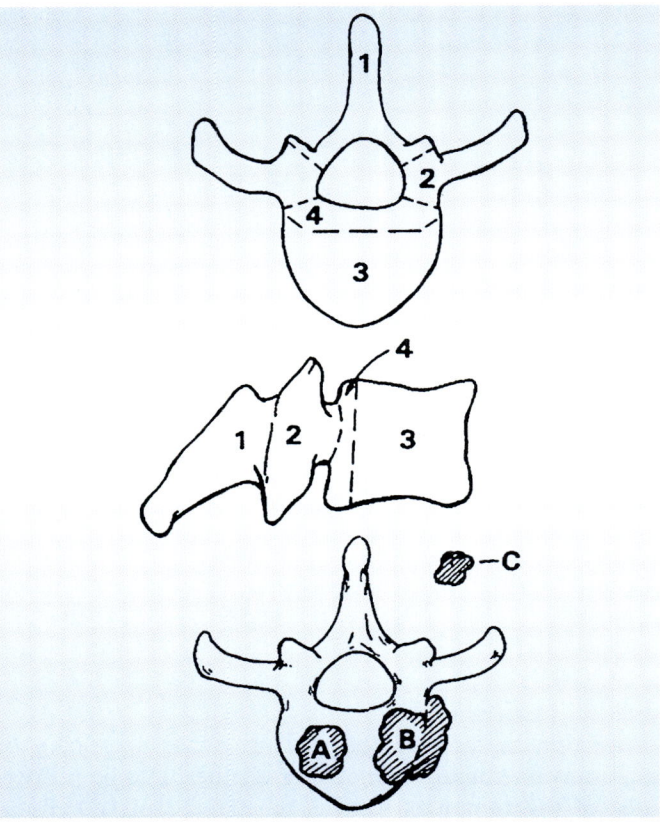

Figure 3 Tumor staging. Axial (*top*) and lateral (*center*) views of the vertebral body showing four zones of tumor involvement and three stages of tumor progression (*bottom*). Stage A = intraosseous; stage B = extraosseous; stage C = distant metastasis. (*Reproduced from Beaty JH (ed):* Orthopaedic Knowledge Update 6. *Rosemont, IL, American Academy of Orthopaedic Surgeons, 1999, pp 723-736.*)

rior body is mobilized by transecting the disks and anterior and posterior longitudinal ligaments. En bloc resection of the vertebral body is performed posterolaterally. A combined anterior and posterior reconstruction is then performed.

Spinal Stabilization
The goal of spinal stabilization is to help compensate for the resulting instability caused by resection and permit postoperative imaging (CT and MRI) so that tumor recurrence can be monitored. Posterior segmental fixation with hooks and screws can stabilize the spine. The use of titanium implants allows improved imaging because there is less metal artifact on both CT and MRI.

When a vertebral body resection is performed, an anterior weight-bearing strut reconstruction is required to provide necessary axial, torsional, and sagittal rigidity. Untreated anterior column deficiencies expose both anterior and posterior fixation devices to cantilever loads that will lead to construct failure. When a total vertebrectomy is performed, combined anterior and posterior reconstruction is necessary to achieve adequate stability.

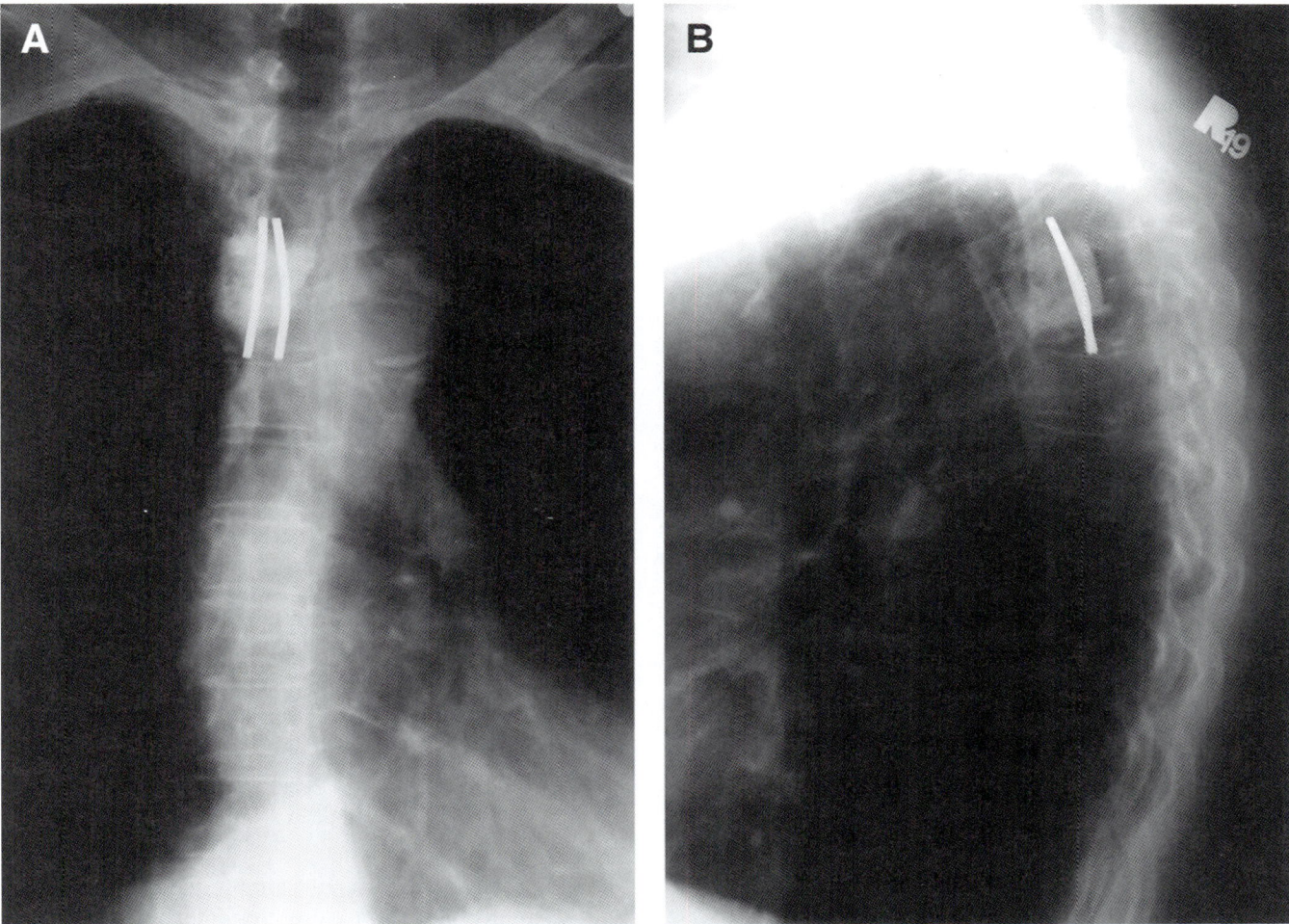

Figure 4   **A** and **B,** AP and lateral radiographs of cement reconstruction of metastatic breast carcinoma in the thoracic spine.

In cases that will require adjuvant radiation therapy, there is very poor potential for incorporation of biologic struts (iliac crest grafts) placed at the time of surgery; therefore, a nonbiologic strut should be considered. Polymethylmethacrylate (PMMA) reconstruction with pins or rods placed into the adjacent vertebrae can serve as an inexpensive reconstruction, but this method offers no potential for biologic healing (Fig. 4). However, in patients with limited life expectancy, this option can provide immediate stability. The PMMA construct can be protected with a posterior bony fusion in those patients with expected survival of more than 12 to 18 months. Several other anterior strut devices have been designed to stabilize the anterior spine and can be called vertical cages. These devices are adjustable and can be bone grafted to offer the potential for biologic incorporation. In cases for which adjuvant radiation is not required, these devices or structural bone grafts (iliac crest or structural allograft) can provide the initial load-sharing capacity of an anterior strut as well as the possibility for biologic fusion. In a

few centers, bioceramic or foam metal implants, which have some osteoconductive potential to reconstruct these defects, are being used.

Tumor Types

Metastatic Tumors

Because surgical treatment cannot cure metastatic carcinoma, it is only undertaken after conservative therapies have failed. Grading scales have been developed to help predict a patient's expected survival and chance of recovery based on individual characteristics of the patient and tumor; however, the reliability of these scores still needs to be demonstrated. Treatment of recurrent tumors is more difficult; therefore, an adequate resection and stabilization should be performed initially.

In most patients with symptomatic spinal metastases, treatment with external bracing and irradiation is successful. Advanced bony destruction often requires surgical stabilization to either restore spinal stability or prevent instability. Surgical stabilization with a posterior spinal instrumentation can be followed by adjuvant radiotherapy to gain local control of radiosensitive tumors. If the tumor is not radiosensitive or there is significant thecal sac compression from an anterior tumor, then either a circumferential or posterolateral reconstruction can combine neural decompression with spinal stabilization.

The primary goal of treatment for metastatic tumors with neurologic involvement is decompression of the neurologic elements. Radiation therapy is the treatment of choice for radiosensitive tumors with gradual onset of compression. Surgical decompression and reconstruction via the most direct approach should be undertaken when progression of symptoms is rapid and the tumor is unresponsive to radiation or due to bony compression from a pathologic fracture. When there is an isolated metastasis from a tumor with the potential for long-term survival, or when radiosensitivity is poor, then complete en bloc resection with wide excision of the lesion should be considered.

Special considerations must be given when treating renal cell metastases. These tumors can be extremely vascular and catastrophic hemorrhage can occur during attempted resections or biopsy procedures. If a primary renal tumor is identified, then angiography and embolization of the neovascular tumor should be performed within 24 hours of the planned resection.

Benign Primary Tumors

These tumors are treated with intralesional curettage and excision for tumors with a limited potential for local recurrence, such as aneurysmal bone cyst, osteoblastoma, osteoid osteoma, or osteochondroma via the most direct surgical approach. Although curettage and bone grafting may be adequate for many of these tumors, spinal reconstruction may be necessary if the resection causes a focal instability. Because of the proximity of vital structures such as the aorta and vena cava, the recurrence of benign tumors can be lethal. Therefore, en bloc excision should be considered in tumors with higher risk of local recurrence.

Osteochondroma

Although these tumors rarely are symptomatic, symptoms can occur with impingement of neural tissues by the osteochondroma. Eighty percent of symptomatic osteochondromas occur in the cervical and upper thoracic spine. The expanding cartilage cap seen on MRI can compress upon either the spinal cord or nerve root. En bloc or piecemeal excision can provide adequate neural decompression with little risk of local recurrence. When the chondral cap is greater than 2 cm thick, it is possible

that the tumor may represent a chondrosarcoma and not just a simple osteochondroma.

Osteoid Osteoma

An osteoid osteoma frequently will present as a painful and progressive scoliosis, and is often difficult to detect on plain radiographs because of the overlying soft tissue and bony shadows around the spinal column. A bone scan is the most reliable means to localize these tumors. The tumor can be defined with a follow-up fine cut CT scan of the suspected area. Complete surgical excision of the tumor nidus will relieve pain. Radiofrequency ablation of these lesions under CT guidance is being used in some centers to effectively treat patients.

Osteoblastoma

This tumor is large (72 cm) and is histologically indistinguishable from an osteoid osteoma. A characteristic cortical expansion with a rim of reactive bone can be seen at the tumor margin on either plain radiographs or CT scan. Osteoblastomas typically involve the posterior spinal elements and a reactive and progressive scoliosis can often be seen. Either en bloc excision or curettage and bone grafting can provide acceptable long-term results. Recurrence is uncommon, but is usually cured by repeated resection and bone grafting.

Hemangioma

Hemangiomas of the spinal column are quite common and normally asymptomatic, characterized by prominent vertical trabeculae seen as vertical striations on plain radiographs and as a stippled pattern on CT scan. Most hemangiomas are discovered as an incidental finding on MRI, where a bright T2 lesion will be seen within the vertebral body. Progressive bony destruction and deformity are rare with these tumors. For the few lesions that cause progressive bone destruction that will lead to neural compression and vertebral collapse, surgical decompression and reconstruction through an anterior approach is normally effective (Fig. 5). Over the past decade, vertebroplasty (the placement of PMMA into a vertebral body) has been used in France to treat these lesions and reinforce the vertebral body via a percutaneous route.

Eosinophilic Granuloma

This tumor is commonly seen in children younger than 10 years of age. Involvement in the spine usually is associated with an isolated eosinophilic granuloma, Hand-Schüller-Christian syndrome, or Letterer-Siwe disease. Radiographs usually will demonstrate a vertebrae plana; however, infection and Ewing's sarcoma also can be present. Percutaneous needle biopsy will establish the diagnosis. Except in the case of neuro-

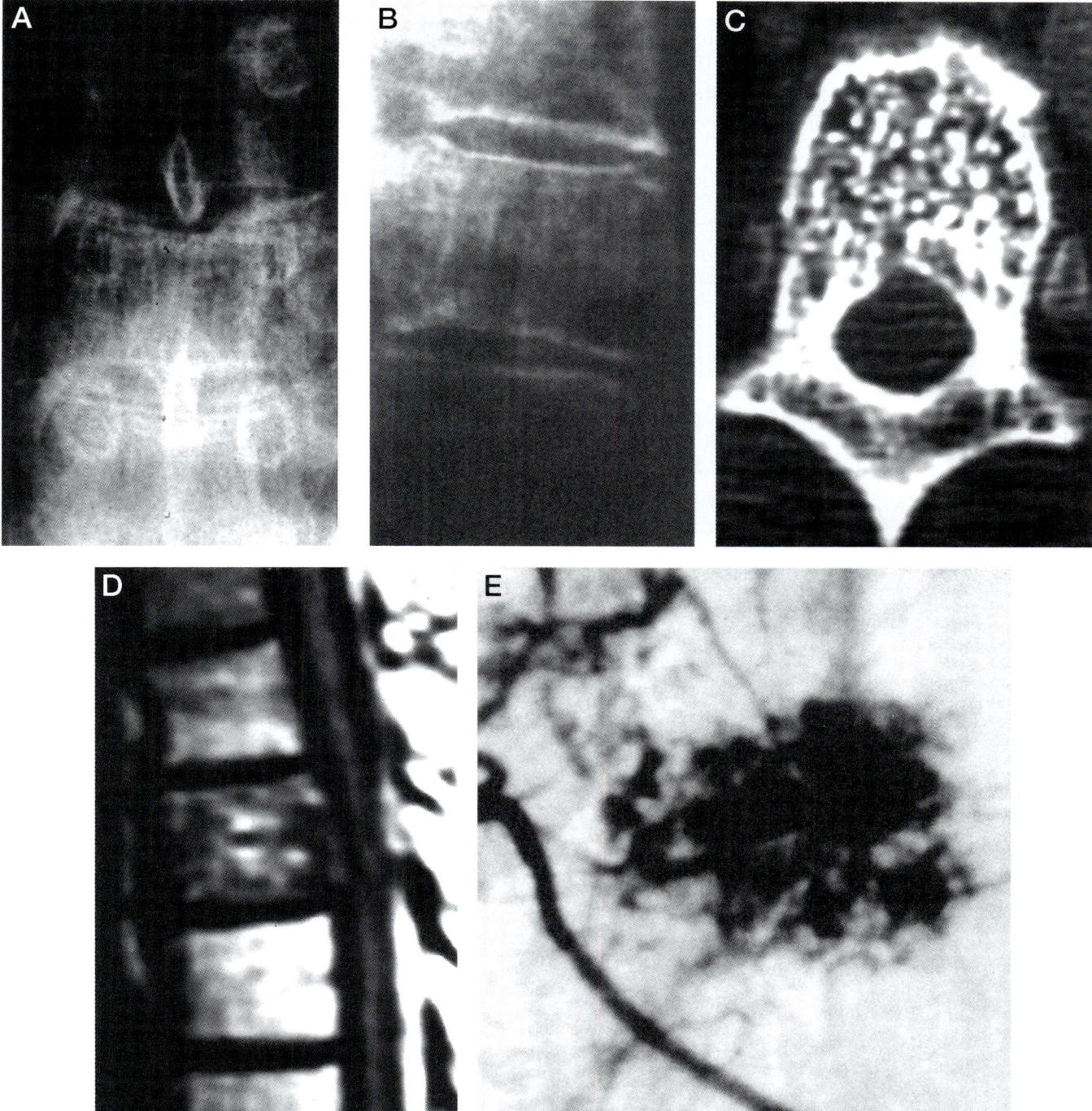

Figure 5 Vertebral hemangioma in a 48-year-old man. **A,** AP and **B,** lateral radiographs with coarse trabeculae. **C,** Typical CT scan showing trabeculae. **D,** Heterogenous T1 MRI study. **E,** Typical angiogram.

logic symptoms, patients can be treated with bracing and observation, which often result in reconstitution of vertebral body height as spinal growth proceeds. In the face of neurologic compromise, surgical decompression, strut grafting, and immobilization may be necessary. Radiation therapy is now reserved for any recurrent lesions.

Aneurysmal Bone Cysts

Although common in the posterior elements of the lumbar spine, aneurysmal bone cysts can be seen in any portion of the spine. An expansile lesion with an osteolytic center is seen on imaging studies. The cortical bone is often disrupted, with strands of bone within the lesion giving a typical bubbly appearance. Curet-

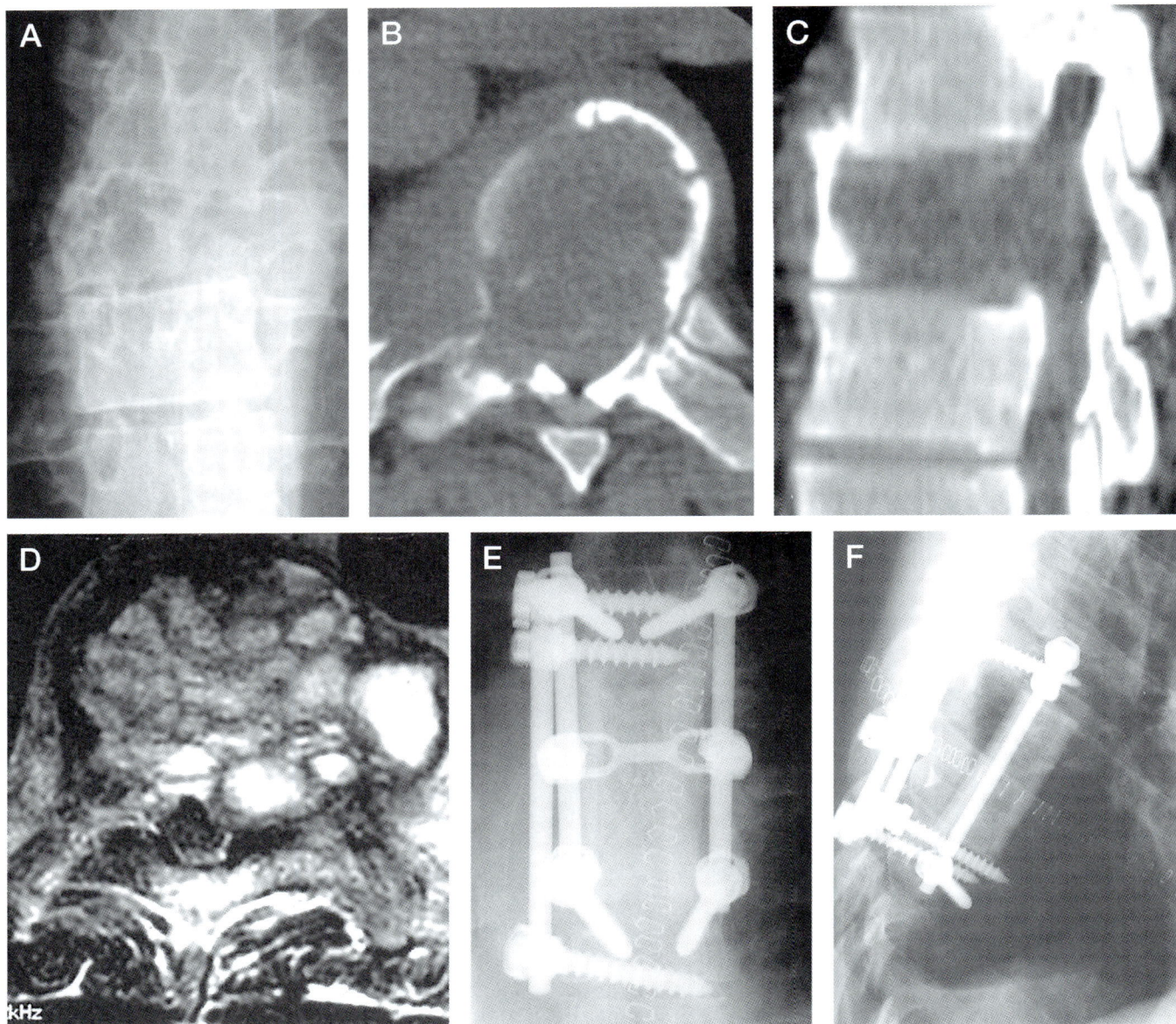

Figure 6 T8 aneurysmal bone cyst and pathologic fracture in a 37-year-old man. **A,** AP radiograph with pathologic fracture. **B** and **C,** Axial CT scan and reconstruction showing bone destruction. **D,** T2 Axial MRI study with fluid-filled lesion. **E** and **F,** AP and lateral radiographs after corpectomy and combined AP reconstruction.

tage is sufficient for most primary and recurrent lesions located in the posterior spinal elements. When lesions involve the anterior spinal elements, a more formal excision and reconstruction should be considered because of the proximity of vital structures that could be affected by a recurrence (Fig. 6).

Locally Aggressive Tumors

In the treatment of a tumor that demonstrates a locally aggressive biology, a more rigorous approach must be undertaken because of the proximity of vital structures and the spinal cord. Local invasion of the primary lesion or recurrence into the aorta, vena cava, or dura

can lead to death or paralysis. Therefore, the optimal treatment for a benign or malignant locally aggressive tumor is an en bloc excision with a clear surgical margin when possible.

Locally Aggressive Benign Tumors
Giant Cell Tumors

Giant cell tumors are most commonly seen in the third and fourth decade of life and appear lytic on plain radiographs with marginal sclerosis and a geographic pattern of bone destruction. They arise most commonly in the vertebral body and the vertebral cortex expands as they grow. Because of the locally aggressive nature of these tumors and the difficulty with achieving clean margins in revision surgery, every effort must be made to perform an en bloc excision when possible. Even though they rarely metastasize and demonstrate a benign histology, giant cell tumors of the spine can often cause death if local control of the tumor is not achieved. Total vertebrectomy through a combined anterior and posterior approach allows for a clear margin and a stable reconstruction. If preoperative vertebral body fracture precludes a clean margin, then adjuvant local therapies such as cryotherapy, intraoperative or postoperative brachytherapy, or standard postoperative radiotherapy should be considered to obtain a clean tumor bed.

Primary Malignant Tumors
Stage A Tumors
Stage A tumors have not yet extended beyond the bone. Thus, when a posterior-based tumor must be excised, a longitudinal posterior approach incorporating any previous biopsy wound can be performed. The entire biopsy tract and a cuff of normal surrounding muscle are excised en bloc with the tumor. Laminectomy at the level above and below the tumor allows isolation and resection of the involved elements by cutting through the uninvolved lamina or pedicles. The spine can then be reconstructed with a posterior instrumentation and fusion.

For stage A anterior column lesions, a combined anterior and posterior approach is required to obtain a surgical margin. First, the posterior elements, pedicles, and posterior anulus are resected to free the vertebral body for removal via an anterior approach. Posterior stabilization of the spine and then an anterior en bloc corpectomy are performed. After freeing the great vessels, adjacent disks are excised back through the posterior longitudinal ligament and then the vertebral body removed en bloc. Excision of any involved dura can be done, if needed, and repair with a fascial graft can be performed to gain local control. Reconstruction of the anterior column with a structural graft or cage and fixation can then be performed. Total spondylectomy has been recently performed via a single posterior approach, with posterolateral dissection used to free the great vessels from the vertebral body before removing the vertebral body from the posterior incision.

Stage B Tumors
Stage B tumors have locally extended beyond the osseous confines, resulting in mechanical instability. As the deformity progresses pain will develop and the neural elements will be threatened. The principles of treatment of these lesions are the same as those for stage A tumors. A surgical margin through normal tissues is still the goal of treatment. Because of the extraosseous tumor extension, excision margins must include extraosseous tissues. Adjuvant therapies play an even larger role in treatment of stage B tumors. Intraoperative or perioperative radiotherapy can be used to enhance local control of the tumor bed. In addition, the surgical reconstruction must also treat a deformity or residual instability from the resection.

Stage C Tumors
Stage C tumors are characterized by extensive collapse and metastatic lesions at the time of patient presentation; a surgical margin is not always possible. Local and systemic control of disease will depend on the success of adjuvant therapy. An intralesional resection can debulk a radiosensitive tumor (such as chondrosarcoma or chordoma) and prepare the area for reconstruction. However, a surgical margin still should be attempted whenever possible.

Lesions of the distal sacrum will require a partial sacral amputation through a combined anterior and posterior approach. The exiting nerve roots at the involved segments are sacrificed; for higher sacral lesions, this may cause the loss of bowel or bladder function. Bowel and bladder continence can be maintained if the S2 roots can be preserved bilaterally, or the S2 and S3 root can be spared on one side. The involvement of a colorectal general surgeon in the assessment of these patients is critical. If the tumor has spread from the sacrum and invaded the rectum, then the tumor must be excised through a combined sacrectomy and low anterior resection.

Low-Grade Primary Malignancies
Chordoma
Chordoma is a rare, slow-growing tumor of the axial skeleton that arises from notochordal stem cell nests within either the base of the skull, sacrococcygeal region, or a vertebral segment. These tumors are most often found in the spine and sacrum and demonstrate a tendency for unyielding local progression and aggressive recurrences. The histology is more aggressive in younger patients. Because of the anatomic location of most chordomas, they can reach remarkable size before detection and patients may experience progressive pain, sitting intolerance, and constipation for 1 year or longer.

Chordoma is generally unresponsive to radiation or chemotherapy; therefore, surgical margin is critical to local control and long-term survival. Approximately 5% of patients with a spinal chordoma develop metastases; however, almost 70% die as a result of local tumor extension and recurrence. Biopsy to confirm the diagnosis should never be done through the rectal vault, because this will necessitate colectomy at the time of resection. Total en bloc corpectomy is required for vertebral lesions.

Chondrosarcoma

Almost 10% of all chondrosarcomas are in either the spinal column or sacrum. Chondosarcoma is typically resistant to radiation and chemotherapy and can be difficult to remove from the spinal column. The key to long-term patient survival is gaining local control of the tumor. Chondrosarcoma produces extensive bony destruction and prominent soft-tissue mass that are best seen with CT and MRI. If possible, an extralesional resection with a wide margin should be performed (Fig. 7). Intraoperative radiotherapy or perioperative high-dose brachytherapy may provide improved local tumor control when a clear margin is not possible. In some centers, proton beam radiation has shown some promise in these difficult cases.

High-Grade Primary Malignancies

Osteosarcoma

Spinal osteosarcoma arises from the vertebral body in 95% of cases. Median survival of patients with osteosarcoma of the spine ranges from 6 to 18 months following diagnosis regardless of the surgical approach. When local control can be obtained with a surgical margin, then patient survival is comparable to that of an extremity lesion. Unfortunately, complete excision is possible in less than half of all spinal osteosarcomas.

Plain radiographs will reveal cortical destruction, soft-tissue calcification, and periosteal reactions. Pathologic fractures and vertebral collapse may be present in some patients. Paraspinal soft-tissue involvement can involve vascular, neural, and other contiguous structures. Before either biopsy or surgical resection is attempted, CT and MRI can delineate the extent of a tumor. Adjuvant chemotherapy and extensive anterior and posterior resection are examples of treatment protocols that have improved local tumor control, neurologic function, and patient survival.

Ewing's Sarcoma

Ewing's sarcoma of the spine may present as either a primary or metastatic lesion with 3.5% of all lesions arising primarily in the spine. These tumors are characterized by a permeative destructive pattern that is often difficult to detect on plain radiographs, with vertebral collapse and vertebra plana on the first radiographic findings. Neurologic symptoms may occur as a result of intraspinal tumor extension before findings are identified on plain radiographs. MRI shows the frequently significant extraspinal involvement seen in these tumors that is usually present at initial diagnosis and is a result of the tumor's rapid growth. Fortunately, Ewing's sarcomas can be successfully treated with a combination of multiagent chemotherapy and radiation therapy. Surgery is indicated only to confirm diagnosis as well as decompress neural tissues or stabilize the spinal column. Laminectomies in the thoracic and thoracolumbar spine often place children at high risk to develop kyphosis. The prognosis for Ewing's sarcoma of the spine is generally worse than that for extremity lesions, but promising results have been obtained using current chemotherapy and radiation regimen, resulting in almost 50% 5-year survival.

Solitary Plasmacytoma

Although both are B cell lymphoproliferative diseases, solitary plasmacytoma and multiple myeloma tend to behave in biologically different ways. Multiple myeloma is a quickly progressing and often lethal disseminated disease that normally affects the spine. Although recent advances in treatment regimens offer hopes of improved survival, spinal involvement with multiple myeloma is typically treated in the same manner as a metastatic carcinoma (Fig. 8). Solitary plasmacytoma will frequently degenerate into disseminated myeloma, but nearly 60% of patients remain disease free at 5 years.

Recommended therapy for plasmacytoma, which is radiosensitive, is a course of radiation therapy. Surgery plays a role in diagnosis of these lesions or decompression of neural structures and stabilization of the spinal column in cases of severe destruction. Surgery is the treatment of choice for recurrent lesions in which en bloc resection and prophylactic reconstruction with repeat radiotherapy may provide extended disease-free survival.

Lymphoma

Lymphoma of the spine can occur as an isolated lesion or as a focal involvement of disseminated disease. Surgery may be used in conjunction with chemotherapy and radiation therapy. In cases of solitary lymphoma, local control can be enhanced if an en bloc resection is possible. In the presence of widespread disease, surgical decompression or spinal stabilization may be indicated if neurologic compromise or instability is present.

Pediatric Tumors

Neuroblastoma

Neuroblastoma is a highly aggressive malignancy that can spread to the spine via either vascular dissemination or contiguous spread from the retroperitoneal space, and is responsible for nearly one third of all pediatric spinal tumors. Treatment is with excision, chemotherapy, and radiation therapy, and overall prognosis is poor. Because of the effects of radiation on a young growing spine, patients who survive

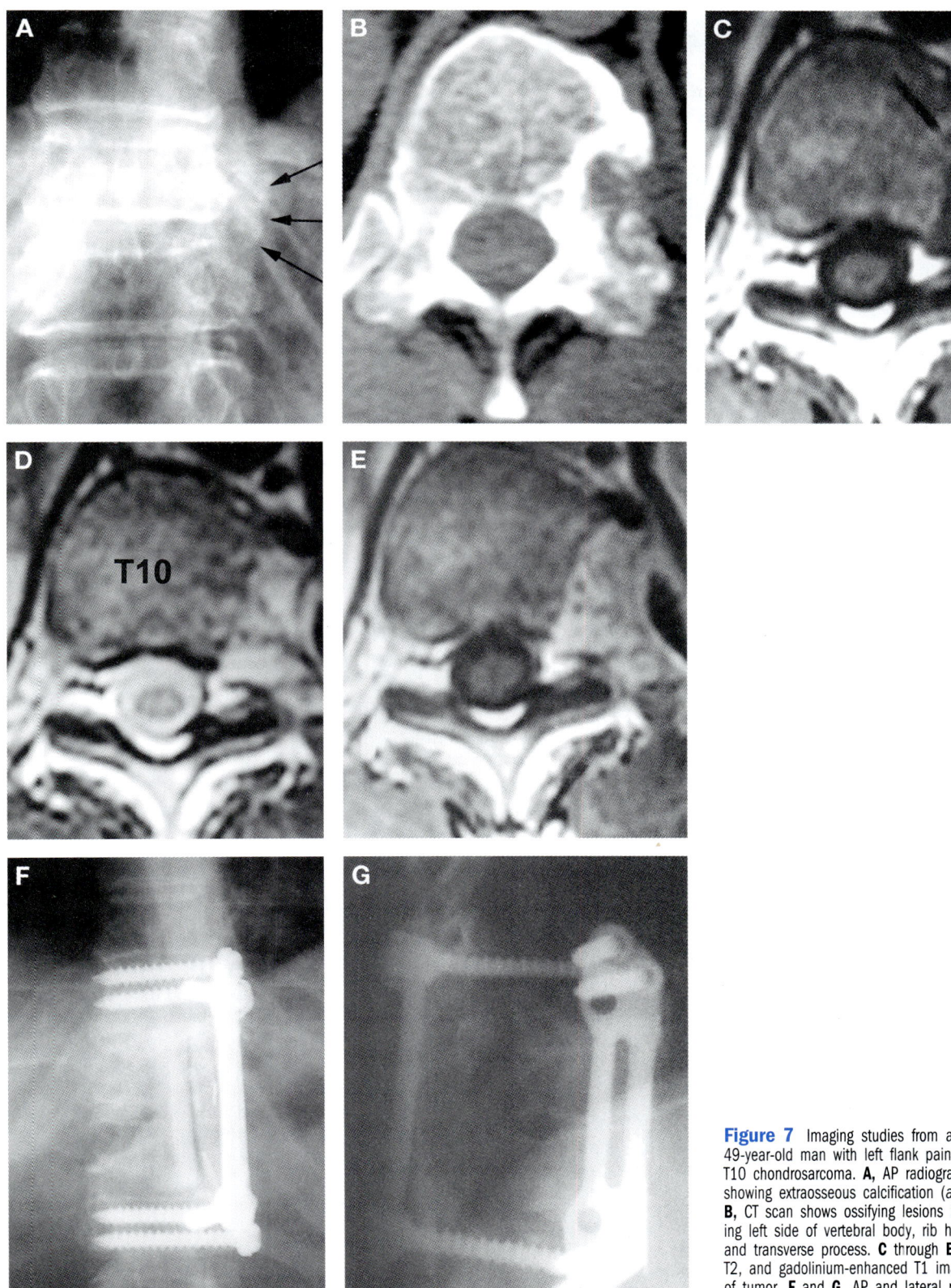

Figure 7 Imaging studies from a 49-year-old man with left flank pain and T10 chondrosarcoma. **A,** AP radiograph showing extraosseous calcification (*arrows*). **B,** CT scan shows ossifying lesions involving left side of vertebral body, rib head, and transverse process. **C** through **E,** T1, T2, and gadolinium-enhanced T1 images of tumor. **F** and **G,** AP and lateral radiographs following en bloc tumor excision and reconstruction with negative margin.

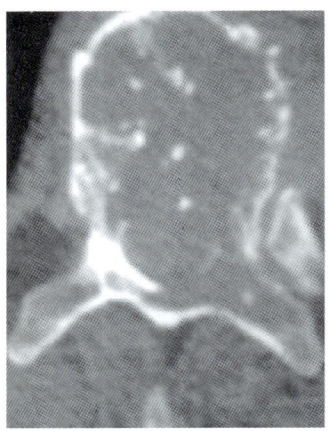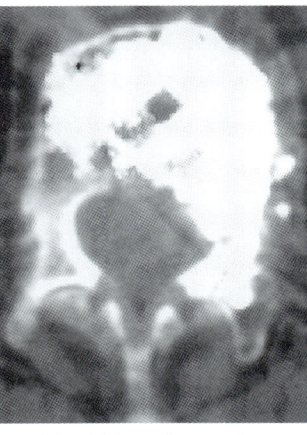

Figure 8 CT scans of a 57-year-old woman with multiple myeloma and severe pain. Lytic lesion in L1 vertebral body before **(A)** and after **(B)** vertebroplasty. Cement filling was performed with CT guidance to allow careful filling of entire lesion and pedicle area.

are at high risk for developing a rapidly progressive scoliosis.

Leukemia

Leukemia may result in single or multiple vertebral lesions in patients with systemic disease. Back pain is common and can lead to vertebral collapse. The primary treatment for the spinal lesion (and simultaneously, the systemic disease), is chemotherapy and radiation therapy. If spinal instability or neural compression is present, then surgery may be performed.

Emerging Technology

Physicians have recently begun to use percutaneous procedures to treat a variety of spinal conditions. Vertebroplasty has been used to treat osteoporotic compression fractures in the United States. In a few centers, lytic lesions from multiple myeloma or metastatic carcinoma are being cemented to restore local stability and avoid the need for open reconstruction. This technique is associated with a 10% chance of neurologic complication. With future advances in materials and imaging, these techniques play an increasing role in the treatment of spinal tumors. In addition, better methods of focal radiation such as intraoperative radiotherapy, perioperative brachytherapy, and confocal proton beam radiation have been proposed that will enhance the ability to gain local control of spinal tumors and improve patient survival. Total en bloc vertebrectomy, once considered a radical procedure, is now starting to be associated with increased patient survival as compared with intralesional excision.

Annotated Bibliography

Bergh P, Kindblom LG, Gunterberg B, Remotti F, Ryd W, Meis-Kindblom JM: Prognostic factors in chordoma of the sacrum and mobile spine: A study of 39 patients. *Cancer* 2000;88:2122-2134.

Thirty sacral and nine spine chordoma were treated surgically. Twenty-three wide surgical margins and 16 marginal/intralesional margins were obtained. At a mean 8.1 years follow-up, 44% of patients developed a recurrence. Estimated 5-, 10-, 15-, and 20-year survival rates were 84%, 64%, 52%, and 52%, respectively.

Boriani S, De Iure F, Bandiera S, et al: Chondrosarcoma of the mobile spine: Report on 22 cases. *Spine* 2000;25:804-812.

In 22 cases of chondrosarcoma of the mobile spine treated with either en bloc excision or curettage, 3 recurrences occurred in 14 en bloc excisions while 8 of 10 patients treated with piecemeal excision died of disease. En bloc excision with a clean surgical margin is the suggested management for chondrosarcoma.

Durr HR, Maier M, Pfahler M, Baur A, Refior HJ: Surgical treatment of osseous metastases in patients with renal cell carcinoma. *Clin Orthop* 1999;367: 283-290.

In 45 patients who underwent surgical treatment for osseous renal cell metastasis, wide resections were performed in 7 and palliative or diagnostic procedures in 38. Overall survival was 49% at 1 year, 39% at 2 years, and 15% at 5 years. Nine patients with solitary bone metastasis more than 12 months after primary tumor resection showed a 5-year survival of 54%.

Kanayama M, Ng JT, Cunningham BW, Abumi K, Kaneda K, McAfee PC: Biomechanical analysis of anterior versus circumferential spinal reconstruction for various anatomic stages of tumor lesions. *Spine* 1999;24:445-450.

The authors studied anterior, posterior, and circumferential reconstructions for spinal defects simulating corpectomy, subtotal spondylectomy, and total spondylectomy at the T12 level in human cadaveric spines. All reconstructions except for anterior-only instrumentation for total spondylectomy returned the stiffness to a level equal or higher than that of the intact spine.

Kawahara N, Tomita K, Matsumoto T, Fujita T: Total en bloc spondylectomy for primary malignant vertebral tumors. *Chir Organi Mov* 1998;83:73-86.

The authors report on a new surgical technique for en bloc excision of primary malignant spinal tumors via a single surgical approach. Seven patients underwent en bloc spondylectomy and at final follow-up there were no local recurrences; however, one patient did die of mediastinal tumor at 3 months.

Wise JJ, Fischgrund JS, Herkowitz HN, Montgomery D, Kurz LT: Complication, survival rates, and risk factors of surgery for metastatic disease of the spine. *Spine* 1999;24:1943-1951.

The authors retrospectively reviewed the risk factors for complication, complication rates, and survival rates in patients with metastatic disease of the spine. Eighty patients surgically treated for spinal metastasis demonstrated a mean survival time of 16 months and a 25% complication rate. Seventy-five percent of patients maintained neural function, 20% improved one Frankel grade, and 5% of patients experienced a decrease in neural function.

Classic Bibliography

Bohlman HH, Sachs BL, Carter JR, Riley L, Robinson RA: Primary neoplasms of the cervical spine: Diagnosis and treatment of twenty-three patients. *J Bone Joint Surg Am* 1986;68:483-494.

Boriani S, Biagini R, De Iure F, et al: En bloc resections of bone tumors of the thoracolumbar spine: A preliminary report of 29 patients. *Spine* 1996;21:1927-1931.

Freiberg AA, Graziano GP, Loder RT, Hensinger RN: Metastatic vertebral disease in children. *J Pediatr Orthop* 1993;13:148-153.

Grubb MR, Currier BL, Pritchard DJ, Ebersold MJ: Primary Ewing's sarcoma of the spine. *Spine* 1994;19:309-313.

Harrington KD: Anterior decompression and stabilization of the spine as a treatment for vertebral collapse and spinal cord compression from metastatic malignancy. *Clin Orthop* 1988;233:177-197.

Kostuik JP, Errico TJ, Gleason TF, Errico CC: Spinal stabilization of vertebral column tumors. *Spine* 1988;13:250-256.

McLain RF, Weinstein JN: Solitary plasmacytomas of the spine: A review of 84 cases. *J Spinal Disord* 1989;2:69-74.

Pettine KA, Klassen RA: Osteoid-osteoma and osteoblastoma of the spine. *J Bone Joint Surg Am* 1986;68:354-361.

Samson IR, Springfield DS, Suit HD, Mankin HJ: Operative treatment of sacrococcygeal chordoma: A review of twenty-one cases. *J Bone Joint Surg Am* 1993;75:1476-1484.

Shives TC, Dahlin DC, Sim FH, Pritchard DJ, Earle JD: Osteosarcoma of the spine. *J Bone Joint Surg Am* 1986;68:660-668.

Simpson AH, Porter A, Davis A, Griffin A, McLeod RS, Bell RS: Cephalad sacral resection with a combined extended ilioinguinal and posterior approach. *J Bone Joint Surg Am* 1995;77:405-411.

Sundaresan N, Steinberger AA, Moore F, et al: Indications and results of combined anterior-posterior approaches for spine tumor surgery. *J Neurosurg* 1996;85:438-446.

Turcotte RE, Sim FH, Unni KK: Giant cell tumor of the sacrum. *Clin Orthop* 1993;291:215-221.

Chapter 57

Inflammatory Arthritis of the Spine

William M. Oxner, MD, FRCSC

James D. Kang, MD

Introduction

Rheumatoid arthritis is a systemic inflammatory disease that affects the entire musculoskeletal system. It is the most common inflammatory disorder affecting the cervical spine, with clinically significant disease occurring in up to 80% of patients after 10 years. The prevalence data on rheumatoid arthritis in the United States suggest that the disease occurs in 0.3% to 1.5% of the general population, with women being more likely affected than men. Up to 85% of patients may develop symptomatic cervical instability as a result of their disease and about 7% to 13% of these patients develop neurologic deficit secondary to bony subluxations and spinal cord or brainstem compression.

Biology

Certain individuals are genetically susceptible to rheumatoid arthritis and begin to produce a new antigen, which stimulates the immune system to produce an autoimmune inflammatory response. The antigenic stimulus triggers the body to produce rheumatoid factor, which is an immunoglobulin (IgM) directed against the Fc portion of the IgG antibody. Immune complexes are then formed and deposited within the synovium, resulting in complement activation and polymorphonucleocyte infiltration and beginning a cycle of inflammation. Histologically, the response somewhat resembles granulation tissue within the synovium. This tissue is populated by fibroblasts and other inflammatory cells and is called rheumatoid pannus. The pannus itself is a destructive mass that is full of collagenase and other proteolytic enzymes capable of destroying cartilage, ligaments, and bone. The rheumatoid process can affect any joint in which there is a synovial lining. The biologic destruction is just one of the mechanisms that initiates the subluxations seen in rheumatoid arthritis. There may be a biomechanical basis for cervical subluxation, which perpetuates the disease. A recent cineradiographic analysis of cervical motion showed that the normal cervical motion pattern consists of a well-regulated stepwise pattern that is initiated at the C1-2 level and is transmitted to the lower cervical spine. In rheumatoid arthritis, the motion is initiated at the unstable cervical levels. In patients with atlantoaxial instability, the motion starts at C1-2 significantly earlier than the C2-3 segment; in spines with subaxial subluxation, the motion in the unstable segment precedes that in the upper stable segments. These abnormal biomechanics show that motion stresses are concentrated at the unstable segments and probably contribute to the progression of the slip.

Rheumatoid arthritis very rarely has a clinical effect on the thoracic and lumbar spines. The cervical spine is most commonly affected, particularly occiput-C1 and C1-2 levels. The anatomy of the upper cervical region leaves it most susceptible to symptomatic subluxations and its complications. The occiput-C1 joint is a saddle joint and is actually much more stable than the C1-2 joint. Fifty percent of flexion and extension motion in the cervical spine occurs through the occiput-C1 articulation and 50% of the cervical spine's axial rotation occurs through C1-2. These joints, in combination with the rheumatoid destruction of the ligaments such as the transverse atlantoaxial ligament and the apical alar ligaments, leave the upper segments susceptible to translation in the sagittal plane. The translation in the sagittal plane may result in spinal stenosis. It is unclear whether the myelopathy that results from rheumatoid arthritis is the result of the degree of static canal stenosis or whether it is the result of excessive motion or dynamic instability. For example, some patients will present with myelopathy and no significant stenosis but with considerable motion detectable on flexion-extension films. Substantial bony destruction of the C1 lateral masses is often present, allowing the second cervical vertebra to migrate cephalad. In a recent study, a finite element model of the craniocervical junction in rheumatoid arthritis predicted that transverse atlantoaxial ligament failure is an essential part of increasing subluxation. The model also predicted that with the loss of transverse ligament stiffness, the loads transmitted to the odontoid process and the lateral masses of the atlas are decreased. Therefore, bone loss in these areas may not be caused by the destructive pannus alone but also may be secondary to the unloading that occurs with the mechanical environment created by loss of the transverse ligament. Pathologic studies of the spinal cord in patients with rheumatoid arthritis show that the spinal cord is thin and atrophic. There is evidence of axonal retraction balls in the white matter, as well as nuclear chromatolysis in the anterior horn cells. Some investigators believe that these pathologic changes are representative of the chronic abnormal motion that occurs in this state.

Types of Cervical Involvement

Three clinical conditions are common in the cervical spine affected by rheumatoid arthritis. The first is atlantoaxial instability (AAI), which is noted in up to 50% of patients with symptomatic rheumatoid subluxations. Most of these subluxations are anterior and are the result of the attenuation of the transverse atlantoaxial ligament as well as the apical ligaments, which allow the atlas to move forward on the axis. In 20% of cases the subluxation may be lateral and in 7% it may be posterior. The posterior subluxation is the result of complete destruction of the anterior aspect of the ring of the atlas, which allows the atlas to migrate posteriorly on the axis.

The second most common type of cervical subluxation is superior migration of the odontoid, also called cranial settling, atlantoaxial impaction, or basilar invagination. This condition represents about 40% of rheumatoid subluxations and can lead to direct compression of the brainstem. As the atlas migrates up through the foramen magnum, the head drifts into kyphosis and results in direct compression of the brainstem by the odontoid. The settling occurs due to the destruction of the lateral masses and erosions of the occipital condyles. This type of subluxation commonly occurs in conjunction with atlantoaxial instability and may represent a continuum of the disease process.

The third most common type is subaxial subluxation, which occurs as the result of destruction of facets, interspinous ligaments, and the intervertebral disks. This condition represents about 20% of the subluxations in the cervical spine and at times is seen at multiple levels, causing a stepladder deformity that often is associated with kyphosis. Each of these patterns of subluxations may occur in isolation or in conjunction with one of the other types of subluxation and must be carefully evaluated radiographically (on both static and flexion-extension films). Failure to identify basilar invagination on preoperative radiographs could result in disastrous consequences.

Natural History

The key to treatment of any disease is knowing the natural history of the disease process and recognizing the best time for some form of surgical or nonsurgical intervention. Unfortunately, the complete natural history of patients with rheumatoid subluxations is not well known, particularly because almost all patients have had some form of intervention. The prevalence of cervical involvement is estimated at 25% to 80%, depending on the inclusion criteria used. Cervical involvement usually begins early in the disease process and has been closely correlated with the extent of peripheral joint involvement. A recent study showed that the level of C-reactive protein (CRP), the number of joints with erosions, and the carpal height ratio significantly correlate with the stage and the natural history of upper cervical lesions and the development of subaxial subluxations. The average CRP levels in patients with progressive cervical lesions were significantly higher in those patients with nonprogressive lesions. Elevation of serum CRP could be a marker of the beginning of cervical subluxation. Seropositivity, history of steroid use, male sex, and greater hand deformity have been correlated with more extensive cervical involvement. It is well known that the longer a patient has rheumatoid arthritis the greater is the likelihood that cervical disease will develop. What is unknown, however, is what percentage of patients who develop cervical disease will progress to paralysis. In patients with neck symptoms, progression of subluxation has been observed in 35% to 85% of patients. A recent study has shown that rheumatoid arthritis of the neck typically progresses from isolated AAI to AAI with superior migration of the odontoid and finally to superior migration of the odontoid alone. With the final stage, the amount of atlantoaxial instability actually decreases; this phenomenon has been called pseudostabilization.

Cervical myelopathy has been noted to occur in 11% to 58% of patients with rheumatoid arthritis of the neck. In addition, a postmortem study has indicated that medullary compression may be the cause of death in approximately 10% of patients with rheumatoid arthritis. Once paralysis develops, most studies have shown that it is progressive and death is a common outcome if the condition is left untreated. A 1997 study showed that the cumulative expected survival in patients with untreated rheumatoid myelopathy is 7% in the first 7 years after the onset of myelopathy. Clinical manifestations of patients with rheumatoid disease

TABLE 1 | Ranawat Classification of Neurologic Deficit

Class I	Pain, no neurologic deficit
Class II	Subjective weakness, hyperreflexia, dysesthesias
Class III	Objective weakness, long tract signs
Class III A	Ambulatory
Class III B	Nonambulatory

(Reproduced with permission from Ranawat CS, O'Leary P, Pellicci P, et al: Cervical fusion in rheumatoid arthritis. J Bone Joint Surg Am 1979;61:1003–1010.)

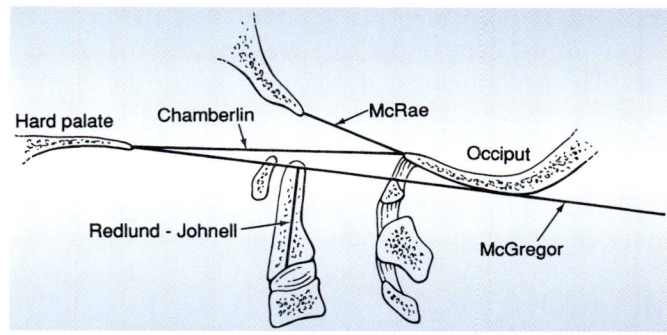

Figure 1 Schematic of the upper cervical spine showing some of the reference lines for measuring basilar invagination. *(Reproduced with permission from Boden SC, Clark CR: Rheumatoid arthritis of the cervical spine, in Clark CR (ed): The Cervical Spine, ed 3. Philadelphia, PA, Lippincott-Raven, 1998, pp 693-703.)*

of the cervical spine can be quite varied and many patients (50%) may remain asymptomatic despite instability noted on flexion-extension films. Neck pain is common and may occur in 40% to 80% of patients with AAI and may be associated with occipital headaches. Ear pain, occipital neuralgia, and facial pain all can occur secondary to compression of the C2 posterior ramus. Patients may also report myelopathic symptoms such as weakness, gait disturbance, loss of dexterity, and paresthesias in the hands. Some patients complain of a feeling of their head falling forward in flexion. Later in the myelopathic process there may be urinary retention or incontinence. Shock-like sensations in the torso or extremities (Lhermitte's sign) may be reported. Vertebrobasilar insufficiency has been reported but is uncommon. Similar symptoms such as visual disturbance, loss of equilibrium, vertigo, tinnitus, and dysphagia also may be caused by brainstem compression. In the end stage, patients become bedridden.

The examination of the rheumatoid patient is often difficult. As a group they do not display the classic signs of cervical myelopathy because their disease process is chronic and debilitating. Many of the patients have progressive peripheral disease, and peripheral joint, tendon, and nerve diseases may mask identification of subtle neurologic signs. Late signs of brainstem compression include nystagmus and Cheyne-Stokes respirations. Another emerging modality that may be an adjunct to the physical examination in the diagnosis of patients with early rheumatoid myelopathy is somatosensory-evoked potentials (SSEP). A recent study of this patient population showed that myelopathy was detectable by SSEP findings even in the absence of overt clinical findings. The authors recommend routine use of electrodiagnostic studies in the evaluation of these patients. The combination of the history and physical examination can be used to classify the patient according to the Ranawat criteria of rheumatoid myelopathy. This classification is useful in planning treatment, predicting recovery, and examining results (Table 1).

Imaging

Radiography is the standard imaging modality used for diagnosing and classifying rheumatoid cervical disease. Neutral position lateral radiographs have a low sensitivity. In a recent study of 65 rheumatoid patients with unstable atlantoaxial subluxation, lateral cervical radiographs taken in the neutral position were compared with the flexion-extension views. The neutral position radiograph would have failed to confirm the diagnosis in 48% of cases and would have failed to identify the severity in 66%. The standard series should include AP, lateral, and flexion-extension views of the cervical spine. Periodic radiographic evaluations should be performed on all patients with rheumatoid arthritis because up to 50% of affected patients may be asymptomatic. A retrospective study in rheumatoid patients undergoing total hip or knee arthroplasty found cervical spine abnormalities in 61% of patients on routine radiographic analysis (Fig. 1).

There are several common measurements that are used to diagnose and classify those patients with rheumatoid subluxations. The classic measurement is the anterior atlantodental interval (AADI). This measurement is taken from the posterior aspect of the anterior ring of C1 to the anterior aspect of the dens on lateral radiographs. The normal value is 3 mm or less in an adult and 4 mm or less in a child. In the past, surgeons used values of 8, 9, or 10 mm as a cutoff point for surgical intervention in patients with symptomatic atlantoaxial subluxation. However, this measurement has been found to have a relatively low specificity and sensitivity and a relatively low negative predictive value of paralysis. Some apparent differences between this value and the space available for the cord are that some patients have different canal diameters, there may be a variable amount of pannus (up to 3 mm) behind the odontoid, and in some patients the odontoid itself may be decreased in diameter secondary to the erosive disease. The posterior atlantodental interval (PADI) measurement is taken from the posterior aspect of the dens to the anterior aspect of the C1 lamina. This measurement has been shown to be a much better predictor of paralysis than the AADI. Using a PADI of 14 mm or less yields 97% sensitivity for predicting patients with paralysis. Ninety-four percent of patients with a PADI of greater than 14 mm had no neurologic deficit in a large retrospective study. The same study found that the AADI did not correlate with paralysis.

Superior migration of the odontoid can be measured in one of several different ways on lateral cervical radiographs. One of the difficulties in measuring these numbers on radiographs is that there can be marked destruction and osteopenia of bone in the proximal cervical spine, making identification of anatomic landmarks difficult. McGregor's line becomes one of the more reliable measurements because often the hard palate and the most caudal point of the occiput can still be identified, even late in the disease process. Vertical settling of the occiput has been defined as migration of the odontoid more than 4.5 mm above McGregor's line. The station of the atlas in relation to the axis can be measured as described by Clark. Another useful measurement is the Redlund-Johnell criterion. A value of less than 34 mm in men or 29 mm in women is considered abnormal and diagnostic of vertical settling. If any doubt remains regarding vertical migration of the odontoid, then MRI should be obtained. Radiographs can be difficult to interpret and MRI currently is the gold standard for documentation of vertical migration (Fig. 2).

Subaxial subluxation can usually be detected on the lateral flexion and extension radiographs. Traditionally, the slip has been quantified as a number of millimeters of olisthesis or as a percentage of slip in relation to the vertebral body's sagittal diameter. In this scheme more than 4 mm of translation or 20% slip has been considered a significant amount of olisthesis. More recently, investigators have identified that the sagittal diameter of the spinal canal correlates with the presence and degree of paralysis. Patients with canal diameters of 13 mm or less in the subaxial region are at high risk of developing paralysis.

MRI has surpassed CT-myelography and tomography as a diagnostic tool. A recent comparative study of conventional tomography with MRI showed that MRI more consistently revealed cystic changes in the odontoid process and the lateral masses of C1 and was better at detecting vertical migration. However, tomography was superior at detecting lateral subluxation, probably because coronal imaging was not used. MRI can reveal retrodental pannus and accurately quantify the space available for the cord. Spinal cord compres-

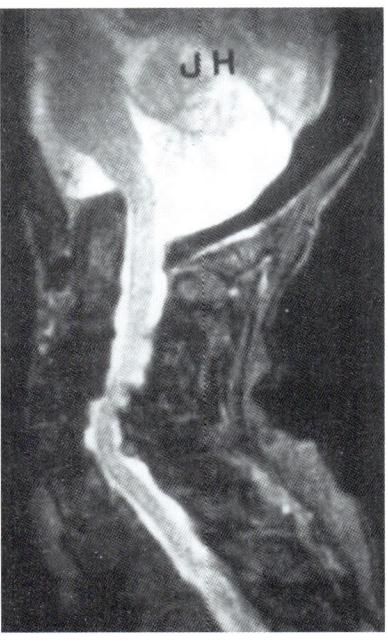

Figure 2 MRI scan of a patient with rheumatoid arthritis. Basilar invagination and subaxial subluxation with stenosis are apparent.

sion has been noted to be present in all rheumatoid patients with space available for the cord on MRI of 13 mm or less. MRI is also accurate at assessing the degree of superior migration of the odontoid and surpasses all other diagnostic tools at assessing the cervicomedullary angle, the angle measured between the long axis of the cervical cord and the brainstem. The normal measurement should be between 135° and 175°, and values of less than 135° have been shown to be closely correlated with myelopathy. In addition, an angle of less than 135° may mean that decompression of the cord may not be attainable from a posterior procedure alone. Flexion and extension MRI is a new test that is being investigated as an imaging modality for the rheumatoid cervical spine. A study of 42 rheumatoid arthritis patients undergoing flexion MRI revealed that the subarachnoid space is significantly narrowed at the atlantoaxial level and in the subaxial spine in flexion. However, there were no patients with a normal subarachnoid space in the neutral position and compression of the spinal cord in the flexed position. Another study showed that a space available for the cord of less than 6 mm in flexion correlates with paralysis. Adding a dynamic flexion MRI study to the sequence of a patient with a neurologic deficit and cord compression on the neutral MRI may be superfluous and potentially dangerous.

Nonsurgical and Surgical Treatment

The goals of nonsurgical treatment of patients with rheumatoid involvement of the cervical spine are threefold. The first goal is to avoid the development of an irreversible neurologic deficit. Patients with more severe neurologic deficits tend to show less potential for recovery and have a high rate of morbidity and mortality with surgical intervention. The second goal is to prevent sudden death by unrecognized brainstem compression, which has been noted at autopsy as the cause of death in up to 10% of cases. The third goal is to avoid unnecessary surgery. Fifty percent of patients with cervical involvement are asymptomatic and the natural history of their subluxations is unknown. In fact, many of these subluxations will stabilize in time.

The nonsurgical treatment of rheumatoid arthritis is mostly supportive. The severity of the subluxation in the cervical spine is correlated with the severity of the peripheral disease, and systemic treatment of the disease process by a rheumatologist is essential. It is unknown whether good medical management of the disease will halt or decrease the amount of cervical subluxations. Cervical collars may provide comfort in some patients with neck pain, but they may not protect against progressive subluxation or neurologic deficit. Cervical collars can reduce instability in patients with AAI. The effect is greatest if reduction is performed in the neutral position. However, rigid orthoses are poorly tolerated in this patient population because of temporomandibular subluxation and skin sensitivity. In some patients, the subluxations will stabilize with time and supportive care may be the definitive treatment. In others, the deterioration in function may be slow and insidious with subtle signs of myelopathy developing over several months or years. As such, careful observation and serial radiographic examination should be the mainstay of conservative care. In general, surgical stabilization has traditionally been indicated in the patient with intractable pain or clear-cut neurologic deficit. In addition, other high-risk patients, including those with radiographic evidence of superior migration of the odontoid, PADI of 14 mm or less, or subaxial canal diameter of 14 mm or less, should probably be included in this group.

Atlantoaxial Subluxation

In patients with isolated rheumatoid atlantodental instability and no neurologic deficit, nonsurgical management can be done safely provided that the PADI is more than 14 mm on the lateral radiograph. If the PADI is less than 14 mm, then an MRI study should be done to assess the true space available for the cord. If the MRI study shows significant retrodental pannus with a space available for the cord of 13 mm or less, a cervicomedullary angle of less than 135°, or a cord diameter in flexion of less than 6 mm, then a posterior C1-2 fusion should be strongly considered. If there is also an element of basilar invagination, then the fusion

should be extended to the occiput. If the subluxation is reducible or can be reduced with a short trial of preoperative traction, then the fusion can be performed with the Gallie or Brooks technique, posterior transarticular screws, or a combination of screws and wiring. In these osteoporotic patients, depending on the quality of the fixation, a halo vest may be used. If the deformity is irreducible, then it would be unsafe to pass wires under the arch of C1, and a C1 laminectomy should be performed in conjunction with the fusion. Laminectomy of C1 necessitates extending the fusion to the occiput. Posterior atlantoaxial facet fixation coupled with C1-2 wiring and bone grafting was shown to have a 92% union rate at 2 years. MRI studies have shown that when fusion is obtained, the retrodental pannus will resorb in the majority of patients. If the anterior compression is bony, then consideration should be given to performing transoral decompression prior to the posterior fusion (Fig. 3).

Basilar Invagination

Patients with basilar invagination have a high surgical morbidity and poor potential for neurologic recovery. Therefore, they should be treated with a more aggressive surgical approach than the patients with AAI. If basilar invagination is revealed radiographically, then an MRI scan should be performed. The MRI can be used to measure the cervicomedullary angle and to determine the degree of spinal cord compression. It is suggested that if there is any evidence of basilar invagination on either radiographs or MRI, or if there is evidence of cord compression or neurologic deficit, surgery is recommended. The role of preoperative traction in these patients is unclear, but it is often recommended to reduce the deformity and possibly spare an anterior procedure. An option for traction in these patients is halo wheelchair traction, which appears to be relatively well tolerated. The surgical procedure of choice in these patients is an occipitocervical fusion. Devices such as wires, loops, mesh, and plates have been used in occipitocervical fusion. Some studies have demonstrated superior results using modern plating techniques, with higher rates of neurologic improvement and lower rates of pseudarthrosis. Occipitocervical fusion using cervical pedicle screws in the axis and in the subaxial spine has recently been reported with good results. If reduction of the deformity is not obtained and there is still significant compression of the anterior brainstem, then the fusion should also be accompanied by a decompressive procedure such as a C1 laminectomy with enlargement of the foramen magnum, or an anterior transoral odontoid resection. If anterior transoral decompression is performed, then measures should be taken to avoid the division of the

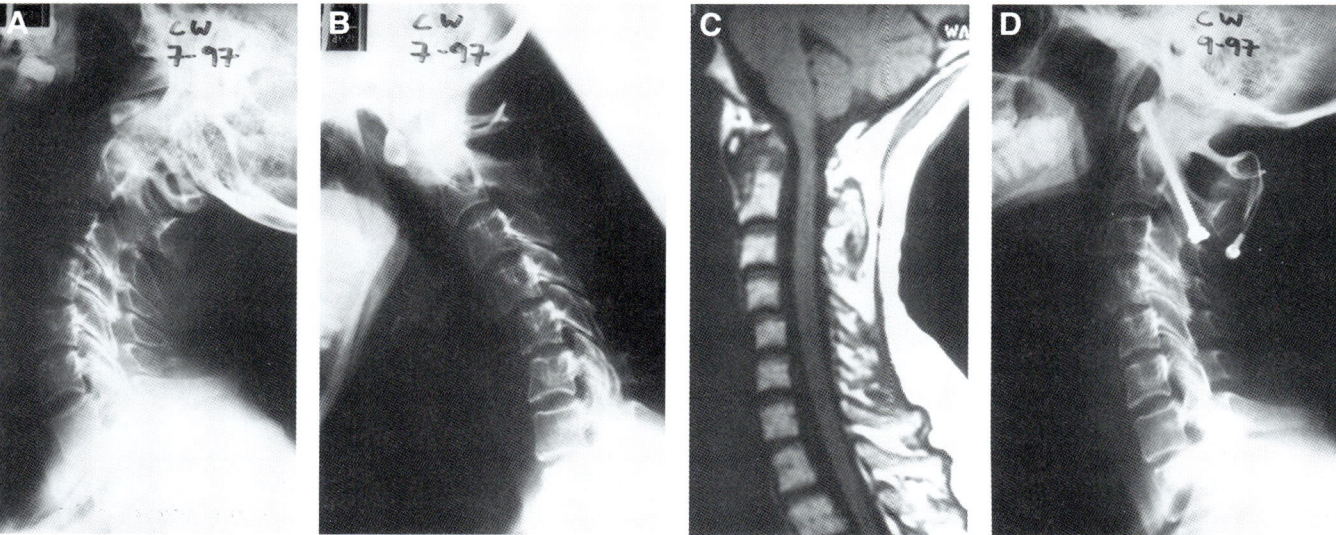

Figure 3 Radiographs and MRI scans of a 65-year-old woman with rheumatoid arthritis who presents with subtle signs of myelopathy. There is atlantoaxial instability (**A** and **B**) but cord signal change is not apparent on MRI (**C**). Atlantoaxial fusion with transarticular C1-2 screws and posterior wiring and bone graft were performed (**D**), with neurologic improvement noted postoperatively.

soft palate if possible. Division of the soft palate is associated with substantial increases in surgical morbidity. The decision of whether or not to perform a transoral decompression can be made by careful review of the preoperative MRI study. It is important to note that most of the compression in this type of subluxation is bony, and significant postoperative resorption will not occur as it does when the compression is secondary to pannus. However, there is some evidence that realigning the upper cervical spine and holding it there with rigid instrumentation may obviate the need for anterior decompressive surgery. A recent follow-up study of occipitocervical fusions showed that the incidence of cervical or nuchal pain is decreased in almost all cases. Myelopathy is relieved in about 67% of cases with improvement of one or more levels in the *Ranawat criteria*. No serious postoperative complications were seen except for one case of nonunion. The cumulative survival was 79.5% in the first 5 years and 27.5% after 10 years. The authors concluded that occipitocervical fusion using loops and wires is an acceptable method of relieving cervical myelopathy. Another recent report on occipitocervical fusions showed that there are some technical difficulties with fixation to the lateral occipital region with screws. Anatomic studies show that the bone in this area of the skull may be as little as 3 mm in thickness. In 17 patients treated with a custom T-plate that involved fixation with screws to the midline of the occiput where the thickness can be 11 mm to 17 mm, the fusion rate was 100% with no failures of instrumentation.

Subaxial Subluxation

Patients with subaxial subluxation and no neurologic deficit can be observed and managed with serial lateral flexion and extension radiographs. If the subaxial canal diameter is less than 14 mm, then an MRI should be ordered and if the space available for the cord on the MRI is 13 mm or less, then surgical arthrodesis should be strongly considered. On occasion, preoperative traction will reduce subaxial subluxation and make the surgical procedure safer. In most cases posterior cervical fusion is the procedure of choice. The amount of space available for the cord in the subaxial spine after surgery for myelopathy has been shown to be correlated with neurologic recovery. Efforts should be made to ensure that the subaxial canal will be reconstituted to a diameter of 14 mm or greater for optimum recovery. Achieving this goal may require a decompressive procedure such as a laminectomy or an anterior cervical procedure, especially if the patient has drifted into kyphosis. It is also important to remember that subaxial subluxation can occur in conjunction with C1-2 instability or occiput-C1 instability. Subaxial subluxation also has been noted as a complication of upper cervical fusion in long-term studies. The traditional preoperative plan includes addressing all unstable segments at the time of arthrodesis to avoid junctional problems. In a recent review of 15 patients with rheumatoid myelopathy and radiographically stable subluxations, all patients were treated with laminectomy without concomitant fusion. Ten of the 15 patients noted improvement in neurologic function; the condition of five patients remained unchanged. During the median follow-up of 43 months, four patients experienced progression of the slip despite stable preoperative radiographs. Three of these patients were unaffected by the slip progression, but one patient developed sudden onset of tetraplegia because of missed basilar invagination with progression. This patient responded favorably to traction, decompression, and occipitocervical fusion, thereby illustrating the need to watch for the presence of basilar invagination on preoperative films.

Results of Surgery

Several debilitating issues complicate the surgical management of cervical subluxation in rheumatoid patients. Patients with rheumatoid arthritis are usually taking several antimetabolic medications and tend to have poor skin quality, poorly healing wounds, and osteoporotic bone. However, relief of neck pain is quite reliable and has been reported in up to 90% of patients. A recent study of the medical and surgical treatment of cervical spine disease in rheumatoid patients identified 111 patients who underwent MRI investigation of their cervical spine. The indications for the MRI were cervical spine pain unresponsive to nonsurgical measures, signs or symptoms suggestive of myelopathy, or progressive subluxation. Twenty-seven patients required surgery within the study period. There was very little correlation between the MRI findings and the clinical features. The authors found that compared to their previous cohort of study patients, fewer patients in the present study had severe myelopathy in the surgical group (34% versus 7%), early postoperative mortality improved from 9% to 0, and surgical complications fell from 50% to 22%. Eighty-nine percent of patients reported subjective improvement in overall function. The results of surgery with regard to neurologic improvement have not been quite so consistent. Neurologic deterioration as the result of surgery is extremely uncommon in this patient group. The rates of neurologic improvement have been quoted as anywhere from 27% to 100%. A recent 10-year follow-up of patients treated surgically for rheumatoid myelopathy showed that the myelopathy improved in 75% of cases by at least one Ranawat class. In particular, 60% of the class IIIB patients improved neurologically. All those who underwent surgery within 3 months of the onset of paralysis had neurologic improvement whereas those who presented with paralysis lasting 1 year or longer had no improvement in neurologic status. The survival rate at 10 years was 38% and all patients had relief of their neck pain. Vertical translation returned to its preoperative position despite reduction with traction, but the atlantodental interval remained the same as it did immediately post-

operatively. Age, gender, duration of paralysis, preoperative atlantodental interval, and degree of slippage are not related to neurologic recovery. The location of the disease seems to be an important factor, with patients suffering from basilar invagination carrying a significantly poor prognosis than isolated subaxial or atlantoaxial instability. The degree of preoperative neurologic deficit correlates closely with postoperative recovery. The more profound the neurologic deficit preoperatively, the less likely are the patients to recover. When the PADI was less than 10 mm before surgery, the prognosis for motor recovery was poor. Clinically significant neurologic recovery occurred only when the PADI was greater than 13 mm before surgery in patients with basilar invagination. Also important in achieving a good neurologic result is ensuring that the postoperative sagittal canal diameter will be 14 mm or greater after the surgical procedure. This factor has been seen in patients with AAI and in the subaxial spine as well. Ranawat class IIIB patients have had a particularly poor rate of neurologic improvement and a high mortality rate. It has been suggested that, because of the high complication rate of surgical intervention, surgery should not be attempted in these bedridden patients. On the other hand, functional improvement has been noted in these patients, and making the case for aggressive surgical treatment. Approximately 50% of ambulatory patients will improve by one or two grades after surgery, whereas only 20% of Ranawat class IIIB patients will improve to class I or II.

Nonunion and Bone Graft

A recent study questioned the use of autogenous iliac crest bone graft in the treatment of occipitocervical fusions in rheumatoid patients. One hundred fifty patients who underwent posterior cervical stabilization with the use of a contoured Ransford loop fixed with sublaminar wires were compared with 30 patients with and 120 patients without bone graft. There was no significant difference in outcome between the two groups, and it was concluded that autogenous bone grafting is unnecessary in this group of patients. The surgical mortality rate was 10% in the first month after surgery, and approximately two thirds of the patients had at least one level of improvement in the Ranawat scale. Excluded from this study were those patients with isolated AAI in whom bone graft was routinely used in an effort to achieve union. Another report showed an 88% radiographic fusion rate in 25 adults with rheumatoid arthritis undergoing occipitocervical fusion using local calvarial split-thickness bone graft; no hardware failures occurred in any of the 25 patients. This procedure avoids many of the problems associated with bone graft harvesting, such as donor site pain, bleeding, and lack of good quality bone graft in these osteopenic patients.

Complications

Complications resulting from surgery of the rheumatoid spine include death, infection, wound dehiscence, nonunion, and instability below a previously fused segment. The death rate after spine surgery, at 5% to 10%, has been markedly diminished in the past few years, mostly as a result of better screening programs. Patients are receiving treatment earlier in the disease process (before Ranawat class IIB) where significant gain can be made without undue risk. Management of the airway is an important factor. Airway complications with routine intubations for posterior cervical fusions approach 14% in the rheumatoid patient. In addition, losing access to the airway in the postoperative period can be disastrous in these patients, because reintubation is difficult. Routine use of fiberoptic intubation decreased airway complications to less than 1%. Nonunion rates, at 5% to 20%, are quite high in the rheumatoid patient and may correlate with a lack of neurologic improvement. The high nonunion rate may in part be related to the administration of immunosuppressive drugs and poor nutritional status. Whenever possible, nutritional deficiencies should be dealt with prior to surgical intervention. Meticulous surgical technique with redundant fixation also should be used in an attempt to reduce the rates of nonunion. Neurologic deterioration should be an uncommon complication of surgery if care is taken to prevent overcorrection of the deformities and to avoid passing sublaminar wires into a stenotic canal. A minimum canal diameter of 14 mm should be the goal in order to maximize postoperative recovery of neurologic deficit.

Juvenile Rheumatoid Arthritis

Juvenile rheumatoid arthritis (JRA), a disease somewhat like its adult counterpart, is characterized by chronic synovitis and systemic involvement. There are three identifiable types of JRA: pauciarticular, polyarticular, and systemic. Cervical spine involvement is uncommon in the pauciarticular type but can occur in polyarticular disease. Neck stiffness occurs in 46% to 60% of patients. Neck pain is seen in only 2% to 17% of patients and radiographic changes are seen only in the late stages of the disease in children with severe involvement. Neurologic complications are uncommon in JRA. Myelopathy develops in about 2% of patients with symptomatic cervical involvement. Torticollis may occur and has been reported as the initial presenting symptom of JRA. Growth disturbances may arise sec-

ondary to spontaneous posterior cervical fusions, but subluxations are uncommon. Surgical treatment is reserved for patients with severe instability or those with neurologic involvement. As with adult patients with rheumatoid arthritis, surgical intervention can be complicated by instrumentation failure. Children with JRA experience a decrease in bone mineral content that probably occurs secondary to the disease process and the systemic therapy. The cortical appendicular skeleton is affected more than is the axial trabecular bone mass, and the severity of the osteopenia is directly correlated with the severity of peripheral involvement. A recent study has shown that if the disease goes into remission by the third decade of life, normal bone mineral density can be achieved. In adults with a disease-free interval of at least 6 months, bone mineral density was shown to be within the limits of normal controls.

Seronegative Spondyloarthropathies

The seronegative spondyloarthropathies are arthritides that typically cause inflammation and ossification of the entheses (sites of ligament and tendon insertion) of the spine and sacroiliac joints. This group of conditions includes ankylosing spondylitis, psoriatic arthritis, enteropathic arthropathies, and Reiter's syndrome. HLA-B27 is an autosomal dominant gene of the MHC gene complex that plays some role in the immune system and self-recognition. The B27 allele is detected in about 8% of the general population in the United States but is present in 90% of those with ankylosing spondylitis and those with spinal involvement and one of the other seronegative spondyloarthropathies. Children of female patients with ankylosing spondylitis may get the disease more frequently than children of male patients. The net result of the autoimmune disease is the production of antibodies against host tissues. Why the entheses and the sacroiliac joints are targeted and why the inflammatory response stimulates ankylosis of the spine rather than the destructive changes seen in other inflammatory arthritides such as rheumatoid arthritis is unknown.

Extraskeletal Manifestations of Ankylosing Spondylitis

Anterior uveitis is the most common extraskeletal manifestation of ankylosing spondylitis. It occurs in approximately 25% to 30% of patients with ankylosing spondylitis, and exacerbations of this process can be extremely painful. Flare-ups are treated with topical corticosteroids or other anti-inflammatory medications under the supervision of an ophthalmologist. Loss of vision occurs only if chronic inflammatory cells and fibrin are deposited in the vitreous and cause opacity. Restrictive pulmonary disease is a common process that occurs as a result of ankylosis of the ribs with the thoracic spine, which eliminates chest wall expansion during inspiration. Although only mild symptoms are exhibited clinically and pulmonary function tests are not severely affected, pulmonary complications are a frequent cause of morbidity and mortality in patients undergoing surgery. The cardiovascular system is also affected with aortic valve incompetence, aortitis, and cardiac conduction disturbances occurring in 3% to 10% of patients. Amyloidosis, frequently seen in ankylosing spondylitis, can cause renal failure.

Radiographic Evaluation

In patients with ankylosing spondylitis, the disease is always localized to the sacroiliac joint. The sacroiliac joint involvement is the radiographic hallmark of the disease, as are bridging syndesmophytes that represent ossification of the anulus fibrosus of the intervertebral disk. Eventually, the spine takes on the radiographic appearance of the so-called bamboo spine. Spinal and sacroiliac ankylosis is usually manifested by age 30 years in most patients with ankylosing spondylitis, and by age 60 years in the other seronegative spondyloarthropathies; the hips and shoulders are often affected by the disease as well. In patients with ankylosing spondylitis and hip disease, spinal disease is more severe than in those without hip involvement, and spinal disease is more severe in men than in women. Osteoporosis is a common finding and is often underestimated by standard bone density studies because of artifact from the formation of bridging osteophytes. Bone density studies should be done in the proximal femur to prevent falsely elevated results from spondylitic osteophytes. Loss of bone mass in patients with ankylosing spondylitis occurs mainly in those with persistently active disease.

The treatment of the disease, usually based on symptoms, is with nonsteroidal anti-inflammatory medications. Calcium and vitamin D supplementation should be considered in an effort to reduce the amount of osteoporosis that will occur. Physical therapy should be used and the patients instructed to abstain from smoking, exercise regularly, and avoid placing large pillows under the head at night in order to try to prevent the development of kyphosis. These patients should be instructed to avoid contact sports or any sport that will put them at risk of spine fracture, which can occur with trivial trauma. The severity of the symptoms and the disability associated with the disease is extremely variable. As the disease progresses over many years, the back and neck pain improve secondary to the loss of motion as the spine spontaneously fuses. Unfortu-

nately, as the spine fuses it usually does so in a kyphotic position. With complete ankylosis, the pain subsides, and other issues such as management of fractures and deformity become important.

Fractures

Spine fractures are a feared complication of ankylosis and they occur rather frequently. Fractures have received much attention in the literature because of the difficulty in management and frequent neurologic complications that occur both before and after the initiation of treatment. The long segments of ankylosis result in stress concentrations in weakened or fractured areas and the marked osteoporosis that occurs in this disease state leaves the spine susceptible to injury, even from trivial trauma. In some cases the patient has such a trivial injury that the fractures may go unnoticed until adverse consequences develop. A high index of suspicion must be maintained in treating these patients because of the difficulty in obtaining radiographs and the high rate of neurologic injury with unrecognized fractures. The prevalence of fractures is greater in the patient group with ankylosing spondylitis than in the general population, and fractures tend to occur in the sixth to eighth decade of life. Multiple spine fractures are more common than in a similar cohort of patients without the disease. When fractures do occur there are two complications that are somewhat unique to this disease. Because of the long segments of ankylosis, motion is concentrated in the fractured segment. Even nondisplaced fractures have been noted to displace completely despite appropriate nonsurgical care. In addition, these patients are prone to the development of epidural hematoma for several hours, days, or even weeks after the initial trauma. The collection of blood in the epidural space is probably related to the fact that there is micromotion at the fracture site despite adequate attempts at immobilization. Careful surveillance by the patient, doctors, and nurses is essential to quickly identify this complication. Neurologic compromise is common after the development of this complication. Unfortunately, complete deficits below the lesion are common and lead to a grave prognosis for recovery. Early detection of an epidural hematoma can lead to a more favorable result.

Regarding cervical spine fractures, management is quite difficult and is associated with high rates of morbidity and mortality with surgical and nonsurgical treatment. Good results have been reported with closed treatment consisting of skeletal traction followed by halo vest application in patients with nondisplaced injuries and no neurologic deficit. Care must be taken to put the traction in line with the patient's spine. Weights of 10 lb or less should be used because overdistraction can cause neurologic deficit. Fusion rates have been uniformly high, with bony union occurring in 12 to 18 weeks. These patients should be handled with extreme care because simply positioning the patient supine on the bed in a CT scanner can result in neurologic deterioration. If the patient has a fractured neck and complete neurologic deficit, traction should be used to realign the spine, which can be followed by the application of a halo vest at a later date. If the fracture is grossly unstable in the halo vest, surgery should be considered because ascending paralysis has been reported to occur with this scenario. If the patient is neurologically intact, or has a partial deficit and shows signs of neurologic deterioration, surgery should be performed immediately. The neurologic decline may be caused by displacement of the fracture but is more likely related to epidural hematoma, which is common in this condition. Epidural hematoma is best seen on an MRI study and is best treated by laminectomy. Some form of internal fixation should accompany laminectomy in order to prevent translation, which is not well controlled by a halo vest alone. Surgical intervention can be bloody and internal fixation can be very difficult in this osteopenic bone. Instrumentation of several segments above and below the fracture site should be attempted. Use of a halo vest may be necessary postoperatively unless the fixation is extremely solid. Rigid internal fixation of thoracic and lumbar spine fractures should be considered. Another relatively common complication of ankylosing spondylitis is the occurrence of spondylodiskitis. This complication occurs in 5% to 23% of patients and is believed to result from a missed fracture through a disk space that went unrecognized and failed to heal on its own. In many patients this process is noticed on routine radiographs obtained after a fall. The treatment is usually bed rest or immobilization. Many patients will go on to develop a spontaneous fusion at this site, but surgical treatment should be considered in persistently symptomatic patients or those who develop a progressive neurologic deficit.

The principal deformity seen in patients with ankylosing spondylitis is kyphosis. Kyphosis can occur in the cervical spine, usually at the cervicothoracic junction, and in the thoracolumbar spine. Kyphosis in both of these areas is probably caused by spondylodiskitis, which sets up a cycle of anterior loading that accentuates the deformity in these markedly osteoporotic spines. As the deformities increase, the patients will have difficulty with forward gaze without the use of reflective mirrors in their glasses and standing with their knees bent. With time the deformity can progress to a chin-on-chest deformity. Thoracolumbar kyphotic deformity can be so severe that the patient cannot sit, stand, or lie in comfort, and personal hygiene tasks become difficult to perform. If there is ankylosis of the hips, then total hip arthroplasty should be considered prior to spinal osteotomy. The severity of the kyphosis and the functional impact can be measured by the chin-brow vertical angle. This angle can be useful because it can be used as an estimate of how much surgical correction is needed to result in the patient being able to see straight ahead. Cervical thoracic osteotomy can significantly improve the quality of life of these patients. The optimal location of the osteotomy is between C7 and T1 because the canal is widest at this level and the vertebral arteries enter the spine above this level. Osteotomy at a higher level may interfere with the vertebral arteries and should be avoided. The operation is usually done under local anesthesia with the patient awake in the sitting position, but it may be done under general anesthesia with good quality spinal cord monitoring. Wide laminectomy with removal of the lateral masses and exposure of the C8 nerve roots bilaterally is undertaken at the C7-T1 region. A manual osteoclasis is then performed after which internal fixation can be applied with the head in an adequate position. A halo vest is also applied at this time (Fig. 4).

If the deformity is localized to the thoracic spine, then it is most effectively treated by lumbar osteotomy at or below the second lumbar vertebra. The mean age at the time of surgery is 41 years, with a male to female ratio of 7.5:1. The lumbar spine is chosen primarily because it is below the level of the spinal cord, allowing the osteotomy to be performed more safely and allowing greater correction than would be obtained in the thoracic spine, correction would be strongly limited by ankylosis of the costovertebral joints. The best correction is obtained when the osteotomy is carried out at the lowest possible level. The classic operation for this condition is the Smith-Petersen osteotomy, which involves performing a posterior wedge resection of the laminae and facets at the osteotomy site after which a forced osteoclasis is performed, hinging on the posterior aspect of the vertebral body. The anterior column is wedged open anteriorly through the disk space. The mortality rate has been reported as high as 10%. Although corrections of up to 75° are possible with this technique, the lengthening of the anterior column that occurs has been occasionally associated with a tear of the aorta, which may be calcified. Vascular injury has been reported, most commonly with the opening wedge type of osteotomy, with an overall incidence of about 1% in a recent review of the literature. Multiple osteotomies also have been performed in combination with secure instrumentation. The latest technique to be advocated is a pedicle subtraction osteotomy. This technique involves removing the lamina, facets,

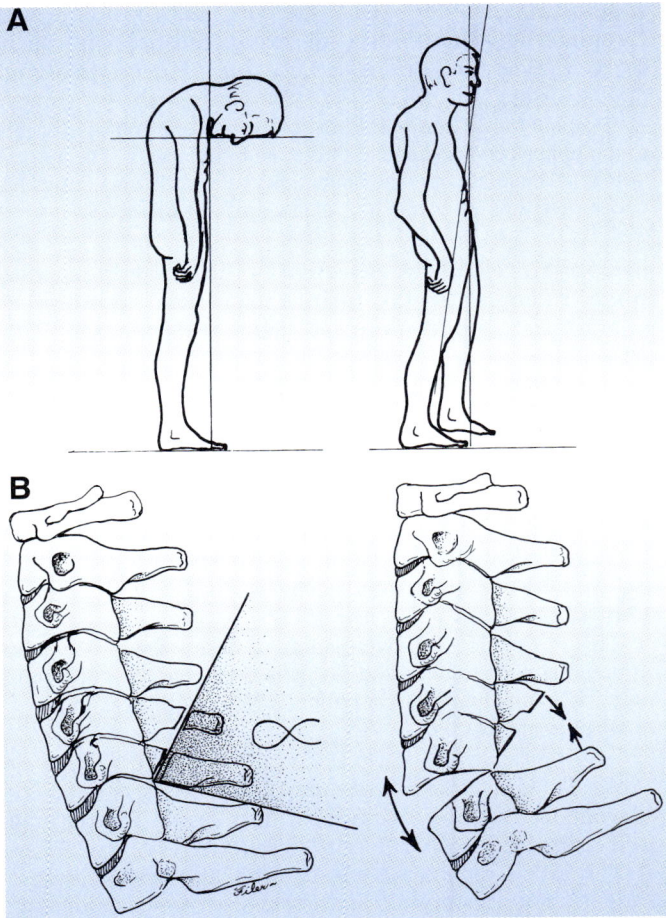

Figure 4 **A,** Schematic of a man with a cervical kyphotic deformity. The chin-brow vertical angle can help in deciding how much correction of the deformity is required. *(Reproduced with permission from Simmons EH: Kyphotic deformity of the spine in ankylosing spondylitis. Clin Orthop 1977;128:65-77.)* **B,** The osteotomy is centered at C7-T1, which is below the level of the vertebral artery.

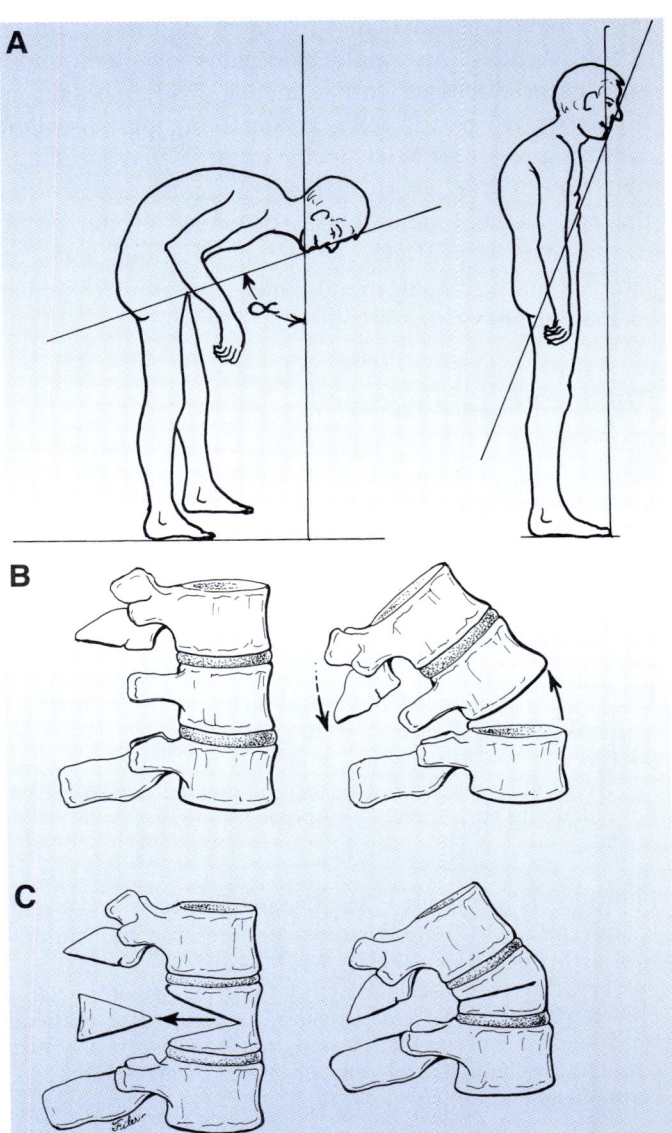

Figure 5 **A,** Schematic of a man with kyphotic deformity in the thoracolumbar spine. The chin-brow vertical angle is measured to give some indication of the amount of correction necessary to restore horizontal gaze. It is important not to overcorrect the deformity or the patients will have an upward gaze and will not be able to see their feet. *(Reproduced with permission from Simmons EH: Kyphotic deformity of the spine in ankylosing spondylitis. Clin Orthop 1977;128:65-77.)* **B** and **C,** Smith-Petersen and pedicle subtraction osteotomies, respectively.

pedicles, and a wedge out of the posterior aspect of the vertebral body where the osteotomy is to be centered. The osteotomy can be centered at L3 or L4 and instrumentation should extend two or three levels above and below the osteotomy. Correction of about 45° is possible and on occasion can be performed at both L3 and L4 if more correction is needed. Several authors have reported good results with this demanding technique. The advantages of this technique over the other osteotomies are that it is more stable, does not open the anterior column, and allows for a more controlled correction of deformity as opposed to a forced osteoclasis. In addition, it brings together two cancellous surfaces of bone that should aid in healing of the osteotomy. There was a trend toward less serious complications in the patients undergoing pedicle subtraction osteotomy (Fig. 5).

Psoriatic Arthritis and Reiter's Syndrome

Psoriatic arthritis and Reiter's syndrome are two common seronegative spondyloarthropathies that also may affect the spine, with up to 70% of patients with psoriatic arthritis having spinal involvement. Classic marginal syndesmophytes represent calcification of the outer fibers of the anulus fibrosus of the intervertebral disk and are the predominant form of involvement of the spine in the seronegative spondyloarthropathies. The syndesmophytes that occur in psoriatic arthritis are often bulkier and broader. In addition, psoriatic arthritis can affect the spine in a way that tends to be more like that seen in rheumatoid arthritis, with bony erosions and subluxations. There may occasionally be AAI and marked pannus around the odontoid, resulting in neurologic deficit. Treatment of this condition should follow the same guidelines as rheumatoid arthritis as discussed earlier in this chapter. A recent report on a case of AAI in a patient with psoriatic arthritis presented MRI documentation that periodontoid pannus will resorb in these patients as well after the achievement of a solid arthrodesis. Reiter's syndrome can also affect the spine in about 3.4% of patients and its biologic and clinical behavior is similar to that of ankylosing spondylitis.

Annotated Bibliography

Christensson D, Saveland H, Zygmunt S, Jonsson K, Rydholm U: Cervical laminectomy without fusion in patients with rheumatoid arthritis. *J Neurosurg* 1999; 90(suppl 4):186-190.

The authors studied 15 patients with rheumatoid arthritis with spinal cord compression and stable flexion-extension films. Cervical laminectomy was performed without fusion, with satisfactory results.

Dreyer SJ, Boden SD: Natural history of rheumatoid arthritis of the cervical spine. *Clin Orthop* 1999;366: 98-106.

A review of the natural history of rheumatoid arthritis is presented and the predictors of paralysis are discussed in this article.

Fujiwara K, Fujimoto M, Owaki H, et al: Cervical lesions related to the systemic progression in rheumatoid arthritis. *Spine* 1998;23:2052-2056.

This is a cross-sectional study of cervical involvement in rheumatoid arthritis. One hundred seventy-three patients were studied and results showed that cervical involvement correlated with CRP level, number of joints with erosions, and carpal height ratio.

Haugen M, Lien G, Flato B, et al: Young adults with juvenile arthritis in remission attain normal peak bone mass at the lumbar spine and forearm. *Arthritis Rheum* 2000;43:1504-1510.

The authors studied 229 patients with JRA and found that bone mineral density returns to normal for young adults if the disease goes into remission.

Hino H, Abumi K, Kanayama M, Kaneda K: Dynamic motion analysis of normal and unstable cervical spines using cineradiography: An in vivo study. *Spine* 1999;24: 163-168.

This study compared normal subjects and rheumatoid patients with cervical involvement. Motion was initiated in the unstable motion segments earlier than in normal subjects. This phenomenon may be responsible for stress concentration at diseased motion segments and deterioration clinically.

Jones DC, Hayter JP, Vaughan ED, Findlay GF: Oropharyngeal morbidity following transoral approaches to the upper cervical spine. *Int J Oral Maxillofac Surg* 1998;27:295-298.

Oropharyngeal complications following transoral approaches to the upper cervical spine are assessed in this study. The authors noted a decrease in the infection rate following transoral decompressions when the soft palate was not divided.

Kauppi M, Neva MH: Sensitivity of lateral view cervical spine radiographs taken in the neutral position in atlantoaxial subluxation in rheumatic diseases. *Clin Rheumatol* 1998;17:511-514.

In 65 rheumatoid patients with cervical involvement, the lateral cervical radiograph was only 52% sensitive in diagnosing atlantoaxial subluxation. Routine flexion-extension films are recommended.

Matsunaga S, Ijiri K, Koga H: Results of a longer than 10-year follow-up of patients with rheumatoid arthritis treated by occipitocervical fusion. *Spine* 2000;25: 1749-1753.

This is a clinical follow-up study of occipitocervical fusions in patients with rheumatoid arthritis. There was a good relief of neck pain and 75% of patients had neurologic improvement postoperatively.

Mori T, Matsunaga S, Sunahara N, Sakou T: 3- to 11-year followup of occipitocervical fusion for rheumatoid arthritis. *Clin Orthop* 1998;351:169-179.

This article reports the results of a long-term follow-up of patients who underwent decompressive laminectomy and fusion with a ring for irreducible rheumatoid subluxations.

Moskovich R, Crockard HA, Shott S, Ransford AO: Occipitocervical stabilization for myelopathy in patients with rheumatoid arthritis: Implications of not bone-grafting. *J Bone Joint Surg Am* 2000;82:349-365.

In this clinical study, 150 patients with multilevel cervical involvement who underwent cervical fusion were studied. There was no difference in the outcome between the patients treated with and without bone graft. The authors excluded isolated AAI, which they believe should be bone grafted.

Puttlitz CM, Goel VK, Clark CR, Traynelis VC, Scifert JL, Grosland NM: Biomechanical rationale for the pathology of rheumatoid arthritis in the craniovertebral junction. *Spine* 2000;25:1607-1616.

This is the first finite element analysis model of rheumatoid arthritis of the upper cervical spine. The results suggest that disruption of the transverse atlantoaxial ligament results in stress shielding in the lateral masses of C1 and may contribute to the erosive changes seen in these areas.

Reijnierse M, Breedveld FC, Kroon HM, Hansen B, Pope TL, Bloem JL: Are magnetic resonance flexion views useful in evaluating the cervical spine of patients with rheumatoid arthritis? *Skeletal Radiol* 2000;29: 85-89.

This study examined the role of dynamic flexion MRI in 42 rheumatoid patients and found that the subarachnoid space is narrowed in flexion.

Robertson SC, Menezes AH: Occipital calvarial bone graft in posterior occipitocervical fusion. *Spine* 1998;23: 249-255.

In this clinical study the use of local calvarial split-thickness graft in 25 patients resulted in stable fusion in 22 of the 25 patients.

Sivri A, Guler-Uysal F: The electroneurophysiological findings in rheumatoid arthritis patients. *Electromyogr Clin Neurophysiol* 1999;39:387-391.

The authors of this study performed neurophysiologic monitoring in patients with rheumatoid neck involvement and found a high incidence of neurologic problems without overt clinical myelopathy.

Vale FL, Oliver M, Cahill DW: Rigid occipitocervical fusion. *J Neurosurg* 1999;91(suppl 2):144-150.

This study reports the results of occipitocervical fusion with a custom T plate in 24 patients with rheumatoid necks. The fusion rate with this new technique was 100%.

Van Royen BJ, De Gast A: Lumbar osteotomy for correction of thoracolumbar kyphotic deformity in ankylosing spondylitis: A structured review of three methods of treatment. *Ann Rheum Dis* 1999;58:399-406.

This study is a review of the literature, which identifies 41 articles with 856 patients who underwent thoracolumbar osteotomy for ankylosing spondylitis. The authors did not notice any significant difference between three types of osteotomy but there was a trend toward less complications associated with the closing wedge osteotomy.

Classic Bibliography

Boden SD, Dodge LD, Bohlman HH, Rechtine GR: Rheumatoid arthritis of the cervical spine: A long-term analysis with predictors of paralysis and recovery. *J Bone Joint Surg Am* 1993;75:1282-1297.

Boden SD: Rheumatoid arthritis of the cervical spine: Surgical decision making based on predictors of paralysis and recovery. *Spine* 1994;19:2275-2280.

Casey AT, Crockard HA, Bland JM, Stevens J, Moskovich R, Ransford AO: Surgery on the rheumatoid cervical spine for the non-ambulant myelopathic patient: Too much, too late? *Lancet* 1996;347:1004-1007.

Collins DN, Barnes CL, FitzRandolph RL: Cervical spine instability in rheumatoid patients having total hip or knee arthroplasty. *Clin Orthop* 1991;272:127-135.

Crockard HA, Calder I, Ransford AO: One-stage transoral decompression and posterior fixation in rheumatoid atlanto-axial subluxation. *J Bone Joint Surg Br* 1990;72:682-685.

Crockard HA: Surgical management of cervical rheumatoid problems. *Spine* 1995;20:2584-2590.

Grob D, Wursch R, Grauer W, Sturzenegger J, Dvorak J: Atlantoaxial fusion and retrodental pannus in rheumatoid arthritis. *Spine* 1997;22:1580-1584.

Hensinger RN, DeVito PD, Ragsdale CG: Changes in the cervical spine in juvenile rheumatoid arthritis. *J Bone Joint Surg Am* 1986;68:189-198.

Kraus DR, Peppelman WC, Agarwal AK, DeLeeuw HW, Donaldson WF: Incidence of subaxial subluxation in patients with generalized rheumatoid arthritis who have had previous occipital cervical fusions. *Spine* 1991;16(suppl 10):486-489.

Pellicci PM, Ranawat CS, Tsairis P. Bryan WJ: A prospective study of the progression of rheumatoid arthritis of the cervical spine. *J Bone Joint Surg Am* 1981; 63:342-350.

Ranawat CS, O'Leary P, Pellicci P, Tsairis P, Marchisello P, Dorr L: Cervical spine fusion in rheumatoid arthritis. *J Bone Joint Surg Am* 1979;61:1003-1010.

Simmons EH: Kyphotic deformity of the spine in ankylosing spondylitis. *Clin Orthop* 1977;128:65-77.

van Royen BJ, Slot GH: Closing-wedge posterior osteotomy for ankylosing spondylitis: Partial corporectomy and transpedicular fixation in 22 cases. *J Bone Joint Surg Br* 1995;77:117-121.

Wattenmaker I, Concepcion M, Hibberd P, Lipson S: Upper-airway obstruction and perioperative management of the airway in patients managed with posterior operations on the cervical spine for rheumatoid arthritis. *J Bone Joint Surg Am* 1994;76:360-365.

Zeidman SM, Ducker TB: Rheumatoid arthritis: Neuroanatomy, compression, and grading of deficits. *Spine* 1994;19:2259-2266.

Chapter 58

Spine Instrumentation

Steven D. Glassman, MD

John R. Dimar, MD

Introduction

Spinal fusion surgery has a long history, beginning with the management of spinal tuberculosis in 1911. However, the field of spinal surgery was relatively static until 1960, until the revolutionary introduction of Harrington rod instrumentation. Over the subsequent 40 years, refinements in instrumentation technique and technology have expanded the capability of spine surgeons to optimize outcome in the management of routine fusion procedures and to manage complex spinal pathology.

A wide array of techniques using spine instrumentation systems currently are available to address the unique anatomic and pathologic characteristics of the cervical, thoracic, and lumbar spines. In addition, certain systems are intended for implantation specifically via an anterior or posterior approach to the spine. For every generic instrumentation concept there are multiple brands and iterations available, each with potential advantages in terms of performance or ease of application. It is critical to remember that despite the focus on instrumentation, the factors that determine the ultimate success of a particular procedure are proper patient selection and fusion healing.

Cervical Spine Instrumentation

Occipitocervical Junction

Fusion across the occipitocervical junction is an infrequently performed procedure that presents unique problems in terms of fixation at the base of the skull. Indications for occipitocervical fusion include basilar invagination or C1-C2 instability with a congenital or traumatic deficiency of the posterior C1 arch. In some cases this difficulty is compounded by poor bone quality, such as in patients with rheumatoid arthritis. The traditional method of fixation is the use of a rectangular frame affixed to the spine and occiput using multiple wires. Drill holes are placed proximally in the occi-

put and wires passed through the foramen magnum. Sublaminar wires serve as the distal anchor in the upper cervical spine. More recently, plates have become available that allow screw fixation in the occiput coupled to screw, sublaminar wire, or hook fixation in the cervical spine. Proximal plate fixation is enhanced by selecting screw sites central to and directly below the inion where bone stock is greatest. Regardless of instrumentation technique, the occipitocervical junction is an area of increased force concentration, and supplemental external fixation using a halo vest may be advisable (Fig. 1).

Upper Cervical Spine

Fixation of the upper cervical spine is most frequently performed for management of traumatic injury or ligamentous instability. Posterior wiring techniques have been widely accepted because of their relative simplicity and efficacy. The Gallie fusion involves placement of an H-shaped iliac crest graft secured between C1 and C2 with a wire passed under the arch of C1 and behind the spinous process at C2. The Gallie technique is effective in limiting flexion and extension but provides limited rotatory stability. With the Brooks technique, bilateral sublaminar wires are passed under the arches of both C1 and C2. The Brooks technique is stronger than the Gallie technique and effectively resists both flexion/extension and rotational forces. However, it is more technically demanding and was avoided in the past because of the neurologic risks in passing a wire under the span of two laminar arches. More recently, flexible cable technology has significantly offset this risk because the cable can be passed sequentially under each of the two arches and then tightened and fixed over the entire span (Fig. 2).

Screw fixation techniques for the upper cervical spine include posterior transarticular facet screw placement for C1-C2 fusion, anterior odontoid screw insertion for C2 fracture fixation, and C2 pedicle fixation.

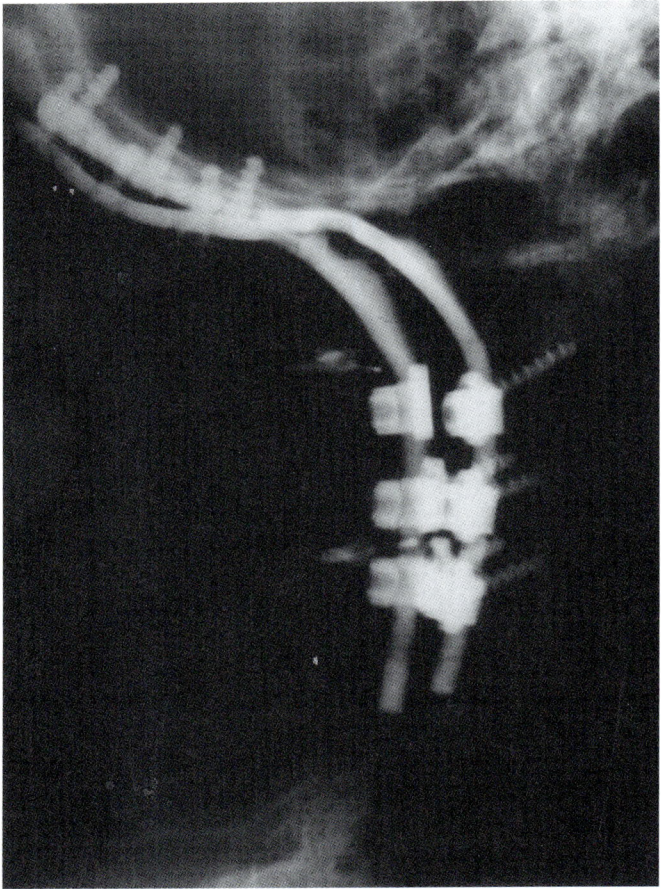

Figure 1 Lateral radiograph of the occipitocervical plate. Occipitocervical fixation including screw fixation to the occiput, C2 pedicle screws, and C3 and C4 lateral mass screws are shown.

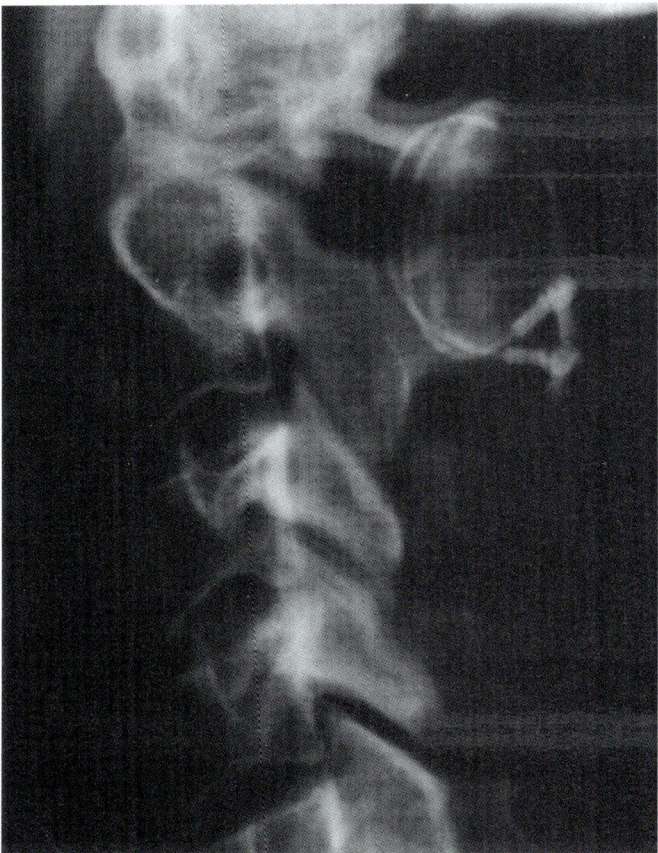

Figure 2 Brooks fusion technique involves passing bilateral flexible cables under the laminar arches of C1 and C2, resulting in stable fixation in both flexion/ extension and rotation.

These techniques have been used less frequently than wiring techniques because of the perceived risk of neurologic or vascular injury and the requirement for high-quality biplanar fluoroscopic guidance. Posterior transarticular C1-C2 facet screw fixation is particularly useful in cases where associated laminar arch fracture or absence limits the use of a sublaminar wire. Bilateral screw placement provides good rotational control and C1-C2 facet fusion can be achieved even in the absence of an intact posterior C1 arch. Risk of injury to the vertebral artery must be minimized by careful evaluation of preoperative CT or MRI studies (Fig. 3).

Odontoid screw fixation is advantageous because it theoretically preserves C1-C2 motion, which is critical for cervical rotation. Odontoid fixation can be achieved with either one or two screws. Although two screws provide better rotational control at the fracture site, one screw can be placed centrally within the odontoid, therefore simplifying the technique. Odontoid screw fixation requires good bone stock and is most appropriate for younger patients with acute fractures. The technique appears less effective in older patients, and

in those with osteoporosis and established nonunions. Risks of odontoid screw fixation include screw misplacement with resultant neurologic or vascular injury, loss of fixation, or distraction at the fracture site with screw insertion.

For anterior and posterior screw fixation, the degree of risk is proportional to the accuracy of biplanar fluoroscopic visualization. These techniques may therefore become more widely accepted if the advent of computer-guided surgical navigational technology provides more accurate intraoperative anatomic detail that should reduce the risk of screw misplacement.

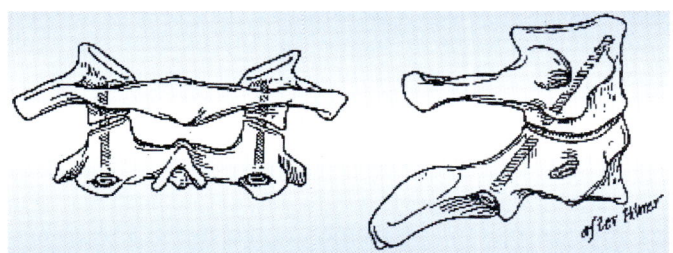

Figure 3 Placement of bilateral transarticular facet screws and the importance of careful preoperative delineation of the vascular anatomy.

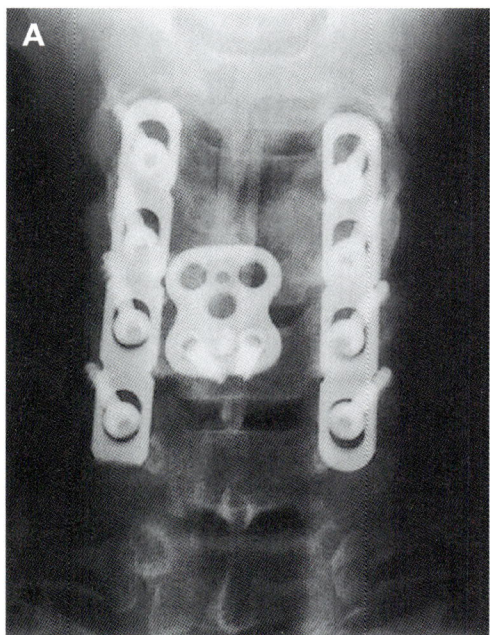
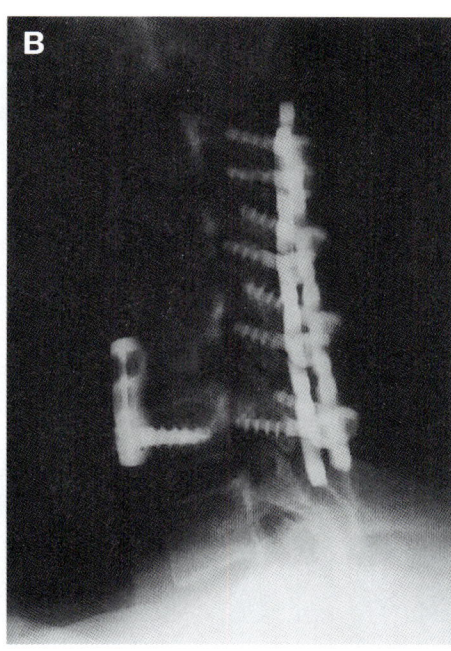

Figure 4 **A** and **B,** An anterior buttress plate is used to prevent graft dislodgement in conjunction with posterior lateral mass fixation.

Lower Cervical Spine: Anterior Fixation

The use of both anterior and posterior instrumentation in the mid and lower cervical spine has increased. Anterior fusions have traditionally been done without internal fixation, relying instead on halo fixation for multilevel or complex cases. Subsequently, anterior cervical plates became popular because their use decreased the need for halo placement and improved postoperative mobilization.

The appropriate indications for anterior cervical plating are controversial. Plates are often used to augment the fusion rate in association with anterior cervical decompression and fusion, for disk herniation or degenerative disk disease. Improved fusion rates have been documented in multilevel procedures; however, plates are being used with increasing frequency in single-level fusions as well. The rationale is both a potential increase in fusion rate and decreased postoperative immobilization. At the other end of the spectrum, anterior plating for two-level or multilevel corpectomy has been associated with a greater incidence of complications and nonunions. A recent biomechanical study suggests that a long anterior plate may actually increase the forces at the graft-end plate interface in extension. This raises the question as to whether supplementary posterior fixation is advisable in these cases.

Early plate designs used bicortical screw fixation with the attendant risk of spinal cord impingement. Newer designs have generally relied on unicortical cancellous screw fixation, which has afforded a greater margin of safety and has not been associated with an unacceptable rate of plate dislodgement. At present,

the major issues in plate design revolve around variability in angulation for screw insertion, locking mechanisms to prevent screw backout, and plate thickness to provide adequate strength with minimal impingement on the overlying pharyngeal structures.

An alternative technique of anterior plating is to use a short plate affixed to only the cephalad or caudad vertebral body. This buttress plate is intended to prevent graft dislodgment after channel corpectomy and fibular strut grafting. In general, this construct should be supplemented with posterior fixation (Fig. 4).

Regardless of the specific indications or technique of anterior cervical plating, several consistent pitfalls must be avoided. First, the extended soft-tissue dissection required for plate placement mandates extreme care in soft-tissue handling and retraction. Second, attention to detail is needed with regard to screw placement because radiographic identification of the bony landmarks may be difficult, particularly in the distal cervical spine. Finally, patients will frequently experience a transient discomfort with swallowing and should be warned to expect this problem.

Lower Cervical Spine: Posterior Fixation

Indications for posterior fixation in the lower cervical spine include fracture fixation, stabilization in conjunction with posterior decompression, and repair of an anterior nonunion. Historically, posterior cervical fixation was performed using various posterior wiring techniques. The Dewar or Compere wire procedure uses threaded pins driven across a corticocancellous iliac strut, the base of a spinous process, then a second iliac strut. This construct is reinforced with figure-of-8 wir-

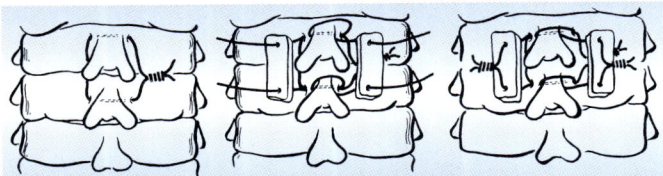

Figure 5 In the Bohlman triple wire technique, after placement of an initial cerclage wire for reduction, corticocancellous struts are wired to the spinous processes to add stability and promote fusion.

ing and provides excellent stability. The Bohlman triple wire technique (Fig. 5) provides similar although slightly less rigid fixation with relative safety and reproducible clinical results. The difficulty with these techniques is that they rely on intact posterior elements and therefore may require extension of the fusion to an otherwise uninvolved level.

Currently, posterior cervical fixation is often achieved using lateral mass plates. Lateral mass fixation is most useful from C3 through C6 and is often combined with fixation via pedicle screws at the cervicothoracic junction. Lateral mass plates provide excellent fixation; however, screw placement is technically demanding because of risks for neurologic or vascular injury. Careful assessment of individual anatomic variation using a preoperative CT scan can be helpful in avoiding complications secondary to screw misplacement.

Lateral mass screw insertion is done using 25° of lateral inclination and a minimum of 30° of cephalad inclination after starting 1 mm medial to the center of the lateral mass. A high-speed burr is used to start a pilot hole followed by drilling and tapping of the lateral mass. Once the distal cortex is engaged, the depth of the hole is measured and a 3.5-mm cancellous screw is placed through the plate, which has been previously contoured to accommodate cervical lordosis. Meticulous decortication of the facet and lamina for bone graft placement, preferably autogenous, is crucial prior to plate placement. The use of lateral mass screw-rod systems offers the increased benefit of being able to decorticate and place bone graft into the facet and over the lamina prior to or after rod placement. The average screw length is between 12 and 15 mm. In addition, a flexible wire may be used to anatomically reduce a fracture, thus allowing for simpler application of lateral mass fixation or to augment construct stability. Intraoperative radiographs are essential to confirm levels and accurate screw placement.

The C7 vertebra is the transitional vertebra between the cervical and thoracic spine and has a lateral mass that is generally so thin that it cannot accommodate a lateral mass screw. Fortunately, the C7 pedicle is well developed and can usually accommodate a 3.5-mm pedicle screw without difficulty. The starting point for a C7 pedicle screw is different than for the lateral mass and is determined by either drawing a line vertically from the center of the C7-T1 facet until it intersects with one drawn from the center of the C7 transverse process or 3 to 5 mm medial to the lateral vertebral notch. In a similar drilling technique used within the lateral masses, the drill is angled in a 20° medial inclination and drilled to a depth of 16 to 18 mm. A small laminotomy may be created if there is any difficulty in either identifying the correct drill angle or advancing the drill. The pedicle is easily palpated for orientation with a blunt nerve hook. Confirmatory radiographs of screw placement always should be done. When posterior element disruption includes a fracture of the lateral mass, alternative fixation techniques must be considered. Options include extension of the plate and fusion to an intact level, pedicle screw fixation at the level of the fractured lateral mass, and unilateral plate fixation in conjunction with spinous process wiring. Whenever the ultimate fixation construct is deemed suboptimal, supplemental halo immobilization should be considered.

In addition to lateral mass plates, there are systems that combine lateral mass or cervical pedicle screw fixation with small rod constructs. These systems in general are somewhat more bulky but may provide an advantage in flexibility, accommodating the divergent angulations required for screw placement, particularly when crossing the cervicothoracic junction (Fig. 6).

A recently expanded indication for posterior cervical instrumentation is the use of small fracture fragment plates as part of a laminaplasty procedure. Laminaplasty has been used with increasing frequency for management of multilevel cervical spinal stenosis; however, care must be taken to ensure that a minimum of three cervical levels are involved and that a reasonable cervical lordosis is present. Although a variety of laminaplasty techniques have been reported, the use of small fracture fragment plates to hold open the laminar osteotomies is often advantageous.

Thoracolumbar Spine Instrumentation
Anterior Thoracolumbar Spine Instrumentation
The thoracolumbar spine is routinely accessed through both anterior and posterior approaches. Historically the anterior approach was used primarily for diskectomy or corpectomy and bone grafting with a subsequent posterior approach for instrumentation. More recently, based in part on improved instrumentation systems, anterior spinal fixation is frequently sufficient to allow a single-stage procedure for decompression and stabilization. Anterior instrumentation in the thoracolumbar spine is most often used for management of fracture or scoliosis. In some instances a single-stage

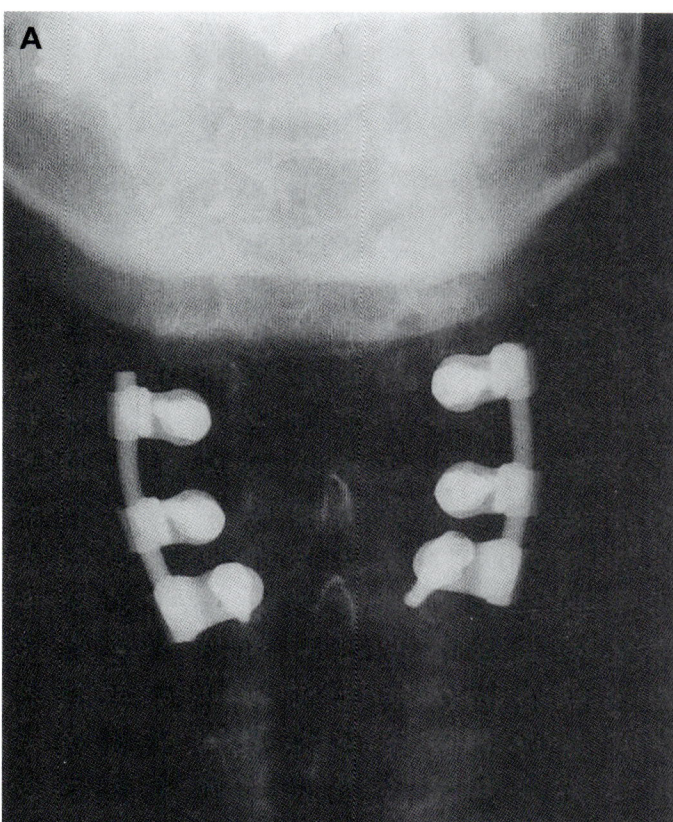
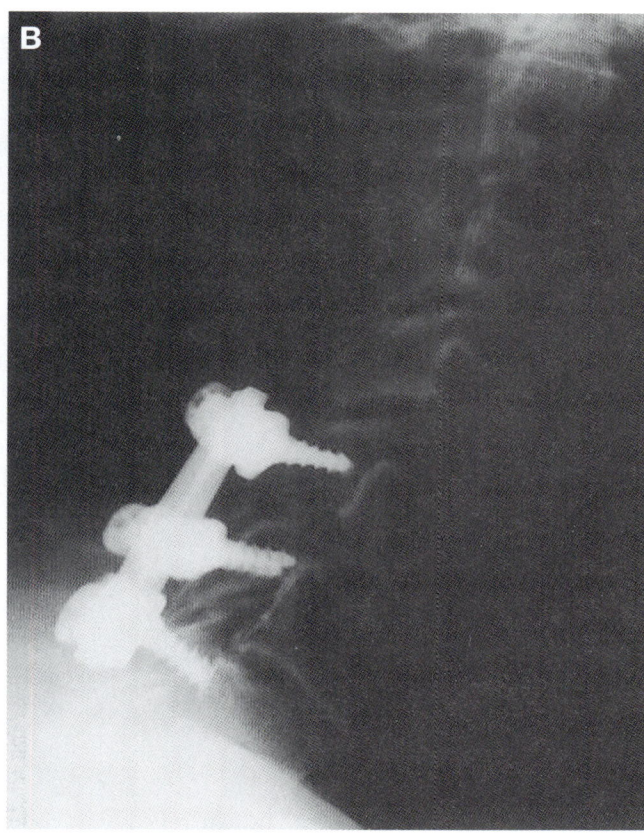

Figure 6 **A** and **B,** Posterior cervicothoracic junction fixation. Newer screw rod systems offer greater flexibility in the linkage mechanism facilitating fixation combining lateral mass and pedicle screws at the cervicothoracic junction.

resection and stabilization is also appropriate for treatment of a spinal tumor.

Fracture plating systems have been specifically designed for anterior thoracolumbar fixation and involve placement of two screws in the vertebral bodies above and below the fracture (Fig. 7). After corpectomy, an iliac crest graft or graft-filled mesh cage is inserted and secured with the application of a lateral plate or rod system in compression. Isolated anterior decompression and stabilization is ideally suited to injuries with marked canal compromise but retained posterior column stability. Although anterior plating systems maintain alignment reasonably well, they are less effective for reduction of deformity and therefore better suited to new injuries than established malunions.

Important technical issues in anterior fracture fixation include patient selection, grafting technique, and instrumentation profile. Isolated anterior instrumentation relies on fixation in the cancellous bone of a vertebral body and thus requires reasonable bone quality. Anterior fixation also provides less rigid stabilization than supplemental posterior fixation and therefore must be used cautiously in the presence of a significant posterior ligamentous injury. A common pitfall associ-

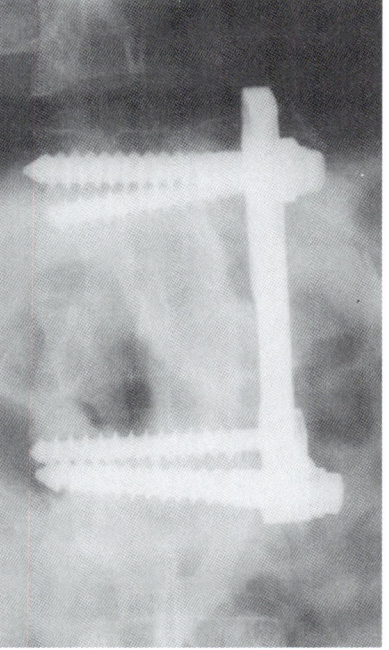

Figure 7 Anterior thoracolumbar plate fixation. Fracture plate fixation, here using autologous iliac crest graft, can also be applied in conjunction with cage or allograft reconstruction.

ated with anterior fracture fixation is the assumption that plating diminishes the importance of an appropriately sized strut graft. A well fixed graft prior to plat-

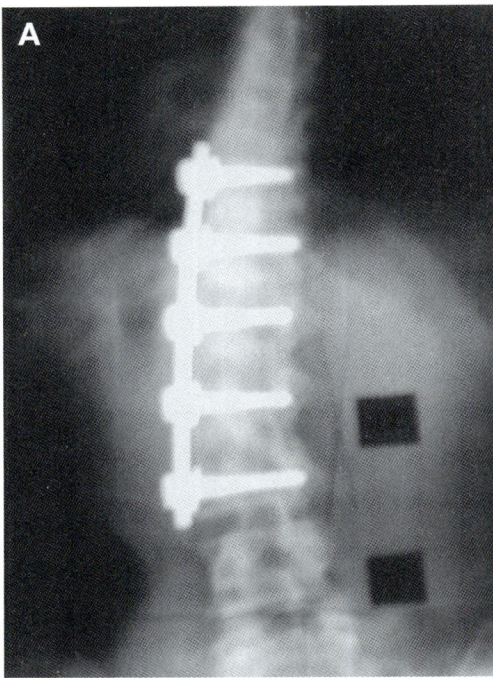
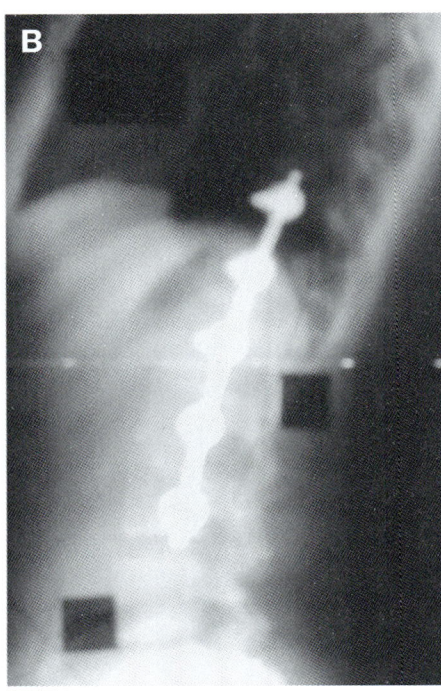

Figure 8 **A** and **B**, Anterior thoracolumbar rod fixation. The use of a top-loading solid rod system facilitates scoliosis correction and offers improved control of the sagittal plane.

ing greatly reduces the likelihood of subsidence and plate or screw failure.

Anterior instrumentation and fusion has become popular for management of isolated lumbar or thoracolumbar scoliosis. The success of this procedure has been enhanced with the advent of solid rod systems, which offer improved fixation and sagittal plane control as compared with the traditional Zielke flexible rod technique. The stronger rod also facilitates postoperative mobilization and reduces the reliance on external bracing. In addition, top-loading solid rod systems are much more user-friendly, thus expediting the procedure (Fig. 8).

The increased rotational control afforded by a solid anterior rod has broadened the surgeon's options for selection of fusion level and reduction technique. The traditional technique of instrumentation over the entire curve can be modified in some cases to limit the distal extent of the fusion. Some authors have advocated a short segment technique in which instrumentation and fusion is limited to the apex of the curvature, which is then overcorrected to balance the spine.

Recently, more user friendly dual rod anterior systems have been introduced. This technique offers the advantage of improved vertebral body fixation but the disadvantage of increased bulk and reduced margin for error in screw placement. This tradeoff may be worthwhile in adult deformity where osteopenia makes bone quality and screw fixation a particularly crucial issue.

Posterior Thoracolumbar Spine Instrumentation

Posterior thoracolumbar fixation is frequently achieved using hook/rod systems, pedicle screw systems, or both. Indications for posterior thoracolumbar instrumentation include fracture fixation, correction of scoliosis or kyphosis, and stabilization following laminectomy for decompression or tumor resection. Supplemental fixation with sublaminar or spinous process wires is generally reserved for special circumstances such as neuromuscular scoliosis. Since the introduction of Cotrel-Dubousset segmental hook/rod instrumentation in the early 1980s, changes in system design have focused primarily on ease of application and reducing implant bulk. Most present systems offer top or side loading access and the ability to interchange hook or screw anchors.

Hook systems have proven extremely effective in managing deformity in the thoracic spine or at the thoracolumbar junction. Hook designs vary depending on the intended attachment site and include supralaminar, sublaminar, pedicle, and transverse process hooks. Although both supralaminar and sublaminar hooks are placed within the spinal canal, supralaminar hook insertion requires a laminotomy and particular care to protect the underlying neural elements. Pedicle hooks are bifid in design and engage the pedicle laterally to the spinal canal. Pedicle hooks are generally used in the thoracic spine at or cephalad to the T10 level. Transverse process hooks are frequently used at the most cephalad aspect of an instrumentation construct

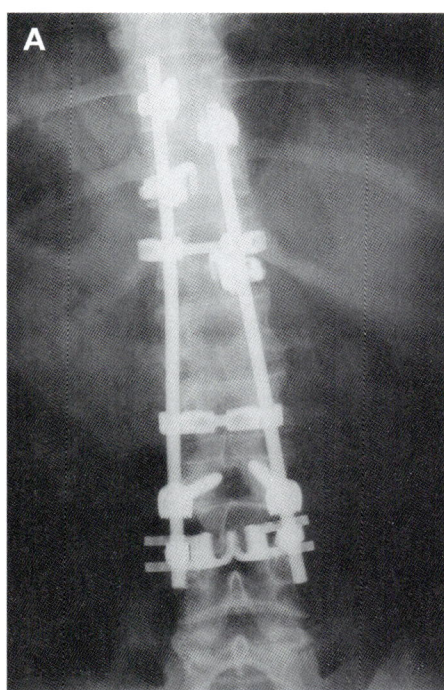

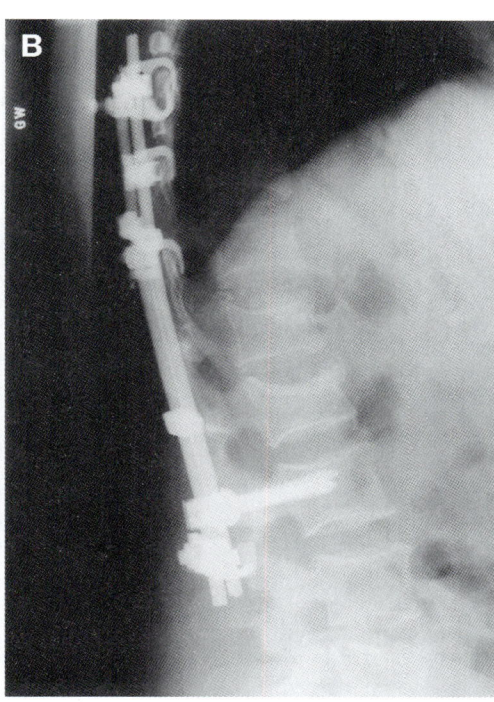

Figure 9 **A,** AP and **B,** lateral posterior thoracolumbar fracture fixation. Posterior rod systems offer the ability to use various anchors, including this combination of hooks and pedicle screws.

and may be combined with a pedicle hook in a claw configuration. Transverse process fixation is usually weaker than supralaminar fixation and therefore more appropriate in situations where significant force is not required at the involved level.

Use of pedicle screws in the thoracic spine is more common outside of the United States and currently seems to offer little advantage except in situations such as prior laminectomy for tumor. Thoracic pedicle screw advocates cite the advantages of improved fixation; however, loss of fixation is an infrequent problem in scoliosis surgery. Although computer-based surgical navigation systems may improve the safety margin for screw insertion in the future, it remains questionable as to whether this technique offers sufficient benefit to assume the increased risk of thoracic pedicle screws on a routine basis.

Application of pedicle screws for the extension of a thoracic instrumentation construct into the lumbar spine is widespread. The risk of lumbar pedicle screw placement is well defined and relatively minimal. There are several reasons to use screws as the distal anchor in deformity constructs. First, distal hooks are the most likely to dislodge if they are not well seated, a risk that is exacerbated in cases of significant sagittal plane deformity such as Scheuermann's kyphosis. Second, screws may facilitate increased rotational correction and thus limit lumbar fusion levels without the need for an anterior release. Although screw fixation in the pedicle is usually adequate, it may be augmented by

sublaminar hook fixation at the same level in a construct termed pediculolaminar fixation (Fig. 9).

Pedicle screws are also used for management of thoracolumbar or lumbar fractures. Use of screws rather than hooks may allow a shorter segment fusion, but careful attention must be given to the extent of anterior column injury. Posterior screw failure is a significant potential problem unless the anterior column is relatively intact or is reconstructed by corpectomy and strut grafting (Fig. 10).

Lumbar Spine Instrumentation

Despite the development of stronger and more versatile instrumentation systems, fixation in the lumbar spine and at the lumbosacral junction has remained a significant challenge. The difficulty is magnified in long fusion constructs or in cases with significant sagittal plane deformity. Instrumentation failures may result from either inadequate initial fixation or prolonged loading as a result of problems with fusion healing. Lumbar fusion techniques are used most frequently for treatment of degenerative disorders. Instrumentation options include posterior pedicle screw fixation, cages inserted either anteriorly, posteriorly, or transforaminally, and machined bone dowels which mimic cage geometry. Less frequently used techniques such as transarticular facet screws may be indicated in isolated instances.

The use of pedicle screw instrumentation is well established, with fusion rates approaching 90% in non-

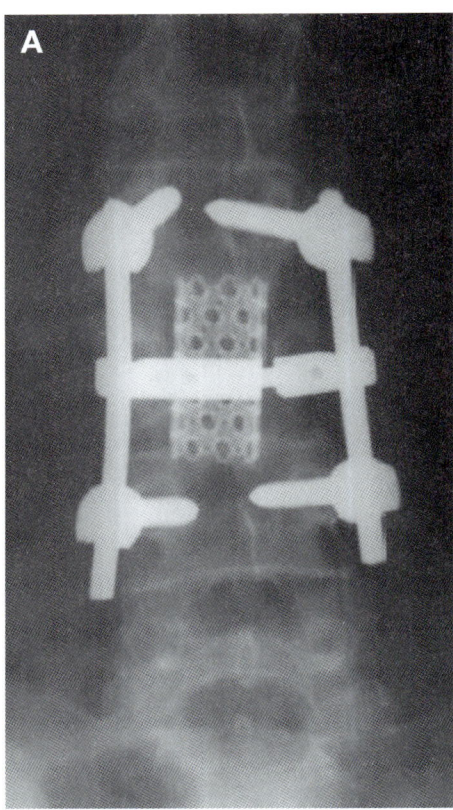

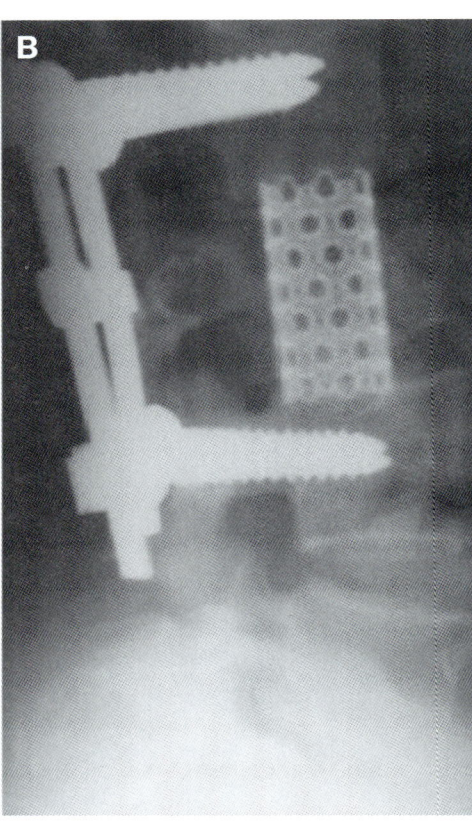

Figure 10 **A** and **B**, Posterior pedicle screw fracture fixation. Short segment pedicle screw constructs can be used provided there is adequate anterior column support or if the anterior column is reconstructed as in this L3 fracture.

smokers undergoing one- or two-level fusion procedures. Recent changes in instrumentation design have focused on decreasing the size and bulk of the implant construct. Many systems also use multiaxial screw heads or a multiaxial rod/screw interface for ease of insertion. There has also been a trend toward the use of titanium implants to facilitate subsequent MRI evaluation if necessary (Fig. 11).

Lumbar pedicle screw insertion techniques can be divided into five general categories, with three being based on anatomic landmarks and two using newer navigational aides. The first anatomic technique uses the transverse process, which generally exhibits consistent anatomy. The transverse process is bisected and an entry hole is created at its insertion into the lateral aspect of the facet. As with all techniques the pedicle is then probed 35 to 45 mm with a blunted instrument. Taping of the pedicle may be beneficial when dense bone is encountered. This preparation is followed by pedicle screw placement. This technique is advantageous because the facet anatomy is preserved.

The second anatomic technique is used at the level of decompression where the facet capsule is removed and the facet is prepared for decortication and fusion. A rongeur is used to remove the dorsal portion of the superior articulating facet near the insertion of the transverse process. This triangular area is then probed and leads directly to the pedicle. The entry to the pedi-

cle with this technique is more medial, therefore, less lateral angular screw insertion is required.

The third technique of anatomic insertion relies on the presence of a preexisting laminotomy that exposes the medial pedicle wall to direct probing to determine its orientation. Once the pedicle dimensions and orientation are determined, regardless of the anatomic variances encountered, an insertion portal can be created into the top of the pedicle for probing and pedicle screw insertion. This technique is particularly useful in an area of preexisting fusion where frequently the anatomic landmarks have been obliterated. All of the techniques can be used in combination to increase the precision of free hand pedicle screw insertion. Nevertheless, these anatomically based techniques require a great degree of technical training and surgical expertise.

Traditional navigational aides for pedicle screw insertion include intraoperative anterior/posterior and lateral radiographs along with biplanar fluoroscopy. Although these techniques have proved useful they have failed to consistently prevent pedicle screw misplacement and may result in the false impression that the pedicle screws are well placed. Intraoperative electromyographic stimulation has proved to be an essential adjunct in identifying inferior and medially misplaced screws that might lead to postoperative neurologic complications. As a result of shortfalls in

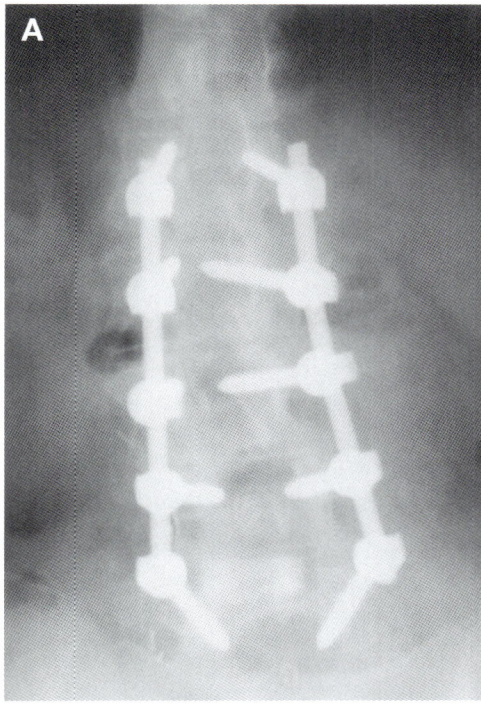
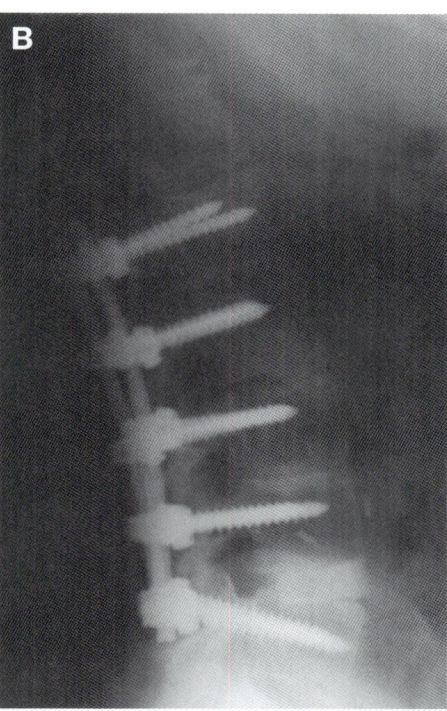

Figure 11 **A** and **B,** Multilevel posterior lumbar pedicle screw fixation combined with distal anterior interbody grafting to increase maintenance of sagittal plane correction.

traditional imaging technique, a new generation of more technically advanced image guidance systems have evolved.

The first stereotactic navigational system, of which there are several that are commercially available, uses the combination of fine cut CT images, infrared targeting using light-emitting diodes, and sophisticated computer analysis to accurately identify orientation and guide the insertion of a special probe under direct visualization on a video monitor into the pedicle. In most instances the computer will display a two- or three-dimensional representation of the spine and concurrently place a cursor overlay at the pedicle insertion point, thus orienting the surgeon to the entry point and direction of screw insertion. These systems, when used properly, will accurately target to within 1 to 2 mm but still require specific expertise by the surgeon and surgical team. Because reference points on the spine are critical to orienting the probe in space, a prior fusion, laminectomy, or motion, or any other factor that alters these points of reference will significantly affect the accuracy of targeting. Nevertheless, these systems can provide an accurate three-dimensional video presentation of the spine to target the pedicle for screw insertion and are particularly useful in spines with significant rotatory deformities and in the cervical spine.

The second navigational aide recently introduced combines fluoroscopy with a targeting grid along with computer analysis. This system results in a greatly enhanced fluoroscopic targeting system to pinpoint the pedicle for screw insertion. This system appears to be as accurate as the light-emitting diode systems and may be adaptable to existing fluoroscopic units.

Despite the overall success of pedicle screw instrumentation in achieving fusion, there is concern that the extensive dissection required for posterior instrumentation and fusion results in a significant deterioration in the lumbar musculature termed "fusion disease." In addition, pedicle screw instrumentation has been only marginally successful in restoring and maintaining physiologic lumbar lordosis. To offset these shortcomings of pedicle screw fixation, and potentially to improve fusion rates, there has been in the last several years a dramatic increase in the use of interbody fusion devices.

Lumbosacral Fixation Techniques

All instrumentation at the lumbosacral junction is exposed to significant force and therefore subject to implant loosening or failure. For management of spinal deformity, fixation to the sacrum can be augmented with sacral alar screws or intrasacral rods. Conversely, pelvic fixation via the ilium can be obtained with rods or screws between the tables of the iliac crest, or by iliosacral screw fixation. None of these techniques provide sufficient strength to offset the forces generated unless reasonable coronal and sagittal balance exists or the posterior fixation is supplemented with an anterior load-sharing construct. This region is subject to a high nonunion rate and therefore adequate grafting and physiologic measures to encourage healing are critical to the long-term success of any instrumentation construct.

Lumbosacral fixation techniques are technically demanding. The three most frequently used sites for posterior fixation of the spine are the first sacral pedicles, the iliac crests, and the sacral ala. Historically important and still used in specific situations is the Luque-Galveston segmental instrumentation technique. With this technique, the cephalad rods used in the spinal fusion are anchored between the tables of the iliac crest, and expert rod bending and fixation skills are required. As originally described, these rods were secured to the spine via sublaminar wires and in the pelvis by friction. Several modifications of this technique have been offered, with most obviating the need for a one-piece rod by allowing for the use of modular rods that can be coupled via strong connectors. The traditional use of sublaminar wires for fixation to the spine has generally been supplanted in favor of the modular approach of hooks and pedicle screw systems, which are more easily applied to the spine and offer greater flexibility.

The current method of iliac fixation uses iliac bolts that are screwed between the iliac tables using a similar technique as the Luque/Galveston. After lumbar fixation with pedicle screws and/or hooks, a subcutaneous plane is developed over both iliac crests where the fascia is divided, exposing the top of the iliac crest and the outer iliac table to allow for screw placement orientation. A notch is then made in the crests to recess the iliac bolts and couplers followed by the development of a subfascial tunnel to connect the iliac bolts via a rod or connector to the cephalad lumbar construct. A probe is then passed between the iliac tables in a directly ventral direction, taking care to avoid the sciatic notch. Finally, a long 50- to 70-mm screw is threaded between the iliac tables and connected to the main lumbar construct via a variety of multiaxial connectors. The use of iliac bolts compromises the ability to obtain the usual quantity of autogenous iliac bone graft because more aggressive removal would destroy the fixation sites (Fig. 12).

The second method of lumbosacral fixation used involves the S1 sacral pedicle. The technique is similar to previously described lumbar pedicle fixation and may use the same anatomic and/or navigational aides. The transverse process is, however, replaced by the sacral ala. Therefore, use of the superior facet decortication or a laminotomy to establish the pedicle borders and orientation may be beneficial. One additional landmark is the first dorsal sacral foramen, which delineates the inferior border of the S1 pedicle. Although the sacral pedicle is generally quite large, the anterior cortex must be engaged to improve fixation.

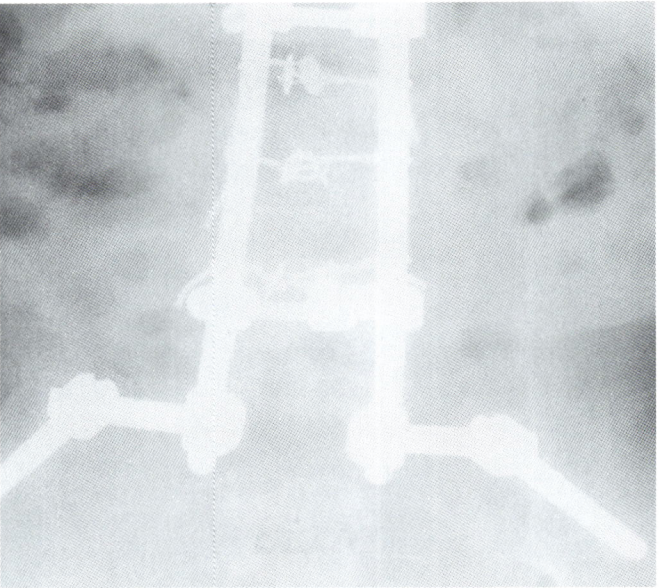

Figure 12 Iliac bolt fixation is one option for pelvic fixation that involves the application of large diameter screws driven between the tables of the iliac crests and subsequently fixed by variable angle connectors to a posterior spinal instrumentation system.

Isolated sacral pedicle fixation is frequently satisfactory but certain situations may require supplemental anterior structural augmentation and/or iliac screws, particularly with a refusion or with the long constructs above the lumbosacral junction that result in increased stress on the fusion and thus a higher pseudarthrosis rate.

Alar screws supplement S1 pedicle screws and represent a third anatomic site that can be used for lumbosacral fixation. Placement is lateral to the S1 pedicle, inferior to the top of the ala and angulated away from the midline 45°, engaging both cortices. Care must be taken to preserve the sacroiliac joint and stay lateral to the L5 nerve root running on the anterior surface of the ala. However, even with multiaxial pedicle screws, connecting the alar screws to the S1 and lumbar pedicle screws remains a technical challenge.

Cage Instrumentation

With cage instrumentation, it is important to delineate between cylindrical screw-in cages and vertical mesh reconstruction cages because there are significant conceptual and functional differences between these instrumentation designs (Fig. 13). Anterior column reconstruction following diskectomy or corpectomy can be performed using mesh cages, which offer structural support and are filled with cancellous bone for fusion. These cages are an alternative to structural allograft or larger structural autologous iliac crest grafts. The advantages of a cage over structural grafts include ease of application, variability in sizing and some increase in

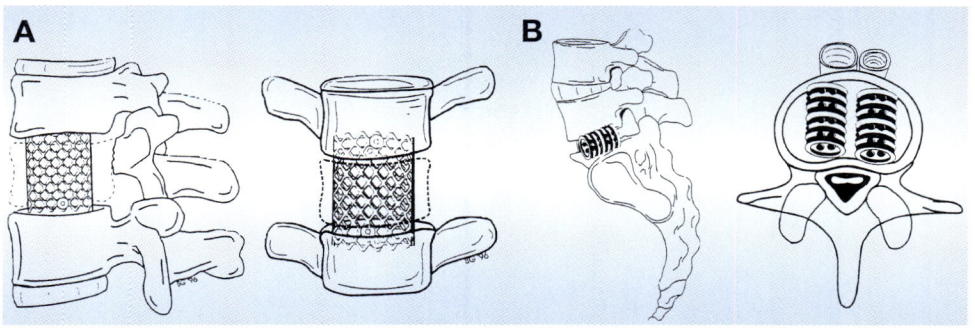

Figure 13 Fusion cage designs. **A,** Mesh fusion cages provide structural support similar to that of a tricortical iliac crest graft or structural allograft. They are available in multiple diameters and can be cut to adjust length as needed. **B,** Screw-in cylindrical cages are used primarily for lumbar interbody fusion. Cage size is limited by access in a posterior lumbar interbody fusion technique and by disk space width in an anterior lumbar interbody fusion technique.

end plate fixation. The obvious disadvantage is that the cage cannot remodel or incorporate over time. Additionally, cage removal when necessary may be technically difficult in comparison to bone resection.

The use of reconstruction cages is ideal in instances of tumor resection where the defect may be large and the nature of the pathology makes subsequent incorporation of a bone graft unlikely. After corpectomy for fracture, the advantage of the cage over autologous iliac crest graft is primarily the avoidance of morbidity related to the graft site. Smaller cages can be used following multilevel disk excision in the management of spinal deformity. Varying cage size and position may aid in correction of the deformity and the use of anterior structural support has been shown to improve long-term sagittal alignment and fusion.

Cylindrical screw-in cages were initially tested and advocated as stand-alone devices, whether inserted via an anterior or posterior approach. In theory, distraction of the disk space and insertion of the cage under tension would provide both fixation and a conduit for bone healing. In contrast, mesh cages are used as an interbody spacer in a load-sharing capacity. They provide significantly greater surface area for fusion but require supplementary fixation, usually with pedicle screw or posterior hook/rod instrumentation.

A critical observation regarding both cylindrical and mesh cages is that present techniques of radiographic evaluation are ineffective in assessing fusion following cage placement. Neither radiographs and flexion/extension films as used in the initial studies, nor reconstructive fine-cut CT scans have accurately predicted fusion status. In some instances, fusion can be determined by the presence of bridging bone surrounding the cage, although care must be taken to differentiate bridging fusion from nonbridging osteophyte. Because unfused cages restrict motion and limit effective evaluation, standard 2-year follow-up may be insufficient to accurately assess fusion status, particularly if the patient has symptoms consistent with nonunion.

As more extended follow-up studies of cylindrical cage fusion procedures become available, positive out-

comes are being reported, but many of the initial application concepts are being revised. Both clinical experience and laboratory studies suggest that cages placed via a posterior lumbar interbody fusion approach do not provide sufficient stability to be used as stand-alone devices in most cases. The inherent difficulty is that placement of a cage of adequate size to provide fixation via distraction requires either extensive posterior element resection or excessive retraction of the neural elements (Fig. 14). If undersized cages are used, they may augment fusion but are unlikely to provide stability. Although pedicle screw fixation will restore stability, the need for posterior instrumentation largely offsets the potential advantage of cage placement.

Cylindrical cages placed via an anterior approach are more likely to provide stable fixation because cage size can be increased to generate annular tension. This technique is better suited to partially collapsed disk spaces because cage size is ultimately limited by disk space width. Disk spaces that are very tall or distract significantly on implantation may still be problematic. Early insertion techniques using a trephine approach left surrounding disk, which limited distraction and improved fixation. Unfortunately, the limited bony surface area generated by this technique leads to an increased nonunion rate. At this time, most surgeons advocate a radical diskectomy, which allows graft to be packed around the cages for fusion but reduces the tension band effect of the surrounding disk and anulus. Despite concern that fixation may diminish soon after implantation, secondary to stress relaxation in the annular fibers, anterior cylindrical cages are more successful than posterior cages as a stand-alone fixation technique.

Although cylindrical cages are used primarily for degenerative disorders, mesh cages placed via an anterior approach might be used for either degenerative disease or management of lumbar spine deformity. Varying the location of the cage within the interbody space facilitates deformity correction and subsequent maintenance of alignment, particularly in the sagittal plane. Although cylindrical cages designed with a lor-

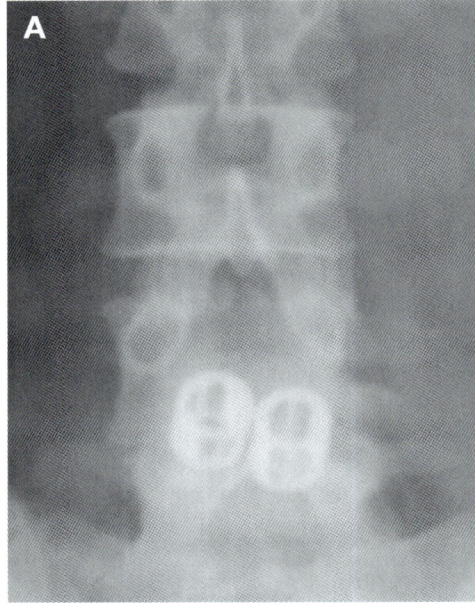 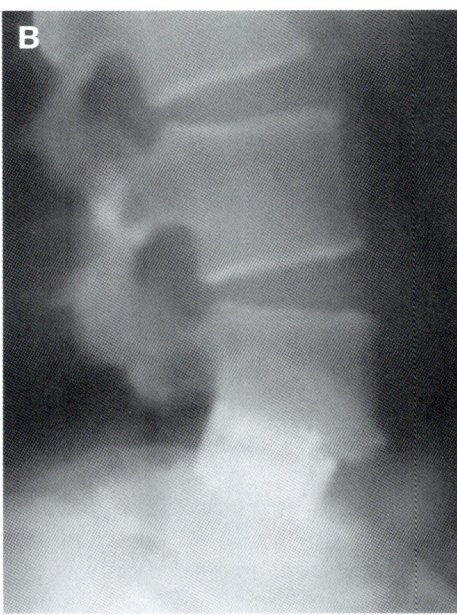

Figure 14 **A** and **B,** Posterior lumbar interbody fusion cages. Significant posterior bone resection was performed to facilitate bilateral cylindrical cage placement via a posterior approach.

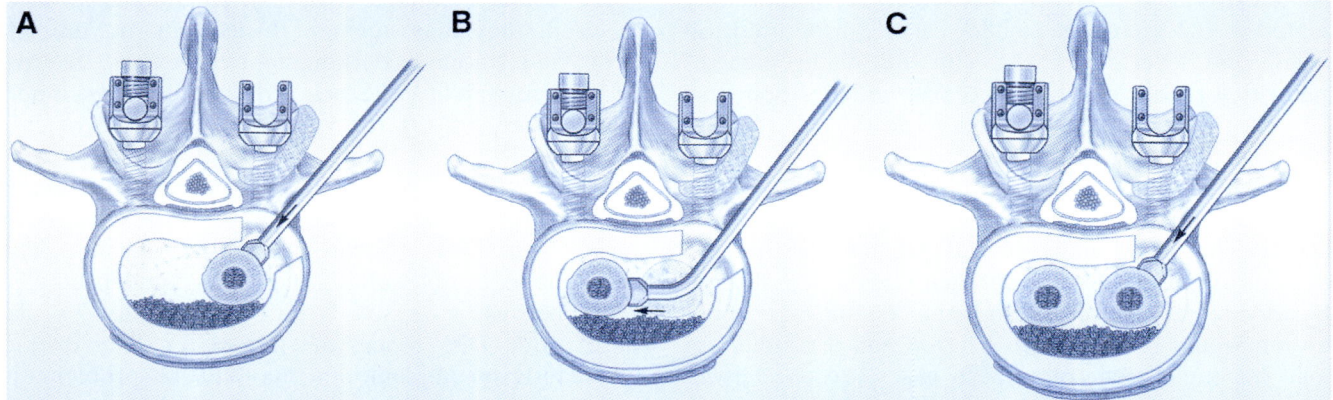

Figure 15 **A** through **C,** Transforaminal interbody fusion. Through access achieved via unilateral facetectomy, small mesh cages or structural bone graft is inserted to provide anterior column support. Pedicle screws are inserted prior to diskectomy and interbody fusion such that the disk space can be distracted for access and then subsequently compressed for stability.

dotic component are available, they do not provide the degree of variability offered by mesh cages, which can be cut individually for each disk space.

Mesh cages are also used via a posterior approach. They can be inserted with a bilateral posterior lumbar interbody fusion approach, similar to the cylindrical cages, or by a more lateral transforaminal approach (Fig. 15). The advantage of the transforaminal fusion approach is that the entire interbody space can be accessed through a unilateral facetectomy exposure without significant neural retraction. The mesh cages can be "rolled" into any quadrant of the disk space, allowing some correction of deformity. However, the technique requires supplemental posterior pedicle screw instrumentation.

For all of the cage techniques previously described, bone dowels or bone plugs with geometries very simi-

lar to the metallic implant are available. In some instances the insertion systems will allow interchange between the metallic or cadaveric bone implants. The relative advantages of a metallic implant include ease of handling for insertion, wider variety in available implant sizes, low risk of disease transmission, and maintenance of structural integrity over time. Advantages of cadaveric bone implants include the potential for remodeling and eventual incorporation, better capacity to visualize fusion healing, and the availability of effective removal techniques should revision become necessary.

Frequently Asked Questions

Several issues are commonly raised by patients who have undergone an instrumented spinal fusion procedure, including the need for eventual instrumentation removal and the need for antibiotic prophylaxis with minor procedures such as dental work. Patients may be concerned regarding the effect of the instrumentation if they need to undergo MRI evaluation or the possibility of setting off the metal detector at the airport. Overall, patients should be assured that their concerns are unlikely to present major problems. Provided that the fusion heals successfully, modern low-profile instrumentation has greatly reduced the need for instrumentation removal. With regard to MRI studies, metal artifact may degrade the images in the region of the instrumentation. The presence of spinal implants is not an impediment to imaging studies focused elsewhere. Additionally, titanium implants produce less MRI artifact and allow limited visualization in the region of the spinal instrumentation. Although some disagreement exists, no literature validates the need for antibiotic prophylaxis for minor procedures based on the presence of spinal instrumentation. Patients with spinal implants usually will not set off airport metal detectors at normal sensitivity levels.

Annotated Bibliography

Cervical Spine Instrumentation

DiAngelo DJ, Foley KT, Vossel KA, Rampersaud YR, Jansen TH: Anterior cervical plating reverses load transfer through multilevel strut-grafts. *Spine* 2000;25:783-795.

This biomechanical study demonstrates that multilevel anterior cervical plating increases graft loading in extension. The authors postulate that this force may result in graft pistoning and failure of multilevel constructs.

Graham AW, Swank ML, Kinard RE, Lowery GL, Dials BE: Posterior cervical arthrodesis and stabilization with a lateral mass plate: Clinical and computed tomographic evaluation of lateral mass screw placement and associated complications. *Spine* 1996;21:323-329.

This study analyzes screw position and associated complication rates in 21 patients after lateral mass plate fixation.

McCullen GM, Garfin SR: Spine update: Cervical spine internal fixation using screw and screw-plate constructs. *Spine* 2000;25:643-652.

This review article highlights indications and pitfalls for the most widely used current techniques in cervical spinal instrumentation.

Wang JC, McDonough PW, Endow KK, Delamarter RB: Increased fusion rates with cervical plating for two-level anterior cervical discectomy and fusion. *Spine* 2000;25:41-45.

This retrospective review of 60 patients undergoing two-level anterior cervical diskectomy and fusion demonstrates a significant reduction in pseudarthrosis rate with the addition of plate fixation.

Thoracolumbar Spine Instrumentation

Eck KR, Bridwell KH, Ungacta FF, Lapp MA, Lenke LG, Riew KD: Analysis of titanium mesh cages in adults with minimum two-year follow-up. *Spine* 2000;25:2407-2415.

This retrospective study of 66 consecutive adult patients examines the role of structural titanium mesh implanted in the anterior column in conjunction with a posterior instrumented fusion. Follow-up longer than 2 years revealed maintenance of sagittal alignment and a high rate of radiographic incorporation. The authors conclude that anterior structural grafting with titanium mesh is a viable option for maintaining sagittal alignment in patients being treated for adult spinal disorders and in particular spinal deformity.

Lenke LG, Bridwell KH, Blanke K, Baldus C, Weston J: Radiographic results of arthrodesis with Cotrel-Dubousset instrumentation for the treatment of adolescent idiopathic scoliosis: A five to ten-year follow-up study. *J Bone Joint Surg Am* 1998;80:807-814.

This retrospective review of 76 patients followed up for 5 years or longer after scoliosis fusion with Cotrel-Dubousset instrumentation demonstrates reliable outcome and high patient satisfaction.

Molinari RW, Bridwell KH, Klepps SJ, Baldus C: Minimum 5-year follow-up of anterior column structural allografts in the thoracic and lumbar spine. *Spine* 1999;24:967-972.

This study showed that the use of structural allografts in combination with posterior fusion and instrumentation effectively maintained postoperative sagittal plane correction for a minimum of 5 years.

Lumbar Spine Instrumentation

Kornblum MB, Fischgrund JS, Herkowitz HN, Abraham DA, Berkower DL, Ditkoff JS: Abstract: *Degenerative Lumbar Spondylolisthesis with Spinal Stenosis: A Prospective Long-Term Study Comparing Fusion and Pseudarthrosis.* Rosemont, IL, American Academy of Orthopaedic Surgeons, 2000.

In this study, the authors present more extended (average, 7 years and 8 month) follow-up on patients with lumbar spondylolisthesis and spinal stenosis managed by decompression and fusion. In a prior study the authors reported that clinical outcome was unrelated to fusion status. In the present study, however, patients with solid fusion reported less pain than patients with pseudarthrosis. The authors conclude that fusion status is in fact important in long-term outcome and recommend the addition of spinal instrumentation as an adjunct to fusion in those patients at risk for pseudarthrosis.

Lonstein JE, Denis F, Perra JH, Pinto MR, Smith MD, Winter RB: Complications associated with pedicle screws. *J Bone Joint Surg Am* 1999;81;1519-1528.

This study of 915 surgical procedures involving the insertion of 4,790 pedicle screws showed a low rate of screw-related complications.

Cage Instrumentation

Brantigan JW, Steffee AD, Lewis ML, Quinn LM, Persenaire JM: Lumbar interbody fusion using the Brantigan I/F cage for posterior lumbar interbody fusion and the variable pedicle screw placement system: Two-year results from a Food and Drug Administration investigational device exemption clinical trial. *Spine* 2000;25:1437-1446.

In this study of posterior lumbar interbody fusion supplemented with pedicle screw fixation, a high rate of successful bony arthrodesis was shown.

Classic Bibliography

Albert TJ, Klein GR, Joffe D, Vaccaro AR: Use of cervicothoracic junction pedicle screws for reconstruction of complex cervical spine pathology. *Spine* 1998;23:1596-1599.

Anderson PA, Henley MB, Grady MS, Montesano PX, Winn HR: Posterior cervical arthrodesis with AO reconstruction plates and bone graft. *Spine* 1991;16(suppl 3):S72-S79.

Brooks AL, Jenkins EB: Atlanto-axial arthrodesis by the wedge compression method. *J Bone Joint Surg Am* 1978;60:279-284.

Fischgrund JS, Mackay M, Herkowitz HN, Brower R, Montgomery DM, Kurz LT: Degenerative lumbar spondylolisthesis with spinal stenosis: A prospective, randomized study comparing decompressive laminectomy and arthrodesis with and without spinal instrumentation. *Spine* 1997;22:2807-2812.

Glassman SD, Johnson JR, Raque G, Puno RM, Dimar JR: Management of iatrogenic spinal stenosis complicating placement of a fusion cage: A case report. *Spine* 1996;21:2383-2386.

Haher TR, Merola A, Zipnick RI, Gorup J, Mannor D, Orchowski J: Meta-analysis of surgical outcome in adolescent idiopathic scoliosis: A 35-year English literature review of 11,000 patients. *Spine* 1995;20:1575-1584.

Heller JG, Estes BT, Zaouali M, Diop A: Biomechanical study of screws in the lateral masses: Variables affecting pull-out resistance. *J Bone Joint Surg Am* 1996;78:1315-1321.

Kaneda K, Shono Y, Satoh S, Abumi K: New anterior instrumentation for the management of thoracolumbar and lumbar scoliosis: Application of the Kaneda two-rod system. *Spine* 1996;21:1250-1262.

Kaneda K, Taneichi H, Abumi K, Hashimoto T, Satoh S, Fujiya M: Anterior decompression and stabilization with the Kaneda device for thoracolumbar burst fractures associated with neurological deficits. *J Bone Joint Surg Am* 1997;79:69-83.

Liljenqvist UR, Halm HF, Link TM: Pedicle screw instrumentation of the thoracic spine in idiopathic scoliosis. *Spine* 1997;22:2239-2245.

McLain RF, Sparling E, Benson DR: Early failure of short-segment pedicle instrumentation for thoracolumbar fractures: A preliminary report. *J Bone Joint Surg Am* 1993;75:162-167.

Ranawat CS, O'Leary P, Pellicci P, Tsairis P, Marchisello P, Dorr L: Cervical spine fusion in rheumatoid arthritis. *J Bone Joint Sug Am* 1979;61:1003-1010.

Ray CD: Threaded titanium cages for lumbar interbody fusions. *Spine* 1997;22:667-680.

Smith MD, Anderson P, Grady MS: Occipitocervical arthrodesis using contoured plate fixation: An early report on a versatile fixation technique. *Spine* 1993;18:1984-1990.

Steffee AD, Brantigan JW: The variable screw placement spinal fixation system: Report of a prospective study of 250 patients enrolled in Food and Drug Administration clinical trials. *Spine* 1993;18:1160-1172.

Turi M, Johnston CE, Richards BS: Anterior correction of idiopathic scoliosis using TSRH instrumentation. *Spine* 1993;18:417-422.

Vaccaro AR, Rizzolo SJ, Balderston RA, et al: Placement of pedicle screws in the thoracic spine: Part II. An anatomical and radiographic assessment. *J Bone Joint Surg Am* 1995;77:1200-1206.

Yuan HA, Garfin SR, Dickman CA, Mardjetko SM: A historical cohort study of pedicle screw fixation in thoracic, lumbar, and sacral spinal fusions. *Spine* 1994;19(suppl 20):2279S-2296S.

Zdeblick TA: A prospective, randomized study of lumbar fusion: Preliminary results. *Spine* 1993;18:983-991.

Chapter 59

Minimally Invasive Techniques for Thoracic and Lumbar Spine Procedures

John J. Regan, MD

Introduction

Minimally invasive techniques in spine surgery gained popularity with percutaneous endoscopic diskectomy. Although technology has improved since its inception, percutaneous techniques for disk removal have not demonstrated a significant improvement in outcome over microdiskectomy. Recent interest in what should be called "minimal access spine surgery" has been rekindled as a result of advances in laparoscopy.

The modern era of thoracoscopy or video-assisted thoracic spine surgery (VATS) began as a direct result of early success of laparoscopy with the addition of video to standard endoscopic techniques. Application of thoracoscopy for diseases of the spine was described in 1993. More recently, several authors have reported results of laparoscopic fusion of the lumbar spine using a threaded fusion cage. Titanium cylinders that engage both end plates of the disk space to be fused are packed with iliac crest bone graft. This approach is gaining acceptance specifically in anterior lumbar fusion at the L5-S1 disk space. The Food and Drug Administration's approval of threaded cages has also resulted in a general surge of interest in anterior access to the spine with open minilaparotomy, and retroperitoneal exposure has become the most popular anterior technique for exposure of the lumbar spine.

Anterior endoscopic spine procedures require advanced training and are associated with a steep learning curve. To achieve the best results, a spine surgeon should work with a thoracic surgeon during this procedure.

Video-Assisted Thoracic Spine Surgery

During VATS, modified long, narrow instruments are passed through small incisions in the chest. The area is viewed through a 10-mm diameter endoscope and with high-resolution video imaging. Lung deflation and optimal placement of trocar sites allow endoscopic spinal intervention to achieve the same goals as open surgery.

The need for CO_2 insufflation is avoided because the thoracic cavity allows a large working space. Thoracoscopy is advantageous because of the improved view of the entire thoracic spine, decrease in incisional pain and postoperative intercostal neuralgia, fewer pulmonary complications, early rehabilitation, improved cosmesis, and decrease in overall cost of the procedure. In addition, it is possible to perform surgery on the upper thoracic spine through the axilla without rib or clavicle resection, which is necessary in open approaches. Potential disadvantages are the steep learning curve associated with the procedure and the difficulty placing anterior endoscopic spinal fixation hardware. Procedures that can be done with the anterior endoscopic approach include, in order of increasing difficulty, incisional biopsy, anterior release and fusion for rigid kyphosis or scoliosis, thoracoplasty, thoracic diskectomy, corpectomy, and anterior endoscopic scoliosis instrumentation. Endoscopic anterior instrumentation of the thoracic spine after corpectomy and for deformity has been described, and progress is being made in this area. However, the problems of endoscopic distraction, compression, and rod rotation as well as maintaining fixation and preventing screw pullout are the main challenges associated with anterior instrumentation.

Preliminary results indicate that thoracoscopy for anterior releases is a safe and effective alternative to open thoracotomy for the treatment of certain types of pediatric and adolescent spinal deformity. Although curve correction, blood loss, and complication rates were similar between thoracoscopic and open methods, length of hospital stay was not reduced and the cost of thoracoscopy was higher.

Thoracoscopic techniques have been successful in the surgical treatment of clinically significant disk herniation from T1-T2 to T12-L1. The excellent view of the anterior thoracic spine permits safe decompression of central and paracentral disk herniations. The experienced surgeon can remove calcified disks and large osteophytes located behind the vertebral body. Ossification of the posterior longitudinal ligament and calcified disk herniation are commonly associated with dural adherence or confluence with a risk of dural tear. Preoperative CT myelogram may be indicated to further define the nature of the calcified or ossified material. Although minimal resection of normal disk and adjacent vertebral body can sometimes be achieved using VATS, rib head resection, which is necessary to see the pedicle and spinal canal, may result in instability. Rib graft can be harvested if anterior strut graft fusion is necessary. Also, laterally placed threaded fusion cages, initially developed for upper lumbar disk disease, have been successfully used for thoracic fusion.

Thoracic vertebrectomy and reconstruction using an endoscopic technique has been described for the treatment of osteomyelitis, tumors, and compression fractures. The same amount of spinal dissection and decompression is achieved as with open spinal procedures, with a better view of the exposed dura by using the 30° angle endoscope. Thoracoscopic vertebrectomy at T3 and T4 avoids the morbidity of the transclavicular approach or high thoracotomy, which requires transection of the rhomboid muscles and mobilization of the scapula. Tumor seeding in primary malignant lung tumors has been reported in the literature. Placement of tumor material in an endoscopic bag is recommended to avoid chest wall seeding.

In a report on 100 consecutive anterior endoscopic spinal procedures, transient intercostal neuralgia and atelectasis were the most common complications. Flexible trocars have significantly reduced the incidence of intercostal neuralgia, compared with that of open thoracotomy procedures. Perforation of the diaphragm and parenchymal lung injury can occur in VATS and these complications are best avoided by seeing the instruments as they are introduced into the chest cavity (Fig. 1).

Anterior Endoscopic Scoliosis Instrumentation

The endoscopic technique of instrumentation, correction, and fusion has undergone several modifications since the first few cases. Surgical times are greater than open techniques, and decrease with surgeon experience. Average correction is 68% in flexible idiopathic pediatric curves. Screw pullout at the top of the corrected curve occurs as a result of poor screw placement and unicortical purchase, leading to the need for bicortical screw placement and use of staples to improve pullout strength. Curves must be fused to the Cobb angle. Fusion short of this angle yields poor results.

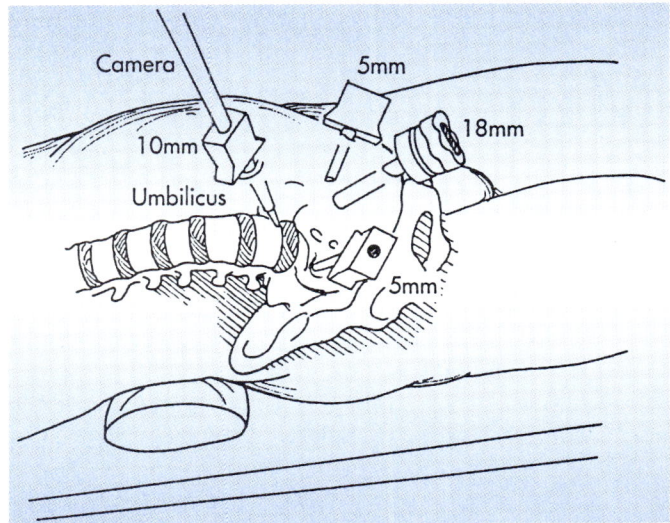

Figure 1 Drawing of the lateral video-assisted approach to the thoracic spine. *(Reproduced with permission from Regan JJ, McAfee PC, Guyer RD, Aronoff RJ: Laparoscopic fusion of the lumbar spine in a multicenter series of the first 34 consecutive patients. Surg Laparosc Endosc 1996;6:459-468.)*

The primary advantage of anterior endoscopic scoliosis instrumentation over open techniques is cosmesis and possible faster recovery. Current disadvantages are prolonged surgery time and potential problems achieving multilevel fusion.

Instrumented Laparoscopic Fusion of the Spine

Transabdominal and retroperitoneal approaches for anterior lumbar interbody fusions are widely accepted, effective tools for the management of painful degenerative disk disease unresponsive to nonsurgical measures. Recent advances in interbody fusion cage technology have generated a great deal of interest in their application with laparoscopic techniques. There are several potential advantages of a spinal fusion system that can be inserted laparoscopically. This approach avoids posterior incisions and the associated trauma to the paraspinal musculature. Epidural scarring, traction on nerve roots with injury, and dural lacerations are common problems related to posterior lumbar interbody fusion and can be avoided with the anterior approach. Surgical anatomy is easier to see and greater participation of the entire operating team is possible because the monitor can be watched during the surgical procedure. Laparoscopic technology is now merging with robotics, voice activation, and image guidance systems that may lead to improved surgical efficiency, accuracy, and lower patient morbidity.

A team approach and appropriate patient selection are essential to the success of this technology. The ideal candidate is a patient with discogenic pain related to isolated disk space collapse following a previous laminectomy. Assessment of vascular anatomy on preoperative MRI and identification of anomalies or vascular disease are essential. Monopolar cautery is avoided during surgery and blunt dissection is used to avoid injury to the superior hypogastric plexus. The laparoscopic experience should begin at the L5-S1 disk space. Patients with significant osteoporosis should be excluded from interbody fusion surgery. Achieving appropriate distraction with the cages and packing bone anterior to the cages may improve fusion success. Using this technique, radiologic identification of the "sentinel fusion sign" and the bridging bone anterior to the cage can be seen on a lateral spine radiograph.

Indications

Laparoscopic fusion techniques are indicated for use in patients with single-level symptomatic degenerative disk disease, internal disk disruption, and pseudarthrosis. Stable grade I spondylolisthesis and two-level degenerative disk disease are technically challenging and should be performed by an experienced surgeon. The ideal patient for laparoscopic fusion is one who has radiographic degenerative disk changes such as disk space narrowing, end plate sclerosis, and osteophyte formation. Symptomatic degenerative disk disease can be diagnosed in a patient with a strong history of mechanical back pain who has isolated degenerative changes at one spinal level on radiographs and MRI. The diagnosis is best made in a patient younger than 45 years of age with normal disk intensity signal on MRI at adjacent disks. In older patients the diagnosis may be less clear because of the naturally occurring degenerative changes in the intervertebral disks.

In a patient with single-level disk disease and end plate sclerotic changes confirmed on MRI, diskography is not always necessary. Patients with a strong history of mechanical back pain who have participated in a physical therapy program for 4 months without relief are good candidates for the procedure. Patients who have underlying psychological conditions, a positive Waddell's sign, and habitual narcotics users are not candidates for fusion surgery.

Patients with internal disk disruption are not ideal candidates for laparoscopic fusion. Radiographic examinations are relatively normal, there is decreased signal on MRI and concordant pain response and morphology are evident on diskography. They can be treated with laparoscopic techniques, but because of a tall disk height, it is more difficult to obtain the disk distraction required for stability. Anatomic fit is more difficult because larger cages are required.

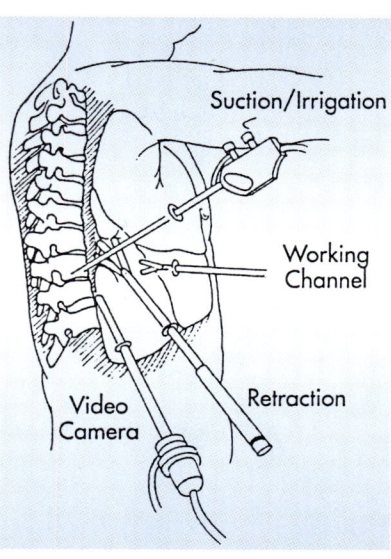

Figure 2 Drawing of the laparoscopic approach with portals. *(Reproduced with permission from Regan JJ: Percutaneous endoscopic thoracic discectomy. Neurosurg Clin North Am 1996;7:87-98.)*

Patients with extensive peritoneal adhesions from previous surgery or those with inflammatory or infectious diseases affecting the peritoneum should be excluded from the laparoscopic transperitoneal approach. Radiographs and MRI should also be assessed for vascular calcifications, aneurysms, and anomalies that may exclude the anterior approach altogether.

Surgical Technique
L5-S1 Approach
As a general rule of laparoscopy, all trocars are inserted under direct vision and 5-mm trocars are used whenever possible to avoid the need for fascial closure, which is required for trocars larger than 10 mm. Four incisions are used with a periumbilical trocar placed for the endoscope at 0° followed by placement of two 5-mm trocars lateral to the inferior epigastric arteries that run along the ventrolateral border of the rectus abdominus muscle. After insertion of the periumbilical trocar and establishment of the pneumoperitoneum, other trocar placements are made under direct vision (Fig. 2). The patient is positioned into a 20° to 30° Trendelenburg position and graspers are placed in the 5-mm portals to facilitate packing the intestines into the superior portion of the abdomen. Manual traction on the bowel is avoided to minimize the risk of postoperative ileus. The location of the aortic bifurcation is identified, and the sigmoid colon mesentery is approached from the right side. The right ureter coursing over the right iliac artery must be identified prior to making this incision in the posterior peritoneum. Electrocautery is not used in making the incision to avoid injury to the superior hypogastric plexus that will result in retrograde ejaculation. Blunt dissection using Kidner wands is then used to sweep the retroperito-

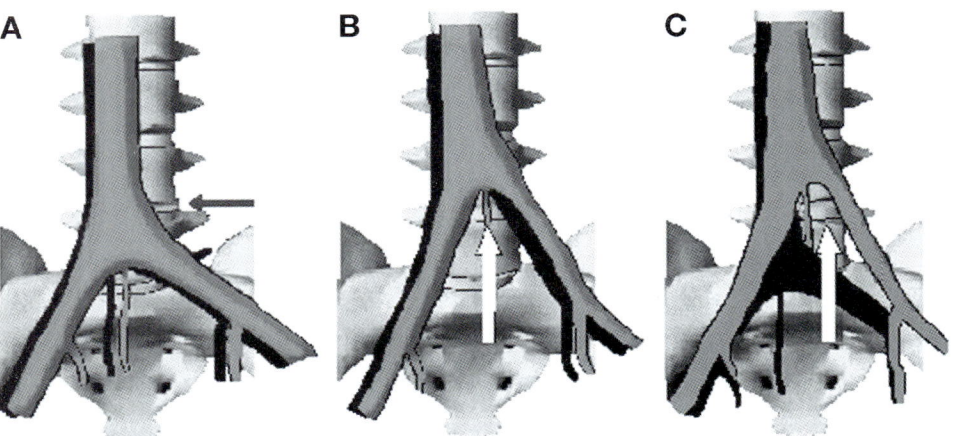

Figure 3 Three variations of vascular anatomy are identified in anterior approaches to the L4-5 disk space. The most common is bifurcation at L4-5, which requires that the left iliac artery and vein be mobilized from left to right (**A**). The second most common variation occurring almost 30% of the time is bifurcation above the L4-5 space, where the disk can be approached under the bifurcation (**B**). The least common variation is where the artery bifurcates above the L4-5 disk space and the vein at or below the space (**C**). Preferred approach is between the artery and vein to avoid excessive traction on the left iliac vein. *(Reproduced with permission from Regan JJ, Aronoff RJ, Ohnmeiss DD, Sengupta DK: Laparoscopic approach to L4-L5 for interbody fusion using BAK cages: Experience in the first 58 cases. Spine 1999;24: 2171-2174.)*

neal tissue from right to left. The sigmoid colon may travel close to the midline requiring retraction. A preoperative laxative and a light dinner the day before surgery should result in colon evacuation, which will improve handling of the bowel.

After incising the peritoneum and mobilizing the sigmoid colon, the L5-S1 disk space is viewed with the middle sacral vessels traveling close to the midline across the disk space. The median sacral vein and artery should be mobilized and ligated. The vessels are mobilized until the sympathetic plexus can be seen on either side. At L5-S1 the left iliac vein may pass over the disk space close to the midline. In cases of severe disk degeneration and anterior disk herniation, the iliac vein may be adherent to the anulus and must be carefully dissected to avoid laceration. Wide visualization of the disk space combined with a true AP-lordotic fluoroscopic image (Ferguson view) of the L5-S1 disk space is essential in locating the true midline of the disk space. Complications of lateral cage placement with resulting nerve root irritation or injury are most commonly associated with problems identifying the midline.

The process of disk evacuation has been a source of debate. Although it is clear that simple channel reaming without thorough disk removal may lead to a higher rate of pseudarthrosis, it may not be necessary or desirable to remove the entire anterior anulus and anterior longitudinal ligament. Disk removal can be accomplished using ring curettes and angled and straight pituitary rongeurs.

L4-5 Approach

The four key points regarding exposure to the L4-5 disk space all relate to vascular anatomy. A preoperative MRI study that includes the vascular anatomy anterior to the spine is important in deciding on the surgical approach, depending on the location of the

bifurcation of the great vessels (Fig. 3). The ascending lumbar vein must be identified during surgery and ligated prior to retracting the left iliac vein to the right. Gentle handling of the left iliac artery and avoidance of prolonged traction is recommended to avoid arterial thromboembolism. Clear visualization of the vessels at all times during the preparation and insertion of spinal instrumentation is most important and is necessary to avoid inadvertent vascular injury.

The L4-5 disk space is viewed by making an incision in the posterior peritoneum to the right of the sigmoid mesocolon after viewing the bifurcation of the aorta and vena cava. Preoperative MRI studies are evaluated to determine the location of the vascular bifurcation. The L5-S1 disk space is identified and the dissection is carried in a cephalad direction between the bifurcation. At this point it may be possible to approach the L4-5 disk space from below the bifurcation. Depending on the vascular anatomy, the L4-5 disk space may be approached by retracting the left iliac artery and vein from left to right or between the left iliac artery and vein.

Above the Bifurcation of the Vessels

This approach should be feasible in most patients, unless the bifurcation of the vessels is extremely high. However, the issue of autonomic nerve dysfunction is a concern. One critical step needed in order to successfully view the interspace is to identify and divide the ascending iliolumbar vein, which may be a single large vessel taking off obliquely from the left iliac vein or vena cava above or below the L4-5 disk space, or up to three or four small venous branches arising from the left iliac vein. Loss of control of segmental vessels can often be recovered, but loss of control of the ascending lumbar vein often requires suture-ligature closure and may lead to conversion of the procedure to open surgery. The dissection is complete when either the sympathetic plexus is seen on the patient's right side. Reported results in 58 consecutive patients indicate that 50% required this approach.

Below the Bifurcation of the Vessels

This approach provides the easiest access to the L4-5 disk space, minimizes retraction on the vessels, and obviates the need to ligate the ascending lumbar vein. However, surgery below the bifurcation of the vessels involves the most dissection and possibly retraction in the area of the superior hypogastric plexus. All dissection is done with scissors and no monopolar cautery is used at any time. The bifurcation is elevated and retraction of the left and right iliac vessels is performed using a 5-mm vessel retractor. It is helpful to elevate the vessels off the surface of the vertebral body to facilitate drill tube insertion. In the recent series of 58 patients, the L4-5 disk space was approached by going under the bifurcation 33% of the time.

Between the Artery and Vein

This procedure gives excellent exposure with minimal retraction on the iliac artery. Of concern is that during procedures on the disk, both the artery and vein can be injured and must be protected. Therefore, more diligence is required when performing this approach. With diseased arteries or difficult exposure, this approach is an option that minimizes traction on the left iliac artery. This approach was used 16% of the time in the series of 58 patients.

Lateral Endoscopic Fusion L1-L5

Retroperitonoscopy was initially described in 1992 for urologic procedures. Endoscopic retroperitoneal access for spine fusion was first performed in 1995. The first series to describe lumbar spine fusion using a lateral fusion cage inserted through a lateral endoscopic retroperitoneal approach was reported in 1998. Retroperitoneal lumbar fusion and stabilization offers several advantages over conventional anterior transperitoneal laparoscopic approaches to the lumbar spine. Retroperitoneal approaches eliminate the risk of small bowel adhesions and reduce the risk of autonomic plexus dysfunction. The patient is placed in the lateral decubitus position, which facilitates exposure of the lumbar spine as the intra-abdominal contents fall away anteriorly away from the spine. The lateral approach to the disk space minimizes retraction of the great vessels and, in cases of single level fusion, the segmental vessels and sympathetic plexus can be spared. The surgeon can "dial in" the lordosis by using a drill tube with lordosis-producing paddles. Small degrees of scoliosis can be corrected with distraction plugs. With the lateral approach the disk space preparation and cage insertion are directed toward the opposite psoas

muscle rather than the spinal canal as is the cage for transperitoneal cage insertion.

There are several potential disadvantages associated with the minimally invasive retroperitoneal approach. A large psoas muscle containing the lumbosacral roots may need to be mobilized laterally. Prolonged retraction may cause neurapraxia of the genitofemoral nerve or pressure on the lumbosacral plexus. A muscle-splitting approach to the psoas with constant vigilance of the lumbosacral plexus provides a direct lateral approach to the spine and minimizes traction injury to the genitofemoral nerve. A large psoas or the iliac crest may hamper the approach to L4-5. The surgeon must decide if this approach is preferable to the transperitoneal approach to L4-5, which requires mobilization of the left iliac artery and vein.

The patient is placed under general anesthesia and turned in the lateral decubitus position on a radiolucent table. A 1-cm incision is made at the anterior portion of the 12th rib for approaching L1 or L2. A c-arm fluoroscopic image is obtained, marking the skin directly over the midaxillary line. A working portal is then placed directly over the disk scheduled for surgery to facilitate orthogonal drill tube positioning and lateral cage insertion. The three techniques to dissect the retroperitoneal space are finger dissection, balloon insufflation, or use of an optical, transparent, dissecting trocar. Three secondary trocars are placed after the peritonium is dissected away from the anterior abdominal wall. The endoscope is inserted into the anteroinferior site. An anterosuperior site is used for exposing the lumbar spine and a posterior portal is used for retraction on the psoas muscle. The ureter, aorta, and vena cava are identified and dissected anterior to the spine. Retraction of these structures is not necessary. The sympathetic plexus can be mobilized anteriorly and the anterior portion of the psoas muscle is split if necessary to access the lateral aspect of the disk space. The genitofemoral nerve is identified on the surface of the psoas and retraction is avoided to prevent neurapraxia, which will result in dysesthesia of the anterior thigh and groin. Segmental vessels can be protected when a drill tube is used for lateral cage placement at the disk space. Long distraction plugs produce symmetric distraction and will correct a minor degenerative scoliosis. This technique is most useful in single-level disk instability from L1-L4, and can also be used as an anterior step in the correction of a kyphotic deformity (Fig. 4).

Results and Complications

Patient hospital stays following laparoscopic fusion have shortened dramatically. In one study, the mean

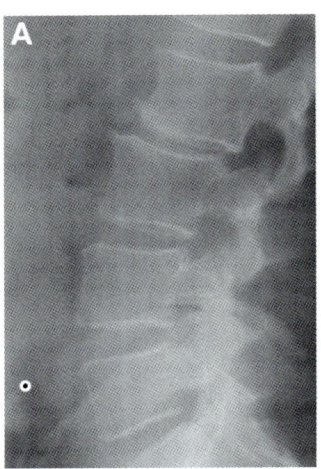
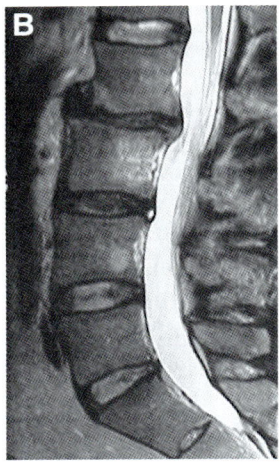
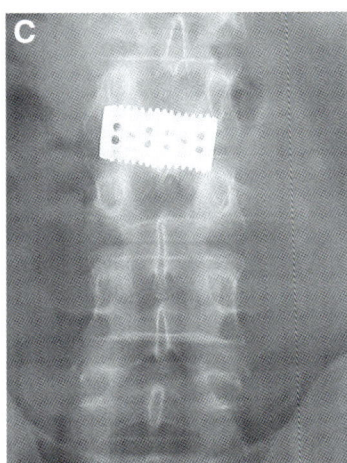
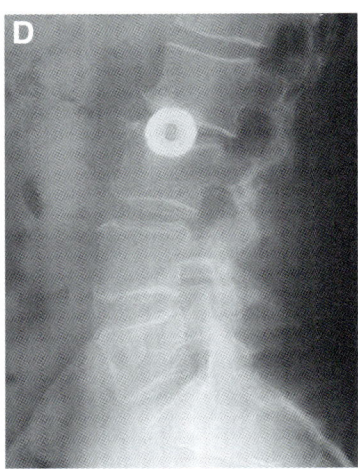

Figure 4 **A,** Lateral radiograph demonstrates severe degenerative collapse and retrolisthesis at L2-3 in a patient with intractable mechanical back pain unresponsive to nonsurgical measures. **B,** MRI confirms isolated disk degeneration at L2-3 with minimal central disk herniation caused by retrolisthesis. The patient underwent lateral endoscopic retroperitoneal diskectomy and placement of lateral fusion cage at L2-3 (**C** and **D**).

hospital stay was 1.7 days, ranging from up to 2 days in 20 consecutive patients. Nine of the 18 procedures were performed on an outpatient basis. Time for surgery averaged 125 minutes (range, 70 to 160 minutes). In a prospective study, the results of laparoscopic fusion (group I) to posterolateral fusion with pedicle screws (group II) and posterior interbody fusion with pedicle fixation (group III) were compared. Thirty-nine patients were randomized to these three groups for the treatment of L5-S1 degenerative disk disease. The hospital stay was 1.8 days for group I, 5 days for group II, and 5.1 days for group III. The average time to return to work in the posterior fusion groups with pedicle fixation was 21 and 23 weeks compared with 11 weeks for the laparoscopic group. Good to excellent clinical results were reported in 100% of the laparoscopic group compared with 73% for group II and 91% for group III.

Long-term survival of threaded fusion devices implanted as stand-alone devices at one or two levels was evaluated at a medical center where 190 procedures were performed by five surgeons. In a retrospective analysis with average follow-up of 33 months (range, 24 to 61 months) in patients undergoing surgery between 1994 and 1997, three patients (1.6%) required posterior revision for pseudarthrosis and three (1.6%) needed cage removal for nerve impingement by cage or displaced disk material. There were 6 patients (3.2%) who required revision surgery at the same level and 6 patients (3.2%) had procedures at adjacent levels. There was no statistically significant difference in the revision rate of the laparoscopic group, which consisted of 80 patients (42%).

In a prospective, multicenter study evaluating open and laparoscopic lumbar fusion in over 500 patients, there were no major complications (such as great vessel damage, pulmonary embolism, implant migration, death) in the laparoscopic group, which consisted of 215 patients treated by 19 surgeons at 10 medical centers. Preliminary experience indicated a small conversion rate to open fusion resulting from preoperative scarring, bleeding, and poor view of the surgical site. Instruments and technique changed from the earliest experience and no further conversions occurred. Intraoperative disk herniation from reaming and lateral cage placement with nerve irritation requiring posterior surgery was reported in 3.2% of the laparoscopic cases. Postoperative ileus was reported in 4.7%, and incisional hernia did not occur. Retrograde ejaculation occurred in 5.1% of laparoscopic cases, twice the rate of open cases. Almost all of these cases occurred early in the series as a result of monopolar cauterization. Approximately 50% of the cases in both groups resolved spontaneously with permanent cases associated with use of monopolar cautery and multilevel cases where bleeding occurred. The elimination of monopolar cautery and use of blunt dissection after incising the peritonium to the right of the midline has significantly decreased this problem.

Vertebroplasty and Kyphoplasty

Approximately 700,000 osteoporotic compression fractures occur yearly; almost one third of these become chronically painful. Primary osteoporosis accounts for 85% of these fractures, which are associated with a

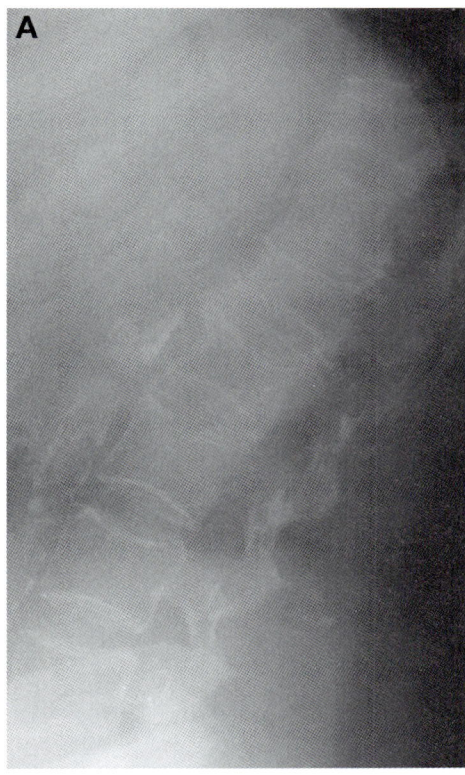
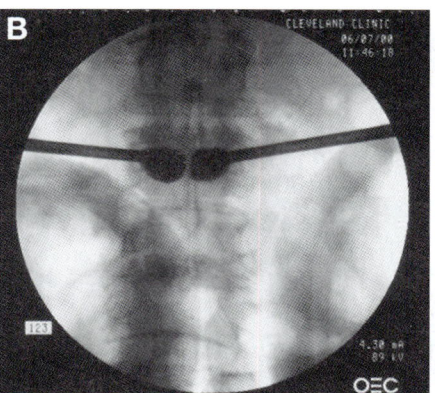
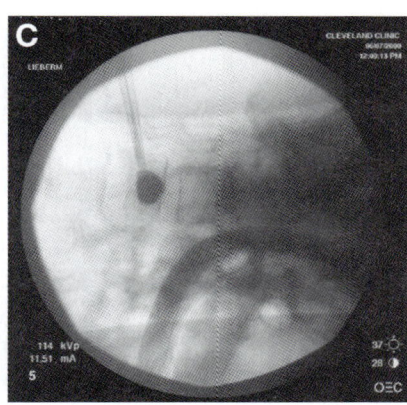
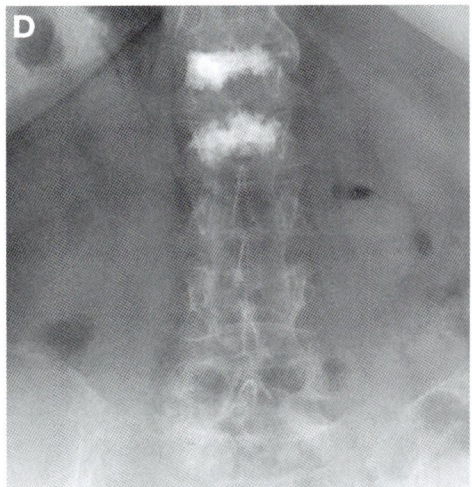
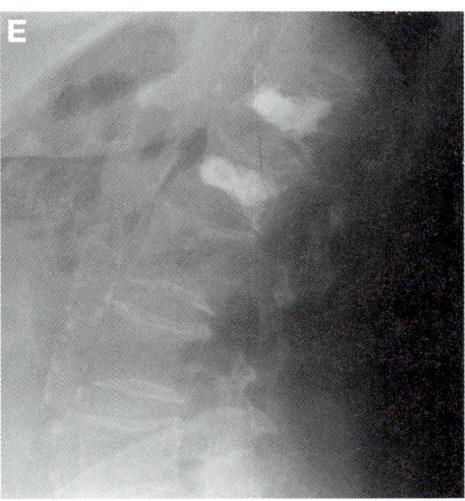

Figure 5 Imaging studies of a 71-year-old woman with a 4-week-old osteoporotic compression fracture that causes continued intractable pain. Preoperative lateral radiograph **(A)** confirmed compression fractures at L1 and L2. Percussion over the L1 and L2 spinous process confirmed location of maximal pain. The patient underwent kyphoplasty. Intraoperative fluoroscopic images demonstrate balloon insufflation using contrast **(B** and **C)**. Restoration of vertebral body height occurs with balloon insufflation in the anterior vertebral body. Postoperative anteroposterior **(D)** and lateral **(E)** radiographs show polymethylmethacrylate cement in the vertebral bodies at L1 and L2. The patient had excellent pain relief after the procedure.

fivefold increase in subsequent fractures, increased spinal deformity, reduced pulmonary function, and increased mortality. The occurrence of multilevel fractures leads to progressive kyphosis with resulting pulmonary compromise and reduced ambulatory status. Vertebroplasty has been performed in the United States for over 8 years with a goal of pain relief. Kyphoplasty involves the use of a balloon catheter inserted through the pedicle using a percutaneous technique and fluoroscopy (Fig. 5). By inflating the balloon, proponents of the technique believe that the kyphosis is corrected and long-term complications of progressive kyphosis are avoided. Two balloons are inserted, one through each pedicle, and polymethylmethacrylate is injected into the anteroinferior vertebral body after each balloon is removed. Preliminary results indicate excellent pain relief and functional improvement following the procedure, and that height restoration occurred in 70% of the patients studied, with an average improvement of 47%. Cement extravasation occurred in 8.6% of 100 patients and was not associated with complications. These complications are technique dependent and are minimized by fluoroscopic imaging during cement placement and delivering the cement in a doughy state with minimal pressurization.

Annotated Bibliography

Video-Assisted Thoracic Spine Surgery

Regan JJ, Ben-Yishay A, Mack MJ: Video-assisted thoracoscopic excision of herniated thoracic disc: Description of technique and preliminary experience in the first 29 cases. *J Spinal Disord* 1998;11:183-191.

At 12- to 24-month follow-up, 75.8% of patients had satisfactory outcomes with relief of myelopathic and radicular symptoms. The postoperative complication rate was 13.8%. Complications included excessive bleeding, atelectasis, pleural effusion, and diaphragm puncture. Video-assisted thoracoscopic excision resulted in decreased hospitalization time, less use of postoperative narcotics, and early recovery.

Laparoscopic Fusion of the Lumbar Spine

McAfee PC, Regan JJ, Geis WP, Fedder IL: Minimally invasive anterior retroperitoneal approach to the lumbar spine: Emphasis on the lateral BAK. *Spine* 1998;23:1476-1484.

This technical report on the lateral approach to the lumbar spine details preliminary results of single lateral cages.

Regan JJ, Aronoff RJ, Ohnmeiss DD, Sengupta DK: Laparoscopic approach to L4-L5 for interbody fusion using BAK cages: Experience in the first 58 cases. *Spine* 1999;24:2171-2174.

In 58 consecutive patients operated on by the same surgical team, 50% of the time the exposure of the L4-5 disk was achieved by retracting the iliac artery and vein from left to right. Unexpectedly, 33% of the approaches were successful below the bifurcation of the great vessels, the typical approach to L5-S1. Two cages were placed in all but two patients, where only one cage was placed as a result of inability to mobilize the iliac vein as a result of adhesions.

Regan JJ, Yuan H, McAfee PC: Laparoscopic fusion of the lumbar spine: Minimally invasive spine surgery. A prospective multicenter study evaluating open and laparoscopic lumbar fusion. *Spine* 1999;24:402-411.

In this prospective series of over 500 patients, results of laparoscopic fusion were compared with those of the open minilaparotomy approach. Postoperative ileus was noted in 4.7% of patients, nerve irritation from lateral cage placement in 3.2%, and retrograde ejaculation in 5.2% in the laparoscopic group. These complication rates were similar to those reported for the open approach with the exception of retrograde ejaculation. Most of the complications occurred early in the series and were thought to be a result of using monopolar cautery and difficulty identifying the midline, resulting in lateral cage placement.

Classic Bibliography

Blackman RG, Picetti GD, O'Neal K, et al: Surgical technique for endoscopic anterior correction of idiopathic scoliosis, in *Spinal Instrumentation Techniques Manual: Scoliosis Research Society*. Chicago, IL, Lippincott, 2000, vol 2.

Dickman CA, Rosenthal D, Karahalios DG, et al: Thoracic vertebrectomy and reconstruction using a microsurgical thoracoscopic approach. *Neurosurgery* 1996;38:279-293.

Gaur DD: Laparoscopic operative retroperitoneoscopy: Use of a new device. *J Urol* 1992;148:1137-1139.

Hazelrigg SR, Landreneau RJ, Boley TM, et al: The effect of muscle-sparing versus standard posterolateral thoracotomy on pulmonary function, muscle strength, and postoperative pain. *J Thorac Cardiovasc Surg* 1991;101:394-401.

Horowitz MB, Moossy JJ, Julian T, Ferson PF, Huneke K: Thoracic discectomy using video assisted thoracoscopy. *Spine* 1994;19:1082-1086.

Landreneau RJ, Dowling RD, Ferson PF: Thoracoscopic resection of a posterior mediastinal neurogenic tumor. *Chest* 1992;102:1288-1290.

Mack MJ, Regan JJ, Bobechko WP, Acuff TE: Application of thoracoscopy for diseases of the spine. *Ann Thorac Surg* 1993;56:736-738.

Mack MJ, Regan JJ, McAfee PC, Picetti G, Ben-Yishay A, Acuff TE: Video-assisted thoracic surgery for the anterior approach to the thoracic spine. *Ann Thorac Surg* 1995;59:1100-1106.

Mathews HH, Evans MT, Molligan HJ, Long BH: Laparoscopic discectomy with anterior lumbar interbody fusion: A preliminary review. *Spine* 1995;20:1797-1802.

McAfee PC, Regan JR, Fedder IL, Mack MJ, Geis WP: Anterior thoracic corpectomy for spinal cord decompression performed endoscopically. *Surg Laparosc Endosc* 1995;5:339-348.

McAfee PC, Regan JJ, Zdeblick T, et al: The incidence of complications in endoscopic anterior thoracolumbar spinal reconstructive surgery: A prospective multicenter study comprising the first 100 consecutive cases. *Spine* 1995;20:1624-1632.

Modic MT, Steinberg PM, Ross JS, Masaryk TJ, Carter JR: Degenerative disk disease: Assessment of changes in vertebral marrow with MR imaging. *Radiology* 1988;166:193-199.

Newton PO, Wenger DR, Mubarak SJ, Meyer RS: Anterior release and fusion in pediatric spinal deformity: A comparison of early outcome and cost of thoracoscopic and open thoracotomy approaches. *Spine* 1997;22:1398-1406.

Obenchain TG: Laparoscopic lumbar discectomy: Case report. *J Laparoendosc Surg* 1991;1:145-149.

Reddick EJ, Olsen DO: Laparoscopic laser cholecystectomy: A comparison with mini-lap cholecystectomy. *Surg Endosc* 1989;3:131-133.

Regan JJ, Mack MJ, Picetti GD III: A technical report on video-assisted thoracoscopy in thoracic spinal surgery: Preliminary description. *Spine* 1995;20:831-837.

Regan JJ, McAfee PC, Guyer RD, Aronoff RJ: Laparoscopic fusion of the lumbar spine in a multicenter series of the first 34 consecutive patients. *Surg Laparosc Endosc* 1996;6:459-468.

Regan JJ, McAfee PC, Mack MJ (eds): *Atlas of Endoscopic Spine Surgery*. St Louis, MO, Quality Medical Publishing, 1995.

Regan JJ, Yuan H, McCullen G: Minimally invasive approaches to the spine. *Instr Course Lect* 1997;46: 127-141.

Rosenthal D, Marquardt G, Lorenz R, Nichtweiss M: Anterior decompression and stabilization using a microsurgical endoscopic technique for metastatic tumors of the thoracic spine. *J Neurosurg* 1996;84: 565-572.

Rosenthal D, Rosenthal R, de Simone A: Removal of a protruded thoracic disc using microsurgical endoscopy: A new technique. *Spine* 1994;19:1087-1091.

Zdeblick TA: A prospective, randomized study of lumbar fusion: Preliminary results. *Spine* 1993;18:983-991.

Zucherman JF, Zdeblick TA, Bailey SA, Mahvi D, Hsu KY, Kohrs D: Instrumented laparoscopic spinal fusion: Preliminary results. *Spine* 1995;20:2029-2035.

Index